KT-130-696

# KAPLAN'S CLINICAL HYPERTENSION

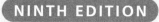

NINTH EDITION

# KAPLAN'S CLINICAL HYPERTENSION

**NORMAN M. KAPLAN**, M.D.
Clinical Professor of Medicine
Department of Internal Medicine
University of Texas Southwestern Medical School
Dallas, Texas


with a chapter by
**JOSEPH T. FLYNN**, M.D.
Director, Pediatric Hypertension Program
Children's Hospital at Montefiore
Bronx, NY

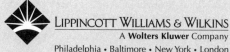

LIPPINCOTT WILLIAMS & WILKINS
A **Wolters Kluwer** Company
Philadelphia • Baltimore • New York • London
Buenos Aires • Hong Kong • Sydney • Tokyo

*Acquisitions Editor:* Frances Destefano
*Managing Editor:* Joanne Bersin
*Project Manager:* Alicia Jackson
*Senior Manufacturing Manager:* Benjamin Rivera
*Marketing Manager:* Kathy Neely
*Cover Designer:* Larry Didona
*Production Service:* Schawk, Inc.
*Printer:* Quebecor World -Taunton

© 2006 by LIPPINCOTT WILLIAMS & WILKINS
530 Walnut Street
Philadelphia, PA 19106 USA
LWW.com

8th Edition, ©2000 Lippincott Williams & Wilkins
7th Edition, ©1998 Lippincott Williams & Wilkins
6th Edition, ©1994 Williams & Wilkins
5th Edition, ©1990 Williams & Wilkins
4th Edition, ©1986 Williams & Wilkins
3rd Edition, ©1982 Williams & Wilkins
2nd Edition, ©1978 Williams & Wilkins
1st Edition, © 1973 Williams & Wilkins

All rights reserved. This book is protected by copyright. No part of this book may be reproduced in any form by any means, including photocopying, or utilized by any information storage and retrieval system without written permission from the copyright owner, except for brief quotations embodied in critical articles and reviews. Materials appearing in this book prepared by individuals as part of their official duties as U.S. government employees are not covered by the above-mentioned copyright.

Printed in the USA

Library of Congress Cataloging-in-Publication Data
Kaplan, Norman M., 1931-
  Kaplan's clinical hypertension / Norman M. Kaplan ; with a chapter by Joseph T.
Flynn.— 9th ed.
    p. ; cm.
  Includes bibliographical references and index.
  ISBN 13: 978-0-7817-6198-7 (alk. paper)
  ISBN 10: 0-7817-6198-0 (alk. paper)
  1. Hypertension. I. Flynn, Joseph T. II. Title. III. Title: Clinical hypertension.
  [DNLM: 1. Hypertension. WG 340 K17k 2006]
  RC685.H8K35 2006
  616.1'32—dc22
                                                    2005017049

Care has been taken to confirm the accuracy of the information presented and to describe generally accepted practices. However, the authors, editors, and publisher are not responsible for errors or omissions or for any consequences from application of the information in this book and make no warranty, expressed or implied, with respect to the currency, completeness, or accuracy of the contents of the publication. Application of the information in a particular situation remains the professional responsibility of the practitioner.

The authors, editors, and publisher have exerted every effort to ensure that drug selection and dosage set forth in this text are in accordance with current recommendations and practice at the time of publication. However, in view of ongoing research, changes in government regulations, and the constant flow of information relating to drug therapy and drug reactions, the reader is urged to check the package insert for each drug for any change in indications and dosage and for added warnings and precautions. This is particularly important when the recommended agent is a new or infrequently employed drug.

Some drugs and medical devices presented in the publication have Food and Drug Administration (FDA) clearance for limited use in restricted research settings. It is the responsibility of the health care provider to ascertain the FDA status of each drug or device planned for use in their clinical practice.

To purchase additional copies of this book, call our customer service department at (800) 639-3030 or fax orders to (301) 824-7390. International customers should call (301) 714-2324.

Visit Lippincott Williams & Wilkins on the Internet: at LWW.com. Lippincott Williams & Wilkins customer service representatives are available from 8:30 am to 6 pm, EST.

10 9 8 7 6 5 4 3

*To those such as:*
*Goldblatt and Groilman,*
*Braun-Menéndez and Page,*
*Lever and Pickering,*
*Mancia, Brenner, and Laragh,*
*Julius, Hansson, and Freis,*
*And the many others, whose work has made it possible for me to put*
*together what I hope will be a useful book on clinical hypertension*

# Contents

# Preface to the Ninth Edition

As befits my age, prior to preparation of this ninth edition, I developed isolated systolic hypertension. As I struggled with its control–and it has been a struggle–a number of useful insights were learned and these insights have been incorporated into this text.

This book represents the distillation of a tremendous volume of literature, filtered through the receptive and, I trust, discriminating awareness of a single author. When I wrote the first edition in 1973, the task was challenging, mainly because few had tried a synthesis of what was then known. But–as most who read this book are well aware–in the ensuing 35 years, the task has become much more difficult, mainly because the literature on hypertension has grown so that it is almost beyond the grasp of any one person. I continue to be a single author (with the important exception of the chapter on children) for two reasons:

- First, a single-authored text offers more cohesion and completeness, and, at the same time, brevity and lack of repetition, compared to most multiauthored but rarely edited megabooks.
- Second, I have the time, energy, and interest to keep up with the literature, and this book has become the major focus of my professional life. The success of the previous editions and the many compliments received from both clinicians in the field and investigators from the research bench have prompted me to do it again.

The very reason that a single-authored text has become such a rarity explains the need for a new edition fairly often. I am amazed at the tremendous amount of hypertension-related literature published over the past 4 years. A considerable amount of significant new information is included in this edition, presented in a manner that I hope enables the reader to grasp its significance and place it in perspective. Almost every page has been revised, using the same goals:

- Give more attention to the common problems; primary hypertension takes up almost half the book.
- Cover every form of hypertension at least briefly, providing references for those seeking more information. Additional coverage is provided on some topics that have recently assumed importance.
- Include the latest data, even if available only in abstract form.
- Provide enough pathophysiology to permit sound clinical judgment.
- Be objective and clearly identify biases. Although my views may differ from those of others, I have tried to give reasonable attention to those with whom I disagree.

Dr. Joseph T. Flynn, head of the Pediatric Hypertension Program at Children's Hospital at Montefiore in the Bronx, has contributed a chapter on hypertension in children and adolescents. I have been fortunate in being in an academic setting wherein such endeavors are nurtured, and where colleagues such as Dr. Ronald G. Victor provide coverage for time spent in writing a book. I am also thankful for the diligent and timely work of my secretary, Ms. Vicki Martin, as well as the publisher's staff who worked on this edition. And last, the forbearance of Audrey, my wife, can be acknowledged only by the promise that I will not do it again–at least for another 4 years.

*Norman M. Kaplan, MD*

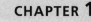

# Hypertension in the Population at Large

Hypertension provides both despair and hope. Despair because it is quantitatively the largest risk factor for cardiovascular diseases, is growing in prevalence, and is poorly controlled virtually everywhere. Hope because prevention is possible (though rarely achieved) and because treatment can control hypertension in almost all patients with consequent marked reductions in stroke and heart attack.

Although most of this book addresses hypertension in the United States and other developed countries, it should be noted that cardiovascular diseases are the leading cause of death worldwide, more so in the economically developed countries but also in the developing world (Kearney et al., 2005).

In turn, hypertension is overall the major contributor to the risks for cardiovascular diseases. When the total global impact of known risk factors on the overall burden of disease is calculated, hypertension comes behind only undernutrition and unsafe sex (Ezzati et al., 2003). Of all the potentially modifiable risk factors for myocardial infarction in 52 countries, hypertension is exceeded only by smoking (Yusuf et al., 2004). As reviewed by Kearney et al. (2005), the overall worldwide prevalence of hypertension is approximately 26% of the adult population, with marked differences between countries.

The second contributor to our current despair is the growing prevalence of hypertension as seen in the ongoing survey of a representative sample of the U.S. population (Fields et al., 2004). According to the analysis, the prevalence of hypertension in the United States has increased from 50 million in 1990 to 65 million in 2000. This increased prevalence primarily is a consequence of the population becoming older and more obese.

The striking impact of aging was seen among participants in the Framingham Heart Study: Among those who remained normotensive at either age 55 or 65 (providing 2 cohorts) over a 20-year follow-up, hypertension developed in almost 90% of those who were now aged 75 or 85 (Vasan et al., 2002).

The impact of aging and the accompanying increased prevalence of hypertension on both stroke and ischemic heart disease (IHD) mortality has been clearly portrayed in a metaanalysis of data from over one million adults in 61 prospective studies by the Prospective Studies Collaboration (Lewington et al., 2002). As seen in Figure 1–1, the absolute risk for IHD mortality was increased at least twofold at every higher decade of age, with similar lines of progression for both systolic and diastolic pressure in every decade.

At the same time as populations are growing older, obesity has become epidemic in the United States (Hedley et al., 2004) and is increasing rapidly wherever urbanization is occurring (Yusuf et al., 2001). With weight gain, blood pressure (BP) usually increases, and the increased prevalence of overweight is likely responsible for the significant increase in the BP of children and adolescents in the United States over the past 12 years (Muntner et al., 2004).

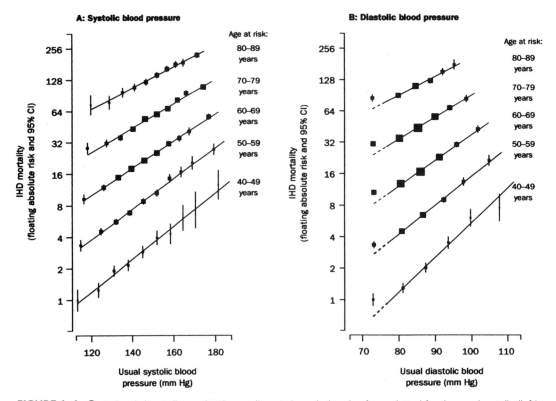

**FIGURE 1–1** ● Ischemic heart disease (IHD) mortality rate in each decade of age plotted for the usual systolic *(left)* and diastolic *(right)* blood pressures at the start of that decade. Data from almost one million adults in 61 prospective studies. (Modified from Lewington S, Clarke R, Qizilbash N, et al. Age-specifc relevance of usual blood pressure to vascular mortality: a meta-analysis of individual data for one million adults in 61 prospective studies. *Lancet* 2002;360:1903–1913.)

The third contributor to our current despair is the inadequate control of hypertension virtually everywhere. According to similar surveys in the 1990s, with control defined at the 140/90 mm Hg threshold, control has been achieved in 29% of hypertensives in the United States, 17% in Canada, but in fewer than 10% in five European countries (England, Germany, Italy, Spain, and Sweden) (Wolf-Maier et al., 2004). Some improvement in the U.S. control rate has subsequently been found but the percentage has reached only 34% (Chobanian et al., 2003) (Table 1–1). As expected, even lower rates of control have been reported from less developed countries such as Ghana (Cappuccio et al., 2004) and developing nations such as China and Egypt (Whelton et al., 2004). But the poor control rates in countries with high socioeconomic status and universal access to health care, such as Sweden (Li et al., 2005), are more difficult to understand. In particular, control rates among the most commonly afflicted, the elderly, are significantly lower than among younger hypertensives (Primatesta & Poulter, 2004).

Thus, despair seems appropriate. However, there is hope, which starts with impressive evidence of decreased mortality from cardiovascular diseases, at least in the United States (Fox et al., 2004) and England (Unal et al., 2004). However, as well as can be ascertained, control of hypertension has played a very small role in the decreased mortality from coronary disease in England and Wales between 1981 and 2000 (Unal et al., 2004).

Nonetheless, there is also hope relative to hypertension. Primary prevention has been found to be possible (Whelton et al., 2002), though the rising number of the obese seriously questions the ability to implement the necessary lifestyle changes in today's world of faster foods and slower physical activity. Therefore, controlled trials of primary prevention of hypertension using antihypertensive drugs have begun (Julius et al., 2004).

On the other hand, the ability to provide protection against stroke and heart attack by antihypertensive therapy in those who have hypertension has been overwhelmingly documented (Turnbull & Blood Pressure Trialists, 2003). There is no longer argument as to the benefits of lowering BP, even though uncertainty persists as to the most cost-effective way to achieve the lower BP. Meanwhile, the unraveling of the human genome has given rise to the hope that gene manipulation or transfer can prevent

## TABLE 1–1

### Trends in Awareness, Treatment, and Control of High Blood Pressure, 1976–2000

| | National Health and Nutrition Examination Survey, % | | | |
|---|---|---|---|---|
| | 1976–1980 | 1988–1991 | 1991–1994 | 1990–2000 |
| Awareness | 51 | 73 | 68 | 70 |
| Treatment | 31 | 55 | 54 | 59 |
| Control | 10 | 29 | 27 | 34 |

Percentage of adults aged 18 to 74 years with systolic blood pressure of 140 mm Hg or greater, diastolic blood pressure of 90 mm Hg or greater, or taking antihypertensive medication who were aware of the diagnosis, on antihypertensive treatment, or with BP controlled to less than 140/90 mm Hg. Adapted from Chobanian et al. Seventh report of the Joint National Committee on the Prevention, Detection, Evaluation, and Treatment of High Blood Pressure. *Hypertension* 2003;42:1206–1252.

hypertension. As of now, that hope seems extremely unlikely beyond the very small number of patients with monogenetic defects that have been discovered.

All in all, hope about hypertension seems overshadowed by despair. However, healthcare providers must, by nature, be optimistic and there is an inherent value in considering the despairs about hypertension to be a challenge rather than an acceptance of defeat. As portrayed by Nolte and McKee (2003), the most realistic way to measure the health of nations is to analyze the mortality that is amenable to health care. By this criterion, the United States ranks sixteenth among the 19 developed countries analyzed. This sobering fact can be looked upon as a failure of the vastly wasteful, disorganized U.S. healthcare system. I prefer to look upon this poor rating as a challenge: Current health care is inadequate, obviously including the management of hypertension, but the potential to improve has never been greater. The path to improvement has been plotted: greater awareness (Mosca et al., 2005) and patient participation (Canzanello et al., 2005).

This book summarizes and analyzes the work of thousands of clinicians and investigators worldwide who have advanced our knowledge about the mechanisms behind hypertension and who have provided increasingly effective therapies for its control. Despite their continued efforts, however, hypertension will almost certainly never be totally conquered, because it is one of those diseases that, in the words of a *Lancet* editorialist (Anonymous, 1993):

. . . afflict us from middle age onwards [that] might simply represent "unfavorable" genes that have accumulated to express themselves in the second half of our lives. This could never be corrected by any evolutionary pressure since such

pressures act only on the first half of our lives: once we have reproduced, it does not greatly matter that we grow "sans teeth, sans eyes, sans taste, sans everything."

In this chapter, the overall problems of hypertension for the population at large are considered. I define the disease, quantify its prevalence and consequences, classify its types, and describe the current status of detection and control. In the remainder of the book, these generalities will be amplified into practical ways to evaluate and treat hypertension in its various presentations.

## CONCEPTUAL DEFINITION OF HYPERTENSION

The following will examine the definition of hypertension. As important as that definition has been in directing clinical practice, we must get away from our current focus on blood pressure *per se* to determine the need for active therapy. The level of BP is rarely, if ever, the only risk but is almost always part of a multifaceted pattern of risk. Jackson et al. (2005) go so far as to recommend that "terms such as hypertension (and hypercholesterolemia) be removed from our clinical vocabulary [and] the next generation of clinicians should treat risk, not risk factors" (Jackson et al., 2005). In a similar vein, MacMahon et al. (2005) insist that the overall degree of cardiovascular risk and not the level of blood pressure be used to determine the need for antihypertensive therapy. Noting that "although non-optimum blood pressure is the leading cause of death worldwide, less than 40% of this burden is due to hypertension as currently defined." MacMahon et al. (2005) conclude: "A change in paradigm is long overdue—the world needs comprehensive programmes to prevent blood-pressure-related diseases and not just programmes concerned with the diagnosis, classification, and treatment of hypertension."

These experts are undoubtedly correct. They remind us of two oft forgotten facts. First, as Sir George Pickering said in 1972, "There is no dividing line [between normal and high BP]. The relationship between arterial pressure and mortality is quantitative; the higher the pressure, the worse the prognosis" (Pickering, 1972).

Second, as another wise Englishman, Geoffrey Rose, said, "The operational definition of hypertension is the level at which the benefits of action exceed those of inaction" (Rose, 1980). Fortunately, more intensive therapy with less bothersome drugs has lowered the level of pressure wherein benefit is seen and diminished the risks and costs of such therapy (Table 1–2).

Therefore, our focus must shift from a narrow view of hypertension as a certain level of BP to a broader view of blood pressure as a part of overall cardiovascular risk, a part that can and should be treated wherein the benefits of action exceed those of inaction. In the words of MacMahon et al. (2005): "Evidence from randomised trials does not provide any rationale for maintenance of present definitions of hypertension, especially in those at high absolute risk of blood-presure-related cardiovascular events. Indeed, the evidence shows that any definition restricting the use of blood-pressure-lowering therapy in high-risk, non-hypertensive individuals would deny them a potentially life-saving treatment" (MacMahon et al., 2005).

Nonetheless, practitioners need precise criteria for the diagnosis of hypertension, even if the criteria are arbitrary. To consider a BP of 138/88 as normal and not in need of treatment and one of 140/90 as abnormal and in need of treatment is obviously inappropriate but medical practice (and third-party payers) require that some criteria be used to determine the need for workup and therapy. The need to put BP into the context of overall cardiovascular risk is obvious but practitioners do not usually consider risk (Mosca et al., 2005) and are often confused as to the best way to determine absolute treatment benefits (Jackson et al., 2005).

## Risks of Inaction: Increased Risk of Cardiovascular Disease

The risks of elevated BP have been determined from large-scale epidemiologic surveys. The Prospective Studies Collaboration (Lewington et al., 2002) obtained data on each of 958,074 participants in 61 prospective observational studies of blood pressure and mortality. Over a mean time of 12 years, there were 11,960 deaths attributed to stroke; 32,283 attributed to IHD; 10,092 attributed to other vascular causes; and 60,797 attributed to nonvascular causes. Mortality during each decade of age at death was related to the estimated usual blood pressure at the start of that decade. The relation between usual systolic and diastolic blood pressure and the absolute risk for IHD mortality is shown in Figure 1–1. From ages 40 to 69, each increase of 20 mm Hg BP or 10 mm Hg diastolic BP is associated with a twofold increase in mortality rates from IHD and more than a twofold increase in stroke mortality.

## TABLE 1–2

### Factors Involved in the Conceptual Definition of Hypertension

| Action | Benefits | Risks and Costs |
|---|---|---|
| Action | Reduce risk of cardiovascular disease, debility, and death | Assume psychological burdens of "the hypertensive patient" |
| | | Interfere with quality of life |
| | Decrease monetary costs of catastrophic events | Require changes in lifestyle |
| | | Add risks and side effects from therapy |
| | | Add monetary costs of health care |
| Inaction | Preserve "nonpatient" role | |
| | Maintain current lifestyle and quality of life | Increase risk of cardiovascular disease, debility, and death |
| | Avoid risks and side effects of therapy | Increase monetary costs of catastrophic events |
| | Avoid monetary costs of health care | |

These proportional differences in vascular mortality are about half as great in the 80–89 decade than in the 40–49 decade, but the annual absolute increases in risk are considerably greater in the elderly. As is evident from the straight lines in Figure 1–1, there is no evidence of a threshold wherein BP is not directly related to risk down to as low as 115/75 mm Hg.

As the authors conclude: "Not only do the present analyses confirm that there is a continuous relationship with risk throughout the normal range of usual blood pressure, but they demonstrate that within this range the usual blood pressure is even more strongly related to vascular mortality than had previously been supposed." They conclude that a 10 mm Hg higher usual systolic BP or 5 mm Hg higher usual diastolic BP would, in the long term, be associated with about a 40% higher risk of death from stroke and about a 30% higher risk of death from IHD.

These data clearly incriminate levels of BP below the level usually considered as indicative of hypertension, i.e., 140/90 or higher. Data from the closely observed participants in the Framingham Heart Study confirm the increased risks of cardiovascular disease with BP levels previously defined as *normal* (120–129/80–84) or *high-normal* (130–139/85–89) compared to those with *optimal* BP (less than 120/80) (Vasan et al., 2001b) (Figure 1–2). The data of Lewington et al. (2002) and Vasan et al. (2001b) are the basis of a new classification of BP levels, as will be described later in this chapter.

A similar relation between levels of BP and cardiovascular diseases has been seen in eight Asian Pacific countries, although the association is even stronger for stroke and somewhat less for coronary disease than seen in the Western world (Lawes et al., 2003). Some of these differences in risk and BP levels can be explained by obvious factors such as socioeconomic differences and variable access to health care (Isaacs & Schroeder, 2004).

Beyond the essential contribution of blood pressure *per se* to cardiovascular risk, a number of other associations may influence the relationship.

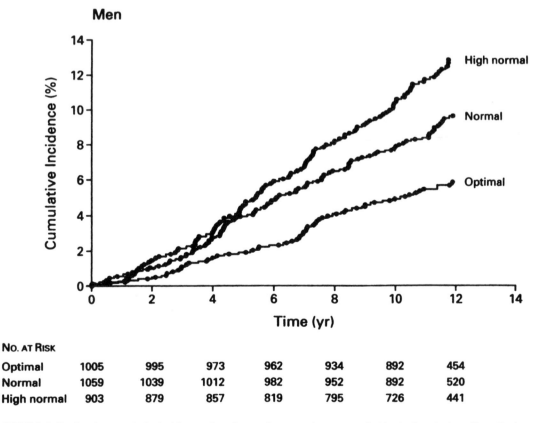

**FIGURE 1–2** ● The cumulative incidence of cardiovascular events in men enrolled in the Framingham Heart Study with initial blood pressures classified as optimal (below 120/80), normal (120–129/80–84), or high-normal (130–139/85–89) over a 12-year follow-up. (Modified from Vasan RS, Larson MG, Leip EP, et al. Impact of high-normal blood pressure on the risk of cardiovascular disease. *N Engl J Med* 2001b;345:1291–1297.)

## Gender and Risk

Although some studies of women have shown that they tolerate hypertension better than do men and have lower coronary mortality rates with any level of hypertension (Barrett-Connor, 1997), the Prospective Studies Collaboration found the age-specific associations of IHD mortality with BP to be slightly greater for women than for men and concluded that "for vascular mortality as a whole, sex is of little relevance" (Lewington et al., 2002).

## Race and Risk

As shown in Figure 1–3, U.S. Blacks tend to have higher levels of BP than do non-Blacks (Hajjar & Kotchen, 2003) and overall hypertension-related mortality rates are higher among Blacks (Gillum, 1996). In the Multiple Risk Factor Intervention Trial, which involved more than 23,000 Black men and 325,000 White men who were followed up for 10 years, an interesting racial difference was confirmed: The mortality rate for coronary heart disease (CHD) was lower in Black men with a diastolic exceeding 90 mm Hg than in White men (relative risk, 0.84), but the mortality rate for cerebrovascular disease was higher (relative risk, 2.0) (Neaton et al., 1989).

The greater risk of hypertension among Blacks suggests that more attention must be given to even lower levels of hypertension among this group, but there seems little reason to use different criteria to diagnose hypertension in Blacks than in Whites. The special features of hypertension in Blacks are discussed in more detail in Chapter 4.

The relative risk of hypertension differs among other racial groups as well. In particular, hypertension rates in U.S. Hispanics of Mexican origin are lower than those for Whites (Lorenzo et al., 2002). Despite their higher prevalence of obesity

and diabetes, U.S. Hispanics have lower rates of cardiovascular disease than do Whites (Ramirez, 1996).

## Age and Risk: The Elderly

The number of people older than 65 years is rapidly increasing and, in fewer than 30 years, one of every five people in the United States will be older than 65 (Spillman & Lubitz, 2000). Systolic BP rises progressively with age (Burt et al., 1995) and elderly people with hypertension are at greater risk for cardiovascular disease (Figure 1–4).

## Pulse Pressure

As seen in Figure 1–4, systolic levels rise progressively with age, whereas diastolic levels typically start to fall beyond age 50 (Burt et al., 1995). Both of these changes reflect increased aortic stiffness and pulse-wave velocity with a more rapid return of the reflected pressure waves (Asmar et al., 2001), as are described in more detail in Chapter 3. It comes as no surprise that the progressive widening of pulse pressure is a prognosticator of cardiovascular risk, as both the widening pulse pressure and most of the risk come from the same pathology—atherosclerosis and arteriosclerosis (de Simone et al., 2005).

Awareness of the critical nature of the widened pulse pressure began in the late 1980s (Darne et al., 1989) but, as Swales (2000) pointed out, the risk of rising systolic BP in the elderly actually was recognized in the early 1900s. For somewhat obscure reasons, most of the risks of hypertension were ascribed soon thereafter to the higher diastolic levels typically seen in the younger population. From the 1920s until the mid-1980s, the diastolic levels "ruled" (Ramsay & Waller, 1986), even though the Framingham data were shown in 1971 to document the greater predictive value of systolic levels for cardio-

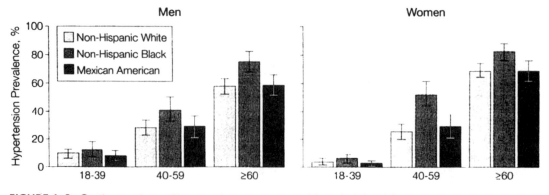

**FIGURE 1–3** ● The prevalence of hypertension among 5,448 adults included in the 1999–2000 NHANES survey classified by race/ethnicity, age, and gender. Data are weighted to the U.S. population. (Modified from Hajjar I, Kotchen TA. Trends in prevalence, awareness, treatment, and control of hypertension in the United States, 1988–2000. *JAMA* 2003;290:199–206.)

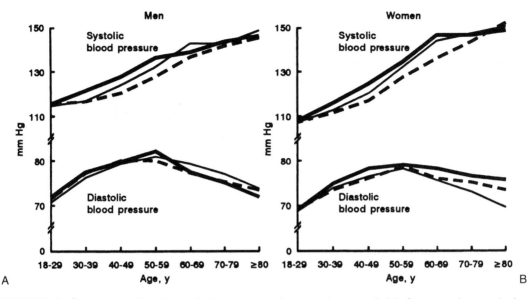

**FIGURE 1–4** ● Mean systolic and diastolic blood pressures by age and race or ethnicity for men and women in the U.S. population 18 years of age or older. *Thick solid line*, non-Hispanic blacks; *dashed line*, non-Hispanic whites; *thin solid line*, Mexican-Americans. Data from the NHANES III survey. (Modified from Burt VL, Whelton P, Roccella EJ, et al. Prevalence of hypertension in the U.S. adult population. Results from the Third National Health and Nutrition Examination Survey, 1988–1991. *Hypertension* 1995;25:305–313.)

vascular disease (Kannel et al., 1971). Now, systolic levels are recognized to be a far better predictor of cardiovascular risk in those over age 50 to a degree that some question whether diastolic levels are worth measuring after middle age (Beevers, 2004).

There is disagreement, however, over the relative value of systolic and diastolic levels versus pulse pressure. The massive Prospective Studies Collaboration found that, for people aged 40 to 89 years, systolic BP was slightly more predictive of death from IHD than was diastolic but pulse pressure was much less predictive than either systolic or diastolic BPs (Lewington et al., 2002). However, investigators from the Framingham Heart Study found that pulse pressure is more predictive than is systolic BP of risk of IHD (Franklin et al., 2003) as well as the risk of congestive heart failure (Haider et al., 2003). These investigators and other expert cardiovascular epidemiologists have gone so far as to recommend that pulse pressure replace the systolic BP in the Framingham risk score among middle-aged and older individuals (Nawrot et al., 2004).

However, the use of pulse pressure across all age groups would be problematic. In the Framingham study participants, a gradual shift from diastolic BP to systolic BP and pulse pressure as predictors of coronary risk was noted with increasing age of the participants (Franklin et al., 2001b). At less than age 50, diastolic BP was the strongest predictor of CHD risk. From age 50 to 59, all three indices were comparable predictors. From age 60 on, diastolic BP

was negatively associated with risk so that the pulse pressure then became superior to systolic BP.

Similar discordant results have been noted in other observational studies, including the 22-year follow-up of the 340,815 men enrolled in the Multiple Risk Factor Interventional Trial (Domanski et al., 2002) and the 15-year follow-up of 7,830 participants in the second NHANES survey (Pastor-Barriuso et al., 2003). Therefore, as Pastor-Barriuso et al. (2003) conclude: "The complexity of the association of pulse pressure with mortality discourages its use for prognostic or therapeutic decisions."

### Isolated Systolic Hypertension

As expected from Figure 1–4, most hypertension after age 50 is isolated systolic hypertension (ISH), with a diastolic BP of less than 90 mm Hg. In an analysis based on the NHANES III data, Franklin et al. (2001a) found that ISH was the diagnosis in 65% of all cases of uncontrolled hypertension seen in the entire population and in 80% of patients older than 50. It should be noted that, unlike some reports that define ISH as a systolic BP of 160 mm Hg or greater, Franklin et al. (2001a) appropriately use 140 or higher.

Isolated systolic hypertension is associated with increased morbidity and mortality from coronary disease and stroke in patients as old as 94 years (Kannel, 2000a). However, as older patients develop cardiovascular disease and cardiac pump function deteriorates, systolic levels often fall and a U-shaped curve of cardiovascular mortality becomes obvious: Mortality increases both in those with systolic BP of less than 120 and in those with systolic BP of more than 140. Similarly, mortality is higher in those 85 years or older if their systolic BP is lower than 125 or their diastolic BP is lower than 65, both indicative of poor overall health (Boshuizen et al., 1998).

### Isolated Diastolic Hypertension

In people under age 45, isolated systolic hypertension is exceedingly rare but isolated diastolic hypertension (IDH), i.e., systolic below 140 mm Hg, diastolic 90 mm Hg or higher, may be found in 10% or more (Strandberg et al., 2002). Among the 346 such patients with IDH followed for up to 32 years, no increase in cardiovascular mortality was found, whereas mortality was increased 2.7-fold in those with combined systolic and diastolic elevations (Strandberg et al., 2002).

Other studies have found a similar absence of increased risk for IDH, leading Pickering (2003) to conclude: "It would seem reasonable not to prescribe antihypertensive treatment for patients with [IDH] at the present time."

### Relative versus Absolute Risk

The risks of elevated BP are often presented as relative to risks found with lower levels of BP. This way of looking at risk tends to exaggerate its degree, as is described in Chapter 5 when the benefits of therapy and the decision to treat are discussed. For now, a single example should suffice. As seen in Figure 1–5, when the associations among various levels of BP to the risk of having a stroke were examined in a total of 450,000 patients followed for 5 to 30 years, there was a clear increase in stroke risk with increasing levels of diastolic BP (Prospective Studies Collaboration, 1995). In relative terms, the increase in risk was much greater in the younger group (less than 45 years), going from 0.2 to 1.9, which is almost a tenfold increase in relative risk compared to the less than twofold increase in the older group (10.0 to 18.4). But it is obvious that the *absolute* risk is much greater in the elderly, with 8.4% (18.4 minus 10.0) more having a stroke with the higher diastolic BP but only 1.7% (1.9 minus 0.2) more of the younger were afflicted. The importance of this increased risk in the young with higher BP should not be ignored, but the use of the smaller change in absolute risk rather than the larger change in relative risk seems more appropriate when applying epidemiologic statistics to individual patients.

The distinction between the risks for the population and for the individual is important. For the population at large, risk clearly increases with every increment in BP, and levels of BP that are accompanied by significantly increased risks should be called

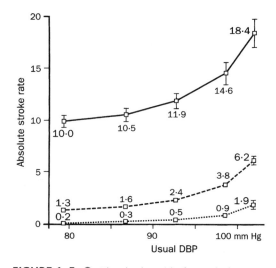

**FIGURE 1–5** ● The absolute risks for stroke by age and usual diastolic blood pressure in 45 prospective observational studies involving 450,000 individuals with 5 to 30 years of follow-up during which 13,397 participants had a stroke. *Dotted line*, <45 years old; *dashed line*, 45–65 years old; *solid line*, ≥65 years old. (Modified from Prospective Studies Collaboration. Cholesterol, diastolic blood pressure, and stroke: 13,000 strokes in 450,000 people in 45 prospective cohorts. *Lancet* 1995;346:1647–1653.)

*high*. As Stamler et al. (1993) note: "Among persons aged 35 years or more, most have BP above optimal (<120/<80 mm Hg); hence, they are at increased CVD [cardiovascular disease] risk, i.e., the BP problem involves most of the population, not only the substantial minority with clinical hypertension." However, for individual patients, the absolute risk from slightly elevated BP may be quite small. Therefore, as noted previously, more than just the level of BP should be used to determine risk and, even more importantly, to determine the need to institute therapy (Jackson et al., 2005).

### Benefits of Action: Decreased Risk of Cardiovascular Disease

We now turn to the major benefit listed in Table 1–2 that is involved in a conceptual definition of hypertension, the level at which it is possible to show the benefit of reducing cardiovascular disease by lowering the BP. Inclusion of this factor is predicated on the assumption that it is of no benefit—and, as we shall see, is potentially harmful—to label a person hypertensive if nothing will be done to lower the BP.

### Natural versus Treatment-Induced Blood Pressure

Before proceeding, one caveat is in order. As noted earlier, less cardiovascular disease is seen in people with low BP who are not receiving antihypertensive therapy. However, that fact cannot be used as evidence to support the benefits of therapy, because naturally low BP may offer a degree of protection not provided by a similarly low BP resulting from antihypertensive therapy.

The available evidence supports that view: Morbidity and mortality rates, particularly those of coronary disease, continue to be higher in many patients at relatively low risk who are undergoing antihypertensive drug treatment than in untreated people with similar levels of BP. This has been shown in follow-up studies of multiple populations (Andersson et al., 1998; Clausen & Jensen, 1992; Thürmer et al., 1994). This issue, too, will be covered in more detail in Chapter 5, but one piece of the evidence will be acknowledged here.

An analysis of all-cause and cardiovascular mortality observed in seven randomized trials of middle-aged patients with diastolic BP from 90 to 114 mm Hg showed a reduction in mortality in the treated half in those trials wherein the population was at fairly high risk, as defined by an all-cause mortality rate of greater than 6 per 1,000 person-years in the untreated population (Hoes et al., 1995). However, in those studies involving patients who started at a lower degree of risk, those who were treated had *higher* mortality rates than were seen in the untreated groups.

These disquieting data should not be taken as evidence against the use of antihypertensive drug therapy. They do not, in any way, deny that protection against cardiovascular complications can be achieved by successful reduction of BP with drugs in patients at risk. They simply indicate that the protection may not be universal or uniform for one or more reasons, including the following: (a) only a partial reduction of BP may be achieved; (b) irreversible hypertensive damage may be present; (c) other risk factors that accompany hypertension may not be improved; and (d) there are dangers inherent to the use of some drugs, in particular the high doses of diuretics used in the earlier trials covered by Hoes et al. (1995). Whatever the explanation, these data document a difference between natural and induced levels of BP.

In contrast to these data, considerable experimental, epidemiologic, and clinical evidence indicates that reducing elevated BP is beneficial, particularly in high-risk patients (Turnbull & Blood Pressure Lowering, 2003).

### Rationale for Reducing Elevated Blood Pressure

Table 1–3 presents the rationale for lowering elevated BP. The reduction in cardiovascular disease and death (listed last in the table) has been

## TABLE 1–3

### Rationale for the Reduction of Elevated Blood Pressure

1. Morbidity and mortality as a result of cardiovascular diseases are directly related to the level of blood pressure.
2. Blood pressure rises most in those whose pressures are already high.
3. In humans, there is less vascular damage where the blood pressure is lower: beneath a coarctation, beyond a renovascular stenosis, and in the pulmonary circulation.
4. In animal experiments, lowering the blood pressure has been shown to protect the vascular system.
5. Antihypertensive therapy reduces cardiovascular disease and death.

used as the primary reason to use antihypertensive therapy, but data are not available to document the level of BP at which therapy is needed for the majority of patients.

During the past 40 years, controlled therapeutic trials have included patients with diastolic BP levels as low as 90 mm Hg. Detailed analyses of these trials are presented in Chapter 5. For now, it is enough to say that there is no question that protection against cardiovascular disease has been documented for reduction of diastolic BP levels that start at or above 95 mm Hg, but there is continued disagreement about whether protection has been shown for those whose diastolic BP starts at or above 90 mm Hg who are otherwise at low risk. Similarly, protection for the elderly with ISH has been documented with systolic BP ≥160 but there are no data for the large elderly population with BP between 140 and 160 mm Hg. Therefore, expert committees have disagreed about the minimum level of BP at which drug treatment should begin.

These disagreements have highlighted the need to consider more than the level of BP in making that decision. As will be noted in Chapter 5, the consideration of other risk factors, target organ damage, and symptomatic cardiovascular disease allows a more rational decision to be made about whom to treat.

### Prevention of Progression of Hypertension

Another benefit of action is the prevention of progression of hypertension, which should be looked on as a surrogate for reducing the risk of cardiovascular disease. Evidence of that benefit is strong, based on data from multiple, randomized, placebo-controlled clinical trials. In such trials, the number of patients whose hypertension progressed from their initially less severe degree to more severe hypertension, defined as BP >200/110 mm Hg, increased from only 95 of 13,389 patients on active treatment to 1,493 of 13,342 patients on placebo (Moser & Hebert, 1996).

## Risks and Costs of Action

The decision to label a person hypertensive and begin treatment involves assumption of the role of a patient, changes in lifestyle, possible interference with the quality of life, risks from biochemical side effects of therapy, and financial costs. As will be emphasized in the next chapter, the diagnosis should not be based on one or only a few readings since there is often an initial white-coat effect, which frequently dissipates after a few weeks.

### Assumption of the Role of a Patient and Worsening Quality of Life

Merely labeling a person hypertensive may cause negative effects as well as enough sympathetic nervous system activity to change hemodynamic measurements (Rostrup et al., 1991). People who know they are hypertensive may have considerable anxiety over the diagnosis of "the silent killer" and experience multiple symptoms as a consequence (Kaplan, 1997). The adverse effects of labeling were identified in a population-based study of 466 Spanish subjects who had careful assessment of their blood pressure status and health-related quality of life (QOL) with the SF-36 Health Survey (Mena-Martin et al., 2003). Those with known hypertension had significantly poorer QOL measures including physical functioning, general health, vitality, and mental health than did those who were hypertensive with similar levels of BP but who were unaware of their condition. Quality-of-life measures were similar in the unknown hypertensives and the normotensives. Fortunately, hypertensive people who receive appropriate counseling and comply with modern-day therapy usually have no impairment and may have improvements in overall QOL measures (Degl'Innocenti et al., 2004; Grimm et al., 1997).

### Risks from Biochemical Side Effects of Therapy

Biochemical risks are less likely to be perceived by the patient than the interferences with quality of life, but they may actually be more hazardous. These risks are discussed in detail in Chapter 7. For now, only two will be mentioned: hypokalemia, which develops in 5% to 20% of diuretic-treated patients, and elevations in blood triglyceride and glucose levels, which may accompany the use of β-blockers.

## Overview of Risks and Benefits

Obviously, many issues are involved in determining the level of BP that poses enough risk to mandate the diagnosis of hypertension and to call for therapy, despite the potential risks that appropriate therapy entails. An analysis of issues relating to risk factor intervention by Brett (1984) clearly defines the problem:

> Risk factor intervention is usually undertaken in the hope of long-term gain in survival or quality of life. Unfortunately, there are sometimes trade-offs (such as inconvenience, expense, or side effects) and something immediate must be sacrificed. This tension between benefits and liabilities is not necessarily resolved by appealing to statements of medical fact, and it is highlighted by the fact that many persons at risk are asymptomatic. Particularly when proposing drug therapy, the physician cannot make an asymptomatic person feel any better, but might make him feel worse, since most drugs have some incidence of adverse effects. But how should side effects be quantitated on a balance sheet of net drug benefit? If a successful antihypertensive drug causes impotence in a patient, how many months or years of potentially increased survival make the side effect acceptable? There is obviously no dogmatic answer; accordingly, global statements such as "all patients with asymptomatic mild hypertension should be treated" are inappropriate, even if treatment were clearly shown to lower morbidity or mortality rates.

On the other hand, as noted in Figures 1–1 and 1–2, the risks related to blood pressure are directly related to the level, progressively increasing with every increment of blood pressure. Therefore, the argument has been made that, with current available antihypertensive drugs, which have few if any side effects, therapy should be provided even at BP levels lower than 140/90 mm Hg, to prevent both the progression of BP and target organ damages that occur at "high-normal" levels (Julius, 2000). Julius and co-workers are conducting a controlled trial of placebo versus active drug therapy in such patients in an attempt to prove the principle that drug therapy can prevent or at least delay progression (Julius et al., 2004).

An even more audacious approach toward prevention of cardiovascular consequences of hypertension has been proposed by the English epidemiologists Wald and Law (2003). They recommend a "Polypill" composed of low doses of a statin, a diuretic, an ACEI, a β-blocker, folic acid, and aspirin to be given to all people from age 55 on and everyone with existing cardiovascular disease, regardless of pretreatment levels of cholesterol or blood pressure. Wald and Law conclude that the use of the Polypill in this manner would reduce IHD events by 88% and stroke by 80%, with one-third of people benefiting and gaining an average 11 years of life free from IHD or stroke. They estimate side effects in from 8% to 15% of people, depending on the exact formulation.

Although on the surface such a broad attack seems counter to conventional wisdom, it may take much more than our current cautious step-by-step approach. In fact, such a Polypill provides all of the medications deemed necessary in a "practical and evidence-based approach to cardiovascular disease risk reduction" in addition to smoking cessation, diet and weight control, and physical activity (Gluckman et al., 2004). The protective value of three of the five components—aspirin, statin and β-blocker (but not the ACEI)—has been noted among patients with known IHD (Hippisley-Cox & Coupland, 2005). Whether such a combination would provide primary prevention has not been tested.

Yet another proposal has been made by another group of investigators—the Polymeal—perhaps less audacious than the Polypill but certainly more tongue-in-cheek (Franco et al., 2004). The Polymeal offers a 75% or greater reduction in CVD when the published reductions of CVD risk provided by each of its individual components are added up:

- Wine, 150 ml/day                    32%
- Fish, 114 g four times/week         14%
- Dark chocolate, 100 g/day           21%
- Fruit and vegetables, 400 g/day     21%
- Garlic, 2.7 g/day                   25%
- Almonds, 68 g/day                   12%
  Combined Effect  =  76%

In subsequent letters to the *British Medical Journal* editors, claims were made that such a diet, particularly the chocolate, could relieve impotence and depression. Could this be the next Atkins? As the *British Medical Journal* editors predict: "Finding happiness in a frugal, active lifestyle can spare us a future of pills and hypochondria" (Franco et al., 2004). Oh, that it would be so.

## OPERATIONAL DEFINITIONS OF HYPERTENSION

### Seventh Joint National Committee Criteria

In recognition of the data shown in Figures 1–1 and 1–2, the Seventh Joint National Committee report (JNC-7) has introduced a new classification—prehypertension—for those whose blood pressures range from 120 to 139 systolic and/or 80 to 89 diastolic, as opposed to the JNC-6 classification

## TABLE 1–4

### Changes in Blood Pressure Classification

| JNC 6 Category | SBP/DBP | JNC 7 Category |
|---|---|---|
| Optimal | < 120/80 | → Normal |
| Normal | 120–129/80–84 | → Prehypertension |
| Borderline | 130–139/85–89 | |
| Hypertension | ≥ 140/90 | → Hypertension |
| Stage 1 | 140–159/90–99 | → Stage 1 |
| Stage 2 | 160–179/100–109 | → Stage 2 |
| Stage 3 | ≥ 180/110 | |

Sources: The sixth report of the Joint National Committee on Prevention, Detection, Evaluation, and Treatment of High Blood Pressure. *Arch Intern Med* 1997;157:2413–2446.
The seventh report of the Joint National Committee on Prevention, Detection, Evaluation, and Treatment of High Blood Pressure. *JAMA* 2003;289:2560–2572.

of such levels as "normal" and "high-normal" (Chobanian et al., 2003) (Table 1–4). In addition, the former stages two and three have been combined into a single stage two category since management of all patients with BP above 160/100 is similar.

## CLASSIFICATION OF BLOOD PRESSURE

### Prehypertension

The JNC-7 report (Chobanian et al., 2003) states:

> Prehypertension is not a disease category. Rather it is a designation chosen to identify individuals at high risk of developing hypertension, so that both patients and clinicians are alerted to this risk and encouraged to intervene and prevent or delay the disease from developing. Individuals who are prehypertensive are not candidates for drug therapy on the basis of their level of BP and should be firmly and unambiguously advised to practice lifestyle modification in order to reduce their risk of developing hypertension in the future. . . . Moreover, individuals with prehypertension who also have diabetes or kidney disease should be considered candidates for appropriate drug therapy if a trial of lifestyle modification fails to reduce their BP to 130/80 mm Hg or less. . . . The goal for individuals with prehypertension and no compelling indications is to lower BP to normal with lifestyle changes and prevent the progressive rise in BP using the recommended lifestyle modifications.

The guidelines from the European (Guidelines Committee, 2003), World Health Organization-International Society of Hypertension (WHO/ISH Writing Group, 2003), and the British Hypertension Societies (Williams et al., 2004) continue to classify BP below 140/90 as did JNC-6 into normal and high-normal. However, the JNC-7 classification seems appropriate, recognizing the significantly increased risk for patients with above-optimal levels. Since for every increase in blood pressure by 20/10 mm Hg the risk of CVD doubles, a level of 135/85, with a double degree of risk, is better called prehypertension than high-normal.

Not surprisingly, considering the bell-shaped curve of blood pressure in the U.S. adult population (Figure 1–6), the number of people with prehypertension is even greater than those with hypertension, 31% (or 63 million) versus 29% (or 59 million) of the adult population (Greenlund et al., 2004; Wang & Wang, 2004).

It should be remembered that—despite an unequivocal call for health-promoting lifestyle modifications and no antihypertensive drug for such prehypertensives (unless they have a compelling indication such as diabetes or renal insufficiency)—the labeling of prehypertension could cause anxiety and lead to the premature use of drugs that have not yet been shown to be protective at such low levels of elevated blood pressure. Americans are pill happy and doctors often acquiesce to patients' requests even when the doctors know better. So, time will tell: Are Americans too quick or is the rest of the world too slow?

### Systolic Hypertension in the Elderly

In view of the previously noted risks of isolated systolic elevations, JNC-7 recommends that, in the presence of a diastolic BP of less than 90 mm Hg,

a systolic BP level of 140 mm Hg or higher is classified as ISH. Although risks of such elevations of systolic BP in the elderly have been clearly identified (Franklin et al., 2001b), the value of therapy to reduce systolic levels between 140 and 160 mm Hg in the elderly has not been well documented.

### Hypertension in Children

For children, JNC-7 uses the definition from the *Report of the Second Task Force on Blood Pressure Control in Children* (1996), which identifies *significant hypertension* as BP persistently equal to or greater than the ninety-fifth percentile for age and height and *severe hypertension* as BP persistently equal to or greater than the ninety-ninth percentile for age and height. Hypertension in children is covered in Chapter 16, wherein more recent guidelines are provided.

### Labile Hypertension

As ambulatory readings have been recorded, the marked variability in virtually everyone's BP has become obvious (see Chapter 2). In view of the usual variability of BP, the term *labile* is neither useful nor meaningful.

### Borderline Hypertension

The term *borderline* may be used to describe hypertension in which the BP only occasionally rises above 140/90 mm Hg. Persistently elevated BP is more likely to develop in such people than in those with consistently normal readings. However, this progression is by no means certain. In one study of a particularly fit, low-risk group of air cadets with borderline pressures, only 12% developed sustained hypertension over the subsequent 20 years (Madsen & Buch, 1971). Nonetheless, people with borderline pressures tend to have hemodynamic changes

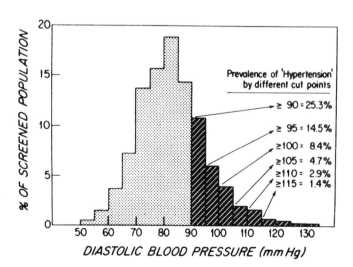

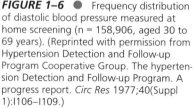

**FIGURE 1–6** ● Frequency distribution of diastolic blood pressure measured at home screening (n = 158,906, aged 30 to 69 years). (Reprinted with permission from Hypertension Detection and Follow-up Program Cooperative Group. The hypertension Detection and Follow-up Program. A progress report. *Circ Res* 1977;40(Suppl 1):I106–I109.)

indicative of early hypertension and greater degrees of other cardiovascular risk factors, including greater body weight, dyslipidemia, and higher plasma insulin levels (Julius et al., 1990) and should, therefore, be followed more closely and advised to modify their lifestyle.

## PREVALENCE OF HYPERTENSION

As previously noted, the prevalence of hypertension is increasing worldwide because of both increasing longevity and increasing obesity from more fast foods and less physical activity.

### Prevalence in the U.S. Adult Population

The best sources of data for the U.S. population are the previously noted NHANES studies, which have examined a large representative sample of the U.S. adult population aged 18 and older approximately every 10 years. Unfortunately, methodological differences between surveys have resulted in variable estimates of the prevalence of hypertension based on these surveys.

The presence of hypertension has been defined in the NHANES as having a measured systolic BP of 140 mm Hg or higher, a measured diastolic BP of 90 mm Hg or higher, or taking antihypertensive drug therapy, or having been told by a physician two or more times that they were hypertensive. The overall number of U.S. adults with hypertension defined by these criteria decreased from nearly 58 million during 1976 to 1980 to approximately 50 million during 1988 to 1994 (Wolz et al., 2000). One probable explanation for this decrease in the prevalence of hypertension involves the setting in which the BP measurements were made in these surveys. In NHANES II (1976–1980), BPs were measured at one visit to special clinics, whereas in NHANES III (1986–1994), three readings were taken at the subjects' homes and three at the clinic several weeks later, and the mean of the six readings was used. In the NHANES IV data, the mean of only three readings taken in the clinic was used, which may partly explain the higher prevalence in the latest survey.

Data from the NHANES IV (1999–2000) reveal a significant increase from the NHANES III (1986–1994) data. Hajjar and Kotchen (2003) estimate an overall prevalence of hypertension of 28.7%, which translates into 58.4 million U.S. adults; Fields et al. (2004) estimate an overall prevalence of 31.3%, translating to 65.2 million U.S. adults.

Despite these discrepancies, the two analyses of the 1999–2000 data show a definite increase in the prevalence of hypertension in the United States. And, even though the totals may differ, the distributions within the total population by gender and race are quite similar. As seen in Figure 1–3, the prevalence rises in both genders with age, more so in older women than in older men. The prevalence among U.S. Blacks is higher than in Whites and Mexican-Americans in both genders and at all ages. Compared to their proportion of the total population, U.S. Whites comprise the same proportion of the hypertensive population whereas U.S. Blacks comprise 21.2% more and Mexican-Americans 33.8% less than expected (Fields et al., 2004). Part of the lower overall rates in Mexican-Americans reflects their younger average age. With age-adjustment, Mexican-Americans had prevalence rates similar to U.S. Whites.

U.S. women had 20% more hypertension overall and 74% more after age 65 compared to men. Women displayed a progressive increased prevalence with age, whereas the prevalence peaked in men aged 45 to 54 and then progressively declined.

Other subpopulations, including American Indian, Alaskan Native, or Asian Pacific Islander, comprised 9.1% of the NHANES 1999–2000 total population and contributed 8.1% of the hypertensive population, 11.0% lower than expected.

These increases in prevalence over the past 10 years are attributed to a number of factors, including:

- The increased number of older people: 81% of all U.S. hypertensive adults are 45 years of age or older, though this group comprised only 46% of the U.S. population (Fields et al., 2004).
- The increase in obesity; Hajjar and Kotchen (2003) calculate that more than half of the increase in prevalence can be attributed to the increase in body mass index.
- An increased number of hypertensives who live longer as a result of improved lifestyles or more effective drug therapy.
- An increased rate of new-onset hypertension not attributable to older age or obesity; the prevalence rates increased in all groups except those aged 18 to 34.

### Populations Outside the United States

In national surveys performed in the 1990s using similar sampling and reporting techniques, significantly higher prevalences of hypertension were noted in six European countries (England, Finland, Germany, Italy, Spain, and Sweden) compared to the United States and Canada (Wolf-Maier et al., 2003). The age- and sex-adjusted prevalence of hypertension was 28% in the United States and Canada and 44% in the six European countries. The overall 60%

higher prevalence of hypertension was closely correlated with stroke mortalities in the various countries, adding to the validity of the findings.

Rather marked differences in the prevalence of hypertension among similar populations that cannot be easily explained have also been noted. For example, Shaper et al. (1988) reported a threefold variation among 7,735 middle-aged men in 24 towns throughout Great Britain, with higher rates in northern England and Scotland. Some of the variation could be explained by such obvious factors as body weight or alcohol and sodium and potassium intake, but most of the variation remains unexplained (Bruce et al., 1993).

Equally striking are the major differences in mortality due to coronary disease as related to levels of BP in various countries (van den Hoogen et al., 2000). Rates of CHD mortality at any level of BP were more than three times higher in the United States and northern Europe than in Japan and southern Europe; however, the relative increase in CHD mortality for a given increase in BP is similar in all countries.

## INCIDENCE OF HYPERTENSION

Much less is known about the incidence of newly developed hypertension than about its prevalence. The Framingham study provides one database (Vasan et al., 2001a) and the National Health Epidemiologic Follow-up Study another (Cornoni-Huntley et al., 1989). In the latter study, 14,407 participants in NHANES I (1971 to 1975) were followed an average of 9.5 years. Unfortunately, BP was measured only once for each participant at the beginning of the study, and only the first of three measured during follow-up was used in the analysis to provide comparability. Therefore, the rates provided by this

survey are likely considerably higher than would be found with a more careful assessment based on several readings.

Nonetheless, as seen in Figure 1–7, comparison of the incidence of hypertension (systolic BP >160 mm Hg; diastolic BP >95 mm Hg) in White men and women shows an approximate 5% increase for each 10-year interval of age at baseline, except in the 65- to 74-year-old group. The incidence among Blacks was at least twice that among Whites. The high incidence in the 55- to 64-year-old and 65- to 74-year-old groups likely represents a considerable proportion of cases of isolated systolic hypertension, because the diagnosis was based on elevations in either systolic BP or diastolic BP.

As seen in Table 1–5, the incidence of hypertension in the Framingham cohort over four years was directly related to the prior level of BP and to age with similar rates among men and women (Vasan et al., 2001a). Obesity and weight gain also contributed to progression. A 5% weight gain after four years was associated with 20% to 30% increased odds of hypertension.

## CAUSES OF HYPERTENSION

The list of causes of hypertension (Table 1–6) is quite long; however, the cause of more than 90% of the cases of hypertension is unknown, i.e., primary or essential. The proportion of cases secondary to some identifiable mechanism has been debated considerably, as more specific causes have been recognized. Claims that one cause or another is responsible for up to 20% of all cases of hypertension repeatedly appear from investigators who are particularly interested in a certain category of hypertension and therefore see only a highly selected population.

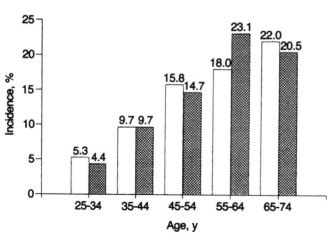

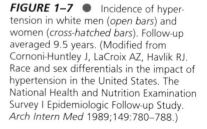

**FIGURE 1–7** ● Incidence of hypertension in white men (*open bars*) and women (*cross-hatched bars*). Follow-up averaged 9.5 years. (Modified from Cornoni-Huntley J, LaCroix AZ, Havlik RJ. Race and sex differentials in the impact of hypertension in the United States. The National Health and Nutrition Examination Survey I Epidemiologic Follow-up Study. *Arch Intern Med* 1989;149:780–788.)

**TABLE 1–5**

### Rates of Progression to Hypertension in Framingham

| Blood Pressure Category | Percentage of 4-yr Progression to Hypertension | | | |
| --- | --- | --- | --- | --- |
| | Men, age 35–64 yr | Men, age 65–74 yr | Women, age 35–64 yr | Women, age 65–94 yr |
| Optimal BP | 5 | 15 | 5 | 16 |
| Normal BP | 18 | 25 | 12 | 26 |
| High Normal BP | 37 | 47 | 37 | 49 |

Data adapted from Vasan RS, Larson MG, Leip EP, et al. Assessment of frequency of progression to hypertension in non-hypertensive participants in the Framingham Heart Study: a cohort study. *Lancet* 2001a;358:1682–1686.

Older data from surveys of various populations are available (Table 1–7). Even though the patients in some of these studies were referred specifically for evaluation of identifiable causes or because they had more severe hypertension wherein identifiable causes are more likely, note that the prevalence of primary (essential) hypertension was 90% or higher.

Perhaps the best data on what could be expected in a usual clinical practice come from the study by Rudnick et al. (1977), which involved 655 hypertensive patients in a family practice in Hamilton, Ontario, Canada. Each patient had a complete workup, including an intravenous pyelogram. Notice again the rarity of identifiable hypertension in this relatively unselected population.

However, improved diagnostic procedures are now available that almost certainly would increase the frequency of various identifiable (secondary) forms than those uncovered in these older surveys. More about this is found in Chapters 9 through 15. In truth, the frequencies of various forms in an otherwise unselected population of hypertensives is unknown.

## POPULATION RISK FROM HYPERTENSION

Now that the definition of hypertension and its classification have been provided, along with various estimates of its prevalence, the impact of hypertension on the population at large can be considered. As noted, for the individual patient, the higher the level of BP, the greater the risk of morbidity and mortality. However, for the population at large, the greatest burden from hypertension occurs among people with only minimally elevated pressures, because there are so many of them. This burden can be seen in Figure 1–8, where 12-year cardiovascular mortality rates observed with each increment of BP are plotted against the distribution of the various levels of BP among the 350,000 35- to 57-year-old men screened for the Multiple Risk Factor Intervention Trial (National High Blood Pressure Education Program Working Group, 1993). Although the mortality rates climb progressively, most deaths occur in the much larger proportion of the population with minimally elevated pressures. By multiplying the percentage of men at any given level of BP by the relative risk for that level, it can be seen that more cardiovascular mortality will occur in those with a diastolic BP of 80 to 84 than among those with a diastolic BP of 95 mm Hg or greater.

### Strategy for the Population

This disproportionate risk for the population at large from relatively mild hypertension bears strongly on the question of how to achieve the greatest reduction in the risks of hypertension. In the past, most effort has been directed at the group with the highest levels of BP. However, this "high-risk" strategy, as effective as it may be for those affected, does little to reduce total morbidity and mortality if the "low-risk" patients, who make up the largest share of the population at risk, are ignored (Rose, 1985).

Many more people with mild hypertension are now being treated actively and intensively with antihypertensive drugs. However, as emphasized by Rose (1992), a more effective strategy would be to lower the BP level of the entire population, as might be accomplished by reduction of sodium

## TABLE 1-6

### Types and Causes of Hypertension

**Systolic and diastolic hypertension**
Primary, essential, or idiopathic
Identifiable causes
  Renal
    Renal parenchymal disease
      Acute glomerulonephritis
      Chronic nephritis
      Polycystic disease
      Diabetic nephropathy
      Hydronephrosis
    Renovascular disease
      Renal artery stenosis
      Other causes of renal ischemia
    Renin-producing tumors
    Renoprival
    Primary sodium retention: Liddle's syndrome, Gordon's syndrome
  Endocrine
    Acromegaly
    Hypothyroidism
    Hyperthyroidism
    Hypercalcemia (hyperparathyroidism)
    Adrenal disorders
      Cortical disorders
        Cushing's syndrome
        Primary aldosteronism
        Congenital adrenal hyperplasia
      Medullary tumors: pheochromocytoma
    Extra-adrenal chromaffin tumors
    11-$\beta$-hydroxysteroid dehydrogenase deficiency or inhibition (licorice)
  Carcinoids
  Exogenous hormones
    Estrogen
    Glucocorticoids
    Mineralocorticoids
    Sympathomimetics
    Erythropoietin
Foods containing tyramine with monamine oxidase inhibitors
Coarctation of the aorta and aortitis
Pregnancy-induced
Neurological disorders
  Increased intracranial pressure
  Sleep apnea
  Quadriplegia
  Acute porphyria
  Familial dysautonomia
  Lead poisoning
  Guillain-Barré syndrome
Acute stress
  Psychogenic hyperventilation
  Hypoglycemia
  Burns
  Alcohol withdrawal
  Sickle cell crisis
  After resuscitation
  Perioperative
Increased intravascular volume (polycythemia)
Alcohol
Nicotine
Cyclosporine, tacrolimus
Other agents (see Table 15–5)

**Systolic hypertension**
Increased cardiac output
  Aortic valvular insufficiency
  Arteriovenous fistula, patent ductus
  Thyrotoxicosis
  Paget's disease of bone
  Beriberi
Arterial rigidity

---

intake. Rose estimated that lowering the entire distribution of BP by only 2 to 3 mm Hg would be as effective in reducing the overall risks of hypertension as prescribing current antihypertensive drug therapy for all people with definite hypertension.

This issue is eloquently addressed by Stamler (1998):

The high-risk strategy of the last 25 years— involving detection, evaluation, and treatment

## TABLE 1-7

### Frequency of Various Diagnoses in Hypertensive Subjects

| Diagnosis | Frequency of Diagnosis (%) | | | | |
|---|---|---|---|---|---|
| | Gifford (1969) | Berglund et al. (1976) | Rudnick et al. (1977) | Danielson & Dammström (1981) | Sinclair et al. (1987) |
| *Number of patients* | *4,339* | *689* | *665* | *1,000* | *3,783* |
| Essential hypertension | 89 | 94 | 94 | 95.3 | 92.1 |
| Chronic renal disease | 5 | 4 | 5 | 2.4 | 5.6 |
| Renovascular disease | 4 | 1 | 0.2 | 1.0 | 0.7 |
| Coarctation of the aorta | 1 | 0.1 | 0.2 | – | – |
| Primary aldosteronism | 0.5 | 0.1 | – | 0.1 | 0.3 |
| Cushing's syndrome | 0.2 | – | 0.2 | 0.1 | 0.1 |
| Pheochromocytoma | 0.2 | – | – | 0.2 | 0.1 |
| Oral contraceptive use | – | – | 0.2 | 0.8 | 1.0 |

(usually including drug therapy) of tens of millions of people with already established high BP—useful as it has been, has serious limitations: It is late, defensive, mainly reactive, time-consuming, associated with adverse effects (inevitable with drugs, however favorable the mix of benefit and risk), costly, only partially successful, and endless. It offers no possibility of ending the high BP epidemic.

However, present knowledge enables pursuit of the additional goal of the primary prevention of high BP, the solution to the high BP epidemic. For decades, extensive concordant evidence has been amassed by all research disciplines showing that high salt intake, obesity, excess alcohol intake, inadequate potassium intake, and sedentary lifestyle all have adverse effects on population

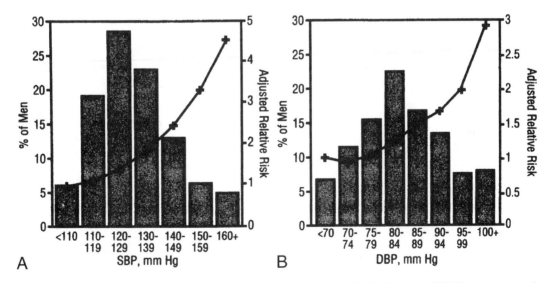

**FIGURE 1–8** ● (**A**) The bars indicate the percentage distribution of systolic blood pressure (SBP) for men screened for the MRFIT who were 35 to 57 years old and had no history of myocardial infarction (*n* = 347,978). The curves show the corresponding 12-year rates of cardiovascular mortality by SBP level adjusted for age, race, total serum cholesterol level, cigarettes smoked per day, reported use of medication for diabetes mellitus, and imputed household income (using census tract for residence). (**B**) Same as part (**A**) showing the distribution of diastolic blood pressure (DBP) (*n* = 356,222). (Modified from National High Blood Pressure Education Program Working Group. National High Blood Pressure Education Program Working Group report on primary prevention of hypertension. *Arch Intern Med* 1993;153:186–208.)

BP levels. This evidence is the solid scientific foundation for the expansion in the strategy to attempt primary prevention of high BP by improving lifestyles across entire populations.

The broader approach is almost certainly correct on epidemiologic grounds. Easier, more effective and cost-beneficial approaches have been proposed: The Polypill given to all people over age 55 regardless of their pretreatment risk status (Wald & Law, 2003) or, even tastier, the advocacy of a Polymeal for everyone (Franco et al., 2004). However, until (and if) such mass strategies can be implemented, we are left with the need to better treat those with established hypertension.

## DETECTION AND CONTROL OF HYPERTENSION IN THE POPULATION

As seen in Table 1–1, the percentages of people in the United States who are aware of their hypertension, who are receiving treatment, and whose hypertension is controlled have risen progressively over the past 25 years. However, using the threshold level of 140/90 mm Hg, the percentage of people in the United States with controlled hypertension as of 2000 was only 34%. Similarly poor or even worse rates of adequate control have been noted worldwide (Whelton et al., 2004; Wolf-Maier et al., 2004).

## Benefits of Improved Control of Hypertension

Nonetheless, at least partly as a result of the somewhat improved control of hypertension, there has been a steady decrease in the mortality rate of CHD and an even greater decrease in that of stroke in the United States since 1960 (Figure 1–9). The decline in mortality due to these two diseases has been steeper than for noncardiovascular disease and has been observed in men and women, Blacks and Whites.

The explanation for the reduced mortality rate of cardiovascular disease in the United States remains uncertain. However, the total contribution from all improvements in risk factors, including the control of hypertension, appears to explain about half of the decline. Among three groups of subjects in the Framingham Heart Study who were 50 to 59 years old in 1950, 1960, or 1970, the decline in cardiovascular mortality over the subsequent 20-year intervals was 59% in the female cohorts and 53% in the male cohorts (Sytkowski et al., 1996a). More than half of the decline in CHD mortality in women and from one-third to one-half

of the decline in men would be attributed to improvements in risk factors, including reductions in hypercholesterolemia, smoking, and hypertension. The effect of the treatment of hypertension was an important part of the overall reduction in risk, with a 60% reduction in the 10-year risk of mortality from cardiovascular diseases in patients with hypertension who were treated as compared to those who were not treated (Sytkowski et al., 1996b).

With a computer simulation model of the entire U.S. population between the ages of 35 and 84, Hunink et al. (1997) devised these estimates of the reasons for the decline in CHD mortality from 1980 to 1990: 43% by improvements in treatment (e.g., bypass surgery) in patients with CHD; 29% by reduction of risk factors, including smoking, hypercholesterolemia, and hypertension, in patients with CHD; and 25% by primary prevention of these risk factors in people without preexisting CHD. Thus, the overall contribution of reductions in risk factors was slightly more than 50%.

In a careful analysis of the causes for the similar relative reduction in CHD mortality in England and Wales between 1981 and 2000 as seen in the United States, Unal et al. (2004) found similar results as the prior U.S. analysis: 42% of the decrease is attributable to treatment of individuals and 58% to reductions in population-wide risk factors. Better control of hypertension was credited with only a 3.1% contribution to individual treatment but the 7.7% lower population level of blood pressure contributed 9.5% of the effects of risk factor reduction (Unal et al., 2004).

Since hypertension plays an even greater role in stroke than in CHD and since reductions in stroke have been greater than reductions in CHD in the therapeutic trials of antihypertensive therapy (see Chapter 5), it is likely the reduction of individualized and population blood pressure has contributed even more to the decreases in stroke mortality than CHD mortality. A comparison of follow-up from NHANES surveys from the 1970s compared to the 1980s showed an even greater reduction in the incidence of stroke than of coronary disease in the United States (Ergin et al., 2004), supporting a major contribution of primary and secondary prevention.

Whatever the impact of hypertensive therapy has been, the United States continues to rank fifteenth of 19 developed countries in life expectancy and sixteenth in amenable mortality (Nolte & McKee, 2003). Moreover, we should not lose sight of the continued increase in the incidence of two major hypertension-related problems: congestive heart failure and end-stage renal disease (Chobanian et al., 2003). Therefore, we have a long way to go in reducing hypertension-related morbidity and mortality.

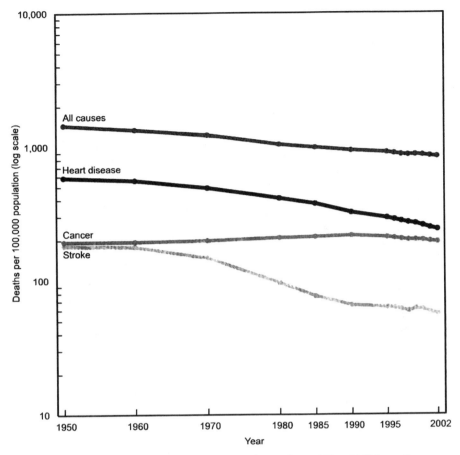

**FIGURE 1–9** ● Changes in age-adjusted U.S. death rates from 1950 to 2002 from all causes, heart disease, cancer, and stroke on a log scale. (From Centers for Disease Control and Prevention, National Center for Health Statistics. Figure 25 in Health, United States, 2004. http://www.cdc.gov/hchs/hus.htm.)

## Continued Problems

Multiple reasons have been given for poor rates of control, including the following:

- The inherent nature of hypertension: a lifelong condition that is usually asymptomatic for many years but that requires daily therapy that may induce symptoms and can be expensive.
- Poor perception of patients' risk by physicians (Mosca et al., 2005).
- Unwillingness of both practitioners and patients to accept the need for treatment of levels of blood pressure that are clearly associated with significantly increased risk, particularly in the elderly with systolic hypertension (Egan et al., 2003).
- Failure to intensify therapy to achieve adequate control (Hicks et al., 2004).
- Inability of patients to modify unhealthy lifestyles, particularly excess calories and inadequate physical activity leading to obesity (Hedley et al., 2004).

- Inadequate access to a regular source of health care (He et al., 2002).

## Individual Solutions

These and other reasons are behind our current failure to control hypertension. Population-wide changes must be encouraged but, in the meantime, the individual patient must be better protected. The patient and his or her practitioner must take hypertension seriously, as seriously as insulin-taking diabetics take their disease. The currently typical, *laissez-faire*, indulgent attitude includes:

- go to the doctor every six months for a blood pressure check,
- avoid the discipline needed to improve lifestyle, and
- take the same pills every morning

Such an approach may work for some but likely never has worked for most and that is why even "well-controlled" hypertensives still suffer more strokes and die earlier than nonhypertensives.

These issues are addressed more fully in the next chapter (the need for closer monitoring), Chapter 6 (the need for lifestyle changes), and Chapter 7 (the need for more tailored, tighter control).

## Practitioner Solutions

The major need now is not to screen or evaluate but to improve continuation of treatment by maintaining contact and encouraging follow-up care. Improvements in long-term management can be made by both large-scale approaches and individual providers (Asch et al., 2004; Canzanello et al., 2005). At least among patients of a higher socioeconomic status improved rates of control have been achieved by provision of good access to health care, a progressive treatment regimen, and self-monitoring by home BPs (Borzecki et al., 2003; Chen et al., 2003; Hicks et al., 2004; Mancia et al., 2004; Szirmai et al., 2005).

JNC-7 (Chobanian et al., 2003) details multifaceted approaches to improve control, including:

- Increasing clinician's awareness of patients' nonadherence to therapy.
- Organizing healthcare delivery systems to efficiently manage hypertensives.
- Individualizing and simplifying the antihypertensive regimen.
- Educating patients about the intricacies of effective treatment.
- Utilizing multiple healthcare professionals.
- Promoting social support systems.

Only a few specific maneuvers have been proven effective in increasing long-term adherence to therapy. These include home BP monitoring, once-a-day therapy, and involvement of ancillary personnel to maintain close follow-up (Canzanello et al., 2005; Schroeder et al., 2004). More details about improving adherence and achieving control of hypertension are provided in Chapter 7.

At the same time, guidelines for improving cardiovascular health in addition to the control of hypertension have been provided by U.S. (Pearson et al., 2003) and international (Smith et al., 2004) expert guidelines.

## POTENTIAL FOR PREVENTION

A greater awareness of the causes and accelerators of hypertension may provide insights into the real goal: prevention. Despite more intensive treatment of millions of people with hypertension, we have done little to prevent its onset with an older

and more obese population, of which the incidence (Vasan et al., 2001a) and prevalence of hypertension are increasing (Fields et al., 2004).

Nonetheless, increasingly strong evidence documents the ability to delay, if not to prevent, the onset of hypertension (Whelton et al., 2002). Crucial to that effort is the prevention of obesity. In the Framingham population, 70% of hypertension in men and 61% in women were directly attributable to excess adiposity (Kannel, 2000b). Unfortunately, the prevalence of obesity in the United States has risen progressively both in adults and, even more disturbingly, in children, who are also developing more obesity-related hypertension (Muntner et al., 2004).

## The Issue of Prehypertension

The introduction by JNC-7 of "prehypertension" covering an additional 60 million people in the United States alone poses both an opportunity and a problem: the opportunity to alert practitioners and patients to the need for primary prevention, and the problem of placing additional burdens on an already harried healthcare profession.

The issue was nicely addressed by Tom Pickering (2004). First, he reminds us of the data from the Chicago Heart Association Detection Program in Industry, which enrolled 10,874 men who were originally aged 18 to 39 and followed them for 25 years (Miura et al., 2001). Mortality was the same in those with a systolic BP between 120 and 129 as it was in those with a systolic BP below 120. Mortality was 33% higher in those with a systolic BP between 130 and 139 but in absolute terms, the mortality rate increased from 6.1 per 10,000 person years to 8.7 per 10,000 person years. As Pickering says: "Put another way, in 100 patients with a systolic pressure <120 mm Hg, there would be 1.5 CV deaths over 25 years; in individuals with pressures in the 'high prehypertensive' range (130-139 mm Hg) the number would be 2.2 deaths."

Second, Pickering considers the consequences of caring for the many millions of prehypertensives whose level of risk is still quite small. He asks:

If, as physicians, we are successful in lowering a patient's BP from 134 mm Hg to 119 mm Hg, what have we achieved? The answer is in the numbers. If we could do it for the whole population of prehypertensives, the benefits would be huge, but if we can only do it for a small number of our patients, they would be negligible. Physician time is limited and expensive, and a good principle for the best use of it would be to achieve the "biggest possible bang for your bucks." We are doing a conspicuously bad job of controlling BP in our hypertensive patients who are at genuinely high risk, and we all know that persuading patients to take pills is much easier than convincing them to change their lifestyles. Therefore, if we need to start setting BP goals for our prehypertensive patients, we are going to have less time to attend to more urgent matters.

## The Purveyors of Prevention

As Pickering (2004) notes: "If we could do it for the whole population of prehypertensives, the benefits would be huge." From that truth, I would take a different reading. We, the healthcare providers, are not the ones to do this, other than to become much more vocal in demanding that others do their job. The task belongs to others, including:

- City planners to provide sidewalks and bicycle paths.
- School administrators to require physical activity in school time and to get rid of soft drinks and candy bars.
- Food processors and marketers to quit preparing and pushing high calorie, high fat, high salt products. (The argument that they should be allowed to sell what consumers want falls down with cigarettes for children.)
- Television programmers to quit assaulting young children with unhealthy choices of food.
- Parents to take responsibility for their children's level of physical activity.
- Adults to forgo instant pleasures (Krispy Kremes) for future benefits.
- Society to protect immature young adults—old enough to die in Iraq—who will surely continue to smoke, drink, and have unprotected sex. Ways to help include enforcing selling restrictions on cigarettes and alcohol, providing chaperones at student drinking parties, and ensuring availability of condoms and morning-after pills to prevent unwanted pregnancies. Adults may not like what hot-blooded young people do but "just saying no" isn't enough.

Until (and if) such nirvana arrives, it may take active drug therapies, either in the slow, measured approach being taken by Julius et al. (2004) or the broad, unmeasured use of a Polypill as advocated by Wald and Law (2003). In whatever way it may be accomplished, we need to keep the goal of prevention in mind as we consider the overall problems of hypertension for the individual patient in the ensuing chapters.

## REFERENCES

Andersson OK, Almgren T, Persson B, et al. Survival of treated hypertension. *BMJ* 1998;317:167–171.

Anonymous. Rise and fall of diseases [Editorial]. *Lancet* 1993;341:151–152.

Asch SM, McGlynn EA, Hogan MM, et al. Comparison of quality of care for patients in the Veterans Health Administration and patients in a national sample. *Ann Intern Med* 2004;141:938–945.

Asmar R, Rudnichi A, Blacher J, et al. Pulse pressure and aortic pulse wave are markers of cardiovascular risk in hypertensive populations. *Am J Hypertens* 2001;14:91–97.

Barrett-Connor E. Sex differences in coronary heart disease. *Circulation* 1997;95:252–264.

Beevers DG. Epidemiological, pathophysiological and clinical significance of systolic, diastolic and pulse pressure. *J Human Hypertens* 2004;18:531–533.

Berglund G, Anderson O, Wilhelmsen L. Prevalence of primary and secondary hypertension. *BMJ* 1976;2:554–556.

Borzecki AM, Wong AT, Hickey EC, et al. Hypertension control: how well are we doing? *Arch Intern Med* 2003;163:2705–2711.

Boshuizen HC, Izaks GJ, van Buuren S, Ligthart GJ. Blood pressure and mortality in elderly people aged 85 and older. *BMJ* 1998;316:1780–1784.

Brett AS. Ethical issues in risk factor intervention. *Am J Med* 1984;76:557–561.

Bruce NG, Wannamethee G, Shaper AG. Lifestyle factors associated with geographic blood pressure variations among men and women in the UK. *J Hum Hypertens* 1993;7:229–238.

Burt VL, Whelton P, Roccella EJ, et al. Prevalence of hypertension in the US adult population. Results from the Third National Health and Nutrition Examination Survey, 1988–91. *Hypertension* 1995;25:305–313.

Canzanello VJ, Jensen PL, Schwartz LL, et al. Improved blood pressure control with a physician-nurse team and home blood pressure measurement. *Mayo Clin Proc* 2005;80:31–36.

Cappuccio FP, Micah FB, Emmett L, et al. Prevalence, detection, management, and control of hypertension in Ashanti, West Africa. *Hypertension* 2004;43:1017–1022.

Chen R, Tunstall-Pedoe H, Morrison C, et al. Trends and social factors in blood pressure control in Scottish MONICA surveys 1986–1995: the rule of halves revisited. *J Human Hypertens* 2003;17:751–759.

Chobanian AV, Bakris GL, Black HR, et al. Seventh report of the Joint National Committee on the Prevention, Detection, Evaluation, and Treatment of High Blood Pressure. *Hypertension* 2003;42:1206–1252.

Clausen J, Jensen G. Blood pressure and mortality: an epidemiological survey with 10 years follow-up. *J Hum Hypertens* 1992;6:53–59.

Cornoni-Huntley J, LaCroix AZ, Havlik RJ. Race and sex differentials in the impact of hypertension in the United States. *Arch Intern Med* 1989;149:780–788.

Danielson M, Dammström B-G. The prevalence of secondary and curable hypertension. *Acta Med Scand* 1981;209:451–455.

Darne B, Girerd X, Safar M, et al. Pulsatile versus steady component of blood pressure. *Hypertension* 1989;13:392–400.

Degl'Innocenti A, Elmfeldt D, Hofman A, et al. Health-related quality of life during treatment of elderly patients with hypertension: results from the Study on Cognition and Prognosis in the Elderly (SCOPE). *J Human Hypertens* 2004;18:239–245.

de Simone G, Roman MJ, Alderman MH, et al. Is high pulse pressure a marker of preclinical cardiovascular disease? *Hypertension* 2005;45:575.

Domanski M, Mitchell G, Pfeffer M, et al. Pulse pressure and cardiovascular disease-related mortality: follow-up study of the Multiple Risk Factor Intervention Trial (MRFIT). *JAMA* 2002;287:2677–2683.

Egan BM, Lackland DT, Cutler NE. Awareness, knowledge, and attitudes of older Americans about high blood pressure: implications for health care policy, education, and research. *Arch Intern Med* 2003;163:681–687.

Ergin A, Muntner P, Sherwin R, He J. Secular trends in cardiovascular disease mortality, incidence, and case fatality rates in adults in the United States. *Am J Med* 2004; 117:219–227.

Ezzati M, Vander Hoorn S, Rodgers A, et al. Estimates of global and regional potential health gains from reducing multiple major risk factors. *Lancet* 2003;362:271–280.

Fields LE, Burt VL, Cutler JA, et al. The burden of adult hypertension in the United States 1999 to 2000. A rising tide. *Hypertension* 2004;44:398–404.

Fox CS, Evans JC, Larson MG, et al. Temporal trends in coronary heart disease mortality and sudden cardiac death from 1950 to 1999: the Framingham Heart Study. *Circulation* 2004;110:522–527.

Franco OH, Bonneux L, de Laet C, et al. The Polymeal: a more natural, safer, and possibly tastier (than the Polypill) strategy to reduce cardiovascular disease by more than 75%. *BMJ* 2004;329:1447–1150.

Franklin SS, Jacobs MJ, Wong ND, et al. Predominance of isolated systolic hypertension among middle-aged and elderly U.S. hypertensives. *Hypertension* 2001a;37:869–874.

Franklin SS, Larson MG, Khan SA, et al. Does the relation of blood pressure to coronary heart disease change with aging? *Circulation* 2001b;103:1245–1249.

Franklin SS, Wong ND, Kannel WB. Age-specific relevance of usual blood pressure to vascular mortality. *Lancet* 2003;361:1389–1392.

Gifford RW. Evaluation of the hypertensive patient with emphasis on detecting curable causes. *Milbank Memorial Fund Q* 1969;47:170–186.

Gillum RF. The epidemiology of cardiovascular disease in black Americans. *N Engl J Med* 1996;335:1597–1599.

Gluckman TJ, Baranowski B, Ashen MD, et al. A practical and evidence-based approach to cardiovascular disease risk reduction. *Arch Intern Med* 2004;164:1490–1500.

Greenlund KJ, Croft JB, Mensah GA. Prevalence of heart disease and stroke risk factors in persons with prehypertension in the United States, 1999–2000. *Arch Intern Med* 2004;164:2113–2118.

Grimm RH Jr, Grandits GA, Cutler JA, et al. Relationships of quality-of-life measures to long-term lifestyle and drug treatment in the Treatment of Mild Hypertension Study. *Arch Intern Med* 1997;157:638–648.

Guidelines Committee. 2003 European Society of Hypertension-European Society of Cardiology guidelines for the management of arterial hypertension. *J Hypertens* 2003;21:1011–1053.

Haider AW, Larson MG, Franklin SS, Levy D. Systolic blood pressure, diastolic blood pressure, and pulse pressure as predictors of risk for congestive heart failure in the Framingham Heart Study. *Ann Intern Med* 2003;138:10–16.

Hajjar I, Kotchen TA. Trends in prevalence, awareness, treatment, and control of hypertension in the United States, 1988–2000. *JAMA* 2003;290:199–206.

He J, Muntner P, Chen J, et al. Factors associated with hypertension control in the general population of the United States. *Arch Intern Med* 2002;162:1051–1058.

Hedley AA, Ogden CL, Johnson CL, et al. Prevalence of overweight and obesity among US children, adolescents, and adults, 1999–2002. *JAMA* 2004;291:2847–2850.

Hicks LS, Fairchild DG, Horng MS, et al. Determinants of JNC VI guidelines adherence, intensity of drug therapy,

and blood pressure control by race and ethnicity. *Hypertension* 2004;44:429–434.

Hippisley-Cox J, Coupland C. Effect of combinations of drugs on all cause mortality in patients with ischaemic heart disease: nested case-control analysis. *BMJ* 2005; 1059–1063.

Hoes AW, Grobbee DE, Lubsen J, et al. Diuretics, beta-blockers, and the risk for sudden cardiac death in hypertensive patients. *Ann Intern Med* 1995;123:148–487.

Hunink MGM, Goldman L, Tosteson ANA, et al. The recent decline in mortality from coronary heart disease, 1980–1990. *JAMA* 1997;277:535–542.

Isaacs SL, Schroeder SA. Class—the ignored determinant of the nation's health. *N Engl J Med* 2004;351:1137–1142.

Jackson R, Lawes CM, Bennett DA, et al. Treatment with drugs to lower blood pressure and blood cholesterol based on an individual's absolute cardiovascular risk. *Lancet* 2005;365:434–441.

Joint National Committee. The sixth report of the Joint National Committee on Detection, Evaluation, and Treatment of High Blood Pressure (JNC VI). *Arch Intern Med* 1997;157:2413–2446.

Julius S. Trials of antihypertensive treatment. *Am J Hypertens* 2000;13:11S–17S.

Julius S, Jamerson K, Mejia A, et al. The association of borderline hypertension with target organ changes and higher coronary risk. *JAMA* 1990;264:354–358.

Julius S, Nesbitt S, Egan B, et al. Trial of preventing hypertension: design and 2-year progress report. *Hypertension* 2004;44:146–151.

Kannel WB. Elevated systolic blood pressure as a cardiovascular risk factor. *Am J Cardiol* 2000a;85:251–255.

Kannel WB. Risk stratification in hypertension. *Am J Hypertens* 2000b;13:3S–10S.

Kannel WB. Hypertensive risk assessment: cardiovascular risk factors and hypertension. *J Clin Hypertens* 2004; 6:393–399.

Kannel WB, Gordon T, Schwartz MJ. Systolic versus diastolic blood pressure and risk of coronary heart disease. *Am J Cardiol* 1971;27:335–346.

Kaplan NM. Anxiety-induced hyperventilation. *Arch Intern Med* 1997;157:945–948.

Kearney PM, Whelton M, Reynolds K, et al. Worldwide prevalence of hypertension: a systematic review. *J Hypertens* 2004;22:11–19.

Kearney PM, Whelton M, Reynolds K, et al. Global burden of hypertension: analysis of worldwide data. *Lancet* 2005;365:217–223.

Lawes CM, Rodgers A, Bennett DA, et al. Blood pressure and cardiovascular disease in the Asia Pacific region. *J Hypertens* 2003;21:707–716.

Lewington S, Clarke R, Qizilbash N, et al. Age-specific relevance of usual blood pressure to vascular mortality: a meta-analysis of individual data for one million adults in 61 prospective studies. *Lancet* 2002;360:1903–1913.

Li C, Engström G, Hedblad B, et al. Blood pressure control and risk of stroke: a population-based prospective cohort study. *Stroke* 2005;36:725–730

Lorenzo C, Serrano-Rios M, Martinez-Larrad MT, et al. Prevalence of hypertension in Hispanic and non-Hispanic white populations. *Hypertension* 2002;39:203–208.

MacMahon S, Neal B, Rodgers A. Hypertension—time to move on. *Lancet* 2005;365:1108–1109.

Madsen RER, Buch J. Long-term prognosis of transient hypertension in young male adults. *Aerospace Med* 1971; 42:752–755.

Mancia G, Pessina AC, Trimarco B, Grassi G. Blood pressure control according to new guidelines targets in low- and high-risk hypertensives managed in specialist practice. *J Hypertens* 2004;22:2387–2396.

Mena-Martin FJ, Martin-Escudero JC, Simal-Blanco F, et al. Health-related quality of life of subjects with known and unknown hypertension: results from the population-based Hortega study. *J Hypertens* 2003;21:1283–1289.

Miura K, Daviglus ML, Dyer AR, et al. Relationship of blood pressure to 25-year mortality due to coronary heart disease, cardiovascular disease, and all causes in young adult men. *Arch Intern Med* 2001;161:1501–1508.

Mosca L, Linfante AH, Benjamin EJ, et al. National Survey of physician awareness and adherence to cardiovascular disease prevention guidelines. *Circulation* 2005;111:449–510.

Moser M, Hebert PR. Prevention of disease progression, left ventricular hypertrophy and congestive heart failure in hypertension treatment trials. *J Am Coll Cardiol* 1996; 27:1214–1218.

Muntner P, He J, Cutler JA, et al. Trends in blood pressure among children and adolescents. *JAMA* 2004; 291:2107–2113.

National High Blood Pressure Education Program Working Group. National High Blood Pressure Education Program Working Group report on primary prevention of hypertension. *Arch Intern Med* 1993;153:186–208.

National High Blood Pressure Education Program Working Group. Update on the 1987 Task Force Report on high blood pressure in children and adolescents. *Pediatrics* 1996;98:649–658.

Nawrot TS, Staessen JA, Thijs L, et al. Should pulse pressure become part of the Framingham risk score? *J Human Hypertens* 2004;18:279–286.

Neaton JD, Wentworth D, Sherwin R, et al. Comparison of 10 year coronary and cerebrovascular disease mortality rates by hypertensive status for black and non-black men screened in the Multiple Risk Factor Intervention Trial (MRFIT) [Abstract]. *Circulation* 1989; 80(Suppl 2):II300.

Nolte E, McKee M. Measuring the health of nations: analysis of mortality amenable to health care. *BMJ* 2003; 327:1129–1133.

Pastor-Barriuso R, Banegas JR, Damián J, et al. Systolic blood pressure, diastolic blood pressure, and pulse pressure: an evaluation of their joint effect on mortality. *Ann Intern Med* 2003;139:731–739.

Pearson TA, Bazzarre TL, Daniels SR, et al. American Heart Association guide for improving cardiovascular health at the community level: a statement for public health practitioners, healthcare providers, and health policy makers from the American Heart Association Expert Panel on Population and Prevention Science. *Circulation* 2003;107:645–651.

Pickering G. Hypertension. Definitions, natural histories and consequences. *Am J Med* 1972;52:570–583.

Pickering TG. Isolated diastolic hypertension. *J Clin Hypertens* 2003;5:411–413.

Pickering TG. Lowering the thresholds of disease—are any of us still healthy? *J Clin Hypertens* 2004;6:672–674.

Primatesta P, Poulter NR. Hypertension management and control among English adults aged 65 years and older in 2000 and 2001. *J Hypertens* 2004;22:1093–1098.

Prospective Studies Collaboration. Cholesterol, diastolic blood pressure, and stroke. *Lancet* 1995;346:1647–1653.

Ramirez AG. Hypertension in Hispanic Americans. *Public Health Rep* 1996;111(Suppl 2):25–26.

Ramsay LE, Waller PC. Strokes in mild hypertension: diastolic rules. *Lancet* 1986;11:854–855.

Rose G. Epidemiology. In: Marshall AJ, Barritt DW, eds. *The Hypertensive Patient.* Kent, UK: Pitman Medical, 1980:1–21.

Rose G. Sick individuals and sick populations. *Int J Epidemiol* 1985;14:32–38.

Rose G. *The Strategy of Preventive Medicine.* Oxford, UK: Oxford University Press, 1992.

Rostrup M, Mundal MH, Westheim A, Eide I. Awareness of high blood pressure increases arterial plasma catecholamines, platelet noradrenaline and adrenergic responses to mental stress. *J Hypertens* 1991;9:159–166.

Rudnick KV, Sackett DL, Hirst S, Holmes C. Hypertension in a family practice. *Can Med Assoc J* 1977;117:492–497.

Schroeder K, Fahey T, Ebrahim S. How can we improve adherence to blood pressure-lowering medication in ambulatory care? Systematic review of randomized controlled trials. *Arch Intern Med* 2004;164:722–732.

Shaper AG, Ashby D, Pocock SJ. Blood pressure and hypertension in middle-aged British men. *J Hypertens* 1988; 6:367–374.

Sinclair AM, Isles CG, Brown I, et al. Secondary hypertension in a blood pressure clinic. *Arch Intern Med* 1987; 147:1289–1293.

Smith SC Jr., Jackson R, Pearson TA, et al. Principles for national and regional guidelines on cardiovascular disease prevention: a scientific statement from the World Heart and Stroke Forum. *Circulation* 2004;109:3112–3121.

Spillman BC, Lubitz J. The effect of longevity on spending for acute and long-term care. *N Engl J Med* 2000; 342:1409–1415.

Stamler J. Setting the TONE for ending the hypertension epidemic. *JAMA* 1998;279:878–879.

Stamler J, Stamler R, Neaton JD. Blood pressure, systolic and diastolic, and cardiovascular risks. *Arch Intern Med* 1993;153:598–615.

Strandberg TE, Salomaa VV, Vanhanen HT, et al. Isolated diastolic hypertension, pulse pressure, and mean arterial pressure as predictors of mortality during a follow-up of up to 32 years. *J Hypertens* 2002;20:399–404.

Swales JD. Systolic versus diastolic pressure. *J Hum Hypertens* 2000;14:477–479.

Sytkowski PA, D'Agostino RB, Belanger A, Kannel WB. Sex and time trends in cardiovascular disease incidence and mortality. *Am J Epidemiol* 1996a;143:338–350.

Sytkowski PA, D'Agostino RB, Belanger AJ, Kannel WB. Secular trends in long-term sustained hypertension, long-term treatment, and cardiovascular mortality. *Circulation* 1996b;93:697–703.

Szirmai LA, Arnold C, Farsang C. Improving control of hypertension by an integrated approach: results of the "Manage it well!" programme. *J Hypertens* 2005;23:203–211.

Thürmer HL, Lund-Larsen PG, Tverdal A. Is blood pressure treatment as effective in a population setting as in controlled trials? Results from a prospective study. *J Hypertens* 1994;12:481–490.

Turnbull F, Blood Pressure Lowering Treatment Trialists' Collaboration. Effects of different blood-pressure-lowering regimens on major cardiovascular events: results of prospectively designed overviews of randomized trials. *Lancet* 2003;362:1527–1545.

Unal B, Critchley JA, Capewell S. Explaining the decline in coronary heart disease mortality in England and Wales between 1981 and 2000. *Circulation* 2004;109:1101–1107.

van den Hoogen PCW, Feskens EJM, Nagelkerke NJD, et al. The relation between blood pressure and mortality due to coronary heart disease among men in different parts of the world. *N Engl J Med* 2000;342:1–8.

Vasan RS, Beiser A, Seshadri S, et al. Residual lifetime risk for developing hypertension in middle-aged women and men: the Framingham Heart Study. *JAMA* 2002; 287:1003–1010.

Vasan RS, Larson MG, Leip EP, et al. Assessment of frequency of progression to hypertension in non-hypertensive participants in the Framingham Heart Study: a cohort study. *Lancet* 2001a;358:1682–1686.

Vasan RS, Larson MG, Leip EP, et al. Impact of high-normal blood pressure on the risk of cardiovascular disease. *N Engl J Med* 2001b;345:1291–1297.

Wald NJ, Law MR. A strategy to reduce cardiovascular disease by more than 80%. *BMJ* 2003;326:1419–1423.

Wang Y, Wang QJ. The prevalence of prehypertension and hypertension among US adults according to the new Joint National Committee guidelines. *Arch Intern Med* 2004; 164:2126–2134.

Whelton PK, He J, Appel LJ, et al. Primary prevention of hypertension: clinical and public health advisory from the National High Blood Pressure Education Program. *JAMA* 2002;288:1882–1888.

Whelton PK, He J, Muntner P. Prevalence, awareness, treatment and control of hypertension in North America, North Africa, and Asia. *J Human Hypertens* 2004;18:545–551.

WHO/ISH Writing Group. World Health Organization (WHO)/International Society of Hypertension (ISH) statement on management of hypertension. *J Hypertens* 2003; 21:1983–1992.

Williams B, Poulter NR, Brown MJ, et al. Guidelines for management of hypertension: report of the fourth working party of the British Hypertension Society, 2004—BHS IV. *J Human Hypertens* 2004;18:139–185.

Wolf-Maier K, Cooper RS, Banegas JR, et al. Hypertension prevalence and blood pressure levels in six European countries, Canada, and the United States. *JAMA* 2003; 289:2363–2369.

Wolf-Maier K, Cooper RS, Kramer H, et al. Hypertension treatment and control in five European countries, Canada, and the United States. *Hypertension* 2004;43:10–17.

Wolz M, Cutler J, Roccella EJ, et al. Statement from the National High Blood Pressure Education Program: prevalence of hypertension. *Am J Hypertens* 2000;13:103–104.

Yusuf S, Hawken S, Ôunpuu S, et al. Effect of potentially modifiable risk factors associated with myocardial infarction in 52 countries (the INTERHEART study): case-control study. *Lancet* 2004;364:937–952.

Yusuf S, Reddy S, Ôunpuu S, Anand S. Global burden of cardiovascular diseases. Part I: general considerations, the epidemiologic transition, risk factors, and impact of urbanization. *Circulation* 2001;104:2746–2753.

# Measurement of Blood Pressure

Now that some of the major issues about hypertension in the population at large have been addressed, we turn to the evaluation of the individual patient with hypertension. This chapter covers the measurement of blood pressure (BP), first considering many aspects of its variability. These, in turn, are involved in a number of special features that are of considerable clinical importance, including the "white-coat" effect, nocturnal dipping, and the early morning surge in pressure.

Over the past few years, BP has become recognized as a continuous variable, impossible to characterize accurately except by multiple readings under various conditions; its measurement is known to be often inaccurate and in need of escaping the physician's office to be fully effective as a tool for the control of hypertension. Multiple out-of-the-office measurements are essential for accurate diagnosis and management. Self-measurements at home are the logical alternative since, at least in the United States, ambulatory monitoring is not generally available.

Excellent review of these and other issues about BP measurements has been provided by committees of experts (O'Brien  et al., 2005; Pickering et al., 2005).

Before going into particulars, a more general comment seems appropriate: Self-monitoring of BP by patients both at home and work must be more widely implemented. The variability of BP covered in the next section is typical. Few patients have steady BP, well controlled on stable medication. Most patients (or at least the ones I see) have variable BP, poorly controlled on multiple medications. Practitioners in their offices cannot solve the problem. In fact, the doctor's office is responsible for a good part of the problem.

The only solution is to have hypertensive patients (and their practitioners) take hypertension more seriously, as seriously as insulin-taking diabetics take their disease, as seriously as breast cancer survivors take the need for careful follow-up. This may sound overly dramatic, but hypertension-related consequences maim and kill many more people than diabetes and cancer. Being asymptomatic, hypertension doesn't demand that patients or physicians pay it much attention.

One of the few ways proven to improve patients' adherence to therapy is home BP monitoring (Canzanello et al., 2005). I believe hypertensives should have a home BP device and monitor their BPs as carefully as diabetics should monitor their blood glucose. As a "brittle" hypertensive, the author knows how variable BP can be, how the morning surge is so difficult to minimize, how the late afternoon can expose orthostatic symptoms from too tightly controlled hypertension the rest of the day.

Unlike the population-wide approach needed to handle "prehypertension" that should only peripherally involve the practitioner (discussed at the end of the previous chapter), the practitioner must take direct responsibility for the individual hypertensive patient. And I know of nothing more helpful in achieving good control of an individual patient's hypertension than the home monitoring of BP. In the best of worlds, the patient could alter his or her antihypertensive regimen based on his or her home BP readings just as diabetics are allowed to alter their insulin dosage based on their home glucose readings. Such self-modification may be too much to ask, but phones, faxes, and emails can easily send the readings to an office assistant or practitioner who can then provide appropriate advice.

For too long, practitioners have kept patients out of the loop, either too proud to give up some of their power or too suspicious of the ability of their patients to help themselves. We need to recognize the potential of home monitoring and use it to our patients' benefit. An appreciation of the variability of BP is a good place to start.

## VARIABILITY OF BLOOD PRESSURE

The variability of the BP on repeated measurements, both at a single visit and on separate occasions, is much greater than most practitioners realize (Reeves, 1995; Kario, 2005a).

The adverse consequences of not recognizing and dealing with this variability are obvious: Individual patients may be falsely labeled as hypertensive or normotensive (Turner et al., 2004). If falsely labeled as normotensive, needed therapy

may be denied. If falsely labeled as hypertensive, the label itself may provoke ill effects, and unnecessary therapy will likely be given. Moreover, variability per se may be associated with greater degrees of target organ damage (Gómez-Angelats et al., 2004; Zakopoulos et al., 2005).

The typical variability of the BP through the 24-hour day is easily recognized by ambulatory BP monitoring (ABPM) (Figure 2–1). This printout of readings taken in a single patient every 15 minutes during the day and every 30 minutes at night displays the large differences in daytime readings, the typical dipping during sleep, and the abrupt increase on arising.

### Sources of Variation

Blood pressure readings are often variable because of problems involving the observer (measurement variation) or factors working within the patient (biologic variation) (Beevers et al., 2001a; Pickering et al., 2005).

### *Measurement Variations*

An impressively long list of factors that can affect the immediate accuracy of office measurements has

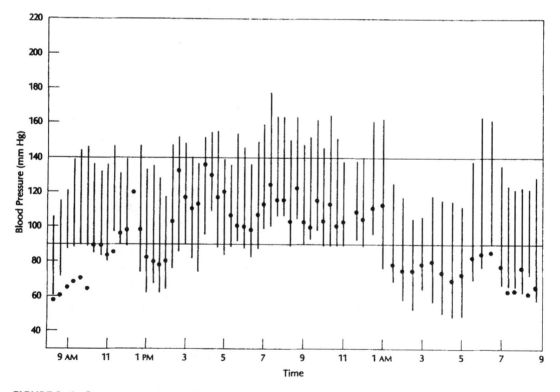

**FIGURE 2–1** ● Computer printout of blood pressures obtained by ambulatory blood pressure monitoring over 24 hours, beginning at 9 a.m., in a 50-year-old man with hypertension receiving no therapy. The patient slept from midnight until 6 a.m. *Solid circles*, heart rate in beats per minute. (From Zachariah PK, Sheps SG, Smith RL. Defining the roles of home and ambulatory monitoring. *Diagnosis* 1988;10:39–50, with permission.)

been compiled and referenced by Reeves (1995) (Table 2–1). These errors are more common than most realize and regular, frequent retraining of personnel is needed to prevent them (Ostchega et al., 2003).

### Biologic Variations

Biologic variations in BP may be either random or systematic. Random variations are uncontrollable but can be reduced simply by repeating the measurement as many times as needed. Systematic variations are introduced by something affecting the patient and, if recognized, are controllable; however, if not recognized, they cannot be reduced by multiple readings. An example is a systematic variation related to environmental temperature: Higher readings usually are noted in the winter, particularly in thin people, who often display systolic BPs

10 mm Hg or higher than they do in the summer (Kristal-Boneh et al., 1996).

As seen in Figure 2–1, considerable differences in readings can be seen at different times of the day, whether or not the subject is active (Cavelaars et al., 2004a). Beyond these, between-visit variations in BP can be substantial. Even after three office visits, the standard deviation of the difference in BP from one visit to another in 32 subjects was 10.4 mm Hg for systolic BP and 7.0 mm Hg for diastolic BP (Watson et al., 1987).

### Types of Variation

Variability in BP arises from different sources: short-term, daytime, diurnal, and seasonal. *Short-term* variability at rest is affected by respiration and heart rate, which are under the influence of the

## TABLE 2–1

### Factors Affecting the Immediate Accuracy of Office Blood Pressure (BP) Measurements

| Increases BP | Decreases BP | No Effect on BP |
|---|---|---|
| Examinee | Examinee | Examinee |
| Soft Korotkoff sounds | Soft Korotkoff sounds | Menstrual phase |
| Pseudohypertension | Recent meal | Chronic caffeine ingestion |
| White-coat reaction | Missed auscultatory gap | Cuff self-inflation |
| Paretic arm (due to stroke) | High stroke volume | Examinee and examiner |
| Pain, anxiety | Setting, equipment | Discordance in gender or race |
| Acute smoking | Noisy environs | Examination |
| Acute caffeine | Faulty aneroid device | Thin shirtsleeve under cuff |
| Acute ethanol ingestion | Low mercury level | Bell vs. diaphragm |
| Distended bladder | Leaky bulb | Cuff inflation per se |
| Talking, signing | Examiner | Hour of day (during work hours) |
| Setting, equipment | Reading to next lowest 5 or 10 mm Hg, or expectation bias | |
| Cold environment | Impaired hearing | |
| Leaky bulb valve | Examination | |
| Examination | Resting for too long | |
| Cuff too narrow | Arm above heart level | |
| Arm below heart level | Too rapid deflation | |
| Too-short rest period | Excess bell pressure | |
| Arm, back unsupported | Parallax error (aneroid) | |
| Parallax error | | |
| Using phase IV (adult) | | |

Modified from Reeves RA. Does this patient have hypertension? *JAMA* 1995;273:1211–1218.

autonomic nervous system. *Daytime* variability is mainly determined by the degree of mental and physical activity. *Diurnal* variability is substantial, with an average fall in BP of approximately 15% during sleep. As noted, *seasonal* variations can be considerable.

The overriding influence of activity on daytime and diurnal variations was well demonstrated in a study of 461 untreated hypertensive patients whose BP was recorded with an ambulatory monitor every 15 minutes during the day and every 30 minutes at night over 24 hours (Clark et al., 1987). In addition, five readings were taken in the clinic before and another five after the 24-hour recording. When the mean diastolic BP readings for each hour were plotted against each patient's mean clinic diastolic BP, considerable variations were noted, with the lowest BPs occurring during the night and the highest near midday (Figure 2–2A). The patients recorded in a diary the location at which their BP was taken (e.g., at home, work, or other location) and what they were doing at the time, selecting from 15 choices

of activity. When the effects of the various combinations of location and activity on the BP were analyzed, variable effects relative to the BP recorded while relaxing were seen (Table 2–2). When the estimated effects of the various combinations of location and activity then were subtracted from the individual readings obtained throughout the 24-hour period, little residual effect related to the time of day was found (Figure 2–2B). The authors concluded that "there is no important circadian rhythm of BP which is independent of activity" (Clark et al., 1987).

## Additional Sources of Variation

Beyond the level of activity and the stresses related to the measurement, a number of other factors affect BP variability, including the sensitivity of baroreflexes and the level of BP, with more variability occurring with higher BPs (Ragot et al., 2001). This latter relationship probably is responsible for the widespread perception that the elderly have more variable BP. When younger and older

---

### TABLE 2–2

**Average Changes in Blood Pressure Associated with Commonly Occurring Activities, Relative to Blood Pressure while Relaxing**

| Activity | Systolic Blood Pressure (mm Hg) | Diastolic Blood Pressure (mm Hg) |
|---|---|---|
| Meetings | +20.2 | +15.0 |
| Work | +16.0 | +13.0 |
| Transportation | +14.0 | +9.2 |
| Walking | +12.0 | +5.5 |
| Dressing | +11.5 | +9.5 |
| Chores | +10.7 | +6.7 |
| Telephone | +9.5 | +7.2 |
| Eating | +8.8 | +9.6 |
| Talking | +6.7 | +6.7 |
| Desk work | +5.9 | +5.3 |
| Reading | +1.9 | +2.2 |
| Business (at home) | +1.6 | +3.2 |
| Television | +0.3 | +1.1 |
| Relaxing | 0.0 | 0.0 |
| Sleeping | −10.0 | −7.6 |

Data adapted from Clark LA, Denby L, Pregibon D, et al. A quantitative analysis of the effects of activity and time of day on the diurnal variations of blood pressure. *J Chronic Dis* 1987;40:671–679.

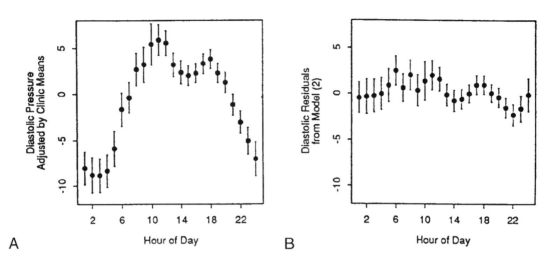

**FIGURE 2–2** ● **(A)** Plot of diastolic blood pressure readings adjusted by individual clinic means. **(B)** Plot of the diastolic blood pressure hourly mean residuals after adjustments for various activities by a time-of-day model. The hourly means (*solid circles*) ± 2 standard errors of the mean (*vertical lines*) are plotted versus the corresponding time of day. (Modified from Clark LA, Denby L, Pregibon D, et al. A quantitative analysis of the effects of activity and time of day on the diurnal variations of blood pressure. *J Chronic Dis* 1987;40:671–679.)

hypertensives with comparable BP levels were studied, variability was not consistently related to age (Brennan et al., 1986).

It is important to minimize the changes in BP that arise because of variations within the patient. Even little things can have an impact: Both systolic BP and diastolic BP may rise 10 mm Hg or more with a distended urinary bladder (Fagius & Karhuvaara, 1989) or during ordinary conversation (Le Pailleur et al., 1998). Just the presence of a medical student was found to increase BP an average of 6.4/2.4 mm Hg (Matthys et al., 2004). Those who are more anxious or elated tend to have higher levels (Jacob et al., 1999). Particularly in the elderly, eating may lower the BP (Smith et al., 2003). Two common practices may exert significant pressor effects: smoking (Groppelli et al., 1992) or drinking caffeinated beverages (Hartley et al., 2004).

One last issue about BP variability is whether it is, by itself, harmful. Over an average 8.5-year follow-up of 1,542 subjects, a significant increase in cardiovascular mortality was found with increased daytime systolic BP variability noted on ambulatory monitoring (Kikuya et al., 2000). Greater BP variability was associated with increased carotid artery thickness (Zakopoulos et al., 2005) and the risk of stroke was increased with greater variability in nighttime systolic BP but not with daytime variability (Pringle et al., 2003). Therefore, it seems likely that the damage induced by hypertension is related not only to the average BP level but also to the magnitude of its variability. Moreover, some of the protective effect of antihypertensive

drug therapy may reflect a decrease in BP variability (Frattola et al., 2000).

## Blood Pressure During Sleep and on Awakening

### Normal Pattern

The usual fall in BP at night is largely the result of sleep and inactivity rather than the time of day (Sternberg et al., 1995). Whereas the nocturnal fall averages approximately 15% in those who are active during the day, it is only about 5% in those who remain in bed for the entire 24 hours (Casiglia et al., 1996).

The nocturnal dip in pressure is normally distributed with no evidence of bimodality in either normotensive or hypertensive people (Staessen et al., 1997). Therefore, the separation between "dippers" and "nondippers" is, in a sense, artefactual. Therefore, to improve the diagnostic reliability of dipping status, some recommend at least two 24-hour ambulatory monitorings (Cuspidi et al., 2004a); others define nondipping as the presence of a nocturnal BP above 125/80 (White & Larocca, 2003).

The usual falls in BP and heart rate that occur with sleep reflect a decrease in sympathetic nervous tone. In healthy young men, plasma catecholamine levels fell during rapid-eye-movement sleep, whereas awakening immediately increased epinephrine, and subsequent standing induced a marked increase in norepinephrine (Dodt et al., 1997).

What appears to be nondipping may be simply a consequence of getting up to urinate (Perk et al.,

2001) or a reflection of obstructive sleep apnea (Peltari et al., 1998). Moreover, the degree of dipping during sleep is affected by the amount of dietary sodium in those who are salt-sensitive: Sodium reduction restores their dipping status (Higashi et al., 1997; Uzu et al., 1999). Furthermore, dipping is more common among people who are more physically active during the day (Cavelaars et al., 2004b).

## Associations with Nondipping

Even though there is no clear separation between dippers and nondippers in large populations, a number of associations have been noted with a lesser fall than usual in nocturnal BP. These include:

- Older age (Staessen et al., 1997)
- Cognitive dysfunction (van Boxtel et al., 1998)
- Diabetes (Björklund et al., 2002)
- Obesity (Kotsis et al., 2005)
- African Americans and Hispanics (Agyemang et al., 2005; Hyman et al., 2000)
- Impaired endothelium-dependent vasodilation (Higashi et al., 2002)
- Elevated levels of markers of cellular adhesion and inflammation (von Känel et al., 2004)
- Left ventricular hypertrophy (Cuspidi et al., 2004a)
- Loss of renal function (Fukuda et al., 2004)
- Mortality from cardiovascular disease (Ohkubo et al., 2002)

## Associations with Excessive Dipping

Just as a failure of the BP to fall during sleep may reflect or contribute to cardiovascular damage, there may also be danger from too great a fall in nocturnal BP. Floras (1988) suggested that nocturnal falls in BP could induce myocardial ischemia in hypertensives with left ventricular hypertrophy and impaired coronary vasodilator reserve, contributing to the J-curve of increased coronary events when diastolic BP is lowered below 85 mm Hg (see Chapter 5).

The first objective evidence for this threat from too much dipping was the finding by Kario et al. (1996) that more silent cerebrovascular disease (identified by brain magnetic resonance imaging) was found among extreme dippers who had a greater than 20% fall in nocturnal systolic BP. Subsequently, Kario et al. (2001a), in a 41-month follow-up of 575 elderly hypertensives, found the lowest stroke risk to be at a sleep diastolic BP of 75 mm Hg, with an increased risk below 75 mm Hg that was associated with their intake of antihypertensive drugs. Similarly, in a smaller group of hypertensives with stable coronary artery disease, myocardial ischemia occurred during the night more frequently in untreated nondippers and in treated overdippers (Pierdomenico et al., 1998). Despite the multiple adverse associations with too little or too much nocturnal

dipping, Pickering (2005a) concludes that the routine performance of ABPM that is needed to identify the dipping status in not currently warranted.

## Early Morning Surge

Even more ominous is the usual abrupt rise in BP that occurs after arising from sleep, whether it be in the early morning (Gosse et al., 2004) or after a midafternoon siesta (Bursztyn et al., 1999). As amply described, the early morning hours after 6 a.m. are accompanied by an increased prevalence of all cardiovascular catastrophes as compared to the remainder of the 24-hour period (Giles, 2005; Muller, 1999). Early morning increases have been noted for stroke (Kario et al., 2003), cardiac arrest (Peckova et al., 1998; Soo et al., 2000), rupture of the abdominal aorta (Manfredini et al., 1999), and epistaxis (Manfredini et al., 2000).

These abrupt changes are likely mediated by heightened sympathetic activity after hours of relative quiescence (Dodt et al., 1997; Panza et al., 1991), which may be accentuated in subjects with a great deal of hostility (Pasic et al., 1998). The surge may be aggravated by increased physical activity (Leary et al., 2002), but simply arising from sleep may significantly raise BP even in patients with hypertension under apparently good control (Redón et al., 2002). As will be noted, home BP measurements are the only practical way to recognize and then modulate this surge (Kario, 2005b).

Similar sudden sympathetic nervous surges are likely involved in the increased frequency of heart attack within 1 hour of driving in heavy traffic (Peters et al., 2004).

## White-Coat Effect

Measurement of the BP may invoke an alerting reaction, a reaction that is only transient in most patients but persistent in some. It usually is seen more often in people who have a greater rise in BP under psychological stress (Palatini et al., 2003), but the majority of people have higher office BP than out-of-the-office BP (O'Brien et al., 2003).

### Environment

There is a hierarchy of alerting: least at home, more in the clinic or office, most in the hospital. Measurements by the same physician were higher in the hospital than in a health center (Enström et al., 2000). Whether taken by the physician or an automatic device, readings obtained in the office were higher than those taken out of the office (Little et al., 2002).

### Measurer

Figure 2–3 demonstrates that the presence of a physician usually causes a rise in BP that is sometimes very impressive (Mancia et al., 1987). The data in Figure 2–3 were obtained from patients who underwent a 24-hour intraarterial recording after 5 to 7 days in the hospital. When the intraarterial readings were stable, the BP was measured in the noncatheterized arm by both a male physician and a female nurse, half of the time by the physician first, the other half by the nurse first. The patients had not met the personnel but had been told that they would be coming. When the physician took the first readings, the BPs rose an average of 22/14 mm Hg and as much as 74 mm Hg systolic. The readings were approximately half that much above baseline at 5 and 10 minutes. Similar rises were seen during three subsequent visits. When the nurses took the first set of readings, the rises were only half as great as those noted by the physician, and the BP usually returned to near-baseline when measured again after 5 and 10 minutes. The rises were not related to patient age, gender, overall BP variability, or BP levels. These marked differences are not limited to handsome Italian doctors or their excitable patients. Similar nurse-physician differences have been repeatedly noted elsewhere (Little et al., 2002).

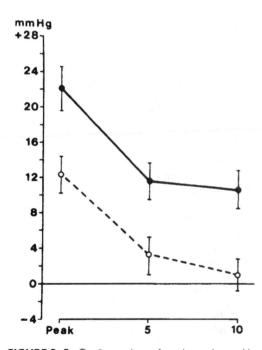

**FIGURE 2–3** ● Comparison of maximum (or peak) rises in systolic blood pressure in 30 subjects during visits with a physician (*solid line*) and a nurse (*dashed line*). The rises occurring at 5 and 10 minutes into the visits are shown. Data are expressed as mean (± standard error of the mean) changes from a control value taken 4 minutes before each visit. (Modified from Mancia G, Paroti G, Pomidossi G, et al. Alerting reaction and rise in blood pressure during measurement by physician and nurse. *Hypertension* 1987;9:209–215.)

These findings are in keeping with a large amount of data that indicates a marked tendency in most patients for BP to fall after repeated measurements, regardless of the time interval between readings (Pickering, 1994). They strongly suggest that nurses and not physicians should measure the BP and that at least three sets of readings should be taken before the patient is labeled hypertensive and the need for treatment is determined (Graves & Sheps, 2004).

## White-Coat Hypertension

*White-coat hypertension* is the presence of usual office readings above 140/90 mm Hg but average out-of-office daytime readings below 135/85 (O'Brien et al., 2003) or below 130/80 (Verdecchia et al., 2003).

Most patients have higher BP levels when taken in the office than when taken out of the office, as shown in a comparison between the systolic BPs obtained by a physician versus the average daytime systolic BPs obtained by ambulatory monitors (Pickering, 1996) (Figure 2–4). In the figure, all the points above the diagonal line represent higher office readings than out-of-office readings, indicating that a majority of patients demonstrate the white-coat effect.

Whereas most patients exhibiting a white-coat effect also had elevated out-of-office readings, so that they are hypertensive in all settings (Figure 2–4, group 2), a smaller but significant number of patients had normal readings outside the office—that is, white-coat hypertension (Figure 2–4, group 1). Pickering et al. (1988) had previously found that among 292 untreated patients with persistently elevated office readings over an average of 6 years, the out-of-office readings recorded by a 24-hour ambulatory monitor were normal in 21%. Since that observation, the prevalence of white-coat hypertension has been found to be approximately 20% in multiple groups of patients with office hypertension (Høegholm et al., 1992; Owens et al., 1999; Staessen et al., 1993; Verdecchia et al., 1995).

It is important to avoid confusion between the white-coat effect and white-coat hypertension. As Pickering (1996) emphasized, "White coat hypertension is a measure of blood pressure level, whereas the white coat effect is a measure of change. A large white coat effect is by no means confined to patients with white coat hypertension, and indeed is often more pronounced in patients with severe hypertension."

The clinical recognition of white-coat hypertension may eventually be easier since reimbursement for ambulatory BP monitoring (although at a woefully inadequate level) for "patients with suspected white-coat hypertension" has been approved

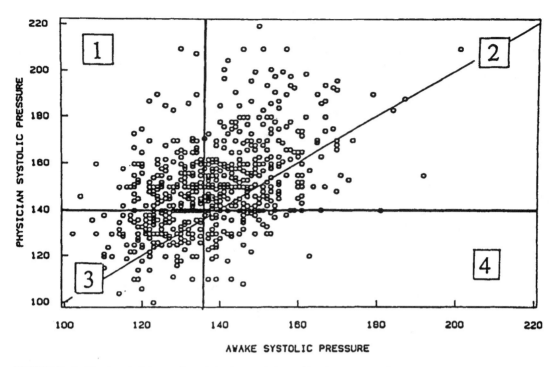

**FIGURE 2–4** ● Plot of clinic systolic and daytime ambulatory blood pressure readings in 573 patients. *1*, patients with white-coat hypertension; *2*, patients with sustained hypertension; *3*, patients with normal blood pressure; *4*, patients whose clinic blood pressure underestimates ambulatory blood pressure (masked hypertension). The majority of sustained hypertensives and normotensives had higher clinic pressures than awake ambulatory pressures. (Adapted from Pickering TG. Ambulatory monitoring and the definition of hypertension. *J Hypertens* 1992;10:401–409.)

by the U.S. Medicare payment system (Centers for Medicare, 2001).

As interest in white-coat hypertension has grown, a number of its features have become apparent, including:

- The prevalence depends largely on the definition of the upper limit of normal for daytime out-of-office readings; depending on the level chosen, the prevalence has been shown to vary from as low as 12% to as high as 53.2% (Verdecchia et al., 1995).
- The prevalence of white-coat hypertension may be reduced if the office readings are based on at least five separate visits (Pearce et al., 1992). The less the elevation in office BP, the greater the frequency of white-coat hypertension (Verdecchia et al., 2001).
- Obviously, only daytime ambulatory readings should be used to define white-coat hypertension, as nighttime readings are typically lower.
- Multiple self-obtained home readings are as good as ambulatory readings to document white-coat hypertension (Den Hond et al., 2003).
- The prevalence rises with the age of the patient (Mansoor et al., 1996) and is particularly high in elderly patients with isolated systolic hypertension (Aihara et al., 1998).

- Women are more likely to have white-coat hypertension (Verdecchia et al., 2003).
- Some patients considered to have resistant or uncontrolled hypertension on the basis of office readings instead have white-coat hypertension and, therefore, may not need more intensive therapy (Redon et al., 1998). However, most treated hypertensives with persistently high office readings also have high out-of-office readings so that their inadequate control cannot be attributed to the white-coat effect (Mancia et al., 1997).
- Antihypertensive therapy has been shown to reduce office BP to the same extent in patients with sustained and white-coat hypertension but lowered the ambulatory BP in only those with sustained hypertension (Pickering et al., 1999).

Beyond these features, two more important and inter-related issues remain: What is the natural history of white-coat hypertension, and what is its prognosis?

### Natural History

Too few patients have been followed long enough to be sure of the natural history of white-coat hypertension (Verdecchia et al., 2001). Whereas Bidling-meyer et al. (1996) found that 60 of 81 patients had a progression to a daytime ambulatory BP greater than 140/90 mm Hg over a 5- to 6-year follow-up, others have found that only 10% to 30% become hypertensive over 3 to 5 years (Pickering et al., 1999). Whereas this transition may suggest that white-coat hypertension is a prehypertensive state, it may also reflect regression to the mean, with a fall in the initially high office readings and a rise in the initially low ambulatory values. This explanation is supported by the finding that among 90 patients initially found to have white-coat hypertension, repeated ambulatory monitoring 3 months later revealed higher readings in 52 so that only 38 were still classified as having white-coat hypertension (Palatini et al., 1998).

### Prognosis

Uncertainty remains about the risks of white-coat hypertension. Some investigators find that white-coat hypertensives are at relatively little risk when identified and remain so over variable periods of follow-up (Kario et al., 2001b; Verdecchia et al., 2001). Others find considerably more risk, as great or greater than in patients with elevated ambulatory readings (Gustavsen et al., 2003).

The major determinant of prognosis, of course, is the morbidity and mortality experience of white-coat hypertensives as compared to normotensives and sustained hypertensives. Here again, the data are inadequate to allow certainty. In five prospective studies of patients with white-coat hypertension, defined with varying criteria, who were followed up for 3 to 9 years, the cardiovascular event rate was found to be relatively low, intermediate between that seen in normotensive and hypertensive patients (Khattar et al., 1998; Perloff et al., 1991; Pierdomenico et al., 2004; Redon et al., 1998; Verdecchia et al., 1996).

Until recently, the best evidence came from the continuing follow-up of 1,522 hypertensive subjects for up to 10 years by Verdecchia et al. (1996). With a conservative definition of white-coat hypertension (i.e., daytime ambulatory BP <130/80 mm Hg), the rate of major cardiovascular morbid events in such patients was 0.67 per 100 patient-years, little beyond what was seen in normotensives but far less than the 2.71 per 100 patient-years rate seen in those with ambulatory hypertension (daytime BP >131/86 mm Hg in women, >136/ 87 mm Hg in men).

However, in a more recent report (Verdecchia et al., 2005), the data are much less reassuring. In an analysis of data from four prospective cohort studies from the United States, Italy, and Japan that used comparable methodology for 24-hour ABPM in 1,549 normotensives and 4,406 essential hypertensives, the prevalence of white-coat hypertension was 9%. Over the first 6 years of follow-up, the risk of stroke in a multivariate analysis was a statistically insignificant 1.15 in the WCH group versus 2.01 in the ambulatory hypertensive group compared to the normotensive group. However, the incidence of stroke began to increase after the sixth year in the WCH group and, by the ninth year, crossed the hazard curve of the ambulatory hypertensive group (Figure 2–5).

Therefore, more long-term follow-up data are needed. The prognosis may be benign over the short term but much less benign later.

Obviously, close follow-up of patients carefully diagnosed with white-coat hypertension is mandatory. At the least, they should be encouraged to modify lifestyle in an appropriate manner and continue to monitor their blood pressure status.

**FIGURE 2–5** ● The cumulative hazard for stroke over follow-up for as long as 14 years (median of 5.4 years) after 24-hour ambulatory blood pressure monitoring (ABPM) in 4,406 subjects with ambulatory hypertension, 1,549 normotensive controls, and 398 with white-coat hypertension (defined as average daytime level of less than 130/80). The analysis included individual data from 4 prospective cohort studies from the U.S., Italy, and Japan that used similar ABPM methodology. (Modified from Verdecchia P, Reboldi GP, Angeli F, et al. Short- and long-term incidence of stroke in white-coat hypertension. *Hypertension* 2005;45:203–208.)

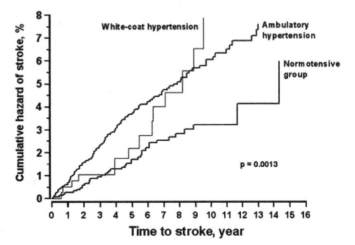

## Masked Hypertension

As seen in the lower right portion of Figure 2–4, labeled as #4, some patients have normal office BP but elevated ambulatory readings. These "masked hypertensives" may comprise a significant portion, 5% or more, of the general population (Pickering, 2003) and young people (Lurbe et al., 2005). Higher daytime ambulatory BPs than clinic readings were found in more than 20% of 713 elderly hypertensives (Wing et al., 2002) and in 13.8% of never-treated stage 1 hypertensives (Palatini et al., 2004). Such patients have increased rates of cardiovascular morbidity, almost as high as seen in those with both clinic and ambulatory hypertension (Björklund et al., 2003; Bobrie et al., 2004). To identify masked hypertension, ABPM should be obtained in patients with normal office BP but one or more of these features: occasional high office BP, family history of early onset hypertension, obesity, fast pulse rate or left ventricular hypertrophy (O'Brien, 2005).

## OFFICE MEASUREMENT OF BLOOD PRESSURE

In the everyday practice of medicine, office measurements of blood pressure may be the least accurately performed procedure which, at the same time, has the greatest impact on patient care. Under the best of circumstances, all of the previously described causes of variability are different to control. Therefore, we must do what can be done to improve current practice (Beevers et al., 2001b). Use of the guidelines shown in Table 2–3 will prevent most measurement errors. The American Heart Association (Pickering et al., 2005) and the European Society of Hypertension (O'Brien et al., 2005) provide more detailed instructions.

### Patient and Arm Position

The patient should be seated comfortably with the arm supported and positioned at the level of the heart (Figure 2–6). Measurements taken with the arm hanging at the patient's side or supported on the armrests of a chair averaged 10 mm Hg higher than those taken with the arm supported in a horizontal position at heart level (Netea et al., 2003). When sitting upright on a table without support, readings may be as much as 10 mm Hg higher because of the isometric exertion needed to support the body and arm (Cushman et al., 1990). Systolic readings are approximately 8 mm Hg higher in the supine than in the seated position even when the arm is at the level of the right atrium (Netea et al., 2003).

### Differences between Arms

Initially, the BP should be measured in both arms to ascertain the differences between them; if the reading is higher in one arm, that arm should be used for future measurements. In two series of patients, the mean absolute levels of systolic and diastolic BPs were higher in the right arm, 6.3/5.1 mm Hg, in 400 subjects measured while seated (Lane et al., 2002) and 4.9/3.7 mm Hg in 1,090 people measured while supine (Kimura et al., 2004). Absolute differences greater than 10 mm Hg in systolic levels were found in 9% of subjects by Kimura et al. (2004) and in 20% by Lane et al. (2002). Lower BP in the left arm is seen in patients with subclavian steal caused by reversal of flow down a vertebral artery distal to an obstructed subclavian artery, as noted in 9% of 500 patients with asymptomatic neck bruits (Bornstein & Norris, 1986). On the other hand, BP may be either higher or lower in the paretic arm of a stroke patient (Dewar et al., 1992).

### Standing Pressure

Readings should be taken immediately on standing and after standing at least 2 minutes to check for spontaneous or drug-induced postural changes, particularly in the elderly and in diabetics. If no fall in BP is seen in patients with suggestive symptoms, the time of quiet standing should be prolonged to at least 5 minutes. In most people, systolic BP falls and diastolic BP rises by a few millimeters of mercury on changing from the supine to the standing position. In the elderly, significant postural falls of 20 mm Hg or more in systolic BP are more common, occurring in approximately 10% of ambulatory people older than 65 years and in more than half of frail nursing-home residents, particularly in those with elevated supine systolic BP (Ooi et al., 1997) (see Chapter 4).

### Leg Pressure

If the arm reading is elevated, particularly in a patient younger than 30, the BP should be taken in one leg to rule out coarctation.

### Sphygmomanometer

Independent evaluations of BP device accuracy and performance are available at http://www.dableducational.com, but there are no obligatory standards which must be met. In a survey of hospitals and physicians' offices in São Paulo, 21% of the mercury sphygmomanometers and more than 50% of the aneroid manometers were inaccurate (Mion & Pierin, 1998).

## TABLE 2–3

### Guidelines for Measurement of Blood Pressure

Patient Conditions
  Posture
  - Initially, particularly >65 years, with diabetes, or receiving antihypertensive therapy, check for postural changes by taking readings after 5 min supine, then immediately and 2 min after standing
  - For routine follow-up, the patient should sit quietly for 5 min with the arm bared and supported at the level of the heart and the back resting against a chair
  Circumstances
  - No caffeine or smoking within 30 min preceding the reading
  - A quiet, warm setting
Equipment
  Cuff size
  - The bladder should encircle at least 80% of the circumference and cover two-thirds of the length of the arm
  - A too small bladder may cause falsely high readings
  Manometer
  - Either a mercury, recently calibrated aneroid or validated electronic device
  Stethoscope
  - The bell of the stethoscope should be used
  - Avoid excess bell pressure
  Infants
  - Use ultrasound (e.g., the Doppler method)
Technique
  Number of readings
  - On each occasion, take at least two readings, separated by as much time as is practical; if readings vary >5 mm Hg, take additional readings until two are close
  - For diagnosis, obtain three sets of readings at least 1 week apart
  - Initially, take pressure in both arms; if the pressures differ, use the arm with the higher pressure
  - If the arm pressure is elevated, take the pressure in one leg, particularly in patients <30 years old
  Performance
  - Inflate the bladder quickly to a pressure 20 mm Hg above the systolic pressure, recognized by disappearance of radial pulse, to avoid an auscultatory gap
  - Deflate the bladder 3 mm Hg/s
  - Record the Korotkoff phase I (appearance) and phase V (disappearance)
  - If the Korotkoff sounds are weak, have the patient raise the arm and open and close the hand 5–10 times, then inflate the bladder quickly
  Recordings
  - Note the pressure, patient position, the arm, and cuff size (e.g., 140/90, seated, right arm, large adult cuff)

If mercury manometers are to be phased out because of the toxic potential of mercury spills and with the inaccuracies of aneroid manometers, automated electronic devices will increasingly be used. Attention to the equipment and technique improves the accuracy of the procedure (Beevers et al., 2001b; Pickering et al., 2005).

### Bladder Size

The width of the bladder should be equal to approximately two-thirds the distance from the axilla to the antecubital space; a 16-cm-wide bladder is adequate for most adults. The bladder should be long enough to encircle at least 80% of the arm.

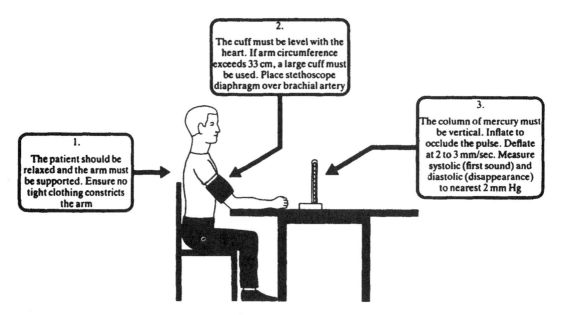

**FIGURE 2–6** ● Technique of blood pressure measurement recommended by the British Hypertension Society. (From British Hypertension Society. Standardization of blood pressure measurement. *J Hypertens* 1985;3:29–31.)

Erroneously high readings may occur with use of a bladder that is too short (Aylett et al., 2001) and erroneously low readings with a bladder that is too wide (Bakx et al., 1997).

An alert family doctor, Ronald D. Reynolds, MD, identified an inexplicable design problem with the Walgreens BC200W Large Arm Cuff, manufactured by Samsung. The bladder, approximately sized at 15 cm, had been sealed longitudinally into two 7.5 cm bladders, causing markedly false high readings. Despite Dr. Reynolds' pleas to the FDA and the manufacturer, the cuff remains on the market.

Most sphygmomanometers sold in the United States have a cuff with a bladder that is 12 cm wide and 22 cm long, which is too short for patients with an arm circumference greater than 26 cm, whether fat or muscular (Aylett et al., 2001). The British Hypertension Society recommends longer cuff size (12 x 40 cm) for obese arms (O'Brien et al., 2003). The American Heart Association recommends progressively larger cuffs with larger arm circumference:

- Arm circumference 22–26 cm, 12 × 22 cm cuff (small adult)
- Arm circumference 27–34 cm, 16 × 30 cm cuff (adult)
- Arm circumference 35–44 cm, 16 × 36 cm cuff (large adult)
- Arm circumference 45–52 cm, 16 × 42 cm cuff (adult thigh)

Children require smaller cuffs depending on their size (Clausen et al., 1999). Meanwhile, a triple-bladder cuff (tricuff) which automatically selects the appropriate size in relation to the arm circumference and an adjustable cuff has been marketed (O'Brien et al., 2003).

### Cuff Position

If the bladder within the cuff does not completely encircle the arm, particular care should be taken to ensure that the bladder is placed over the brachial artery. The lower edge of the cuff should be approximately 2.5 cm above the antecubital space. In extremely obese people, a thigh cuff may be used with the wide bladder folded on itself if necessary, or the bladder may be placed on the forearm and the sounds heard over the radial artery. However, the forearm readings may be higher (Pierin et al., 2004).

### Manometer

Despite the pleas that they be retained (Jones, et al., 2001), mercury manometers are being phased out because of concern over toxicity from spills (O'Brien et al., 2001). At the least, a few should be kept in every facility as standards for other manometers. Aneroid manometers are less reliable than mercury manometers but their accuracy can easily be ascertained (Pickering et al., 2005).

Electronic devices are rapidly taking over the home market and will most likely become standard in offices and hospitals. Fortunately, their accuracy and reliability are improving, and more have passed the protocols of the U.S. Association for the

Advancement of Medical Instrumentation (AAMI) and the British Hypertension Society (BHS) (O'Brien et al., 2001; Verdecchia et al., 2001). Under the supervision of W.J. Rickard and Professor Erin O'Brien, a wonderful website (http://www.dableducational.com) has been established to provide all of the available information needed about the devices being marketed.

Most of the newer electronic devices are based on oscillometry, which detects initial (systolic) and maximal (mean arterial pressure) oscillations in the brachial artery and calculates the diastolic BP based on proprietary algorithms. In general, the readings obtained by auscultatory and oscillometric devices are closely correlated (Yarows & Brook, 2000; Yarows et al., 2000). The oscillometric devices are faster to use, and they minimize the common terminal digit preference wherein the last number is rounded off to 0 or 5 (de Lusignan et al., 2004). Some of the electronic devices inflate automatically, which is especially useful for patients with arthritis. Others have a printer attached, and some can have the data downloaded after storing a number of readings. Devices are available for automatic transmission of data to a central location (Møller et al., 2003). An adequate device can be purchased for less than $40. To ensure its proper use and accuracy, the electronic device should be checked by having the patient use it on one arm while the pressure is simultaneously taken in the office with a sphygmomanometer on the other arm.

### Wrist and Finger Devices

Most wrist oscillometric devices, such as the Omron HEM-637, have not provided acceptable reproducibility (http://www.dableducational.com) and should always be checked against a device with an upper arm cuff (Zweiker et al., 2000).

Finger devices measure the pressure in the finger by volume-clamp plethysmography. The Finapres finger cuff may be used for continuous BP monitoring under carefully controlled conditions (Silke & McAuley, 1998), but it is not suitable for intermittent readings (Lal et al., 1995). Home finger units are not recommended for self-monitoring (White et al., 1999).

### Automated Devices

The automated oscillometric devices increasingly used in offices, emergency rooms, and hospitals are often inaccurate. Devices such as the Dinamapp 8100 (Park et al., 2001) and the IVAC 4200 (Shuler et al., 1998) usually overestimate BP by 10/5 mm Hg. Nonetheless, these and other automated devices such as the Accutorr and Paramed usually provide readings that are satisfactory for most clinical

settings (Lehmann et al., 1998). The Welch Allyn Vital Signs bedside monitor has been validated (Jones, Taylor, et al., 2001).

On the other hand, community-based automated machines may be even more inaccurate, particularly in patients with arm sizes smaller or larger than average (Van Durme et al., 2000). For those who cannot use more accurate (and more easily validated) home devices, readings obtained by such an automated machine are better than nothing, but patients should not be managed solely on the basis of the readings from such machines.

## Technique for Measuring Blood Pressure

As noted in Table 2–3, care should be taken to raise the pressure in the bladder approximately 20 mm Hg above the systolic level, as indicated by disappearance of the radial pulse, because patients may have an auscultatory gap (a temporary disappearance of the sound after it first appears), which is related to increased arterial stiffness (Cavallini et al., 1996).

The measurement may be repeated after as little a span as 15 seconds without significantly affecting accuracy. The cuff should be deflated at a rate of 2 to 4 mm Hg/s; either a slower or faster rate may cause falsely higher readings (Bos et al., 1992).

Disappearance of the sound (phase V) is a more sensitive and reproducible end point than muffling (phase IV) (de Mey, 1995). In some patients with a hyperkinetic circulation (e.g., anemia), the sounds do not disappear, and the muffled sound is heard well below the expected diastolic BP, sometimes near zero. This phenomenon can also be caused by pressing the stethoscope too firmly against the artery. If arrhythmias are present, additional readings with either auscultatory or oscillometric devices may be required to estimate the average systolic and diastolic BP (Lip et al., 2001).

### Pseudohypertension

In some elderly patients with very rigid, calcified arteries, the bladder may not be able to collapse the brachial artery, giving rise to falsely high readings, or pseudohypertension (Spence, 1997). The possibility of pseudohypertension should be suspected in elderly people whose vessels feel rigid; who have little vascular damage in the retina or elsewhere, despite markedly high BP readings; and who suffer inordinate postural symptoms despite cautious therapy.

If one is suspicious, an automatic oscillometric recorder or finger BP measurement should settle the issue (Zweifler & Shahab, 1993), but a direct intraarterial reading may be needed.

### Ways to Amplify the Sounds

The loudness and sharpness of the Korotkoff sounds depend in part on the pressure differential between the arteries in the forearm and those beneath the bladder. To increase the differential and thereby increase the loudness of the sounds, either the amount of blood in the forearm can be decreased or the capacity of the vascular bed can be increased. The amount of blood can be decreased by rapidly inflating the bladder, thereby shortening the time when venous outflow is prevented but arterial inflow continues, or by raising the arm for a few seconds to drain venous blood before inflating the bladder. The vascular bed capacity can be increased by inducing vasodilation through muscular exercise, specifically by having the patient open and close the hand ten times before the observer inflates the bladder. If the sounds are not heard well, the balloon should be emptied and reinflated; otherwise, the vessels will have been partially refilled and the sounds thereby muffled.

### Taking Blood Pressure in the Thigh

A large (thigh) cuff should be used to avoid factitiously elevated readings. With the patient lying prone and the leg bent and cradled by the observer, the observer listens with the stethoscope for the Korotkoff sounds in the popliteal fossa. This should be done as part of the initial workup of every young hypertensive, in whom coarctation is more common. Normally, the systolic BP is higher and the diastolic BP a little lower at the knee than in the arm because of the contour of the pulse wave (Hugue et al., 1988).

### Taking Blood Pressure in Children

If the child is calm, the same technique that is used with adults should be followed; however, smaller, narrower cuffs must be used (see Chapter 16). Korotkoff phase V is more reliable than phase IV (Penny et al., 1996). If the child is upset, the best procedure may be simply to determine the systolic BP by palpating the radial pulse as the cuff is deflated. In infants, the use of ultrasound techniques is much easier (Laaser & Labarthe, 1986).

### Recording of Findings

Regardless of which method is used to measure BP, notation should be made of the conditions so that others can compare the findings or interpret them properly. This is particularly critical in scientific reports, yet many articles about hypertension fail to provide this information.

### Blood Pressure during Exercise

An exaggerated response of BP during or immediately after graded exercise has been found to predict the development of hypertension in normotensives (Matthews et al., 1998; Miyai et al., 2000; Singh et al., 1999) and their subsequent morbidity or mortality from cardiovascular disease (Kjeldsen et al., 2001; Laukkanen et al., 2004; Mundal et al., 1996). Different upper limits for a normal response to exercise have been used in various series, but an exaggerated response to a systolic level above 200 mm Hg at a 100W workload increases the likelihood of the onset of hypertension from two- to fourfold over the subsequent 5 to 10 years as compared with that seen with nonexaggerated responses. Even a rise in BP of more than 30/15 mm Hg in anticipation of an exercise test has been found to predict the onset of hypertension over the next 4 years (Everson et al., 1996).

Because most patients who have a supernormal response do not develop hypertension if they are normotensive nor develop cardiovascular mortality if they are hypertensive, exercise tests should not be performed for prognostic purposes. If, however, exercise tests are undertaken for appropriate reasons and the BP response is supernormal, the normotensive patient should be advised to modify his or her lifestyle (including gradual institution of an aerobic exercise program), and the hypertensive patient should be advised to achieve better control of existing hypertension. Hypertensives may have an impaired capacity to exercise (Lim et al., 1996), but they should be advised to continue the effort, because a low level of cardiorespiratory fitness is a strong predictor of future mortality, comparable to smoking (Blair et al., 1998).

### Importance of Office Blood Pressures

Even if all the guidelines listed in Table 2–3 are followed, routine office measurements of BP by sphygmomanometry will continue to show considerable variability. However, before discounting even single casual BP readings, recall that almost all the data on the risks of hypertension described in Chapter 1 are based on only one or a few readings taken in large groups of people. There is no denying that such data have epidemiologic value, but a few casual office readings are usually not sufficient to determine the status of an individual patient. Two actions minimize variability. First, at least two readings should be taken at every visit, as many as needed to obtain a stable level with less than a 5-mm Hg difference; second, at least three and, preferably, more sets of readings, weeks apart, should be taken unless the initial value is so high (e.g., >180/120 mm Hg) that immediate therapy is needed.

The closer the initial readings are to 140/90 mm Hg, the more repeated readings are needed to allow determination of a patient's usual status (Perry & Miller, 1992). Although multiple carefully taken office readings may be as reliable as those taken by ambulatory monitors (Pearce et al., 1992; Reeves, 1995), out-of-office readings provide additional data, both to confirm the diagnosis and, more important, to document the adequacy of therapy.

## HOME MEASUREMENTS

From the preceding, it is clear that BPs recorded in the hospital or office often are affected by both acute and chronic alerting reactions that tend to accentuate variability and raise the BP, giving rise to a significant white-coat effect. Two techniques—home measurements and ABPM—minimize these problems. Whereas ABPM will likely continue to have more limited applications, the use of home measurements will likely continue to expand (Pickering et al., 2005; Stergiou et al., 2004) (Table 2–4).

The main reason why the use of home BP measurements will expand is the need to first recognize and then modulate the increase in cardiovascular events and deaths occurring in the first few hours after arising from sleep (Gosse et al., 2004). Some morning surge is inevitable since the sympathetic nerves must be activated when rising from overnight sleep and ambulating; otherwise, orthostatic falls would occur. By measuring the BP soon after arising, the degree of surge can be identified and, if it is to a level above 160/100, changes made in the timing of antihypertensive therapy (Mosenkis & Townsend, 2004). Rather than taking the presumably long-acting, once-a-day pills soon after awakening, as is usually recommended, two options are available: Split the dosage to twice a day or change the time of the once a day to 6 p.m. or bedtime or to around 3 a.m. when the almost invariable nocturia strikes.

Concerns have arisen about the reliability of both the performance and the reporting of home BP measurements. In multiple small groups of patients, unaware that their readings were being stored electronically for later surveillance, the self-recorded values have been found to differ by more than 10 mm Hg from the actual measurement in 15% to 25% of the readings (Johnson et al., 1999; Nordmann et al., 1999). It should be noted that similar or worse inaccuracies in reporting home blood

## TABLE 2–4

### Indications for Home Blood Pressure Monitoring

For diagnosis
  To recognize initial, short-term elevations in blood pressure
  To identify persistent white-coat hypertension
  To determine usual blood pressure levels
For prognosis
  To ascertain cardiovascular risk
For therapy
  To monitor response to therapy
    To ensure adequate blood pressure control during waking hours
    To evaluate effects of increasing or decreasing amounts of therapy
    To ascertain whether poor office blood pressure response to increased treatment represents true resistance
    To identify periods of poor control when office readings are normal but target organ damage progresses
    To identify relation of blood pressure levels to presumed side effects of therapy
  To involve patient and improve adherence

glucose measurements have long been recognized without diminishing its acceptance as a critical element in the management of diabetes (Mazze et al., 1984). Nonetheless, the problem could be minimized by teletransmission of automatically stored readings to a computer monitor (Møller et al., 2003).

### Uses for Home Measurements

#### Diagnosis

From multiple surveys of large populations, a reasonable upper limit of normal for home BP is 135/85 mm Hg (O'Brien et al., 2003).

Multiple home recordings overcome much of the error caused by the acute and persistent alerting reaction that is responsible for most white-coat hypertension (Hozawa et al., 2001; Staessen et al., 2004) and can be used to make the diagnosis of hypertension as efficient as ambulatory monitoring can (Den Hond et al., 2003; Yarows et al., 2000). The data in Table 2–5 document the significantly lower average of the 32 home readings per patient obtained during the 2 weeks between the first and second clinic visits of 268 patients having a BP above 160/95 mm Hg on three consecutive occasions before the first clinic reading (Hall et al., 1990). The home readings were lower in 80% of the patients, by more than 20/10 mm Hg in 40%, so that therapy was deemed unnecessary in 38% of untreated patients and reducible in 16% of treated patients. The accuracy of the home readings taken with the electronic devices is evident by the identical readings taken with that device and the mercury sphygmomanometer at the second clinic visit.

Over a one-year follow-up, home monitoring of 203 patients being treated identified 25.6% to have white-coat hypertension and thereby able to discontinue therapy (Staessen et al., 2004). These two sets of data attest to the ability of home monitoring to identify the significant number of patients with white-coat hypertension.

### Prognosis

Considerable data documenting the validity of self-recorded home measurements for ascertainment of long-term prognosis has come from an ongoing follow-up of 1,913 subjects in Ohasama, Japan (Asayama et al., 2004; Ohkubo et al., 2004). After a mean follow-up of 8.6 years, the risks of cardiovascular mortality have been documented for isolated systolic and combined systolic-diastolic hypertension diagnosed by home measurements (Hozawa et al., 2000). In other populations, home readings have been found to be closely correlated to the presence of left ventricular hypertrophy and albuminuria (Jula et al., 1999), to the progression of diabetic nephropathy (Kamoi et al., 2002), and to mortality (Sega et al., 2005).

The most impressive evidence for a greater prognostic reliability for home readings than for office readings comes from a study of 4,939 treated hypertensives followed for a mean of 3.2 years (Bobrie et al., 2004). The hazard ratio of a cardiovascular event was increased by a statistically significant 2.06-fold in those with elevated home readings but normal office readings but only a statistically insignificant 1.18-fold in those with normal home readings but elevated office readings.

### Therapy

Home recordings should be used to monitor therapy (Canzanello et al., 2005; Cuspidi et al., 2004a). When patients are followed only by infrequent office visits, their responses may be either underestimated by the white-coat effect or overestimated when the BP is taken near the peak of the effect of medications. As a consequence, they may be either overtreated or undertreated.

The problem of overtreatment is encountered occasionally with patients whose office readings do not seem to be responding to increasing therapy but whose out-of-office readings are well controlled (pseudoresistance) (Redon et al., 1998). Other patients who seem properly controlled in the office may have too low pressures at home, a particular danger for the elderly, who may not be able to withstand such low BPs (Raccaud et al., 1992).

When only office readings are taken, the problem of undertreatment may be even more of a danger. Recall that in the large study by Bobrie et al. (2004), those patients with normal clinic pressures

## TABLE 2-5

### Blood Pressure Recorded at Home between Clinic Visits

| Patient Group | First Clinic Reading (Mercury Manometer) | | Home Series (Electronic Device) | | Second Clinic Reading | | | |
|---|---|---|---|---|---|---|---|---|
| | | | | | Electronic Device | | Mercury Manometer | |
| | SBP (mm Hg) | DBP (mm Hg) | SBP (mm Hg) | DBP (mm Hg) | SBP (mm Hg) | DBP (mm Hg) | SBP (mm Hg) | DBP (mm Hg) |
| Untreated (n = 114) | 174 | 103 | 148 | 90 | 165 | 95 | 164 | 97 |
| Treated (n = 154) | 177 | 104 | 147 | 87 | 163 | 95 | 164 | 95 |

DBP, diastolic blood pressure; SBP, systolic blood pressure. Data from Hall CL, Higgs CMB, Notarianni L. Home blood pressure recording in mild hypertension. *J Hum Hypertens* 1990;4:501–507.

but elevated home pressures, i.e., masked hypertensives, had more than a twofold increased risk of a cardiovascular event than did those with normal clinic and home pressures.

Moreover, those who perform home measurements are more likely to remain under management (Elliott, 1995) and to achieve better control of their hypertension (Canzanello et al., 2005; Cuspidi et al., 2004b). In an analysis of 18 randomized controlled trials involving a total of 2,700 hypertensives, those who performed home BP monitoring had an average 4.2/2.4 mm Hg lower blood pressure than did those who had only office monitoring (Cappuccio et al., 2004). Those who used home readings had a 10% increased likelihood of reaching the goal of therapy.

### Technique

All the instructions that are needed for office readings (Table 2–3) must be followed with home readings as well, and patients should always be given instructions to supplement those provided with the device. These points should be made to the patient:

- Check the device and the patient's technique by simultaneous measurements in the office against a mercury manometer.
- The first few readings may reflect an alerting reaction similar to that usually experienced in the physician's office. Most patients overcome this anxiety and can obtain "nonstressed" readings after a few days (Celis et al., 1997). However, a few people continue to be frightened by the prospect of finding a high reading that could reflect impending doom, further raising their home readings. If such anxiety cannot be allayed, the patient should not take home measurements.
- Do not be concerned by fluctuations of even 20 mm Hg, but do inform the physician's office if the pressures are going up progressively over a period of 1 week or longer.
- If the home readings are being taken to determine the average BP for diagnostic purposes, the readings should be made at different times (e.g., when the patient is either relaxed or stressed, anytime throughout the day or evening). It is not appropriate to use a few "relaxed" BP readings that are lower than office readings to diagnose white-coat hypertension (Stergiou et al., 2000).
- If the readings are being taken to determine the adequacy of antihypertensive therapy, they should be taken at the same time of day, preferably in the early morning soon after the patient arises from bed, to ensure 24-hour control with the regimen being prescribed. Readings should

occasionally be taken repeatedly throughout the day to ascertain both the peak effect and the duration of effect, particularly after changes in therapy.

## AMBULATORY MONITORING

Although some of the same information provided by noninvasive ABPM may be obtained by multiple office or home measurements, ABPM is being advocated for multiple additional reasons (Table 2–6). The U.S. JNC-7 report (Chobanian et al., 2003) is less enthusiastic in its recommendations for ABPM than is the European Society of Hypertension (O'Brien et al., 2003), but all expert groups recognize its special benefits. Unfortunately, lack of adequate reimbursement by third-party payers has limited its clinical use in the United States. Moreover, routine ABPM on all patients is not cost-effective (Lorgelly et al., 2003), so it should be used only for specific indications.

### Equipment

The noninvasive 24-hour ABPM systems now available use a standard arm cuff that is inflated at predetermined intervals, usually every 15 to 30 minutes during the day and every 30 to 60 minutes during the night, by a small pump. The individual BPs measured throughout the 24 hours are stored in the unit worn by the patient and later are read by a computer that prints all of the readings (Figure 2–1), along with the mean plus or minus standard deviations for whatever intervals are desired.

As more of these devices are being marketed, the BHS and the AAMI have established protocols for accuracy and performance. The website http://www.dableducational.com should be accessed to

---

## TABLE 2–6

### Situations where Ambulatory Blood Pressure Monitoring Is Helpful

Excluding white-coat hypertension in patients with office hypertension but no target organ damage

Deciding on treatment of elderly patients

Identifying nocturnal hypertension (dipping status)

Assessing apparent resistance to therapy

Assuring efficacy of treatment over entire 24 hours

Managing hypertension during pregnancy

Evaluating hypotension and episodic hypertension

ascertain the types and validations of the devices now marketed.

## Technique

Those who wish to perform ABPM would do well to read the consensus views on the technique published by a group of experts from the British (O'Brien et al., 2000) and European Societies of Hypertension (O'Brien et al., 2003).

### Effects of Activity

To monitor the effects of activity, patients should keep a diary of activities during the 24-hour period because of the often marked associated changes in BP (Table 2–2). In addition, an initial alerting reaction may be seen for the first few hours of ABPM, so a 48-hour procedure may give more valid data (Calvo et al., 2003).

### Analyzing the Data

To analyze 24-hour data, in the past most investigators used the average value of all readings obtained throughout the 24-hour period. Recognizing that readings during sleep are normally considerably lower than daytime readings, making the 24-hour average lower than the daytime average, there is increasing use of the mean of all daytime (awake) and nighttime (sleep) readings, a procedure that seems sensible and appropriate (Table 2–7). The average daytime value more closely approximates that found by multiple office or home readings and, by this method, the nighttime readings receive the attention they deserve. One continuing source of confusion is the timing of the awake and sleeping intervals. To resolve the issue, O'Brien et al. (2003) recommend setting the daytime period at 0900 to 2100 (9 a.m. to 9 p.m.) and the nighttime at 0100 to 0600 (1 a.m. to 6 a.m.).

Because virtually all normotensive people have occasional high readings and virtually all fixed hypertensive patients have some normal readings, some clinicians advocate use of the load (i.e., the percentage of ambulatory BPs higher than 140 mm Hg systolic or 90 mm Hg diastolic) to diagnose hypertension (Zachariah & Sumner, 1993) and to ascertain the response to therapy (White, 1996).

## Uses for Ambulatory Monitoring

### Diagnosis

As noted earlier, the definitions of normal and high BP levels obtained by routine sphygmomanometry are arbitrary and still not universally agreed on. Because ABPM has been performed on far fewer people and because long-term follow-up is not yet

### TABLE 2–7

**Recommended Thresholds for Ambulatory Blood Pressure Measurements in Adults**

|          | Optimal  | Normal   | Abnormal |
|----------|----------|----------|----------|
| Awake    | <130/80  | <135/85  | >140/90  |
| Asleep   | <115/65  | <120/70  | >125/75  |

Adapted from O'Brien et al. European Society of Hypertension recommendations for conventional, ambulatory and home blood pressure measurement. *J Hypertens* 2003;21:821–848.

available to establish the prognostic meaning of different BP levels, the definition of *normal* by ABPM remains uncertain. However, data from multiple studies have been used as the basis for the thresholds shown in Table 2–7.

As expected, higher readings are usual in older people. In 685 untreated men 70 years of age, the ninety-fifth percentile for daytime levels was 153/85 mm Hg and for nighttime was 132/73 mm Hg (Björklund et al., 2000). Nocturnal dipping is reduced in those over age 80 (O'Sullivan et al., 2003).

### Decision to Treat

Most expert committees continue to recommend that the decision to treat hypertension should be based on multiple office readings since ABPM is not universally available and there are relatively little long-term follow-up data on the relation between various ABPM levels and cardiovascular events (Meyers, 2005). However, ABPM values, particularly the nighttime readings, have been correlated with concurrent cardiovascular damage (Cuspidi et al., 2004a) and prediction of future levels of blood pressure (Georgiades et al., 2004). Moreover, in placebo-treated patients followed beyond 6 months, the incidence of cardiovascular events was significantly related to the baseline ambulatory BP but not to subsequent clinic pressures (Fagard et al., 2004).

At this time, perhaps the major values of ABPM are to identify those with white-coat hypertension who likely do not need immediate antihypertensive drug therapy and to ascertain nocturnal dipping status.

### Prognosis

Ambulatory BP monitoring has been found to be superior to office readings in assessing the current status of target organ damage, in particular left ventricular hypertrophy (Cuspidi et al., 2004), and in predicting the future prognosis of any level of hypertension (Björklund et al., 2004; Clement et al., 2003; Hansen et al., 2005; Khattar et al., 1999; Kikuya et al., 2005; Perloff et al., 1991; Verdecchia et al., 1996). A striking example of the closer relation to subsequent cardiovascular risk of ABPM levels than of conventional office readings are the data from the placebo-treated half of a group of 808 older patients enrolled in the Systolic Hypertension in Europe trial (Staessen et al., 1999). As seen in Figure 2–7, the various elements of the ABPM recording were much more closely correlated to the two-year incidence of cardiovascular events than was the office (conventional) BP.

Another specific situation wherein ABPM provides better prognostic information than do office readings is the presence of hypertension during pregnancy (Bellomo et al., 1999). Ambulatory BP monitoring also was found to predict the development of preeclampsia in pregnant diabetic women (Flores et al., 1999).

### Response to Therapy

A seeming paradox is noted in the relation between ABPM and the response to antihypertensive therapy: The blood pressure does not fall as much with ABPM as with office readings but the cardiovascular protection is more closely related to the changes in ABPM.

As to the first part of the paradox, Mancia and Parati (2004) analyzed 23 studies of 6 months or longer duration that examined the effect of various therapies on both office and ABPM readings. In all but a few, the office systolic and diastolic levels fell more than the ABPM readings, averaging –24.9/–14.5 mm Hg by office and –14.6/–9.2 mm Hg by ABPM. Most of this difference is likely related to the initially higher office readings, reflecting a white-coat effect. The authors also discuss other possible reasons for the disparity.

As to the second part, there are increasingly impressive data showing that cardiovascular protection is more closely related to changes in ABPM than office readings. Among 790 hypertensives followed an average of 3.7 years, the relative risk of cardiovascular events was reduced by 64% in those with controlled ABPM (below 135/85) but only by 37% in those with controlled office readings (to below 140/90) (Verdecchia et al., 2002). Similar closer associations between cardiovascular events and ABPM than office readings have been reported by Hansen et al. (2005), Ohkubo et al. (2002), and Redon et al. (1998).

Beyond the better predictive value of ABPM, such readings are useful in assuring the 24-hour effectiveness of therapy (Neutel et al., 1993) and assessing apparent resistance to increased therapy (Pickering, 2005b) (Figure 2–8). If, in the absence of target organ damage, office BP remains high despite more and more therapy, either home or ambulatory readings may identify pseudoresistance.

In addition, the use of ABPM, by avoiding the initial white-coat response and placebo effect, can markedly reduce the number of patients needed in studies of antihypertensive drug efficacy (Mancia & Parati, 2004).

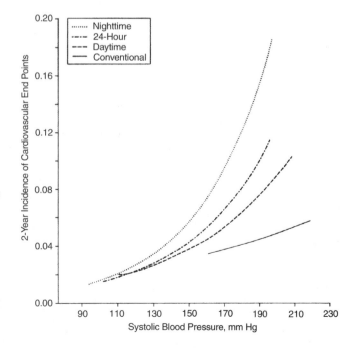

**FIGURE 2–7** ● The relation of systolic blood pressure by conventional (office) or 24-hour daytime and nighttime ambulatory measurements at entry as predictors of the two-year incidence of cardiovascular end points in the placebo-treated older patients with systolic hypertension. Incidence is given as a fraction (i.e., 0.02 is an incidence of 2 events per 100 people). Using multiple Cox regression, the event rate was standardized to female gender, mean age of 69.6 years, no previous cardiovascular complications, nonsmoking status, and residence in western Europe. (Modified from Staessen JA, Thijs L, Fagard R, et al. Predicting cardiovascular risk using conventional vs ambulatory blood pressure in older patients with systolic hypertension. *JAMA* 1999;282:539–546.)

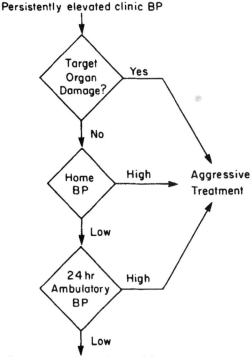

Persistently elevated clinic BP

**FIGURE 2-8** ● Proposed schema of blood pressure (BP) measurement for patients with apparently resistant hypertension. (Adapted from Pickering TG. Blood pressure monitoring outside the office for the evaluation of patients with resistant hypertension. *Hypertension* 1988; 11(Suppl 2):96–100.)

## CONCLUSION

Despite all the reasons that home and ambulatory measurements are better than office readings, for now office sphygmomanometry will continue to be the primary tool for diagnosing and monitoring hypertension. Home readings should be routinely used both to confirm the diagnosis and to provide better assurance of appropriate therapy. Ambulatory monitoring should be increasingly used to look for white-coat hypertension, to evaluate apparent resistance to therapy, and to determine the adequacy of therapy, particularly during sleep and the early morning hours.

We next turn to the mechanisms responsible for elevated BP in 95% of those with hypertension, i.e., those with primary (essential) hypertension.

## REFERENCES

Agyemang C, Bhopal R, Bruijnzeels M, Redekop WK. Does nocturnal blood pressure fall in people of African and South Asian descent differ from that in European white populations? A systematic review and meta-analysis. *J Hypertens* 2005;23:913–920.

Aihara A, Imai Y, Sekino M, et al. Discrepancy between screening blood pressure and ambulatory blood pressure. *Hypertens Res* 1998;21:127–136.

Asayama K, Ohkubo T, Kikuya M, et al. Prediction of stroke by self-measurement of blood pressure at home versus casual screening blood pressure measurement in relation to the Joint National Committee 7 classification: the Ohasama study. *Stroke* 2004;35:2356–2361.

Aylett M, Marples G, Jones K, Rhodes D. Evaluation of normal and large sphygmomanometer cuffs using the Omron 705CP. *J Hum Hypertens* 2001;15:131–134.

Bakx C, Oerlemans G, van den Hoogen H, et al., The influence of cuff size on blood pressure measurement. *J Hum Hypertens* 1997;11:439–445.

Beevers G, Lip GYH, O'Brien E. Blood pressure measurement. Part I—sphygmomanometry: factors common to all techniques. *BMJ* 2001a;322:981–985.

Beevers G, Lip GYH, O'Brien E. Blood pressure measurement. Part II—conventional sphygmomanometry: technique of auscultatory blood pressure measurement. *BMJ* 2001b;322:1043–1046.

Bellomo G, Narducci PL, Rondoni F, et al. Prognostic value of 24-hour blood pressure in pregnancy. *JAMA* 1999;282:1447–1452.

Bidlingmeyer I, Burnier M, Bidlingmeyer M, et al. Isolated office hypertension: a prehypertensive state? *J Hypertens* 1996;14:327–332.

Björklund K, Lind L, Andren B, Lithell H. The majority of nondipping men do not have increased cardiovascular risk: a population-based study. *J Hypertens* 2002;20:1501–1506.

Björklund, Lind L, Lithell H. Twenty-four hour ambulatory blood pressure in a population of elderly men. *J Intern Med* 2000;248:501–510.

Björklund K, Lind L, Zethelius B, et al. Prognostic significance of 24-h ambulatory blood pressure characteristics for cardiovascular morbidity in a population of elderly men. *J Hypertens* 2004;22:1691–1697.

Björklund K, Lind L, Zethelius B, et al. Isolated ambulatory hypertension predicts cardiovascular morbidity in elderly men. *Circulation* 2003;107:1297–1302.

Blair SN, Wei M, Lee CD. Cardiorespiratory fitness by exercise heart rate as a predictor of mortality in the Aerobics Center Longitudinal Study. *J Sports Sci* 1998;16:S47–S55.

Blood-pressure monitors. *Consum Rep* 2003;68:22–24.

Bobrie G, Chatellier G, Genes N, et al. Cardiovascular prognosis of "masked hypertension" detected by blood pressure self-measurement in elderly treated hypertensive patients. *JAMA* 2004;291:1342–1349.

Bornstein NM, Norris JW. Subclavian steal: a harmless haemodynamic phenomenon? *Lancet* 1986;2:303–305.

Bos WJW, van Goudoever J, van Montfrans GA, Wesseling KH. Influence of short-term blood pressure variability on blood pressure determinations. *Hypertension* 1992;19:606–609.

Brennan M, O'Brien E, O'Malley K. The effect of age on blood pressure and heart rate variability in hypertension. *J Hypertens* 1986;4(Suppl 6):S269–S272.

British Hypertension Society. Standardization of blood pressure measurement. *J Hypertens* 1985;3:293.

Bursztyn M, Ginsberg G, Hammerman-Rozenberg R, Stessman J. The siesta in the elderly. Risk factor for mortality? *Arch Intern Med* 1999;159:1582–1586.

Calvo C, Hermida RC, Ayala DE, et al. The "ABPM effect" gradually decreases but does not disappear in successive sessions of ambulatory monitoring. *J Hypertens* 2003;21:2265–2273.

Canzanello VJ, Jensen PL, Schwartz LL, et al. Improved blood pressure control with a physician-nurse team and home blood pressure measurement. *Mayo Clin Proc* 2005; 80:31–36.

Cappuccio FP, Kerry SM, Forbes L, Donald A. Blood pressure control by home monitoring: meta-analysis of randomised trials. *BMJ* 2004;329:145–150.

Casiglia E, Palatini P, Colangeli G, et al. 24 h rhythm of blood pressure and forearm peripheral resistance in normotensive and hypertensive subjects confined to bed. *J Hypertens* 1996;14:47–52.

Cavallini MC, Roman MJ, Blank SG, et al. Association of the auscultatory gap with vascular disease in hypertensive patients. *Ann Intern Med* 1996;124:877–883.

Cavelaars M, Tulen JH, van Bemmel JH, et al. Reproducibility of intra-arterial ambulatory blood pressure: effects of physical activity and posture. *J Hypertens* 2004a;22:1105–1112.

Cavelaars M, Tulen JHM, van Bemmel JH, van den Meiracker AH. Physical activity, dipping and haemodynamics. *J Hypertens* 2004b;22:2303–2309.

Celis H, De Cort P, Fagard R, et al. For how many days should blood pressure be measured at home in older patients before steady levels are obtained? *J Hum Hypertens* 1997;11:673–677.

Centers for Medicare & Medicaid Services. Medicare coverage policy—decisions. Ambulatory blood pressure monitoring (CAG-00067N), 2001. http://www.hefa.gov/coverage/8b3-ff.htm.

Chobanian AV, Bakris GL, Black HR, et al. Seventh report of the Joint National Committee on Prevention, Detection, Evaluation, and Treatment of High Blood Pressure. *Hypertension* 2003;42:1206–1252.

Clark LA, Denby L, Pregibon D, et al. A quantitative analysis of the effects of activity and time of day on the diurnal variations of blood pressure. *J Chronic Dis* 1987;40:671–679.

Clausen LR, Olsen CA, Olsen JA, et al. Influence of cuff size on blood pressure among schoolchildren. *Blood Pressure* 1999;8:172–176.

Clement DL, De Buyzere ML, De Bacquer DA, et al. Prognostic value of ambulatory blood-pressure recordings in patients with treated hypertension. *N Engl J Med* 2003; 348:2407–2415.

Cushman WC, Cooper KM, Horne RA, Meydrech EF. Effect of back support and stethoscope head on seated blood pressure determinations. *Am J Hypertens* 1990; 3:240–241.

Cuspidi C, Meani S, Salerno M, et al. Cardiovascular target organ damage in essential hypertensives with or without reproducible nocturnal fall in blood pressure. *J Hypertens* 2004a;22:273–280.

Cuspidi C, Meani S, Fusi V, et al. Home blood pressure measurement and its relationship with blood pressure control in a large selected hypertensive population. *J Hum Hypertens* 2004b;18:725–731.

De Lusignan S, Belsey J, Hague N, Dzregah B. End-digit preference in blood pressure recordings of patients with ischaemic heart disease in primary care. *J Hum Hypertens* 2004;18:261–265.

De Mey C. Method specificity of the auscultatory estimates of the inodilatory reduction of diastolic blood pressure based on Korotkoff IV and V criteria. *Br J Clin Pharmacol* 1995;39:485–490.

Den Hond E, Celis H, Fagard R, et al. Self-measured versus ambulatory blood pressure in the diagnosis of hypertension. *J Hypertens* 2003;21:717–722.

Dewar R, Sykes D, Mulkerrin E, et al. The effect of hemiplegia on blood pressure measurement in the elderly. *Postgrad Med J* 1992;68:888–891.

Dodt C, Breckling U, Derad I, et al. Plasma epinephrine and norepinephrine concentrations of healthy humans associated with nighttime sleep and morning arousal. *Hypertension* 1997;30:71–76.

Elliott WJ. Methods of measuring blood pressure and dropouts in a tertiary hypertension clinic [Abstract]. *Am J Hypertens* 1995;8:100A.

Enström I, Pennert K, Lindholm LH. Difference in blood pressure, but not in heart rate, between measurements performed at a health centre and at a hospital by one and the same physician. *J Hum Hypertens* 2000;14:355–358.

Everson SA, Kaplan GA, Goldberg DE, Salonen JT. Anticipatory blood pressure response to exercise predicts future high blood pressure in middle-aged men. *Hypertension* 1996;27: 1059–1064.

Fagard RH, Staessen JA, Thijs L, et al. Relationship between ambulatory blood pressure and follow-up clinic blood pressure in elderly patients with systolic hypertension. *J Hypertens* 2004;22:81–87.

Fagius J, Karhuvaara S. Sympathetic activity and blood pressure increases with bladder distension in humans. *Hypertension* 1989;14:511–517.

Floras JS. Antihypertensive treatment, myocardial infarction, and nocturnal myocardial ischaemia. *Lancet* 1988;2: 994–996.

Flores L, Levy I, Aguilera E, et al. Usefulness of ambulatory blood pressure monitoring in pregnant women with type 1 diabetes. *Diabetes Care* 1999;22:1507–1511.

Frattola A, Parati G, Castiglioni P, et al. Lacicipine and blood pressure variability in diabetic hypertensive patients. *Hypertension* 2000;36:622–628.

Fukuda M, Munemura M, Usami T, et al. Nocturnal blood pressure is elevated with natriuresis and proteinuria as renal function deteriorates in nephropathy. *Kidney Int* 2004;65:621–625.

Georgiades A, de Faire U, Lemne C. Clinical prediction of normotension in borderline hypertensive men—a 10 year study. *J Hypertens* 2004;22:471–478.

Giles T. Relevance of blood pressure variation in the circadian onset of cardiovascular events. *J Hypertens* 2005;23(Suppl 1):S35–S39.

Gómez-Angelats E, de La Sierra A, Sierra C, et al. Blood pressure variability and silent cerebral damage in essential hypertension. *Am J Hypertens* 2004;17:696–700.

Gosse P, Lasserre R, Minifié C, et al. Blood pressure surge on rising. *J Hypertens* 2004;22:1113–1118.

Graves JW, Sheps SG. Does evidence-based medicine suggest that physicians should not be measuring blood pressure in the hypertensive patient? *Am J Hypertens* 2004;17:354–360.

Groppelli A, Giorgi DMA, Omboni S, et al. Persistent blood pressure increase induced by heavy smoking. *J Hypertens* 1992;10:495–499.

Gustavsen PH, Høegholm A, Bang LE, Kristensen KS. White coat hypertension is a cardiovascular risk factor: a 10-year follow-up study. *J Hum Hypertens* 2003;17:811–817.

Hall CL, Higgs CMB, Notarianni L. Home blood pressure recording in mild hypertension. *J Hum Hypertens* 1990; 4:501–507.

Hansen TW, Jeppesen J, Rasmussen S, et al. Ambulatory blood pressure and mortality: a population based study. *Hypertension* 2005;45:499–504.

Hartley TR, Lovallo WR, Whitsett TL. Cardiovascular effects of caffeine in men and women. *Am J Cardiol* 2004; 93:1022–1026.

Higashi Y, Nakagawa K, Kimura M, et al. Circadian variation of blood pressure and endothelial function in patients with essential hypertension: a comparison of dippers and nondippers. *J Am Coll Cardiol* 2002;40:2039–2043.

Higashi Y, Oshima T, Ozono R, et al. Nocturnal decline in blood pressure is attenuated by NaCl loading in salt-sensitive patients with essential hypertension. *Hypertension* 1997; 30:163–167.

Høegholm A, Kristensen KS, Madsen NH, Svendsen TL. White coat hypertension diagnosed by 24-h ambulatory monitoring. *Am J Hypertens* 1992;5:64–70.

Hozawa A, Ohkubo T, Nagai K, et al. Factors affecting the difference between screening and home blood pressure measurements. The Ohamasa study. *J Hypertens* 2001; 19:13–19.

Hozawa A, Ohkubo T, Nagai K, et al. Prognosis of isolated systolic and isolated diastolic hypertension as assessed by self-measurement of blood pressure at home. *Arch Intern Med* 2000;160:3301–3306.

Hugue CJ, Safar ME, Aliefierakis MC, et al. The ratio between ankle and brachial systolic pressure in patients with sustained uncomplicated essential hypertension. *Clin Sci* 1988;74:179–182.

Hyman DJ, Ogbonnaya K, Taylor AA, et al. Ethnic differences in nocturnal blood pressure decline in treated hypertensives. *Am J Hypertens* 2000;13:884–891.

Jacob RG, Thayer JF, Manuck SB, et al. Ambulatory blood pressure responses and the circumplex model of mood. *Psychosomatic Med* 1999;61:319–333.

Johnson KA, Partsch DJ, Rippole LL, McVey DM. Reliability of self-reported blood pressure measurements. *Arch Intern Med* 1999;159:2689–2693.

Jones CR, Taylor K, Poston L, Shennan AH. Validation of the Welch Allyn "Vital Signs" oscillometric blood pressure monitor. *J Hum Hypertens* 2001;15:191–195.

Jones DW, Frohlich ED, Grim CM, et al. Mercury sphygmomanometers should not be abandoned: an advisory statement from the Council for High Blood Pressure Research, American Heart Association. *Hypertension* 2001; 37:185–186.

Jula A, Puukka P, Karanko H. Multiple clinic and home blood pressure measurements versus ambulatory blood pressure monitoring. *Hypertension* 1999;34:261–266.

Kamoi K, Miyakoshi M, Soda S, et al. Usefulness of home blood pressure measurement in the morning in type 2 diabetic patients. *Diabetes Care* 2002;25:2218–2223.

Kario K. Morning surge and variability in blood pressure: a new therapeutic target? *Hypertension* 2005a;45:485–486.

Kario K. Time for focus on morning hypertension: pitfall of current antihypertensive medication. *Am J Hypertens* 2005b; 18:149–151.

Kario K, Matsuo T, Kobayashi H, et al. Nocturnal fall of blood pressure and silent cerebrovascular damage in elderly hypertensive patients. *Hypertension* 1996; 27:130–135.

Kario K, Pickering TG, Matsuo T, et al. Stroke prognosis and abnormal nocturnal blood pressure falls in older hypertensives. *Hypertension* 2001a;38:852–857.

Kario K, Pickering TG, Umeda Y, et al. Morning surge in blood pressure as a predictor of silent and clinical cerebrovascular disease in elderly hypertensives: a prospective study. *Circulation* 2003;107:1401–1406.

Kario K, Shimada K, Schwartz JE, et al. Silent and clinically overt stroke in older Japanese subjects with white-coat and sustained hypertension. *J Am Coll Cardiol* 2001b; 38:238–245.

Khattar RS, Senior R, Lahiri A. Cardiovascular outcome in white-coat versus sustained mild hypertension. *Circulation* 1998;98:1892–1897.

Khattar RS, Swales JD, Banfield A, et al. Prediction of coronary and cerebrovascular morbidity and mortality by direct continuous ambulatory blood pressure monitoring in essential hypertension. *Circulation* 1999;100:1071–1076.

Kikuya M, Hozawa A, Ohokubo T, et al. Prognostic significance of blood pressure and heart rate variabilities. *Hypertension* 2000;36:901–906.

Kikuya M, Ohkubo T, Asayama K, et al. Ambulatory blood pressure and 10-year risk of cardiovascular and noncardiovascular mortality: the Ohasama study. *Hypertension* 2005;45:240–245.

Kimura A, Hashimoto J, Watabe D, et al. Patient characteristics and factors associated with inter-arm difference of blood pressure measurements in a general population in Ohasama, Japan. *J Hypertens* 2004;22:2277–2283.

Kjeldsen SE, Mundal R, Sandvik L, et al. Supine and exercise systolic blood pressure predict cardiovascular death in middle-aged men. *J Hypertens* 2001;19:1343–1348.

Kotsis V, Stabouli S, Bouldin M, et al. Impact of obesity on 24-hour ambulatory blood pressure and hypertension. *Hypertension* 2005;45:602–607.

Kristal-Boneh E, Harari G, Green MS, Ribak J. Body mass index is associated with differential seasonal change in ambulatory blood pressure levels. *Am J Hypertens* 1996; 9:1179–1185.

Laaser U, Labarthe R. Recommendations for blood pressure measurement in children and adolescents. *Clin Exp Hypertens* 1986;A8:903–911.

Lal SKL, Henderson RJ, Cejnar M, et al. Physiological influences on continuous finger and simultaneous intra-arterial blood pressure. *Hypertension* 1995;26:307–314.

Lane D, Beevers M, Barnes N, et al. Inter-arm differences in blood pressure: when are they clinically significant? *J Hypertens* 2002;20:1089–1095.

Laukkanen JA, Kurl S, Salonen R, et al. Systolic blood pressure during recovery from exercise and the risk of acute myocardial infarction in middle-aged men. *Hypertension* 2004;44:820–825.

Le Pailleur C, Helft G, Landais P, et al. The effects of talking, reading, and silence on the "white coat" phenomenon in hypertensive patients. *Am J Hypertens* 1998;11:203–207.

Leary AC, Struthers AD, Donnan PT, et al. The morning surge in blood pressure and heart rate is dependent on levels of physical activity after waking. *J Hypertens* 2002;20: 865–870.

Lehmann KG, Gelman JA, Weber MA, Lafrades A. Comparative accuracy of three automated techniques in the noninvasive estimation of central blood pressure in men. *Am J Cardiol* 1998;81:1004–1012.

Lim PO, MacFadyen RJ, Clarkson PBM, MacDonald TM. Impaired exercise tolerance in hypertensive patients. *Ann Intern Med* 1996;124(1 pt 1):41–55.

Lip GYH, Zarifis J, Beevers DG. Blood pressure monitoring in atrial fibrillation using electronic devices. *Arch Intern Med* 2001;161:294.

Little P, Barnett J, Barnsley L, et al. Comparison of agreement between different measures of blood pressure in primary care and daytime ambulatory blood pressure. *BMJ* 2002;325:254–257.

Lorgelly P, Siatis I, Brooks A, et al. Is ambulatory blood pressure monitoring cost-effective in the routine surveillance of treated hypertensive patients in primary care? *Br J Gen Pract* 2003;53:794–796.

Lurbe E, Torro I, Alvarez V, et al. Prevalence, persistence, and clinical significance of masked hypertension in youth. *Hypertension* 2005;45:493–498.

Mancia G, Parati G. Office compared with ambulatory blood pressure in assessing response to antihypertensive treatment: a meta-analysis. *J Hypertens* 2004; 22:435–445.

Mancia G, Parati G, Pomidossi G, et al. Alerting reaction and rise in blood pressure during measurement by physician and nurse. *Hypertension* 1987;9:209–215.

Mancia G, Sega R, Milesi C, et al. Blood pressure control in the hypertensive population. *Lancet* 1997;349:454–457.

Manfredini R, Portaluppi F, Salmi R, et al. Circadian variation in onset of epistaxis. *BMJ* 2000;321:1112.

Manfredini R, Portaluppi F, Zamboni P, et al. Circadian variation in spontaneous rupture of abdominal aorta. *Lancet* 1999;353:643–644.

Mansoor GA, McCabe EJ, White WB. Determinants of the white-coat effect in hypertensive subjects. *J Hum Hypertens* 1996;10:87–92.

Matthews CE, Pate RR, Jackson KL, et al. Exaggerated blood pressure response to dynamic exercise and risk of future hypertension. *J Clin Epidemiol* 1998;51:29–35.

Matthys J, De Meyere M, Mervielde I, et al. Influence of the presence of doctors-in-training on the blood pressure of patients: a randomised controlled trial in 22 teaching practices. *J Hum Hypertens* 2004;18:769–773.

Mazze RS, Shamoon H, Rasmantier R, et al. Reliability of blood glucose monitoring by patients with diabetes mellitus. *Am J Med* 1984;77:211–217.

Mion D, Pierin AMG. How accurate are sphygmomanometers? *J Hum Hypertens* 1998;12:245–248.

Miyai N, Arita M, Morioka I, et al. Exercise BP response in subjects with high-normal BP. *J Am Coll Cardiol* 2000; 36:1626–1631.

Møller DS, Dideriksen A, Sørensen S, et al. Accuracy of telemedical home blood pressure measurement in the diagnosis of hypertension. *J Hum Hypertens* 2003;17:549–554.

Mosenkis A, Townsend RR. What time of day should I take my antihypertensive medications? *J Clin Hypertens* 2004; 6:593–597.

Muller JE. Circadian variation in cardiovascular events. *Am J Hypertens* 1999;12:35S–42S.

Mundal R, Kjeldsen SE, Sandvik L, et al. Exercise blood pressure predicts mortality from myocardial infarction. *Hypertension* 1996;27:324–329.

Myers MG. Ambulatory blood pressure monitoring for routine clinical practice. *Hypertension* 2005;45:483–484.

Netea RT, Lenders JW, Smits P, Thien T. Influence of body and arm position on blood pressure readings: an overview. *J Hypertens* 2003;21:237–241.

Neutel JM, Smith DHG, Ram CVS, et al. Application of ambulatory blood pressure monitoring in differentiating between antihypertensive agents. *Am J Med* 1993;94:181–187.

Nordmann A, Frach B, Walker T, et al. Reliability of patients measuring blood pressure at home. *BMJ* 1999;319:1172.

O'Brien E. Unmasking hypertension. *Hypertension* 2005;45: 481–482.

O'Brien E, Asmar R, Beilin L, et al. European Society of Hypertension recommendations for conventional, ambulatory and home blood pressure measurement. *J Hypertens* 2003;21:821–848.

O'Brien E, Asmar R, Beilin L, et al. Practice guidelines of the European Society of Hypertension for clinic, ambulatory and self blood pressure measurement. *J Hypertens* 2005; 23:697–701.

O'Brien E, Coats A, Owens P, et al. Use and interpretation of ambulatory blood pressure monitoring: recommendations of the British Hypertension Society. *BMJ* 2000;320: 1128–1134.

O'Brien E, Waeber B, Parati G, et al. Blood pressure measuring devices: recommendations of the European Society of Hypertension. *BMJ* 2001;322:531–536.

Ohkubo T, Asayama K, Kikuya M, et al. How many times should blood pressure be measured at home for better prediction of stroke risk? Ten-year follow-up results from the Ohasama study. *J Hypertens* 2004;22:1099–1104.

Ohkubo T, Hozawa A, Yamaguchi J, et al. Prognostic significance of the nocturnal decline in blood pressure in individuals with and without high 24-h blood pressure: the Ohasama study. *J Hypertens* 2002;20:2183–2189.

Ooi WL, Barrett S, Hossain M, et al. Patterns of orthostatic blood pressure change and their clinical correlates in a frail, elderly population. *JAMA* 1997;277:1299–1304.

Ostchega Y, Prineas RJ, Paulose-Ram R, et al. National Health and Nutrition Examination Survey 1999-2000: effect of observer training and protocol standardization on reducing blood pressure measurement error. *J Clin Epidemiol* 2003;56:768–774.

O'Sullivan C, Duggan J, Atkins N, O'Brien E. Twenty-four-hour ambulatory blood pressure in community-dwelling elderly men and women, aged 60–102 years. *J Hypertens* 2003;21:1641–1647.

Owens P, Atkins N, O'Brien E. Diagnosis of white coat hypertension by ambulatory blood pressure monitoring. *Hypertension* 1999;34:267–272.

Palatini P, Dorigatti F, Roman E, et al. White-coat hypertension: a selection bias? *J Hypertens* 1998;16:977–984.

Palatini P, Palomba D, Bertolo O, et al. The white-coat effect is unrelated to the difference between clinic and daytime blood pressure and is associated with greater reactivity to public speaking. *J Hypertens* 2003; 21:545–553.

Palantini P, Winnicki M, Santonastaso M, et al. Prevalence and clinical significance of isolated ambulatory hypertension in young subjects screened for stage 1 hypertension. *Hypertension* 2004;44:170–174.

Panza JA, Epstein SE, Quyyumi AA. Circadian variation in vascular tone and its relation to alpha-sympathetic vasoconstrictor activity. *N Engl J Med* 1991;325:986–990.

Park MK, Menard SW, Yuan C. Comparison of auscultatory and oscillometric blood pressures. *Arch Pediatr Adolesc Med* 2001;155:50–53.

Pasic J, Shapiro D, Motivala S, Hui KK. Blood pressure morning surge and hostility. *Am J Hypertens* 1998; 11:245–250.

Pearce KA, Grimm RH Jr, Rao S, et al. Population-derived comparisons of ambulatory and office blood pressures. *Arch Intern Med* 1992;152:750–756.

Peckova M, Fahrenbruch CE, Cobb LA, Hallstrom AP. Circadian variations in the occurrence of cardiac arrests. *Circulation* 1998;98:31–39.

Pelttari LH, Hietanen EK, Salo TT, et al. Little effect of ordinary antihypertensive therapy on nocturnal high blood pressure in patients with sleep disordered breathing. *Am J Hypertens* 1998;11:272–279.

Penny J, Shennan A, de Swiet M. The reproducibility of Korotkoff 4 and 5. *Am J Hypertens* 1996;9:839.

Perk G, Ben-Arie L, Mekler J, Bursztyn M. Dipping status may be determined by nocturnal urination. *Hypertension* 2001;37:749–752.

Perloff D, Sokolow M, Cowan R. The prognostic value of ambulatory blood pressure monitoring in treated hypertensive patients. *J Hypertens* 1991;9(Suppl 1):S33–S40.

Perry HM Jr, Miller JP. Difficulties in diagnosing hypertension. *J Hypertens* 1992;10:887–896.

Peters A, von Klot S, Heier M, et al. Exposure to traffic and the onset of myocardial infarction. *New Engl J Med* 2004; 351:1721–1730.

Pickering TG. Blood pressure monitoring outside the office for the evaluation of patients with resistant hypertension. *Hypertension* 1988;11:(Suppl 2):96–100.

Pickering TG. Blood pressure measurement and detection of hypertension. *Lancet* 1994;344:31–35.

Pickering TG. White coat hypertension. *Curr Opin Nephrol Hypertens* 1996;5:192–198.

Pickering TG. Effects of stress and behavioral interventions in hypertension: what is masked hypertension? *J Clin Hypertens* 2003;5:171–176.

Pickering TG. Should we be evaluating blood pressure dipping status in clinical practice? *J Clin Hypertens* 2005a;7: 178–182.

Pickering TG. Measurement of blood pressure in and out of the office. *J Clin Hypertens* 2005b;7:123–129.

Pickering TG, Coats A, Mallion JM, et al. White-coat hypertension. *Blood Pres Monit* 1999;4:333–341.

Pickering TG, Hall JE, Appel LJ, et al. Recommendations for blood pressure measurement in humans and experimental animals. Part 1: blood pressure measurement in humans: a statement for professionals from the Subcommittee of Professional and Public Education of the American Heart Association Council on High Blood Pressure Research. *Hypertension* 2005;45:142–161.

Pickering TG, James GD, Boddie C, et al. How common is white coat hypertension? *JAMA* 1988;259:225–228.

Pierdomenico SD, Bucci A, Costantini F, et al. Circadian blood pressure changes and myocardial ischemia in hypertensive patients with coronary artery disease. *J Am Coll Cardiol* 1998;31:1627–1634.

Pierdomenico SD, Lapenna D, Bucci A, et al. Cardiovascular and renal events in uncomplicated mild hypertensive patients with sustained and white coat hypertension. *Am J Hypertens* 2004;17:876–881.

Pierin AMG, Alavarce DC, Gusmão JL, et al. Blood pressure measurement in obese patients: comparison between upper arm and forearm measurements. *Blood Press Monit* 2004;9:101–105.

Pringle E, Phillips C, Thijs L, et al. Systolic blood pressure variability as a risk factor for stroke and cardiovascular mortality in the elderly hypertensive population. *J Hypertens* 2003;21:2251–2257.

Raccaud O, Waeber B, Petrillo A, et al. Ambulatory blood pressure monitoring as a means to avoid overtreatment of elderly hypertensive patients. *Gerontology* 1992; 38:99–104.

Ragot S, Herpin D, Siché JP, et al. Relationship between short-term and long-term blood pressure variabilities in essential hypertensives. *J Hum Hypertens* 2001;15:41–48.

Redon J, Campos C, Narciso ML, et al. Prognostic value of ambulatory blood pressure monitoring in refractory hypertension. *Hypertension* 1998;31:712–718.

Redon J, Roca-Cusachs A, Mora-Macia J. Uncontrolled early morning blood pressure in medicated patients: the ACAMPA study. *Blood Press Monit* 2002;7:111–116.

Reeves RA. Does this patient have hypertension? *JAMA* 1995;273:1211–1218.

Sega R, Facchetti R, Bombelli M, et al. Prognostic value of ambulatory and home blood pressures compared with office blood pressure in the general population: follow-up results from the Pressioni Arteriose Monitorate e Loro Associazioni (PAMELA) study. *Circulation* 2005;111:1777–1783.

Shuler CL, Allison N, Holcomb S, et al. Accuracy of an automated blood pressure device in stable inpatients. *Arch Intern Med* 1998;158:714–721.

Silke B, McAuley D. Accuracy and precision of blood pressure determination with the Finapres. *J Hum Hypertens* 1998;12:403–409.

Singh JP, Larson MG, Manolio TA, et al. Blood pressure response during treadmill testing as a risk factor for new-onset hypertension. *Circulation* 1999;99:1831–1836.

Smith NL, Psaty BM, Rutan GH, et al. The association between time since last meal and blood pressure in older adults: the cardiovascular health study. *J Am Geriatr Soc* 2003;51:824–828.

Soo LH, Gray D, Young T, Hampton JR. Circadian variation in witnessed out of hospital cardiac arrest. *Heart* 2000;84:370–376.

Spence JD. Pseudo-hypertension in the elderly. *J Hum Hypertens* 1997;11:621–623.

Staessen JA, Bieniaszewski L, O'Brien E, et al. Nocturnal blood pressure fall on ambulatory monitoring in a large international database. *Hypertension* 1997;29:30–39.

Staessen JA, Den Hond E, Celis H, et al. Antihypertensive treatment based on blood pressure measurement at home or in the physician's office: a randomized controlled trial. *JAMA* 2004;291:955–964.

Staessen JA, O'Brien ET, Atkins N, et al. Short report: ambulatory blood pressure in normotensive compared with hypertensive subjects. *J Hypertens* 1993;11:1289–1297.

Staessen JA, Thijs L, Fagard R, et al. Predicting cardiovascular risk using conventional vs ambulatory blood pressure in older patients with systolic hypertension. *JAMA* 1999;282:539–546.

Stergiou G, Mengden T, Padfield PL, et al. Self-monitoring of blood pressure at home: is an important adjunct to clinical measurements. *BMJ* 2004;329:870–871.

Stergiou GS, Skeva II, Baibas NM, et al. Diagnosis of hypertension using home or ambulatory blood pressure monitoring. *J Hypertens* 2000;18:1745–1751.

Sternberg H, Rosenthal T, Shamiss A, Green M. Altered circadian rhythm of blood pressure in shift workers. *J Hum Hypertens* 1995;9:349–353.

Turner MJ, Baker AB, Kam PC. Effects of systematic errors in blood pressure measurements on the diagnosis of hypertension. *Blood Press Monit* 2004;9:249–253.

Uzu T, Fujii T, Nishimura M, et al. Determinants in circadian blood pressure rhythm in essential hypertension. *Am J Hypertens* 1999;12:35–39.

Van Boxtel MPJ, Gaillard C, Houx PJ, et al. Is nondipping in 24 h ambulatory blood pressure related to cognitive dysfunction? *J Hypertens* 1998;16:1425–1432.

Van Durme DJ, Goldstein M, Pal N, et al. The accuracy of community-based automated blood pressure machines. *J Fam Pract* 2000;49:449–452.

Verdecchia P, O'Brien E, Pickering T, et al. When can the practicing physician suspect white coat hypertension? Statement from the Working Group on Blood Pressure Monitoring of the European Society of Hypertension. *Am J Hypertens* 2003;16:87–91.

Verdecchia P, Palatini P, Schillaci G, et al. Independent predictors of isolated clinic ("white-coat") hypertension. *J Hypertens* 2001;19:1015–1020.

Verdecchia P, Reboldi GP, Angeli F, et al. Short- and long-term incidence of stroke in white-coat hypertension. *Hypertension* 2005;45:203–208.

Verdecchia P, Reboldi G, Porcellati C, et al. Risk of cardiovascular disease in relation to achieved office and ambulatory blood pressure control in treated hypertensive subjects. *J Am Coll Cardiol* 2002;39:878–885.

Verdecchia P, Schillaci G, Boldrini F, et al. White coat hypertension. *Lancet* 1996;348:1443–1445.

Verdecchia P, Schillaci G, Borgioni C, et al. White coat hypertension and white coat effect. *Am J Hypertens* 1995; 8:790–798.

Von Känel R, Jain S, Mills PJ, et al. Relation of nocturnal blood pressure dipping to cellular adhesion, inflammation and hemostasis. *J Hypertens* 2004;22:2087–2093.

Watson RDS, Lumb R, Young MA, et al. Variation in cuff blood pressure in untreated outpatients with mild hypertension—implications for initiating antihypertensive treatment. *J Hypertens* 1987;5:207–211.

White WB. Relevance of the trough-to-peak ratio to the 24h blood pressure load. *Am J Hypertens* 1996;9:91s–96s.

White WB, Asmar R, Imai Y, et al. Self-monitoring of the blood pressure. *Blood Pres Monit* 1999;4:343–351.

White WB, Larocca GM. Improving the utility of the nocturnal hypertension definition by using absolute sleep blood pressure rather than the "dipping" proportion. *Am J Cardiol* 2003;92:1439–1441.

Wing LM, Brown MA, Beilin LJ, et al. "Reverse white-coat hypertension" in older hypertensives. Second Australian National Blood Pressure Study. *J Hypertens* 2002; 20:639–644.

Yarows SA, Brook RD. Measurement variation among 12 electronic home blood pressure monitors. *Am J Hypertens* 2000;13:276–282.

Yarows SA, Julius S, Pickering TG. Home blood pressure monitoring. *Arch Intern Med* 2000;160:1251–1257.

Zachariah PK, Sheps SG, Smith RL. Defining the roles of home and ambulatory monitoring. *Diagnosis* 1988; 10:39–50.

Zachariah PK, Sumner WE III. The clinical utility of blood pressure load in hypertension. *Am J Hypertens* 1993; 6:194S–197S.

Zakopoulos NA, Tsivgoulis G, Barlas G, et al. Time rate of blood pressure variation is associated with increased common carotid artery intima-media thickness. *Hypertension* 2005;45:505–512.

Zweifler AJ, Shahab ST. Pseudohypertension. *J Hypertens* 1993;11:1–6.

Zweiker R, Schumacher M, Fruhwald FM, et al. Comparison of wrist blood pressure measurement with conventional sphygmomanometry at a cardiology outpatient clinic. *J Hypertens* 2000;18:1013–1018.

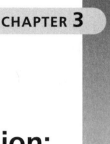

# Primary Hypertension: Pathogenesis

$A$s I review the extensive literature on the pathogenesis of primary hypertension published over the past 4 years since composing the previous edition of this book, a sense of futility arises. Hundreds of papers have been published describing the work of thousands of investigators who have spent many millions, perhaps billions, of dollars. Yet the pathogenesis of primary[1] hypertension is as elusive and enigmatic as ever. The enthusiasm released by the elucidation of the human genome has

quickly been dampened by the reality, as Sir George Pickering warned over 40 years ago (1964) that "elevated blood pressure is not a function of one gene, but rather a host of genes, each contributing a small effect."

This overall pessimism should be lightened by the knowledge that a few new components, e.g., leptin, and a number of older ones, e.g., aldosterone and uric acid, have been added to the mosaic. However, these and other advances to be described seem only small pieces that will not solve the larger puzzle. Moreover, the puzzle may be unsolvable. In the words of Coggon and Martyn (2005):

> Diseases that entail amplification of a microscopic or molecular event tend to be "all or none" in nature. Anyway, it is not difficult to separate cases of the disorder from most people who show no evidence whatsoever of disease. But for many other conditions, there is no clear dichotomy between those who have them and those that do not. Such cases, exemplified by hypertension, sensorineural deafness, and osteoporosis, represent the extreme of a physiological state whose variability is described by a continuous unimodal frequency distribution. Here, case definition is somewhat arbitrary, and understanding of causation amounts to identification of factors that modify this physiological state one way or the other. A full understanding of causation would mean the ability to predict

---

[1] Since as much as 95% of all hypertension is of unknown cause, there is no obvious name for the disease. Essential may be mistakenly interpreted to infer an essential need for higher pressure to push blood through vessels narrowed by age. The term benign has been buried along with the millions of unfortunate victims of uncontrolled hypertension. Idiopathic seems a bit unwieldy; so I have chosen primary simply to distinguish it from all the remaining hypertensive diseases, which are "secondary" to known causes or "identifiable."

accurately an individual's physiological state— their systolic blood pressure or bone mineral density, for example—from a knowledge of these modifying factors. However, the fact that these physiological states exist in a continuum in the population suggests that they are determined by the combination of factors, many of which might have only a small individual effect. This multiplicity means that complete understanding of causation is unlikely to be feasible, although it may be possible to identify some factors whose effects are large enough to offer scope for prevention.

## GENERAL CONSIDERATIONS

Before considering the specific genetic and environmental factors that may be responsible for hypertension, a few generalizations are in order:

- A separation is necessary between primary, i.e., systolic and diastolic hypertension, and isolated systolic hypertension. As here defined, primary hypertension is the elevation of blood pressure (BP) seen in younger people which has a genetic foundation and is shaped by many environmental factors and which tends to be progressive if not treated but can usually be controlled. Isolated systolic hypertension (ISH), on the other hand, is the elevation of systolic pressure which is almost exclusively seen in the elderly, which has no obvious genetic foundation, and is more loosely shaped by the same environmental factors that induce primary hypertension. Isolated systolic hypertension appears to be both less progressive and less responsive to treatment, in part because its duration is usually fairly short.

   The distinction may be even simpler: Primary hypertension reflects both an increase in cardiac output and a functional, i.e., reversible, constriction of peripheral resistance vessels. Isolated systolic hypertension mainly reflects a stiffness of proximal, capacitance vessels (Safar, 2005).

   Different precursors of these forms of hypertension can be identified in large populations (Franklin et al., 2005), but the multiple factors considered in this chapter mainly relate to primary hypertension.

- As noted by Coggon and Martyn (2005), although the concept of a single underlying abnormality that begins the hemodynamic cascade toward sustained hypertension is attractive, there may be no such single defect. In view of the multiple factors involved in the control of the BP, the concept of a multifaceted mosaic, introduced by

Page (1963), may be more appropriate, as unattractive as it may be to those who prefer to believe that for every biologic defect there should be a single, specific cause.

- The relevance of data from animal models is highly questionable. Even though 70% of current research on hypertension is being done on rats or other small animals (Kwitek-Black & Jacob, 2001; Sugiyama et al., 2001), the relevance of such data to the human condition is suspect. For example, transgenic hypertensive rats develop fulminant hypertension at an early age despite low levels of renin in the plasma and kidney (Lee et al., 1996), quite unlike what is seen in humans. Therefore, this discussion will almost exclusively examine data from human studies.

- Few analytic techniques are available to measure accurately and repetitively small changes in various hemodynamic functions involved in the development of hypertension that may occur over many years. Cross-sectional observations may never be able to uncover the sequential changes that could be revealed by longitudinal studies.

- Even when studies are performed among adolescent and borderline hypertensives, the beginnings of the disease may have already been missed. In the absence of a marker to identify the prehypertensive individual, before the BP has risen, we may be viewing the process after the initiating factors are no longer recognizable, obscured by adaptations invoked by the rising pressure. An editorial some time ago in the *Lancet* (Anonymous, 1977) describes the situation aptly:

   Blood pressure is a measurable end product of an exceedingly complex series of factors including those which control blood vessel calibre and responsiveness, those which control fluid volume within and outside the vascular bed, and those which control cardiac output. None of these factors is independent: They interact with each other and respond to changes in blood pressure. It is not easy, therefore, to dissect out cause and effect. Few factors which play a role in cardiovascular control are completely normal in hypertension: Indeed, normality would require explanation since it would suggest a lack of responsiveness to increased pressure.

As we shall see, more and more differences are being identified within the population of patients with primary hypertension. For now, however, unifying hypotheses seem appropriate, with the recognition that there may be considerable variations in the role of various components at different times and stages and in different people. Before examining the specific hypotheses that may explain the development of hypertension, the role of genetics will be considered.

## ROLE OF GENETICS

### Family History

In the rush to discover specific genetic mutations responsible for hypertension, the relatively simple ascertainment of a family history is often neglected but should not be (Guttmacher et al., 2004). Former estimates of heritability based on office BPs were in the range of 20% to 40% (Dominiczak et al., 2000). More recent estimates based on ambulatory BPs are higher (Fava et al., 2004), reaching 61% in a large sample of twins (Kupper et al., 2005).

### Genetic Associations

The current situation of the search for hypertension genes was characterized by Castellano (2004):

> . . . several different strategies have been adopted to dissect the genetic contribution to blood pressure, including investigations of specific candidate genes, genome-wide searches, the use of intermediate phenotypes, gene expression studies, comparative genomics and synteny in animal models. Overall, the candidate gene approach has been the main strategy utilized for searching for hypertension loci. . . . Recent studies conducted using another major strategy for identifying loci contributing to a complex trait (i.e. genome-wide scanning) strongly suggest that the genetics of human essential hypertension is probably characterized by many rare, recent-onset, population-specific alleles, carrying a genotype relative risk as little as 1.2–1.5. This scenario closely resembles the "geneticist's nightmare," as hypothesized for other common diseases such as diabetes mellitus, and some scientists believe that, under these conditions, finding genotype-phenotype correlations is an almost impossible task. To give one example, assuming an odds ratio of 1.2 for the variant genotype in the development of hypertension, an 80% statistical power to detect an association with a $P$-value of 0.05 could be achieved only by studying close to 20,000 subjects (cases plus controls).

Lest Castellano be considered too pessimistic, Lohmueller et al. (2003) analyzed all of the 18 studies of the polymorphisms of the α-adducin gene described first by Cusi et al. (1997). They found only seven to be statistically significant and of those, five were of the same direction as the original report, the other two to be in the opposite direction. It seems apparent that "we are not there yet" in demonstrating specific genetic causation in complex diseases (Page et al., 2003) but the search will surely go on (de Lange et al., 2004) (Table 3–1).

### Pharmacogenetics

Since individual patients' responses to any given monotherapy is so variable, pharmacogenetic approaches are being intensively pursued to predict the basis for response and thereby provide greater individualization and efficacy of antihypertensive therapy (Turner & Schwartz, 2005). As of now, a few tentative successes have been reported, as with polymorphism of the β-adrenergic receptor genes and response to β-blockers (Filigheddu et al., 2004). However, discrepancies abound. For example, the presence of the α-adducin Gly460→Trp polymorphism was found by one group to provide an odds ratio of 15.75 of being a responder to hydrochlorothiazide (Sciarrone et al., 2003) but the same polymorphism made no contribution to the BP response to

## TABLE 3–1

### Some of the Candidate Genes for Which Polymorphisms Have Been Reported in Human Hypertension

Adrenosine type $A_{2a}$ receptor

α-Adducin

$β_2$-Adrenergic receptor

Angiotensin type 1 receptor

Angiotensinogen

Atrial natriuretic peptide and receptor

Bradykinin type 2 receptor

Dopamine D1 receptor

Endothelial nitric oxide synthase

Endothelin 1 and 2

Epithelial sodium channel, β-subunit

G-Protein, $β_3$ subunit

11β-Hydroxysteroid dehydrogenase type 2

Insulin growth factor 1

Insulin receptor substrate 1

Neutral endopeptidase

Prostacyclin synthase

Prostaglandin EP2 receptor

Renin

Sodium amiloride-sensitive channel

Sodium-chloride thiazide-sensitive cotransporter

Sodium-potassium-chloride cotransporter

Sodium-proton exchanger 3

Transforming growth factor - $β_1$

20-HETE-synthase

diuretics by another group (Turner et al., 2003). Nonetheless, carriers of this particular polymorphism were found to have a lower risk of combined stroke and myocardial infarction (MI) with diuretic therapy than with other antihypertensive therapies (Psaty et al., 2002).

The field looks promising, but as Califf (2004) notes: "The promise of genomics and proteomics is largely built on the theory that these technologies will be able to judge the risks and benefits of therapies in much smaller, focused groups of patients. While a few notable successes have occurred, progress has been slow, and many heralded advances have not been replicated in validation studies."

### Monogenic Hypertension

Unlike the problems of identifying the genes responsible for primary hypertension and those related to responses to drugs, the study of rare medelian forms of hypertension in which mutations in single genes caused marked rises in blood pressure has been very informative (Nabel, 2003; Wilson et al., 2004). These are described in Chapters 12, 13, and 14 and most involve increased sodium reabsorption (Staessen et al., 2003). They include:

• Glucocorticoid-remediable aldosteronism
• Apparent mineralocorticoid excess
• Liddle's syndrome
• Hypertension exacerbated by pregnancy
• Pseudohypoaldosteronism, type 2
• Congenital adrenal hyperplasia (11β and 17α hydroxylase)
• Hypertension with bachydactyly
• PPARγ missense mutations
• Multiple endocrine neoplasia-2 with pheochromocytoma
• Polycystic kidney disease
• Mutation in a mitochondrial tRNA

Scattered reports suggest that one or more of those monogenetic forms of hypertension may be more frequent, particularly in patients resistant to conventional therapies (Oparil et al., 2003) or with low renin levels (Carvajal et al., 2005). In the meantime, caution is advised in accepting such reports as reflecting real genetic differences (Crawford et al., 2004).

### Limitations of Genetics

Even as the scope of genetic research is broadened, cautions about the limitations of what can be expected in the future are bringing the initial overenthusiasm about the "genetic revolution" into a more guarded perspective (Castellano, 2004). In addition

to the fundamental problems of the complexity of BP regulation, Weatherall (1999) notes that "the complexity of the genotype-phenotype relationship has undoubtedly been underestimated. . . . It is far from certain that we will ever reach a stage in which we can accurately predict the occurrence of some of the common disorders of Western society at any particular stage in an individual's life."

### Genes versus Environment

As the complexities of the genotype-phenotype relationships are being addressed, a simple portrayal of the underlying interactions have been described by Carretero and Oparil (2000):

> Theoretically, in a population unaffected by hypertensinogenic factors, BP will have a normal distribution; it will be skewed to the right and will have a narrow base or less variance [Figure 3–1, *continuous line*]. When one hypertensinogenic factor is added to this population, such as increased body mass, one would expect the normal distribution curve to be further skewed to the right; consequently the base will be wider (more variance) and the curve will be flatter [Figure 3–1, *broken line*]. If a second hypertensinogenic factor such as alcohol intake is added to increased body mass, the curve will be skewed more to the right and the variance will increase further, with more subjects classified as hypertensive [Figure 3–1, *dotted line*].
>
> Discovering which genetic variations place BP on the left or right side of the distribution curve is of both theoretical and practical importance because it could help the physician to better treat or cure hypertension. Recognition of the hypertensinogenic factors may allow nonpharmacological prevention, treatment, or cure of hypertension.

As will be noted in greater detail, the boundaries between genes and environment have been blurred further by the recognition of intrauterine growth retardation as an apparently strong predictor of subsequent hypertension. Obviously, it would be easy to mistake prenatal influences for genetic defects.

### Promise of Genetics

Although a complete unraveling of the genotype-phenotype relationships involved in human hypertension may never be achieved, a great deal of good may come along the way. We can hope for another discovery such as the low-density lipoprotein receptor mutations underlying familial hypercholesterolemia that led to the development of the remarkably effective statin drugs. However, as Luft (2004) observes:

> Compared with hypertension, lipid metabolism is a "no brainer." Low-density lipoprotein cholesterol

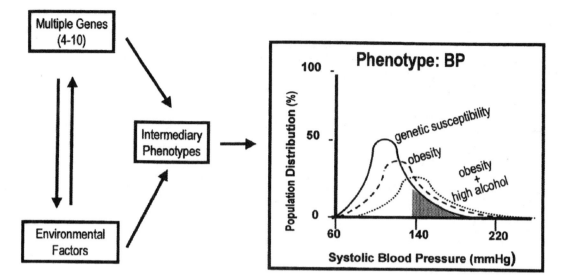

**FIGURE 3–1** ● Interaction among genetic and environmental factors in the development of hypertension. The left side of the figure shows how environmental factors and multiple genes responsible for high blood pressure (BP) interact and affect intermediary phenotypes. The result of these intermediary phenotypes is BP with a normal distribution skewed to the right. *Continuous line* indicates the theoretic BP of the population that is not affected by hypertensinogenic factors; *shaded area* indicates systolic BP in the hypertensive range. *Broken lines* and *dotted lines* indicate populations in which one (obesity) or two (obesity plus high alcohol intake) hypertensinogenic factors have been added. (Modified from Carretero OA, Oparil S. Essential hypertension. *Circulation* 2000;101:329–335.)

(LDL) and high-density cholesterol (HDL) can be easily measured, are relatively constant, and can be sent through the mail, in contrast to blood pressure measurements. . . . We are able to account for almost all the genetic variance in the clinically relevant LDL/HDL ratio. These findings give us some grounds for optimism in terms of tackling complex genetic traits. However, lipid metabolism is a trivial academic pursuit compared with blood pressure.

My colleagues at the University of Texas Southwestern Medical School, Drs. Michael Brown and Joe Goldstein, might take exception to the "no-brainer" depiction of lipid genetics, but it may still be possible to use gene therapy for complications of hypertension, as is being applied to patients with peripheral vascular disease (Morishita et al., 2004). Perhaps closer to practical application is the use of pharmacogenetics.

We will now examine various environmental factors, including stress, obesity, and electrolyte intake, that likely interact with multiple genes. These factors will be considered as part of a construct that covers multiple possible pathways to hypertension.

## OVERVIEW OF PATHOGENESIS

The pressure required to move blood through the circulatory bed is provided by the pumping action of the heart [cardiac output (CO)] and the tone of the arteries [peripheral resistance (PR)]. Each of these primary determinants of the BP is, in turn, determined by the interaction of the "exceedingly complex series of factors" (Anonymous, 1977) displayed in part in Figure 3–2.

Hypertension has been attributed to abnormalities in virtually every one of these factors. Each will be examined and attempts will be made along the way to integrate them into logical hypotheses. It is unlikely that all these factors are operative in any given patient; but multiple hypotheses may prove to be correct, because the hemodynamic hallmark of primary hypertension—a persistently elevated vascular resistance—may be reached through a number of different paths. Before the final destination, these may converge into either structural thickening of the vessel walls or functional vasoconstriction. Moreover, individual factors often interact, and the interactions are proving to be increasingly complex.

We will follow the outline shown in Figure 3–2, recognizing that the position of each factor in the outline is not necessarily in the order that the hemodynamic cascade follows in the pathogenesis of hypertension. Without knowing what starts the process, we can lay out only a preliminary blueprint that can be used by beginning at multiple sites.

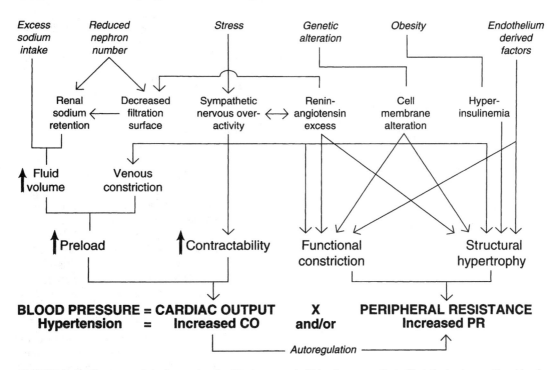

**FIGURE 3–2** ● Some of the factors involved in the control of blood pressure that affect the basic equation: blood pressure = cardiac output × peripheral resistance.

## CARDIAC OUTPUT

An increased CO has been found in some young, borderline hypertensives who may display a hyperkinetic circulation. If it is responsible for the hypertension, the increase in CO could logically arise in two ways: either from an increase in fluid volume (preload) or from an increase in contractility from neural stimulation of the heart (Figure 3–2). However, even if it is involved in the initiation of hypertension, the increased CO likely does not persist, because the typical hemodynamic finding in established hypertension is an elevated PR and lower or normal CO (Taler et al., 2004a).

### Heart Rate

Although an increased heart rate may not simply be a reflection of a hyperdynamic circulation or an indicator of increased sympathetic activity, multiple epidemiologic surveys have shown that an elevated heart rate is an independent predictor of the development of hypertension (Palatini & Julius, 1999). Moreover, both an elevated heart rate and decreased heart rate variability are predictors of cardiovascular mortality, at least in part because they are associated with other cardiovascular risk factors (Palatini et al., 2002).

### Hyperkinetic Hypertensives

Numerous investigators have described hypertensives, mostly young, who definitely have high CO (Finkielman et al., 1965; Jiang et al., 1995). Using echocardiography to study young borderline hypertensives (average age, 33 years), 37 of 99 subjects were found to have increased heart rate, cardiac index, and forearm blood flow caused by an excessive autonomic drive (Julius et al., 1991c).

It should be noted that most of these features could reflect anxiety over both the knowledge that they were hypertensive (Rostrup et al., 1991) and the procedures used in the studies (Marshall et al., 2002; Palatini et al., 1996). Moreover, these features have not been observed either in small groups of normotensive children who are likely to develop hypertension because both their parents were hypertensive (van Hooft et al., 1993) or in almost 500 participants in the Framingham Heart Study who developed hypertension (Post et al., 1994). In this echocardiographic follow-up in Framingham, initially increased heart rate and cardiac index were related to the subsequent onset of hypertension, but none of the hemodynamic evidences of a hyperkinetic circulation was a significant predictor of the development of hypertension after controlling for age and baseline BP.

## Cardiac Contribution

Nonetheless, significant increases in left ventricular mass have been recognized in the still-normotensive children of hypertensive parents (Koren & Devereux, 1993; van Hooft et al., 1993). Such left ventricular hypertrophy (described in greater detail in Chapter 4) has generally been considered a compensatory mechanism to an increased vascular resistance (afterload). However, it could also reflect a primary response to repeated neural stimulation and, thereby, could be an initiating mechanism for hypertension (Julius et al., 1991c) as well as an amplifier of CO that reinforces the elevation of BP from arterial stiffening (Segers et al., 2000).

## Increased Fluid Volume

A second mechanism that could induce hypertension by increasing CO would be an increased circulating fluid volume (preload). However, in most studies, subjects with high BP have a lower blood volume and total exchangeable sodium than do normal subjects (Harrap et al., 2000).

### Relation of Blood Volume to Blood Pressure

When the BP was correlated to the total blood volume in 48 healthy subjects and 106 patients with fairly early and mild primary hypertension, an interesting relationship was observed (London et al., 1977) (Figure 3–3). A negative correlation was found in the healthy subjects but not in the hypertensives, with 80% of the hypertensives being outside the 95% confidence limits of the normal curve. The authors interpret their data as indicating a quantitative disturbance in the pressure-volume relationship in primary hypertension (i.e., a plasma volume that is inappropriately high for the level of BP). Thus, even if absolute values are reduced, a relatively expanded blood volume may be involved in the maintenance of hypertension.

Even if CO is involved in the initiation of hypertension, once hypertension is established, CO usually is not increased, but PR is elevated (Taler et al., 2004a).

## Autoregulation

### Definition and Description

The pattern of initially high CO giving way to a persistently elevated PR has been observed in a few people and many animals with experimental hypertension. When animals with markedly reduced renal tissue are given volume loads, the BP rises initially as a consequence of the high CO but, within a few days, PR rises and CO returns to near the basal level (Guyton, 1992) (Figure 3–4). This changeover has been interpreted as reflecting an intrinsic property of the vascular bed to regulate the flow of blood, depending on the metabolic need of tissues. This process, called *autoregulation*, was described by Borst and Borst-de Geus (1963) and demonstrated experimentally by Guyton and Coleman (1969). With increased CO, more blood flows through the tissues than is required, and the increased flow delivers extra nutrients or removes additional metabolic products; in response, the vessels constrict, decreasing blood flow and returning the balance of supply and demand to normal. Thus, PR increases and remains high by the rapid induction of structural thickening of the resistance vessels, as described in the section Peripheral Resistance.

Similar conversion from an initially high CO to a later increased PR has been shown in hypertensive people (Andersson et al., 1989; Julius, 1988b; Lund-Johansen, 1989). In Lund-Johansen's (1989) study, younger (17- to 29-year-old) mild hypertensives were restudied both at rest and during exercise

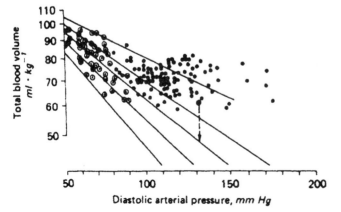

**FIGURE 3–3** ● Relation between diastolic blood pressure and total blood volume in 48 normotensive (*open circles*) and 106 hypertensive (*solid circles*) subjects. Only 20% of the hypertensive patients fell within the 95% confidence limits of the normal curve. The total blood volume definition (*solid circles with arrow*) represents the degree of the pressure-volume disturbance. (Modified from London GM, Safer ME, Weiss YA, et al. Volume-dependent parameters in essential hypertension. *Kidney Int* 1997;11:204–208.)

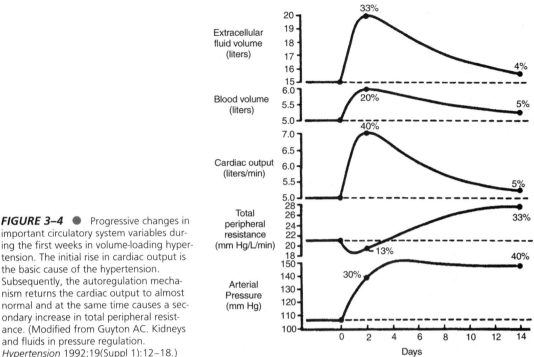

**FIGURE 3–4** ● Progressive changes in important circulatory system variables during the first weeks in volume-loading hypertension. The initial rise in cardiac output is the basic cause of the hypertension. Subsequently, the autoregulation mechanism returns the cardiac output to almost normal and at the same time causes a secondary increase in total peripheral resistance. (Modified from Guyton AC. Kidneys and fluids in pressure regulation. *Hypertension* 1992;19(Suppl 1):12–18.)

after 10 years on no treatment and then after 20 years following withdrawal of intervening therapy. As the overall BPs rose, the CO fell and PR increased (Figure 3–5).

### Problems with the Autoregulation Model

Julius (1988b) considers autoregulation to be an unlikely explanation for the switch from high CO to increased PR and offers another: structural changes that decrease the cardiac responses to nervous and hormonal stimuli but enhance the vascular responses. His proposal states that the "hemodynamic transition can be explained by a secondary response to elevated blood pressure. The heart becomes less responsive as a result of altered receptor responsiveness and decreased cardiac compliance, whereas the responsiveness of arterioles increases because of vascular hypertrophy, which leads to changes in the wall-to-lumen ratio" (Julius, 1988b).

Nonetheless, the autoregulatory model does explain the course of hypertension in volume-expanded animals and people, particularly in the presence of reduced renal mass (Figure 3–4). Ledingham (1989) defends autoregulation as the "dominant factor" leading to the rise in PR in hypertension. Moreover, there is additional evidence in favor of

volume expansion in the pathogenesis of the disease, reflecting the effect of too much sodium coming in and not enough going out, the latter because of a less-than-normal number of nephrons.

## EXCESS SODIUM INTAKE

Figure 3–2 shows excess sodium intake inducing hypertension by increasing fluid volume and preload, thereby increasing CO. As will become obvious, sodium excess may increase BP in multiple other ways also.

### Overview

After reviewing the available evidence relating sodium intake to hypertension, most investigators determine that "there is conclusive evidence that dietary salt is positively associated with BP and that BP can be lowered with reductions in sodium intake of 40 to 50 mmol [per day] in both hypertensive and non-hypertensive persons" (Chobanian & Hill, 2000). Some authors, reviewing the same evidence, do not agree (Brown et al., 1984), whereas others accept a role for sodium but question the wisdom of advocating sodium restriction in view of potential hazards (Alderman, 2004).

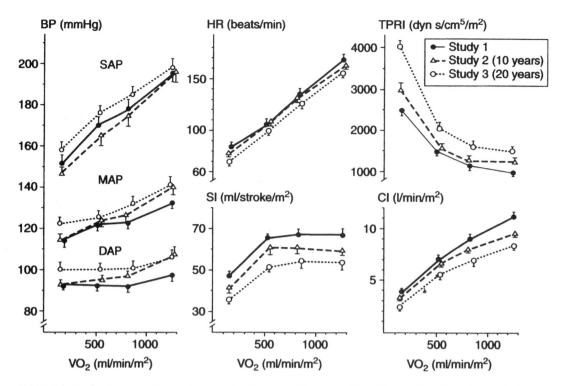

**FIGURE 3–5** ● Overview of hemodynamic alterations over 20 years in 17- to 29-year-old males at first study. Mean values. Note the marked increase in TPRI and fall in SI and CI. (Adapted from Lund-Johansen. Central haemodynamics in essential hypertension at rest and during exercise. *J Hypertens* 1989;7(Suppl 6):S52–S55.)

The basis for the generally accepted necessary but not, in itself, sufficient role of sodium excess was stated by Denton (1997):

> Human prehistory as hunter-gatherers with inland savannah existence involved a paucity of salt. The hedonistic liking for it, physiologically apt in those circumstances, is maladaptive in Western metropolitan existence with processed food and cheap abundant salt sources. Above a threshold of 70–100 mmol Na per day, sodium intake may be directly causal of BP increase in sensitive individuals, and permissive of action of other factors such as low K and Ca intake, stress, obesity and alcohol to influence BP.

As will be noted, diets in industrialized societies contain many times the daily adult sodium requirement, an amount that is beyond the threshold level needed to induce hypertension (Figure 3–6). Only part of the population may be susceptible to the deleterious effects of this high sodium intake, presumably because these individuals have an additional renal defect in sodium excretion. As portrayed in Figure 3–6, because almost everyone in industrialized societies ingests an excess of sodium beyond the threshold needed to induce hypertension, it may not be possible to show a relationship between sodium intake and BP in these populations. The absence of such a relationship in

no way detracts from the possible role of excess dietary sodium in causing hypertension.

### Dietary Chloride

Chloride, and not just sodium, may be involved in causing hypertension. In two classic rat models of sodium-dependent hypertension, hypertension could

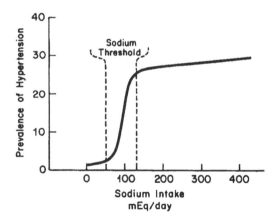

**FIGURE 3–6** ● Probable association between usual dietary sodium intake and the prevalence of hypertension in large populations. (Modified from Kaplan NM. Dietary salt intake and blood pressure. *JAMA* 1984;251:1429–1430. Copyright 1984, American Medical Association.)

be induced with sodium chloride but not with sodium bicarbonate or ascorbate (Kurtz & Morris, 1983; Whitescarver et al., 1984). In people, too, the BP rises more with NaCl than with nonchloride salts of sodium (Schorr et al., 1996). This issue is largely academic, as chloride is the major anion accompanying sodium in the diet and in body fluids.

## Epidemiologic Evidence

The epidemiologic evidence incriminating an excess of sodium includes the following points:

- Primitive people from widely different parts of the world who do not eat sodium have no hypertension, and their BP does not rise with age, as it does in all industrialized populations (Denton, 1997; Page et al., 1981). For example, the Yanomamo Indians of northern Brazil, who excrete only approximately 1 mmol of sodium per day, have an average BP of 107/67 mm Hg among men and 98/62 mm Hg among women aged 40 to 49 (Oliver et al., 1975).
- The lack of hypertension may be attributable to other differences in lifestyle, but comparisons made in groups living under similar conditions relate the BP most directly to the level of dietary sodium intake (Lowenstein, 1961; Page et al., 1981). Moreover, when primitive peoples who are free of hypertension adopt modern lifestyles, including increased intake of sodium, their BP rises and hypertension appears (Klag et al., 1995; Poulter et al., 1990).
- Significant correlations between the level of salt intake and the levels of BP and frequency of hypertension have been found in most large populations (Beard et al., 1997; du Cailar et al., 2004; Khaw et al., 2004; Stamler et al., 1996) but not in all (Smith et al., 1988). The strongest data come from the Intersalt study, which measured 24-hour urine electrolytes and BP in 10,079 men and women aged 20 to 59 years in 52 places around the world (Elliott et al., 1996; Intersalt Cooperative Research Group, 1988). For all 52 centers, there was a positive correlation between sodium excretion and both systolic BP and diastolic BP but an even more significant association between sodium excretion and the changes in BP with age (Figure 3–7). Few populations were found whose levels of sodium intake were in the 50- to 100-mmol per day range, wherein the threshold for the sodium effect on BP likely resides. However, the virtual absence of either hypertension or a progressive rise in BP with advancing age in populations with an average sodium ingestion of only about 50 mmol per day supports the concept of a threshold.

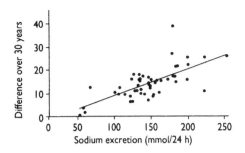

**FIGURE 3–7** ● Plot of the difference in systolic blood pressure over 30 years (age 55 minus age 25) in relation to median urinary sodium excretion across 52 populations. (Modified from Stamler J, Elliott P, Dyer AR, et al. Commentary: sodium and blood pressure in the Intersalt study and other studies. *BMJ* 1996;312:1285–1287.)

As noted by Denton (1997), our current high sodium-low potassium intake is a recent phenomenon in the span of human existence, beginning only a few hundred years ago and accelerated by modern food processing, which adds sodium and removes potassium. Table 3–2 shows that our herbivorous ancestors probably consumed less than 10 mmol of sodium per day, whereas our carnivorous ancestors might have eaten 30 mmol per day (Eaton et al., 1996). Human physiology evolved in a low-sodium/high-potassium environment, and we seem ill equipped to handle the current exposure to high sodium and low potassium.

Our current preference for a high sodium intake likely is an acquired taste, one that may develop early in childhood (Zinner et al., 2002). In the typical diet of industrialized societies, as little as 15% of total sodium consumption is discretionary, and even less is inherent to the food, with more than 75% being added in the processing (Engstrom et al., 1997). This increase in sodium intake from processed foods has been so recent that genetic adaptation has not been possible. Because evolutionary changes to preserve Darwinian fitness are not needed if new environmental factors produce disability or death only after the reproductive years, modern humans may simply not be able to adapt successfully to their high sodium exposure (Trowell, 1980).

## Experimental Evidence

The experimental evidence for a role of sodium excess in hypertension development includes the following:

- When hypertensives are sodium-restricted, their BP falls. As described more fully in Chapter 6, dramatic falls in BP may follow rigid sodium restriction (Kempner, 1948), whereas less rigid

## TABLE 3-2

### Estimated Diet of Late Paleolithic Humans versus That of Contemporary Americans

| Nutrient | Late Paleolithic Diet (Assuming 35% Meat) | Current American Diet |
| --- | --- | --- |
| Total dietary energy, % | | |
| Protein | 30 | 12 |
| Carbohydrate | 45–50 | 46 |
| Fat | 20–25 | 42 |
| Polyunsaturated:saturated fat ratio | 1.41 | 0.44 |
| Fiber, g/day | 86 | 10–20 |
| Sodium, mg | 604 | 3400 |
| Potassium, mg | 6970 | 2400 |
| Potassium-sodium ratio | 12:1 | 0.7:1 |
| Calcium, mg | 1520 | 740 |

Data from Eaton SB, Eaton SB III, Konner MJ, Shostak M. An evolutionary perspective enhances understanding of human nutritional requirements. *J Nutr* 1996;126:1732–1740.

restriction to a level of 75 to 100 mmol per day has been found to lower BP modestly in most studies (He & MacGregor, 2003).

- Short periods of increased NaCl intake have been shown to raise BP in some normotensive subjects (Luft et al., 1979; Mascioli et al., 1991) but not in others (Heer et al., 2000; Houben et al., 2005). Whereas it may never be possible to show conclusively that salt intake causes hypertension in people, it is fairly easy to do so in genetically predisposed animals (Dahl, 1972; Tobian, 1997). As seen in Figure 3–8, the most impressive evidence comes from the study on free-living chimpanzees, half of whom were given progressively increasing amounts of sodium in their food, while the other half remained on their usual low-sodium diet (Denton et al., 1995). During the 89 weeks in which the chimps received extra sodium, the BP rose an average of 33/10 mm Hg, returning to baseline after 20 weeks without added sodium. In keeping with varying sodium sensitivity, the BP rose in only seven of ten chimpanzees on the added sodium.

- Although long-term intervention studies that start with infants and children to confirm that sodium restriction can prevent hypertension in humans or that sodium excess can cause it are not feasible, a short-term 6-month study involving almost 500 newborn infants showed that the half whose sodium intake was reduced by nearly 50% had a 2.1-mm Hg lower systolic BP at the end of the 6 months than did the half who were on normal sodium intake (Hofman et al., 1983). Among the 35% of the participants who could be located 15 years later, those originally on the low-sodium diet had 3.6/2.2-mm Hg lower BP (Geleijnse et al., 1997). In another study, higher BPs were observed at 6 months in neonates given increased sodium in their drinking water for the first 8 weeks of life (Pomeranz et al., 2002). Moreover, in randomized controlled studies of hundreds of patients with high-normal BP, those patients who moderately restricted their sodium intake for 30 months or longer had lower BP and a decreased incidence of hypertension than did the patients who did not reduce their sodium intake (Stamler et al., 1989; Trials of Hypertension Prevention, 1997; Whelton et al., 1998).

- A high sodium intake may activate a number of pressor mechanisms (O'Shaughnessy & Karet, 2004). These include increases in intracellular calcium (Resnick et al., 1994), insulin resistance (Suzuki et al., 2000), a paradoxical rise in atrial natriuretic peptide (Melander et al., 2002), and an upregulation of angiotensin type 1 receptors (Nickenig et al., 1998). In animals, high sodium intake accelerates the development of hypertension along with increased oxidative stress in the vasculature and renal damage (Dobrian et al., 2003).

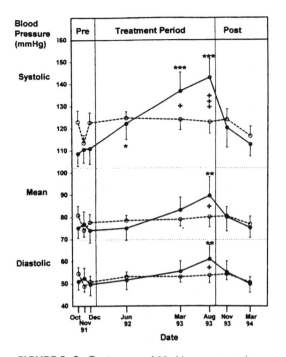

**FIGURE 3–8** ● A group of 22 chimpanzees maintained in small, long-term, stable social groups and fed a vegetable-fruit diet with the addition of infant formula were studied. The 12 control animals (*open circles, dotted line*) experienced no change in conditions over 2.4 years and no significant change of systolic, diastolic, or mean blood pressure (mean ± standard error of the mean). For the 10 experimental animals (*solid circles, solid line*), 5 g per day NaCl was added to the infant formula for 19 weeks, 10 g per day for 3 weeks, and 15 g per day for 67 weeks. A 20-week period without salt addition followed. Significance values of the increase in blood pressure relative to the mean of the three baseline determinations were as follows: *p <.05, **p <.0021; significance values of the difference between the experimental and control groups: *p <.05, ***p <.001. (Modified from Denton D, Weisinger R, Mundy NI, et al. The effect of increased salt intake on blood pressure of chimpanzees. *Nat Med* 1995;1:1009–1016.)

Parenthetically, additional damages may be associated with high sodium intake that are not mediated by the effects of sodium on BP (de Wardener & MacGregor, 2002; du Cailar et al., 2002). Both in animals (Tobian & Hanlon, 1990) and in humans (Sasaki et al., 1995), a high intake of sodium increases the risk of stroke, independent of the effect on BP. Other adverse effects of high-sodium intake include left ventricular hypertrophy and more rapid deterioration of renal function through hyperfiltration (du Cailar et al., 2002). Both osteoporosis and renal stones accompany the increase in calcium excretion that occurs with increased sodium excretion (Stamler & Cirillo, 1997). As if these damages were not enough,

dietary sodium intake also is strongly correlated with stomach cancer mortality (Joossens et al., 1996) and the incidence of cataracts (Cummings et al., 2000).

## Interventional Evidence

More than 100 trials exploring the effect of dietary sodium reduction on BP have been published, which demonstrate an average reduction of 5/2 mm Hg in hypertensives who lower their sodium intake to approximately 100 mmol per day (Cutler et al., 1997). Unfortunately, most interventional trials find little persistence of sodium reduction after 6 months and, not surprisingly, little effect on BP (Hooper et al., 2002). More about this evidence is provided in Chapter 6.

## Sensitivity to Sodium

Because almost everyone in industrialized societies ingests a high-sodium diet, the fact that only about half will develop hypertension suggests a variable degree of BP sensitivity to sodium, although obviously both heredity and interactions with other environmental exposures may be involved (Weinberger, 1996). Since Luft et al. (1977) and Kawasaki et al. (1978) described varying responses of BP to short periods of low- and high-sodium intake, numerous protocols have been used to determine so-called sodium sensitivity with variable results (de la Sierra et al., 2002). Weinberger et al. (1986) defined sodium sensitivity as a 10-mm Hg or greater decrease in mean BP from the level measured after a 4-hour infusion of 2 L normal saline as compared to the level measured the morning after 1 day of a 10-mmol sodium diet, during which three oral doses of furosemide were given at 10 a.m., 2 p.m., and 6 p.m. Using this criterion, these researchers found that 51% of hypertensives and 26% of normotensives were sodium-sensitive. They noted that sodium sensitivity displays a typical bell-shaped distribution, with a shift in those who are hypertensive. These investigators observed a further shift with increasing age both in normotensives and, even more markedly, in hypertensives (Weinberger & Fineberg, 1991) (Figure 3–9). The prevalence of sodium sensitivity was similar in White and Black subjects (Wright et al., 2003).

Multiple mechanisms for sodium sensitivity have been proposed, including:

- A defect in renal sodium excretion manifested by renal vasoconstriction (Johnson et al., 2005c), perhaps in turn secondary to hyperuricemia (Watanabe et al., 2002).

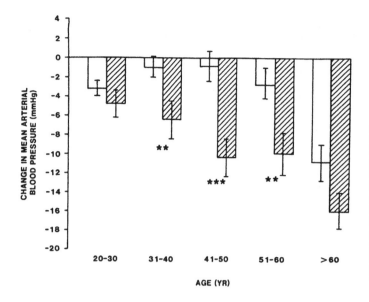

**FIGURE 3–9** ● This bar graph shows changes in mean arterial pressure in response to maneuvers used to define salt responsiveness as a function of age in normotensive (*open bars*) and hypertensive (*hatched bars*) patients. Brackets represent standard deviation of the mean. Significance values between hypertensive and normal subjects were as follows: **p <.01, ***p <.001. (Modified from Weinberger MH, Fineberg NS. Sodium and volume sensitivity of blood pressure. *Hypertension* 1991;18:67–71.)

- Increased activity of the sodium-hydrogen exchanger in the proximal tubule (Siffert & Düsing, 1995).
- Impaired natriuretic response to 20-HETE (Laffer et al., 2003b).
- A higher level of sympathetic nervous system (SNS) activity and greater pressor reactivity (Campese et al., 1993).
- Endothelial dysfunction (Bragulat et al., 2001) related to a decreased nitric oxide response to sodium loads (Cubeddu et al., 2000).

The number of proposed mechanisms underscores the lack of certainty about which of these are involved (Weinberger, 2004). Regardless of how it occurs, greater sodium sensitivity is related to a higher incidence of cardiovascular events (Morimoto et al., 1997) and mortality (Weinberger et al., 2001).

Whatever the mechanism, sodium sensitivity is likely heritable, with close mother-offspring resemblance in BP change with sodium restriction (Miller et al., 1987). Moreover, greater sodium sensitivity has been noted in two populations in those persons who have the 235T allele of the angiotensinogen gene, which is associated with higher blood angiotensinogen levels (Hunt et al., 1999).

## RENAL SODIUM RETENTION

With more than enough sodium in the diet and many mechanisms to explain sodium sensitivity, we turn to the evidence that "essential hypertension is due primarily to an abnormal kidney which has an unwillingness to excrete sodium" (de Wardener,

1996). Literally thousands of investigators have brought us to our current understanding of the role of the kidneys in primary hypertension. Of these, the hypotheses of four investigators (and their co-workers) will be described: those of Guyton, Laragh, Brenner, and the trio of Dahl, de Wardener, and Blaustein. Although their concepts do not meld into a unifying hypothesis and often are in conflict, a case can be built for what each has proposed to be a logical explanation for abnormal renal sodium retention as the initiating event for hypertension. Each of the four hypotheses will now be described.

### Importance of Pressure-Natriuresis

In healthy people, when BP rises, renal excretion of sodium and water increases, shrinking fluid volume and returning the BP to normal—the phenomenon of *pressure-natriuresis*. On the basis of animal experiments and computer models, Guyton (1961, 1992) considered the regulation of body fluid volume by the kidneys to be the dominant mechanism for the long-term control of BP, the only one of many regulatory controls to have sustained and infinite power. Therefore, if hypertension develops, he reasoned that something must be amiss with the pressure-natriuresis control mechanism; otherwise, the BP would return to normal. The evidence has been nicely summarized by Cowley and Roman (1996).

### Experimental Support

The concept is based on a solid foundation: When BP is raised, the normal kidney excretes more

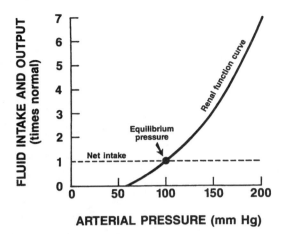

**FIGURE 3–10** ● Graphic analysis of arterial pressure regulation by the kidney-fluid volume pressure control system. Pressure continually approaches the point at which the renal function curve intersects the net intake line (i.e., equilibrium pressure). (Modified from Guyton AC. Kidneys and fluids in pressure regulation. *Hypertension* 1992; 19(Suppl 1):I2–I8.)

salt and water—that is, pressure-natriuresis occurs (Selkurt, 1951). The curve relating BP to sodium excretion is steep (Figure 3–10). A small change in renal perfusion pressure causes a large change in the rate of sodium and water excretion, acting as a powerful negative-feedback stabilizer of systemic BP. As BP rises, the elevation in renal perfusion pressure leads to a decrease in sodium reabsorption in the proximal tubule (Yip et al., 2000) and, perhaps, in the loop of Henle. As a consequence, body fluid volumes would shrink enough to lower the BP back to its previous level.

### Resetting of Pressure-Natriuresis

In patients with primary hypertension, as in every genetic form of experimental hypertension, a resetting of the pressure-sodium excretion curve prevents the return of BP to normal so that fluid balance is maintained only in the presence of an increased BP (Palmer, 2001). As a consequence of the resetting, when BP is lowered by nondiuretic drugs, reactive sodium retention occurs. In a study by Omvik et al. (1980), 12 hypertensive patients were given nitroprusside while sodium excretion was continually monitored. The slope of the pressure-natriuresis curve was directly related to the severity of the hypertension, and when the BP was reduced, sodium excretion immediately fell. Moreover, in two forms of secondary hypertension—primary aldosteronism and renovascular hypertension—resetting has been shown to shift back toward normal when the hypertension is relieved (Kimura et al., 1987).

As seen in Figure 3–11, Guyton and co-workers have shown that either the entire curve can be shifted to the right or the slope can be depressed, depending on the type of renal insult, which is, in turn, reflected by varying sensitivity to sodium (Hall et al., 1996). Kimura and Brenner (1993) have hypothesized that a rightward shift follows preglomerular (i.e., afferent arteriolar) vasoconstriction as in primary hypertension, whereas a depressed slope is the consequence of a decrease in glomerular ultrafiltration or an increase in tubular sodium reabsorption as in primary aldosteronism (Table 3–3).

### Mechanisms of Resetting

The pressure-natriuresis relationship can be modified by neural and humoral factors including the renin-angiotensin system (RAS), sympathetic nervous activity, atrial natriuretic factor, metabolites of arachidonic acid (Laffer et al., 2003b), and intrarenal nitric oxide, which increases renal interstitial guanosine cyclic 3', 5'-monophosphate (Jin et al., 2004). The RAS is likely the major modifier (Hall et al., 1999; van Paassen et al., 2000), with an increase in renal sodium reabsorption occurring at concentrations of angiotensin II (AII) much below those needed for peripheral vasoconstriction. In normotension, RAS is suppressed when sodium intake is increased and stimulated when sodium intake is reduced, allowing sodium excretion to be adjusted without changes in BP. Suppression of the RAS by angiotensin-converting enzyme inhibitors (ACEIs) or AII receptor blockers (ARBs) allows sodium excretion to be maintained at reduced BP while decreasing the slope of pressure-natriuresis (i.e., BP becomes more sodium-sensitive). Stimulation of the RAS reduces renal sodium excretion and impairs pressure-natriuresis, necessitating a higher BP to maintain sodium balance. Clinically, such persistent stimulation of the RAS is seen in chronic edematous states, such as cirrhosis with ascites, wherein sodium excretion is limited because BP cannot rise from an inability to fill the circulation; the RAS remains elevated despite progressive fluid retention.

In hypertension, as will be noted, RAS activity is "inappropriately normal"; that is, it is not suppressed as expected from higher pressure against the juxtaglomerular apparatus. The inappropriately high RAS level reduces renal sodium excretory ability and shifts pressure-natriuresis to the right, necessitating an increased level of BP to maintain sodium balance. Blockade of the RAS in hypertension allows pressure-natriuresis to shift back toward normal so that renal sodium excretion is increased at a lower BP, thereby maintaining sodium balance without an expansion of fluid volume.

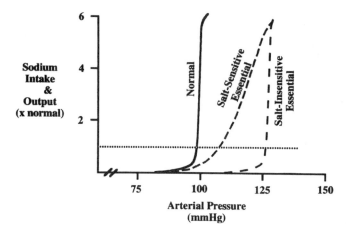

**FIGURE 3–11** ● Schematic of steady-state relationships between arterial pressures and sodium excretion (equal to intake) in both salt-sensitive and salt-insensitive essential hypertension. (Modified from Hall JE, Brands MW, Henegar JR. Angiotensin II and long-term arterial pressure regulation. *J Am Soc Nephrol* 1999;10:S258–S265.)

The primacy of the RAS in resetting pressure-natriuresis has been questioned, particularly by DiBona (2004), who has worked long and hard to support a major role for increased renal sympathetic nervous activity as the mechanism to decrease renal excretory function and to thereby reset the pressure-natriuresis relation. More about this is in the section on the Sympathetic Nervous System later in this chapter.

### Inherited Defect in Renal Sodium Excretion

In certain animal models, the alteration in renal function responsible for the resetting of the pressure-natriuresis curve is inherited. Using rats bred to be either sensitive or resistant to the hypertensive action of dietary sodium, Dahl and Heine (1975) demonstrated the primacy of the kidney in the development of hypertension by a series of transplant experiments. As shown in Figure 3–12, the BP follows the kidney: When a kidney from a normotensive donor was transplanted to a hypertensive host, the BP of the recipient fell to normal. Conversely, when a hypertensive kidney was transplanted into a normotensive host, the BP rose. Moreover, transplantation of a kidney from a hypertensive rat that has been briefly made normotensive with an ACEI causes the blood pressure to normalize in a hypertensive host (Smallegange et al., 2004).

### Evidence in Humans

An acquired glomerulopathy that results from a high sodium intake and maintains an elevated blood pressure has been postulated as the mechanism for the increased prevalence of both hypertension and progressive renal damage in Blacks (Aviv et al., 2004) (Figure 3–13). This scheme involves a failure of tubular glomerular feedback, leading to increased glomerular capillary hydraulic pressure and glomerular damage.

## TABLE 3–3

### Renal Mechanisms of Hypertension (Hypothesis)

| Pressure-Natriuresis Relationship | Glomerular Hemodynamics | Examples of Human Hypertension |
|---|---|---|
| Rightward shift (non–sodium-sensitive) | Preglomerular; (afferent arteriolar) vasoconstriction | Renovascular hypertension; essential hypertension |
| Depressed slope (sodium-sensitive) | Decrease in ultrafiltration coefficient;[a] increase in tubule sodium reabsorption | Hypertension in blacks; glomerulonephritis; primary aldosteronism; diabetes mellitus |

[a]The ultrafiltration coefficient can be expressed as the product of the number of glomeruli, the glomerular filtration surface area per glomerulus, and the hydraulic conductivity of the glomerular capillary walls.

Reprinted with permission from Kimura G, Brenner BM. A method for distinguishing salt-sensitive from non–salt-sensitive forms of human and experimental hypertension. *Curr Opin Nephrol Hypertens* 1993;2:341–349.

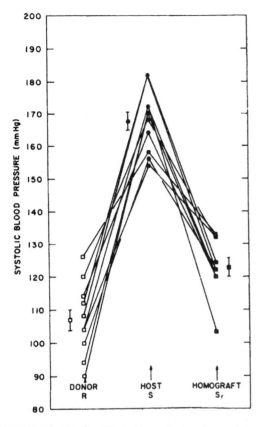

**FIGURE 3–12** ● Effect of transplanting "normotensive" kidneys from resistant rats (donor R; *open squares*) to hypertensive sensitive rats (host S; *closed circles*). The resultant blood pressure levels at a median time of 17 weeks after surgery are shown on the right (*closed squares*). The mean blood pressure plus or minus the standard error is indicated for each group. (Modified from Dahl LK, Heine M. Primary role of renal homographs in setting chronic blood pressure and levels in rats. *Circ Res* 1975;36:692–696.)

The possibility of an inherited defect in renal function is supported further by transplantation studies in humans. Curtis et al. (1983) observed long-term remission of hypertension after renal transplantation in six Black male patients who likely developed renal failure solely as a consequence of primary hypertension. Because five of these patients had remained hypertensive after removal of their native kidneys, their hypertension was presumably not of renal pressor origin. The most likely explanation for the reversal of hypertension in these patients was the implantation of normal renal tissue, which provided control of body fluid volume, something their original kidneys had been unable to manage. Moreover, hypertension develops more frequently in recipients of renal transplants from hypertensive donors

than in recipients from normotensive donors (Guidi et al., 1996).

### Nocturia and Natriuresis

A more benign but bothersome aspect of the shift in pressure-natriuresis is nocturia. A reversal of the normal circadian rhythm of urine output occurs with aging and is further accentuated with hypertension. In normotensives, nocturnal urine flow accounts for 53% of urine output in 60- to 80-year-olds as compared to 25% in 25- to 35-year-olds (McKeigue & Reynard, 2000). Hypertensives have even more nocturia, presumably reflecting the resetting of the pressure-natriuresis relationship (Fukuda et al., 2004). Fluid retained during the day, accentuated by upright posture, is then excreted during the night. Relief should be provided by a morning dose of a diuretic such as hydrochlorothiazide that prevents fluid retention during the day.

### Induced Natriuretic Hormone

The Guyton hypothesis allows for a normal or slightly contracted blood volume despite an elevated pressure, in keeping with most volume measurements in hypertensive patients (Harrap et al., 2000). The next hypothesis requires an initially expanded plasma volume that, after an inhibition of renal sodium reabsorption, is allowed to return to normal.

The concept began with another set of Dahl's experiments in rats (Dahl et al., 1967). A chronic parabiotic union was made between sodium-sensitive and sodium-resistant rats. The authors observed that "the animal from the strain that normally fails to develop salt hypertension rapidly developed chronic hypertension provided that a high NaCl diet was consumed by the pair. This response has been interpreted as being compatible with the transfer of a humoral influence from one parabiotic animal to the other" (Dahl et al., 1967). Soon thereafter, Dahl et al. (1969) provided evidence that this "humoral influence" worked as a "sodium-excreting hormone."

The search for the nature of this sodium-excreting hormone, made in the salt-sensitive animal and transferred to the salt-resistant one, actually had begun in 1961 when de Wardener et al. showed that plasma from sodium-loaded animals contains a natriuretic substance. In 1976, Haddy and Overbeck proposed that the BP of volume-expanded hypertension was raised by a circulating inhibitor of the $Na^+/K^+$-ATPase pump. The next year, Blaustein (1977) provided evidence that such an inhibitor could induce hypertension by inhibiting sodium-calcium exchange in vascular tissue, increasing intracellular calcium and thereby raising peripheral resistance. De Wardener and MacGregor (1980) then suggested

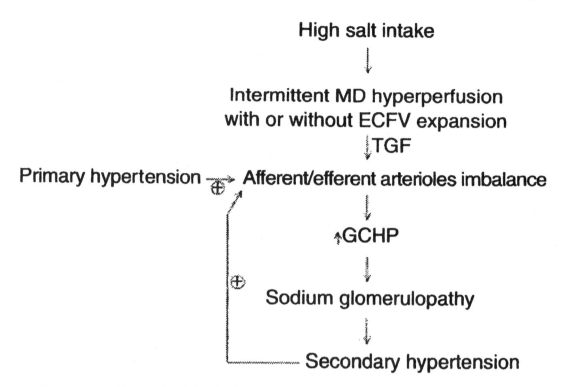

FIGURE 3-13 ● Schematic description of sodium glomerulopathy in African Americans. The model centers on hyperperfusion of the macula densa (MD) with or without expansion of the extracellular fluid volume (ECFV) as the cause, through tubular glomerular feedback (TGF), of an imbalance between the afferent and the efferent arterioles. The model also suggests a positive feedback loop through which hypertension caused by either sodium glomerulopathy (secondary hypertension) or hypertension due to other causes (primary hypertension) exacerbates the renal damage caused by an imbalance between the afferent and efferent arterioles. + denotes an amplifying effect; GCHP, glomerular capillary hydrostatic pressure. (Modified from Aviv A, et al. Sodium glomerulopathy: tubuloglomerular feedback and renal injury in African Americans. *Kidney Int* 2004;65:361–368.)

that the increase in the sodium transport inhibitor (Dahl's saluretic substance) might be a consequence of an inherited defect in the kidney's ability to excrete sodium.

The search for the natriuretic hormone that arises when plasma volume is expanded, perhaps from an inherited defect in renal sodium excretion, has gone on for more than 40 years (de Wardener, 1996). (This natriuretic hormone is functionally and chemically entirely distinct from the atrial and brain natriuretic peptides that were identified more recently.) Endogenous inhibitors of $Na^+/K^+$- ATPase pump activity have been found in sodium-sensitive rats. Some believe that ouabain is the endogenous pump inhibitor (Zhang et al., 2004), others an isomer of a steroid (bufenolide) structure found in human placenta (McKinnon et al., 2003). In mice arteries, ouabain acts upon sodium pumps with $\alpha2$ subunits to increase myogenic tone and BP (Zhang, 2005).

In keeping with the experimental evidence that ouabain increases intracellular sodium and thereby mobilizes calcium from intracellular stores (Borin et al., 1994), Blaustein (1996) formulated an overall scheme for this acquired compensatory mechanism for renal sodium retention, which could be a cause of primary hypertension. The latest evidence for this pathway to sodium-sensitive hypertension is the reversal of ouabain-induced cytosolic calcium elevation and arterial constriction by SEA0400, a specific inhibitor of calcium entry through the sodium-calcium exchange type 1 (NCX1) (Iwamoto et al., 2004) (Figure 3–14). This evidence may provide the opening to an exciting new therapy for hypertension (Zhang et al., 2004).

As will be covered later in this chapter, numerous other defects in sodium and calcium transport and intracellular binding have been postulated to be involved in the pathogenesis of hypertension.

### Renin and Nephron Heterogeneity

For more than 40 years, Laragh (2001) has explored the RAS, adding immensely to our understanding of both the mechanisms and treatment of hypertension.

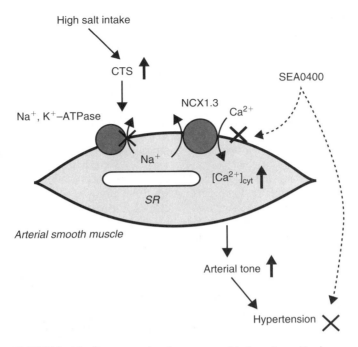

**FIGURE 3–14** ● Proposed pathway responsible for salt-sensitive hypertension. High salt intake causes the levels of endogenous CTS to rise in the plasma. This results in the increase in subplasma membrane ($Na^+$) of arterial smooth muscle. The restricted ($Na^+$) accumulation elevates ($Ca^{2+}$)cyt by vascular NCX1 isoform-mediated $Ca^{2+}$ entry. This enhances arterial tone and causes hypertension. SEA0400 blocks this $Ca^{2+}$ entry and exerts an antihypertensive effect in salt-sensitive hypertension. *NCX*, sodium-calcium exchange; *CTS*, cardiotonic steroids. (Modified from Iwamoto T, et al. Salt-sensitive hypertension is triggered by $Ca^{2+}$ entry via Na+/$Ca^{2+}$ exchanger type-1 in vascular smooth muscle. *Nat Med* 2004;10:1193–1199.)

As part of these labors, Sealey et al. (1988) have provided another hypothesis for the renal contribution to the pathogenesis of primary hypertension, based on the presence of ". . . a subpopulation of nephrons that is ischemic from either afferent arteriolar vasoconstriction or from an intrinsic narrowing of the lumen. Renin secretion from this subgroup of nephrons is tonically elevated. This increased renin secretion then interferes with the compensatory capacity of intermingled normal nephrons to adaptively excrete sodium and, consequently, perturbs overall blood pressure homeostasis."

This hypothesis is similar to that proposed by Goldblatt (1958), who believed that "the primary cause of essential hypertension in humans is intrarenal obliterative vascular disease, from any cause, usually arterial and arteriolar sclerosis, or any other condition that brings about the same disturbance of intrarenal hemodynamics." Although investigators were unable to place minuscule clamps on small arterioles, Goldblatt's experimental concept nonetheless is the basis for the more modern model proposed by Sealey et al. (1988). The elevated renin levels from the ischemic population of nephrons, although diluted in the systemic circulation, become the "normal" renin levels that are usual in patients early in the course of primary hypertension (Harrap et al., 2000), in whom suppression of renin secretion and demonstration of low circulating levels would otherwise be expected. The diluted levels are still high enough to impair sodium excretion in the non-ischemic hyperfiltering nephrons but are too low to support efferent tone in the ischemic nephrons, thereby reducing sodium excretion in them as well.

Sealey et al. (1988) expanded their model to explain the varying plasma renin levels seen both in healthy individuals at different ages and in patients with primary hypertension as well as the high renin levels seen with renovascular hypertension and the low renin levels seen with primary aldosteronism. Even the low-renin form of primary hypertension presumably involves a few ischemic nephrons, because "*any* renin secretion in the presence of arterial hypertension is abnormal and it works in the same way to impair salt excretion and raise BP" (Sealey et al., 1988).

Additional discussion of the multiple roles of the RAS will come later in this chapter, after we review the last of the four models for renal sodium retention.

## Reduced Nephron Number

Brenner et al. (1988) proposed that hypertension may arise from a congenital reduction in the number of nephrons or in the filtration surface area per glomerulus, thereby limiting the ability to excrete sodium, raising the BP, and setting off a vicious circle whereby systemic hypertension begets glomerular hypertension, which begets more systemic hypertension (Brenner & Chertow, 1994) (Figure 3–15). These investigators point out that as many as 40% of individuals younger than 30 years have fewer than the presumably normal number of nephrons (600,000 per kidney) and "speculate that those individuals whose congenital nephron numbers fall in the lower range constitute the population subsets that exhibit enhanced susceptibility to the development of essential hypertension."

Brenner and Anderson (1992) invoke this congenital decrease in filtration surface as a possible explanation for observed differences in susceptibility to hypertension among certain populations such as in Blacks, women, and older people, all of whom may have smaller kidneys or fewer functioning nephrons than other populations. As is described in Chapter 9, these investigators have developed a similar hypothesis for the progression of renal damage that is commonly observed among diabetics and patients with most forms of acquired kidney disease (Brenner & Mackenzie, 1997).

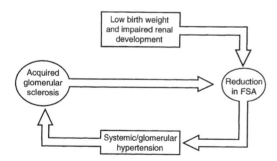

**FIGURE 3–15** ● A diagram of the hypothesis that the risks of developing essential hypertension and progressive renal injury in adult life are increased as a result of congenital oligonephropathy, or an inborn deficit of filtration surface area (FSA), caused by impaired renal development. (Modified from Brenner BM, Chertow GM. Congenital oligonephropathy and the etiology of adult hypertension and progressive renal injury. *Am J Kidney Dis* 1994;23:171–175.)

The Brenner hypothesis received major affirmation from a careful analysis of total nephron numbers in kidneys from 10 previously hypertensive patients and 10 previously normotensive people, all of whom died in accidents (Keller et al., 2003). The two groups were matched for age, gender, height, and weight. The median number of glomeruli in the hypertensives was less than half of the number in the normotensives. Moreover, the glomerular volume in the hypertensives was greater, suggesting that they were hyperfiltering. The likelihood that the lower number of glomeruli in the hypertensives was from birth was supported by the absence of obsolescent glomeruli as would be seen if they had been present but dropped out.

### Congenital Oligonephropathy

The Brenner hypothesis invokes a reduced number of nephrons from congenital oligonephropathy, i.e., fewer nephons as a result of intrauterine growth retardation (Mackenzie & Brenner, 1995). As first reported by Barker et al. (1989) on the basis of epidemiological studies, infants born small for gestational age, i.e., low birth weight, are at increased risk for development of hypertension, diabetes, and cardiovascular diseases later in life. The concept of "perinatal programming" has focused on maternal protein restriction (Woods et al., 2004) as responsible for the shunting of necessary fuels to the developing brain at the expense of less vital organs including the kidneys and pancreas, a hypothesis described as "thrifty-phenotype" (Hales & Barker, 2001).

The presence of congenital oligonephropathy in human babies born with intrauterine growth retardation was first shown by Hinchliffe et al. (1992) and confirmed by Konje et al. (1996), Mañalich et al. (2000), and Hughson et al. (2003). The latter group found an average of 260,000 fewer nephrons with each kilogram of decrease in birth weight. The reduced number of nephrons at birth in low-birth-weight babies cannot be replenished later by adequate postnatal nutrition since most nephrons are formed in the first part of the last trimester and no further nephrogenesis occurs after 34 to 36 weeks of gestation (Lucas & Morley, 1994).

The subsequent scenario has been described by Mackenzie and Brenner (1995):

Deficiencies in the total nephron supply, by limiting total renal excretory capacity and thereby influencing the point at which steady-state conditions between BP and sodium excretion are achieved, could profoundly affect long-term BP regulation. When renal mass is greatly reduced, as in the case of extensive experimental ablation of the kidney in rodents, BP increases in the systemic arterial circulation and in the glomerular capillaries, thus increasing glomerular filtration rate and promoting fluid excretion. However, sustained elevations in glomerular capillary hydraulic pressure are associated with the development of focal and segmental glomerular sclerosis leading to further loss of nephrons and a self-perpetuating vicious cycle of hypertension and progressive glomerular injury. . . . Given the association between low birth weight and fewer nephrons . . . it is naturally tempting to speculate that the origins of hypertension in adults who were of low birth weight lie in a deficient endowment of nephrons secondary to intrauterine growth retardation.

The Barker and Brenner hypotheses have been generously supported by a large amount of epidemiological evidence including an association of low birth weight not only with adult hypertension (Irving et al., 2004) but also with increased sympathetic nerve activity (Boguszewski et al., 2004), endothelial dysfunction (Norman & Martin, 2003), abnormal retinal vascular morphology (Hellström et al., 2004), aortic wall thickness (Skilton et al., 2005), and stroke mortality (Barker & Lackland, 2003). In addition, more diabetes (with hypertension) (Fagerudd et al., 2004), hyperuricemia (Feig et al., 2004), and even suicides (Mittendorfer-Rutz et al., 2004) have been reported subsequent to low birth weight.

### Postnatal Weight Gain

Despite all of the evidence supporting a role of low birth weight with adult hypertension, its contribution may be quantitatively small (Falkner et al., 1998; Huxley et al., 2002). An even greater contribution has more recently been shown for the rapid postnatal "catch-up" in body weight that such infants typically undergo, referred to by Singhal and Lucas (2004) as "growth acceleration." These researchers have summarized a great deal of their own and others' convincing evidence for a critical period— the first two weeks after birth—where overfeeding programs the infant for later obesity, insulin resistance, and endothelial dysfunction, which, in turn, results in diabetes, hypertension, and coronary disease (Singhal et al., 2004).

Their evidence includes multiple observations on the benefits of feeding with breast milk (with lower caloric content and lower initial volume) rather than formula milk (with higher caloric content and larger volume) on subsequent adult health (Martin et al., 2004; Stettler et al., 2005).

Thus, the combination of low birth weight and postnatal growth acceleration sets the stage for a great amount of poor health in later life (Primatesta et al., 2005). The implications are obvious: Provide good prenatal care to prevent intrauterine growth retardation, and encourage mothers to breast-feed their newborns.

The opportunity for overcoming most of these contributing factors may be obvious but has not yet been tested (Sperling, 2004). Moreover, recent cutbacks in support for teenage contraception, maternal nutrition, and postnatal care in the United States suggest that we will continue to pay billions for the eventual care of hypertension-related end-stage renal disease, strokes, and heart attacks instead of millions for preventive care of the disadvantaged.

### An Adaptation to Growth

Another view of the relation between BP and renal function has been provided by Weder and Schork (1994). Having observed an intimate linkage in rats between somatic growth and BP, these investigators "propose that blood pressure rises during childhood to subserve homeostatic needs of the organism," specifically renal function. They believe that because modern diet and lifestyle stimulate earlier and greater somatic growth, rising BP is a necessary, but also eventually harmful, compensation for maintaining renal function.

Their hypothesis can be viewed as the body's response both to postnatal growth acceleration and to the pressure-natriuresis relationship and the inability to expand the number of nephrons postnatally: As more sodium is ingested and more demands are placed on the fixed renal capacity, higher BP is needed to maintain natriuresis and overall renal excretory function. Hypertension is the unfortunate price paid to preserve homeostasis.

Now that numerous mechanisms for renal sodium retention have been reviewed, we will return to an examination of the RAS.

## RENIN-ANGIOTENSIN SYSTEM

More than 100 years since the discovery of renin by Tigerstedt and Bergman (Phillips & Schmidt-Ott, 1999), our knowledge of the many roles of the RAS continues to expand (Fuchs et al., 2004; Navar, 2004). Figure 3–16 is a schematic overview of the RAS, showing its major components, the regulators of renin release, and the primary effects of AII, excluding the AII receptors. In addition, several alternate or degradation products of AII may have biologic functions (Ferrario & Chappell, 2004).

### Properties and Control of Renin

Renin is stored and secreted from the renal juxtaglomerular cells located in the wall of the afferent arteriole, which is contiguous with the macula densa

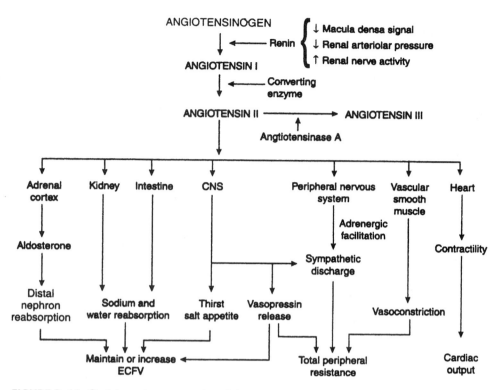

**FIGURE 3–16** ● Schematic representation of the renin-angiotensin system, showing the major regulators of renin release, the biochemical cascade leading to angiotensin II, and the major effects of angiotensin II. CNS, central nervous system; ECFV, extracellular fluid volume.

portion of the same nephron (Schnermann & Briggs, 1999). The multiple factors that can alter renin secretion include those shown in Figure 3–16, with changes in pressure within the afferent arterioles and sodium concentration in the macula densa likely playing the most important roles.

Expression and regulation of the human renin gene and the structure of the enzyme have been elucidated (Pan & Gross, 2005).

### Prorenin

The first product of the translation of renin messenger RNA is preprorenin, which is processed in the endoplasmic reticulum to the 47-kDa prorenin. Although prorenin constitutes 80% to 90% of the renin in human plasma (Danser et al., 1996), its physiologic or pathogenic role has not yet been established. High plasma prorenin levels are present in type 1 diabetics, particularly in those with microvascular complications (Wilson & Luetscher, 1990). Sealey and co-workers have presented an imaginative scheme for an active *vasodilatory* role for prorenin, believing that it acts as a balance to the vasoconstrictive effects of renin-AII (Halimi & Sealey, 1992). Thus, high levels of vasodilatory prorenin could contribute to the hyperperfusion

seen in diabetes mellitus, whereas high levels of renin would explain the ischemic vascular injury of high-renin hypertensive states.

### Extrarenal Renin-Angiotensin

The RAS acts within both the circulation and various tissues (Re, 2004). Most workers in this field now accept the presence of a functional cardiac RAS (de Mello, 2004). Although most cardiac renin is likely derived from plasma renin of renal origin, most cardiac AII is likely produced within the heart by conversion of locally synthesized rather than blood-derived angiotensin I (AI) (van Kats et al., 1998).

## Components of the System

Renin acts as an aspartyl proteinase that catalyzes the hydrolytic release of the decapeptide AI from its α-globulin substrate, angiotensinogen (Figure 3–16). Renin itself probably is without effect other than by its generation of AI.

### Angiotensinogen

The amount of the renin substrate (angiotensinogen) in the plasma may vary considerably, and its level may play some role in the overall function of the RAS (Bohlender et al., 2000). Estrogens and other stimulators of hepatic microsomal enzyme activity will increase renin substrate levels.

### Angiotensin-Converting Enzyme

The two end-amino acids, histidyl and leucine, of AI are removed, forming the 8-amino acid polypeptide AII, by a converting enzyme present in plasma but mainly bound to tissues (Esther et al., 1997). Conversion occurs throughout the body, particularly in the lung (Erdös, 1990). ACE may play additional roles in angiogenesis, tumor growth, and diabetes (Fuchs et al., 2004).

### Chymase

Chymase, a serine protease that also converts AI to AII, has been identified in various sites but particularly in the heart (Wei et al., 1999) and arteries (Richard et al., 2001). Obviously, the presence of an ACE-independent pathway could support additional benefits of AII receptor blockers over ACEIs (see Chapter 7).

### Angiotensin Receptors and Effects

Most, if not all, of the effects of the RAS are mediated by the 8-amino acid AII, but angiotensin-(1-7) may be a modulator of the system (Ferrario & Chappell, 2004), and smaller fragments may play a role (Watanabe et al., 2005).

In a manner comparable with that of other peptide hormones, the action of AII is triggered by its interaction with receptors on the plasma membrane of the tissues responsive to the hormone (Figure 3–17). Two receptors have been cloned. $AT_1$ receptors are found in the vasculature, kidney, adrenals, heart, liver, and brain. The $AT_2$ receptor is widely distributed in the fetus but in adults is found only in the adrenal medulla, uterus, ovary, vascular endothelium, and distinct brain areas (Brewster & Perazella, 2004).

Considerable effort has been directed at the possible role of the AII type 2 receptor ($AT_2$), whose activation likely stimulates vasodilation via bradykinin and nitric oxide and perhaps has other effects that oppose those of activation of the

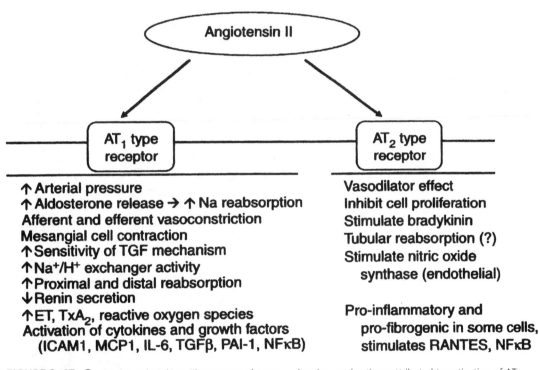

**FIGURE 3–17** ● Angiotensin II (Ang II) receptor subtypes and major renal actions attributed to activation of $AT_1$ and $AT_2$ receptors. Na, sodium; TGF, tubular glomerular feedback; ET, endothelin; $TxA_2$, thromboxane $A_2$; ICAM1, intracellular adhesion molecule-1; MCP1, monocyte chemoattractant protein-1; IL-6, interleukin-6; TGFβ, transforming growth factor beta; PAI-1, plasminogen-activated inhibitor-1; NFκB, nuclear factor kappaB; RANTES, regulated upon activation, normal T cell expressed and excreted. (Modified from Navar LG. The intrarenal renin-angiotensin system in hypertension. *Kidney Int* 2004;65:1522–1532.)

AT$_1$ receptor (Carey, 2005; Hannan & Widdop, 2004). The cardiac actions of stimulation of AT$_2$ receptors appear to be different depending upon changes in the ratio of AT$_1$ to AT$_2$ receptors, which can change considerably (Booz, 2004). Levy (2004) has forcefully argued that the high level of AT$_2$ receptor stimulation that occurs when AT$_1$-receptor blockers (ARBs) are given could have deleterious effects. As will be described more in Chapter 7, there is clinical evidence that ARBs have been associated with lesser protection against myocardial infarction than seen with ACE inhibitors (Verma & Strauss, 2004).

As the multiple actions of AII continue to be revealed, including its stimulation of oxidative stress (Imanishi et al., 2005), its necessary interaction with multiple cytokines and growth factors listed in Figure 3–17 have become apparent (Arenas, 2004; Kelly et al., 2004; Nabah et al., 2004). Moreover, the effects of AII often are mediated through other factors including aldosterone (Xiao et al., 2004) and osteopontin (Matsui et al., 2004).

### Effects of Inhibition of Renin-Angiotensin

Figure 3–18 shows the sites at which interruption of the RAS is now feasible. In the future, direct renin inhibition will likely be added. The mechanisms by which agents can act to inhibit the system will be covered in detail in Chapter 7, along with practical considerations about their use to treat hypertension and its complications.

Evidence derived from these inhibitors has helped to define the role of the RAS in primary hypertension. This role will be examined after a brief review of the measurements of these hormones.

### Plasma Renin Activity

Direct assays of plasma renin are now commercially available (Ferrari et al., 2004) so that the use of measurements of plasma renin activity (PRA) will likely diminish. Plasma renin activity is measured by incubating a patient's plasma, which contains both angiotensinogen and renin, to generate AI, which then is measured by radioimmunoassay

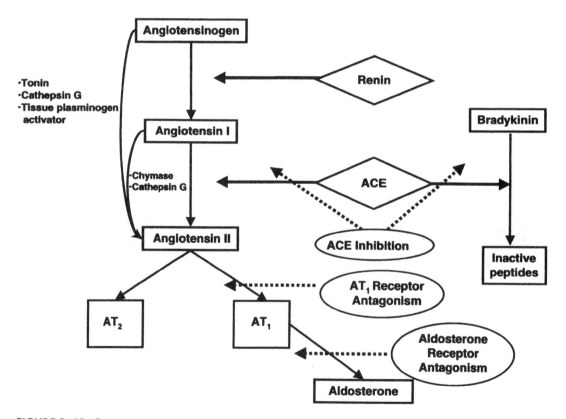

FIGURE 3–18 ● The renin-angiotensin-aldosterone system and its inhibitors. ACE, angiotensin-converting enzyme; AT$_1$, angiotension II type 1 receptor; AT$_2$, angiotensin II type 2 receptor. (Modified from Brewster UC, Perazella MA. The renin-angiotensin-aldosterone system and the kidney: effects on kidney disease. *Am J Med* 2004;116:263–272.)

(Sealey et al., 1995). The amount of AI generated is proportional to the amount of renin present. Care must be taken to prevent generation of AI by cryoactivation of prorenin (Sealey et al., 2005).

Considering all the factors affecting the level of renin, the agreement noted in the literature is rather surprising: Almost all patients with primary aldosteronism have suppressed values, most patients with renovascular or accelerated malignant hypertension have elevated levels, and the incidence of suppressed values among patients with primary hypertension is surprisingly similar in different series (Figure 3–19). Specific information about the use of PRA assays in the evaluation of various identifiable forms of hypertension is provided in subsequent chapters.

The listing in Table 3–4 is not intended to cover every known condition and disease in which a renin assay has been performed, but the more clinically important ones are listed in an attempt to categorize them by mechanism. Some conditions could fit in two or more categories; for example, upright posture may involve a decreased effective plasma volume, a decreased renal perfusion or sympathetic activation.

### Role in Primary Hypertension

In keeping with the effects of higher perfusion pressure at the juxtaglomerular cell and the high-normal blood volume seen in primary hypertension, suppression of renin release and low levels of PRA are expected. In fact, patients with primary hypertension tend to have lower PRA levels than do age- and gender-matched normotensives (Helmer, 1964; Meade et al., 1983). However, the majority of patients with primary hypertension do not have low, suppressed renin-angiotensin levels, stimulating a large amount of clinical research to explain the "inappropriately" normal or even elevated PRA levels seen in most patients (Figure 3–19). Two logical explanations have been presented: the proposal of Sealey et al. (1988) of nephron heterogeneity, with a population of ischemic nephrons contributing excess renin (as described earlier in this chapter), and Julius's (1988a) concept of a state of increased sympathetic drive (explored later in this chapter).

### Nonmodulation

A third explanation for inappropriately normal renin levels has been proposed by Hollenberg, Williams, and colleagues on the basis of a series of studies indicating that as many as half of normal-renin and high-renin hypertensive patients have defective feedback regulation of the RAS within the kidney and the adrenal glands (Williams et al., 2000). The study of modulation continues to provide useful insights (Hurwitz et al., 2003) but has not received clinical application.

If the ability to use genotyping to identify modulation fulfills its promise (Kosachunhanun et al., 2003) as a substitute for the complicated phenotyping needed until now, the identification of nonmodulation may find wider clinical use.

### Primary Hypertension with Low Renin

Clearly, there are numerous possible explanations for normal levels of renin in hypertension, which is the usual finding. Although low renin levels are expected in the absence of one or another of the previously described circumstances (Alderman et al., 2004), a great deal of work has been done to uncover special mechanisms, prognoses, and therapy for hypertensives with low renin, in particular for the twofold greater prevalence of low renin in Blacks than in non-Blacks (Sagnella, 2001).

*Mechanisms*

One of the possible mechanisms for low-renin hypertension is volume expansion with or without mineralocorticoid excess, but the majority of careful analyses fail to indicate volume expansion (Sagnella, 2001) or increased levels of mineralocorticoids (Pratt et al., 1999). In keeping with normal levels of aldosterone despite the low renin levels, low-renin hypertensives showed a lesser rise in aldosterone secretion on a low-sodium diet (Fisher et al., 1999).

Genetically determined impairment of renal sodium excretion has been associated with low-renin hypertension. In a study of 279 hypertensives, Grant

**FIGURE 3–19** ● Schematic representation of plasma renin activity in various hypertensive diseases. The approximate number of patients with each type of hypertension is indicated along with their proportion of low, normal, or high renin levels. (Modified from Kaplan NM. Renin profiles. *JAMA* 1977;238:611–613. Copyright 1977, American Medical Association.)

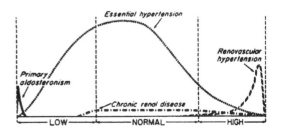

## TABLE 3-4

### Clinical Conditions Affecting Plasma Renin Activity (PRA)

| Decreased PRA | Increased PRA |
|---|---|
| Expanded fluid volume | Shrunken fluid volume |
|   Salt loads, oral or intravenous |   Sodium restriction |
|   Primary salt retention |   Fluid losses |
|     Liddle's syndrome |     Diuretic induced |
|     Gordon's syndrome |     Gastrointestinal losses |
| Mineralocorticoid excess |     Hemorrhage |
|   Primary aldosteronism | Decreased effective plasma volume |
|   Cushing's syndrome |   Upright posture |
|   Congenital adrenal hyperplasia |   Cirrhosis with ascites |
|   Deoxycorticosterone (DOC), 18-hydroxy-DOC excess |   Nephrotic syndrome |
|   $11\beta$-Hydroxysteroid dehydrogenase inhibition (licorice) | Decreased renal perfusion pressure |
| Sympathetic inhibition |   Renovascular hypertension |
|   Autonomic dysfunction |   Accelerated-malignant hypertension |
|   Therapy with adrenergic neuronal blockers |   Chronic renal disease (renin dependent) |
|   Therapy with $\beta$-adrenergic blockers |   Juxtaglomerular hyperplasia |
| Hyperkalemia | Sympathetic activation |
| Decreased renin substrate (?) |   Therapy with direct vasodilators |
|   Androgen therapy |   Pheochromocytoma |
| Decrease in renal tissue |   Stress: exercise, hypoglycemia |
|   Hyporeninemic hypoaldosteronism |   Hyperthyroidism |
|   Chronic renal disease (volume dependent) |   Sympathomimetic agents (caffeine) |
|   Anephric | Hypokalemia |
|   Increasing age | Increased renin substrate |
| Unknown |   Pregnancy |
|   Low renin primary hypertension |   Estrogen therapy |
|   Black race | Autonomous renin hypersecretion |
| |   Renin-secreting tumors |
| | Acute damage to juxtaglomerular cells |
| |   Acute glomerulonephritis |
| | Decreased feedback inhibition |
| |   Low AII levels (ACEI therapy) |
| | Unknown |
| |   High renin primary hypertension |

et al. (2002) found 19% to have the 460 Trp polymorphism of the α-adducin gene and nine of the subjects were homozygous for the allele. The homozygous nine had multiple defects in sodium excretion, were sodium sensitive, and had low renin levels.

As described in Chapters 13 and 14, new forms of low-renin hypertension have recently been recognized, one with increased amounts of 18-hydroxylated steroids, the other with high levels of cortisol from inhibition of the 11β-hydroxysteroid dehydrogenase enzyme. Not surprisingly, subtle degrees of these defects have been looked for in low-renin hypertensives, with only equivocal results (Carvajal et al., 2005; Rossi et al., 2001; Soro et al., 1995; Williams et al., 2005). There is limited evidence for the presence of a mutation in the epithelial sodium channel (ENaC), as is responsible for Liddle's syndrome (see Chapter 13): Among Black hypertensives in London, 8.3% had a heterozygous T594M mutation of the ENaC, as compared with 2.1% of the Black normotensives (Baker et al., 1998).

*Prognosis*

A retrospective analysis over a 7-year interval showed that patients with low-renin hypertension had no strokes or heart attacks, whereas 11% of normal-renin and 14% of high-renin patients had experienced one of these cardiovascular complications (Brunner et al., 1972). High renin levels most likely indicate more severe intrarenal vascular damage, so the higher rate of complications among the high-renin group is not surprising. However, the data of Brunner et al. posed the possibility of vasculotoxic effects of presumably normal levels of renin.

Although a number of subsequent studies failed to document an improved prognosis in low-renin hypertension, Alderman et al. (1991) prospectively tested the prognostic value of the renin-sodium profile in 1,717 hypertensive subjects followed up for as long as 8 years while being treated. The incidence of myocardial infarction was 14.7 per 1,000 person-years in the 12% with high renin levels, 5.6 per 1,000 person-years in the 56% with a normal level, and 2.8 per 1,000 person-years in the 32% with a low renin level. The incidence of stroke was not correlated with renin status, but the association with heart attack remained significant after adjustment for various possible confounders. In an expanded population followed up for as long as 3.6 years, the relation between PRA levels and myocardial infarction remained independent and direct, but only in those with an initial BP above 95 mm Hg (Alderman et al., 1997).

Conversely, Meade et al. (1993) found no association between PRA levels and ischemic heart disease in a 20-year follow-up of 803 White, normotensive men. Similarly, total plasma renin concentration was not found to be a risk factor for coronary disease in a 4.9-year prospective study of White men (Singh et al., 2000), and no increase in carotid artery disease was found among high-renin patients (Rossi et al., 2000). Some have noted direct relation between renin levels and left ventricular hypertrophy (Aronow et al., 1997; Koga et al., 1998), whereas others have not (Vakili et al., 2000).

*Therapy*

In keeping with their presumed but unproved volume excess, patients with low-renin primary hypertension have been found by some investigators (Preston et al., 1998; Vaughan et al., 1973), but not by others (Ferguson et al., 1977; Holland et al., 1979; Hunyor et al., 1975), to experience a greater fall in BP when given diuretics than do normal-renin patients.

If low-renin hypertensive patients do respond better to diuretics, the response does not necessarily indicate a greater volume load. Patients with low renin, by definition, are less responsive to stimuli that increase renin levels, including volume depletion, and they therefore experience a lesser rise in PRA with diuretic therapy. This would result in less compensatory vasoconstriction and aldosterone secretion, so that volume depletion would proceed and the BP would fall further in low-renin hypertensive patients given a diuretic than in those with greater renin responsiveness.

Despite the attractiveness of basing therapeutic choices on the renin profile (Laragh & Sealey, 2003), age and race were better predictors of response to various drugs (Preston et al., 1998) and, in some studies, the renin status simply did not reflect the response at all (Weir & Saunders, 1998).

## Summary

Although low renin levels are expected in primary hypertension, the presence of normal or high levels in most patients has generated a search for an involvement of such inappropriate levels in the pathogenesis of the disease. It seems likely that this mechanism is abnormally activated in many patients with primary hypertension, and at least three mechanisms have been offered: nephron heterogeneity, nonmodulation, and increased sympathetic drive.

Laragh (1973) and colleagues (Laragh & Sealey, 2003) have long attached a great deal of significance to the various PRA levels found in patients with primary hypertension. According to this view, the levels of renin can identify the relative contributions of vasoconstriction (PR) and body fluid volume expansion to the pathogenesis of hypertension. According to the "bipolar vasoconstriction-volume analysis," arteriolar vasoconstriction by AII is predominantly responsible for the hypertension in patients with high renin, whereas volume expansion is predominantly responsible in those with low renin.

As imaginative and logical as this construct may be, in clinical practice most practitioners have not found renin profiling to be necessary for establishing prognosis or determining therapy. As will be noted in subsequent chapters, renin profiling is often used in the diagnosis of low- and high-renin forms of hypertension.

## THE SYMPATHETIC NERVOUS SYSTEM AND STRESS

As shown in Figure 3–2, an excess of renin and angiotensin activity could interact with the sympathetic nervous system (SNS) to mediate most of its effects. In contrast, stress may activate the SNS directly; and SNS overactivity, in turn, may interact with high sodium intake, the RAS, and insulin resistance, among other possible mechanisms. Considerable evidence supports increased SNS activity in early hypertension (Grassi & Mancia, 2004) and, even more impressively, in the still-normotensive offspring of hypertensive parents, among whom a large number are likely to develop hypertension.

Before considering further some of the evidence, a brief review of the pertinent physiology of the SNS will be provided.

### Normal Physiology

Figure 3–20 shows the two major neural reflex acts that are involved in the regulation of BP: the high-pressure baroreceptors of the aortic arch and carotid

sinus and the low-pressure cardiopulmonary baroreceptors (Chapleau, 2003). After the afferent signals enter the vasomotor center in the brainstem, efferent impulses traverse the parasympathetic and sympathetic nerves to the heart and vasculature. Sympathetic nerves and their catecholamine secretions induce their effects by multiple interactions with both presynaptic and postsynaptic receptors (Goldstein & Eisenhofer, 2003).

### Role in Primary Hypertension

As succinctly summarized by Grassi and Mancia (2004), the evidence for a significant role of the sympathetic nervous system in the pathogenesis of primary hypertension includes:

- The hyperkinetic circulation seen in some, usually young hypertensives, that could reflect a blunted parasympathetic and an enhanced sympathetic drive (Julius & Nesbitt, 1996).
- Plasma norepinephrine levels, an indirect marker of sympathetic function, are significantly elevated in hypertensives compared with normotensives (Goldstein, 1983).
- The rate of turnover of radiolabeled norepinephrine from the sympathetic neuroeffector junctions is increased in young hypertensives, particularly from the kidney and heart (Esler et al., 1989).

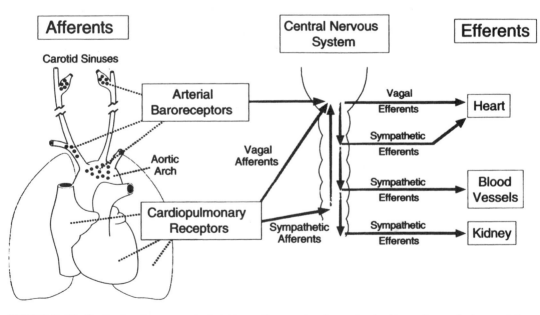

**FIGURE 3–20** ● Cardiopulmonary and arterial baroreflex neural pathways involved in cardiovascular homeostatis and blood pressure regulation. *Filled circles,* locations of arterial baroreceptors. (Modified from Chapleau MW. Arterial baroreflexes. In: Izzo JL, Black HR, eds. *Hypertension Primer: Essentials of High Blood Pressure,* 3rd Ed. Philadelphia: Lippincott Williams & Wilkins, 2003.)

- The uptake of a radiolabeled catecholamine mimic into the heart is lower and its washout rate is greater in hypertensives than in normotensives, suggesting enhanced adrenergic drive to the heart (Sakata et al., 1998). Schlaich et al. (2004a) also found reduced cardiac neuronal noepinephrine reuptake in hypertensives.
- With direct microneurographic measurement, efferent postganglionic sympathetic nerve traffic to the skeletal muscle is increased in primary but not secondary forms of hypertension, in parallel with the degree of hypertension (Anderson et al., 1988). This, too, was reaffirmed by Schlaich et al. (2004a) as by many other investigators.

Grassi and Mancia (2004) state: "Taken together, these findings therefore strongly support the notion that an increase in sympathetic cardiovascular drive participates in the development, maintenance, and progression of the hypertensive state and imply that sympathetic deactivation should represent a major goal of the antihypertensive pharmacologic treatment."

### Baroreceptor Malfunction

The arterial baroreceptors acutely respond to increases in blood pressure by parasympathetic activation and sympathetic inhibition, so that heart rate is slowed and vascular resistance decreased, buffering the rise in BP (Chapleau, 2003). Conversely, baroreceptor activity decreases when BP falls, producing reflex-mediated increases in heart rate and PR. Marked BP variability is seen in patients with baroreceptor denervation (Sharabi et al., 2003).

Baroreceptor activity is generally thought to be reset during sustained increases in BP so that baroreceptors are not thought to play a role in long-term control of BP. However, in conscious dogs, stimulation of baroreceptors for 7 days maintained a lower BP (Lohmeier et al., 2004), so perhaps baroreceptors may play a more persistent role in human BP control. Moreover, the reset baroreceptors still buffer changes in BP so that most hypertensives maintain normal baroceptor function (Schlaich et al., 2004b). Baroreceptor insensitivity or blunting, manifested as a diminished change in heart rate as BP changes, may occur in long-standing hypertension, presumably from arteriosclerotic stiffness of the large arteries wherein the receptors are located. The decreased baroreceptor sensitivity would permit elevated BP to remain high while simultaneously leading to the propensity to postural hypotension often seen in elderly patients with systolic hypertension (see Chapter 4).

### Brainstem Compression

In rats, lesions of the nucleus tractus solitarius in the medulla produce a labile form of hypertension. A connection between the experimental and clinical evidence has been claimed by Jannetta et al. (1985) and others (Naraghi et al., 1994) who have performed vascular decompression of looping arteries at the lateral aspect of the medulla. Further coverage of this contentious issue is provided in Chapter 6.

### Faulty Norepinephrine Reuptake

Esler and co-workers (Schlaich et al., 2004a) have found also an impairment of the neuronal reuptake of norepinephrine as a cause of the increased norepinephrine spillover seen in hypertensives, pointing to a peripheral rather than central nervous system origin of sympathetic overactivity.

### Renal Effects of Sympathetic Activity

Hypertensive patients decrease renal sodium excretion in response to mental stress (Schneider et al., 2001). This response, according to some, could also be a persistent part of the resetting of the pressure-natriuresis relation wherein decreased sodium excretion persists in the face of hypertension. In particular, Di Bona has spent much of his academic career providing evidence for a specifically activated renal sympathetic nerve activity (RSNA) as having a role in the pathogenesis of primary hypertension. He has recently summarized this evidence, along with a defense against some objections to this concept (DiBona, 2004). Despite this admirable dedication to this concept, DiBona admits that "acceptance [of increased RSNA] has been slow and incomplete."

## Changes with Age

Various indices of sympathetic nerve hyperreactivity are seen mainly in younger patients, including higher plasma levels of norepinephrine and epinephrine (Reims et al., 2004), norepinephrine spillover (Ferrier et al., 1993), and increased epinephrine release (Jacobs et al., 1997). Julius (1990) explains the tendency for previously elevated plasma norepinephrine levels to fall as hypertension becomes established by a negative feedback of the elevated BP per se on the central nervous system. This same explanation is offered for the transition from a high CO to an elevated vascular resistance. As stated by Julius and Nesbitt (1996):

> As hypertension escalates, the hemodynamic pattern changes from a high cardiac output to a high resistance pattern. This hemodynamic change is best explained by an alteration in the structure

and responsiveness of the heart and blood vessels. Decreased cardiac compliance and diminished α-adrenergic responsiveness tend to decrease cardiac output, whereas the development of vascular hypertrophy increases vascular resistance. In parallel, the sympathetic tone is down-regulated, since, with emerging vascular hyperresponsiveness, less sympathetic drive is needed to maintain the elevated blood pressure.

The concept seems logical, but sympathetic nerve traffic by microneurography (MSNA) increases with age (Narkiewicz et al., 2005), so more evidence is needed.

## Stress

Stress not only decreases sodium excretion by activation of the sympathetic nervous system (Schneider et al., 2001), but it may be involved in the pathogenesis of primary hypertension by a number of other mechanisms as well (Brydon & Steptoe, 2005).

### Relation Between Stress and Hypertension

Multiple studies suggest that people exposed to repeated psychogenic stresses may develop hypertension more frequently than would otherwise similar people who are not stressed.

- As an extreme example, the BP remained normal among nuns in a secluded order over a 30-year period, whereas it rose with age in women living nearby in the outside world (Timio et al., 1999).
- Air traffic controllers, who work under high-level psychological stress, annually develop hypertension at a rate 5.6 times greater than that of nonprofessional pilots who were initially comparable to the controllers in physical characteristics (Cobb & Rose, 1973). However, no differences in ambulatory BP were seen between 80 air traffic controllers in Milan and age-matched men in a nearby town (Sega et al., 1998).
- Among healthy employed men, job strain (defined as high psychological demands and low decision latitude on the job) is associated with higher awake ambulatory BP (Cesana et al., 2003; Steptoe & Willemsen, 2004), an increased risk for developing hypertension, and an increased left ventricular mass index by echocardiography (Pickering, 1997), at least partly mediated by an increased heart rate in response to stress (Vrijkotte et al., 2000).
- Exposure to major catastrophes such as earthquakes and massive explosions leads to higher levels of BP that may persist for months (Gerin et al., 2005).
- Multiple populations living in small, cohesive, protected societies have been found to have low BPs that do not rise with aging, whereas individuals who abandon such an environment and migrate to more urbanized, modern, disorganized societies have higher BPs that do rise with age (Kaufman et al., 1996; Poulter et al., 1990). Environmental factors such as weight gain and increased sodium intake may be responsible, but there is considerable evidence that social disorganization, as would be expected with migration, is associated with more hypertension.
- The relatively high prevalence of hypertension among Blacks has been attributed to their increased level of anger and social stresses (Shapiro et al., 1996) and greater pressor response to them (Knox et al., 2002). However, Blacks may not be unique in this regard: Whites with lower socioeconimc status (Diez Roux et al., 2002; Matthews et al., 2002) who are more anxious (Markovitz et al., 1993), who are unemployed (Brackbill et al., 1995), or who have less formal education (Stamler et al., 1992) also experience more hypertension and the higher mortality associated with it than do Whites with higher socioeconomic status.

## Reactivity to Stress

Even healthy young people display transient endothelial dysfunction after mental stress (Ghiadoni et al., 2000). However, greater cardiovascular and SNS reactivities to various ordinary life experiences (Mancia et al., 2003) and laboratory stresses have been documented in hypertensives and in normotensives at higher risk for developing hypertension (Borghi et al., 2004; Schneider et al., 2003; Steptoe & Marmót, 2005). extending even to a greater anticipatory BP response while awaiting an exercise stress test (Everson et al., 1996).

Some investigators, however, do not find increased responses to laboratory stresses among the offspring of hypertensives (de Visser et al., 1995; Manuck et al., 1996). Although the evidence for a different psychological substrate in prehypertensive people is impressive, it should be remembered that, with fewer exceptions (Armario et al., 2003; Matthews et al., 2004), most of the data are short-term, cross-sectional observations that may not relate to the underlying pathogenesis of hypertension. Julius et al. (1991b) found that hyperreactivity to mental stress was seen more often in the offspring of hypertensive parents, but that such hyperreactivity was unrelated to the future development of hypertension. In particular, there is a need to study patients' reactivity before they are aware of their diagnosis, as they may display increases in various measures of SNS activity in response to mental stress after becoming aware of their diagnosis

(Rostrup et al., 1991) or as a result of an alerting reaction to the examinations (Palatini et al., 1996).

Nonetheless, numerous studies show a greater intensity of anger and hostility (Knox et al., 2004) but, at the same time, a greater suppression of the expression of anger among hypertensives (Schneider et al., 1986), patients whose BP rises over time (Yan et al., 2003), and normotensive offspring of hypertensive parents (Perini et al., 1990).

Part of the explanation for the inconsistent findings of an enhanced pressor response to laboratory stress as a predictor of future hypertension may be the failure to consider both the genetic predisposition to hypertension and the level of life stress. In a 10-year follow-up of 103 young men, Light et al. (1999) found the highest rises in BP over time among those who responded most to laboratory stresses and who also had a positive family history of hypertension and were exposed to higher levels of daily stress.

Obviously, stress and hypertension are not always connected in isolation. As Pickering (1997) wrote:

> There is emerging evidence that the various stimuli that lead to hypertension are not independent of each other, but tend to interact in clusters. Thus exposure to stress may not only raise BP itself, but also lead to increased alcohol and fat intake. A final common pathway for many of these factors is the sympathetic nervous system, which is involved in the development of essential hypertension in its early stages, and in the hypertensive effects of salt, obesity, physical inactivity, and possibly stress as well.

### Summary

These various pieces of evidence add up to make a fairly strong case for a role of increased SNS activity in the pathogenesis of hypertension (Grassi & Mancia, 2004). This role may be even greater in magnitude when hypertension and obesity coexist, as they so often do (Daniels et al., 2005). Therefore, catecholamines are leading candidates to be both the pressor mechanism that initiates the rise in BP and the trophic mechanism that maintains hypertension via vascular hypertrophy.

Whatever the specific role of SNS activity in the pathogenesis of hypertension, it is likely involved in the development of hypertension-related target organ damages, including carotid atherosclerosis (Jennings et al., 2004), strokes (Waldstein et al., 2004), and heart attacks (Rosengren et al., 2004). In turn, SNS activation is almost certainly involved in the increased cardiovascular morbidity and mortality that afflicts hypertensive patients during the early morning hours. Epinephrine levels begin to increase after awakening and norepinephrine rises sharply on standing (Dodt et al., 1997). As a consequence of the increased SNS activity, BP rises abruptly and markedly and, as detailed in Chapter 2, this rise is at least partly responsible for the increase in sudden death, heart attack, and stroke during the early morning hours.

### PERIPHERAL RESISTANCE

The preceding sections have covered the major elements that could induce hypertension primarily by increasing CO. Although many variables can influence CO, the preceding discussion of fluid volume and myocardial contractility seems adequate to explain the primary mechanisms. However, when we turn to the second part of the equation BP = CO·PR, the situation becomes inherently more complicated. The multiple factors affecting PR that are shown in Figure 3–2 make up only a superficial listing of what may be involved (Simon, 2004).

For greater clarity, endothelial function and cell membrane alterations are considered separately, recognizing their close interactions. A continued problem of the use of various methodologies to measure endothelial function persists (Deanfield et al., 2005).

### Causes and Consequences

Beyond the complexities of what may influence PR is a fundamental problem: The major consequences of hypertension afflict the larger capacitance arteries, which are also the only ones that can be directly visualized and easily studied; however, the major cause of hypertension—elevated PR—resides in the distal resistance arteries and arterioles, with diameters of less than 1 mm, whose contribution can be studied only by biopsy and *in vitro* techniques (Park & Schiffrin, 2001). Therefore, most of the literature covers the larger arteries, both because they are more easily studied and because they are involved in the major complications induced by hypertension. Even the microcirculation, studied indirectly, plays a role in hypertension and its sequelae (Strain et al., 2005).

Another caveat is in order: Changes in vascular structure and function may be either the cause or the consequence of elevated BP. For example, even acute rises in BP disturb endothelial function (Mitchell et al., 2004), but endothelial dysfunction clearly can be responsible for rises in BP.

The atherosclerotic and arteriosclerotic consequences of hypertension are addressed in the next chapter. Here, however, as the role of PR in the pathogenesis of hypertension is considered, we should not lose sight of the primacy of the microcirculation in the genesis and maintenance of hypertension (Levy et al., 2001). This contribution of the microcirculation may involve even the capillary bed, because capillary rarefaction is present early in the course of hypertension (Ciuffetti et al., 2003), even in normotensive offspring of hypertensive parents (Noon et al., 1997).

## Vascular Changes in Hypertension

Hypertension, however it begins, is maintained by increased PR, largely due to decreased arterial lumen size or radius (Schiffrin, 2004). According to Poiseuille's law, vascular resistance is positively related to both the viscosity of blood and the length of the arterial system and inversely proportional to the radius of the fourth power. Because neither viscosity nor length is much, if at all, altered, and because small changes in the luminal radius can have a major effect, it is apparent that the increased vascular resistance seen in established hypertension must reflect changes in the caliber of the small resistance arteries and arterioles (Folkow et al., 1970; Safar, 2004). In studies of small resistance vessels from subcutaneous tissue of hypertensive subjects as compared to normotensives, increases in the ratio of media thickness to internal diameter of 26% to 62% have been recorded (Heagerty et al., 1993; Park et al., 2001). Because of the increased wall thickness–lumen diameter ratio, higher wall stress and intraluminal pressure develop when resistance vessels are stimulated.

### Remodeling

In response to flow, pressure, and vasoconstrictive factors (Figure 3–21), the structure of small arteries remodel, the process taking different patterns under different conditions (Mulvany, 2004) (Figure 3–22). In human primary hypertension, the pattern is inward eutrophic remodeling, a rearrangement of otherwise normal cells around a smaller diameter.

The determinants of remodeling have been described by Mulvany (2002) as shown in Figure 3–21:

> An increase in intravascular pressure causes an increase in the wall stress, which then stimulates a hypertrophic process leading to an increase in wall thickness. Increases in flow can also lead to increases in wall thickness. Here the mechanism is likely due, at least in part, to increased flow causing endothelial-mediated vasodilation, which—according to the Laplace relation—leads to increased wall stress, and again to increase in wall thickness. Hypertrophic processes are also thought to be initiated through growth factors, including angiotensin.

### Large-Vessel Hypertrophy

Unlike the eutrophic remodeling process in smaller resistance vessels, hypertrophic remodeling clearly develops in larger arteries as an early manifestation of primary hypertension (Schiffrin, 2004), with close symmetry between vascular and cardiac hypertrophy (Vaudo et al., 2000).

Much of our current knowledge about vascular hypertrophy has come from the study of certain

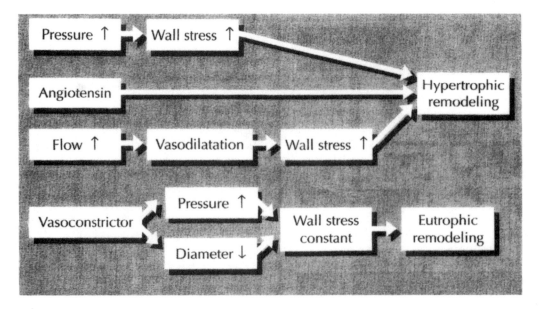

**FIGURE 3–21** ● Some determinants of small artery remodeling. (Modified from Mulvany MJ. Small artery remodeling in hypertension. *Curr Hypertens Rep* 2002;4:49–55.)

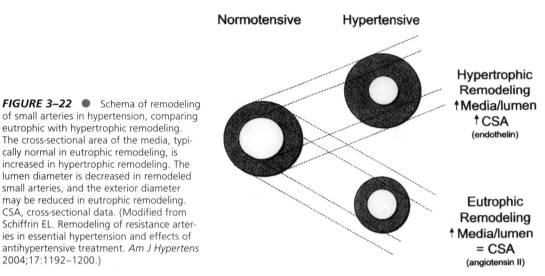

**FIGURE 3–22** ● Schema of remodeling of small arteries in hypertension, comparing eutrophic with hypertrophic remodeling. The cross-sectional area of the media, typically normal in eutrophic remodeling, is increased in hypertrophic remodeling. The lumen diameter is decreased in remodeled small arteries, and the exterior diameter may be reduced in eutrophic remodeling. CSA, cross-sectional data. (Modified from Schiffrin EL. Remodeling of resistance arteries in essential hypertension and effects of antihypertensive treatment. *Am J Hypertens* 2004;17:1192–1200.)

forms of endocrine hypertension, including pheochromocytoma, primary aldosteronism, and renovascular disease. Each of these secondary forms of hypertension is known to arise from the direct effect of a specific pressor hormone. What has now become obvious is that, regardless of the initial hormonal effect, whether it be volume retention (as with primary aldosteronism) or vasoconstriction (as with pheochromocytoma or renovascular disease), maintenance of hypertension derives from vascular hypertrophy that increases PR. As summarized by Lever and Harrap (1992):

> Most forms of secondary hypertension have two pressor mechanisms; a primary cause, e.g., renal clip, and a second process, which is slow to develop, capable of maintaining hypertension after removal of the primary cause, and probably self-perpetuating in nature. We suggest that essential hypertension also has two mechanisms, both based upon cardiovascular hypertrophy: (a) a growth-promoting process in children (equivalent to the primary cause in secondary hypertension); and (b) a self-perpetuating mechanism in adults.

### Sustaining Hypertrophic Response

As seen in Figure 3–23, Lever and Harrap (1992) start with the original proposal of Folkow (1990), wherein hypertension is initiated by a minor overactivity of a specific fast-acting pressor mechanism (e.g., AII) that raises BP slightly and initiates a positive feedback loop that induces vascular hypertrophy and maintains the hypertension. The amplification (or feedback loop) is "slowly progressive, ultimately large and probably nonspecific. Thus different forms of chronic hypertension may resemble each other because part of the hypertension in each has the same mechanism" (Lever, 1986). In the second and

third hypotheses, two other elements are added: a genetically determined, reinforced hypertrophic response and the direct contribution of one or more trophic mechanisms for hypertrophy.

This scheme, involving both an immediate pressor action and a slow hypertrophic effect, may be common to the action of various pressor-growth promoters. In the majority of hypertensive patients, no marked excess of any of the known pressor hormones is identifiable. Nonetheless, a lesser excess of one or more may have been responsible

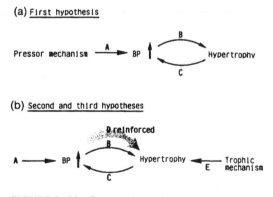

**FIGURE 3–23** ● Hypotheses for the initiation and maintenance of hypertension. (**A**) Folkow's first proposal that a minor overactivity of a pressure mechanism (A) raises blood pressure (BP) slightly, initiating positive feedback (*B* to *C* to *B*) and a progressive rise in blood pressure. (**B**) Second and third hypotheses, which are similar to the first, with two additional signals: an abnormal or "reinforced" hypertrophic response to pressure (*D*) and an increase of a humoral agent (*E*) that causes hypertrophy directly. (Adapted from Lever AF, Harrap SB. Essential hypertension: a disorder of growth with origins in childhood? *J Hypertens* 1992;10:101–120.)

for initiation of the process that is sustained by the positive feedback postulated by Folkow (1990) and the trophic effects emphasized by Lever and Harrap (1992). This sequence encompasses a variety of specific initiating mechanisms that accentuate and maintain the hypertension by a nonspecific feedback-trophic mechanism. If this double process is involved in the pathogenesis of primary hypertension, as seems likely, the difficulty in recognizing the initiating, causal factor is easily explained. In the words of Lever (1986):

> The primary cause of hypertension will be most apparent in the early stages; in the later stages, the cause will be concealed by an increasing contribution from hypertrophy. . . . A particular form of hypertension may wrongly be judged to have "no known cause" because each mechanism considered is insufficiently abnormal by itself to have produced the hypertension. The cause of essential hypertension may have been considered already but rejected for this reason.

## Mechanisms of Vascular Changes

The mechanisms that generate the narrowed lumen size of hypertension can involve either structural remodeling or a functional increase in vascular tone. In addition, increased mechanical stiffness of arteries occurs, attributable both to structural and functional changes.

As described by Touyz (2003):

> Functional alterations include enhanced reactivity or impaired relaxation, and reflect changes in excitation–contraction coupling, altered electrical properties of vascular smooth muscle cells, or endothelial dysfunction. Major structural changes include remodelling due to increased cell growth, extracellular matrix deposition and inflammation. . . . Vascular changes in hypertension are associated with humoral and mechanical factors that modulate signalling events, resulting in abnormal function and growth of cellular components of the media. Among the humoral factors that regulate arteries in hypertension are vasoconstrictor agents such as angiotensin II, endothelin-1, catecholamines and vasopressin; vasodilator agents such as nitric oxide, endothelium-derived hyperpolarizing factor and natriureic peptides; growth factors such as insulin-like growth factor-1, platelet-derived growth factor (PDGF), epidermal growth factor (EGF) and basic fibroblast growth factor; and cytokines such as transforming growth factor-β, tumour necrosis factor and interleukins. Mechanical factors that influence the vasculature in hypertension include shear stress, wall stress and direct actions of pressure itself.

Touyz (2003) emphasizes the major role of angiotensin II signaling through tyrosine kinases that can lead to inflammation, contraction, adhesion, migration, and cell growth (Imanishi et al., 2005). She also focuses on the role of reactive oxygen species (ROS), acting as inter- and intrasignaling molecules, thereby regulating vascular tone and structure.

### Oxidative Stress

Reactive oxygen species , undesirable byproducts of aerobic metabolism, include superoxide, hydroxyl radical, hydrogen peroxide, and other oxidants. Under usual conditions, ROS formation and elimination are balanced in the vessel wall. However, enhanced activity of oxidant enzymes or reduced activity of antioxidant enzymes can lead to oxidative stress (Lassègue & Griendling, 2004; Touyz, 2004; Wassmann et al., 2004) (Figure 3–24). Moreover, AII increases ROS by stimulating NAD(P)H oxidase activity (Imanishi et al., 2005).

Evidence of increased ROS production has been found in patients with severe (Lip et al., 2002) but not in milder degrees of hypertension (Cracowski et al., 2003). Nonetheless, multiple trials of antioxidants have been performed in hopes of preventing or treating cardiovascular disease, but such trials have been largely negative (Touyz, 2004). The disappointing outcomes could reflect the wrong types or doses of antioxidants or inclusion of patients with irreversible cardiovascular disease. In the meantime, the benefits of currently used antihypertensive drugs may be at least partly mediated by reducing oxidative stress (Ghiadoni et al., 2003). The combination of a NO donor and an antioxidant significantly reduced mortality in Blacks with congestive heart failure (CHF) (Taylor et al., 2004), posing the possible use of such therapy for hypertension.

### Arterial Stiffness

These interacting factors affect arterial structure and function differently throughout the arterial bed, which has been roughly divided into proximal and distal compartments. As Safar et al. (2003) state:

> The proximal compartment (the aorta and its main branches) is characterized by low stiffness and is composed of VSM cells originating from the neural crest and involving prominent secretory properties (elastin and collagen). This compartment is highly sensitive to age and changes in BP. It differs substantially from the distal compartment, which is characterized by a higher stiffness. The distal compartment is the major source of wave reflections, and is mainly composed of [vascular smooth muscle] cells with contractile properties, which are highly sensitive to vasoactive substances, particularly those of endothelial origin. . . . The 2

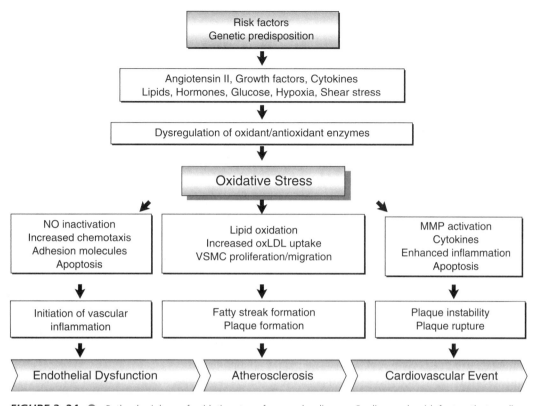

**FIGURE 3–24** ● Pathophysiology of oxidative stress for vascular disease. Cardiovascular risk factors that predispose to atherogenesis are associated with oxidative stress. Oxidative stress promotes pathological cellular events, which are involved in the development and progression of atherosclerosis at all stages of the disease. oxLDL, oxidized low-density lipoprotein; MMP, matrix metalloproteinase. (Modified from Wassmann S, Wassmann K, Nickenig G. Modulation of oxidant and antioxidant enzyme expression and function in vascular cells. *Hypertension* 2004;44:381–386.)

compartments of the arterial tree are interconnected by an information system that consists of BP propagation, from which frequency-dependent mechanical signals arise independently of and in addition to conventional neurohumoral signals. This information system is based on arterial stiffness, wave reflections, and PP. Their message is related to CV survival and longevity.

Over the past few years, large artery stiffness has been the focus of increasing attention, mainly because of its primary role in the progressive rise in systolic BP with age (Tomiyama et al., 2004). Stiffness, in the words of Mitchell (2004):

. . .depends on three basic properties of the artery—wall stiffness, wall thickness, and lumen diameter. Because these individual arterial properties are often difficult or impossible to measure in vivo, an alternative approach is to consider the functional implications of increased arterial stiffness and then establish methods to evaluate this functionality. In addition to delivering blood to the periphery (the "conduit" function), two key elements of aortic functionality are to minimize the pulsatile pressure generated

by a given ventricular flow wave and to keep waveform propagation velocity or pulse wave velocity (PWV) relatively low. The first requirement serves to limit the amplitude of the forward pressure wave ($P_f$) that is generated by a given flow wave in the central aorta [Figure 3–25]. The second requirement (low PWV) arises because of the presence of reflected pressure waves in the arterial system.

A forward traveling pressure wave is partially reflected at branch points and other areas where arterial properties change quickly, including the interface between muscular arteries and arterioles. The innumerable tiny reflections from these various reflecting sites summate to form a relatively discrete composite reflected wave that returns to the central aorta in late systole or early diastole when PWV is low [Figure 3–25A]. The presence of wave reflection in the arterial system is normally favorable because it returns a substantial component of the pulsatile energy of the advancing pressure wave to the central circulation, where it is dissipated, thus protecting the microcirculation from exposure to excessive pressure pulsatility. Furthermore, a properly timed reflected wave augments coronary

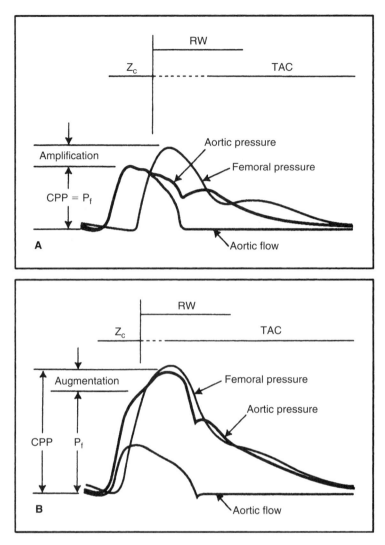

**FIGURE 3–25** ● Carotid (*thick black line*) and femoral (*thin black line*) pressures and central aortic flow (*gray line*) in normotensive (**A**) and hypertensive (**B**) individuals. Horizontal lines at the top of each panel represent phases of the cardiac cycle when characteristic impedance ($Z_c$), the reflected wave (RW), and total arterial compliance (TAC) have their predominant effects on the pressure waveform shape. In **A**, flow was rescaled to similar units as pressure (using $Z_c$) to illustrate the marked similarity between pressure and flow in a normal arterial system. In **B**, flow is plotted on approximately the same scale as in **A**. Note the much greater increase in pressure in early systole in the hypertensive individual, despite a lower peak flow. (Modifed from Mitchell GF. Arterial stiffness and wave reflection in hypertension: pathophysiologic and therapeutic implications. *Curr Hypertens* Rep 2004;6:436–441.)

perfusion pressure in diastole, when the bulk of coronary perfusion normally occurs. If PWV is elevated, the reflected wave can return to the heart prematurely during systole. Premature reflected waves increase central pulse pressure (CPP), which increases pulsatile load on the heart and cyclic stress on the proximal aorta [Figure 3–25B].

### Clinical Applications

These arterial properties are being measured in a variety of different ways (Table 3–5) providing indices of different qualities of function (Table 3–6). Despite considerable enthusiasm over their clinical usefulness (O'Rourke et al., 2002), two caveats remain: First, as noted by McVeigh et al. (2002):

## TABLE 3–5

### Methods of Assessing Arterial Stiffness

| Method | Advantages | Disadvantages |
| --- | --- | --- |
| Pulse pressure | Simple | Less accurate than other methods |
|  | Equipment readily available | Central pulse pressure more useful than peripheral pulse pressure |
| Pulse wave velocity | Relatively simple | Relatively expensive |
|  | Portable equipment | Some training required |
| Ultrasound | Can measure distensibility | Operator-dependent |
|  |  | Expensive, nonportable equipment |
| MRI | Can measure distensibility | Very expensive |
|  |  | Limited availability |
| Waveform analysis | Relatively simple | Relatively expensive |
|  | Portable | Some training required |
| Oscillometric blood pressure measurement | Simple | May be less accurate than other methods, especially in the elderly |

"All techniques have theoretical, technical, and practical limitations that impact on their widespread applications in the clinical setting and use as measurement tools to improve cardiovascular risk stratification." Second, no outcome data are available on their diagnostic or predictive value (Davies & Struthers, 2003).

Despite these caveats, measures of stiffness and pressure wave indices have been amply documented to be related to clinical cardiovascular disease (O'Rourke, 2004). In particular, the easiest to measure—pulse pressure—has been closely correlated with both cardiovascular morbidity and mortality (Safar & Smulyan, 2004).

Recently presented data suggest that arterial stiffness is not simply the result of hypertension but may be its cause. In the words of Franklin (2005): "the relationship may be bidirectional." Liao et al. (1999) were the first to show that increased stiffness (measured by ultrasonography of the carotid artery) was associated with an increased risk of future hypertension, independent of the level of BP or the presence of other traditional risk factors. The same predictive power has

## TABLE 3–6

### Indices of Arterial Stiffness

| | |
| --- | --- |
| Elastic modulus | The pressure step required for (theoretical) 100% stretch from resting diameter at fixed vessel length |
| Arterial distensibility | Relative diameter (or area) change for a pressure increment; the inverse of elastic modulus |
| Arterial compliance | Absolute diameter (or area) change for a given pressure step at fixed vessel length |
| Volume elastic modus | Pressure step required for (theoretical) 100% increase in volume |
| Young's modulus | Elastic modulus per unit area; the pressure step per square centimeter required for (theoretical) 100% stretch from resting length |
| Pulse wave velocity | Speed of travel of the pulse along an arterial segment |
| Characteristic impedance | Relationship between pressure change and flow velocity in the absence of wave reflections |
| Stiffness index | Ratio of logarithm (systolic/diastolic pressures) to relative change in diameter |

Modified from O'Rourke M. Mechanical principles in arterial disease. *Hypertension* 1995;26:2–9.

been shown by Dernellis and Panaretou (2005) and Najjar et al. (2004).

Hopefully, therapies can be developed that will specifically reduce stiffness, both for prevention and treatment (Safar, 2005). Currently available drugs, including diuretics and ACEIs, improve large artery function but most of their effort is on pressure *per se* and not on intrinsic properties of the vessel walls (Mitchell, 2004). Meanwhile, a most impressive effect upon large artery compliance in older patients with systolic hypertension has been seen with dietary sodium restriction (Gates et al., 2004).

Even more impressively, among otherwise healthy young adults, weight loss of 4.6 kg or more per year was associated with a significant reduction in arterial stiffness measured by pulse wave velocity, whereas weight gain of 4.5 kg or more was associated with a significant increase in stiffness (Wildman et al., 2005). In addition, poor fitness is associated with stiffness, and physical activity can reduce it (Boreham et al., 2004).

## ENDOTHELIAL FUNCTION

The factors affecting arterial stiffness include a number arising from the endothelium (Calles-Escandon & Cipolla, 2001) (Table 3–7). By the release of a variety of relaxing and contracting factors shown in Figure 3–26, endothelial cells regulate vascular tone and reactivity. Pertubations in one or more of these endothelial-derived factors leads to endothelial dysfunctions that can reduce vasodilation, add to inflammation, and incite thrombosis (Endemann & Schiffrin, 2004a). Of these, nitric oxide (NO) is most frequently implicated (Wilkinson et al., 2004).

A deficiency of circulating endothelial progenitor cells derived from the bone marrow, which are used for ongoing repair of endothelial injury, has been shown to be associated with a higher level of the overall cardiovascular risk profile and a greater degree of endothelial dysfunction (Hill et al., 2003).

## Nitric Oxide

In 1980, Furchgott and Zawadzki showed that, in vessels constricted by norepinephrine, the normal relaxing response to acetylcholine was abolished if the endothelial lining was rubbed off, depriving the cells of an endothelium-derived relaxing factor. Seven years later, Palmer et al. (1987) identified the endothelium-derived relaxing factor as NO, now known to be the primary endogenous vasodilator.

## TABLE 3–7

### Endothelial Cell Functions

| Functional Targets | Specific Cellular or Physiological Action (mediators are listed in *italics*) | |
|---|---|---|
| Lumen | Vasoconstriction | Vasodilation |
| | *Endothelin* | *Nitric oxide* |
| | *Angiotensin II* | *Bradykinin* |
| | *Thromboxane A$_2$* | *Hyperpolarizing factor* |
| | *Prostaglandin H$_2$* | |
| Growth | Stimulation | Inhibition |
| | *Platelet growth-derived factor* | *Nitric oxide* |
| | *Fibroblast growth factor* | *Prostaglandin I$_2$* |
| | *Insulin growth factor-1* | *Transforming growth factor* |
| | *Endothelin* | |
| | *Angiotensin II* | |
| Inflammation | Proinflammatory | Antiinflammatory |
| | *Adhesion molecules (ELAM, VCAM, ICAM)* | |
| Hemostatis | Prothrombotic | Antithrombotic |
| | *PAI-1* | *Prostacyclin* |
| | | *Tissue plasminogen activator* |

Modified from Calles-Escandon J, Cipolla M. Diabetes and endothelial dysfunction. *Endocrine Rev* 2001;22:36–52.

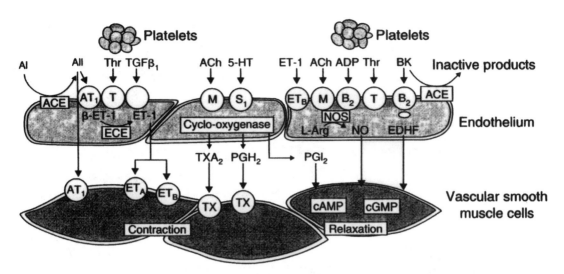

**FIGURE 3–26** ● Endothelium-derived vasoactive substances. NO is released from endothelial cells in response to shear stress and to activation of a variety of receptors. NO exerts vasodilating and antiproliferative effects on smooth muscle cells and inhibits thrombocyte aggregation and leukocyte adhesion. Endothelin-1 (ET-1) exerts its major vascular effects—vasoconstriction and cell proliferation—through activation of specific $ET_A$ receptors on vascular smooth muscle cells. In contrast, endothelial $ET_B$ receptors mediate vasodilatation via release of NO and prostacyclin ($PGI_2$). Additionally, $ET_B$ receptors in the lung were shown to be a major pathway for the clearance of ET-1 from plasma. ACE, angiotensin-converting enzymes; ACh, acetylcholine; ADP, adenosine diphosphate; AI, angiotensin I; AII, angiotensin II; $AT_1$, angiotensin 1 receptor; $B_2$, bradykinin receptor; BK, bradykinin; ECE, endothelin-converting enzyme; EDHF, endothelium-derived hyperpolarizing factor; $ET_A$ and $ET_B$, endothelin A and B receptor; L-Arg, L-arginine; M, muscarinergic receptor; $PGH_2$, prostaglandin $H_2$; S, serotoninergic receptor; Thr, thrombin; T, thromboxane receptor; $TXA_2$, thromboxane $A_2$; 5-HT, 5-hydroxytryptamine; TGF, tumor growth factor; cGMP, cyclic guanosine monophosphate; cAMP, cyclic adenosine monophosphate. (Modified from Cosentino F, Lüscher TF. Effects of blood pressure and glucose on endothelial function. *Curr Hypertens Rep* 2001;3:79–88.)

The synthesis of NO is controlled by the enzyme endothelial NO synthase and is induced by calcium-mobilizing agents and fluid shear stress (Govers & Rabelink, 2001). The intravascular half-life of NO is approximately 2 milliseconds, but its extravascular half-life is up to 2 seconds, depending on tissue oxygen concentration (Thomas et al., 2001).

### Physiologic Role

NO has been characterized as the perfect messenger (Madison, 1993): fast, because it is not stored in vesicles; short-lived; easily passable through and between cells; and economically produced from an abundant and recyclable substrate. In addition, it uses ubiquitous regulatory machinery (e.g., guanylate cyclase). Basal generation of NO keeps the arterial circulation in an actively dilated state (Vallance, 1998). When the inhibitor of NO synthesis, *N*-monomethyl-L- arginine, is infused, BP rises (Rees et al., 1989). Beyond its major role in controlling the cardiovascular system, NO is a principal factor involved in the antiatherosclerotic properties of the endothelium, inhibiting platelet-vessel wall interaction, endothelial permeability, and proliferation of vascular smooth muscle cells (Wilkinson et al., 2004).

### Pathologic Role

Under basal conditions, whole-body NO production is diminished in patients with essential hypertension (Forte et al., 1997), and impaired NO synthesis may play a role in hypertension and atherosclerosis that develop with aging, hypercholesterolemia, diabetes, homocystinemia, smoking, and physical inactivity. With few exceptions (Cockcroft et al., 1994), hypertensives have been shown to have an impaired vasodilative response (usually measured as forearm blood flow) to NO stimulants (usually acetylcholine) but not to endothelium-independent vasodilators such as nitroprusside, as first reported by Panza et al. (1990) and Linder et al. (1990). The impairment, also demonstrated by ultrasonography in response to reactive hyperemia (Iiyama et al., 1996), may reflect more than just reduced synthesis of NO (Kelm et al., 1996; Panza et al., 1995) but is not related to decreased availability of substrate (Panza et al., 1993). As noted by Hare (2004), an imbalance between NO availability and reactive oxygen species, i.e., the nitroso-redox balance, may be involved in CHF and other cardiovascular diseases.

The evidence for a role of defective NO-mediated vasodilation in the pathogenesis of hypertension has been further strengthened by its recognition in the still-normotensive children of hypertensive parents (McAllister et al., 1999). Impaired L-arginine transport may be the link between defective NO production and primary hypertension (Schlaich et al., 2004b). However, the fact that even transient rises in BP significantly impair endothelium-dependent vasodilation (Paniagua et al., 2000) raises the fundamental question: Is defective endothelium-dependent vasodilation that is mediated by NO the cause or the consequence of hypertension? The answer is likely a causal connection since changes in flow-mediated vasodilation precede and predict the future development of hypertension (Rossi et al., 2004).

### Effects of Therapy

Drugs that contribute NO, such as nitroglycerin, have been the cornerstone of antianginal therapy for centuries, and nitroprusside is the most potent antihypertensive agent. As of now, the only long-acting NO donor for treatment of hypertension is isosorbide mono- or dinitrate, but no large-scale trials to prove its efficacy are anticipated since it is generic. However, the remarkable benefit of a combination of isosorbide dinitrate and hydralazine in Blacks with CHF (Taylor et al., 2004) may provide the impetus for testing of nitrates with an antioxidant for hypertension.

Variable effects of various classes of antihypertensive drugs on endothelium-dependent vasodilation have been reported (Spieker & Lüscher, 2004), but reduction of BP per se does not seem to restore endothelial function (Endemann & Schiffrin, 2004a).

### Aging, Hypercholesterolemia, and Diabetes

A progressive reduction in NO-availability and endothelium-dependent vasodilation with increasing age has been seen in cross-sectional studies of both normotensive and hypertensive patients (Taddei et al., 2001).

Hypercholesterolemia, in addition to promoting atherosclerosis, may aggravate hypertension by impairing vasodilation, as seen in coronary arteries and forearm resistance vessels (Creager et al., 1990). Lipid-lowering therapy has been shown to restore bioavailability of NO (John & Schmieder, 2000), an effect that occurs with statins even without lowering of blood lipid levels (Wilson et al., 2001).

Diabetes may engender its vascular havoc through impaired endothelial function (Calles-Escandon & Cipolla, 2001; Cosentino & Lüscher, 2001). It is likely that every major cardiovascular risk factor may work, at least in part, through endothelial dysfunction (Glasser et al., 1996).

### Other Vasodilators

In the excitement over NO, the roles of other putative relaxing factors, shown in Figure 3–26, are seldom mentioned. Prostacyclin and a still-unidentified endothelium-derived hyperpolarizing factor, which may be potassium (Savage et al., 2003), may also be involved (Cohen, 2005).

### Endothelin

The left of Figure 3–26 shows a number of endothelium-derived contracting factors. Of these, endothelin has been increasingly emphasized since its discovery in 1988 (Yanagisawa et al., 1988). Now known to be composed of four distinct peptides, the endothelins have been shown to have a wide range of biologic actions that may involve them in numerous pathologic conditions (Savoia & Schiffrin, 2004). Endothelin-1 is the predominant endothelium-derived isoform, exerting its major vascular effect—vasoconstriction and cell proliferation—through activation of specific endothelin A receptors on vascular smooth muscle cells (Aiello et al., 2005). Although plasma endothelin-1 levels were not related to hypertension (Hirai et al., 2004), obese hypertensives showed an enhanced vasoconstrictor response to endogenous endothelin-1 (Cardillo et al., 2004). Moreover, in some hypertensive patients, enhanced endothelial expression of the endothelin-1 gene has been seen in small resistance arteries, suggesting a possible role in vascular hypertrophy (Schiffrin et al., 1997), whereas polymorphisms of the gene were associated with lower BP (Dong et al., 2004). The role of endothelin may be most critical in maintaining sodium balance (Perez del Villar et al., 2005).

As effective endothelin blockers become available, they may turn out to be useful in the treatment of heart failure (Hürlimann et al., 2002) and perhaps hypertension (Nakov et al., 2002).

### Other Vasoconstrictors

Through the action of cytochrome P-450 and other enzymes, arachidonic acid is converted to a number of epoxyeicosatrienoic acids (EETs) and hydroxyeicosatetraenoic (HETEs) acids (Fleming, 2005). Of these, 20-HETE acts as both a vasoconstrictor and a natriuretic. A variant of the gene controlling production of 20-HETE has been associated with hypertension in human subjects, presumably by a decrease in the synthase of 20-HETE (Gainer et al., 2005). Laffer et al. (2003a) have shown that decreases in 20-HETE were involved with the reduced natriuresis in salt-sensitive patients in response to diuretics.

## INFLAMMATORY MARKERS

Inflammation is associated with endothelial dysfunction and, in turn, with elevations in blood pressure even in the prehypertensve (<140/90 mm Hg) stage (Chrysohoou et al., 2004). C-reactive protein (CRP) has been most frequently used as the marker of inflammation (Venugopal et al., 2005). Increased serum levels of other markers including interleukin-6, soluble intracellur adhesion molecule-1, and monocyte chemotactic protein-1 have also been found (Bautista et al., 2005) and shown to be associated with reduced brachial artery vasodilation in response to hyperemia in the Framingham Offspring Study (Vita et al., 2004). As a likely consequence of the inflammatory process as reflected in CRP levels, the incidence of hypertension was 52% higher among women with initially normal BP and no traditional coronary risk factors but whose CPR levels were in the higher quintile (above 3.5 mg/L) (Sesso et al., 2003).

Granger et al. (2004) pose this sequence:

Risk factors for CVD [cardiovascular disease] cause endothelial cells throughout the vascular tree to assume an inflammatory phenotype. These activated endothelial cells characteristically exhibit oxidative stress and increased adhesiveness for circulating leukocytes. . . . Recent work has implicated a variety of additional factors that can modulate the magnitude and/or nature of the inflammatory responses in CVD. Platelets, angiotensin II, and the CD40/CD40 ligand signaling system are gaining recognition as contributors to the pathogenesis of CVD. These factors appear to converge with known pathways that link oxidative stress with adhesion molecule expression and help to explain the apparent integration of

coagulation with inflammation in CVD. These factors also hold the promise of offering multiple sites for therapeutic intervention in CVD.

## CELL MEMBRANE ALTERATIONS

The preceding sections reviewed the possible role of various factors acting through presumably normal cell membranes. There is, however, a body of evidence that shows that the cell membranes of hypertensive animals and, less convincingly, of hypertensive people are altered in a primary manner, allowing abnormal movement of ions and thereby changing the intracellular environment to favor contraction and growth (Swales, 1990a) (Figure 3–27). These primary alterations are differentiated from the secondary inhibition of the $Na^+/K^+$-ATPase pump by a putative natriuretic hormone secreted after volume expansion, described earlier in this chapter, that may be a mechanism for renal sodium retention.

### Ion Transport across Membranes

Figure 3–28 portrays some of the transport systems present in the cell membrane of erythrocytes that control the movement of sodium and potassium to maintain the marked differences in concentration of these ions on the outside and inside of cells, differences which, in turn, provide the electrochemical gradients needed for various cell functions (Jiang et al., 2004). Abnormalities of the physical properties of the membrane and of multiple transport systems have been implicated in the pathogenesis of hypertension (Russo et al., 1997). Most of what follows relates to vascular smooth muscle cells but, because such human

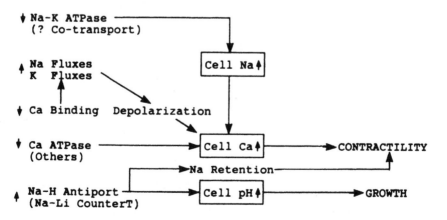

**FIGURE 3–27** ● Hypotheses linking abnormal ionic fluxes to increased peripheral resistance through increases in cell sodium (Na), calcium (Ca), or pH. ATPase, adenosine triphosphatase; CounterT, countertransport; K, potassium; Li, lithium. (Modified from Swales JD. Functional disturbance of the cell membrane in hypertension. *J Hypertens* 1990a;8(Suppl 7): S203–S211.)

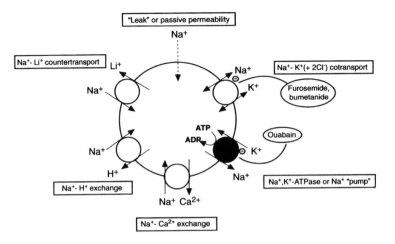

**FIGURE 3–28** ● Abnormalities of one or more of the sodium ($Na^+$) transport pathways depicted are thought to contribute to the development of essential hypertension. Solid circle, active transport; *open circles*, passive transport; *open ovals*, inhibitors; ADP, adenosine diphosphate; ATP, adenosine triphosphate; $Ca^{2+}$, calcium; $Cl^-$, chlorine; $H^+$, hydrogen; $K^+$, potassium; $Li^+$, lithium. (Modified from Weder AB. Membrane sodium transport. In: Izzo JL, Black HR, eds. *Hypertension Primer*, 2nd Ed. Dallas: American Heart Association, 1999;52.)

cells are not readily available for study, surrogates such as red and white blood cells have been used. There are serious reservations about the pertinence of these in vitro measurements to in vivo changes (Swales, 1991), but at least some of these in vitro findings have also been seen in vascular smooth muscle cells of hypertensive rats and humans (Orlov et al., 1999).

It has become obvious that none of these defects is present in all or even the majority of hypertensives, and Swales in particular questioned their pathogenetic role. He concluded that "the best unifying hypothesis is that all the reported abnormalities are markers for a disturbance of physicochemical properties of the cell membrane lipids of hypertensive patients" (Swales, 1990b). Because the active transport of sodium is a fundamental property of all cells, even minor changes in the properties of cell membranes could lead to secondary alterations in sodium transport (Swales, 1991).

### Intracellular Sodium

Most measurements of intracellular sodium have found higher concentrations in cells from hypertensives than in those from normotensives (Lijnen, 1995). However, a number of technical, environmental, and racial factors have been recognized to affect red blood cell sodium concentration.

### Sodium-Hydrogen Exchange

An increased $Na^+/H^+$ exchanger could play a significant role in the pathogenesis of hypertension, both by stimulating vascular tone and cell growth and, possibly, by increasing sodium reabsorption in renal proximal tubule cells (Soleimani & Singh, 1995). In 12 of 27 hypertensives, high $Na^+/H^+$ exchanger activity was associated with lower fractional sodium excretion and inappropriately low levels of plasma renin activity (Díez et al., 1995).

### Sodium-Lithium Countertransport

To simplify measurements without using radioisotopes, under appropriate conditions intracellular $H^+$ can be replaced by $Li^+$, and the exchange for external $Na^+$ can be measured as sodium-lithium countertransport (SLC) (Canessa, 1995). SLC is under genetic control and is increased in many hypertensives and patients with diabetic nephropathy. Whatever its role, SLC has been noted to be the most frequent and persistent measure of abnormal red blood cell sodium transport in hypertensives. Over 6- to 8-year follow-up periods, high SLC was significantly associated with the incidence of hypertension (Laurenzi et al., 1997; Strazzullo et al., 1998) and rising BP over 10 years in Chinese children (Mu et al., 2004).

### Alterations in Cell Membranes

Red blood cell membranes from hypertensives have an increased cholesterol-phospholipid ratio in association with high SLC (Villar et al., 1996) and increased ratios of fatty acid metabolites to precursors as compared to those from age-matched normotensives (Russo et al., 1997). Such changes in lipids produce a high membrane microviscosity and decrease in fluidity (Carr et al., 1995), which may be responsible for increased permeability to sodium and other alterations in sodium transport (Zicha et al., 1999).

### Calcium Transport and Binding

Even mild mechanical perturbation of cultured endothelial cells causes a rapid increase of intracellular calcium (Sigurdson et al., 1993). It is easy to visualize a major contribution of increased membrane calcium concentrations to the heightened vascular tone that is involved in the increased PR of hypertension. A significantly increased calcium content was found in the membranes of red blood cells in 39 untreated hypertensives as compared to 40 normotensives (Kosch et al., 2001). Both plasma and intracellular calcium concentrations were similar in the two groups. Even without increases in calcium concentration, vasoactive stimuli may act through calcium signaling. In some manner, two endothelium-derived vasoconstrictors, endothelin and thromboxane $A_2$, increased the calcium sensitivity of the contractile apparatus of arteriolar smooth muscle so that similar increases in intracellular calcium elicited greater myogenic constriction (Ungvari & Koller, 2000).

### Ion Channels

The functions of ion channels across cell membranes are fundamental determinants of vascular tone (Jackson, 2000). Mechanosensitive channels in vascular smooth muscle cells are likely responsible for the signal transduction of a mechanical stimulus, i.e., stretch, to a cellular response, i.e., vasoconstriciton. Drummond et al. (2004) have provided evidence that degenerin/epithelial sodium channel (DEG/ENaC) proteins may serve as the mechanosensor in vascular cells.

Now that various mechanisms that may induce hypertension either through CO or PR have been covered, consideration will be given to some clinical conditions that are associated with a higher incidence of hypertension.

## OBESITY

The first and foremost of these clinical conditions is the triad of obesity, the metabolic syndrome, and type 2 diabetes, both because they contribute so much to the prevalence of hypertension but also because they are growing at a phenomenal rate in young people (Ferreira et al., 2005). The evidence about obesity includes:

- Over 65% of the U.S. adult population is overweight (BMI >25), 30% are obese (BMI >30), and 5.1% are massively obese (BMI >40) (Hedley et al., 2004).
- Over 42 years of observations, 40-year-old male obese nonsmokers lost 5.8 years of life expectancy, and 40-year-old obese female nonsmokers lost 7.1 years (Peeters et al., 2003).
- The highest rate of growth of obesity is among U.S. children aged 6 through 19, with 16% overweight (defined as BMI >95 percentile) (Hedley et al., 2004).
- Among 16-year-olds in Quebec, Canada, 30% had high-normal or elevated systolic BPs closely associated with BMI (Paradis et al., 2004).

### Association with Hypertension

Weight gain, even to levels not considered to be a problem, increases the incidence of hypertension. This was clearly shown in a cohort study of more than 80,000 women participating in the Nurses' Health Study (Huang et al., 1998) (Figure 3–29). Those women, now in midlife, who had gained as little as 5 kg over their weight at age 18 had a 60% higher relative risk of developing hypertension than did those whose weight had not changed more than 2 kg. Those who gained 10 kg or more had a 2.2-fold greater risk. In a cross-sectional study, adults with a BMI >40 had a 6.38 times greater odds ratio for hypertension (Mokdad et al., 2003). A further estimate of the association comes from the Framingham Study: Seventy percent of hypertension in men and 61% in women were directly attributable to excess adiposity; a 4.5-mm Hg average increase in systolic BP was seen with every 10-pound weight gain (Kannel et al., 1993).

Moreover, obesity is accompanied by an increased incidence of hypertension-related outcomes, including stroke (Jood et al., 2004), coronary disease (Widlansky et al., 2004), heart failure (Kenchaiah et al., 2002), and restrictive cardiomyopathy (Pilz et al., 2004).

### Mechanisms of Hypertension with Obesity

The hemodynamic pattern of obesity-related hypertension is volume expansion, increased cardiac output, and systemic vascular resistance that fails to fall enough to balance the higher cardiac output (Taler et al., 2004b).

A large number of mechanisms are supported by data from animal and human observations

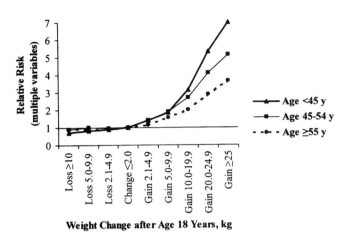

**Weight Change after Age 18 Years, kg**

**FIGURE 3–29** ● Multivariate relative risk for hypertension according to weight change after 18 years within strata of age among U.S. women enrolled in the Nurses' Health Study. Adjusted for age, body mass, index at age 18 years, height, family history of myocardial infarction, parity, oral contraceptive use, menopausal status, postmenopausal use of hormones, and smoking status. (Modified from Huang Z, Willett WC, Manson JE, et al. Body weight, weight change, and risk of hypertension in women. *Ann Intern Med* 1998;128:81–88.)

(Rahmouni et al., 2005) (Figure 3.30). Recent references for each include:

- Increased sympathetic nervous activity (Landsberg, 2001)
- Increased renin-angiotensin activity (Gorzelniak et al., 2002)
- Increased aldosterone (Ehrhart-Bornstein et al., 2003)
- Increased leptin from selective leptin resistance (Correia & Haynes, 2004)
- Increased insulin (Sowers & Frohlich, 2004)
- Increased free fatty acids (Nielsen et al., 2004a)
- Decreased nitric oxide (Perticone et al., 2001)
- Increased endothelin-1 (Cardillo et al., 2004)

Figure 3–30 does not exhaust the potential mechanisms for obesity-related hypertension. Fat cells are literally factories, turning out a large number of proteins with endocrine functions (Kershaw & Flier, 2004). Many of these have been implicated as pro-hypertensive, including leptin, angiotensinogen, and 11β-hydroxysteroid hydrogenase-1 (Kannisto et al., 2004). On the other hand, Unger (2005) has made a persuasive case for a protective effect of the hyperleptinemia against lipid-induced damages seen in diet-induced obesity.

As a consequence of whatever is responsible, weight gain is accompanied by increased arterial stiffness as measured by pulse wave velocity (Wildman et al., 2005). Those who are obese have impaired microvascular function (de Jongh et al., 2004).

## Prevention of Obesity Hypertension

The lifestyle changes and drug therapy of obesity-related hypertension are covered in Chapters 6 and 7, respectively. However, in view of its importance, a few comments about the need and the possible methods for prevention of obesity seem appropriate.

The problem, as noted earlier in this chapter, starts during the first 2 postnatal weeks from too rapid weight gain, particularly in low-birth-weight babies (Stettler et al., 2002). Thereafter, a number of environmental barriers are imposed on physical activity and healthful diet (Ebbeling et al., 2002). A common sense approach to preventing and treating childhood obesity (Table 3–8) would improve the currently "toxic" environment we have imposed on our children.

Once developed, significant obesity is almost impossible to overcome save by gastric surgeries. Despite a lot of good advice, e.g., Klein et al. (2004a), Manson et al. (2004), and Willett et al. (1999), many practitioners do not even advise obese patients to lose weight (Galuska et al., 1999), and those who really try have little success (Moore et al., 2003).

Acupuncture doesn't work (Lacey et al., 2003), but drinking more cool water may help by generating heat before absorption (Boschmann et al., 2003). More drugs are being advocated (McTigue et al., 2003; Van Gaal et al., 2005), but most provide small and short-term effects. Bariatric surgery does work (Cummings et al., 2004), with increasingly less danger (Steinbrook, 2004). However, the even more popular liposuction does not improve patients' risk factors (Klein et al., 2004b).

The same aggressive, multifaceted strategies used against tobacco will likely be needed to force the large multinational companies that are responsible for pushing energy dense foods on a willing public, particularly children (Chopra & Darnton-Hill, 2004). Until or if that campaign works, people increasing just their daily level of physical activity can make a major impact on the prevention of obesity (Blair & Church, 2004). Perhaps we can walk up that flight of stairs, just as an example to our patients.

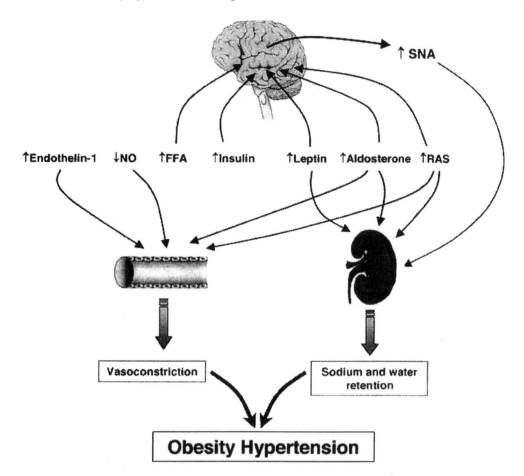

**FIGURE 3–30** ● Summary of mechanisms and hormonal systems involved in obesity-associated hypertension. FAA, free fatty acids; SNA, sympathetic nerve activity. (Modified from Rahmouni K, Correia ML, Haynes WG, Mark AL. Obesity-associated hypertension: new insights into mechanisms. *Hypertension* 2005;45:9–14.)

## THE METABOLIC SYNDROME

Obesity in the periphery is not as bad as obesity localized in the upper body, i.e., visceral or abdominal or masculine obesity (Ferreira et al., 2004; Tankó et al., 2003). This difference was observed by Jean Vague (1956) (actually in 1947 but in a French paper that received little attention) and has been so well confirmed that an increased waist circumference is a principal component of the Metabolic Syndrome (Eckel et al., 2005) (Table 3–9). This simple set of criteria is a better determinant of risk than those used by other groups (Hunt et al., 2004). To label a patient as having the syndrome, three of the five features need to be present.

The role of abdominal obesity is critical, both for the presence of the other elements (Nieves et al., 2003; Sironi et al., 2004) and for its independent role in the consequences of the syndrome (Empana et al., 2004; Nicklas et al., 2004).

### Prevalence

Among the adult U.S. population, more than 20% have the Metabolic Syndrome. The prevalence differs between men and women in the three major ethnic categories (Park et al., 2003) (Figure 3–31). Using a definition analagous to the adult criteria, 9.2% of U.S. adolescents aged 12 to 19 had the syndrome (de Ferranti et al., 2004). Among European adults, a 15% prevalence has been found (Hu et al., 2004).

### Mechanisms

Most patients who develop the full syndrome start with obesity (Palaniappan et al., 2004), which congregates in the abdomen under both genetic and environmental influences (Reilly & Rader, 2003) (Figure 3–32).

## TABLE 3-8

### A Common Sense Approach to Prevention and Treatment of Childhood Obesity

| | |
|---|---|
| Home | Set aside time for |
| |    Healthy meals |
| |    Physical activity |
| | Limit television viewing and computer gaming |
| School | Fund mandatory physical education |
| | Establish stricter standards for school lunch programs |
| | Eliminate unhealthful foods—e.g., soft drinks and candy—from vending machines |
| | Provide healthy snacks through concession stands and vending machines |
| Urban design | Protect open spaces |
| | Build pavements (sidewalks), bike paths, parks, playgrounds, and pedestrian zones |
| Health care | Improve insurance coverage for effective obesity treatment |
| Marketing and media | Consider a tax on fast food and soft drinks |
| | Subsidize nutritious foods—e.g., fruits and vegetables |
| | Require nutrition labels on fast-food packaging |
| | Prohibit food advertisement and marketing directed at children |
| | Increase funding for public-health compaigns for obesity prevention |
| Politics | Regulate political contributions from the food industry |

Modified from Ebbeling et al.,Childhood obesity: public-health crisis, common sense cure. *Lancet* 2002;360:473–482.

Once there, abdominal fat cells and elements of innate immunity set off various adipokines, cytokines, and inflammatory markers that induce the lipid, glucose/insulin, and blood pressure abnormalities that comprise the full syndrome (Eckel et al., 2005). Thereby, atherosclerosis is accelerated,

eventuating in increased risks for coronary disease (McNeill et al., 2004), stroke (Suk et al., 2003), and cardiovascular mortality (Malik et al., 2004) that are greater than those seen with individual components of the syndrome.

### Insulin Resistance

Insulin resistance and consequent hyperinsulinemia are not part of the five elements that make up the Metabolic Syndrome as defined by the NCEP expert panel (2002) (Table 3–9).

Nonetheless, insulin resistance is virtually ubiquitous in the presence of abdominal obesity and is directly involved with the other elements: the primary mechanism for glucose intolerance and/or diabetes, and dyslipidemia, a secondary mechanism for hypertension (Reaven, 1988). As seen in Figure 3–32, Reilly and Rader (2003) have put insulin resistance in place of diabetes. Moveover, they (Reilly et al., 2004) and virtually

## TABLE 3-9

### Diagnostic Criteria for the Metabolic Syndrome

Abdominal girth, >35 inches (88 cm) in women, >40 inches (102 cm) in men

HDL-C, <40 mg/dL in men, <50 mg/dL in women

Triglycerides, fasting, >150 mg/dL (1.69 mmol/L)

Blood pressure, >130/85 mm Hg

Fasting glucose, ≥110 mg/dL (>6.1 mmol/L)

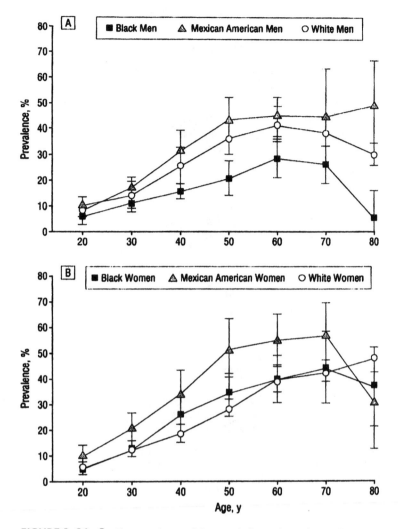

***FIGURE 3–31*** ● The prevalence of the metabolic syndrome by age in men (**A**) and women (**B**) in the Third NHANES sample. Error bars represent the 95% confidence interval, expressed as the mean ± 1.96 SE. (Modified from Park YW, et al. The metabolic syndrome: prevalence and associated risk factor findings in the US population from the Third National Health and Nutrition Examination Survey, 1988-1994. *Arch Intern Med* 2003;163:427–436.)

all investigators in this field recognize that insulin resistance per se adds incremental value to the clinical diagnosis of the Metabolic Syndrome in determining cardiovascular risk (Eckel et al., 2005).

## Hypertension

The presence of abdominal obesity is associated with an increased incidence of hypertension beyond what is seen with generalized obesity in multiple populations (Canoy et al., 2004; Ding et al., 2004; Gus et al., 2004; Hayashi et al., 2004). The presence of the syndrome amplifies the risk seen with hypertension alone (Schillaci et al., 2004; Scuteri et al., 2004).

### Mechanisms for Hypertension

The evidence for a causal relationship between insulin resistance and hypertension includes:

- Hyperinsulinemia is directly correlated with blood pressure in multiple populations (Reaven, 2003).
- Hyperinsulinemia often presages the development of hypertension and is often found in the still normotensive children of hypertensive parents.
- Insulin resistance is present in about 50% of patients with primary hypertension (Reaven, 2003) but is rarely seen in secondary forms of hypertension.
- Hyperinsulinemia can induce a number of pro-hypertensive mechanisms, including endothelial

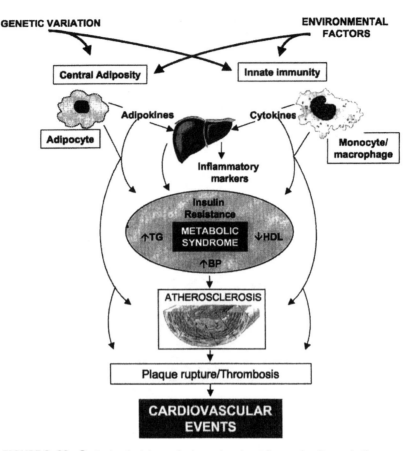

**FIGURE 3-32** ● Pathophysiology of atherosclerotic cardiovascular disease in the Metabolic Syndrome. Central adiposity and innate immunity play key roles in the development of insulin resistance, chronic inflammation, and Metabolic Syndrome features through the effects of the adipokines (e.g., leptin, adiponectine, resistin) and cytokines (e.g., tumor necrosis factor-α, interleukin-6) on liver, skeletal muscle, and immune cells. In addition, monocyte/macrophage and adipocyte-derived factors may have direct atherothrombotic effects that promote the development of atherosclerotic cardiovascular events. (Modified from Reilly MP, Rader DJ. The metabolic syndrome: more than the sum of its parts? *Circulation* 2003;108:1546–1551.)

dysfunction (Arcaro et al., 2004), endogenous angiotensin II production (Tuck et al., 2004), and activation of the sympathetic nervous system (Haffner & Taegtmeyer, 2003).

- The normal vasodilatory effect of insulin, mediated through increased nitric oxide (NO) production is impaired in patients with primary hypertension (Baron et al., 2000), which in turn may be mediated by impaired NO synthesis (Kashyap et al., 2005).
- Reduction in insulin resistance/hyperinsulinemia by physical activity and weight loss or drugs can lower blood pressure (Matthaei et al., 2000).

The relation looks solid but there are a few holes:

- In some ethnic groups, neither insulin resistance nor hyperinsulinemia were related to

hypertension in those with type 2 diabetes (Saad et al., 2004).
- Insulin resistance and the Metabolic Syndrome are occasionally seen separately in patients with high-normal BP (Egan et al., 2004).
- In dogs with obesity-induced hypertension, insulin resistance is not directly related to the rise in BP (Rocchini et al., 2004).

Beyond insulin resistance, other mechanisms suggested by the higher prevalence and greater risk of hypertension as part of the Metabolic Syndrome include:

- Increased renin-angiotensin activity (Prasad & Quyyumi, 2004) and responsiveness (Nielsen et al., 2004b)
- More intense inflammation (Rutter et al., 2004)

- Increased renal sodium retention (Strazzullo et al., 2001)
- Increased sympathetic nervous system activity (Egan, 2003)

Most, if not all of these, could reflect insulin resistance and hyperinsulinemia.

### Management

As with all forms of hypertension, lifestyle changes are useful but difficult to achieve (Eckel et al., 2005). Intensive control of diabetes and dyslipidemia should be provided and one of the glitazones may provide additional benefit (Grassi, 2004). Treatment of the hypertension should avoid high doses of diuretic and β-blockers.

## DIABETES

Type 2 diabetes is growing rapidly in prevalence as obesity increases and is becoming a major source of end-stage renal failure, strokes, heart failure, and heart attacks as it starts earlier in life and persists for many years (Almdal et al., 2004). In the United States, the lifetime risk of developing diabetes for people born in 2000 is 32.8% for men and 38.5% for women (Narayan et al., 2003). If diagnosed at age 40, diabetic men will lose 11.6 years of life, women 14.3 years. The global prevalence of diabetes is expected to increase from 171 million people in 2000 to 366 million in 2030 (Wild et al., 2004).

### Hypertension

The usual suspects—hyperglycemia, insulin resistance, and hyperinsulinemia, as well as increased free fatty acids—are involved in the oxidative stress and reduced nitric oxide availability that leads to the vasoconstriction, inflammation, and thrombosis that characterize diabetes (Creager et al., 2003; Endemann & Schiffrin, 2004b). Hyperglycemia adds additional insults (Tropeano et al., 2004) and is independently associated with the development of hypertension (Bjørnholt et al., 2003).

### Prevalence

Diabetes mellitus and hypertension coexist more commonly than is predicted by chance, perhaps three times more commonly. In those with insulin-dependent diabetes (type 1), hypertension is seen in most of the 40% who develop nephropathy but is seen no more frequently in those who escape nephropathy than in the nondiabetic population (Nørgaard et al., 1993). In those with insulin-independent diabetes (type 2), almost all of whom are obese, hypertension is more common than among obese people without diabetes (Hypertension in Diabetes Study Group, 1993). As noted earlier, the connection between hypertension, diabetes, and obesity is even stronger in those whose obesity is predominantly in the upper body, comprising the major components of the Metabolic Syndrome.

### Mechanisms

In both type 1 and type 2 diabetics, hyperinsulinemia is present: in type 1, because the amount of exogenous insulin given is larger than the normal endogenous levels; in type 2, because of obesity-induced insulin resistance with resultant increased secretion of insulin in the eventually futile attempt to maintain euglycemia.

The hypertension seen in type 2 diabetics is characterized by both volume expansion and increased vascular resistance, the latter related to the accelerated atherosclerosis that is common with long-standing hyperglycemia (Hackam et al., 2004). Even when the BP is reduced, resistance arteries from diabetic hypertensives show greater remodeling than seen in untreated hypertensives (Endemann et al., 2004).

The consequences of the coexistence of diabetes and hypertension are covered in Chapter 4 and the treatment of the diabetic hypertensive in Chapter 7. Here, mention will only be made of the potential advantages of peroxisome proliferator-activated ligands (PPARs), i.e., the glitazones, in blocking some of the underlying pathophysiology of diabetes (Villareal & Asbun, 2004). The special problems of diabetic nephropathy are described in Chapter 9.

### Hyperuricemia

The steadily growing evidence for a causal role of hyperuricemia in primary hypertension has been largely marshalled by Johnson et al. (2005). In brief, their evidence includes:

- The initial description of an association between uric acid and hypertension by Mahomed in 1879 was followed by many similar observations over the next 100 years (Klein et al., 1973).
- The induction of hypertension in rats made hyperuricemic (Mazzali et al., 2001). This has been found to reflect renal afferent thickening and vasoconstriction (Sánchez-Lozada et al., 2005).
- The publication of nine studies showing that an increased uric acid level predicts the development of hypertension (Johnson et al., 2004). These include data from the Bogalusa Heart Study wherein childhood uric acid levels predicted hypertension over an average 12 year follow-up (Alper et al.,

# Johnson et al's Pathogenesis of Hypertension

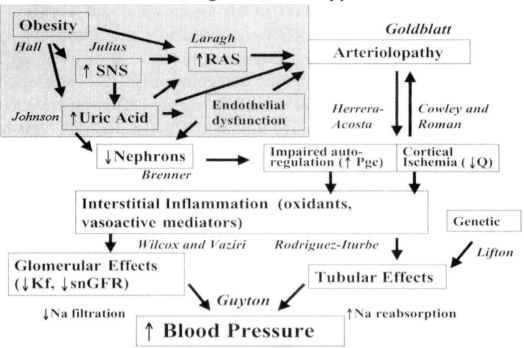

**FIGURE 3–33** ● A schema for the pathogenesis of primary hypertension incorporating a role for hyperuricemia, proposed by Johnson et al. (2005b). The upper left shaded area represents the initial phase which is sodium-resistant and which progresses into a sodium sensitive form of hypertension through a shift in pressure-natriuresis. (Modified from Johnson RJ, Rodriguez-Iturbe B, Kang D-H, et al. A unifying pathway for essential hypertension. *Am J Hypertens* 2005b;18:431–440.)

2005) and from the Framingham Study wherein uric acid level was an independent predictor of hypertension (Sundström et al., 2005).

- Recognition of impaired endothelial function with hyperuricemia that was improved when uric acid levels were reduced (Mercuro et al., 2004).
- Recognition of an elevated uric acid level as a strong independent predictor of cardiovascular mortality (Niskanen et al., 2004).

Johnson et al. (2005c) provide an overall scheme for the pathogenesis of primary hypertension which includes hyperuricemia (Figure 3–33). Obviously, more will be forthcoming including results of a proper trial to see if reducing uric acid levels will reduce blood pressure.

## OTHER POSSIBLE MECHANISMS FOR PRIMARY HYPERTENSION

The preceding exposition of the multiple factors shown in Figures 3–2 and 3–33 does not, unfortunately, exhaust the possible mechanisms for primary hypertension. The evidence for the mechanisms that

follow is less impressive, and some of these factors seem to affect only a portion of the larger hypertensive population.

## Abnormal Steroid Metabolism

In addition to the known monogenic forms of hypertension involving mineralocorticoid effects mentioned at the beginning of this chapter and described more fully in Chapters 13 and 14, claims have been made for a number of abnormal patterns of adrenocortical response to stimulation and types of hormones secreted in addition to aldosterone as described in the next paragraph. These include:

- Increased level of urinary free cortisol in sodium-resistant hypertensives (Litchfield et al., 1998)
- A relation between cortisol and left ventricular mass independent of BP (Duprez et al., 1999)
- Slightly elevated corticosterone levels (Soro et al., 1996)
- Increased vasoconstrictor sensitivity to glucocorticoids (Walker et al., 1996)

- Increased levels of ACTH from the left ventricle (Mizuno et al., 2005)

## Aldosterone

After lying almost dormant for 40 years, only rising for the putatively rare patient with primary aldosteronism, aldosterone has become the designer hormone in primary hypertension over the past few years (Freel & Connell, 2004). The reasons are multiple, including:

- Increased aldosterone levels, still within the "normal" range, predispose people to hypertension (Vasan et al., 2004). Such slight elevations require higher levels of sodium intake to cause mischief (Sato & Saruta, 2004).
- Even higher levels of aldosterone (and renin-angiotensin) have been found in normotensive type 1 diabetics (Hollenberg et al., 2004).
- Aldosterone receptors are present on human vascular smooth muscle cells (Jaffe & Mendelsohn, 2004) and rat cardiac myocytes (Mano et al., 2004).
- Aldosterone is produced in the heart (Wasywich et al., 2004).
- Aldosterone has rapid damaging effects on vascular endothelial and smooth muscle cells and cardiac fibroblasts and myocytes in vitro, effects that are not blocked by aldosterone receptor blockers (Lösel et al., 2004).
- Aldosterone acts in concert with angiotensin II (Michel et al., 2004; Xiao et al., 2004).
- Aldosterone induces myocyte apoptosis through calcineurin-dependent pathways (Mano et al., 2004).
- Aldosterone induces a "proinflammatory vascular phenotype" with changes in intracellular Mg, Ca, and $H_2O_2$ (Ahokas et al., 2005). Moreover, increased levels of the inflammatory markers in SHR animals are normalized by aldosterone antagonists but not by other anti-hypertensive drugs (Sanz-Rosa et al., 2005).

An excellent review of the pathophyiology of aldosterone in the cardiovascular system has been written by two of the investigators responsible for the development of the new aldosterone receptor blocker eplerenone (Rocha & Funder, 2002). Although some of the mischief induced by aldosterone may not work through its receptor, most does, and the deleterious effects can be prevented by receptor blockers (Martinez et al., 2002).

## Vasoactive Peptides

Some of these—the natriuretic peptide family (Talwar et al., 2000), adrenomedullin (Charles et al., 1999), calcitonin gene-related peptide (Supowit et al., 2005)—are likely little involved with the pathogenesis of primary hypertension.

### Kallikrein-Bradykinin

One group, the kallikrein-bradykinin system, has primarily been of interest because of its likely role in inducing the cough and angioedema that often accompany angiotensin-converting enzyme inhibitor (ACEI) therapy as well as probably contributing to its antihypertensive efficacy (Watanabe et al., 2005). Because the kininase that inactivates bradykinin is inhibited by ACEIs, the subsequent higher levels of bradykinin induce vasodilation by endothelium-dependent hyperpolarization (Batenburg et al., 2004) and increased prostacyclin synthesis (Yamasaki et al., 2000).

Whether contributing only to the benefits of ACEIs or providing additional benefits, including a major role in regulation of renal hemodynamics by vasodilation of efferent aterioles (Ren et al., 2002), bradykinin may play a greater role in human hypertension than was previously recognized (Sànchez et al., 2003).

### Other Vasoactive Peptides

Less is known about the role of a number of other vasoactive peptides in human hypertension. These include:

- Adenosine (Ledent et al., 1997)
- Dopamine (Kuchel, 1999)
- Melatonin (Arangino et al., 1999)
- Neuropeptide Y (Michel & Rascher, 1995)
- Opioid peptides (McCubbin et al., 1998)
- Parathyroid hormone-related peptide (Schlüter & Piper, 1998)
- Serotonin (Missouris et al., 1998)
- Substance P (Newby et al., 1997)
- Vasopressin (Mohr & Richter, 1994)

## Prostaglandins

Various prostaglandins have different sites of origin and different effects on BP. Platelet-derived thromboxanes promote platelet aggregation, constrict vascular smooth muscle, and may inhibit sodium excretion. Prostacyclin, synthesized within the blood vessel wall, inhibits platelet aggregation; relaxes vascular smooth muscle; and, by reducing renal vascular resistance, promotes natriuresis. Prostaglandin $E_2$ is vasodilative, and prostaglandin $F_2\alpha$ is vasoconstrictive. As autocrine or paracrine hormones, they may be involved in both contraction and relaxation of vascular smooth muscle (Figure 3–26).

Despite numerous findings that suggest a role for prostaglandins, the general impression is that prostaglandins probably are not major players in primary hypertension. Prostacyclin biosynthesis, assessed by urinary excretion of metabolites, was not correlated with BP, either treated or untreated (Ritter et al., 1996). However, prostaglandins may be needed to sustain the renal circulation in the face of any situation in which it is threatened (Imig, 2000). The inhibition of renal prostaglandins may be responsible for the slight rise in BP and the more impressive inhibition of the action of various antihypertensive agents with the use of nonsteroidal antiinflammatory drugs (Whelton, 2001). As previously noted, changes in other arachidonic acid derivatives may be involved (Fleming, 2005).

### Medullipin: The Renomedullary Vasodepressor Lipid

After 40 years of persistent work, Muirhead (1993) and co-workers documented both the existence and the role of a substance secreted from renal medullary cells that appears to function as a counterbalance to the effects of AII. The renomedullary hormone, called *medullipin I*, requires activation by the cytochrome P-450-dependent enzyme system of the liver into medullipin II.

The structure of this substance remains unknown, but its existence has been strongly inferred from multiple experiments in animals, wherein a rise in renal perfusion causes BP to fall (Göthberg, 1994). This hypotensive response depends on an intact renal medulla and is not altered by renal denervation or the inhibition of RAS or autonomic nervous function (Cowley, 1994). A patient with persistent hypotension associated with elevated medullipin levels has been described (Muirhead et al., 1993). Whether medullipin functions under normal circumstances and is involved in various human hypertensive diseases remains to be ascertained.

## CONTRIBUTING FACTORS

A number of secondary features may contribute to the role of the primary mechanisms of hypertension covered earlier in this chapter—for example, the major impact of physical inactivity on obesity and diabetes. Beyond these primary and secondary mechanisms, a variety of factors may raise the BP in those who are exposed and susceptible to them. Either because they do not impact the majority of individuals who develop hypertension or because they have only a minimal effect, these factors are considered to be contributing rather than causal. Most of modern society's major lifestyle faults can be included among the contributors: smoking, alcohol abuse, stress, physical inactivity, excessive caloric intake

that causes obesity, and reduced intake of fresh fruits and vegetables (Hajjar et al., 2001). Some of these are more likely directly implicated, and they have been given more emphasis earlier in this chapter.

### Fetal Environment

As noted earlier in the section Reduced Nephron Number, the development of hypertension may begin in utero: Low birth weight, from intrauterine growth retardation, and rapid post-natal weight gain are associated with the subsequent development of hypertension in most surveys.

### Calcium and Parathyroid Hormone

Beyond the probability that increased intracellular calcium is involved in the pathogenesis of hypertension, as noted earlier in this chapter, there are other aspects of the relationship between calcium and hypertension.

The following findings usually are noted in uncomplicated, untreated primary hypertension:

- Lower dietary intake of calcium (McCarron et al., 1984).
- Increased urinary calcium excretion (McCarron et al., 1980), which is likely the reason for an increased incidence of kidney stones (Borghi et al., 1999) and perhaps, eventually, for lesser bone density (Cappuccio et al., 1999).
- Lower plasma ionized calcium levels (Hvarfner et al., 1990).
- Increased levels of parathyroid hormone in some, likely related to reduced intake of calcium (Jorde et al., 2000). Parathyroid hormone levels are even higher in Blacks than Whites and are potentially able to raise BP (Fliser et al., 1997).

One way to put the various components into a logical sequence is depicted in Figure 3–34 (MacGregor & Cappuccio, 1993). The starting point has long been known: Whenever intravascular volume is expanded and sodium excretion is increased, calcium excretion increases (Suki et al., 1968). Intake of more sodium leads directly to an increase in calcium excretion (Breslau et al., 1982). The remainder of the scheme fits with the known associations and strongly supports a reduction in dietary sodium intake rather than an increase in dietary calcium intake to help overcome the consequences.

### Other Minerals

#### Potassium

Considerable data suggest that a lower intake of potassium is involved in hypertension (Tobian,

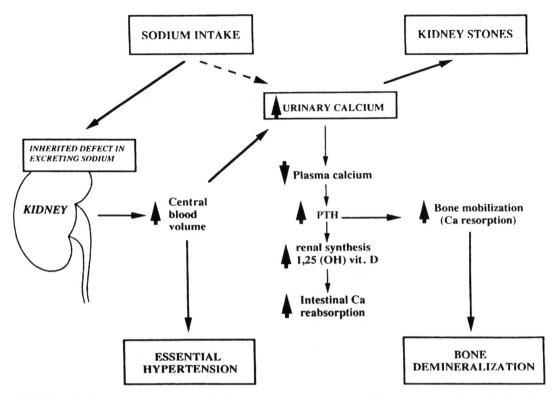

**FIGURE 3–34** ● Hypothesis on the possible link between the kidney, essential hypertension, and bone demineralization. 1,25 (OH) vit. D, 1,25-dihydroxyvitamin D; Ca, calcium; PTH, parathyroid hormone. (Modified from MacGregor GA, Cappuccio FP. The kidney and essential hypertension: a link to osteoporosis? *J Hypertens* 1993;11:781–785.)

1988) and stroke mortality (Fang et al., 2000). These include population surveys showing an inverse relation between dietary potassium intake and BP (Hajjar et al., 2001; Stamler et al., 1997), particularly in Blacks (Veterans Administration Cooperative Study Group, 1987) and extending to children (Geleijnse et al., 1990). Blacks and sodium-sensitive hypertensives may have impaired ability to conserve potassium (Aviv et al., 2005). Skeletal muscle potassium is decreased in untreated hypertensives (Ericsson, 1984). As noted in Chapter 6, potassium depletion will raise BP, whereas potassium supplementation may lower the BP. The overall potassium intake of modern people has certainly been reduced below that of our ancestors (Table 3–2), so there are logical reasons to advocate a return to a more "natural" higher-potassium/lower-sodium diet.

### Magnesium

Magnesium, beyond its role in activation of many critical enzymes involved in intermediary metabolism and phosphorylation, works as a natural antagonist to many of the actions of calcium (Howard et al., 1995). Concentrations of serum and intracellular free magnesium are generally normal in hypertensives (Delva et al., 1996). A family with hypertension, hypercholesterolemia, and hypomagnesemia was found to have a maternally linked mutation in the mitochondrial genome (Wilson et al., 2004). As the authors conclude: "These findings may have implications for the common clustering of these metabolic disorders."

### Lead

Long-term exposure to even low levels of lead may lead to hypertension, perhaps by increased production of reactive oxygen species (Ding et al., 2001). Increased blood lead levels were associated with higher BPs among Blacks and postmenopausal women examined in the third National Health and Nutrition Examination Survey (Nash et al., 2003; Vupputuri et al., 2000). These data fit with an association between low-level lead exposure and accelerated renal damage in patients with chronic renal disease (Lin et al., 2003).

### Other Trace Metals

More hypertension has been seen in association with long-term exposure to arsenic (Chen et al.,

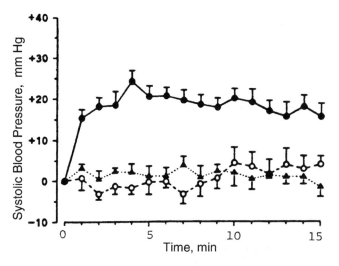

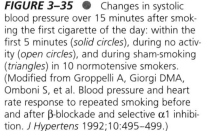

FIGURE 3–35 ● Changes in systolic blood pressure over 15 minutes after smoking the first cigarette of the day: within the first 5 minutes (*solid circles*), during no activity (*open circles*), and during sham-smoking (*triangles*) in 10 normotensive smokers. (Modified from Groppelli A, Giorgi DMA, Omboni S, et al. Blood pressure and heart rate response to repeated smoking before and after β-blockade and selective α1 inhibition. *J Hypertens* 1992;10:495–499.)

1995) and carbon disulfide (Egeland et al., 1992). In a 6-year follow-up of healthy children in Finland, no association was noted between BP and dietary, blood, or tissue levels of copper, zinc, or selenium (Taittonen et al., 1997). No association was found with exposure to environmental cadmium (Staessen et al., 2000).

## Smoking

The nicotine in cigarette smoke acutely raises BP, even in addicted smokers (Groppelli et al., 1992) (Figure 3–35). No tolerance develops, so the BP remains high as long as the patient continues to smoke (Verdecchia et al., 1995). However, the effect of each cigarette is transient and is over within 30 minutes; if the BP is taken in a smoke-free environment, as in most physicians' offices and clinics, the pressor effect may be missed. Cigars, if inhaled, and smokeless tobacco also raise BP (Bolinder & de Faire, 1998), but nicotine replacement therapies do not appear to do so (Rigotti et al., 2002).

Cross-sectional data on smokers and nonsmokers are not consistent: Some studies find smokers to have a higher BP (Poulsen et al., 1998), whereas others find smokers to have a lower BP (Mikkelsen et al., 1997). Regardless, all who smoke should be strongly advised to quit (Pardell & Rodicio, 2005). Smoking is associated with insulin resistance (Rönnemaa et al., 1996) and an attenuation of endothelium-dependent relaxation (Celermajer et al., 1996). These multiple adverse effects obviously add to the major cardiovascular damage induced by smoking (Doll et al., 2004).

## Caffeine

Acutely, consumption of the caffeine contained in 3 cups of coffee will raise BP an average of 4/3 mm Hg (Hartley et al., 2004). Some develop tolerance to this effect (Lovallo et al., 2004), and only an average 2.4/1.2 mm Hg higher pressure has been noted in those who drink 5 cups or more of coffee per day compared to nondrinkers. In contrast, increasing caffeine intake, ascertained by multiple careful dietary recalls, was associated with *lower* BP among the participants in the Multiple Risk Factor Intervention Trial (Stamler et al., 1997). Three cups of black tea raised the BP even more than seen with 3 cups of coffee, but the pressor effect was prevented when the tea was accompanied with food (Hodgson et al., 2005).

## Alcohol

The possible role of alcohol, in amounts consumed by a large part of the overall population, needs special emphasis. In contrast to its immediate vasodepressor effect (Kawano et al., 1996), chronic consumption, even of only moderate quantities, may raise the BP; in larger quantities, alcohol may be responsible for a significant amount of hypertension (Thadhani et al., 2002).

### Nature of the Relationship

The association between alcohol and hypertension was reported in 1915 by Lian, but not until Klatsky et al. (1977) documented it in a large population was alcohol recognized as a pressor substance. The association has been seen in more than 50 population studies (Estruch et al., 2005): Some show a linear relationship throughout the entire range of consumption; others show a J-shaped relationship, with slightly less hypertension in individuals who consume fewer than two drinks per day as compared to those who abstain (Shaper et al., 1988) (Figure 3–36). As much as 10% of hypertension in

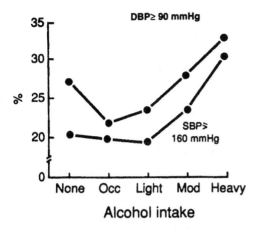

**FIGURE 3–36** ● Age-adjusted prevalence rates (%) of measured systolic and diastolic hypertension by levels of alcohol intake in drinks. DBP, diastolic blood pressure; Occ, occasional drinking; Light, one or two drinks daily; Mod, moderate (three to six drinks daily); Heavy, more than six drinks daily; SBP, systolic blood pressure. (Modified from Shaper AG, Wannamethee G, Whincup P. Alcohol and blood pressure in middle-aged British men. *J Hum Hypertens* 1988;2:71S–78S.)

men can be attributed directly to alcohol excess (MacMahon, 1987). Those who drink large quantities of alcohol only on weekends have a higher 24-hour ambulatory BP on Monday than on Thursday, whereas those who drink daily have similar BPs on both days (Rakic et al., 1998). More hypertension was found among people who drank without food consumption than in those who drank with food (Stranges et al., 2004). When heavy drinkers quit or reduce their intake, their BP usually goes down (Xin et al., 2001).

The J-shaped pattern shown in Figure 3–36 parallels the association with total and coronary mortality. Moderate consumption has been associated with less cardiovascular morbidity and mortality (Mukamal et al., 2003), and this protection applies to hypertensive men as well (Malinski et al., 2004).

### Physical Inactivity

The critical importance of physical activity to prevent obesity and insulin resistance was noted earlier in this chapter. This protection may reflect the finding that regular aerobic exercise prevents and restores age-related declines in endothelium-dependent vasodilation (DeSouza et al., 2000).

People who are physically active and fit are less likely to develop hypertension, and those who are hypertensive may lower their BP by regular isotonic exercise (Blumenthal et al., 2000). Normotensive people who were at a low level of physical fitness, as assessed by maximal treadmill

testing, had a 52% greater relative risk for developing hypertension over the following 1 to 12 years as compared to people who were initially at a high level of physical fitness (Blair et al., 1984).

### Temperature and Altitude

Blood pressure tends to be higher in colder weather (Jansen et al., 2001), which may play a role in the increase in cardiovascular mortality seen during the winter months (Khaw, 1995). Similarly, ascent to higher altitude may raise the BP (Wolfel et al., 1994), and more hypertension may be seen among those who live at higher altitudes (Khalid et al., 1994).

## ASSOCIATIONS WITH HYPERTENSION

In addition to all of these possible mechanisms, surveys of large populations reveal a number of associations with hypertension that are likely not directly causal but are reflective of shared mechanisms or of consequences of the hypertension.

### Hematologic Findings

Lee (2002) has summarized the observational evidence for a possible causal role of various hemorheological factors. Some of these changes could reflect reactions to inflammation.

### Red Cells

Probably related to decreased plasma volume, higher hematocrits are found in hypertensives and are associated with abnormal left ventricular filling on echocardiography (Schunkert et al., 2000). In the young subjects in the Tecumseh study, higher hematocrits were associated with higher BP, weight, cholesterol, glucose, and insulin levels (Smith et al., 1994). In middle-aged subjects in England, the risk of stroke was three times higher in hypertensives with a hematocrit above 51% than in those with a lower hematocrit (Wannamethee et al., 1994).

### White Cells

Elevated white blood cell counts are predictive of the development of hypertension (Shankar et al., 2004) and are likely related to insulin resistance and hyperinsulinemia (Facchini et al., 1992). In the Framingham population, higher white blood cell counts were associated with an increased risk of cardiovascular disease (Kannel et al., 1992).

## Platelets

Platelet counts usually are normal, but hypertensives with existing target organ damage often have changes in platelet structure and function (Nadar et al., 2004).

## Fibrinogen

Elevated plasma fibrinogen levels are a major risk factor for coronary heart disease (Yarnell et al., 1991) and have been noted in hypertensives with insulin resistance (Landin et al., 1990) or reduced renal function (Catena et al., 2000).

## Hypofibrinolysis

Decreased fibrinolytic activity, reflected by increased levels of plasminogen activator inhibitor and tissue plasminogen activator antigen, was directly related to BP levels in the Framingham offspring population (Poli et al., 2000). Such impaired fibrinolysis obviously could increase the likelihood of thrombotic complications (Lee, 2002).

## Viscosity

Not surprisingly, in view of the findings just noted, whole-blood viscosity is increased by approximately 10% in untreated mild hypertensives, comparable to the increase in their PR (Devereux et al., 2000). Increased blood viscosity along with increased hematocrits and thrombogenic factors may be involved in the greater threats of thrombotic rather than hemorrhagic complications in hypertensive patients.

## Sex Hormones

### Menopause

Women have a rising incidence of hypertension after menopause, which is associated with a major increase in cardiovascular risk (Kitler, 1992). A likely too simple explanation for the increased incidence of hypertension after menopause is that the monthly menses keeps fluid volume slightly lower in women before menopause so that the hemodynamic cascade toward hypertension is slowed (Seely, 1976).

### Estrogen

Premenopausal women with hypertension usually have a higher heart rate and CO and a lower PR than do men with similar degrees of hypertension (Messerli et al., 1987). These differences could reflect higher estrogen levels, which have been found to be even higher in premenopausal hypertensive women than in normotensive subjects (Hughes et al., 1989). In that same study, estrogen levels were also higher in hypertensive than in normotensive men, although still well below those in women.

### Testosterone

Hypertensive men have been reported to have lower testosterone levels than normotensive men (Liu et al., 2003).

## Other Associations

The following conditions have been found to have an increased association with hypertension:

- Acute intermittent porphyria (O'Mahoney & Wathen, 1996)
- Ambient air pollution (Zanobetti et al., 2004)
- Aortic stenosis (Ie et al., 1996)
- Birth date in autumn (Banegas et al., 2000)
- Blood group MN (Delanghe et al., 1995)
- Color blindness (Morton, 1975)
- Exposure to radio-frequency electromagnetic field (Braune et al., 1998)
- HIV infection (Jung et al., 2004)
- Hypoalgesia (Ghione, 1996)
- Hypertensive spouse (Hippisley-Cox & Pringle, 1998)
- Keloids (Dustan, 1995)
- Open-angle glaucoma (Fraser et al., 1996)
- Poor quality sleep (Redline et al., 2004)
- Pseudoxanthoma elasticum (Parker et al., 1964)
- Reduced forced vital capacity (Selby et al., 1990)
- Rofecoxib use (Solomon et al., 2004)
- Senile cataracts (Clayton et al., 1980)
- Serum IgG levels (Khraibi, 1991)
- Shrinking body stature (Tabara et al., 2005)
- Turner syndrome (Sybert & McCauley, 2004)

Claims for an increased incidence of cancer have not been substantiated (Batty et al., 2003). A number of other diseases in which accompanying hypertension frequently is noted are described in Chapter 15.

## CONCLUSION

The preceding coverage may not exhaust the possible mechanisms for primary hypertension, but it at least touches on all that have received serious attention to date. It should be reemphasized that multiple defects likely are involved, and some of the initiating factors may no longer be discernible, having been dampened as hypertension develops. Without specific genetic markers, it is impossible to know whether a normotensive person, even with a strongly positive family history, will definitely develop hypertension, so that long-term prospective studies are difficult to design and perform.

In the absence of certainty about the pathogenesis of hypertension, it will be difficult to convince many patients that preventive measures should be undertaken. However, there seems no possible harm and a great deal of potential good to be gained from moderation in intake of sodium, calories, and alcohol; maintenance of good physical condition; and avoidance of unnecessary stress. As is described in Chapter 6, the value of these preventive measures has been demonstrated.

Now that the possible causes of primary hypertension have been examined, we turn to the natural history and clinical consequences of the disease. Regardless of cause, its consequences must be addressed.

## REFERENCES

Ahokas RA, Sun Y, Bhattacharya SK, et al. Aldosteronism and a proinflammatory vascular phenotype: role of Mg2+, Ca2+, and $H_2O_2$ in peripheral blood mononuclear cells. *Circulation* 2005;111:51–57.

Aiello EA, Villa-Abrille MC, Dulce RA, et al. Endothelin-1 stimulates the Na+/Ca2+ exchanger reverse mode through intracellular Na+ (Na+i)-dependent and Na+i-independent pathways. *Hypertension* 2005:288–293.

Alderman MH. Dietary sodium and cardiovascular health in hypertensive patients: the case against universal sodium restriction. *J Am Soc Nephrol* 2004;15(Suppl 1):S47–S50.

Alderman MH. Salt, blood pressure, and human health. *Hypertension* 2000;36:890–893.

Alderman MH, Cohen HW, Sealey JE, Laragh JH. Plasma renin activity levels in hypertensive persons: their wide range and lack of suppression in diabetic and in most elderly patients. *Am J Hypertens* 2004;17:1–7.

Alderman MH, Madhavan S, Ooi WL, et al. Association of the renin-sodium profile with the risk of myocardial infarction in patients with hypertension. *N Engl J Med* 1991;324:1098–1104.

Alderman MH, Ooi WL, Cohen H, et al. Plasma renin activity. *Am J Hypertens* 1997;10:1–8.

Almdal T, Scharling H, Jensen JS, Vestergaard H. The independent effect of type 2 diabetes mellitus on ischemic heart disease, stroke, and death: a population-based study of 13,000 men and women with 20 years of follow-up. *Arch Intern Med* 2004;164:1422–1426.

Alper AB Jr, Chen W, Yau L, et al. Childhood uric acid predicts adult blood pressure: the Bogalusa Heart Study. *Hypertension* 2005;45:34–38.

Anderson EA, Sinkey CA, Lawton WJ, Mark AL. Elevated sympathetic nerve activity in borderline hypertensive humans. Evidence from direct intraneural recordings. *Hypertension* 1988;14:177–183.

Andersson OK, Beckman-Suurküla M, Sannerstedt R, et al. Does hyperkinetic circulation constitute a pre-hypertensive stage? *J Intern Med* 1989;226:401–408.

Anonymous. Catecholamines in essential hypertension. *Lancet* 1977;1:1088–1099.

Arangino S, Cagnacci A, Angiolucci M, et al. Effects of melatonin on vascular reactivity, catecholamine levels, and blood pressure in healthy men. *Am J Cardiol* 1999; 83:1417–1419.

Arcaro G, Fava C, Dagradi R, et al. Acute hyperhomocysteinemia induces a reduction in arterial distensibility and compliance. *J Hypertens* 2004;22:775–781.

Arenas IA, Xu Y, Lopez-Jaramillo P, Davidge ST. Angiotensin II-induced MMP-2 release from endothelial cells is mediated by TNF-alpha. *Am J Physiol Cell Physiol* 2004;286: C779–C784.

Armario P, del Rey RH, Martin-Baranera M, et al. Blood pressure reactivity to mental stress task as a determinant of sustained hypertension after 5 years of follow-up. *J Hum Hypertens* 2003;17:181–186.

Aronow WS, Ahn C, Kronzon I, Gutstein H. Association of plasma renin activity and echocardiographic left ventricular hypertrophy with frequency of new coronary events and new atherothrombotic brain infarction in older persons with systemic hypertension. *Am J Cardiol* 1997;79: 1543–1545.

Aviv A, Hollenberg NK, Weder AB. Sodium glomerulopathy: tubuloglomerular feedback and renal injury in African Americans. *Kidney Int* 2004;65:361–368.

Aviv A, Hollenberg NK, Weder A. Urinary potassium excretion and sodium sensitivity in blacks (Response: reinterpreting sodium-potassium data in salt sensitivity hypertension: a prospective debate). *Hypertension* 2005;45:e4–e5.

Baker EH, Dong YB, Sagnella GA, et al. Association of hypertension with T594M mutation in β subunit of epithelial sodium channels in black people resident in London. *Lancet* 1998;351:1388–1392.

Banegas JR, Rodríguez-Artalejo F, de la Cruz JJ, et al. Adult men born in spring have lower blood pressure. *J Hypertens* 2000;18:1763–1766.

Barker DJ, Lackland DT. Prenatal influences on stroke mortality in England and Wales. *Stroke* 2003;34:1598–1602.

Barker DJ, Osmond C, Golding J, et al. Growth *in utero*, blood pressure in childhood and adult life, and mortality from cardiovascular disease. *BMJ* 1989;298:564–567.

Baron AD, Tarshoby M, Hook G, et al. Interaction between insulin sensitivity and muscle perfusion on glucose uptake in human skeletal muscle. *Diabetes* 2000;49:768–774.

Batenburg WW, de Vries R, Saxena PR, Danser AH. L-S-nitrosothiols: endothelium-derived hyperpolarizing factors in porcine coronary arteries? *J Hypertens* 2004; 22:1927–1936.

Batty GD, Shipley MJ, Marmot MG, Smith GD. Blood pressure and site-specific cancer mortality: evidence from the original Whitehall study. *Br J Cancer* 2003; 89:1243–1247.

Bautista LE, Vera LM, Arenas IA, Gamarra G. Independent association between inflammatory markers (C-reactive protein, interleukin-6, and TNF-α) and essential hypertension. *J Human Hypertens* 2005;19:149–154.

Beard TC, Blizzard L, O'Brien DJ, et al. Association between blood pressure and dietary factors in the dietary and nutritional survey of British adults. *Arch Intern Med* 1997; 157:234–238.

Bjørnholt JV, Erikssen G, Kjeldsen SE, et al. Fasting blood glucose is independently associated with resting and exercise blood pressures and development of elevated blood pressure. *J Hypertens* 2003;21:1383–1389.

Blair SN, Church TS. The fitness, obesity, and health equation: is physical activity the common denominator? *JAMA* 2004;292:1232–1234.

Blair SN, Goodyear NN, Gibbons LW, Cooper KH. Physical fitness and incidence of hypertension in healthy normotensive men and women. *JAMA* 1984;252:487–490.

Blaustein MP. Sodium ions, calcium ions, blood pressure regulation, and hypertension. *Am J Physiol* 1977;232: C165–C173.

Blaustein MP. Endogenous ouabain. *Kidney Int* 1996; 49: 1748–1753.

Blumenthal JA, Sherwood A, Gullette ECD, et al. Exercise and weight loss reduce blood pressure in men and women with mild hypertension. *Arch Intern Med* 2000;160:1947–1958.

Boguszewski MC, Johannsson G, Fortes LC, Sverrisdottir YB. Low birth size and final height predict high sympathetic nerve activity in adulthood. *J Hypertens* 2004;22: 1157–1163.

Bohlender J, Ménard J, Ganten D, Luft FC. Angiotensin concentrations and renin clearance. *Hypertension* 2000; 35:780–786.

Bolinder G, de Faire U. Ambulatory 24-h blood pressure monitoring in healthy, middle-aged smokeless tobacco users, smokers, and nontobacco users. *Am J Hypertens* 1998;11: 1153–1163.

Booz GW. Cardiac angiotensin $AT_2$ receptor: what exactly does it do? *Hypertension* 2004;43:1162–1163.

Boreham CA, Ferreira I, Twisk JW, et al. Cardiorespiratory fitness, physical activity, and arterial stiffness: the Northern Ireland Young Hearts Project. *Hypertension* 2004;44: 721–726.

Borghi C, Veronesi M, Bacchelli S, et al. Serum cholesterol levels, blood pressure response to stress and incidence of stable hypertension in young subjects with high normal blood pressure. *J Hypertens* 2004;22:265–272.

Borghi L, Meschi T, Guerra A, et al. Essential arterial hypertension and stone disease. *Kidney Int* 1999;55:2397–2406.

Borin ML, Tribe RM, Blaustein MP. Increased intracellular $Na^+$ augments mobilization of $Ca^{2+}$ from SR in vascular smooth muscle cells. *Am J Physiol* 1994; 266:C311–C317.

Borst JGG, Borst-de Geus A. Hypertension explained by Starling's theory of circulatory homeostasis. *Lancet* 1963; 1:677–682.

Boschmann M, Steiniger J, Hille U, et al. Water-induced thermogenesis. *J Clin Endocrinol Metab* 2003;88:6015–6019.

Brackbill RM, Siegel PZ, Ackermann SP. Self-reported hypertension among unemployed people in the United States. *BMJ* 1995;310:568.

Bragulat E, De La Sierra A, Antonio MT, Coca A. Endothelial dysfunction in salt-sensitive hypertension. *Hypertension* 2001;37:444–448.

Braune S, Wrocklage C, Raczek J, et al. Resting blood pressure increase during exposure to a radio-frequency electromagnetic field. *Lancet* 1998;351:1857–1858.

Brenner BM, Anderson S. The interrelationships among filtration surface area, blood pressure, and chronic renal disease. *J Cardiovasc Pharmacol* 1992;19(Suppl 6):S1–S7.

Brenner BM, Chertow GM. Congenital oligonephropathy and the etiology of adult hypertension and progressive renal injury. *Am J Kidney Dis* 1994;23:171–175.

Brenner BM, Mackenzie HS. Nephron mass as a risk factor for progression of renal disease. *Kidney Int* 1997;52(Suppl 63):S124–S127.

Brenner BM, Garcia DL, Anderson S. Glomeruli and blood pressure. Less of one, more the other? *Am J Hypertens* 1988;1:335–347.

Breslau NA, McGuire JL, Zerwekh JE, Pak CY. The role of dietary sodium on renal excretion and intestinal absorption of calcium and on vitamin D metabolism. *J Clin Endocrinol Metab* 1982;55:369–373.

Brewster UC, Perazella MA. The renin-angiotensin-aldosterone system and the kidney: effects on kidney disease. *Am J Med* 2004;116:263–272.

Brown JJ, Lever AF, Robertson JI, et al. Salt and hypertension [Letter]. *Lancet* 1984;2:456.

Brunner HR, Laragh JH, Baer L, et al. Essential hypertension. *N Engl J Med* 1972;286:441–449.

Brydon L, Steptoe A. Stress-induced increases in interleukin-6 and fibrinogen predict ambulatory blood pressure at 3-year follow-up. *J Hypertens* 2005;23:1001–1007.

Califf RM. Defining the balance of risk and benefit in the era of genomics and proteomics. *Health Aff* (Millwood) 2004;23:77–87.

Calles-Escandon J, Cipolla M. Diabetes and endothelial dysfunction. *Endocr Rev* 2001;22:36–52.

Campese VM, Karubian F, Chervu I, et al. Pressor reactivity to norepinephrine and angiotensin in salt-sensitive hypertensive patients. *Hypertension* 1993;21:301–307.

Canessa M. Red cell sodium-lithium countertransport and cardiovascular risk factors in essential hypertension. *Trends Cardiovasc Med* 1995;5:102–108.

Canoy D, Luben R, Welch A, et al. Fat distribution, body mass index and blood pressure in 22,090 men and women in the Norfolk cohort of the European Prospective Investigation into Cancer and Nutrition (EPIC-Norfolk) study. *J Hypertens* 2004;22:2067–2074.

Cappuccio FP, Meilahn E, Zmuda JM, Cauley JA. High blood pressure and bone-mineral loss in elderly white women. *Lancet* 1999;354:971–975.

Cardillo C, Campia U, Iantorno M, Panza JA. Enhanced vascular activity of endogenous endothelin-1 in obese hypertensive patients. *Hypertension* 2004;43:36–40.

Carey RM. Update on the role of the $AT_2$ receptor. *Curr Opin Nephrol Hypertens* 2005;14:67–71.

Carr SJ, Sikand K, Moore D, Norman RI. Altered membrane microviscosity in essential hypertension. *J Hypertens* 1995;13:139–146.

Carretero OA, Oparil S. Essential hypertension. *Circulation* 2000;101:329–335.

Carvajal CA, Romero DG, Mosso LM, et al. Biochemical and genetic characterization of 11 β-hydroxysteroid dehydrogenase type 2 in low-renin essential hypertensives. *J Hypertens* 2005;23:71–77.

Castellano M. Diogenes in the 2000s: searching for hypertension genes. *J Hypertens* 2004;22:1081–1083.

Catena C, Zingaro L, Casaccio D, Sechi LA. Abnormalities of coagulation in hypertensive patients with reduced creatinine clearance. *Am J Med* 2000;109:556–561.

Celemajer DS, Adams MR, Clarkson P, et al. Passive smoking and impaired endothelium-dependent arterial dilatation in healthy young adults. *N Engl J Med* 1996; 334:150–154.

Cesana G, Sega R, Ferrario M, et al. Job strain and blood pressure in employed men and women: a pooled analysis of four northern Italian population samples. *Psychosom Med* 2003;65:558–563.

Chapleau MW. Arterial baroreflexes. In: Izzo JL, Black HR, eds. *Hypertension Primer: Essentials of High Blood Pressure*, 3rd Ed. Philadelphia: Lippincott Williams & Wilkins, 2003.

Charles CJ, Lainchbury JG, Lewis LK, et al. The role of adrenomedullin. *Am J Hypertens* 1999;12:166–173.

Chen CJ, Hsueh Y, Lai M, et al. Increased prevalence of hypertension and long-term arsenic exposure. *Hypertension* 1995;25:53–60.

Chobanian AV, Hill M. National Heart, Lung, and Blood Institute workshop on sodium and blood pressure. *Hypertension* 2000;35:858–863.

Chopra M, Darnton-Hill I. Tobacco and obesity epidemics: not so different after all? *BMJ* 2004;328:1558–1560.

Chrysohoou C, Pitsavos C, Panagiotakos DB, et al. Association between prehypertension status and inflammatory markers related to atherosclerotic disease: the ATTICA Study. *Am J Hypertens* 2004;17:568–573.

Ciuffetti G, Schillaci G, Innocente S, et al. Capillary rarefaction and abnormal cardiovascular reactivity in hypertension. *J Hypertens* 2003;21:2297–2303.

Clayton RM, Cuthbert J, Phillips CI, et al. Analysis of individual cataract patients and their lenses. *Exp Eye Res* 1980;31:553–566.

Cobb S, Rose RM. Hypertension, peptic ulcer, and diabetes in air traffic controllers. *JAMA* 1973;224:489–492.

Cockcroft JR, Chowienczyk PJ, Benjamin N, Ritter JM. Preserved endothelium-dependent vasodilatation in patients with essential hypertension. *N Engl J Med* 1994;330: 1036–1040.

Coggon DIW, Martyn CN. Time and chance: the stochastic nature of disease causation. *Lancet* 2005;365:1434–1437.

Cohen RA. The endothelium-derived hyperpolarizing factor puzzle: a mechanism without a mediator? *Circulation* 2005; 111:724–727.

Correia ML, Haynes WG. Obesity-related hypertension: is there a role for selective leptin resistance? *Curr Hypertens Rep* 2004;6:230–235.

Cosentino F, Lüscher TF. Effects of blood pressure and glucose on endothelial function. *Curr Hypertens Rep* 2001; 3:79–88.

Cowley AW Jr. A tribute to Eric Muirhead. Evolution of the Medullipin concept of blood pressure control. *J Hypertens* 1994;12:S25–S34.

Cowley AW Jr, Roman RJ. The role of the kidney in hypertension. *JAMA* 1996;275:1581–1589.

Cracowski JL, Baguet JP, Ormezzano O, et al. Lipid peroxidation is not increased in patients with untreated mild-to-moderate hypertension. *Hypertension* 2003;41:286–288.

Crawford DC, Carlson CS, Rieder MJ, et al. Haplotype diversity across 100 candidate genes for inflammation, lipid metabolism, and blood pressure regulation in two populations. *Am J Hum Genet* 2004;74:610–622.

Creager MA, Cooke JP, Mendelsohn ME, et al. Impaired vasodilation of forearm resistance vessels in hypercholesterolemic humans. *J Clin Invest* 1990;86:228–234.

Creager MA, Luscher TF, Cosentino F, Beckman JA. Diabetes and vascular disease: pathophysiology, clinical consequences, and medical therapy: part I. *Circulation* 2003; 108:1527–1532.

Cubeddu LX, Alfieri AB, Hoffman IS, et al. Nitric oxide and salt sensitivity. *Am J Hypertens* 2000;13:973–979.

Cummings DE, Overduin J, Foster-Schubert KE. Gastric bypass for obesity: mechanisms of weight loss and diabetes resolution. *J Clin Endocrinol Metab* 2004;89:2608–2615.

Cummings RG, Mitchell P, Smith W. Dietary sodium intake and cataract. *Am J Epidemiol* 2000;151:624–626.

Curtis JJ, Luke RG, Dustan HP, et al. Remission of essential hypertension after renal transplantation. *N Engl J Med* 1983;309:1009–1015.

Cusi D, Barlassina C, Azzani T, et al. Polymorphisms of alpha-adducin and salt sensitivity in patients with essential hypertension. *Lancet* 1997;349:1353–1357.

Cutler JA, Follmann D, Allender PS. Randomized trials of sodium reduction. *Am J Clin Nutr* 1997;65(2 Suppl): 643S–651S.

Dahl LK. Salt and hypertension. *Am J Clin Nutr* 1972; 25:231–244.

Dahl LK, Heine M. Primary role of renal homografts in setting chronic blood pressure and levels in rats. *Circ Res* 1975;36:692–696.

Dahl LK, Knudsen KD, Heine M, Leitl G. Effects of chronic excess salt ingestion. *J Exp Med* 1967;126:687–699.

Dahl LK, Knudsen KD, Iwai J. Humoral transmission of hypertension. *Circ Res* 1969;24:I21–I33.

Daniels SR, Arnett DK, Eckel RH, et al. Overweight in children and adolescents: pathophysiology, consequences, prevention, and treatment. *Circulation* 2005;111:1999–2012.

Danser AH, de Bruin RJ, Derkx FH, et al. Determinants of interindividual prorenin variation in humans [Abstract]. *J Hypertens* 1996;14:S4.

Davies JI, Struthers AD. Pulse wave analysis and pulse wave velocity: a critical review of their strengths and weaknesses. *J Hypertens* 2003;21:463–472.

de Ferranti SD, Gauvreau K, Ludwig DS, et al. Prevalence of the metabolic syndrome in American adolescents: findings from the Third National Health and Nutrition Examination Survey. *Circulation* 2004;110:2494–2497.

de Jongh RT, Serne EH, IJzerman RG, et al. Impaired microvascular function in obesity: implications for obesity-associated microangiopathy, hypertension, and insulin resistance. *Circulation*. 2004;109:2529–2535.

de la Sierra A, Giner V, Bragulat E, Coca A. Lack of correlation between two methods for the assessment of salt sensitivity in essential hypertension. *J Hum Hypertens* 2002; 16:255–260.

de Lange M, Spector TD, Andrew T. Genome-wide scan for blood pressure suggests linkage to chromosome 11, and replication of loci on 16, 17, and 22. *Hypertension* 2004; 44:872–877.

De Mello WC, ed. *Renin Angiotensin System and the Heart.* New York: John Wiley & Sons, 2004.

de Visser DC, van Hooft IMS, van Doornen JP, et al. Cardiovascular response to mental stress in offspring of hypertensive parents. *J Hypertens* 1995;13:901–908.

de Wardener HE. Franz Volhard lecture 1996. Sodium transport inhibitors and hypertension. *J Hypertens* 1996; 14(Suppl 5):S9–S18.

de Wardener HE, MacGregor GA. Dahl's hypothesis that a saluretic substance may be responsible for a sustained rise in arterial pressure. *Kidney Int* 1980;18:1–9.

de Wardener HE, MacGregor GA. Harmful effects of dietary salt in addition to hypertension. *J Hum Hypertens* 2002; 16:213–223.

de Wardener HE, Mills IH, Clapham WF, Hayter CJ. Studies on the efferent mechanism of the sodium diuresis which follows the administration of intravenous saline in the dog. *Clin Sci* 1961;21:249–258.

Deanfield J, Donald A, Ferri C, et al. Endothelial function and dysfunction. Part I: methodological issues for assessments in the different vascular beds: a statement by the Working Group on Endothelin and Endothelial Factors of the European Society of Hypertension. *J Hypertens* 2005;23:7–17.

Delanghe J, Duprez D, de Buyzere M, et al. MN blood group, a genetic marker for essential arterial hypertension in young adults. *Eur Heart J* 1995;16:1269–1276.

Delva PT, Pastori C, Degan M, et al. Intralymphocyte free magnesium in a group of subjects with essential hypertension. *Hypertension* 1996;28:433–439.

Denton D, Weisinger R, Mundy NI, et al. The effect of increased salt intake on blood pressure of chimpanzees. *Nature Med* 1995;1:1009–1016.

Denton D. Can hypertension be prevented? *J Hum Hypertens* 1997;11:563–569.

Dernellis J, Panaretou M. Aortic stiffness is an independent predictor of progression to hypertension in non-hypertensive subjects. *Hypertension* 2005;45:426–431.

DeSouza CA, Shapiro LF, Clevenger CM, et al. Regular aerobic exercise prevents and restores age-related declines in endothelium-dependent vasodilation in healthy men. *Circulation* 2000;102:1351–1357.

Devereux RB, Case DB, Alderman MH, et al. Possible role of increased blood viscosity in the hemodynamics of systemic hypertension. *Am J Cardiol* 2000;85:1265–1268.

DiBona GF. The sympathetic nervous system and hypertension: recent developments. *Hypertension* 2004; 43:147–150.

Díez J, Alonso A, Garciandia A, et al. Association of increased erythrocyte $Na^+/H^+$ exchanger with renal $Na^+$ retention in patients with essential hypertension. *Am J Hypertens* 1995;8:124–132.

Diez Roux AV, Chambless L, Merkin SS, et al. Socioeconomic disadvantage and change in blood pressure associated with aging. *Circulation* 2002;106:703–710.

Ding J, Visser M, Kritchevsky SB, et al. The association of regional fat depots with hypertension in older persons of white and African American ethnicity. *Am J Hypertens* 2004;17:971–976.

Ding Y, Gonick HC, Vaziri ND, et al. Lead-induced hypertension. *Am J Hypertens* 2001;14:169–173.

Dobrian AD, Schriver SD, Lynch T, Prewitt RL. Effect of salt on hypertension and oxidative stress in a rat model of diet-induced obesity. *Am J Physiol Renal Physiol* 2003; 285:F619–F628.

Dodt C, Breckling U, Derad I, et al. Plasma epinephrine and norepinephrine concentrations of healthy humans associated with nighttime sleep and morning arousal. *Hypertension* 1997;30:71–76.

Doll R, Peto R, Boreham J, Sutherland I. Mortality in relation to smoking: 50 years' observations on male British doctors. *BMJ* 2004;328:1519.

Dominiczak AF, Negrin DC, Clark JS, et al. Genes and hypertension. *Hypertension* 2000;35:164–172.

Dong Y, Wang X, Zhu H, et al. Endothelin-1 gene and progression of blood pressure and left ventricular mass: longitudinal findings in youth. *Hypertension* 2004;44:884–890.

Drummond HA, Gebremedhin D, Harder DR. Degenerin/epithelial Na+ channel proteins: components of a vascular mechanosensor. *Hypertension* 2004;44:643–648.

du Cailar G, Mimran A, Fesler P, et al. Dietary sodium and pulse pressure in normotensive and essential hypertensive subjects. *J Hypertens* 2004;22:697–703.

du Cailar G, Ribstein J, Mimran A. Dietary sodium and target organ damage in essential hypertension. *Am J Hypertens* 2002;15:222–229.

Duprez D, De Buyzere M, Paelinck M, et al. Relationship between left ventricular mass index and 24-h urinary free cortisol and cortisone in essential arterial hypertension. *J Hypertens* 1999;17:1583–1588.

Dustan HP. Does keloid pathogenesis hold the key to understanding black/white differences in hypertension severity. *Hypertension* 1995;26:858–862.

Eaton SB, Eaton SB III, Konner MJ, Shostak, M. An evolutionary perspective enhances understanding of human nutritional requirements. *J Nutr* 1996;126:1732–1740.

Ebbeling CB, Pawlak DB, Ludwig DS. Childhood obesity: public-health crisis, common sense cure. *Lancet* 2002; 360:473–482.

Eckel RH, Grundy SM, Zimmet PZ. The metabolic syndrome. *Lancet* 2005;365:1415–1428.

Egan BM. Insulin resistance and the sympathetic nervous system. *Curr Hypertens Rep* 2003;5:247–254.

Egan BM, Papademitriou V, Wofford M, et al. Metabolic syndrome and insulin resistance in the TROPHY substudy: contrasting views in high normal blood pressure *Am J Hypertens* 2005;18:3–12.

Egeland GM, Burkhart GA, Schnorr TM, et al. Effects of exposure to carbon disulphide on low density lipoprotein cholesterol concentration and diastolic blood pressure. *Br J Ind Med* 1992;49:287–293.

Ehrhart-Bornstein M, Lamounier-Zepter V, Schraven A, et al. Human adipocytes secrete mineralocorticoid-releasing factors. *Proc Natl Acad Sci USA* 2003;100:14211–14216.

Elliott P, Stamler J, Nichols R, et al. Intersalt revisited. *BMJ* 1996;312:1249–1253.

Empana JP, Ducimetiere P, Charles MA, Jouven X. Sagittal abdominal diameter and risk of sudden death in asymptomatic middle-aged men: the Paris Prospective Study I. *Circulation* 2004;110:2781–2785.

Endemann DH, Schiffrin EL. Endothelial dysfunction. *J Am Soc Nephrol* 2004a;15:1983–1992.

Endemann DH, Schiffrin EL. Nitric oxide, oxidative excess, and vascular complications of diabetes mellitus. *Curr Hypertens Rep* 2004b;6:85–89.

Endemann DH, Pu Q, De Ciuceis C, et al. Persistent remodeling of resistance arteries in type 2 diabetic patients on antihypertensive treatment. *Hypertension* 2004;43:399–404.

Engstrom A, Tobelmann RC, Albertson AM. Sodium intake trends and food choices. *Am J Clin Nutr* 1997;65(Suppl 2): 704S–707S.

Erdös EG. Angiotensin I converting enzyme and the changes in our concepts through the years. *Hypertension* 1990; 16: 363–370.

Ericsson F. Potassium in skeletal muscle in untreated primary hypertension and in chronic renal failure, studied by x-ray fluorescence technique. *Acta Med Scand* 1984; 215: 225–230.

Esler M, Lambert G, Jennings G. Regional norepinephrine turnover in human hypertension. *Clin Exp Hypertens* 1989;11(Suppl 1):75–89.

Esther CR Jr, Marino EM, Howard TE, et al. The critical role of tissue angiotensin-converting enzyme as revealed by gene targeting in mice. *J Clin Invest* 1997;99:2375–2385.

Estruch R, Coca A, Rodicio JL. High blood pressure, alcohol and cardiovascular risk. *J Hypertens* 2005;23:226–229.

Everson SA, Kaplan GA, Goldberg DE, Salonen JT. Anticipatory blood pressure response to exercise predicts future high blood pressure in middle-aged men. *Hypertension* 1996;27:1059–1064.

Facchini F, Hollenbeck CB, Chen YN, et al. Demonstration of a relationship between white blood cell count, insulin resistance, and several risk factors for coronary heart disease in women. *J Intern Med* 1992;232:267–272.

Fagerudd J, Forsblom C, Pettersson-Fernholm K, et al. Birth weight is inversely correlated to adult systolic blood pressure and pulse pressure in type 1 diabetes. *Hypertension* 2004;44:832–837.

Falkner B, Hulman S, Kushner H. Birth weight versus childhood growth as determinants of adult blood pressure. *Hypertension* 1998;31:145–150.

Fang J, Madhavan S, Alderman MH. Dietary potassium intake and stroke mortality. *Stroke* 2000;31:1532–1537.

Fava C, Burri P, Almgren P, et al. Heritability of ambulatory and office blood pressure phenotypes in Swedish families. *J Hypertens* 2004;22:1717–1721.

Feig DI, Nakagawa T, Karumanchi SA, et al. Hypothesis: uric acid, nephron number, and the pathogenesis of essential hypertension. *Kidney Int* 2004;66:281–287.

Ferguson RK, Turek DM, Rovner DR. Spironolactone and hydrochlorothiazide in normal-renin and low-renin essential hypertension. *Clin Pharmacol Ther* 1977;21:62–69.

Ferrari P, Shaw SG, Nicod J, et al. Active renin versus plasma renin activity to define aldosterone-to-renin ratio for primary aldosteronism. *J Hypertens* 2004;22:377–381.

Ferrario CM, Chappell MC. Novel angiotensin peptides. *Cell Mol Life Sci* 2004;61:2720–2727.

Ferreira I, Snijder MB, Twisk JW, et al. Central fat mass versus peripheral fat and lean mass: opposite (adverse versus favorable) associations with arterial stiffness? The Amsterdam Growth and Health Longitudinal Study. *J Clin Endocrinol Metab* 2004;89:2632–2639.

Ferreira I, Twisk JW, van Mechelen W, et al. Development of fatness, fitness, and lifestyle from adolescence to the age of 36 years: determinants of the metabolic syndrome in young adults. The Amsterdam Growth and Health Longitudinal Study. *Arch Intern Med* 2005;165:42–48.

Ferrier C, Cox H, Esler M. Elevated total body noradrenaline spillover in normotensive members of hypertensive families. *Clin Sci* 1993;84:225–230.

Filigheddu F, Reid JE, Troffa C, et al. Genetic polymorphisms of the beta-adrenergic system: association with essential hypertension and response to beta-blockade. *Pharmacogenomics J* 2004;4:154–160.

Finkielman S, Worcel M, Agrest A. Hemodynamic patterns in essential hypertension. *Circulation* 1965;31:356–368.

Fisher NDL, Hurwitz S, Ferri C, et al. Altered adrenal sensitivity to angiotensin II in low-renin essential hypertension. *Hypertension* 1999;34:388–394.

Fleming I. Cytochrome P-450 under pressure: more evidence for a link between 20-hydroxyeicosatetraenoic acid and hypertension. *Circulation* 2005;111:5–7.

Fliser D, Franek E, Fode P, et al. Subacute infusion of physiological doses of parathyroid hormone raises blood pressure in humans. *Nephrol Dial Transplant* 1997; 12:933–938.

Folkow B. "Structural factor" in primary and secondary hypertension. *Hypertension* 1990;16:89–101.

Folkow B, Halläck M, Lundgren Y, Weiss L. Background of increased flow resistance and vascular reactivity in spontaneously hypertensive rats. *Acta Physiol Scand* 1970; 80:93–106.

Forte P, Copland M, Smith LM, et al. Basal nitric oxide synthesis in essential hypertension. *Lancet* 1997; 349:837–842.

Franklin SS. Arterial stiffness and hypertension: a two-way street? *Hypertension* 2005;45:349–351.

Franklin SS, Pio JR, Wong ND, et al. Predictors of new-onset diastolic and systolic hypertension: The Framingham Heart Study. *Circulation* 2005;111:1121–1127.

Fraser S, Wormald R, Hitchings R. Blood pressure and glaucoma. *Br J Opthalmol* 1996;80:858–859.

Freel EM, Connell JM. Mechanisms of hypertension: the expanding role of aldosterone. *J Am Soc Nephrol* 2004; 15:1993–2001.

Fuchs S, Frenzel K, Xiao HD, et al. Newly recognized physiologic and pathophysiologic actions of the angiotensin-converting enzyme. *Curr Hypertens Rep* 2004;6:124–128.

Fukuda M, Munemura M, Usami T, et al. Nocturnal blood pressure is elevated with natriuresis and proteinuria as renal function deteriorates in nephropathy. *Kidney Int* 2004; 65:621–625.

Furchgott RF, Zawadzki JV. The obligatory role of endothelial cells in the relaxation of arterial smooth muscle by acetylcholine. *Nature* 1980;288:373–376.

Gainer JV, Bellamine A, Dawson EP, et al. Functional variant of CYP4A11 20-hydroxyeicosatetraenoic acid synthase is associated with essential hypertension. *Circulation* 2005; 111:63–69.

Galuska DA, Will JC, Serdula MK, Ford ES. Are health care professionals advising obese patients to lose weight? *JAMA* 1999;282:1576–1578.

Gates PE, Tanaka H, Hiatt WR, Seals DR. Dietary sodium restriction rapidly improves large elastic artery compliance in older adults with systolic hypertension. *Hypertension* 2004;44:35–41.

Geleijnse JM, Grobbee DE, Hofman A. Sodium and potassium intake and blood pressure change in childhood. *BMJ* 1990;300:899–902.

Geleijnse JM, Hofman A, Witteman JCM, et al. Long-term effects of neonatal sodium restriction on blood pressure. *Hypertension* 1997;29:913–917.

Gerin W, Chaplin W, Schwartz JE, et al. Sustained blood pressure increase after an acute stressor: the effects of the 11 September 2001 attack on the New York City World Trade Center. *J Hypertens* 2005;23:279–284.

Ghiadoni L, Donald AE, Cropley M, et al. Mental stress induces transient endothelial dysfunction in humans. *Circulation* 2000;102:2473–2378.

Ghiadoni L, Magagna A, Versari D, et al. Different effect of antihypertensive drugs on conduit artery endothelial function. *Hypertension* 2003;41:1281–1286.

Ghione S. Hypertension-associated hypalgesia. Evidence in experimental animals and humans, pathophysiological mechanisms, and potential clinical consequences. *Hypertension* 1996;28:494–504.

Glasser SP, Selwyn AP, Ganz P. Atherosclerosis. *Am Heart J* 1996;131:379–384.

Goldblatt H. Experimental renal hypertension. *Circulation* 1958;17:642–647.

Goldstein DS. Plasma catecholamines and essential hypertension. An analytical review. *Hypertension* 1983;5:86–99.

Goldstein DS, Eisenhofer GF. Catecholamine synthesis, release, reuptake, and metabolism. In: Izzo JL and Black HR, eds. *Hypertension Primer: The Essentials of High Blood Pressure*, 3rd Ed. Philadelphia: Lippincott Williams & Wilkins, 2003.

Gorzelniak K, Engeli S, Janke J, et al. Hormonal regulation of the human adipose-tissue renin-angiotensin system: relationship to obesity and hypertension. *J Hypertens* 2002; 20:965–973.

Göthberg G. Physiology of the renomedullary depressor system. *J Hypertens* 1994;12:S57–S64.

Govers R, Rabelink TJ. Cellular regulation of endothelial nitric oxide synthase. *Am J Physiol Renal Physiol* 2001;280: F193–F206.

Granger DN, Vowinkel T, Petnehazy T. Modulation of the inflammatory response in cardiovascular disease. *Hypertension* 2004;43:924–931.

Grant FD, Romero JR, Jeunemaitre X, et al. Low-renin hypertension, altered sodium homeostasis, and an alpha-adducin polymorphism. *Hypertension* 2002;39:191–196.

Grassi G. Cardiovascular and sympathetic effects of reversing insulin resistance in hypertension. *J Hypertens* 2004; 22:1671–1672.

Grassi G, Mancia G. Neurogenic hypertension: is the enigma of its origin near the solution? *Hypertension* 2004;43: 154–155.

Groppelli A, Giorgi DM, Omboni S, et al. Persistent blood pressure increase induced by heavy smoking. *J Hypertens* 1992;10:495–499.

Guidi E, Menghetti D, Milani S, et al. Hypertension may be transplanted with the kidney in humans. *J Am Soc Nephrol* 1996;7:1131–1138.

Gus M, Fuchs SC, Moreira LB, et al. Association between different measurements of obesity and the incidence of hypertension. *Am J Hypertens* 2004;17:50–53.

Guttmacher AE, Collins FS, Carmona RH. The family history—more important than ever. *N Engl J Med* 2004; 351: 2333–2336.

Guyton AC. Physiologic regulation of arterial pressure. *Am J Cardiol* 1961;8:401–407.

Guyton AC. Kidneys and fluids in pressure regulation. *Hypertension* 1992;19(Suppl 1):I2–I8.

Guyton AC, Coleman TG. Quantitative analysis of the pathophysiology of hypertension. *Circ Res* 1969;24(Suppl 1) I1–I14.

Hackam DG, Tan MK, Honos GN, et al. How does the prognosis of diabetes compare with that of established vascular disease? Insights from the Canadian Vascular Protection (VP) Registry. *Am Heart J* 2004; 148:1028–1033.

Haddy FJ, Overbeck HW. The role of humoral agents in volume expanded hypertension. *Life Sci* 1976;19:935–948.

Haffner S, Taegtmeyer H. Epidemic obesity and the metabolic syndrome. *Circulation* 2003;108:1541–1545.

Hajjar IM, Grim CE, George V, Kotchen TA. Impact of diet on blood pressure and age-related changes in blood pressure in the U.S. population. *Arch Intern Med* 2001;161:589–593.

Hales CN, Barker DJ. The thrifty phenotype hypothesis. *Br Med Bull* 2001;60:5–20.

Halimi J-M, Sealey JE. Prorenin in diabetes mellitus. *Trends Endocrinol Metab* 1992;3:270–275.

Hall JE, Brands MW, Henegar JR. Angiotensin II and long-term arterial pressure regulation. *J Am Soc Nephrol* 1999; 10:S258–S265.

Hall JE, Brands MW, Shek EW. Central role of the kidney and abnormal fluid volume control in hypertension. *J Hum Hypertens* 1996;10:633–639.

Hannan RE, Widdop RE. Vascular angiotensin II actions mediated by angiotensin II type 2 receptors. *Curr Hypertens Rep* 2004;6:117–123.

Hare JM. Nitroso-redox balance in the cardiovascular system. *N Engl J Med* 2004;351:2112–2114.

Harrap SB, Cumming AD, Davies DL, et al. Glomerular hyperfiltration, high renin, and low-extracellular volume in high blood pressure. *Hypertension* 2000;35:952–957.

Hartley TR, Lovallo WR, Whitsett TL. Cardiovascular effects of caffeine in men and women. *Am J Cardiol* 2004; 93:1022–1026.

Hayashi T, Boyko EJ, Leonetti DL, et al. Visceral adiposity is an independent predictor of incident hypertension in Japanese Americans. *Ann Intern Med* 2004;140:992–1000.

He FJ, MacGregor GA. How far should salt intake be reduced? *Hypertension* 2003;42:1093–1099.

Heagerty AM, Aalkjaer C, Bund SJ, et al. Small artery structure in hypertension. *Hypertension* 1993;21:391–397.

Hedley AA, Ogden CL, Johnson CL, et al. Prevalence of overweight and obesity among US children, adolescents, and adults, 1999–2002. *JAMA* 2004;291:2847–2850.

Heer M, Baisch F, Kropp J, et al. High dietary sodium chloride consumption may not induce body fluid retention in humans. *Am J Physiol Renal Physiol* 2000;278:F585–F595.

Hellström A, Dahlgren J, Marsal K, Ley D. Abnormal retinal vascular morphology in young adults following intrauterine growth restriction. *Pediatrics* 2004;113:e77–e80.

Helmer OM. Renin activity in blood from patients with hypertension. *Can Med Assoc J* 1964;90:221–225.

Hill JM, Zalos G, Halcox JP, et al. Circulating endothelial progenitor cells, vascular function, and cardiovascular risk. *N Engl J Med* 2003;348:593–600.

Hinchliffe SA, Lynch MR, Sargent PH, et al. The effect of intrauterine growth retardation on the development of renal nephrons. *Br J Obstet Gynaecol* 1992;99:293–301.

Hippisley-Cox J, Pringle M. Are spouses of patients with hypertension at increased risk of having hypertension? *Br J Gen Pract* 1998;46:1580–1584.

Hirai Y, Adachi H, Fujiura Y, et al. Plasma endothelin-1 level is related to renal function and smoking status but not to blood pressure: an epidemiological study. *J Hypertens* 2004;22:713–718.

Hodgson JM, Burke V, Puddey IB. Acute effects of tea on fasting and postprandial vascular function and blood pressure in humans. *J Hypertens* 2005;23:47–54.

Hofman A, Hazebroek A, Valkenburg HA. A randomized trial of sodium intake and blood pressure in newborn infants. *JAMA* 1983;250:370–373.

Holland OB, Gomez-Sanchez C, Fairchild C, Kaplan NM. Role of renin classification for diuretic treatment of black hypertensive patients. *Arch Intern Med* 1979; 139:1365–1370.

Hollenberg NK, Stevanovic R, Agarwal A, et al. Plasma aldosterone concentration in the patient with diabetes mellitus. *Kidney Int* 2004;65:1435–1439.

Hooper L, Bartlett C, Davey Smith G, Ebrahim S. Systematic review of long-term effects of advice to reduce dietary salt in adults. *BMJ* 2002;325:628.

Houben AJ, Willemsen RT, van de Ven H, de Leeuw PW. Microvascular adaptation to changes in dietary sodium is disturbed in patients with essential hypertension. *J Hypertens* 2005;23:127–132.

Howard AB, Alexander RW, Taylor WR. Effects of magnesium on nitric oxide synthase activity in endothelial cells. *Am J Physiol* 1995;269:C612–C618.

Hu G, Qiao Q, Tuomilehto J, et al. Prevalence of the metabolic syndrome and its relation to all-cause and cardiovascular mortality in nondiabetic European men and women. *Arch Intern Med* 2004;164:1066–1076.

Huang Z, Willett WC, Manson JE, et al. Body weight, weight change, and risk of hypertension in women. *Ann Intern Med* 1998;128:81–88.

Hughes GS, Mathur RS, Margolius HS. Sex steroid hormones are altered in essential hypertension. *J Hypertens* 1989;7:18⊢–187.

Hughson M, Farris AB 3rd, Douglas-Denton R, et al. Glomerular number and size in autopsy kidneys: the relationship to birth weight. *Kidney Int* 2003;63:2113–2122.

Hunt KJ, Resendez RG, Williams K, et al. National Cholesterol Education Program versus World Health Organization metabolic syndrome in relation to all-cause and cardiovascular mortality in the San Antonio Heart Study. *Circulation* 2004;110:1251–1257.

Hunt SC, Geleijnse JM, Wu LL, et al. Enhanced blood pressure response to mild sodium reduction in subjects with

235T variant of the angiotensinogen gene. *J Hypertens* 1999;12:460–466.

Hunyor SN, Zweifler AJ, Hansson L, et al. Effect of high dose spironolactone and chlorthalidone in essential hypertension. *Aust N Z J Med* 1975;5:17–24.

Hürlimann D, Enseleit F, Noll G, et al. Endothelin antagonists and heart failure. *Curr Hypertens Rep* 2002;4:85–92.

Hurwitz S, Fisher ND, Ferri C, et al. Controlled analysis of blood pressure sensitivity to sodium intake: interactions with hypertension type. *J Hypertens* 2003; 21:951–959.

Huxley R, Neil A, Collins R. Unravelling the fetal origins hypothesis: is there really an inverse association between birth weight and subsequent blood pressure? *Lancet* 2002; 360:659–665.

Hvarfner A, Mörlin C, Präntare H, et al. Calcium metabolic indices, vascular retinopathy, and plasma renin activity in essential hypertension. *Am J Hypertens* 1990;3:906–911.

Hypertension in Diabetes Study Group. Prevalence of hypertension in newly presenting type 2 diabetic patients and the association with risk factors for cardiovascular and diabetic complications. *J Hypertens* 1993; 11:309–317.

Ie E, Mook W, Shapiro AP. Systolic hypertension in critical aortic stenosis and the effect of valve replacement. *J Hum Hypertens* 1996;10:65–67.

Iiyama K, Nagano M, Yo Y, et al. Impaired endothelial function with essential hypertension assessed by ultrasonography. *Am Heart J* 1996;132:779–782.

Imanishi T, Hano T, Nishio I. Angiotensin II accelerates endothelial progenitor cell senescence through induction of oxidative stress. *J Hypertens* 2005;23:97–104.

Imig JD. Eicosanoid regulation of the renal vasculature. *Am J Physiol Renal Physiol* 2000;279:F965–F981.

Intersalt Cooperative Research Group. Intersalt: an international study of electrolyte excretion and blood pressure. *BMJ* 1988;297:319–328.

Irving RJ, Shore AC, Belton NR, et al. Low birth weight predicts higher blood pressure but not dermal capillary density in two populations. *Hypertension* 2004;43:610–613.

Iwamoto T, Kita S, Zhang J, et al. Salt-sensitive hypertension is triggered by $Ca^{2+}$ entry via $Na^+/Ca^{2+}$ exchanger type-1 in vascular smooth muscle. *Nat Med* 2004;10:1193–1199.

Jackson WF. Ion channels and vascular tone. *Hypertension* 2000;35:173–178.

Jacobs M-C, Lenders JWM, Willemsen JJ, Thien T. Adrenomedullary secretion of epinephrine is increased in mild essential hypertension. *Hypertension* 1997;29: 1303–1308.

Jaffe IZ, Mendelsohn ME. Functional mineralocorticoid receptors in human vascular smooth muscle cells [Abstract]. *Circulation* 2004;110(Suppl 3):III–190.

Jannetta PJ, Segal R, Wolfson SK. Neurogenic hypertension: etiology and surgical treatment. *Ann Surg* 1985;201: 391–398.

Jansen PM, Leineweber MJ, Thien T. The effect of a change in ambient temperature on blood pressure in normotensives. *J Hum Hypertens* 2001;15:113–117.

Jennings JR, Kamarck TW, Everson-Rose SA, et al. Exaggerated blood pressure responses during mental stress are prospectively related to enhanced carotid atherosclerosis in middle-aged Finnish men. *Circulation* 2004;110: 2198–2203.

Jiang G, Akar F, Cobbs SL, et al. Blood pressure regulates the activity and function of the Na-K-2Cl cotransporter in vascular smooth muscle. *Am J Physiol Heart Circ Physiol* 2004;286:H1552–H1557.

Jiang X, Srinivasan SR, Urbina E, Berenson GS. Hyperdynamic circulation and cardiovascular risk in children and adolescents. *Circulation* 1995;91:1101–1106.

Jin XH, McGrath HE, Gildea JJ, et al. Renal interstitial guanosine cyclic 3',5'-monophosphate mediates pressure-natriuresis via protein kinase G. *Hypertension* 2004;43: 1133–1139.

John S, Schmieder RE. Impaired endothelial function in arterial hypertension and hypercholesterolemia. *J Hypertens* 2000;18:363–374.

Johnson RJ, Feig DI, Herrera-Acosta J, Kang DH. Resurrection of uric acid as a causal risk factor in essential hypertension. *Hypertension* 2005a;45:18–20.

Johnson RJ, Rodriguez-Iturbe B, Kang D-H, et al. A unifying pathway for essential hypertension. *Am J Hypertens* 2005b;18:431–440.

Johnson RJ, Rodriguez-Iturbe B, Nakagawa T, et al. Subtle renal injury is likely a common mechanism for salt-sensitive essential hypertension. *Hypertension* 2005c;45: 326–330.

Jood K, Jern C, Wilhelmsen L, Rosengren A. Body mass index in mid-life is associated with a first stroke in men: a prospective population study over 28 years. *Stroke* 2004; 35:2764–2769.

Joossens JV, Hill MJ, Elliott P, et al. Dietary salt, nitrate and stomach cancer mortality in 24 countries. *Int J Epidemiol* 1996;25:494–504.

Jorde R, Sundsfjord J, Haug E, Bønaa KH. Relation between low calcium intake, parathyroid hormone, and blood pressure. *Hypertension* 2000;35:1154–1159.

Julius S. Changing role of the autonomic nervous system in human hypertension. *J Hypertens* 1990;8(Suppl 7):S59–S65.

Julius S. Interaction between renin and the autonomic nervous system in hypertension. *Am Heart J* 1988a;116:611–616.

Julius S. Transition from high cardiac output to elevated vascular resistance in hypertension. *Am Heart J* 1988b; 116: 600–606.

Julius S, Nesbitt S. Sympathetic overactivity in hypertension. *Am J Hypertens* 1996;9:113S–120S.

Julius S, Jones K, Schork N, et al. Independence of pressure reactivity from pressure levels in Tecumseh, Michigan. *Hypertension* 1991b;17(Suppl 1):III12–III21.

Julius S, Krause L, Schork NJ, et al. Hyperkinetic borderline hypertension in Tecumseh, Michigan. *J Hypertens* 1991c; 9:77–84.

Jung O, Bickel M, Ditting T, et al. Hypertension in HIV-1-infected patients and its impact on renal and cardiovascular integrity. *Nephrol Dial Transplant* 2004;19:2250–2258.

Kannel WB, Anderson K, Wilson PW. White blood cell count and cardiovascular disease. *JAMA* 1992;267:1253–1256.

Kannel WB, Garrison RJ, Dannenberg AL. Secular blood pressure trends in normotensive persons. *Am Heart J* 1993; 125:1154–1158.

Kannisto K, Pietiläinen KH, Ehrenborg E, et al. Overexpression of 11β-hydroxysteroid dehydrogenase-1 in adipose tissue is associated with acquired obesity and features of insulin resistance: studies in young adult monozygotic twins. *J Clin Endocrinol Metab* 2004;89:4414–4421.

Kaplan NM. Renin profiles. *JAMA* 1977;238:611–613.

Kaplan NM. The current epidemic of primary aldosteronism: causes and consequences. *J Hypertens* 2004;22:2040.

Kashyap SR, Roman LJ, Lamont J, et al. Insulin resistance is associated with impaired nitric oxide synthase (NOS) activity in skeletal muscle of type 2 diabetic subjects. *J Clin Endocrinol Metab* 2005;90:1100–1105.

Kaufman JS, Owoaje EE, James SA, et al. Determinants of hypertension in West Africa. *Am J Epidemiol* 1996; 143: 1203–1218.

Kawano Y, Abe H, Imanishi M, et al. Pressor and depressor hormones during alcohol-induced blood pressure reduction in hypertensive patients. *J Hum Hypertens* 1996; 10:595–599.

Kawasaki T, Delea CS, Bartter FC, Smith H. The effect of high-sodium and low-sodium intakes on blood pressure and other related variables in human subjects with idiopathic hypertension. *Am J Med* 1978;64:193–198.

Keller G, Zimmer G, Mall G, et al. Nephron number in patients with primary hypertension. *N Engl J Med* 2003; 348:101–108.

Kelly DJ, Cox AJ, Gow RM, et al. Platelet-derived growth factor receptor transactivation mediates the trophic effects of angiotensin II *in vivo*. *Hypertension* 2004;44:195–202.

Kelm M, Preik M, Hafner DJ, Strauer BE. Evidence for a multifactorial process involved in the impaired flow response to nitric oxide in hypertensive patients with endothelial dysfunction. *Hypertension* 1996;27:346–353.

Kempner W. Treatment of hypertensive vascular disease with rice diet. *Am J Med* 1948;4:545–577.

Kenchaiah S, Evans JC, Levy D, et al. Obesity and the risk of heart failure. *N Engl J Med* 2002;347:305–313.

Kershaw EE, Flier JS. Adipose tissue as an endocrine organ. *J Clin Endocrinol Metab* 2004;89:2548–2556.

Khalid ME, Ali ME, Elbagir M, et al. Pattern of blood pressures among high and low altitude residents of southern Saudi Arabia. *J Hum Hypertens* 1994;8:765–769.

Khaw K. Temperature and cardiovascular mortality. *Lancet* 1995;345:337–338.

Khaw K-T, Bingham S, Welch A, et al. Blood pressure and urinary sodium in men and women: Norfolk cohort of the European Prospective Investigation into Cancer (EPIC-Norfolk). *Am J Clin Nutr* 2004;80:1397–1403.

Khraibi AA. Association between disturbances in the immune system and hypertension. *Am J Hypertens* 1991;4: 635–641.

Kimura G, Brenner BM. A method for distinguishing salt-sensitive from non-salt-sensitive forms of human and experimental hypertension. *Curr Opin Nephrol Hypertens* 1993;2:341–349.

Kimura G, Saito F, Kojima S, et al. Renal function curve in patients with secondary forms of hypertension. *Hypertension* 1987;10:11–15.

Kitler ME. Differences in men and women in coronary artery disease, systemic hypertension and their treatment. *Am J Cardiol* 1992;70:1077–1080.

Klag MJ, He J, Coresh J, et al. The contribution of urinary cations to the blood pressure differences associated with migration. *Am J Epidemiol* 1995;142:295–303.

Klatsky AL, Friedman GD, Siegelaub AB, Gérard MJ. Alcohol consumption and blood pressure. *N Engl J Med* 1977; 296:1194–1200.

Klein R, Klein BE, Cornoni JC, et al. Serum uric acid. Its relationship to coronary heart disease risk factors and cardiovascular disease, Evans County, Georgia. *Arch Intern Med* 1973;132:401–410.

Klein S, Burke LE, Bray GA, et al. Clinical implications of obesity with specific focus on cardiovascular disease: a statement for professionals from the American Heart Association Council on Nutrition, Physical Activity, and Metabolism. *Circulation* 2004a;110:2952–2967.

Klein S, Fontana L, Young VL, et al. Absence of an effect of liposuction on insulin action and risk factors for coronary heart disease. *N Engl J Med* 2004b;350:2549–2557.

Knox SS, Hausdorff J, Markovitz JH. Reactivity as a predictor of subsequent blood pressure: racial differences in the Coronary Artery Risk Development in Young Adults (CARDIA) Study. *Hypertension* 2002;40:914–919.

Knox SS, Weidner G, Adelman A, et al. Hostility and physiological risk in the National Heart, Lung, and Blood Institute Family Heart Study. *Arch Intern Med* 2004; 164: 2442–2448.

Koga M, Sasaguri M, Miura S, et al. Plasma renin activity could be a useful predictor of left ventricular hypertrophy in essential hypertensives. *J Hum Hypertens* 1998;12:455–461.

Konje JC, Bell SC, Morton JJ, et al. Human fetal kidney morphometry during gestation and the relationship between weight, kidney morphometry and plasma active renin concentration at birth. *Clin Sci* 1996;91:169–175.

Koren MJ, Devereux RB. Mechanism, effects, and reversal of left ventricular hypertrophy in hypertension. *Curr Opin Nephrol Hypertens* 1993;2:87–95.

Kosachunhanun N, Hunt SC, Hopkins PN, et al. Genetic determinants of nonmodulating hypertension. *Hypertension* 2003;42:901–908.

Kosch M, Hausberg M, Westermann G, et al. Alterations of calcium and magnesium content of red cell membranes in patients with primary hypertension. *Am J Hypertens* 2001; 14:254–258.

Kuchel O. Peripheral dopamine in hypertension and associated conditions. *J Hum Hypertens* 1999;13:605–615.

Kupper N, Willemsen G, Riese H, et al. Heritability of daytime ambulatory blood pressure in an extended twin design. *Hypertension* 2005;45:80–85.

Kurtz TW, Morris RC Jr. Dietary chloride as a determinant of "sodium-dependent" hypertension. *Science* 1983; 222: 1139–1141.

Kwitek-Black AE, Jacob HJ. The use of designer rats in the genetic dissection of hypertension. *Curr Hypertens Rep* 2001;3:12–18.

Lacey JM, Tershakovec AM, Foster GD. Acupuncture for the treatment of obesity: a review of the evidence. *Int J Obes Relat Metab Disord* 2003;27:419–427.

Laffer CL, Laniado-Schwartzman M, Wang MH, et al. 20-HETE and furosemide-induced natriuresis in salt-sensitive essential hypertension. *Hypertension* 2003a; 41:703–708.

Laffer CL, Laniado-Schwartzman M, Wang MH, et al. Differential regulation of natriuresis by 20-hydroxyeicosatetraenoic acid in human salt-sensitive versus salt-resistant hypertension. *Circulation* 2003b;107:574–578.

Landin K, Tengborn L, Smith U. Elevated fibrinogen and plasminogen activator inhibitor (PAI-1) in hypertension are related to metabolic risk factors for cardiovascular disease. *J Intern Med* 1990;27:273–278.

Landsberg L. Insulin-mediated sympathetic stimulation: role in the pathogenesis of obesity-related hypertension (or, how insulin affects blood pressure, and why). *J Hypertens* 2001;19:523–528.

Laragh JH. Laragh's lessons in pathophysiology and clinical pearls for treating hypertension. *Am J Hypertens* 2001; 14: 84–89.

Laragh JH. Vasoconstriction-volume analysis for understanding and treating hypertension. *Am J Med* 1973; 55: 261–274.

Laragh JH, Sealey JE. Relevance of the plasma renin hormonal control system that regulates blood pressure and sodium balance for correctly treating hypertension and for evaluating ALLHAT. *Am J Hypertens* 2003;16:407–415.

Lassègue B, Griendling KK. Reactive oxygen species in hypertension; an update. *Am J Hypertens* 2004;17:852–860.

Laurenzi M, Cirillo M, Panarelli W, et al. Baseline sodium-lithium countertransport and 6-year incidence of hypertension. *Circulation* 1997;95:581–587.

Ledent C, Vaugeois JM, Schiffmann SN, et al. Aggressiveness, hypoalgesia and high blood pressure in mice lacking the adenosine $A_{2a}$ receptor. *Nature* 1997;388:674–678.

Ledingham JM. Autoregulation in hypertension. *J Hypertens* 1989;7(Suppl 4):S97–S104.

Lee AJ. Haemorheological, platelet and endothelial factors in essential hypertension. *J Hum Hypertens* 2002; 16:529–531.

Lee MA, Böhm M, Paul M, et al. Physiological characterization of the hypertensive transgenic rat TR (mREN2)27. *Am J Physiol* 1996;270(6 Pt 1):E919–E929.

Lever AF. Slow pressor mechanisms in hypertension: a role for hypertrophy of resistance vessels? *J Hypertens* 1986;4:515–524.

Lever AF, Harrap SB. Essential hypertension: a disorder of growth with origins in childhood? *J Hypertens* 1992;10:101–120.

Levy BI. Can angiotensin II type 2 receptors have deleterious effects in cardiovascular disease? Implications for therapeutic blockade of the renin-angiotensin system. *Circulation* 2004;109:8–13.

Levy BI, Ambrosio G, Pries AR, Struijker-Boudier HA. Microcirculation in hypertension: a new target for treatment? *Circulation* 2001;104:735–740.

Liao D, Arnett DK, Tyroler HA, et al. Arterial stiffness and the development of hypertension. *Hypertension* 1999; 34:201–206.

Light KC, Girdler SS, Sherwood A, et al. High stress responsivity predicts later blood pressure only in combination with positive family history and high life stress. *Hypertension* 1999;33:1458–1464.

Lijnen P. Alterations in sodium metabolism as an etiological model for hypertension. *Cardiovasc Drugs Ther* 1995; 9:377–399.

Lin JL, Lin-Tan DT, Hsu KH, Yu CC. Environmental lead exposure and progression of chronic renal diseases in patients without diabetes. *N Engl J Med* 2003;348:277–286.

Linder L, Kiowski W, Bühler FR, Lüscher TF. Indirect evidence for release of endothelium-derived relaxing factor in human forearm circulation *in vivo. Circulation* 1990; 81:1762–1767.

Lip GY, Edmunds E, Nuttall SL, et al. Oxidative stress in malignant and non-malignant phase hypertension. *J Hum Hypertens* 2002;16:333–336.

Litchfield WR, Hunt SC, Juenemaitre X, et al. Increased urinary free cortisol. *Hypertension* 1998;31:569–574.

Liu PY, Death AK, Handelsman DJ. Androgens and cardiovascular disease. *Endocr Rev* 2003;24:313–340.

Lohmeier TE, Irwin ED, Rossing MA, et al. Prolonged activation of the baroreflex produces sustained hypotension. *Hypertension* 2004;43:306–311.

Lohmueller KE, Pearce CL, Pike M, et al. Meta-analysis of genetic association studies supports a contribution of common variants to susceptibility to common disease. *Nat Genet* 2003;33:177–182.

London GM, Safar ME, Weiss YA, et al. Volume-dependent parameters in essential hypertension. *Kidney Int* 1977; 11:204–208.

Lösel R, Schultz A, Boldyreff B, Wehling M. Rapid effects of aldosterone on vascular cells: clinical implications. *Steroids* 2004;69:575–578.

Lovallo WR, Wilson MF, Vincent AS, et al. Blood pressure response to caffeine shows incomplete tolerance after short-term regular consumption. *Hypertension* 2004;43:760–765.

Lowenstein FW. Blood-pressure in relation to age and sex in the tropics and subtropics. *Lancet* 1961;1:389–392.

Lucas A, Morley R. Does early nutrition in infants born before term programme later blood pressure? *BMJ* 1994; 309:304–308.

Luft FC. Geneticism of essential hypertension. *Hypertension* 2004;43:1155–1159.

Luft FC, Grim CE, Higgins JT Jr, Weinberger MH. Differences in response to sodium administration in normotensive white and black subjects. *J Lab Clin Med* 1977; 90:555–562.

Luft FC, Rankin LI, Block R, et al. Cardiovascular and humoral responses to extremes of sodium intake in normal black and white men. *Circulation* 1979;60:697–706.

Lund-Johansen P. Central haemodynamics in essential hypertension at rest and during exercise. *J Hypertens* 1989; 7(Suppl 6):S52–S55.

MacGregor GA, Cappuccio FP. The kidney and essential hypertension. *J Hypertens* 1993;11:781–785.

Mackenzie HS, Brenner BM. Fewer nephrons at birth: a missing link in the etiology of essential hypertension. *Am J Kidney Dis* 1995;26:91–98.

MacMahon S. Alcohol consumption and hypertension. *Hypertension* 1987;9:111–121.

Madison DV. Pass the nitric oxide. *Proc Natl Acad Sci USA* 1993;90:4329–4331.

Malik S, Wong ND, Franklin SS, et al. Impact of the metabolic syndrome on mortality from coronary heart disease, cardiovascular disease, and all causes in United States adults. *Circulation* 2004;110:1245–1250.

Malinski MK, Sesso HD, Lopez-Jimenez F, et al. Alcohol consumption and cardiovascular disease mortality in hypertensive men. *Arch Intern Med* 2004;164:623–628.

Mañalich R, Reyes L, Herrera M, et al. Relationship between weight at birth and the number and size of renal glomeruli in humans. *Kidney Int* 2000;58:770–773.

Mancia G, Parati G, Castiglioni P, et al. Daily life blood pressure changes are steeper in hypertension than in normotensive subjects. *Hypertension* 2003;42:277–282.

Mano A, Tatsumi T, Shiraishi J, et al. Aldosterone directly induces myocyte apoptosis through calcineurin-dependent pathways. *Circulation* 2004;110:317–323.

Manson JE, Skerrett PJ, Greenland P, VanItallie TB. The escalating pandemics of obesity and sedentary lifestyle. A call to action for clinicians. *Arch Intern Med* 2004;164:249–258.

Manuck SB, Polefrone JM, Terrell DF. Absence of enhanced sympathoadrenal activity and behaviorally evoked cardiovascular reactivity among offspring of hypertensives. *Am J Hypertens* 1996;9:245–255.

Markovitz JH, Matthews KA, Kannel WB, et al. Psychological predictors of hypertension in the Framingham study. *JAMA* 1993;270:2439–2443.

Marshall T, Anantharachagan A, Choudhary K, et al. A randomised controlled trial of the effect of anticipation of a blood test on blood pressure. *J Hum Hypertens* 2002; 16:621–625.

Martin RM, Ness AR, Gunnell D, et al. Does breast-feeding in infancy lower blood pressure in childhood? The Avon

Longitudinal Study of Parents and Children (ALSPAC). *Circulation* 2004;109:1259–1266.

Martinez DV, Rocha R, Matsumura M, et al. Cardiac damage prevention by eplerenone: comparison with low sodium diet or potassium loading. *Hypertension* 2002; 39:614–618.

Mascioli S, Grimm R Jr, Launer C, et al. Sodium chloride raises blood pressure in normotensive subjects. *Hypertension* 1991;17(Suppl 1):I21–I26.

Matsui Y, Jia N, Okamoto H, et al. Role of osteopontin in cardiac fibrosis and remodeling in angiotensin II-induced cardiac hypertrophy. *Hypertension* 2004;43:1195–1201.

Matthaei S, Stumvoll M, Kellerer M, Häring HU. Pathophysiology and pharmacological treatment of insulin resistance. *Endocr Rev* 2000;21:585–618.

Matthews KA, Katholi CR, McCreath H, et al. Blood pressure reactivity to psychological stress predicts hypertension in the CARDIA study. *Circulation* 2004;110:74–78.

Matthews KA, Kiefe CI, Lewis CE, et al. Socioeconomic trajectories and incident hypertension in a biracial cohort of young adults. *Hypertension* 2002;39:772–776.

Mazzali M, Hughes J, Kim YG, et al. Elevated uric acid increases blood pressure in the rat by a novel crystal-independent mechanism. *Hypertension* 2001;38:1101–1106.

McAllister AS, Atkinson AB, Johnston GD, et al. Basal nitric oxide production is impaired in offspring of patients with essential hypertension. *Clin Sci* 1999;97:141–147.

McCarron DA, Morris CD, Henry HJ, Stanton JL. Blood pressure and nutrient intake in the United States. *Science* 1984;224:1392–1397.

McCarron DA, Pingree PA, Rubin RJ, et al. Enhanced parathyroid function in essential hypertension. *Hypertension* 1980;2:162–168.

McCubbin JA, Bruehl S, Wilson JF, et al. Endogenous opioids inhibit ambulatory blood pressure during naturally occurring stress. *Psychosom Med* 1998;60:227–231.

McKeigue PM, Reynard JM. Relation of nocturnal polyuria of the elderly to essential hypertension. *Lancet* 2000; 355:486–488.

McKinnon W, Lord GA, Forni LG, Hilton PJ. Circulating sodium pump inhibitors in five volume-expanded humans. *J Hypertens* 2003;21:2315–2321.

McNeill AM, Rosamond WD, Girman CJ, et al. Prevalence of coronary heart disease and carotid arterial thickening in patients with the metabolic syndrome (the ARIC Study). *Am J Cardiol* 2004;94:1249–1254.

McTigue KM, Harris R, Hemphill B, et al. Screening and interventions for obesity in adults: summary of the evidence for the U.S. Preventive Services Task Force. *Ann Intern Med* 2003;139:933–949.

McVeigh GE, Hamilton PK, Morgan DR. Evaluation of mechanical arterial properties: clinical, experimental and therapeutic aspects. *Clin Sci* 2002;102:51–67.

Meade TW, Cooper JA, Peart WS. Plasma renin activity and ischemic heart disease. *N Engl J Med* 1993;329:616–619.

Meade TW, Imeson JD, Gordon D, Peart WS. The epidemiology of plasma renin. *Clin Sci* 1983;64:273–280.

Melander O, Frandsen E, Groop L, Hulthén UL. Plasma ProANP$_{1-30}$ reflects salt sensitivity in subjects with heredity for hypertension. *Hypertension* 2002; 39:996–999.

Mercuro G, Vitale C, Cerquetani E, et al. Effect of hyperuricemia upon endothelial function in patients at increased cardiovascular risk. *Am J Cardiol* 2004; 94:932–935.

Messerli FH, Garavaglia GE, Schmieder RE, et al. Disparate cardiovascular findings in men and women with essential hypertension. *Ann Intern Med* 1987;107:158–161.

Michel F, Ambroisine ML, Duriez M, et al. Aldosterone enhances ischemia-induced neovascularization through angiotensin II-dependent pathway. *Circulation* 2004;109: 1933–1937.

Michel MC, Rascher W. Neuropeptide Y: a possible role in hypertension? *J Hypertens* 1995;13:385–395.

Mikkelsen KL, Wiinberg N, Høegholm A, et al. Smoking related to 24-h ambulatory blood pressure and heart rate. *Am J Hypertens* 1997;10:483–491.

Miller JZ, Weinberger MH, Chirstian JC, Daugherty SA. Familial resemblance in the blood pressure response to sodium restriction. *Am J Epidemiol* 1987;126:822–830.

Missouris CG, Cappuccio FP, Varsamis E, et al. Serotonin and heart rate in hypertensive and normotensive subjects. *Am Heart J* 1998;135:838–843.

Mitchell GF, Parise H, Vita JA, et al. Local shear stress and brachial artery flow-mediated dilation: the Framingham Heart Study. *Hypertension* 2004;44:134–139.

Mitchell GF. Arterial stiffness and wave reflection in hypertension: pathophysiologic and therapeutic implications. *Curr Hypertens Rep* 2004;6:436–441.

Mittendorfer-Rutz E, Rasmussen F, Wasserman D. Restricted fetal growth and adverse maternal psychosocial and socioeconomic conditions as risk factors for suicidal behaviour of offspring: a cohort study. *Lancet* 2004; 364: 1135–1140.

Mizuno Y, Yasue H, Yoshimura M, et al. Adrenocorticotropic hormone is produced in the ventricle of patients with essential hypertension. *J Hypertens* 2005;23:411–416.

Mohr E, Richter D. Vasopressin in the regulation of body functions. *J Hypertens* 1994;12:345–348.

Mokdad AH, Ford ES, Bowman BA, et al. Prevalence of obesity, diabetes, and obesity-related health risk factors, 2001. *JAMA* 2003;289:76–79.

Moore H, Summerbell CD, Greenwood DC, et al. Improving management of obesity in primary care: cluster randomised trial. *BMJ* 2003;327:1085–1089.

Morimoto A, Uzu T, Fujii T, et al. Sodium sensitivity and cardiovascular events in patients with essential hypertension. *Lancet* 1997;350:1734–1737.

Morishita R, Aoki M, Hashiya N, et al. Safety evaluation of clinical gene therapy using hepatocyte growth factor to treat peripheral arterial disease. *Hypertension* 2004;44: 203–209.

Morton WE. Hypertension and color blindness in young men. *Arch Intern Med* 1975;135:653–656.

Mu J, Liu Z, Yang D, et al. Baseline Na-Li countertransport and risk of hypertension in children: a 10-year prospective study in Hanzhong children. *J Hum Hypertens* 2004;18: 885–890.

Muirhead EE. Renal vasodepressor mechanisms. *J Hypertens* 1993;11:S53–S58.

Muirhead EE, Streeten DH, Byers LW. Lipomedullinpinoma. *Blood Pressure* 1993;2:183–188.

Mukamal KJ, Conigrave KM, Mittleman MA, et al. Roles of drinking pattern and type of alcohol consumed in coronary heart disease in men. *N Engl J Med* 2003; 348: 109–118.

Mulvany MJ. Small artery remodeling in hypertension. *Curr Hypertens Rep* 2002;4:49–55.

Nabah YN, Mateo T, Estellés R, et al. Angiotensin II induces neutrophil accumulation *in vivo* through generation and release of CXC chemokines. *Circulation* 2004; 110: 3581–3586.

Nabel EG. Cardiovascular disease. *N Engl J Med* 2003; 349:60–72.

Nadar SK, Blann AD, Kamath S, et al. Platelet indexes in relation to target organ damage in high-risk hypertensive patients: a substudy of the Anglo-Scandinavian Cardiac Outcomes Trial (ASCOT). *J Am Coll Cardiol* 2004;44: 415–422.

Najjar SS, Scuteri A, Shetty V, et al. Arterial stiffness predicts the development of hypertension in younger normotensive adults: the Baltimore Longitudinal Study of Aging [Abstract]. *Circulation* 2004;110(Suppl 3):III–81.

Nakov R, Pfarr E, Eberle S. Darusentan: an effective endothelin receptor antagonist for treatment of hypertension. *Am J Hypertens* 2002;15:583–589.

Naraghi R, Geiger H, Crnac J, et al. Posterior fossa neurovascular anomalies in essential hypertension. *Lancet* 1994;344:1466–1470.

Narayan KM, Boyle JP, Thompson TJ, et al. Lifetime risk for diabetes mellitus in the United States. *JAMA* 2003; 290:1884–1890.

Narkiewicz K, Phillips BG, Kato M, et al. A gender selective interaction between aging, blood pressure and sympathetic nerve activity. *Hypertension* 2005;45:522–525.

Nash D, Magder L, Lustberg M, et al. Blood lead, blood pressure, and hypertension in perimenopausal and postmenopausal women. *JAMA* 2003;289:1523–1532.

Navar LG. The intrarenal renin-angiotensin system in hypertension. *Kidney Int* 2004;65:1522–1532.

NCEP Expert Panel (Adult Treatment Panel III). Third report of the National Cholesterol Education Program (NCEP) Expert Panel on detection, evaluation, and treatment of high blood cholesterol in adults (Adult Treatment Panel III) final report. *Circulation* 2002; 106:3143–3421.

Newby DE, Sciberras DG, Mendel CM, et al. Intra-arterial substance P mediated vasodilatation in the human forearm. *Br J Clin Pharmacol* 1997;43:493–499.

Nickenig G, Strehlow K, Roeling J, et al. Salt induces vascular AT$_1$ receptor overexpression *in vitro* and *in vivo*. *Hypertension* 1998;31:1272–1277.

Nicklas BJ, Penninx BW, Cesari M, et al. Association of visceral adipose tissue with incident myocardial infarction in older men and women: the Health, Aging and Body Composition Study. *Am J Epidemiol* 2004;160:741–749.

Nielsen S, Guo Z, Johnson CM, et al. Splanchnic lipolysis in human obesity. *J Clin Invest* 2004a;113:1582–1588.

Nielsen S, Halliwill JR, Joyner MJ, Jensen MD. Vascular response to angiotensin II in upper body obesity. *Hypertension* 2004b;44:435–441.

Nieves DJ, Cnop M, Retzlaff B, et al. The atherogenic lipoprotein profile associated with obesity and insulin resistance is largely attributable to intra-abdominal fat. *Diabetes* 2003;52:172–179.

Niskanen LK, Laaksonen DE, Nyyssonen K, et al. Uric acid level as a risk factor for cardiovascular and all-cause mortality in middle-aged men: a prospective cohort study. *Arch Intern Med* 2004;164:1546–1551.

Noon JP, Walker BR, Webb DJ, et al. Impaired microvascular dilatation and capillary rarefaction in young adults with a predisposition to high blood pressure. *J Clin Invest* 1997;99:1873–1879.

Nørgaard K, Rasmussen E, Jensen T, et al. Nature of elevated blood pressure in normoalbuminuric type I diabetic patients. Essential hypertension? *Am J Hypertens* 1993;6:830–836.

Norman M, Martin H. Preterm birth attenuates association between low birth weight and endothelial dysfunction. *Circulation* 2003;108:996–1001.

O'Mahoney D, Wathen CG. Hypertension in porphyria—an understated problem. *QJM* 1996;89:161–164.

Oliver WJ, Cohen EL, Neel JV. Blood pressure, sodium intake, and sodium related hormones in the Yanomamo Indians, a "no-salt" culture. *Circulation* 1975;52:146–151.

Omvik P, Tarazi EC, Bravo EL. Regulation of sodium balance in hypertension. *Hypertension* 1980;2:515–523.

Oparil S, Zaman MA, Calhoun DA. Pathogenesis of hypertension. *Ann Intern Med* 2003;139:761–776.

Orlov SN, Adragna NC, Adarichev VA, Hamet P. Genetic and biochemical determinants of abnormal monovalent ion transport in primary hypertension. *Am J Physiol* 1999; 276(3 Pt 1):C511–C536.

O'Rourke MF, Staessen JA, Vlachopoulos C, et al. Clinical applications of arterial stiffness; definitions and reference values. *Am J Hypertens* 2002;15:426–444.

O'Rourke MF. Ascending aortic pressure wave indices and cardiovascular disease. *Am J Hypertens* 2004;17:721–723.

O'Shaughnessy KM, Karet FE. Salt handling and hypertension. *J Clin Invest* 2004;113:1075–1081.

Page GP, George V, Go RC, et al. "Are we there yet?": deciding when one has demonstrated specific genetic causation in complex diseases and quantitative traits. *Am J Hum Genet* 2003;73:711–719.

Page IH. The nature of arterial hypertension. *Arch Intern Med* 1963;111:103–115.

Page LB, Vandevert DE, Nader K, et al. Blood pressure of Qash' qai pastoral nomads in Iran in relation to culture, diet, and body form. *Am J Clin Nutr* 1981;34:527–538.

Palaniappan L, Carnethon MR, Wang Y, et al. Predictors of the incident metabolic syndrome in adults: the Insulin Resistance Atherosclerosis Study. *Diabetes Care* 2004; 27: 788–793.

Palatini P, Julius S. Relevance of heart rate as a risk factor in hypertension. *Curr Hypertens Rep* 1999;3:219–224.

Palatini P, Thijs L, Staessen JA, et al. Predictive value of clinic and ambulatory heart rate for mortality in elderly subjects with systolic hypertension. *Arch Intern Med* 2002;162: 2313–2321.

Palatini P, Visentin P, Nicolosi G, et al. Supernormal left ventricular performance in young subjects with mild hypertension. *Clin Sci* 1996;91:275–281.

Palmer BF. Impaired renal autoregulation: implications for the genesis of hypertension and hypertension-induced renal injury. *Am J Med Sci* 2001;321:388–400.

Palmer RM, Ferrige AG, Moncada S. Nitric oxide release accounts for the biological activity of endothelium-derived relaxing factor. *Nature* 1987;327:524–526.

Pan L, Gross KW. Transcriptional regulation of renin: an update. *Hypertension* 2005;45:3–8.

Paniagua OA, Bryant MB, Panza JA. Transient hypertension directly impairs endothelium-dependent vasodilation of the human microvasculature. *Hypertension* 2000; 36:941–944.

Panza JA, Casino PR, Badan DM, Quyyumi AA. Effect of increased availability of endothelium-derived nitric oxide precursor on endothelium-dependent vascular relaxation in normal subjects and in patients with essential hypertension. *Circulation* 1993;87:1475–1481.

Panza JA, García CE, Kilcoyne CM, et al. Impaired endothelium-dependent vasodilation in patients with essential hypertension. *Circulation* 1995;91:1732–1738.

Panza JA, Quyyumi AA, Brush JE Jr, Epstein SE. Abnormal endothelium-dependent vascular relaxation in patients with essential hypertension. *N Engl J Med* 1990; 323:22–27.

Paradis G, Lambert M, O'Loughlin J, et al. Blood pressure and adiposity in children and adolescents. *Circulation* 2004;110:1832–1838.

Pardell H, Rodicio JL. High blood pressure, smoking and cardiovascular risk. *J Hypertens* 2005;23:219–221.

Park JB, Charbonneau F, Schiffrin EL. Correlation of endothelial function in large and small arteries in human essential hypertension. *J Hypertens* 2001;19:415–420.

Park JB, Schiffrin EL. Small artery remodeling is the most prevalent (earliest?) form of target organ damage in mild essential hypertension. *J Hypertens* 2001;19:921–930.

Park YW, Zhu S, Palaniappan L, et al. The metabolic syndrome: prevalence and associated risk factor findings in the US population from the Third National Health and Nutrition Examination Survey, 1988–1994. *Arch Intern Med* 2003;163:427–436.

Parker JC, Friedman-Kien AE, Levin S, Bartter FC. Pseudoxanthoma elasticum and hypertension. *N Engl J Med* 1964;271:1204–1206.

Peeters A, Barendregt JJ, Willekens F, et al. Obesity in adulthood and its consequences for life expectancy: a life-table analysis. *Ann Intern Med* 2003;138:24–32.

Perez del Villar C, Garcia Alonso CJ, Feldstein CA, et al. Role of endothelin in the pathogenesis of hypertension. *Mayo Clin Proc* 2005;80:84–96.

Perini C, Müller FB, Rauchfleisch U, et al. Psychosomatic factors in borderline hypertensive subjects and offspring of hypertensive parents. *Hypertension* 1990;16:627–634.

Perticone F, Ceravolo R, Candigliota M, et al. Obesity and body fat distribution induce endothelial dysfunction by oxidative stress: protective effect of vitamin C. *Diabetes* 2001;50:159–165.

Phillips MI, Schmidt-Ott KM. The discovery of renin 100 years ago. *News Physiol Sci* 1999;14:271–274.

Pickering G. Systemic arterial hypertension. In: Fisherman AP, Richards CW, eds. *Circulation of the Blood: Men and Ideas*. Bethesda, MD: American Physiological Society, 1964:487–544.

Pickering TG. The effects of environmental and lifestyle factors on blood pressure and the intermediary role of the sympathetic nervous system. *J Hum Hypertens* 1997; 11(Suppl 1):S9–S18.

Pilz B, Bräsen JH, Schneider W, Luft FC. Obesity and hypertension-induced restrictive cardiomyopathy: a harbinger of things to come. *Hypertension* 2004;43:911–917.

Poli KA, Tofler GH, Larson MG, et al. Association of blood pressure with fibrinolytic potential in the Framingham offspring population. *Circulation* 2000;101:264–269.

Pomeranz A, Dolfin T, Korzets Z, et al. Increased sodium concentrations in drinking water increase blood pressure in neonates. *J Hypertens* 2002;20:203–207.

Post WS, Larson MG, Levy D. Hemodynamic predictors of incident hypertension. The Framingham Heart Study. *Hypertension* 1994;24:585–590.

Poulsen PL, Ebbehøj E, Hansen KW, Mogensen CE. Effects of smoking on 24-h ambulatory blood pressure and autonomic function in normoalbuminuric insulin-dependent diabetes mellitus patients. *Am J Hypertens* 1998;11:1093–1099.

Poulter N, Khaw KT, Hopwood BE, et al. The Kenyan Luo migration study: observations on the initiation of a rise in blood pressure. *BMJ* 1990;300:967–972.

Prasad A, Quyyumi AA. Renin-angiotensin system and angiotensin receptor blockers in the metabolic syndrome. *Circulation* 2004;110:1507–1512.

Pratt JH, Rebhun JF, Zhou L, et al. Levels of mineralocorticoids in whites and blacks. *Hypertension* 1999;34:315–319.

Preston RA, Materson BJ, Reda DJ, et al. Age-race subgroup compared with renin profile as predictors of blood pressure response to antihypertensive therapy. *JAMA* 1998;280:1168–1172.

Primatesta P, Falaschetti E, Poulter NR. Birth weight and blood pressure in childhood: results from the Health Survey for England. *Hypertension* 2005;45:75–79.

Psaty BM, Smith NL, Heckbert SR, et al. Diuretic therapy, the α-adducin gene variant, and the risk of myocardial infarction or stroke in persons with treated hypertension. *JAMA* 2002;287:1680–1689.

Rahmouni K, Correia ML, Haynes WG, Mark AL. Obesity-associated hypertension: new insights into mechanisms. *Hypertension* 2005;45:9–14.

Rakic V, Puddey IB, Burke V, et al. Influence of pattern of alcohol intake on blood pressure in regular drinkers. *J Hypertens* 1998;16:165–174.

Re RN. Tissue renin angiotensin systems. *Med Clin NA* 2004;88:19–38.

Reaven GM. Insulin resistance/compensatory hyperinsulinemia, essential hypertension, and cardiovascular disease. *J Clin Endocrinol Metab* 2003;88:2399–2403.

Reaven GM. Role of insulin resistance in human disease. *Diabetes* 1988;37:1595–1607.

Redline S, Kirchner HL, Quan SF, et al. The effects of age, sex, ethnicity, and sleep-disordered breathing on sleep architecture. *Arch Intern Med* 2004;164:406–418.

Rees DD, Palmer RMJ, Moncada S. Role of endothelium-derived nitric oxide in the regulation of blood pressure. *Proc Natl Acad Sci U S A* 1989;86:3375–3378.

Reilly MP, Rader DJ. The metabolic syndrome: more than the sum of its parts? *Circulation* 2003;108:1546–1551.

Reilly MP, Wolfe ML, Rhodes T, et al. Measures of insulin resistance add incremental value to the clinical diagnosis of metabolic syndrome in association with coronary atherosclerosis. *Circulation* 2004;110:803–809.

Reims HM, Fossum E, Høieggen A, et al. Adrenal medullary overactivity in lean, borderline hypertensive young men. *Am J Hypertens* 2004;17:611–618.

Ren Y, Garvin J, Carretero OA. Mechanism involved in bradykinin-induced efferent arteriole dilation. *Kidney Int* 2002;62:544–549.

Resnick LM, Gupta RK, DiFabio B, et al. Intracellular ionic consequences of dietary salt loading in essential hypertension. *J Clin Invest* 1994;94:1269–1276.

Richard V, Hurel-Merle S, Scalbert E, et al. Functional evidence for a role of vascular chymase in the production of angiotensin II in isolated human arteries. *Circulation* 2001;104:750–752.

Rigotti NA. Treatment of tobacco use and dependence. *N Engl J Med* 2002;346:506–512.

Ritter JM, Brett SE, Woods JD, et al. Prostacyclin biosynthesis in essential hypertension before and during treatment. *J Hum Hypertens* 1996;10:37–42.

Rocchini AP, Yang JQ, Gokee A. Hypertension and insulin resistance are not directly related in obese dogs. *Hypertension* 2004;43:1011–1016.

Rocha R, Funder JW. The pathophysiology of aldosterone in the cardiovascular system. *Ann N Y Acad Sci* 2002; 970:89–100.

Rönnemaa T, Rönnemaa EM, Puukka P, et al. Smoking is independently associated with high plasma insulin levels in nondiabetic men. *Diabetes Care* 1996;19: 1229–1232.

Rosengren A, Hawken S, Ôunpuu S, et al. Association of psychosocial risk factors with risk of acute myocardial infarction in 11119 cases and 13648 controls from 52 countries (the INTERHEART study): case-control study. *Lancet* 2004;364:953–962.

Rossi A, Baldo-Enzi G, Calabrò A, et al. The renin-angiotensin-aldosterone system and carotid artery disease in mild-to-moderate primary hypertension. *J Hypertens* 2000; 18:1401–1409.

Rossi E, Regolisti G, Perazzoli F, et al. -344C/T polymorphism of CYP11B2 gene in Italian patients with idiopathic low renin hypertension. *Am J Hypertens* 2001;14: 934–941.

Rossi R, Chiurlia E, Nuzzo A, et al. Flow-mediated vasodilation and the risk of developing hypertension in healthy postmenopausal women. *J Am Coll Cardiol* 2004; 44: 1636–1640.

Rostrup M, Mundal HH, Westheim A, Eide I. Awareness of high blood pressure increases arterial plasma catecholamines, platelet noradrenaline and adrenergic responses to mental stress. *J Hypertens* 1991;9:159–166.

Russo C, Oliveri O, Girelli D, et al. Increased membrane ratios of metabolite to precursor fatty acid in essential hypertension. *Hypertension* 1997;29:1058–1063.

Rutter MK, Meigs JB, Sullivan LM, et al. C-reactive protein, the metabolic syndrome, and prediction of cardiovascular events in the Framingham Offspring Study. *Circulation* 2004;110:380–385.

Saad MF, Rewers M, Selby J, et al. Insulin resistance and hypertension: the Insulin Resistance Atherosclerosis study. *Hypertension* 2004;43:1324–1331.

Safar ME. Systolic hypertension in the elderly: arterial wall mechanical properties and the renin-angiotensin-aldosterone system. *J Hypertens* 2005;23:673–681.

Safar ME, Levy BI, Struijker-Boudier H. Current perspectives on arterial stiffness and pulse pressure in hypertension and cardiovascular diseases. *Circulation* 2003;107: 2864–2869.

Safar ME, Smulyan H. Coronary ischemic disease, arterial stiffness, and pulse pressure. *Am J Hypertens* 2004;17: 724–726.

Sagnella GA. Why is plasma renin activity lower in populations of African origin? *J Hum Hypertens* 2001;15:17–25.

Sakata K, Shirotani M, Yoshida H, Kurata C. Comparison of effects of enalapril and nitrendipine on cardiac sympathetic nervous system in essential hypertension. *J Am Coll Cardiol* 1998;32:438–443.

Sànchez R, Nolly H, Giannone C, et al. Reduced activity of the kallikrein-kinin system predominates over renin-angiotensin system overactivity in all conditions of sodium balance in essential hypertensives and family-related hypertension. *J Hypertens* 2003;21:411–417.

Sánchez-Lozada LG, Tapia E, Santamaría J, et al. Mild hyperuricemia induces vasoconstriction and maintains glomerular hypertension in normal and remnant kidney rats. *Kidney Int* 2005;67:237–247.

Sanz-Rosa D, Cediel E, de las Heras N, et al. Participation of aldosterone in the vascular inflammatory response of spontaneously hypertensive rats: role of the NFκB/IκB system. *J Hypertens* 2005;23:1167–1172.

Sasaki S, Zhang X-H, Kesteloot H. Dietary sodium, potassium, saturated fat, alcohol, and stroke mortality. *Stroke* 1995;26:783–789.

Sato A, Saruta T. Aldosterone-induced organ damage: plasma aldosterone level and inappropriate salt status. *Hypertens Res* 2004;27:303–310.

Savage D, Perkins J, Hong Lim C, Bund SJ. Functional evidence that K+ is the non-nitric oxide, non-prostanoid endothelium-derived relaxing factor in rat femoral arteries. *Vascul Pharmacol* 2003;40:23–28.

Savoia C, Schiffrin EL. Significance of recently identified peptides in hypertension: endothelin, natriuretic peptides, adrenomedullin, leptin. *Med Clin NA* 2004;88:39–62.

Schiffrin EL, Deng LY, Sventek P, Day R. Enhanced expression of endothelin-1 gene in endothelium of resistance arteries in severe human essential hypertension. *J Hypertens* 1997;15:57–63.

Schiffrin EL. Remodeling of resistance arteries in essential hypertension and effects of antihypertensive treatment. *Am J Hypertens* 2004;17:1192–1200.

Schillaci G, Pirro M, Vaudo G, et al. Prognostic value of the metabolic syndrome in essential hypertension. *J Am Coll Cardiol* 2004;43:1817–1822.

Schlaich MP, Lambert E, Kaye DM, et al. Sympathetic augmentation in hypertension: role of nerve firing, norepinephrine reuptake, and angiotensin neuromodulation. *Hypertension* 2004a;43:169–175.

Schlaich MP, Parnell MM, Ahlers BA, et al. Impaired L-arginine transport and endothelial function in hypertensive and genetically predisposed normotensive subjects. *Circulation* 2004b;110:3680–3686.

Schlüter K-D, Piper HM. Cardiovascular actions of parathyroid hormone and parathyroid hormone-related peptide. *Cardiovasc Rev* 1998;37:34–41.

Schneider GM, Jacobs DW, Gevirtz RN, O'Connor DT. Cardiovascular haemodynamic response to repeated mental stress in normotensive subjects at genetic risk of hypertension: evidence of enhanced reactivity, blunted adaptation, and delayed recovery. *J Hum Hypertens* 2003;17:829–840.

Schneider MP, Klingbeil AU, Schlaich MP, et al. Impaired sodium excretion during mental stress in mild essential hypertension. *Hypertension* 2001;37:923–927.

Schneider RH, Egan BM, Johnson EH, et al. Anger and anxiety in borderline hypertension. *Psychosom Med* 1986; 48:242–248.

Schnermann J, Briggs JP. The macula densa is worth its salt. *J Clin Invest* 1999;104:1007–1009.

Schorr U, Distler A, Sharma AM. Effect of sodium chloride- and sodium bicarbonate-rich mineral water on blood pressure and metabolic parameters in elderly normotensive individuals. *J Hypertens* 1996;14:131–135.

Schunkert H, Koenig W, Bröckel U, et al. Haematocrit profoundly affects left ventricular diastolic filling as assessed by Doppler echocardiography. *J Hypertens* 2000; 18:1483–1489.

Sciarrone MT, Stella P, Barlassina C, et al. ACE and α-adducin polymorphism as markers of individual response to diuretic therapy. *Hypertension* 2003;41:398–403.

Scuteri A, Najjar SS, Muller DC, et al. Metabolic syndrome amplifies the age-associated increases in vascular thickness and stiffness. *J Am Coll Cardiol* 2004;43: 1388–1395.

Sealey JE, Blumenfeld JD, Bell GM, et al. On the renal basis for essential hypertension. *J Hypertens* 1988;6:763–777.

Sealey JE, Blumenfeld J, Laragh JH. Prorenin cryoactivation as a possible cause of normal renin levels in patients with primary aldosteronism. *J Hypertens* 2005;23:459–262.

Sealey JE, Trenkwalder P, Gahnem F, et al. Plasma renin methodology. *J Hypertens* 1995;13:27–30.

Seely S. Possible reasons for the comparatively high resistance of women to heart disease. *Am Heart J* 1976;91:275–280.

Sega R, Cesana GC, Costa G, et al. Ambulatory blood pressure in air traffic controllers. *Am J Hypertens* 1998; 11: 208–212.

Segers P, Stergiopulos N, Westerhof N. Quantification of the contribution of cardiac and arterial remodeling to hypertension. *Hypertension* 2000;36:760–765.

Selby JV, Friedman GD, Quesenberry CP Jr. Precursors of essential hypertension. *Am J Epidemiol* 1990; 131:1017–1027.

Selkurt EE. Effect of pulse pressure and mean arterial pressure modification on renal hemodynamics and electrolyte and water excretion. *Circulation* 1951;4:541–551.

Sesso HD, Buring JE, Rifai N, et al. C-reactive protein and the risk of developing hypertension. *JAMA* 2003; 290: 2945–2951.

Shankar A, Klein BE, Klein R. Relationship between white blood cell count and incident hypertension. *Am J Hypertens* 2004;17:233–239.

Shaper AG, Wannamethee G, Whincup P. Alcohol and blood pressure in middle-aged British men. *J Hum Hypertens* 1988;2:71S–78S.

Shapiro D, Goldstein IB, Jamner LD. Effects of cynical hostility, anger out, anxiety, and defensiveness on ambulatory blood pressure in black and white college students. *Psychosom Med* 1996;58:354–364.

Sharabi Y, Dendi R, Holmes C, Goldstein DS. Baroreflex failure as a late sequela of neck irradiation. *Hypertension* 2003;42:110–116.

Siffert W, Düsing R. Sodium-proton exchange and primary hypertension. *Hypertension* 1995;26:649–655.

Sigurdson WJ, Sachs F, Diamond SL. Mechanical perturbation of cultured human endothelial cells causes rapid increases of intracellular calcium. *Am J Physiol* 1993; 264(6 Pt 2):H1745–H1752.

Simon G. Pathogenesis of structural vascular changes in hypertension. *J Hypertens* 2004;22:3–10.

Singh R, Wardle A, McMahon A, Samani N. Prospective analysis of plasma renin concentration as a risk factor for coronary artery disease [Abstract]. *J Hypertens* 2000; 18(Suppl 4):S22.

Singhal A, Cole TJ, Fewtrell M, et al. Is slower early growth beneficial for long-term cardiovascular health? *Circulation* 2004;109:1108–1113.

Singhal A, Lucas A. Early origins of cardiovascular disease: is there a unifying hypothesis? *Lancet* 2004;363: 1642–1645.

Sironi AM, Gastaldelli A, Mari A, et al. Visceral fat in hypertension: influence on insulin resistance and beta-cell function. *Hypertension* 2004;44:127–133.

Skilton MR, Evans N, Griffiths KA, et al. Aortic wall thickness in newborns with intrauterine growth restriction. *Lancet* 2005;365:1484–1486.

Smallegange C, Hale TM, Bushfield TL, Adams MA. Persistent lowering of pressure by transplanting kidneys from adult spontaneously hypertensive rats treated with brief antihypertensive therapy. *Hypertension* 2004;44:89–94.

Smith S, Julius S, Jamerson K, et al. Hematocrit levels and physiologic factors in relationship to cardiovascular risk in Techumseh, Michigan. *J Hypertens* 1994;12:455–462.

Smith WC, Crombie IK, Tavendale RT, et al. Urinary electrolyte excretion, alcohol consumption, and blood pressure in the Scottish heart study. *BMJ* 1988; 297:329–330.

Soleimani M, Singh G. Physiologic and molecular aspects of the $Na^+/H^+$ exchangers in health and disease processes. *J Invest Med* 1995;43:419–430.

Solomon DH, Schneeweiss S, Levin R, Avorn J. Relationship between COX-2 specific inhibitors and hypertension. *Hypertension* 2004;44:140–145.

Soro A, Glorioso N, Tonolo G, et al. Different plasma corticosteroid patterns in normotensive and hypertensive human subjects [Abstract]. *J Hypertens* 1996;14:S79.

Soro A, Ingram MC, Tonolo G, et al. Evidence of coexisting changes in 11β-hydroxysteroid dehydrogenase and 5α-reductase activity in subjects with untreated essential hypertension. *Hypertension* 1995;25:67–70.

Sowers JR, Frohlich ED. Insulin and insulin resistance: impact on blood pressure and cardiovascular disease. *Med Clin North Am* 2004;88:63–82.

Sperling MA. Prematurity–a window of opportunity? *N Engl J Med* 2004;351:2229–2231.

Staessen JA, Kuznetsova T, Roels HA, et al. Exposure to cadmium and conventional and ambulatory blood pressures in a prospective population study. *Am J Hypertens* 2000;13:146–156.

Staessen JA, Wang J, Bianchi G, Birkenhäger WH. Essential hypertension. *Lancet* 2003;361:1629–1641.

Stamler J, Caggiula AW, Gandits GA. Relation of body mass and alcohol, nutrient, fiber, and caffeine intakes to blood pressure in the special intervention and usual care groups in the Multiple Risk Factor Intervention Trial. *Am J Clin Nutr* 1997;659(Suppl l):338S–365S.

Stamler J, Cirillo M. Dietary salt and renal stone disease. *Lancet* 1997;349:506.

Stamler J, Elliott P, Dyer AR, et al. Sodium and blood pressure in the Intersalt study and other studies—in reply to the Salt Institute. *BMJ* 1996;312:1285–2387.

Stamler J, Rose G, Stamler R, et al. Intersalt study findings. Public health and medical care implications. *Hypertension* 1989;14:570–577.

Stamler R, Shipley M, Elliott P, et al. Higher blood pressure in adults with less education. *Hypertension* 1992;19:237–241.

Steinbrook R. Surgery for severe obesity. *N Engl J Med* 2004;350:1075–1079.

Steptoe A, Marmot M. Impaired cardiovascular recovery following stress predicts 3-year increases in blood pressure. *J Hypertens* 2005;23:529–536.

Steptoe A, Willemsen G. The influence of low job control on ambulatory blood pressure and perceived stress over the working day in men and women from the Whitehall II cohort. *J Hypertens* 2004;22:915–920.

Stettler N, Stallings VA, Troxel AB, et al. Weight gain in the first week of life and overweight in adulthood: a cohort study of European American subjects fed infant formula. *Circulation* 2005;111:1897–1903.

Stettler N, Zemel BS, Kumanyika S, Stallings VA. Infant weight gain and childhood overweight status in a multicenter, cohort study. *Pediatrics* 2002;109:194–199.

Strain WD, Chaturvedi N, Leggetter S, et al. Ethnic differences in skin microvascular function and their relation to cardiac target-organ damage. *J Hypertens* 2005;23:133–140.

Stranges S, Wu T, Dorn JM, et al. Relationship of alcohol drinking pattern to risk of hypertension: a population-based study. *Hypertension* 2004;44:813–819.

Strazzullo P, Barba G, Cappuccio FP, et al. Altered renal sodium handling in men with abdominal adiposity: a link to hypertension. *J Hypertens* 2001;19:2157–2164.

Strazzullo P, Siani A, Cappuccio FP, et al. Red blood cell sodium-lithium countertransport and risk of future hypertension. *Hypertension* 1998;31:1284–1289.

Sugiyama F, Yagami K-I, Paigen B. Mouse models of blood pressure regulation and hypertension. *Curr Hypertens Rep* 2001;3:41–48.

Suk SH, Sacco RL, Boden-Albala B, et al. Abdominal obesity and risk of ischemic stroke: the Northern Manhattan Stroke Study. *Stroke* 2003;34:1586–1592.

Suki WN, Schwettmann RS, Rector FC Jr, Seldin DW. Effect of chronic mineralocorticoid administration on calcium excretion in the rat. *Am J Physiol* 1968;215:71–74.

Sundström J, Sullivan L, D'Agostino RB, et al. Relations of serum uric acid to longitudinal blood pressure tracking and hypertension incidence. *Hypertension* 2005; 45:28–33.

Supowit SC, Rao A, Bowers MC, et al. Calcitonin gene-related peptide protects against hypertension-induced heart and kidney damage. *Hypertension* 2005;45:109–114.

Suzuki M, Kimura Y, Tsushima M, Harano Y. Association of insulin resistance with salt sensitivity and nocturnal fall in blood pressure. *Hypertension* 2000;35:864–868.

Swales JD. Functional disturbance of the cell membrane in hypertension. *J Hypertens* 1990a;8(Suppl 7):S203–S211.

Swales JD. Is there a cellular abnormality in hypertension? *J Cardiovasc Pharmacol* 1991;18(Suppl 2):S39–S44.

Swales JD. Membrane transport of ions in hypertension. *Cardiovasc Drug Ther* 1990b;4:367–372.

Sybert VP, McCauley E. Turner's syndrome. *N Engl J Med* 2004;351:1227–1238.

Tabara Y, Tachibana-Iimori R, Kawamoto R, et al. Shrinking stature: a new risk factor for arterial stiffness [Abstract]. *Am J Hypertens* 2005;18:115A–116A.

Taddei S, Virdis A, Ghiadoni L, et al. Age-related reduction of NO availability and oxidative stress in humans. *Hypertension* 2001;38:274–279.

Taittonen L, Nuutinen M, Räsänen L, et al. Lack of association between copper, zinc, selenium and blood pressure among healthy children. *J Hum Hypertens* 1997;11:429–433.

Taler SJ, Driscoll N, Tibor M, et al. Changes in hemodynamic patterns with age in normotensive patients [Abstract]. *Am J Hypertens* 2004a;17:170A.

Taler SJ, Driscoll N, Tibor M, et al. Obesity raises blood pressure in normal subjects via high cardiac output and impaired vasodilation [Abstract]. *Am J Hypertens* 2004b;17:25A.

Talwar S, Siebenhofer A, Williams B, Ng L. Influence of hypertension, left ventricular hypertrophy, and left ventricular systolic dysfunction on plasma N terminal proBNP. *Heart* 2000;83:278–282.

Tankó LB, Bagger YZ, Alexandersen P, et al. Peripheral adiposity exhibits an independent dominant antiatherogenic effect in elderly women. *Circulation* 2003; 107: 1626–1631.

Taylor AL, Ziesche S, Yancy C, et al. Combination of isosorbide dinitrate and hydralazine in blacks with heart failure. *N Engl J Med* 2004;351:2049–2057.

Thadhani R, Camargo CA Jr, Stampfer MJ, et al. Prospective study of moderate alcohol consumption and risk of hypertension in young women. *Arch Intern Med* 2002; 162: 569–574.

Thomas DD, Liu Z, Kantrow SP, Lancaster JR Jr. The biological lifetime of nitric oxide. *Proc Natl Acad Sci USA* 2001;98:355–360.

Timio M, Saronio P, Venanzi S, et al. Blood pressure in nuns in a secluded order. *Miner Electrolyte Metab* 1999; 25:73–79.

Tobian L, Hanlon S. High sodium chloride diets injure arteries and raise mortality without changing blood pressure. *Hypertension* 1990;15:900–903.

Tobian L. Dietary sodium chloride and potassium have effects on the pathophysiology of hypertension in humans and animals. *Am J Clin Nutr* 1997;65(Suppl 2):606S–611S.

Tobian L. Potassium and sodium in hypertension. *J Hypertens* 1988;6(Suppl 4):S12–S24.

Tomiyama H, Arai T, Koji Y, et al. The age-related increase in arterial stiffness is augmented in phases according to the severity of hypertension. *Hypertens Res* 2004;27: 465–470.

Touyz RM. Reactive oxygen species, vascular oxidative stress, and redox signaling in hypertension: what is the clinical significance? *Hypertension* 2004;44:248–252.

Touyz RM. Recent advances in intracellular signalling in hypertension. *Curr Opin Nephrol Hypertens* 2003;12: 165–174.

Trials of Hypertension Prevention Collaborative Research Group. Effects of weight loss and sodium reduction intervention on blood pressure and hypertension incidence in overweight people with high-normal blood pressure. *Arch Intern Med* 1997;157:657–667.

Tropeano AI, Boutouyrie P, Katsahian S, et al. Glucose level is a major determinant of carotid intima-media thickness in patients with hypertension and hyperglycemia. *J Hypertens* 2004;22:2153–2160.

Trowell HC. Salt and hypertension. *Lancet* 1980;2:88.

Tuck ML, Bounoua F, Eslami P, et al. Insulin stimulates endogenous angiotensin II production via a mitogen-activated protein kinase pathway in vascular smooth muscle cells. *J Hypertens* 2004;22:1779–1785.

Turner ST, Chapman AB, Schwartz GL, Boerwinkle E. Effects of endothelial nitric oxide synthase, α-adducin, and other candidate gene polymorphisms on blood pressure response to hydrochlorothiazide. *Am J Hypertens* 2003;16: 834–839.

Turner ST, Schwartz GL. Gene markers and antihypertensive therapy. *Curr Hypertens Rep* 2005;7:21–30.

Unger RH. Hyperleptinemia: protecting the heart from lipid overload. *Hypertension* 2005;45:1031–1034.

Ungvari Z, Koller A. Endothelin and prostaglandin $H_2$ thromboxane $A_2$ enhance myogenic constriction in hypertension by increasing $Ca^{2+}$, sensitivity of arteriolar smooth muscle. Hypertension 2000;36:856–861.

Vague J. The degree of masculine differentiation of obesities: a factor determining predisposition to diabetes, atherosclerosis, gout, and uric calculous disease. *Am J Clin Nutr* 1956;4:20–34.

Vakili BA, Devereux RB, De Simone G, et al. Relationship of plasma renin activity to left ventricular function in normotensive and hypertensive employed adults [Abstract]. *Circulation* 2000;102(Suppl 2):606.

Vallance P. Nitric oxide in the human cardiovascular system. *Br J Clin Pharmacol* 1998;45:433–439.

Van Gaal LF, Rissanen AM, Scheen AJ, et al. Effects of the cannabinoid-1 receptor blocker rimonabant on weight reduction and cardiovascular risk factors in overweight patients: 1-year experience from the RIO-Europe study. *Lancet* 2005; 365:1389–1397.

van Hooft IM, Grobbee DE, Waal-Manning HJ, Hofman A. Hemodynamic characteristics of the early phase of primary hypertension. *Circulation* 1993;87:1100–1106.

van Kats JP, Danser AH, van Meegen JR, et al. Angiotensin production by the heart. *Circulation* 1998;98:73–81.

van Paassen P, de Zeeuw D, de Jong PE, Navis G. Renin inhibition improves pressure natriuresis in essential hypertension. *J Am Soc Nephrol* 2000;11:1813–1818.

Vasan RS, Evans JC, Larson MG, et al. Serum aldosterone and the incidence of hypertension in nonhypertensive persons. *N Engl J Med* 2004;351:33–41.

Vaudo G, Schillaci G, Evangelista F, et al. Arterial wall thickening at different sites and its association with left ventricular hypertrophy in newly diagnosed essential hypertension. *Am J Hypertens* 2000;13:324–331.

Vaughan ED Jr, Laragh JH, Gavras I, et al. Volume factor in low and normal renin essential hypertension. Treatment with either spironolactone or chlorthalidone. *Am J Cardiol* 1973;32:523–532.

Venugopal SK, Devaraj S, Jialal I. Effect of C-reactive protein on vascular cells: evidence for a proinflammatory, proatherogenic role. *Curr Opin Nephrol Hypertens* 2005; 14:33–37.

Verdecchia P, Schillaci G, Borgioni C, et al. Cigarette smoking, ambulatory blood pressure and cardiac hypertrophy in essential hypertension. *J Hypertens* 1995;13:1209–1215.

Verma S, Strauss M. Angiotensin receptor blockers and myocardial infarction. *BMJ* 2004;329:1248–1249.

Veterans Administration Cooperative Study Group on Antihypertensive Agents. Urinary and serum electrolytes in untreated black and white hypertensives. *J Chronic Dis* 1987;40:839–847.

Villar J, Montilla C, Muniz-Grijalvo O, et al. Erythrocyte Na$^+$-Li$^+$ countertransport in essential hypertension. *J Hypertens* 1996;14:969–973.

Villarreal FJ, Asbun J. Peroxisome proliferator-activated receptors ligands, oxidative stress, and cardiac fibroblast extracellular matrix turnover. *Hypertension* 2004;44:621–622.

Vita JA, Keaney JF Jr, Larson MG, et al. Brachial artery vasodilator function and systemic inflammation in the Framingham Offspring Study. *Circulation* 2004;110:3604–3609.

Vrijkotte TG, van Doornen LJ, de Geus EJ. Effects of work stress on ambulatory blood pressure, heart rate, and heart rate variability. *Hypertension* 2000;35:880–886.

Vupputuri S, He J, Batuman V, et al. Relationship between blood lead and blood pressure among whites and African Americans [Abstract]. *Circulation* 2000;102(Suppl 2):844.

Waldstein SR, Siegel EL, Lefkowitz D, et al. Stress-induced blood pressure reactivity and silent cerebrovascular disease. *Stroke* 2004;35:1294–1298.

Walker BR, Best R, Shackleton CH, et al. Increased vasoconstrictor sensitivity to glucocorticoids in essential hypertension. *Hypertension* 1996;27:190–196.

Wannamethee G, Perry IJ, Shaper AG. Haematocrit, hypertension and risk of stroke. *J Intern Med* 1994;235:163–168.

Wassmann S, Wassmann K, Nickenig G. Modulation of oxidant and antioxidant enzyme expression and function in vascular cells. *Hypertension* 2004;44:381–386.

Wasywich CA, Webster MW, Richards AM, et al. Myocardial production of aldosterone in patients with normal left ventricular systolic function [Abstract]. *Circulation* 2004; 110(Suppl 3):III–360.

Watanabe S, Kang DH, Feng L, et al. Uric acid, hominoid evolution, and the pathogenesis of salt-sensitivity. *Hypertension* 2002;40:355–360.

Watanabe T, Barker TA, Berk BC. Angiotensin II and the endothelium: Diverse signals and effects. *Hypertension* 2005;45:163–169.

Weatherall D. From genotype to phenotype: genetics and medical practice in the new millennium. *Philos Trans R Soc Lond B Biol Sci* 1999;354:1995–2010.

Weder AB, Schork NJ. Adaptation, allometry, and hypertension. *Hypertension* 1994;24:145–156.

Weder AB. Membrane sodium transport. In: Izzo JL, Black HR, eds. *Hypertension Primer*, 2nd Ed. Dallas: American Heart Association, 1999:52.

Wei C-C, Meng QC, Palmer R, et al. Evidence of angiotensin-converting enzyme and chymase-mediated angiotensin II formation in the interstitial fluid space of the dog heart *in vivo*. *Circulation* 1999;99:2583–2589.

Weinberger MH. Salt sensitivity of blood pressure in humans. *Hypertension* 1996;27:481–490.

Weinberger MH. More on the sodium saga. *Hypertension* 2004;44:609–611.

Weinberger MH, Fineberg NS. Sodium and volume sensitivity of blood pressure. *Hypertension* 1991;18:67–71.

Weinberger MH, Fineberg NS, Fineberg SE, Weinberger M. Salt sensitivity, pulse pressure and death in normal and hypertensive humans. *Hypertension* 2001;37: 429–432.

Weinberger MH, Miller JZ, Luft FC, et al. Definitions and characteristics of sodium sensitivity and blood pressure resistance. *Hypertension* 1986;8(Suppl 2):II127–II134.

Weir MR, Saunders E. Renin status does not predict the antihypertensive response to angiotensin-converting enzyme inhibition in African-Americans. *J Hum Hypertens* 1998; 12:189–194.

Whelton A. Renal aspects of treatment with conventional nonsteroidal anti-inflammatory drugs versus cyclooxygenase-2-specific inhibitors. *Am J Med* 2001;110(Suppl 3A): 33S–42S.

Whelton PK, Appel LJ, Espeland MA, et al. Sodium reduction and weight loss in the treatment of hypertension in older persons. *JAMA* 1998;279:839–846.

Whitescarver SA, Ott CE, Jackson BA, et al. Salt-sensitive hypertension: contribution of chloride. *Science* 1984;223: 1430–1432.

Widlansky ME, Sesso HD, Rexrode KM, et al. Body mass index and total and cardiovascular mortality in men with a history of cardiovascular disease. *Arch Intern Med* 2004; 164:2326–2332.

Wild S, Roglic G, Green A, et al. Global prevalence of diabetes: estimates for the year 2000 and projections for 2030. *Diabetes Care* 2004;27:1047–1053.

Wildman RP, Farhat GN, Patel AS, et al. Weight change is associated with change in arterial stiffness among healthy young adults. *Hypertension* 2005;45:187–192.

Wilkinson IB, Franklin SS, Cockcroft JR. Nitric oxide and the regulation of large artery stiffness: from physiology to pharmacology. *Hypertension* 2004;44:112–116.

Willett WC, Dietz WH, Colditz GA. Guidelines for healthy weight. *N Engl J Med* 1999;341:427–434.

Williams SM, Addy JH, Phillips JA III, et al. Combinations of variations in multiple genes are associated with hypertension. *Hypertension* 2000;36:2–6.

Williams TA, Mulatero P, Filigheddu F, et al. Role of HSD11B2 polymorphisms in essential hypertension and the diuretic response to thiazides. *Kidney Int* 2005; 67: 631–637.

Wilson DM, Luetscher JA. Plasma prorenin activity and complications in children with insulin-dependent diabetes mellitus. *N Engl J Med* 1990;323:1101–1106.

Wilson FH, Hariri A, Farhi A, et al. A cluster of metabolic defects caused by mutation in a mitochondrial tRNA. *Science* 2004;306:1190–1194.

Wilson SH, Simari RD, Best PJ, et al. Simvastatin preserves coronary endothelial function in hypercholesterolemia in the absence of lipid lowering. *Arterioscler Thromb Vasc Biol* 2001;21:122–128.

Wolfel EE, Selland MA, Mazzeo RS, Reeves JT. Systemic hypertension at 4,300 m is related to sympathoadrenal activity. *J Appl Physiol* 1994;76:1643–1650.

Woods LL, Weeks DA, Rasch R. Programming of adult blood pressure by maternal protein restriction: role of nephrogenesis. *Kidney Int* 2004;65:1339–1348.

Wright JT Jr, Rahman M, Scarpa A, et al. Determinants of salt sensitivity in black and white normotensive and hypertensive women. *Hypertension* 2003;42:1087–1092.

Xiao F, Puddefoot JR, Barker S, Vinson GP. Mechanism for aldosterone potentiation of angiotensin II-stimulated rat arterial smooth muscle cell proliferation. *Hypertension* 2004;44:340–345.

Xin X, He J, Frontini MG, et al. Effects of alcohol reduction on blood pressure. *Hypertension* 2001;38:1112–1117.

Yamasaki S, Sawada S, Komatsu S, et al. Effects of bradykinin on prostaglandin $I_2$ synthesis in human vascular endothelial cells. *Hypertension* 2000;36:201–207.

Yan LL, Liu K, Matthews KA, et al. Psychosocial factors and risk of hypertension: the Coronary Artery Risk Development in Young Adults (CARDIA) study. *JAMA* 2003;290:2138–2148.

Yanagisawa M, Kurihara H, Kimura S, et al. A novel potent vasoconstrictor peptide produced by vascular endothelial cells. *Nature* 1988;332:411–415.

Yarnell JW, Baker IA, Sweetnam PM, et al. Fibrinogen, viscosity, and white blood cell count are major risk factors for ischemic heart disease. *Circulation* 1991;83:836–844.

Yip K-P, Wagner AJ, Marsh DJ. Detection of apical Na+/H+ exchanger activity inhibition in proximal tubules induced by acute hypertension. *Am J Physiol Regul Integr Comp Physiol* 2000;279:R1412–R1418.

Zanobetti A, Canner MJ, Stone PH, et al. Ambient pollution and blood pressure in cardiac rehabilitation patients. *Circulation* 2004;110:2184–2189.

Zhang J, Chen L, Lee MY, et al. Reduced expression of $Na^+$ pumps with $\alpha$2, but not $\alpha$1, subunits increases myogenic tone and blood pressure [Abstract]. *FASEB* 2005;914. 16(Vol. 2): A-1612.

Zhang J, Lee MY, Lingrel JB, et al. Ouabain antagonist and Na/Ca exchange inhibitor block ouabiain-induced increases in myogenic tone [Abstract]. *Circulation* 2004;110(Suppl 3):III–166.

Zicha J, Kunes J, Devynck M-A. Abnormalities of membrane function and lipid metabolism in hypertension. *Am J Hypertens* 1999;12:315–331.

Zinner SH, McGarvey ST, Lipsitt LP, Rosner B. Neonatal blood pressure and salt taste responsiveness. *Hypertension* 2002;40:280–285.

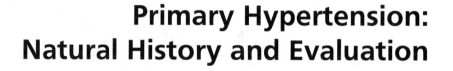

# Primary Hypertension:
# Natural History and Evaluation

Now that the probable causes of primary hypertension have been considered, we turn to its clinical course and complications. We will first view the natural history of the disease if left untreated, examining the specific manner by which hypertension leads to premature cardiovascular damage and how such damage is clinically expressed. Additional coverage is provided for special populations—the elderly, women, Blacks and other ethnic groups, diabetics, the obese—who may follow somewhat different courses. Based on this background, guidelines for evaluating the newly diagnosed hypertensive patient are presented.

As noted in previous chapters, hypertension seems logically divided into two main categories: combined systolic and diastolic hypertension and isolated systolic hypertension (ISH). Table 4–1 delineates some of the main differences between the two. Although the tabulation shows clear separation, the two may overlap. For example, 41% of ISH patients started with diastolic hypertension (Franklin et al., 2005). Most studies on the natural history of hypertension involved younger patients with combined

disease. Only recently has ISH received its deserved recognition (Franklin et al., 2001; Safar, 2005).

## NATURAL HISTORY OF PRIMARY HYPERTENSION

The natural history of hypertension, depicted in Figure 4–1, starts when some combination of hereditary and environmental factors sets into motion transient but repetitive perturbations of cardiovascular homeostasis (*prehypertension*), not enough to raise the blood pressure (BP) to levels defined as abnormal but enough to begin the cascade that, over many years, leads to BPs that usually are elevated (*early hypertension*). Some people, abetted by lifestyle changes, may abort the process and return to normotension. The majority, however, progresses into *established hypertension,* which, as it persists, may induce a variety of complications identifiable as target organ damage and disease, leading to a 4- to 6-year loss of life expectancy (Franco et al., 2005; Miura et al., 2001).

As was noted in Chapter 1, the higher the BP and the longer it remains elevated, the greater the morbidity and mortality. Although some patients with markedly elevated, untreated BP never have trouble, we have no way of accurately identifying in advance those who will have an uncomplicated course, the few who will enter a rapidly progressing, accelerated-malignant phase, and the many who will more slowly but progressively develop cardiovascular complications.

The role of hypertension probably is underestimated from morbidity and mortality statistics, which are largely based on death certificates. When a patient dies from a stroke, a heart attack, or renal failure—all directly attributable to uncontrolled

## TABLE 4–1

### Differences Between Combined Systolic and Diastolic Versus Isolated Systolic Hypertension

|  | Combined | ISH |
|---|---|---|
| **Age of onset** | 30–50 | >55 |
| **Mechanisms** | Multiple | Arterial stiffness |
| **Progression** | Slow, variable | More rapid, continuous |
| **Consequences** | Coronary artery disease, nephrosclerosis | Stroke, CHF |
| **Response to therapy** | Renin-angiotensin blockers more effective | Diuretics, calcium channel blockers more effective |

hypertension—the stroke, the heart attack, or the renal failure, *not* the hypertension, usually is listed as the cause of death.

## PREHYPERTENSION

Prehypertension, defined in the 7th JNC report, is present in 31% of U.S. adults (Svetky, 2005) with BP above 120/80 but still below 140/90 (Chobanian et al., 2003). As the pathogenetic mechanisms start the process that leads to hypertension, certain clues beyond the level of blood pressure may predict that the patient is in the prehypertensive phase. One clue

is low birth weight (Yliharsila et al., 2003); others include:

- *Exaggerated rises of BP during stress or exercise.* Based on an average of 8.8 years' follow-up of healthy normotensive men, it has been noted that those who developed hypertension were three times more likely than matched controls to have had an exaggerated BP response during a graded maximal exercise test (Matthews et al., 1998).
- *BPs that are in the higher ranges of normal.* As perhaps best seen in data from the Framingham cohort shown in Figure 4–2, the BP tends to track

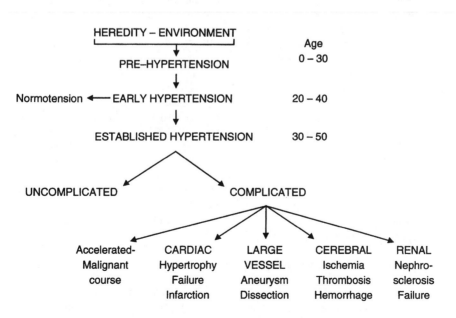

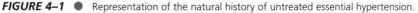

*FIGURE 4–1* ● Representation of the natural history of untreated essential hypertension.

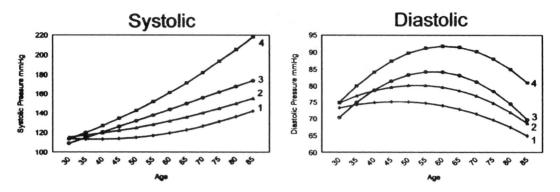

**FIGURE 4-2** ● Tracking systolic and diastolic blood pressures by age for up to 30 years in the Framingham Heart Study. Subjects who were stratified by their systolic BP in middle age: <120, 120–139, 140–159, and ≤160 mm Hg. The curves are derived from averaged individual regression analysis. (Modified from Franklin et al., 1997.)

over many years, remaining in the same relative position over time (Franklin et al, 1997). Subjects in each BP segment tend to remain in that segment, with a slow, gradual rise over the 30 years of follow-up. In a later survey of the Framingham population, hypertension developed over a 4-year interval in only 5% of men and women with a BP of <120/80 mm Hg, in 18% with a BP of 120–129/80–84 mm Hg, and in 37% with a BP of 130–139/85–89 mm Hg (Vasan et al., 2001a).

• *Presence of causal or coincidental features.* In the 30-year observation of the Framingham offspring, the major contributors to the incidence of hypertension beyond age were adiposity, heart rate, alcohol intake, hematocrit; blood glucose; and serum protein, triglyceride, and phosphorus levels, the last having a negative correlation (Garrison et al., 1987). As described in Chapter 3, the distribution of body fat played a significant role, with a markedly higher incidence of hypertension among those with more upper body fat as determined by subscapular skinfold thickness. As in all other populations, the strongest predictor was the previous level of BP, but weight gain was the next strongest predictor, with a 5% weight gain associated with a 20% to 30% increased odds of developing hypertension (Vasan et al., 2001b) (Franklin et al., 2005).

## EARLY HYPERTENSION: COURSE OF THE BLOOD PRESSURE

In most people who become hypertensive, the hypertension persists, but in some the BP returns to normal, presumably not to rise again. As emphasized in Chapter 2, hypertension should be confirmed by multiple readings before the diagnosis is made and therapy is begun. Initial readings may be higher than

subsequent readings because of a greater alerting reaction and, as with all biologic variables, a tendency for initially higher readings to come down from regression toward the mean. If subsequent readings are considerably lower and the patient is free of obvious vascular complications, the patient should be advised to adhere to a healthy lifestyle and either to return every few months for repeat BP measurement or to self-monitor the BP at home.

The wisdom of this course is shown by data from the Australian therapeutic trial (Management Committee, 1982); 12.8% of the patients whose diastolic BPs averaged more than 95 mm Hg on two sets of initial readings obtained 2 weeks apart had a subsequent fall to less than 95 mm Hg that persisted over the next year, such that the patients could not be entered into the trial. An even larger portion (47.5%) of those who entered the trial with a diastolic BP above 95 mm Hg and who received only placebo tablets for the next 3 years maintained their average diastolic BP at less than 95 mm Hg. A significant portion remained below 90 mm Hg while on placebo, including 11% of those whose initial diastolic BP was as high as 105 to 109 mm Hg. Overall, 80% of those on placebo maintained a diastolic BP of less than 100 mm Hg and, during the average 3-year follow-up, had no excess morbidity or mortality. On the other hand, 12.2% of the placebo-treated patients experienced a progressive rise in diastolic BP to more than 110 mm Hg.

In addition, when followed for longer periods, subjects with prehypertension, i.e., BP between 120/80 and 139/89, display an increased risk of cardiovascular disease. In the Framingham cohort, women with prehypertension had a 2.5-fold increased risk of CV disease, and men a 1.6-fold increased risk over 10 years compared to those with BP of 120/80 or below (Vasan et al., 2001a) (see Figure 1–2).

From these data and others that will be described, a number of implications can be made:

- Multiple BP readings over at least 6 weeks may be needed to establish the diagnosis of hypertension.
- Many patients who are not given antihypertensive drugs will have a significant decline in their BP, often to levels considered safe and not requiring therapy.
- Patients who are at low overall cardiovascular risk and free of target organ damage and whose diastolic BPs are lower than 90 mm Hg can safely be left off active drug therapy for at least a few years.
- If not treated, patients must be kept under close observation since a significant number will have a rise in pressure to levels requiring active therapy.

These conclusions form part of the basis of the approach toward initial management of patients with relatively mild hypertension that is presented in Chapter 5.

## ESTABLISHED HYPERTENSION

As delineated in Chapter 1 and shown in Figure 1–1, the long-term effects of progressively higher levels of BP on the incidence of stroke and coronary heart disease (CHD) are clear: In 61 prospective observational studies involving almost 1 million people with BP that started as low as 115/75 who were followed for up to 25 years, the associations were "positive, continuous and apparently independent" (Prospective Studies Collaboration, 2002).

### Uncontrolled Long-Term Observations

In addition to these major studies, smaller groups of patients with fairly severe hypertension were followed up by investigators before effective therapies became available (Bechgaard, 1983). Perera (1955) followed 500 patients with a casual diastolic BP of 90 mm Hg or higher—150 patients from before disease onset and 350 from an uncomplicated phase— until their death. The incidence of complications is given in Table 4–2. The mean age of onset was 32 years, and the mean survival time was 20 years. Perera (1955) summarized his survey of the natural history of hypertension as follows:

> . . . a chronic illness, more common in women, beginning as a rule in early adult life, related little if at all to pregnancy, and persisting for an average period of two decades before its secondary complicating pathologic features cause death at an average age fifteen to twenty years less than

## TABLE 4–2

### Complications in 500 Untreated Hypertensives

| Complication | Percent Affected | Mean Survival After Onset (yr) |
|---|---|---|
| Cardiac | | |
| Hypertrophy seen by radiography | 74 | 8 |
| Hypertrophy seen by electrocardiography | 59 | 6 |
| Congestive heart failure | 50 | 4 |
| Angina pectoris | 16 | 5 |
| Cerebral | | |
| Encephalopathy | 2 | 1 |
| Stroke | 12 | 4 |
| Renal | | |
| Proteinuria | 42 | 5 |
| Elevated blood urea nitrogen | 18 | 1 |
| Accelerated phase | 7 | 1 |

Data from Perera GA. Hypertensive vascular disease. *J Chron Dis* 1955;1:33–42.

the normal life expectancy. Hypertensive vascular disease may progress at a highly variable rate, but on the whole the patient with this disorder spends most of his hypertensive life with insignificant symptoms and without complications.

In more recent times, the loss of life expectancy, though significant, is much less (Franco et al., 2005) likely because most patients start with milder hypertension and more are treated.

### Age of Onset

One additional point about Perera's data is worth emphasizing: Few of his patients experienced the onset of hypertension after age 45. A similar finding was observed in the Cooperative Study of Renovascular Hypertension, wherein the diagnosis of primary hypertension was made with even greater certainty in 1,128 patients (Maxwell, 1975). Of these, the onset of an elevated BP was documented to have occurred at an age younger than 20 years in 12% and older than 50 years in only 7%.

On the other hand, in a more recent prospective study of a large, more representative population than the one followed up by Perera or seen in the Cooperative Study, 20% of people aged 40 to 69 years who developed a diastolic BP of 90 mm Hg or higher over a 5-year period were 60 years of age or older (Buck et al., 1987). In the Framingham study, the mean age of onset of systolic/diastolic hypertension was 53.4 years (Franklin et al., 2005).

### Untreated Patients in Clinical Trials

To those patients left untreated during the 1940s and 1950s, when no effective therapy was readily available, we can add those patients who served as the control populations in the trials of the therapy of hypertension up to the mid-1990s, at which time placebo-controlled trials were no longer considered ethical. Although these trials were not designed to observe the natural history of hypertension, their data can help to define further the course of untreated disease (Table 4–3). The trials involving elderly patients will be considered separately.

The types of patients included in these randomized, controlled trials (RCTs) and the manner in

## TABLE 4–3

### Complications Among Control Groups in Trials of Nonelderly Hypertensives

| Factor | Veterans Administration Cooperative[a] | | USPHS[b] | Australia[c] | Oslo[d] | Medical Research Council[e] |
|---|---|---|---|---|---|---|
| | 1967 | 1970 | | | | |
| Mean age (yr) | 51 | 52 | 44 | 50 | 45 | 52 |
| Range of diastolic blood pressure (mm Hg) | 115–129 | 90–114 | 90–115 | 95–109 | 90–110 | 95–109 |
| Number of subjects on placebo | 70 | 194 | 196 | 1,617 | 379 | 8,654 |
| Average follow-up (yr) | 1.3 | 3.3 | 7.0 | 3.0 | 5.5 | 5.5 |
| Coronary disease[f] | | | | | | |
| Fatal | 1.0 | 6.0 | 2.0 | 0.4 | 0.5 | 1.1 |
| Nonfatal | 3.0 | 1.0 | 26.0 | 4.9 | 2.9 | 1.6 |
| Congestive heart failure[f] | 3.0 | 6.0 | 1.0 | 0.1 | 0.2 | – |
| Cerebrovascular disease[f] | 16.0 | 11.0 | 3.0 | 1.5 | 1.8 | 1.3 |
| Renal insufficiency[f] | 4.0 | 2.0 | 1.0 | 0.1 | – | – |
| Progression of hypertension[f] | 4.0 | 10.0 | 12.0 | 12.1 | 17.2 | 11.7 |
| Total mortality[f] | 6.0 | 10.0 | 2.0 | 1.2 | 2.4 | 2.9 |

USPHS, U.S. Public Health Service. [a]Data from Veterans Administration Cooperative Study Group on Antihypertensive Agents. Effects of treatment on morbidity in hypertension. *JAMA* 1967;202:116–122 and *JAMA* 1970;213:1143–1152. [b]Data from Smith WM. Treatment of mild hypertension. *Circ Res* 1977;40[Suppl 1]:98–115. [c]Data from Management Committee. The Australian therapeutic trial in mild hypertension. *Lancet* 1980;1:1261–1267. [d]Data from Helgeland A. Treatment of mild hypertension. *Am J Med* 1980;69:725–732. [e]Data from Medical Research Council Working Party. Medical Research Council trial of treatment of mild hypertension. *BMJ* 1985;291:97–104. [f]Data reported as rate per 100 patients for the entire trial.

which they were followed up differ considerably, so comparisons between them are largely inappropriate. Moreover, the patients enrolled in these RCTs were, in general, much healthier than the general population. In most, they had to be free of major debilities and, often, any coexisting diseases, such as diabetes. For example, only 1.1% of those screened were eligible for enrollment in the Systolic Hypertension in the Elderly Program (SHEP) trial (SHEP Cooperative Research Group, 1991). Therefore, the rate of complications seen during the few years of follow-up on no therapy can be considered the minimum. In the overall population, much higher rates of cardiovascular diseases would be expected, and the dangers of untreated hypertension would obviously expand over a longer time.

### Veterans Administration Cooperative Study Group on Antihypertensive Agents

Publications of the data of the Veterans Administration Cooperative Study Group on Antihypertensive Agents (1967, 1970, 1972) are landmarks in the field of clinical hypertension. The Veterans Administration (VA) study involved a selected population—male veterans who were reliable and cooperative—but the data probably are applicable to most moderately severe hypertensives.

*Diastolic Blood Pressure Between 115 and 129 mm Hg*

The first VA study described the course of 70 men with an initial diastolic BP between 115 and 129 mm Hg who received only placebo. During their follow-up, which averaged 16 months and ranged up to 3 years, these complications were noted:

• Four patients died, three from ruptured aortic aneurysms.
• Seventeen patients developed accelerated hypertension, cerebral hemorrhage, severe congestive heart failure (CHF), or azotemia.
• Six patients developed myocardial infarction (MI), milder CHF, cerebral thrombosis, or transient ischemic attacks.

Thus, in less than 3 years, almost 40% of the patients with diastolic BP between 115 and 129 mm Hg who were *initially without severe target organ damage* developed complications.

*Diastolic Blood Pressure Between 90 and 114 mm Hg*

As surprising as the results just described were at the time, even more dramatic were the findings in the 194 patients with initial diastolic BP of 90 to 114 mm Hg, a group considered to have mild to moderate hypertension (VA Cooperative Study, 1970, 1972). Their initial BPs averaged 157/101 mm Hg, and just more than half had some evidence

of preexisting hypertensive complications. Maximal follow-up was 5.5 years and averaged 3.3 years. The overall risk to these patients of developing a morbid event in a 5-year period was 55%.

All the various complications except progression into accelerated hypertension occurred more frequently in the patients older than 60 years: Sixty-three percent developed a serious complication during this short interval, as compared to 15% of the patients younger than 50 years. Another 14% of the younger patients had a significant rise in their diastolic BP to more than 124 mm Hg, so that without therapy they would be expected to develop complications quickly.

These results showed a more serious and rapidly progressive course of untreated "mild to moderate" essential hypertension than had been suggested by most previously reported studies. Even among those who had no preexisting target organ damage, 16% developed a complication in only 5 years.

### U.S. Public Health Service Hospital Study

In the U.S. Public Health Service (USPHS) study (Smith, 1977), 389 patients with hypertension milder than that of the patients in the VA study were randomly divided into placebo and drug treatment groups and were followed up for as long as 7 years. At the onset of hypertension, none of the patients had evidence of target organ damage, and their mean BP was only 148/99 mm Hg. During the 7-year follow-up, the complications listed in Table 4–3 were noted among the placebo-treated group of truly mild hypertensives, confirming the conclusions of the VA study.

### Australian Therapeutic Trial

As previously noted, in the Australian therapeutic trial, more than 1,600 adults with diastolic BP of 95 to 109 mm Hg on two sets of readings obtained 2 weeks apart and initially free of known cardiovascular diseases were kept on placebo for an average of 3 years (Management Committee, 1980). Over this relatively short period, significantly increased morbidity and mortality occurred only in those whose diastolic BP averaged 100 mm Hg or higher. Recall, however, that 12.2% of these patients had a progressive rise in diastolic BP to more than 110 mm Hg (Table 4–3).

### Oslo Trial

The smaller Oslo trial (Helgeland, 1980) was similar to the Australian therapeutic trial in that it included only patients with uncomplicated disease who were free of target organ damage with a diastolic BP of less than 110 mm Hg and randomly divided them into nontherapy and drug therapy groups. The two trials differed in that the Oslo trial involved only men younger than 50 years. The results were very similar in both trials. In the Oslo trial, approximately half of the nontreated group experienced a fall in diastolic BP during the first 3 years. Few complications developed among those whose diastolic BP was initially below 100 mm Hg, whereas 16.4% of those whose initial diastolic BP was between 100 and 110 mm Hg had a cardiovascular complication.

### Medical Research Council Trial

For the Medical Research Council trial (1985), half of a large group of men and women aged 35 to 64 years whose diastolic BP ranged from 90 to 109 mm Hg were randomly assigned to placebo tablets

or active drugs for an average of 5.5 years. Their rates of subsequent events and progression to more severe hypertension were similar to those in the other trials of mild to moderate hypertension (Table 4–3).

### Untreated Elderly Patients in Trials

Table 4–4 summarizes data from seven RCTs of elderly hypertensives, two of them [SHEP (1991) and the Systolic Hypertension in Europe Trial (Staessen et al., 1997)] including only patients with ISH, the others including a portion with ISH. The control patients in these trials had much higher

## TABLE 4–4

### Complications Among Control Groups in Trials of Elderly Hypertensives

| Complication | Australian[a] | EWPHE[b] | Coope and Warrender[c] | SHEP[d] | STOP-HT[e] | MRC-2[f] | Syst-Eur[g] |
|---|---|---|---|---|---|---|---|
| Mean age (yr) | 64 | 72 | 69 | 72 | 76 | 70 | 70 |
| Blood pressure at entry (mm Hg) | | | | | | | |
| Systolic | <200 | 160–239 | 190–230 | 160–219 | <180–230 | 160–209 | 160–219 |
| Diastolic | 95–109 | 90–119 | 105–120 | <90 | 90–120 | <115 | <95 |
| Mean | 165/101 | 182/101 | 197/110 | 170/77 | 195/102 | 185/91 | 174/85 |
| Number of subjects on placebo | 289 | 424 | 465 | 2,371 | 815 | 2,113 | 2,297 |
| Average follow-up (yr) | 3.0 | 4.6 | 4.4 | 4.5 | 2.1 | 5.7 | 2.0 |
| Coronary disease[h] | | | | | | | |
| Fatal | 1.3 | 11.8 | 6.0 | 3.4 | 2.5 | 5.2 | 1.8 |
| Nonfatal | 8.3 | 2.8 | 2.2 | 3.4 | 2.7 | 2.3 | 1.4 |
| Congestive heart failure[h] | – | 5.4 | 7.7 | 4.5 | 4.8 | – | 2.1 |
| Cerebrovascular disease[h] | 4.2 | 13.7 | 9.4 | 6.8 | 6.6 | 6.4 | 3.4 |
| Progression of hypertension[h] | – | 6.8 | – | 15.0 | 9.3 | 8.3 | 5.5 |
| Total mortality[h] | 3.1 | 35.1 | 14.8 | 10.2 | 7.9 | 15.0 | 6.0 |

EWPHE, European Working Party on Hypertension in the Elderly; MRC, Medical Research Council; SHEP, Systolic Hypertension in the Elderly Program; STOP-HT, Swedish Trial in Old Patients with Hypertension; Syst-Eur, Systolic Hypertension in Europe Trial. [a]Data from Management Committee. Treatment of mild hypertension in the elderly. *Med J Aust* 1981;2:398–402. [b]Data from Amery A, Birkenäger W, Brixko P, et al. Mortality and morbidity results from the European Working Party on High Blood Pressure in the Elderly Trial. *Lancet* 1985;1:1349–1354. [c]Data from Coope J, Warrender TS. Randomized trial of treatment of hypertension in elderly patients in primary care. *BMJ* 1986;293:1145–1151. [d]Data from SHEP Cooperative Research Group. Prevention of stroke by antihypertensive drug treatment in older persons with isolated systolic hypertension. *JAMA* 1991;265:3255–3264. [e]Data from Dahlöf B, Lindholm LH, Hansson L, et al. Morbidity and mortality in the Swedish Trial in Older Patients with Hypertension. *Lancet* 1991;338:1281–1285. [f]Data from Medical Research Council Working Party. Medical Research Council trial of treatment in older adults. *BMJ* 1992;304:405–412. [g]Data from Staessen JA, Fagard R, Thijs L, et al. Randomized double-blind comparison of placebo and active treatment for older patients with isolated systolic hypertension. *Lancet* 1997;350:757–764. [h]Data reported as rate per 100 patients for the entire trial.

rates of the various end points than were seen in the trials of younger hypertensives listed in Table 4–3.

An additional analysis has examined the experience of patients 80 years and older in all eight trials that included such patients (Gueyffier et al., 1999). Not surprisingly, the untreated hypertensives over age 80 experienced even higher rates of morbidity and mortality than those seen in Tables 4–3 and 4–4 for younger patients. Among the 796 control patients followed for an average 3.5 years, the numbers of events were as follows: 77 strokes, 64 heart failures, and 223 deaths.

### Systolic Versus Diastolic Pressure

A meta-analysis of all published trials of elderly patients (Staessen et al., 2000) reconfirmed what has been repeatedly shown in multiple observational studies: Rises in systolic levels and falls in diastolic levels, with the resultant widening of pulse pressure, are typical changes that occur with aging, and all predict risk. As shown in Figure 4–3, risk of death rises steeply with increasing systolic BP but, at every level of systolic BP, the risk increases further the lower the diastolic BP. Nonetheless, as noted in Chapter 1, the widened pulse pressure is not as predictive of risk as is the higher systolic level.

From these multiple sources, the picture of the natural history of hypertension shown in Figure 4–1 is derived. We now will examine the various complications shown at the bottom of that figure.

## COMPLICATIONS OF HYPERTENSION

The end of the natural history of untreated hypertension is an increased likelihood of premature disability or death from cardiovascular disease. Before considering the specific types of organ damage and the causes of death related to hypertension, the underlying basis for the arterial pathology caused by hypertension and the manner in which this pathology is expressed clinically will be examined.

As described in Chapter 3, the pathogenesis of combined systolic and diastolic hypertension involves structural changes in the resistance arterioles subsumed under the terms *remodeling* and *hypertrophy*. These same changes almost certainly are also involved in the development of the small-vessel arteriosclerosis that is responsible for much of the target organ damage seen in long-standing hypertension. As people age, large artery atherosclerosis becomes an increasing factor, aggravated by the high shear stress of hypertension (Lakatta & Levy, 2003) but involving "several highly interrelated processes, including lipid disturbances, platelet activation, thrombosis, endothelial dysfunction, inflammation, oxidative stress, vascular smooth cell activation, altered matrix metabolism, remodeling, and genetic factors" (Faxon et al., 2004). Small vessel arterial and arteriolar sclerosis may be considered secondary consequences of typical combined systolic-diastolic hypertension, whereas large vessel stiffness is primarily responsible for the

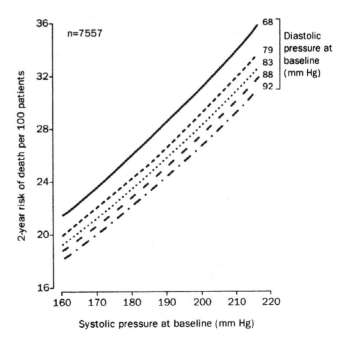

**FIGURE 4–3** ● The 2-year probability of death associated with systolic blood pressure at different levels of diastolic pressure at baseline in untreated elderly women with isolated systolic hypertension but no prior cardiovascular complications enrolled in eight randomized, controlled trials. (Modified from Staessen JA, Gasowski J, Wang JG, et al. Risks of untreated and treated isolated systolic hypertension in the elderly. *Lancet* 2000;355:865–872.)

predominantly systolic hypertension so common among the elderly (O'Rourke & Safar, 2005).

## Types of Arterial Lesions

The more common vascular lesions found in hypertension are:

- Fibrinoid necrosis, seen with acute and severe rises in BP.
- Hyperplastic or proliferative arteriolar sclerosis.
- Hyaline arteriolar sclerosis, with thickening and hyalinization of the intima and media.
- Miliary aneurysms in small cerebral penetration arterioles, usually at their first branching, which represent poststenotic dilations beyond areas of intimal thickening and which, when they rupture, cause the cerebral hemorrhages so typical of hypertension.
- Atherosclerotic plaques where thrombi form and which likely are responsible for the ischemia and infarction of heart, brain, kidney, and other organs that occur more frequently among hypertensives.
- Medial damage in the wall of the aorta may lead to the formation of large plaques with eventual aneurysmal dilation and rupture, as well as aortic dissections.

Most of the premature morbidity and mortality associated with hypertension is related to atherosclerosis. Although usually only one of the multiple risk factors involved, hypertension has an independent role (Agmon et al., 2000) that can be related to subclinical atherosclerosis even in children and adolescents (Berenson et al., 1998; Vos et al., 2003). There are variable rates of atherosclerotic stiffness between genders (Waddell et al., 2001) and ethnic groups (Chaturvedi et al., 2004), which may explain the variability in vascular damage between them. Noninvasive measures of arterial compliance are being used to identify such early atherosclerosis (Herrington et al., 2004).

## Pathogenesis of Atherosclerosis

As reviewed by Ross (1999), "The lesions of atherosclerosis represent a series of highly specific cellular and molecular responses that can best be described, in aggregate, as an inflammatory disease." Rather than the previous concept of a response to injury, "which initially proposed that endothelial denudation was the first step, the most recent version emphasizes endothelial dysfunction rather than denudation." Hypertension is obviously among the possible causes of such endothelial dysfunction.

Hypertension also has proinflammatory actions, increasing the formation of hydrogen peroxide and free radicals. . . . These substances reduce the formation of nitric oxide by the endothelium, increase leukocyte adhesion, and increase peripheral resistance (Ross, 1999).

Ross (1999) ascribes a major role to angiotensin II as contributing to atherogenesis by stimulating the growth of smooth muscle.

As another explanation for the vascular damages seen with hypertension, Hamet et al. (2001) have proposed that "a proliferative process may be primarily involved in hypertension development. . . . with an imbalance of proliferation and apoptosis in later stages. . . . [There is] evidence of a nonlinear, dichotomous process so that cardiovascular cells from hypertensive subjects are subjected to accelerated turnover, potentially culminating in accelerating aging."

## Causes of Death

Death may result when these arterial lesions either rupture or become occluded enough to cause ischemia or infarction of the tissues they supply. The overall increase in mortality associated with hypertension was examined in Chapter 1; Table 4–5 provides a more detailed look at the causes of death in hypertensives, mostly from series published before the availability of effective therapy. The series in the table include different types of patients, so comparisons between them should be avoided.

The following conclusions can be drawn from these data:

- Cardiovascular diseases are responsible for a higher proportion of deaths as the severity of the hypertension worsens (Smith et al., 1950).
- In general, patients with severe, resistant disease die of strokes; those presenting with advanced retinopathy and renal damage die of renal failure; and the majority, with moderately high BP, die of ischemic heart disease.
- Heart disease remains the leading cause of death (Mokdad et al., 2004). Heart failure, included under Heart Disease in Table 4–5, is the fastest growing condition among the elderly (Arnold et al., 2005).

As will be detailed in Chapter 5, with effective therapy of hypertension, strokes are prevented to a greater degree than is coronary disease, and heart failure is at least delayed.

## TARGET ORGAN INVOLVEMENT

Having tabulated the major causes of death resulting from the arterial pathology related to hypertension, we will now examine in more detail the

**TABLE 4–5**

## Causes of Death in Primary Hypertension

| Study | Year | No. of Deaths | Percentage of Deaths Heart Disease[a] | Stroke | Renal Failure | Nonvascular Causes |
|---|---|---|---|---|---|---|
| Untreated | | | | | | |
| Janeway (1913) | 1903–1912 | 212 | 33 | 14 | 23 | 30 |
| Hodge and Smirk (1967) | 1959–1964 | 173 | 48 | 22 | 10 | 20 |
| Bechgaard (1976) | 1932–1938 | 293 | 45 | 16 | 10 | 29 |
| Smith et al. (1950) | 1924–1948 | 376 | | | | |
| Group 1[b] | | 100 | 28 | 9 | 3 | 60 |
| Group 2 | | 100 | 46 | 17 | 2 | 35 |
| Group 3 | | 76 | 52 | 18 | 16 | 14 |
| Group 4 | | 100 | 22 | 16 | 59 | 3 |
| Bauer (1976) | 1955–1974 | 144 | 41 | 34 | 15 | 10 |
| Treated | | | | | | |
| Breckenridge (1970) | 1952–1959 | 87 | 18 | 28 | 44 | 10 |
| Breckenridge et al. (1970) | 1960–1967 | 203 | 38 | 21 | 29 | 11 |
| Strate et al. (1986) | 1970–1980 | 132 | 42 | 7 | 7 | 44 |
| Bulpitt et al. (1986) | 1971–1981 | 410 | 51 | 18 | 3 | 28 |
| Isles et al. (1986) | 1968–1983 | 750 | 52 | 23 | ? | 25 |

[a]Includes ischemic heart disease and congestive failure. [b]Grouping according to Keith-Wagener classification of hypertensive therapy.

pathophysiology and consequences of these various complications. Thereafter, the clinical and laboratory manifestations of the target organ damage will be incorporated into guidelines for evaluating the hypertensive patient.

In general, the complications of hypertension can be considered either hypertensive or atherosclerotic (Table 4–6). Those listed as hypertensive are caused more directly by the increased level of the BP per se, whereas the atherosclerotic complications have multiple causes, with hypertension playing a variable role. The major contribution of hypertension to all cardiovascular diseases is most clearly shown by epidemiologic data, perhaps best from the Prospective Studies Collaboration (Figure 1–1), which includes data from the ongoing Framingham study (Kannel, 1996; Kannel et al., 2004) (Figure 4–4).

### Hypertensive Heart Disease

As seen in Figure 4–4, hypertension more than doubles the risk for symptomatic coronary disease, including acute MI and sudden death, and more than

**TABLE 4–6**

## Complications of Hypertension

Hypertensive complications
    Accelerated-malignant hypertension (grades III and IV retinopathy)
    Encephalopathy
    Cerebral hemorrhage
    Left ventricular hypertrophy
    Congestive heart failure
    Renal insufficiency
    Aortic dissection
Atherosclerotic complications
    Cerebral thrombosis
    Myocardial infarction
    Coronary artery disease
    Claudication syndromes

Data from Smith WM. Treatment of mild hypertension. *Circ Res* 1977;40(Suppl 1):98–105.

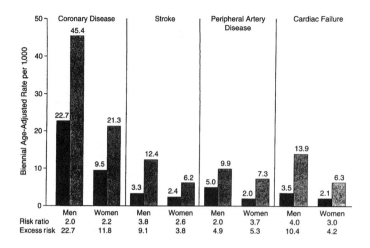

**FIGURE 4–4** ● Risk of cardiovascular events by hypertensive status in subjects aged 35 to 64 years from the Framingham study at 36-year follow-up. Coronary disease includes clinical manifestations such as myocardial infarction, angina pectoris, sudden death, other coronary deaths, and coronary insufficiency syndrome; peripheral artery disease is manifested as intermittent claudication. *Left bars* in each set of columns represent normotensives; *right bars* represent hypertensives. (Modified from Kannel WB. Blood pressure as a cardiovascular risk factor. *JAMA* 1996;275:1571–1576.)

triples the risk for CHF (Kannel, 1996). The consequences reflect an admixture of effects directly induced by the response of the left ventricle to the increased afterload imposed by hypertension, both hypertrophy and stiffening (Kass, 2005), and the acceleration of atherosclerosis through various paths leading to myocardial ischemia (Kostis, 2003).

As shown in Figure 4–5, hypertension, usually in concert with a number of other risk factors, often leads to left ventricular hypertrophy (LVH) and/or myocardial ischemia and/or infarction. These processes, in turn, precipitate systolic and diastolic dysfunction, which often progresses to overt congestive heart failure (Kostis, 2003).

## Left Ventricular Hypertrophy

### Prevalence

Whereas LVH is identified by electrocardiography in only 5% to 10% of hypertensives, LVH is found by echocardiography in nearly 30% of unselected hypertensive adults and in up to 90% of persons with severe hypertension (Schmieder & Messerli, 2000). More LVH is seen with obesity, high dietary sodium intake, anemia of end-stage renal disease, alcohol abuse, diabetes, and hypercholesterolemia (de Simone et al., 2001; Schmieder & Messerli, 2000). On the other hand, cardiac hypertrophy in response to excess load is nonpathologic in three

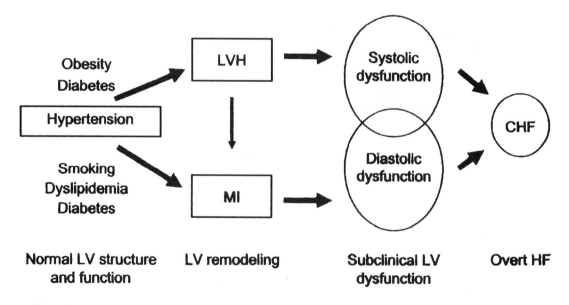

**FIGURE 4–5** ● Progression from hypertension to heart failure. CHF, congestive heart failure; HF, heart failure; LV, left ventricular; LVH, left ventricular hypertrophy; MI, myocardial infarction. (Adapted from Vasan RS, Levy D. The role of hypertension in the pathogenesis of heart failure. A clinical mechanistic overview. *Arch Intern Med* 1996;156:1789–1796.)

circumstances: maturation in infancy and childhood, pregnancy, and high-level exercise (Lorell & Carabello, 2000).

Even with new ECG criteria, only a 25% sensitivity for detection of LVH has been obtained in a population with almost a 40% prevalence of elevated left ventricular mass index by cardiac MRI (Alfakih et al., 2004b).

*Pathogenesis*

In the words of de Simone et al. (2001):

> Myocardial hypertrophy is the chronic adaptation of the left ventricle (LV) to increased cardiac load. Increased wall stress and strain provide a stimulus for signaling to cause mRNA transcription to increase muscular proteins. . . . hemodynamic factors are the basis of molecular changes that eventually yield the cascade of reactions needed to achieve these compensatory goals.

The association between LVH and hypertension is stronger for systolic levels, which contribute most of the relation between pulse pressure and LVH (Mulè et al., 2003). Increased pulse pressure is related to LV mass independent of other pressure components (de Simone et al., 2005). In addition to the stress and strain invoked by increased blood pressure per se, other factors contribute, including:

- Genotype which is the likely mechanism for the higher prevalence of LVH in Black than in White hypertensives (Kizer et al., 2004), although higher levels of poorly controlled blood pressure must also be involved (Hinderliter et al., 2004).
- A polymorphism of the angiotensin type-2 receptor gene (-1332G/A) has been associated with LVH in hypertensives (Alfakih et al., 2004a), as is a deletion polymorphism of the angiotensin converting enzyme gene, the DD genotype.

- An important role of the renin-angiotensin system is supported by the impressive effect of ACEIs and ARBs in causing regression of LVH and preventing remodeling after an MI (Kenchaiah et al., 2004), particularly because all components of the system are in cardiac tissue.
- In women, but not in men, an association between serum aldosterone (Vasan et al., 2004), which could reflect increased renin-angiotensin activity. In view of the pro-fibrotic effects of aldosterone described in Chapter 3, this may be involved in the increased collagen type 1 synthesis noted in patients with hypertensive heart failure (Querejeta et al., 2004).
- Increased cardiac sympathetic nervous activity (Schlaich et al., 2003).

*Patterns*

The patterns of LVH shown in Figure 4–6 differ by the type of hemodynamic load: Volume overload leads to eccentric hypertrophy, whereas pure BP overload leads to an increase in LV wall thickness without concomitant increase in cavity volume, i.e., concentric hypertrophy. The pattern of LVH can also be modified by increased arterial stiffness, increased pulse-wave velocity, and blood viscosity.

In Wachtell et al.'s (2001) series of 913 patients with varying stages of hypertension, these percentages of various patterns were found by echocardiography: 19%, normal geometry; 11%, concentric remodeling; 47%, eccentric hypertrophy; and 23%, concentric hypertrophy.

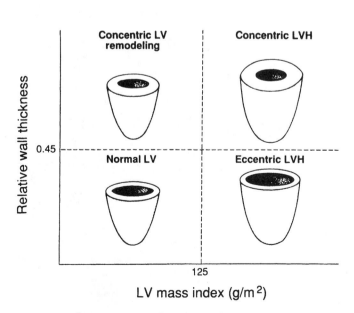

**FIGURE 4–6** ● Schematic diagram showing classification of left ventricular (LV) geometry based on level of its mass and relative wall thickness. Patients with increased LV mass are divided into those with eccentric or concentric LV hypertrophy (LVH), depending on whether they have normal or increased relative wall thickness; those with normal LV mass are similarly divided into groups with normal LV geometry or concentric LV remodeling. (Adapted from Devereux RB, Roman MJ, Ganau A, et al. Cardiac and arterial hypertrophy and atherosclerosis in hypertension. *Hypertension* 1994;23:802–809.)

Most find that concentric hypertrophy is most ominous (Akinboboye et al., 2004), but some find that LVH is a determinant of LV dysfunction independent of chamber geometry (Schillaci et al., 2002b).

*Consequences*

Even without LVH, early hypertensives may have a significantly reduced coronary flow reserve from an impaired capacity for coronary vasodilation (Palombo et al., 2000). The conversion of echocardiographic concentric remodeling to LVH is associated with increased mortality (Milani et al., 2004) and, when present, LVH is consistently and strongly related to subsequent cardiovascular morbidity (mean risk ratio, 2.3) and mortality (mean risk ratio, 2.5) (Vakili et al., 2001). The increased risk for sudden death in hypertensives is likely connected to alterations in ventricular conduction and repolarization associated with LVH (Oikarinen et al., 2004).

*Regression*

Only recently has regression of LVH been shown to improve the prognosis of hypertension (Fagard et al., 2004; Okin et al., 2004). This will be explored further in Chapter 7, in which the effects of various agents are covered.

### Systolic and Diastolic Dysfunction

De Simone et al. (2004) use the term *inappropriate* left ventricular mass (LVM) when the LVM exceeds the theoretical value predicted by gender, body size, and stroke work. Such excessive LVM translates into concentric LV geometry and both systolic and diastolic dysfunction that, in turn, are the predecessors for systolic and diastolic heart failure. Patients with asymptomatic LV systolic dysfunction are at

increased risk of heart failure and death, even with only mildly reduced ejection fractions (Verdecchia et al., 2005). Such LV dysfunction is present in 3 to 6% of the general community, as common as systolic heart failure (Wang et al., 2003).

Similarly, diastolic dysfunction, defined as an echocardiographic normal ejection fraction but abnormal LV filling in an asymptomatic hypertensive with LVH, is a precursor to diastolic heart failure (Aurigemma & Gaasch, 2004).

### Congestive Heart Failure

Hypertension is present in 91% of patients who develop CHF, triple the risk of normotensives (Levy et al., 1996). Hypertension remains the major preventable factor in the disease that is now the leading cause of hospitalization in the United States for adults over age 65 (Lloyd-Jones et al., 2002). It is likely that antihypertensive drugs used in treatment do not completely prevent CHF but postpone its development by several decades and are responsible for the improved survival after onset of CHF (Roger et al., 2004).

Most episodes of CHF in hypertensive patients are associated with systolic dysfunction, as reflected in a reduced ejection fraction. However, approximately 40% of episodes of CHF are associated with diastolic dysfunction and preserved LV systolic function (Table 4–7) (Aurigemma & Gaasch, 2004). Vasan & Benjamin (2001) explain the susceptibility of hypertensives, particularly those with LVH, to diastolic heart failure:

> When hemodynamically challenged by stress (such as exercise, tachycardia, increased afterload, or excessive preload), persons with

---

## TABLE 4–7

### Characteristics of Patients with Systolic or Diastolic Heart Failure

| Characteristics | Systolic Heart Failure | Diastolic Heart Failure |
|---|---|---|
| Age | All ages, typically 50–70 yr | Frequently elderly |
| Sex | More often male | Frequently female |
| Left ventricular ejection fraction | Depressed, approximately 40% or lower | Preserved or normal, approximately 40% or higher |
| Left ventricular cavity size | Usually dilated | Usually normal, often with concentric left ventricular hypertrophy |
| Left ventricular hypertrophy on electrocardiography | Sometimes present | Usually present |
| Chest radiography | Congestion and cardiomegaly | Congestion with or without cardiomegaly |
| Gallop rhythm present | Third heart sound | Fourth heart sound |

hypertension are unable to increase their end-diastolic volume (i.e., they have limited preload reserve), because of decreased LV relaxation and compliance. Consequently, a cascade begins, in which the LV end-diastolic BP rises, left atrial pressure increases, and pulmonary edema develops.

Management of CHF in hypertensive patients is covered in Chapter 7.

### Coronary Heart Disease

As described in Chapter 1, hypertension is quantitatively the largest risk factor for CHD. The development of myocardial ischemia reflects an imbalance between myocardial oxygen supply and demand. Hypertension, by reducing the supply and increasing the demand, can easily tip the balance.

*Clinical Manifestations*

Hypertension may play an even greater role in the pathogenesis of CHD than is commonly realized for two reasons. First, hypertensives suffer more silent ischemia and painless MI (Kannel et al., 1985) than do normotensives, perhaps because they have a lower sensitivity to pain (Hagen et al., 2005). Second, preexisting hypertension may go unrecognized in patients first seen after an MI. Although acute rises in BP may follow the onset of ischemic pain, the BP often falls immediately after the infarct if pump function is impaired.

Once an MI occurs, the prognosis is affected by both the preexisting and the subsequent BP (Kenchaiah et al., 2004). The 28-day case fatality rate among 635 men who had an acute MI was 24.5% in those with a prior systolic BP below 140 mm Hg, 35.6% with a prior systolic BP of 140 to 159 mm Hg, and 48.2% with a prior systolic BP of 160 mm Hg or higher (Njølstad & Arnesen, 1998). On the other hand, an increase in post-MI mortality has been noted among those whose BP fell significantly, presumably a reflection of poor pump function (Flack et al., 1995). If the BP of these subjects remained elevated, the prognosis was even worse, likely representing a severe load on a damaged myocardium, so that care must be taken with patients who have either lower or higher BP after an infarction.

A particular concern when thrombolytic therapy is given for acute MI is the threat for stroke that is imposed by the presence of hypertension. In the Global Utilization of Streptokinase and Tissue Plasminogen Activator for Occluded Coronary Arteries-I (GUSTO-I) trial, the incidence of stroke went from 1.2% for normotensives to 3.4% in those with systolic BP greater than 175 mm Hg (Aylward et al., 1996).

### Atrial Fibrillation

In a 16-year follow-up of 2,482 previously untreated hypertensives, 61 developed atrial fibrillation, a rate of 0.46 per 100 person years (Verdecchia et al., 2003b). The likelihood increased with increasing age, levels of blood pressure, left ventricular mass, and left atrial diameter. The risk of atrial fibrillation was reduced by over 60% in hypertensives treated down to a level below 120/80 (Young-Xu et al., 2004).

### Aortic Stenosis

Among 193 patients with symptomatic aortic stenosis, hypertension was present in 32%, and the additional workload was likely responsible for symptoms developing with larger valve areas and lower stroke work loss (Antonini-Canterin et al., 2003). The presence of aortic stenosis serves as an independent risk for cardiovascular disease in hypertensives (Olsen et al., 2005).

## Large-Vessel Disease

### Abdominal Aortic Aneurysm

The incidence of abdominal aortic aneurysms is increasing, likely as a consequence of the increasing number of elderly people who carry cardiovascular risks from middle age (Rodin et al., 2003). Although hypertension is one of these risk factors, ultrasonography uncovered such an aneurysm in only 3% of mild hypertensives aged 60 to 75 years but in 11% of those with systolic BP above 195 mm Hg and either cerebral or peripheral vascular disease (Simon et al., 1996). One-time ultrasonographic screening is recommended for men over age 65 who have ever smoked (Earnshaw et al., 2004). Aneurysms over 5 cm in diameter are now best repaired endovascularly (Prinssen et al., 2004).

### Aortic Dissection

As many as 80% of patients with aortic dissection have hypertension (Lindsay, 1992). The mechanism of dissection likely involves the combination of high pulsatile wave stress and accelerated atherosclerosis, because the higher the pressure, the greater the likelihood of dissection.

Aortic dissection may occur either in the ascending aorta (proximal, or type A), which requires surgery (Kallenbach et al., 2004), or in the descending aorta (distal, or type B), which usually can be treated medically (Nienaber & Eagle, 2003). Hypertension is more frequently a factor with distal dissections, whereas Marfan's and Ehlers-Danlos syndromes and cystic medial necrosis are seen more frequently with the proximal lesion.

### Peripheral Vascular Disease

The presence of symptomatic peripheral vascular disease (PVD), usually manifested by intermittent claudication, poses a high risk of subsequent cardiovascular mortality (Makin et al., 2001). By measurement of the ankle-arm BP index with a Doppler device, PAD was identified in 4.3% of US adults over age 40, more frequently in those who were older, Black, diabetic, smokers, or hypertensive (Selvin & Erlinger, 2004).

### Takayasu's Arteritis

Hypertension is present in nearly half of patients with Takayasu's disease, an idiopathic, chronic inflammatory disease of large arteries that is reported most frequently in Japan and India (Weaver et al., 2004). Those resistant to glucocorticoids may respond to anti-tumor necrosis factor therapy (Hoffman et al., 2004).

## Cerebrovascular Disease

Stroke is the second leading cause of death worldwide, the leading cause of permanent neurological disability in adults, and the most common indication for use of hospital and chronic care home beds (Rothwell et al., 2004). The stroke death rate is even higher (by approximately 50%) among Blacks who live in the southeastern United States (Obisesan et al., 2000), a rate similar to that noted in numerous other groups with inadequate healthcare worldwide (Sarti et al., 2000). Mortality rates from stroke fell markedly from the 1950s to the 1980s in most industrialized countries, but the long-term decline has since leveled off or reversed (Rothwell et al., 2004).

### Role of Hypertension

Even more than with heart disease, hypertension is the major cause of stroke. About 50% of strokes are attributable to hypertension, the risk rising in tandem with increasing blood pressure (Gorelick, 2002). Hypertensives are at 3–4 times greater risk for stroke and those with blood pressure above 130/85 at 1.5 times greater risk than normotensives.

In hypertensives, nearly 80% of strokes are ischemic, caused by either arterial thrombosis or embolism—15% are caused by intraparenchymal hemorrhage, and another 5% by subarachnoid hemorrhage (Warlow et al., 2003). Transient ischemic attacks—acute episodes of focal loss of cerebral or visual function lasting less than 24 hours and attributed to inadequate blood supply—may arise from emboli from atherosclerotic plaques in the carotids or thrombi in the heart (Flemming et al., 2004) and are followed by a high risk of stroke (Daffertshofer et al., 2004).

Isolated systolic hypertension (ISH) in the elderly is associated with a 2.7 times greater incidence of strokes than is seen in normotensive people of the same age (Qureshi et al., 2002). Elderly hypertensives more often have silent cerebrovascular disease (Vermeer et al., 2002) and cerebral white matter lesions on MRI (van Dijk et al., 2004) which eventually may lead to brain atrophy and vascular dementia.

There is a marked increase in the onset of ischemic stroke in the early morning hours after arising, when BP suddenly increases (Argentino et al., 1990). On the other hand, treated hypertensives whose BP dips during sleep may also be more vulnerable (Morfis et al., 1997). A widening pulse pressure during sleep is associated with a significantly increased risk of stroke (Kario et al., 2004), presumably reflecting the role of arterial stiffness (Laurent et al., 2003).

Whether hypertensive or normotensive before their stroke, the majority of stroke patients at the time they are first seen will have a transient elevation of BP that spontaneously falls within a few days (Vemmos et al., 2004). Therefore, caution is advised in lowering the BP in the immediate post-stroke period, as noted further in Chapter 7. On the other hand, as will be noted, long-term reduction of blood pressure is the most effective protection against both initial and recurrent stroke (Lawes et al., 2004).

### Extracranial Carotid Disease

Increasing thickness of the intima-media of the carotid arteries, usually assessed by ultrasonography, is a measure of preclinical atherosclerosis and is directly associated with both stroke and coronary disease (Chambless et al., 2000). As expected, carotid disease is more common in hypertensives (Parrinello et al., 2004). Those with symptoms or bruits should have noninvasive studies and consideration given to endarterectomy for those with high-grade stenoses (MRC Collaborative Group, 2004).

### Cognitive Impairment and Dementia

Both high and low BP are associated with impaired cognition even in the absence of clinically evident cerebrovascular disease (Waldstein et al., 2005). A similar nonlinear relation has been noted with pulse pressure: both excessively wide pulse pressure (reflecting arterial stiffness) and narrow pulse pressure (reflecting reduced cerebral perfusion) are associated with increased risk for Alzheimer's disease and dementia (Qiu et al., 2003). BP typically begins to decline 3 years before dementia becomes overt and continues to decline thereafter (Qiu et al., 2004).

## Renal Disease

Hypertension plays an important role in renal damage, whether manifested as proteinuria, reduced glomerular filtration rate (GFR), or progression to end-stage renal disease (ESRD). However, the manner by which hypertension injures the kidneys and the frequency of renal damage arising from hypertension are not settled. The most likely sequence is a loss of renal autoregulation which normally attenuates the transmission of increased systemic pressure to the glomeruli (Bidani & Griffin, 2004), leading to glomerular hypertension, glomerulosclerosis and progressive renal dysfunction (Segura et al., 2004). Moreover, reduction of blood pressure can slow if not stop the progression of renal diseases and accompanying cardiovascular events (Ibsen et al., 2005). Much more about more severe forms of renal damage is found in Chapter 9.

A presumably specific form of renal damage is induced by hypertension, *hypertensive nephrosclerosis*. This consists of arteriolar sclerosis and hyalinosis, global and focal glomerular sclerosis, interstitial fibrosis with tubular atrophy, and chronic interstitial inflammation. Blacks develop more of these changes than Whites (Marcantoni et al., 2002), in keeping with their higher incidence of ESRD presumably caused by hypertension (Toto, 2003). A genetic susceptibility may be involved since among African hypertensives, significant hereditability of renal dysfunction has been observed (Bochud et al., 2005).

Although most accept a role of hypertension per se as a cause of ESRD, some believe that only malignant hypertension is responsible (Hsu, 2002) and that most ESRD attributed to nonmalignant hypertension is related to obesity and insulin resistance (Kincaid-Smith, 2004).

### Prevalence

Regardless of its role in producing ESRD, hypertension certainly is associated with proteinuria and reduction of GFR (Daviglus et al., 2005). Microalbuminuria was present in 5% of people without hypertension but in about 16% of those with hypertension in two large population surveys (Hallan et al., 2003; C. Jones et al., 2002). The presence of hypertension increased the risk of a fall of GFR to below 60 ml/min/1.73m$^2$ by 1.57 times among 2,585 participants in the Framingham Heart Study who were free of preexisting kidney disease (Fox et al., 2004). Both high-normal BP (Knight et al., 2003) and systolic hypertension (Young et al., 2002) are associated with increased rates of microalbuminuria and fall in GFR.

### Manifestations and Consequences

Renal involvement usually is asymptomatic, with loss of concentrating ability manifested as nocturia

oftentimes being the first indication. Although in itself perhaps not predictive of persistent hypertension (Palatini et al., 2005), the first objective sign is microalbuminuria, defined as 30 to 300 mg of albuminuria/d, reflecting glomerular hyperfiltration, a marker of altered glomerular barrier integrity, and in turn contributing to progressive tubulointerstitial damage (Schieppati & Remuzzi, 2003). Most easily assessed by measurement of the albumin-creatinine ratio in a random urine sample (Toto, 2004), microalbuminuria is a predictor not only of progressive renal damage but also of overall cardiovascular morbidity (Barzilay et al., 2004; Tsioufis et al., 2004). Heavy proteinuria even to the nephrotic range can occur (Obialo et al., 2002). As proteinuria increases, GFR may fall (Campo et al., 2004) and even small decreases in GFR are associated with more LVH and retinal vascular changes (Leoncini et al., 2004).

The monitoring of renal function by serum creatinine may be misleading, particularly in people with a reduced muscle mass (Swedko et al., 2003). Increasingly, formulae including gender, age, and body weight with serum creatinine are being used to estimate GFR, although they may too underestimate GFR (Rule et al., 2004). Serum cystatin C has been found to be a better proxy for GFR (Shlipak et al., 2005).

As will be emphasized in Chapters 9 and 10, renovascular disease must always be remembered as a not infrequent cause of renal insufficiency and hypertension.

## NATURAL HISTORY OF SPECIAL POPULATIONS

Before turning to evaluation, I will describe groups of people whose hypertension, for various reasons, may follow a different course from that seen in the predominantly male, White, middle-aged populations observed in most clinical trials and long-term observational studies. These special groups include a major part of the hypertensive population: the elderly, women, Blacks and other ethnic groups, diabetics, and the obese.

### Elderly

Two patterns of hypertension are seen in the elderly: combined systolic and diastolic—the carry-over of primary (essential) hypertension common to middle age—and ISH—the more frequent form in those over age 60. However, because the major consequences and, as is noted in Chapter 7, the therapy for both are quite similar, most of this discussion will not make a distinction between the two.

## Prevalence of Hypertension

As noted in Figure 1–4 in Chapter 1, whereas diastolic BPs tend to plateau before age 60 and drop thereafter, systolic BPs rise progressively. Therefore, the incidence of ISH—defined as systolic pressure of 140 mm Hg or more and diastolic pressure of 90 mm Hg or less—progressively rises with age. In the National Health and Nutrition Examination Survey III, the proportion of various types of hypertension seen with advancing age progressively shifted from diastolic and combined hypertension to ISH (Franklin et al., 2001). In those older than 60 years, ISH was the pattern of hypertension in 87% of those who were untreated. In Framingham, only 41% of those who developed ISH had antecedent diastolic hypertension (Franklin et al., 2005). Systolic levels usually continue to rise after age 70 in those who remain healthy but tend to fall if chronic debilitating diseases occur (Starr et al., 1998). Almost 90% of Framingham subjects who were normotensive at age 55 or 65 developed hypertension 20 years later (Vasan et al., 2002).

As described in Chapter 2, two cautions are needed in evaluating BP levels in the elderly, First, the white-coat effect is more common and significant in the elderly than in younger people (Fotherby & Potter, 1993) so out-of-office readings should be obtained if possible. Second, the elderly may have artifactually elevated BPs by usual indirect cuff measurements (i.e., pseudohypertension) because of increased stiffness of the large arteries, which may preclude compression and collapse of the brachial artery by the cuff (Spence, 1997).

## Risks of Hypertension

As seen in Table 4–4 in the data from the placebo-treated half of the elderly patients enrolled in seven RCTs over the past 20 years, mortality in elderly hypertensives is significant, particularly from strokes, even in the brief 2- to 5-year interval of these trials. As noted, the patients enrolled tend to be healthier than the general population, so the risks of both combined systolic-diastolic and ISH are even greater than shown in Table 4–4.

A different pattern appears in the very elderly who have more chronic debility. In the subjects aged 75 to 94 years followed up in the Framingham study, risks for all-cause and cardiovascular mortality increased at the lower levels of systolic BP (<120 mm Hg) (Figure 4–7). Most of this increase occurred in those with existing cardiovascular disease. As Kannel et al. (1997) note:

> There appears to be a different morbidity and mortality rate curve in the elderly that appears to be quadratic (U-shaped) in those who have already had a cardiovascular event and linear in those free of cardiovascular disease. The excess mortality rate at low BP levels could be a reflection of poor ejection fractions rather than the impact of low BP. . . . It is thus likely that BP elevation remains a detrimental risk factor even in the very old.

The validity of this conclusion was shown in a subsequent analysis showing increased cardiovascular risk related to hypertension in those over age 80 compared to those who were younger (Lloyd-Jones et al., 2004).

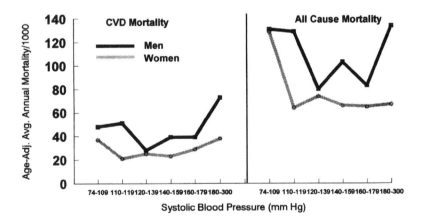

**FIGURE 4–7** ● All-cause and cardiovascular disease (CVD) mortality rates by systolic blood pressure in 75- to 94-year-old subjects in the Framingham Heart Study. (Modified from Kannel WB, D'Agostino RB, Silbershatz H. Blood pressure and cardiovascular morbidity and mortality rates in the elderly. *Am Heart J* 1997;134:758–763.)

In addition to increased mortality seen with either low systolic BP (<120–130 mm Hg) or high systolic BP (>180 mm Hg) in those over age 80, both are associated with the development of cognitive impairment (Waldstein et al., 2005).

## Pathophysiology of Isolated Systolic Hypertension

The basic mechanism for the usual progressive rise in systolic BP with age is the loss of distensibility and elasticity in the large capacitance arteries, a process that was nicely demonstrated more than 50 years ago (Hallock & Benson, 1937) (Figure 4–8). Increasing volumes of saline were infused into the tied-off aortas taken from patients at death whose ages ranged from the twenties to the seventies. The pressure within the aortas from the elderly subjects rose much higher with small increases in volume as compared to that in aortas from the younger subjects, reflecting the rigidity of the vessels.

Subsequently, the progressive rise in systolic pressure with age has been found to reflect a reduced cross-sectional area of the peripheral vascular bed and stiffer aorta and large arteries, producing an increased pulse-wave velocity and an early return of pulse-wave reflection in systole (Safar & Benetos, 2003). The early return of the reflected pressure wave augments aortic pressure throughout systole, increasing both systolic and pulse pressure, further increasing the work of the left ventricle while decreasing the diastolic aortic pressure that supports coronary blood flow (Pierini et al., 2000).

### Postural Hypotension

As is covered in Chapter 7, therapy of hypertension in the elderly is vital but oftentimes must be tempered by the need first to overcome coexisting postural hypotension.

#### Definition and Incidence

A fall in systolic pressure of 20 mm Hg or more after 1 minute of quiet standing is defined as postural hypotension. Postural hypotension was found in 68% of 489 patients with a mean age of 81.6 years in a geriatric ward (Weiss et al., 2002). In the generally healthy population of elderly men and women enrolled in the Systolic Hypertension in the Elderly Program, postural hypotension was found in 10.4% at 1 minute after rising from a seated position and in 12.0% at 3 minutes, with 17.3% having hypotension at one or both intervals (Applegate et al., 1991). The prevalence would likely have been higher if the patients had been tested after rising from a supine position. Although there are multiple, mainly neurological, causes for postural hypotension (Ejaz et al., 2004), the only predisposing factor for postural hypotension found in an unselected elderly population was hypertension (Räihä et al., 1995). As seen in Figure 4–9, the higher the basal supine systolic BP, the greater was the tendency for a postural fall (Lipsitz et al., 1985).

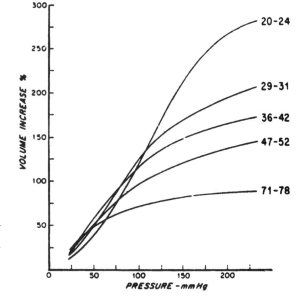

**FIGURE 4–8** ● Curves showing the relation of the percentage of increase in pressure to the increase in volume infused into aortas excised at autopsy from people in five different age groups. The curves were constructed from the mean values obtained from a number of aortas. (Reprinted from Hallock P, Benson IC. Studies of the elastic properties of human isolated aorta. *J Clin Invest* 1937;16:595–602, with permission.)

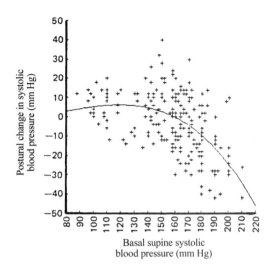

**FIGURE 4–9** ● Relationship between basal supine systolic blood pressure and postural change in systolic blood pressure for aggregate data from older subjects. (Modified from Lipsitz LA, et al. Intra-individual variability in postural BP in the elderly. *Clin Sci* 1985;69:337–341.)

In addition, splanchnic pooling of blood after eating may lead to profound postprandial hypotension (Puisieux et al., 2000).

*Mechanism*

Normal aging is associated with various changes that may lead to postural hypotension. The two most common changes in patients with supine or seated hypertension are venous pooling in the legs and reduced baroreceptor sensitivity (Jones et al., 2003). Even though elderly hypertensives have intact baroreceptor modulation of sympathetic nerve traffic, they have marked impairment of baroreceptor control of heart rate and of cardiopulmonary reflex control of the peripheral circulation (Grassi et al., 2000; Kornet et al., 2005).

## Women

Before age 50, women have a lower prevalence of hypertension than men but, after age 55, women have a greater age-related increase in proximal aortic stiffness which leads to a higher incidence of systolic hypertension in older women (Waddell et al., 2001). In addition, women have two other features which tend to lower diastolic BP and widen pulse pressure: first, shorter stature which causes a more rapid return of the pulse wave to augment the peak systolic pressure; second, a faster heart rate which induces a shorter diastolic period (Safar & Smulyan, 2004).

*Consequences*

Women at all ages have a lower incidence of heart attacks and strokes than men but they maintain a

strong, continuous, and linear association between systolic BP and cardiovascular events (Mason et al., 2004). Their degree of cardioprotection lessens after menopause but, as detailed in Chapter 11, postmenopausal hormone replacement therapy does not reverse this process.

## Blacks

Death from hypertension is the single most common reason for the higher mortality rate for Blacks than for non-Blacks in the United States (Wong et al., 2004). Blacks have more hypertension and suffer more from it because of their lower socioeconomic status and resultant reduced access to necessary health care (Jha et al., 2003). Their higher prevalence of hypertension likely reflects both genetic and environmental factors (El-Gharbawy et al., 2001). If appropriate therapy is provided, most of their excessive morbidity and mortality related to hypertension can be relieved.

### Prevalence of Hypertension

*Blacks in the United States*

The higher BP levels in U.S. Blacks begin during childhood and adolescence and are established by early adulthood. Most of the higher BPs in young Blacks are attributed to a smaller birth weight and greater postnatal weight gain (Cruickshank et al., 2005). Adjustments for age, education, body mass index (BMI), physical activity, and alcohol intake reduced the differences substantially (Liu et al., 1996). In middle age, Blacks and Whites have similar incidences of hypertension given the same baseline BP and BMI (He et al., 1998). However, hypertension in Blacks is a greater risk factor for coronary disease than in Whites (D. Jones et al., 2002). In most studies, Blacks usually have higher sleeping BPs, as recorded by ambulatory monitoring (Harshfield et al., 2002a) but no greater early morning surge in BP (Haas et al., 2003).

*Blacks Outside the United States*

In their survey of Blacks in seven populations of African origin, Cooper et al. (1999) found the rates of hypertension to be 7% in rural Nigeria, 26% in Jamaica, and 33% in the United States. These higher rates were associated with increased BMI and sodium intake.

### Pathophysiology of Hypertension

Table 4–8 lists some of the numerous genotypic and phenotypic features found in Black hypertensives that may explain their higher prevalence and greater degree of target organ damage. Whatever else is responsible, poverty, racial discrimination, and barriers to health care obviously are involved

## TABLE 4 – 8

### Features of Hypertension in Blacks

**Genotype**

Angiotensinogen (Cooper et al., 1999)

Epithelial sodium channel (Pratt et al., 2002)

G protein $\beta_3$-subunit (Dong et al., 1999)

Transforming growth factor-$\beta_1$ (Suthanthiran et al., 2000)

**Intermediate phenotype**

Activation of intrarenal-renin system (Price et al., 2002)

Decreased kallikrein excretion (Song et al., 2000)

Decreased nitric oxide–dependent and –independent vasodilation (Campia et al., 2004)

Decreased potassium intake (Morris et al., 1999)

Diabetes mellitus (Brancati et al., 2000)

Glomerular hyperfiltration (Aviv et al., 2004a)

Increased adrenergic vasoconstriction (Abate et al., 2001)

Increased circulating endothelin-1 (Campia et al., 2004)

Decreased stress-induced pressure natriuresis (Harshfield et al., 2002b)

Increased sodium sensitivity (Aviv et al., 2004b)

Increased retention of sodium load (Palacios et al., 2004)

Obesity (Jones, 1999)

Sodium-induced renal vasoconstriction (Schmidlin et al., 1999)

Lesser fall in nocturnal BP (Hinderliter et al., 2004)

**Phenotype**

Aortic stiffness (Chaturvedi et al., 2004)

Congestive heart failure (Dries et al., 1999)

Left ventricular hypertrophy (Kizer et al., 2004)

Left ventricular systolic dysfunction (Devereux et al., 2001)

Microalbuminuria (Aviv et al., 2004a)

Nephrosclerosis (Toto, 2003)

Stroke (Gillum, 1996)

---

in the higher hypertension-related morbidity and mortality seen in U.S. Blacks (Jha et al., 2003).

*Stress*

As described in Chapter 3, a large body of literature attests to an association between the stresses of low socioeconomic status and hypertension. A good example of the likely interaction between low socioeconomic status and a genetic trait is the finding that BP levels were significantly associated with darker skin color but only in those Blacks in the lower levels of socioeconomic status (Klag et al., 1991).

Beyond low socioeconomic status, James et al. (1996) have long held to an influence of a coping strategy involving an active effort to manage the stressors of life by hard work and determination to succeed. They call this coping strategy *John Henryism,* after a legendary uneducated Black folk hero who defeated a mechanical steam drill in an epic battle but then dropped dead from complete exhaustion.

*Diet*

Particularly among older Black women, the higher prevalence of hypertension is correlated closely with obesity (Jones, 1999). Although they have greater pressor sensitivity to sodium (Palacios et al., 2004), Blacks do not appear to ingest more sodium than do non-Blacks (Ganguli et al., 1999). However, their intake of both potassium and calcium is lower (Langford & Watson, 1990) and they have more unprovoked hypokalemia (Andrew et al., 2002). Moreover, if the hypertension of Blacks is associated with volume expansion, as reflected in their usually lower plasma renin status (Helmer, 1967), a resultant increased excretion of calcium would further lower serum calcium levels and provoke increased parathyroid hormone secretion (Brickman et al., 1993).

*Responsiveness to Growth Factors*

Dustan (1995) hypothesized that the increased prevalence of severe hypertension in Blacks could be due to an increased responsiveness to vascular growth factors comparable to that noted in fibroblasts that form keloids, which are more common in Blacks.

### Complications of Hypertension

Hypertension is not only more common in Blacks, but is also more severe, less well managed and, therefore, more deadly. As best as can be ascertained, Blacks at any given level of BP do not suffer more vascular damage than do non-Blacks; rather, they display a shift to the right of the BP distribution, yielding a higher overall prevalence and a higher proportion of severe disease (Cooper & Liao, 1992).

Much of the excess morbidity and mortality found in U.S. Blacks as compared to U.S. non-Blacks is related to the lower socioeconomic status of Blacks but, at every level of income, Blacks have a higher mortality rate from hypertensive heart disease than do Whites (Mensah et al., 2005). Considerable variation in mortality from cardiovascular causes was found among Blacks living in New York City, depending on their birthplace: Southern-born Blacks had a 30% higher coronary mortality than did northeastern-born Blacks and a four times higher coronary mortality than did Caribbean-born Blacks (Fang et al., 1996).

### Cardiac Disease

Blacks have more LVH than non-Blacks with equal levels of BP and are at a higher risk for progression of systolic dysfunction (Kizer et al., 2004). Although the overall prevalence of CHD may be lower among U.S. Blacks than among non-Blacks, mortality rates from CHD are now higher because of a lesser decline in CHD death rates among Blacks than among Whites in the United States (Gillum, 1996).

### Cerebrovascular Disease

Blacks have more strokes than do non-Blacks, particularly if they are born in the southeastern United States (Lackland et al., 1999). All forms of cerebrovascular disease are more frequent in Blacks, with even greater differences between the Black and non-Black populations in the incidence of strokes that are more tightly connected with hypertension, i.e., small-vessel ischemic stroke (Woo et al., 1999). and intracerebral hemorrhage (Flaherty et al., 2005).

### Renal Disease

As noted earlier in this chapter, hypertensive Blacks are more likely to end up with end-stage renal disease than are hypertensive Whites (Toto, 2003). Much of this increased risk for renal failure results from low socioeconomic status and limited access to health care, but a heightened susceptibility to renal damage is also involved.

## Other Ethnic Groups

Much less is known about the special characteristics of other ethnic groups as compared to Blacks in the United States, so only a few generalizations will be made about them.

### Primitive Versus Industrialized Environment

People of any race living a rural, more primitive lifestyle tend to ingest less sodium, remain less obese, and have less hypertension. When they migrate into urban areas and adopt more modern lifestyles, they ingest more sodium, gain weight, and develop more hypertension (Cooper et al., 1999). Rather dramatic changes in the prevalence of hypertension and the nature of cardiovascular complications have been seen when formerly isolated ethnic groups move to an industrialized environment, as seen among South Asians who move to England (Khattar et al., 2000).

### Persistence of Ethnic Differences

Although environmental changes often alter BP and other cardiovascular traits, some ethnic groups preserve characteristics that presumably reflect stronger genetic influences. Examples include Bedouins in Israel (Paran et al., 1992) and Native Americans in the United States (Howard, 1996). Mexican-Americans in San Antonio have a lesser prevalence of hypertension than Caucasians despite their high prevalence of obesity, diabetes, and insulin resistance (Lorenzo et al., 2002). Nonetheless, they have a higher incidence of hypertension than seen in Mexico City (Lorenzo et al., 2005).

## Diabetes and Hypertension

The combination of diabetes and hypertension poses a major public health challenge:

- The incidence of diabetes is rapidly increasing with a lifetime risk in the United States now estimated to be 33% for men and 39% for women (Narayan et al., 2003). Another 20% have the metabolic syndrome (Park et al., 2003).
- 71% of U.S. adult diabetics have hypertension (Geiss et al., 2002), and a significant number of hypertensives have unrecognized diabetes (Salmasi et al., 2004).
- Even without hypertension, diabetics have a twofold or greater risk for cardiovascular morbidity and mortality (Mooradian, 2003). With hypertension, the risk is even greater (Creager et al., 2003). Moreover, the addition of frequently noted dyslipidemia magnifies coronary heart disease risk in a synergistic interaction (Cohen et al., 2004).
- Coexisting diabetes and hypertension are associated with greater degrees of arterial stiffness (Tedesco et al., 2004) leading to earlier rises in systolic and pulse pressures (Ronnback et al., 2004), the pattern of accelerated arterial aging.
- Even with effective antihypertensive therapy, resistance arteries from diabetic hypertensives have persistently marked remodeling (Endemann et al., 2004).
- The microvascular complications of diabetes, retinopathy in particular, are also increased by hypertension (Stratton et al., 2001).

As will be noted in Chapters 5 and 7, these high risks mandate earlier and more intensive therapy in hypertensives with diabetes.

## Obesity and Hypertension

Even in the absence of type 2 diabetes, obesity is one of the most common factors responsible for hypertension, as discussed in Chapter 3. In the National Health and Nutrition Examination Survey III, a progressive increase in the prevalence of hypertension was seen with increasing BMI at all ages (Thompson et al., 1999) (Figure 4–10). The prevalence is increased further when the obesity is predominantly abdominal (Allemann et al., 2001).

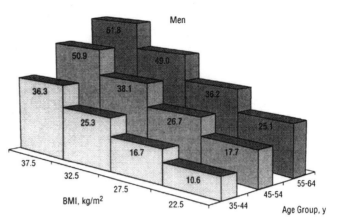

**FIGURE 4–10** ● Estimated risk (%) of hypertension by age group and body mass index (BMI) among men in the National Health and Nutrition Examination Survey III. (Modified from Thompson D, et al. Lifetime health and economic consequences of obesity. *Arch Intern Med* 1999;159:2177–2183.)

The cardiovascular risks of these overweight people are markedly increased in the presence of other features of the metabolic syndrome (Kip et al., 2004). In the elderly, the cardiovascular risks of obesity diminish, but abdominal obesity remains a risk factor for cardiovascular disease mortality (Baik et al., 2000).

## ALTERING THE NATURAL HISTORY

Now that the possible mechanisms, natural history, major consequences, and special populations of untreated primary hypertension have been covered, an additional word about prevention is in order.

Most efforts to alter the natural history of hypertension involve both nondrug and drug therapy of existing disease. However, attempts to *prevent* hypertension must also be more widely promoted and followed. Without knowledge of the specific causes of this disease, no single preventive measure can be promoted with the assurance that it will work. However, to insist that specific causes be known before prevention is attempted is akin to saying that John Snow should not have closed the pump because he had no proof that Vibrio cholera organisms were the cause of death in those who drank the polluted water. The preventive measures likely to help—moderation in sodium intake, reduction of obesity, maintenance of physical conditioning, avoidance of stress, and greater attention to the other coexisting risk factors for premature cardiovascular disease—will do no harm and may do a great deal of good.

Their value has been proved for prevention of diabetes (Tuomilehto et al., 2001; Diabetes Prevention Program, 2002) and strongly supported for prevention of hypertension (Whelton et al., 2002). Nonetheless, with recognition of the difficulty of changing lifestyle habits, trials of antihypertensive drugs are being conducted to prove that they can at least slow, if not stop, the inexorable progress of hypertension (Julius et al., 2004).

## EVALUATION OF THE HYPERTENSIVE PATIENT

Having examined the natural history of various hypertensive populations, we now incorporate these findings into a plan for evaluating the individual hypertensive patient.

There are three main reasons to evaluate patients with hypertension: (a) to determine the type of hypertension, specifically looking for identifiable causes; (b) to assess the impact of the hypertension on target organs; and (c) to estimate a patient's overall risk profile for the development of premature cardiovascular disease. Such evaluation can be accomplished with relative ease and should be part of the initial examination of every newly discovered hypertensive. As Jackson et al. (2005) state: "A quantitative candiovascular risk/benefit assessment should be a routine component of quality clinical practice in middle-aged and older adults." The younger the patient and the higher the BP, the more intensive the search for identifiable causes should be.

### History

The patient history should focus on the duration of the elevated BP and any prior treatment, the current use of various drugs that may cause it to rise, and symptoms of target organ dysfunction (Table 4–9). Attention should also be directed toward the patient's psychosocial status, looking for such information as the degree of knowledge about hypertension, the willingness to make necessary changes in lifestyle and to take medication, and the ability

## TABLE 4-9

### Important Aspects of the Patient's History

Duration of the hypertension
    Last known normal blood pressure
    Course of the blood pressure
Prior treatment of the hypertension
    Drugs: types, doses, side effects
Intake of agents that may interfere
    Nonsteroidal antiinflammatory drugs
    Oral contraceptives
    Sympathomimetics
    Adrenal steroids
    Excessive sodium intake
    Alcohol (>2 drinks/day)
    Herbal remedies
Family history
    Hypertension
    Premature cardiovascular disease or death
    Familial diseases: pheochromocytoma, renal
    disease, diabetes, gout
Symptoms of secondary causes
    Muscle weakness
    Spells of tachycardia, sweating, tremor
    Thinning of the skin
    Flank pain
Symptoms of target organ damage
    Headaches
    Transient weakness or blindness
    Loss of visual acuity
    Chest pain
    Dyspnea
    Edema
    Claudication

Presence of other risk factors
    Smoking
    Diabetes
    Dyslipidemia
    Physical inactivity
Concomitant diseases
Dietary history
    Weight change
    Fresh vs. processed foods
    Sodium
    Saturated fats
Sexual function
Features of sleep apnea
    Early morning headaches
    Daytime somnolence
    Loud snoring
    Erratic sleep

Ability to modify lifestyle and maintain therapy
    Understanding the nature of hypertension
    and the need to follow a regimen
    Ability to perform physical activity
    Source of food preparation
    Financial constraints
    Ability to read instructions
    Need for care providers

to obtain sometimes expensive therapies. An area of great importance is sexual dysfunction, often neglected until it arises after antihypertensive therapy is given. Erectile dysfunction, often attributed to antihypertensive drugs, may be present in as many as one-third of untreated hypertensive men and is most likely related to their underlying vascular disease (see Chapter 7).

A positive family history of hypertension is usually accurate but a negative report is only 33% accurate (Murabito et al., 2004).

### Anxiety-Related Symptoms

Although many, if not most, hypertensives have symptoms that they ascribe to their elevated BP (Kjellgren et al., 1998), most of these symptoms are common to the functional somatic syndromes seen in people who believe they have a serious disease

(Barsky & Borus, 1999). Many believe they can tell when their BP is elevated but, if so, the perception is likely from anxiety which, in turn, may be raising their BP (Cantillon et al., 1997). If questioned before they become aware of being hypertensive, symptoms including headaches, epistaxis, tinnitus, dizziness, and fainting were no more common among those with hypertension than among those with normal BP (Weiss, 1972). Similarly, patients unaware of their hypertension had higher quality of life measures than did those who were aware (Mena-Martin et al., 2003).

This is in keeping with my belief that many of the symptoms described by hypertensives are secondary to anxiety over having "the silent killer" (as hypertension frequently is described), anxiety that often is expressed as recurrent acute hyperventilation or panic attacks (Davies et al., 1999; Smoller et al., 2003). Many of the symptoms described by hypertensives, such as bandlike headaches, dizziness and lightheadedness, fatigue, palpitations, and chest discomfort, reflect recurrent hyperventilation, a common problem among all patients (DeGuire et al., 1992) but likely even more common among hypertensives who are anxious over their diagnosis and its implications (Kaplan, 1997).

The symptoms and signs of panic attack encompass all these same manifestations but go beyond them to include fears of falling apart, losing control, or even more acute anxiety and are associated with increased reactivity of vasoconstricting sympathetic nerves (Lambert et al., 2002). Anxiety and panic attacks are even more common among patients who had nonspecific intolerance to multiple antihypertensive drugs (Davies et al., 2003). In patients who have experienced panic attacks, the BP rises significantly during voluntary hyperventilation, unlike a tendency for the BP to go down during hyperventilation in subjects who have not had panic attacks (Fontana et al., 2003). Moreover, they tend to have more distress and slower recovery from hypocapnia during voluntary hyperventilation (Wilhelm et al., 2001).

The situation is similar for symptoms of depression. Symptoms of depression (and anxiety) were not found to be more common prior to the onset of hypertension (Shinn et al., 2001) but were more common after the diagnosis was made (Scherrer et al., 2003).

### Headache

In cross-sectional surveys, headache is the most common of the symptoms that are reported but, again, mostly in those aware of the diagnosis. Stewart (1953) found that only 17% of patients unaware of their hypertension complained of headache, but among patients with similar levels of BP who were aware of their diagnosis, 71% had headaches. In a prospective 11-year follow-up of 22,685 adults, those who developed hypertension had a 30% *lower* rate of headache (Hagen et al., 2002).

This belief that headache is related not to the level of BP but rather to anxiety over the diagnosis of hypertension is strengthened by the fact that the prevalence of headache among newly diagnosed hypertensives varies little in relation to the level of BP: 15% to 20% had headaches whether their diastolic BPs were as low as 95 mm Hg or as high as 125 mm Hg (Cooper et al., 1989) and headaches were no more common in those with BP above 180/110 than in those with lower levels of BP (Fuchs et al., 2003). Moreover, headaches noted during ambulatory BP monitoring were not associated with simultaneous elevations in BP (Gus et al., 2001; Kruszewski et al., 2000).

However, data from prospective randomized placebo-controlled trials (RCTs) show that the prevalence of headache is often reduced when BP is lowered, irrespective of the drugs used to lower the BP (Law et al., 2005). In this meta-analysis of 97 RCTs involving over 24,000 patients, among those treated to an average 10/5 mm Hg lower BP, headaches were complained about in 7.5% versus 11.1% of those left on placebo, a 33% reduction. These data strongly implicate hypertension as a reversible cause of headache. It should be noted that sleep apnea is common among even minimally obese hypertensives, as described in Chapter 15, so early morning headaches may reflect not hypertension but nocturnal hypoxia.

### Nocturia

Nocturia is more common in hypertensives, often the consequence of coexisting benign prostatic hypertrophy (Blanker et al., 2000) or simply a decreased bladder capacity (Weiss & Blaivas, 2000). At least theoretically, the altered pressure-natriuresis relationship described in Chapter 3 could delay urinary excretion, and a loss of concentrating ability may be an early sign of renal impairment.

### Physical Examination

The physical examination should include a careful search for damage to target organs and for features of various identifiable causes (Table 4–10). Waist circumference should be measured, because values exceeding 88 cm (35 in.) in women and 102 cm (40 in.) in men are indicative of abdominal obesity and the metabolic syndrome (Wilson & Grundy,

---

**TABLE 4–10**

### Important Aspects of the Physical Examination

---

Accurate measurement of blood pressure

General appearance: distribution of body fat, skin lesions, muscle strength, alertness

Funduscopy

Neck: palpation and auscultation of carotids, thyroid

Heart: size, rhythm, sounds

Lungs: rhonchi, rales

Abdomen: renal masses, bruits over aorta or renal arteries, femoral pulses, waist circumference

Extremities: peripheral pulses, edema

Neurologic assessment, including cognitive function

---

2003) and serve as a cardiovascular risk factor independent of weight (Malik et al., 2004).

### Funduscopic Examination

Only in the optic fundi can small blood vessels be seen with ease, but this requires dilation of the pupil, a procedure that should be more commonly practiced using a short-acting mydriatic such as 1% tropicamide. Such routine funduscopy can portray the major changes of hypertensive retinopathy (Figure 4–11) (Pache et al., 2002; Wong & Mitchell, 2004). However, accurate recognition of the more subtle early changes that may appear even before hypertension is manifest requires digitized retinal photography (Wong et al., 2005), now available only in ophthalmology offices but hopefully to become more accessible to all who see hypertensives.

The retinal changes have been most logically classified by Wong and Mitchell (2004) (Table 4–11). The changes progress from the initial vasoconstrictive stage to sclerosis and then to exudation, reflected in the features shown in Figure 4–11. As Wong and Mitchell document, the "mild" changes have been seen even before hypertension is manifest (Wong et al., 2004). The striking association of retinal signs with the risk of stroke and the lesser but still significant association with the risk of CHD make a careful retinal exam an essential part of the initial evaluation of every hypertensive with follow-up exams as indicated. Unfortunately, along with other parts of the physical exam, most practitioners likely do not learn or perform funduscopy very adequately.

### Laboratory Tests

#### Routine Laboratory Testing

For most patients, a hematocrit, urine analysis, automated blood chemistry (glucose, creatinine, electrolytes, and calcium), lipid profile (LDL and HDL cholesterol, triglycerides), and 12-lead electrocardiography are all the routine procedures needed (Chobanian et al., 2003). The blood should be obtained after an overnight fast to improve the diagnostic accuracy of the glucose and triglyceride levels. None of these usually yields abnormal results in the early, uncomplicated phases of primary hypertension, but they should always be obtained for a baseline. The serum creatinine should be used, along with the patient's age, gender, and weight to calculate the GFR using the MDRD formula (Stevens & Levey, 2004).

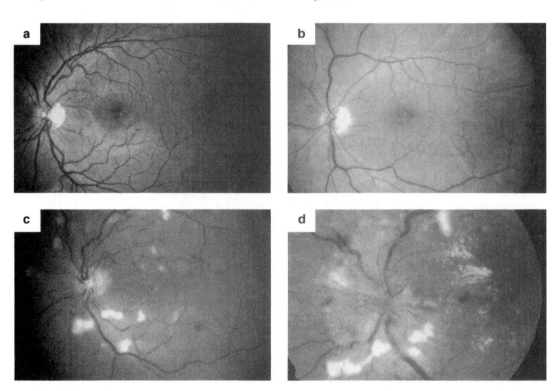

**FIGURE 4–11** ● Retinal photographs of progressively more severe hypertensive retinopathy. (From Pache et al. Do angiographic data support a detailed classification of hypertensive fundus changes? *J Human Hypertens* 2002;16:405–410.)

## TABLE 4–11

### Classification of Hypertensive Retinopathy

| Grade of Retinopathy | Retinal Signs | Systemic Associations |
|---|---|---|
| None | No detectable signs | None |
| Mild | Generalized arteriolar narrowing, focal arteriolar narrowing, arteriovenous nicking, opacity ("copper wiring") of arteriolar wall, or a combination of these signs | Modest association with risk of stroke, coronary heart disease, and death |
| Moderate | Hemmorhage (blot, dot, or flame-shaped), microaneurysm, cotton-wool spot, hard exudate, or a combination of these signs | Strong association with risk of stroke, cognitive decline, and death from cardiovascular causes |
| Malignant | Signs of moderate retinopathy plus bilateral swelling of the optic disk | Strong association with death |

Modified from Wong TY, Mitchell P. Hypertensive retinopathy. *N Engl J Med* 2004;351:2310–2317.

### Dyslipidemia

Hypertriglyceridemia and, even more threatening, hypercholesterolemia are found more frequently in untreated hypertensives than in normotensives (Borghi, 2002). As shown in Figure 4–12, the prevalence of hypercholesterolemia increases with the BP level and contributes to a marked increase in the incidence of fatal coronary disease (Neaton & Wentworth, 1992). Not only is dyslipidemia an important risk factor in established hypertension at all ages (Lloyd-Jones et al., 2003) but it may contribute to the exaggerated pressor response to stress in younger prehypertensives, adding to their risk for developing persistent hypertension (Borghi et al., 2004). Moreover, higher levels of more atherogenic LDL subfractions were found in association with endothelial dysfunction among high-risk hypertensives (Felmeden et al., 2003).

Despite the known additive risks and the known ability of cholesterol reduction to lower blood pressure (Ferrier et al., 2002) and protect against heart attacks and strokes (Sever et al., 2003), few dyslipidemic hypertensives are now being adequately treated (O'Meara et al., 2004).

### Cost Effectiveness

The performance of these few tests seems to be easily justified. In particular, the knowledge that diabetes often coexists with hypertension and that earlier recognition and treatment of diabetes would surely save the health care system money seems to indicate that all hypertensives should have a fasting glucose determination. However, a cost-effectiveness analysis concludes that diabetes screening by fasting capillary blood glucose, requiring an extra 10 minutes at the physician visit and incurring a cost of $24.40 per person screened, if done universally, would cost $360,966 for one quality-adjusted life-year (QALY) (Hoerger et al., 2004). Therefore, these authors recommend screening only for hypertensives from age 55 to 75 years (at a cost of $34,375 for one QALY), since intensive blood pressure control has been shown to quickly reduce cardiovascular complications in older diabetics.

Presumably, if the blood glucose test is done in concert with the other blood tests in a clinic laboratory, the cost per test would be lower and, thereby, more widespread screening would be more cost effective. Meanwhile, blood hemoglobin $A_{1c}$ appears to be an even better determinant of cardiovascular risk and may replace the fasting glucose (Khaw et al., 2004).

Similar analyses of other commonly performed laboratory tests show surprisingly high costs for one QALY (Boulware et al., 2003). Though these cost-effectiveness analyses are increasingly being performed in an attempt to rationalize and justify testing (as well as the use of drugs, surgical procedures, etc.), the results are often contradictory to common practice and, many would say, common sense. Nonetheless, as healthcare costs skyrocket, clinicians must be aware of the true costs of what they often do to individual patients at a relatively small cost when these costs are applied to large populations.

Perhaps an even better reason why testing should be limited is the likelihood of false positive results, particularly in a patient with a low likelihood of having the condition being tested for. In such patients, a positive test result would more likely be a

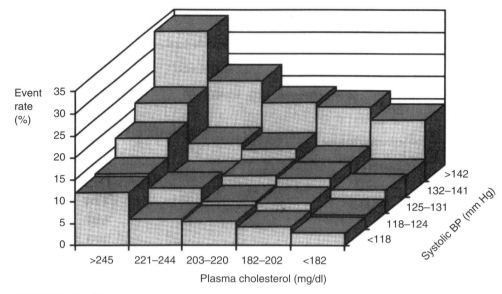

**FIGURE 4–12** ● The associations between systolic BP, plasma cholesterol, and mortality from coronary heart disease over an average 12-year follow-up among the 316,099 men screened for the Multiple Risk Factor Intervention Trial (MRFIT). (Data adapted from Neaton JD, Wentworth D. Serum cholesterol, blood pressure, cigarette smoking, and death from coronary heart disease: overall findings and differences by age for 316,099 White men. *Arch Intern Med* 1992;152:56–64.)

false positive rather than a true positive. Therefore, repeat and additional, ever-more-expensive procedures would need to be done to rule out the diagnosis. As Grimes and Schulz (2002) note:

> Screening has a darker side that is often overlooked. It can be inconvenient, unpleasant, and expensive. . . . A second wave of injury can arise after the initial screening insult: false-positive results and true-positive results leading to dangerous interventions. Although the stigma associated with correct labeling of people as ill might be acceptable, those incorrectly labeled as sick suffer as well. For example, labeling productive steelworkers as being hypertensive led to increased absenteeism and adoption of a sick role, independent of treatment.

The bottom line is that individual practitioners dealing with individual patients must use testing selectively, recognizing both their hidden costs and their potential "darker side." Therefore, the tests that will now be described should be used only if they are known to be cost effective, providing information needed for improved care of patients. Obviously, some tests such as blood glucose and lipids may be justified because they are needed for overall risk assessment; others for uncovering target organ damage, such as an ECG or an analysis for microalbuminuria. But tests should be reserved for recognition of conditions that can be helped by available therapies. As Grimes and Schulz (2002)

ask: "What benefit would accrue (and at what cost) from early diagnosis of Alzheimer's disease, which to date has no effective treatment?"

### Nonroutine Laboratory Testing

*Microalbuminuria*

A measure of urinary albumin excretion is considered an "optional" test in JNC-7 but should be routine. As noted earlier, microalbuminuria is a clear prognostic indicator for renal and cardiovascular risk and could influence the choice of antihypertensive therapy. Moreover, a cost-effectiveness analysis showed a cost of $18,621 per QALY if the test is done on all hypertensives, a very favorable ratio of cost to effectiveness (Boulware et al., 2003).

*Serum Uric Acid*

For many years, elevated uric acid levels have been known to be present in many hypertensives, considered to reflect preexisting renal disease or increased renal urate reabsorption by diuretic therapy. However, largely under the impetus of Richard Johnson and colleagues (2005), the presence of hyperuricemia is now recognized to be a precursor and possible pathogenetic factor for hypertension.

Nonetheless, proof of the ability to ameliorate hypertension by lowering uric acid levels is only now being tested. A glimmer of evidence is now available: the lowering of uric acid by the uricosuric ARB losartan was given credit for 29% of the greater reduction in cardiovascular events in those patients given losartan compared to those given a β-blocker in the LIFE trial (Høieggen et al., 2004).

### Inflammatory Markers

Assessed mainly by measurement of C-reactive protein (CRP), inflammation is emerging as a precursor and predictor of cardiovascular disease in association with the metabolic syndrome and insulin resistance (Rutter et al., 2004). As with homocysteine, which appears to be a marker of inflammation, measures of CRP do not seem to add to the evaluation or management of hypertensives, but they may be helpful in establishing overall cardiovascular risk (Ridker et al., 2005).

### Plasma Insulin

There may be value in the addition of a fasting insulin measurement as a way to assess insulin resistance. Calculation of the "homeostasis model assessment (HOMA)" using fasting glucose and insulin levels has been shown to be a reliable indicator of insulin resistance (Lansang et al., 2001). However, for routine clinical practice, the identification of insulin resistance does not seem necessary, particularly since it is not always synonymous with the metabolic syndrome (Egan et al., 2004).

### Plasma Renin Activity

For many years, Laragh and colleagues (Laragh, 2001) have emphasized the value of ascertaining the plasma renin level coupled with the level of 24-hour urinary sodium excretion, the renin-sodium profile. In various guidelines by expert committees, e.g., JNC-7 (Chobanian et al., 2003), this profile is not recommended as part of the routine evaluation of all hypertensives but rather as a diagnostic tool if other features of low-renin states (e.g., primary aldosteronism) or high-renin states (e.g., renovascular disease) are present.

## Additional Testing for Target Organ Damage

### Cardiac Assessment

All hypertensives should have electrocardiography to identify LVH and conduction defects. Electrocardiography using the Cornell/strain index identifies LVH in 16.3% of hypertensive subjects (Verdecchia et al., 2003a). Echocardiography, although it is much more sensitive in identifying LVH, is recommended only for those patients with an overall low-risk status who meet current criteria for *not* starting antihypertensive therapy (Schillaci et al., 2002a), with the assumption that, if LVH is present, therapy would be indicated. Echocardiography is not recommended for those whose overall risk status necessitates active drug therapy, as it does not appear to be a better guide to therapy than is the level of BP.

Despite the advocacy of some experts (Greenland & Gaziano, 2003), neither exercise treadmill tests (ETT) nor electron-beam computerized tomography (EBCT) scanning for coronary calcification are recommended for adults at low risk for coronary disease (U.S. Preventive Services Task Force, 2004). The recommendation does not address hypertensives per se but, in general, hypertensives without symptoms of coronary disease should not be so tested.

The measurement of hemodynamic indices by impedance cardiography is being recommended, particularly in resistant hypertension (Ventura et al., 2005).

### Cerebral Assessment

Although sensitive testing may show that neurobehavioral function is reduced (Elias et al., 2003), it is not possible to relate cerebral dysfunction to the severity of the BP, unless hypertension has become accelerated with resultant encephalopathy. In the presence of symptoms of cerebral ischemia, particularly transient ischemic attacks, the finding of a carotid bruit indicates the need for carotid ultrasonography in the hope of finding a correctable lesion (Parrinello et al., 2004).

### Renal Assessment

Serum creatinine, preferably converted to an estimate of GFR (Stevens & Levey, 2004), and a measure of albuminuria are the only tests now recommended as routine.

### Vascular Assessment

A low ankle-brachial index (ABI) using a Doppler flow detector is a proven measure of peripheral vascular disease and the risk for cardiovascular events (Murabito et al., 2003). Abdominal palpation should be performed to identify aortic aneurysms, particularly in thin, elderly hypertensives with evidence of vascular disease elsewhere. Ultrasonography is needed for diagnostic certainty (van der Vliet & Boll, 1997). Peripheral vessels should be palpated for diminished pulse and auscultated for bruits.

Safar and associates have used a noninvasive procedure to measure radial artery wall thickness that is closely correlated to pulse pressure and LV mass (Mourad et al., 2000). Carotid intima-media thickening by ultrasonography (Cuspidi et al., 2002) and determination of augmentation index derived by pulse wave analysis have been claimed to be useful markers of cardiovascular risk (Cohn et al., 2005; Nürnberger et al., 2002).

Increasing awareness of the importance of pulsatile phenomena in the pathogenesis of cardiovascular damage has led to attempts to measure arterial compliance, a quantitative measure of the distensibility of the arterial system. A noninvasive diastolic pulse contour analysis from the radial artery pressure wave form has been found to correlate differently from traditional risk factors in men and women (Duprez et al., 2004). Whether such measures provide clinical benefit is not yet known.

## Search for Identifiable Causes

The frequencies of various identifiable causes of hypertension shown in Table 1–7 are likely much too high for the larger population with mild, asymptomatic hypertension. Nonetheless, clues to the presence of an identifiable cause should be sought in the routine evaluation of every new hypertensive. If suggestive clues are found or if the patient has features of "inappropriate" hypertension (Table 4–12), additional workup for an identifiable cause should be performed.

The studies listed in Table 4–13 as initial usually will serve as adequate screening procedures and are readily available to every practitioner. If they are abnormal, the listed additional procedures should be performed, perhaps after referral to a hypertension specialist, along with whatever other tests are needed to confirm the diagnosis. More detail about these procedures is provided in their respective chapters.

## Assessment of Overall Cardiovascular Risk

Once the cause and consequences of the hypertension have been evaluated, it is necessary to assess

### TABLE 4–12

### Features of "Inappropriate" Hypertension

Age of onset: <20 or >50 yr

Level of blood pressure: >180/110 mm Hg

Organ damage

    Funduscopy: moderate or malignant

    Serum creatinine >1.5 mg/dL

    Cardiomegaly or left ventricular hypertrophy as determined by electrocardiography

Presence of features indicative of secondary causes

    Unprovoked hypokalemia

    Abdominal bruit

    Variable pressures with tachycardia, sweating, tremor

    Family history of renal disease

Poor response to generally effective therapy

the patient's overall cardiovascular risk status. The proper management of hypertension should involve attention to all of the risk factors that can be altered. Patients at high risk should be counseled and helped to reduce all of their risk factors. For many patients, the BP may be the easiest of the risks to control, so this may be the first priority. As described more fully in the next chapter, the overall risk profile provides a more rational basis than

### TABLE 4–13

## Overall Guide to Workup for Identifiable Causes of Hypertension

| Diagnosis | Diagnostic Procedure | |
|---|---|---|
| | Initial | Additional |
| Chronic renal disease | Urinalysis; serum creatinine; renal sonography | Isotopic renogram; renal biopsy |
| Renovascular disease | Captopril-enhanced isotopic renogram; duplex sonography | Magnetic resonance or CT angiogram; aortogram |
| Coarctation | Blood pressure in legs | Echocardiogram; aortogram |
| Primary aldosteronism | Plasma and urinary potassium; plasma renin and aldosterone | Plasma or urinary aldosterone after saline load; adrenal CT scans and scintiscans |
| Cushing's syndrome | Morning plasma cortisol after 1 mg dexamethasone at bedtime | Urinary cortisol after variable doses of dexamethasone; adrenal CT scans and scintiscans |
| Pheochromocytoma | Plasma metanephrine; urine metanephrine | Urinary catechols; plasma catechols (basal and after 0.3 mg clonidine); adrenal CT scans and scintiscans |

CT, computed tomography.

an arbitrary BP level for determining whether and when to start treatment and the goal of therapy. For now, the need for a complete assessment of cardiovascular risk—a simple and inexpensive undertaking—should be obvious in the proper management of all hypertensives.

### The Framingham Formula

Most assessments of cardiovascular risk focus on CHD, because that is the most common complication, and some use only "hard" events, excluding angina. Most assessments are based on data from the Framingham Heart Study, the longest and most complete follow-up of a carefully studied, large population (Kannel et al., 2004). Most expert committees use their 10-year risk data, although models using shorter probabilities, either 2 years (D'Agostino et al., 2000) or 5 years (D'Agostino et al., 2001) may be more accurate. The Framingham data have been found to accurately ascertain long-term cardiovascular risks in diverse populations (Kannel et al., 2004) and even the extent of progression of coronary artery plaques over 18 months (von Birgelen et al., 2004).

From a longer list of known risk factors, the Framingham data have used those shown in Table 4–14, which converts gradations in the various risk factors into points. These points then are used to establish the absolute 10-year risk (Table 4–15) which, in turn, is used to ascertain the need for antihypertensive therapy as detailed in the next chapter.

## TABLE 4–14

### Scoring of Risk Factors Used in the Framingham Analyses

| Risk Factors | Risk Points | | Risk Factors | Risk Points | |
|---|---|---|---|---|---|
| | Men | Women | | Men | Women |
| Age (yr) | | | Blood pressure (mm Hg) | | |
| <34 | −1 | −9 | <120 | 0 | −3 |
| 35–39 | 0 | −4 | 120–129 | 0 | 0 |
| 40–44 | 1 | 0 | 130–139 | 1 | 1 |
| 45–49 | 2 | 3 | 140–159 | 2 | 2 |
| 50–54 | 3 | 6 | >160 | 3 | 3 |
| 55–59 | 4 | 7 | Smoker | | |
| 60–64 | 5 | 8 | No | 0 | 0 |
| 65–69 | 6 | 9 | Yes | 2 | 2 |
| 70–74 | 7 | 10 | High-density lipoprotein (HDL) cholesterol (mg/dL) | | |
| Total cholesterol (mg/dL) | | | <35 | 2 | 5 |
| <160 | −3 | −2 | 35–44 | 1 | 2 |
| 160–199 | 0 | 0 | 45–49 | 0 | 1 |
| 200–239 | 1 | 1 | 50–59 | −1 | 0 |
| 240–279 | 2 | 2 | >60 | −2 | −3 |
| >280 | 3 | 3 | Plasma glucose | | |
| | | | <110 | 0 | 0 |
| | | | 110–126 | 1 | 1 |
| | | | >126 | 2 | 2 |

| Adding up the points | |
|---|---|
| Age _____ | Total cholesterol _____ |
| Plasma glucose (diabetes) _____ | HDL cholesterol _____ |
| Smoker _____ | Blood pressure _____ |
| Total _____ | |

Modified from Grundy SM. Cholesterol management in the era of managed care. *Am J Cardiol* 2000;85:3A–9A.

## TABLE 4-15

### Absolute Risk Estimates for Hard Coronary Heart Disease According to Framingham Points

| Framingham Risk Points | Absolute 10-Year Risk (%) | |
|---|---|---|
| | Men | Women |
| 1 | 2 | 1 |
| 2 | 3 | 2 |
| 3 | 4 | 2 |
| 4 | 5 | 2 |
| 5 | 6 | 2 |
| 6 | 7 | 2 |
| 7 | 9 | 3 |
| 8 | 13 | 3 |
| 9 | 16 | 3 |
| 10 | 20 | 4 |
| 11 | 25 | 7 |
| 12 | 30 | 8 |
| 13 | 35 | 11 |
| 14 | 45 | 13 |
| 15 | – | 15 |
| 16 | – | 18 |
| 17 | – | 20 |

Modified from Grundy SM. Cholesterol management in the era of managed care. *Am J Cardiol* 2000;85:3A–9A.

Although age overwhelms all else in increasing risk, the other factors are modifiable and therefore demand attention. Almost all people with clinically significant coronary disease have one or more of these risk factors (Canto & Iskandrian, 2003).

### Other Formulas

A number of other assessments of cardiovascular risks are available, as reviewed by Jackson et al. (2005), including the Sheffield UK (Wallis et al., 2000), the Joint British Society (Williams et al., 2004), and two that apply only to hypertensives (Glynn et al., 2002; Pocock et al., 2001). These and other quantitative risk assessments provide similar sensitivity and specificity.

The Framingham formula seems most appropriate for use in the United States and will be the basis for the decision to start drug therapy in the next chapter. Patients need to be advised in a clear,

understandable manner about their own risk status, both to motivate them to take necessary lifestyle changes and medications and to bring them into the decision-making process, providing them with greater autonomy.

## REFERENCES

Abate NI, Mansour YH, Tuncel M, et al. Overweight and sympathetic overactivity in Black Americans. *Hypertension* 2001;38:379–383.

Agmon Y, Khandheria BK, Meissner I, et al. Independent association of high blood pressure and aortic atherosclerosis. *Circulation* 2000;102:2087–2093.

Akinboboye OO, Chou R-L, Bergmann SR. Myocardial blood flow and efficiency in concentric and essentric left ventricular hypertrophy. *Am J Hypertens* 2004;17:433–438.

Alfakih K, Maqbool A, Sivananthan M, et al. Left ventricle mass index and the common, functional, X-linked angiotensin II type-2 receptor gene polymorphism (-1332 G/A) in patients with systemic hypertension. *Hypertension* 2004a;43:1189–1194.

Alfakih K, Walters K, Jones T, et al. New gender-specific partition values for ECG criteria of left ventricular hypertrophy: recalibration against cardiac MRI. *Hypertension* 2004b;44:175–179.

Allemann Y, Hutter D, Aeschbacher BC, et al. Increased central body fat deposition precedes a significant rise in resting blood pressure in male offspring of essential hypertensive patients: a 5 year follow-up study. *J Hypertens* 2001;19:2143–2148.

Andrew ME, Jones DW, Wofford MR, et al. Ethnicity and unprovoked hypokalemia in the Atherosclerosis Risk in Communities Study. *Am J Hypertens* 2002;15:594–599.

Antonini-Canterin F, Huang G, Cervesato E, et al. Symptomatic aortic stenosis: does systemic hypertension play an additional role? *Hypertension* 2003;41:1268–1272.

Applegate WB, Davis BR, Black RH, et al. Prevalence of postural hypotension at baseline in the Systolic Hypertension in the Elderly Program (SHEP) cohort. *J Am Geriatr Soc* 1991;39:1057–1065.

Argentino C, Toni D, Rasura M, et al. Circadian variation in the frequency of ischemic stroke. *Stroke* 1990;21:387–389.

Arnold AM, Psaty BM, Kuller LH, et al. Incidence of cardiovascular disease in older Americans: the cardiovascular health study. *J Am Geriatr Soc* 2005;53:211–218.

Aurigemma GP, Gaasch WH. Diastolic heart failure. *N Engl J Med* 2004;351:1097–1105.

Aviv A, Hollenberg NK, Weder AB. Sodium glomerulopathy: tubuloglomerular feedback and renal injury in African Americans. *Kidney Int* 2004a;65:361–368.

Aviv A, Hollenberg N, Weder A. Urinary potassium excretion and sodium sensitivity in blacks. *Hypertension* 2004b;43:707–713.

Aylward PE, Wilcox RG, Horgan JH, et al. Relation of increased arterial blood pressure to mortality and stroke in the context of contemporary thrombolytic therapy for acute myocardial infarction. *Ann Intern Med* 1996;125:891–900.

Baik I, Ascherio A, Rimm EB, et al. Adiposity and mortality in men. *Am J Epidemiol* 2000;152:264–271.

Barsky AJ, Borus JF. Functional somatic syndromes. *Ann Intern Med* 1999;130:910–921.

Barzilay JI, Peterson D, Cushman M, et al. The relationship of cardiovascular risk factors to microalbuminuria in older adults with or without diabetes mellitus or hypertension: The Cardiovascular Health Study. *Am J Kidney Dis* 2004;44:25–34.

Bauer GE. Mortality patterns in treated hypertension: results from Sydney Hospital. *Drugs* 1976;11(Suppl 1):39–44.

Bechgaard P. A 40 years' follow-up study of 1000 untreated hypertensive patients. *Clin Sci Mol Med* Suppl 1976; 3:673S-675S.

Bechgaard P. The natural history of arterial hypertension in the elderly. A fifty-year follow-up study. *Acta Med Scand* 1983;(Suppl 676):9–14.

Berenson GS, Srinivasan SR, Bao W, et al. Association between multiple cardiovascular risk factors and atherosclerosis in children and young adults. *N Engl J Med* 1998; 338:1650–1656.

Bidani AK, Griffin KA. Pathophysiology of hypertensive renal damage: implications for therapy. *Hypertension* 2004;44:595–601.

Blanker MH, Bohnen AM, Groeneveld FPMJ, et al. Normal voiding patterns and determinants of increased diurnal and nocturnal voiding frequency in elderly men. *J Urol* 2000;164:1201–1205.

Bochud M, Elston RC, Maillard M, et al. Heritability of renal function in hypertensive families of African descent in the Seychelles (Indian Ocean). *Kidney Int* 2005;67:61–69.

Borghi C. Interactions between hypercholesterolemia and hypertension: implications for therapy. *Curr Opin Nephrol Hypertens* 2002;11:489–496.

Borghi C, Veronisi M, Bacchelli S, et al. Serum cholesterol levels, blood pressure response to stress and incidence of stable hypertension in young subjects with high normal blood pressure. *J Hypertens* 2004;22:265–272.

Boulware LE, Jaar BG, Tarver-Carr ME, et al. Screening for proteinuria in US adults: a cost-effectiveness analysis. *JAMA* 2003;290:3101–3114.

Brancati FL, Kao WHL, Folson AR, et al. Incident type 2 diabetes mellitus in African American and White adults. *JAMA* 2000;283:2253–2259.

Breckenridge A, Dollery CT, Parry EH. Prognosis of treated hypertension. Changes in life expectancy and causes of death between 1952 and 1967. *QJM* 1970;39:411–429.

Brickman AS, Nyby MD, Griffiths RF, et al. Racial differences in platelet cytosolic calcium and calcitropic hormones in normotensive subjects. *Am J Hypertens* 1993;6:46–51.

Buck C, Baker P, Bass M, Donner A. The prognosis of hypertension according to age at onset. *Hypertension* 1987; 9:204–208.

Bulpitt CJ, Beevers DG, Butler A, et al. The survival of treated hypertensive patients and their causes of death: a report from the DHSS hypertensive care computing project (DHCCP). *J Hypertens* 1986;4:93–99.

Campia U, Cardillo C, Panza JA. Ethnic differences in the vasoconstrictor activity of endogenous endothelin-1 in hypertensive patients. *Circulation* 2004;109:3191–3195.

Campo C, Segura J, Roldan C, et al. Correlation between estimated glomerular filtration rate and microalbuminuria in treated essential hypertensive patients [Abstract]. *Am J Hypertens* 2004;17:89A.

Cantillon P, Morgan M, Dundas R, et al. Patients' perceptions of changes in their blood pressure. *J Hum Hypertens* 1997;11:221–225.

Canto JG, Iskandrian AE. Major risk factors for cardiovascular disease: debunking the "only 50%" myth. *JAMA* 2003;290:947–949.

Chambless LE, Folsom AR, Clegg LX, et al. Carotid wall thickness is predictive of incident clinical stroke. *Am J Epidemiol* 2000;151:478–487.

Chaturvedi N, Bulpitt CJ, Leggetter S, et al. Ethnic differences in vascular stiffness and relations to hypertensive target organ damage. *J Hypertens* 2004;22:1731–1737.

Chobanian AV, Bakris GL, Black HR, et al. Seventh report of the Joint National Committee on Prevention, Detection, Evaluation, and Treatment of High Blood Pressure. *Hypertension* 2003;42:1206–1252.

Cohen HW, Hailpern SM, Alderman MH. Glucose-cholesterol interaction magnifies coronary disease risk for hypertensive patients. *Hypertension* 2004;43:983–987.

Cohn JN, Duprez DA, Grandits GA. Arterial elasticity as part of a comprehensive assessment of cardiovascular risk and drug treatment. *Hypertension* 2004;45. Available online at: http:www.hypertensionaha.org. Accessed May 2, 2005.

Cooper RS, Liao Y. Is hypertension among blacks more severe or simply more common [Abstract]? *Circulation* 1992;85:12.

Cooper RS, Rotimmi CN, Ward R. The puzzle of hypertension in African-Americans. *Sci Am* 1999;Feb:56–63.

Cooper WD, Glover DR, Hormbrey JM, Kimber GR. Headache and BP. *J Hum Hypertens* 1989;3:41–44.

Creager MA, Lüscher TF, Cosentino F, Beckman JA. Diabetes and vascular disease: pathophysiology, clinical consequences, and medical therapy. *Circulation* 2003; 108: 1527–1532.

Cruickshank JK, Mzayek F, Liu L, et al. Origins of the "black/white" difference in blood pressure, roles of birth weight, postnatal growth, early blood pressure and adolescent body size; the Bogalusa heart study. *Circulation* 2005;111:1932–1937.

Cuspidi C, Ambrosioni E, Mancia G, et al. Role of echocardiography and carotid ultrasonography in stratifying risk in patients with essential hypertension: The Assessment of Prognostic Risk Observational Study. *J Hypertens* 2002;20:1307–1314.

D'Agostino RB, Grundy S, Sullivan LM, et al. Validation of the Framingham coronary heart disease prediction scores. *JAMA* 2001;286:180–187.

D'Agostino RB, Russell MW, Huse DM, et al. Primary and subsequent coronary risk appraisal. *Am Heart J* 2000;139: 272–281.

Daffertshofer M, Mielke O, Pullwitt A, et al. Transient ischemic attacks are more than "ministrokes." *Stroke* 2004;35: 2453–2458.

Dahlöf B, Lindholm LH, Hansson L, et al. Morbidity and mortality in the Swedish Trial in Older Patients with Hypertension (STOP-Hypertension). *Lancet* 1991;338:1281–1285.

Davies SJC, Ghahramani P, Jackson PR, et al. Association of panic disorder and panic attacks with hypertension. *Am J Med* 1999;107:310–316.

Davies SJC, Jackson PR, Ramsay LE, Ghahramani P. Drug intolerance due to nonspecific adverse effects related to psychiatric morbidity in hypertensive patients. *Arch Intern Med* 2003;163:592–600.

Daviglus ML, Greenland P, Stamler J, et al. Relation of nutrient intake to microalbuminuria in nondiabetic middle-aged men and women: international population study of macronutrients and blood pressure (INTERMAP). *Am J Kidney Dis* 2005;45:256–266.

de Simone G, Kitzman DW, Palmieri V, et al. Association of inappropriate left ventricular mass with systolic and diastolic dysfunction. *Am J Hypertens* 2004;17:828–833.

de Simone G, Pasanisi F, Contraldo F. Link of nonhemodynamic factors to hemodynamic determinants of left ventricular hypertrophy. *Hypertension* 2001;38:13–18.

de Simone G, Roman MJ, Alderman MH, et al. High pulse pressure as a marker of preclinical cardiovascular disease. *Hypertension* 2005;45:575–579.

DeGuire S, Gevirty R, Kawahara Y, Maguire W. Hyperventilation syndrome and the assessment of treatment for functional cardiac symptoms. *Am J Cardiol* 1992;70:673–677.

Devereux RB, Bella JN, Palmieri V, et al. Left ventricular systolic dysfunction in a biracial sample of hypertensive adults. *Hypertension* 2001;38:417–423.

Diabetes Prevention Program Research Group. Reduction in the incidence of type 2 diabetes with lifestyle intervention or metformin. *N Engl J Med* 2002;346:393–403.

Dong Y, Zhu H, Sagnella GA, et al. Association between the C825T polymorphism of the G protein β3-subunit gene and hypertension in blacks. *Hypertension* 1999;34:1193–1196.

Dries DL, Exner DV, Gersh BJ, et al. Racial differences in the outcome of left ventricular dysfunction. *N Engl J Med* 1999;340:609–616.

Duprez DA, Kaiser DR, Whitwam W, et al. Determinants of radial artery pulse wave analysis in asymptomatic individuals. *Am J Hypertens* 2004;17:647–653.

Dustan HP. Does keloid pathogenesis hold the key to understanding Black/White differences in hypertension severity? *Hypertension* 1995;26:858–862.

Earnshaw JJ, Shaw E, Whyman WR, et al. Screening for abdominal aortic aneurysms in men. *Br Med J* 2004;28:1122–1124.

Egan BM, Papademitriou V, Wofford M, et al. Metabolic syndrome and insulin resistance in the TROPHY substudy: contrasting views in high normal blood pressure [Abstract]. *Am J Hypertens* 2004;17:180A.

Ejaz AA, Haley WE, Wasiluk A, et al. Characteristics of 100 consecutive patients presenting with orthostatic hypotension. *Mayo Clin Proc* 2004;79:890–894.

Elias MF, Elias PK, Sullivan LM, et al. Lower cognitive function in the presence of obesity and hypertension: The Framingham heart study. *Int J Obesity* 2003;27:260–268.

El-Gharbawy AH, Kotchen JM, Grim CE, at al. Predictors of target organ damage in hypertensive Blacks and Whites. *Hypertension* 2001;38:761–766.

Endemann DH, Pu Q, De Ciuceis C, et al. Persistent remodeling of resistance arteries in type 2 diabetic patients on antihypertensive treatment. *Hypertension* 2004;43(part 2):399–404.

Fagard RH, Staessen JA, Thijs L, et al. Prognostic significance of electrocardiographic voltages and their serial changes in elderly with systolic hypertension. *Hypertension* 2004;44:459–464.

Fang J, Madhavan S, Alderman MH. The association between birthplace and mortality from cardiovascular causes among black and white residents of New York City. *N Engl J Med* 1996;335:1545–1551.

Faxon DP, Creager MA, Smith SC Jr, et al. Atherosclerotic Vascular Disease Conference: executive summary. *Circulation* 2004;109:2595–2604.

Felmeden DC, Spencer CGC, Blann AD, et al. Low-density lipoprotein subfractions and cardiovascular risk in hypertension: relationship to endothelial dysfunction and effects of treatment. *Hypertension* 2003;41:528–532.

Ferrier KE, Muhlmann MH, Baguet J-P, et al. Intensive cholesterol reduction lowers blood pressure and large artery stiffness in isolated systolic hypertension. *J Am Coll Cardiol* 2002;39:1020–1025.

Flack JM, Neaton J, Grimm R Jr, et al. Blood pressure and mortality among men with prior myocardial infarction. *Circulation* 1995;92:2437–2445.

Flaherty ML, Woo D, Haverbusch M, et al. Racial variations in location and risk of intracerebral hemorrhage. *Stroke* 2005;36:934–937.

Flemming KD, Brown RD Jr, Petty GW, et al. Evaluation and management of transient ischemic attack and minor cerebral infarction. *Mayo Clin Proc* 2004;79:1071–1086.

Fontana F, Bernardi P, Lanfranchi G, et al. Blood pressure response to hyperventilation test reflects daytime pressor profile. *Hypertension* 2003;41:244–248.

Fotherby MD, Potter JF. Reproducibility of ambulatory and clinic blood pressure measurements in elderly hypertensive subjects. *J Hypertens* 1993;11:573–579.

Fox CS, Larson MG, Leip EP, et al. Predictors of new-onset kidney disease in a community-based population. *JAMA* 2004;291:844–850.

Franco OH, Peeters A, Bonneux L, de Laet C. Blood pressure in adulthood and life expectancy with cardiovascular disease in men and women: life course analysis. *Hypertension* 2005;46(in press).

Franklin SS, Gustin W IV, Wong ND, et al. Hemodynamic patterns of age-related changes in blood pressure: The Framingham Heart Study. *Circulation* 1997;96:308–315.

Franklin SS, Jacobs MJ, Wong ND, et al. Predominance of isolated systolic hypertension among middle-aged and elderly US hypertensives: analysis based on National Health and Nutrition Examination Survey (NHANES) III. *Hypertension* 2001;37:869–874.

Franklin SS, Pio JR, Wong ND, et al. Predictors of new-onset diastolic and systolic hypertension: the Framingham heart study. *Circulation* 2005;111:1121–1127.

Fuchs FD, Moreira LB, Moreira WD, et al. Headache is not more frequent among patients with moderate to severe hypertension. *J Human Hypertens* 2003;17:787–790.

Ganguli MC, Grimm RH Jr, Svendsen KH, et al. Urinary sodium and potassium profile of blacks and whites in relation to education in two different geographic urban areas. *Am J Hypertens* 1999;12:69–72.

Garrison RJ, Kannel WB, Stokes J III, Castelli WP. Incidence and precursors of hypertension in young adults. *Prev Med* 1987;16:235–251.

Geiss LS, Rolka DB, Engelgau MM. Elevated blood pressure among U.S. adults with diabetes, 1988–1994. *Am J Prev Med* 2002;22:42–48.

Gillum RF. The epidemiology of cardiovascular disease in black Americans. *N Engl J Med* 1996;335:1597–1599.

Glynn RJ, L'Italien GJ, Sesso HD, et al. Development of predictive models for long-term cardiovascular risk associated with systolic and diastolic blood pressure. *Hypertension* 2002;39:105–110.

Gorelick PB. Stroke prevention therapy beyond antithrombotics: unifying mechanisms in ischemic stroke pathogenesis and implications for therapy: an invited review. *Stroke* 2002;33:862–875.

Grassi G, Seravalle G, Bertinieri G, et al. Sympathetic and reflex alterations in systo-diastolic and systolic hypertension in the elderly. *J Hypertens* 2000;18:587–593.

Greenland P, Gaziano JM. Selecting asymptomatic patients for coronary computed tomography of electrocardiographic exercise testing. *N Engl J Med* 2003;349:465–473.

Grimes DA, Schulz KF. Uses and abuses of screening tests. *Lancet* 2002;359:881–884.

Gueyffier F, Bulpitt C, Boissel J-P, et al. Antihypertensive drugs in very old people. *Lancet* 1999;353:793–796.

Gus M, Fuchs FD, Pimentel M, et al. Behavior of ambulatory blood pressure surrounding episodes of headache in mildly hypertensive patients. *Arch Intern Med* 2001;161:252–255.

Haas DC, Gerber LM, Schwartz JE, et al. A comparison of morning blood pressure surge in blacks and whites [Abstract]. *Circulation* 2003;108(Suppl 4):IV-399.

Hagen K, Stovner LJ, Vatten L, et al. Blood pressure and risk of headache: a prospective of 22,685 adults in Norway. *J Neurol Neurosurg Psychiatry* 2002;72:463–466.

Hagen K, Zwart JA, Holmen J, et al. Does hypertension protect against musculoskeletal complaints? *Arch Intern Med* 2005;165:916–922.

Hallan H, Romundstad S, Kvenild K, Holmen J. Microalbuminuria in diabetic and hypertensive patients and the general population. *Scand J Urol Nephrol* 2003;37:151–158.

Hallock P, Benson IC. Studies of the elastic properties of human isolated aorta. *J Clin Invest* 1937;16:595–602.

Hamet P, Thorin-Trescases N, Moreau P, et al. Excess growth and apoptosis. *Hypertension* 2001;37:760–766.

Harshfield GA, Treiber FA, Wilson ME, et al. A longitudinal study of ethnic differences in ambulatory blood pressure patterns in youth. *Am J Hypertens* 2002a;15:525–530.

Harshfield GA, Wilson ME, Hanevold C, et al. Impaired stress-induced pressure natriuresis increases cardiovascular load in African American youths. *Am J Hypertens* 2002b;15:903–906.

He J, Klag MJ, Appel LJ, et al. Seven-year incidence of hypertension in a cohort of middle-aged African Americans and whites. *Hypertension* 1998;31:1130–1135.

Helgeland A. Treatment of mild hypertension. *Am J Med* 1980;69:725–732.

Helmer OM. Hormonal and biochemical factors controlling BP. In: *Les Concepts de Claude Bernard sur le Milieu Interieur.* Paris: Masson & Cie, 1967;115–128.

Herrington DM, Brown V, Mosca L, et al. Relationship between arterial stiffness and subclinical aortic atherosclerosis. *Circulation* 2004;110:432–437.

Hinderliter AL, Blumenthal JA, Waugh R, et al. Ethnic differences in left ventricular structure: relations to hemodynamics and diurnal blood pressure variation. *Am J Hypertens* 2004;17:43–49.

Hodge JV, Smirk FH. The effect of drug treatment of hypertension on the distribution of deaths from various causes. *Am Heart J* 1967;73:441–452.

Hoerger TJ, Harris R, Hicks KA, et al. Screening for type 2 diabetes mellitus: a cost-effectiveness analysis. *Ann Intern Med* 2004;140:689–699.

Hoffman GS, Merkel PA, Brasington RD, et al. Anti-tumor necrosis factor therapy in patients with difficult to treat Takayasu arteritis. *Arthr Rheum* 2004;50:2296–2304.

Høieggen A, Alderman MH, Kjeldsen SE, et al. The impact of serum uric acid on cardiovascular outcomes in the LIFE study. *Kidney Int* 2004;65:1041–1046.

Howard BV. Blood pressure in 13 American Indian communities. *Pub Health Rep* 1996;111:47–48.

Hsu C-Y. Does non-malignant hypertension cause renal insufficiency? Evidence-based perspective. *Curr Opin Nephrol Hypertens* 2002;11:267–272.

Ibsen H, Olsen MH, Wachtell K, et al. Reduction in albuminuria translates to reduction in cardiovascular events in hypertensive patients: Losartan Intervention for Endpoint Reduction in Hypertension study. *Hypertension* 2005;45:198–202.

Isles CG, Walker LM, Beevers GD, et al. Mortality in patients of the Glasgow Blood Pressure Clinic. *J Hypertens* 1986;4:141–156.

Jackson R, Lawes CMM, Bennett DA, et al. Treatment with drugs to lower blood pressure and blood cholesterol based on an individual's absolute cardiovascular risk. *Lancet* 2005;365:434–441.

James SA, Kaufman JS, Raghunathan TE, et al. Five year hypertension incidence in African Americans: the contribution of socioeconomic status, perceived stress, and John Henryism [Abstract]. *Am J Hypertens* 1996;9:19A.

Janeway TC. A clinical study of hypertensive cardiovascular disease. *Arch Intern Med* 1913;12:755–798.

Jha AK, Varosy PD, Kanaya AM, et al. Differences in medical care and disease outcomes among black and white women with heart disease. *Circulation* 2003;108:1089–1094.

Johnson RJ, Feig DI, Herrera-Acosta J, Kang D-H. The resurrection of uric acid as a causal factor in essential hypertension. *Hypertension* 2005;45:18–20.

Jones CA, Francis ME, Eberhardt MS, et al. Microalbuminuria in the US population: Third National Health and Nutrition Examination Survey. *Am J Kidney Dis* 2002;39:445–459.

Jones DW, Chambless LE, Folsom AR, et al. Risk factors for coronary heart disease in African Americans: The Atherosclerosis Risk in Communities Study, 1987–1997. *Arch Intern Med* 2002;162:2565–2571.

Jones DW. What is the role of obesity in hypertension and target organ injury in African Americans? *Am J Med Sci* 1999;317:147–151.

Jones PP, Christou DD, Jordan J, Seals DR. Baroreflex buffering is reduced with age in healthy men. *Circulation* 2003;107:1770–1774.

Julius S, Nesbitt S, Egan B, et al. Trial of preventing hypertension (TROPHY): design and 2-year progress report. *Hypertension* 2004;44:146–151.

Kallenbach K, Oelze T, Salcher R, et al. Evolving strategies for treatment of acute aortic dissection type A. *Circulation* 2004;110(Suppl):II243-II249.

Kannel WB. Blood pressure as a cardiovascular risk factor. *JAMA* 1996;275:1571–1576.

Kannel WB, D'Agostino RB, Silbershatz H. Blood pressure and cardiovascular morbidity and mortality rates in the elderly. *Am Heart J* 1997;134:758–763.

Kannel WB, D'Agostino RB, Sullivan L, et al. Concept and usefulness of cardiovascular risk profiles. *Am Heart J* 2004;148:16–26.

Kannel WB, Dannenberg AL, Abbott RD. Unrecognized myocardial infarction and hypertension. *Am Heart J* 1985;109:581–585.

Kaplan NM. Anxiety-induced hyperventilation. *Arch Intern Med* 1997;157:945–948.

Kario K, Ishikawa J, Eguchi K, et al. Sleep pulse pressure and awake mean pressure as independent predictors for stroke in older hypertensive patients. *Am J Hypertens* 2004;17:439–445.

Kass, D. Ventricular arterial stiffening, integrating the pathophysiology. *Hypertension* 2005;46. Available online at: http:www.hypertensionaha.org. Accessed May 23, 2005.

Kenchaiah S, David BR, Braunwald E, et al. Antecedent hypertension and the effect of captopril on the risk of adverse cardiovascular outcomes after acute myocardial infarction with left ventricular systolic dysfunction: insights from the Survival and Ventricular Enlargement trial. *Am Heart J* 2004;148:356–364.

Khattar RS, Swales JD, Senior R, Lahiri A. Racial variation in cardiovascular morbidity and mortality in essential hypertension. *Heart* 2000;83:267–271.

Khaw K-T, Wareham N, Bingham S, et al. Association of hemoglobin $A_{1c}$ with cardiovascular disease and mortality in adults: the European prospective investigation into cancer in Norfolk. *Ann Intern Med* 2004;141:413–420.

Kincaid-Smith P. Hypothesis: obesity and the insulin resistance syndrome play a major role in end-stage renal failure attributed to hypertension and labelled "hypertensive nephrosclerosis." *J Hypertens* 2004;22:1051–1055.

Kip KE, Marroquin OC, Kelley DE, et al. Clinical importance of obesity versus the metabolic syndrome in cardiovascular risk in women: a report from the Women's Ischemia Evaluation (WISE) study. *Circulation* 2004;109:706–713.

Kizer JR, Arnett DK, Bella JN, et al. Differences in left ventricular structure between black and white hypertensive adults: The Hypertension Genetic Epidemiology Network Study. *Hypertension* 2004;43:1182–1188.

Kjellgren KI, Ahlner J, Dahlöf B, et al. Perceived symptoms amongst hypertensive patients in routine clinical practice. *J Intern Med* 1998;244:325–332.

Klag MJ, Whelton PK, Coresh J, et al. The association of skin color with blood pressure in U.S. blacks with low socioeconomic status. *JAMA* 1991;265:599–602.

Knight EL, Kramer HM, Curhan GC. High-normal blood pressure and microalbuminuria. *Am J Kidney Dis* 2003; 41:588–595.

Kornet L, Hoeks AP, Janssen BJ, et al. Neural activity of the cardiac baroreflex decreases with age in normotensive and hypertensive subjects. *J Hypertens* 2005;23: 815–823.

Kostis JB. From hypertension to heart failure: update on the management of systolic and diastolic dysfunction. *Am J Hypertens* 2003;16:18S–22S.

Kruszewski P, Bieniaszewski L, Neubauer J, et al. Headache in patients with mild to moderate hypertension is generally not associated with simultaneous blood pressure elevation. *J Hypertens* 2000;18:437–444.

Lackland DT, Egan BM, Jones PJ. Impact of nativity and race on "stroke belt" mortality. *Hypertension* 1999;34:57–62.

Lakatta EG, Levy D. Arterial and cardiac aging: major shareholders in cardiovascular disease enterprises. *Circulation* 2003;107:139–146.

Lambert EA, Thompson J, Schlaich M, et al. Sympathetic and cardiac baroreflex function in panic disorder. *J Hypertens* 2002;20:2445–2451.

Langford HG, Watson RL. Potassium and calcium intake, excretion, and homeostasis in blacks, and their relation to blood pressure. *Cardiovasc Drug Ther* 1990;4:403–406.

Lansang MC, Williams GH, Carroll JS. Correlation between the glucose clamp technique and the homeostasis model assessment in hypertension. *Am J Hypertens* 2001;14: 51–53.

Laragh J. Laragh's lessons in pathophysiology and clinical pearls for treating hypertension. *Am J Hypertens* 2001; 14: 186–194.

Laurent S, Katsahian S, Fassot C, et al. Aortic stiffness is an independent predictor of fatal stroke in essential hypertension. *Stroke* 2003;34:1203–1206.

Law M, Morris J, Jordan R, Wald N. High blood pressure and headaches; results from a meta-analysis of 97 randomised placebo controlled trials with 24000 participants. *Circulation* 2005: (in press).

Lawes CMM, Bennett DA, Feigin VL, Rodgers A. Blood pressure and stroke: an overview of published reviews. *Stroke* 2004;35:776–785.

Leoncini G, Viazzi F, Parodi D, et al. Creatinine clearance and signs of end-organ damage in primary hypertension. *J Hum Hypertens* 2004;18:511–516.

Levy D, Larson MG, Vasan RS, et al. The progression from hypertension to congestive heart failure. *JAMA* 1996; 275:1557–1562.

Lindsay J Jr. Aortic dissection. *Heart Dis Stroke* 1992;Mar-Apr:69–76.

Lipsitz LA, Storch HA, Minaker KL, Rowe JW. Intraindividual variability in postural BP in the elderly. *Clin Sci* 1985;69:337–341.

Liu K, Ruth KJ, Flack JM, et al. Blood pressure in young blacks and whites: relevance of obesity and lifestyle factors in determining differences. *Circulation* 1996;93: 60–66.

Lloyd-Jones DM, Evand JC, Levy D. Epidemiology of hypertension in the old old: data from the community in the 1990s [Abstract]. *Am J Hypertens* 2004;17:200A.

Lloyd-Jones DM, Larson MG, Leip EP, et al. Lifetime risk for developing congestive heart failure: The Framingham Heart Study. *Circulation* 2002;106:3068–3072.

Lloyd-Jones DM, Wilson PWF, Larson MG, et al. Lifetime risk of coronary heart disease by cholesterol levels at selected ages. *Arch Intern Med* 2003;163:1966–1972.

Lorell BH, Carabello BA. Left ventricular hypertrophy. *Circulation* 2000;102:470–479.

Lorenzo C, Serrano-Rios M, Martinez-Larrad MT, et al. Prevalence of hypertension in Hispanic and non-Hispanic white populations. *Hypertension* 2002;39:203–208.

Lorenzo C, Williams K, Gonzalez-Villalpando C, et al. Lower hypertension risk in Mexico City than in San Antonio. *Am J Hypertens* 2005;18:385–391.

Makin A, Lip GYH, Silverman S, Beevers DG. Peripheral vascular disease and hypertension: a forgotten association? *J Human Hypertens* 2001;15:447–454.

Malik S, Wong ND, Franklin SS, et al. Impact of the metabolic syndrome on mortality from coronary heart disease, cardiovascular disease, and all causes in United States adults. *Circulation* 2004;110:1245–1250.

Management Committee. The Australian therapeutic trial in mild hypertension. *Lancet* 1980;1:1261–1267.

Management Committee. Treatment of mild hypertension in the elderly. *Med J Aus* 1981;2:398–402.

Management Committee. Untreated mild hypertension. *Lancet* 1982;1:185–191.

Marcantoni C, Ma L-J, Federspiel C, Fogo AB. Hypertensive nephrosclerosis in African Americans versus Caucasians. *Kidney Int* 2002;62:172–180.

Mason PJ, Manson JE, Sesso HD, et al. Blood pressure and risk of secondary cardiovascular events in women: The Women's Antioxidant Cardiovascular Study (WACS). *Circulation* 2004;109:1623–1629.

Matthews CE, Pate RR, Jackson KL, et al. Exaggerated blood pressure response to dynamic exercise and risk of future hypertension. *J Clin Epidemiol* 1998;51: 29–35.

Maxwell MH. Cooperative study of renovascular hypertension: current status. *Kidney Int Suppl* 1975;8:153–160.

Medical Research Council Working Party. Medical Research Council trial of treatment of mild hypertension. *BMJ* 1985;291:97–104.

Mena-Martin FJ, Martin-Escudero JC, Simal-Blanco F, et al. Health-related quality of life of subjects with known and unknown hypertension: results from the population-based Hortega study. *J Hypertens* 2003;21:1283–1289.

Mensah GA, Mokdad AH, Ford ES, et al. State of disparities in cardiovascular health in the United States. *Circulation* 2005;111:1233–1241.

Milani RV, Lavie CJ, Mehra MR, et al. Impact of changes in left ventricular geometry over time on all-cause mortality [Abstract]. *Clin Sci* 2004;110 (Suppl 3):III-679.

Miura K, Daviglus ML, Dyer AR, et al. Relationship of blood pressure to 25-year mortality due to coronary heart disease, cardiovascular diseases, and all causes in young adult men. *Arch Intern Med* 2001;161:1501–1508.

Mokdad AH, Marks JS, Stroup DF, Gerberding JL. Actual causes of death in the United States, 2000. *JAMA* 2004;291: 1238–1245.

Mooradian AD. Cardiovascular disease in type 2 diabetes mellitus: current management guidelines. *Arch Intern Med* 2003;163:33–40.

Morfis L, Schwartz RS, Poulos R, Howes LG. Blood pressure changes in acute cerebral infarction and hemorrhage. *Stroke* 1997;28:1401–1405.

Morris RC Jr, Sebastian A, Forman A, et al. Normotensive salt sensitivity. *Hypertension* 1999;33:18–23.

Mourad JJ, Hanon O, Girerd X, et al. Effect of hypertension on cardiac mass and radial artery wall thickness. *Am J Cardiol* 2000;86:564–567.

MRC Asymptomatic Carotid Surgery Trial (ACST) Collaborative Group. Prevention of disabling and fatal strokes by successful carotid endarterectomy in patients without recent neurological symptoms: randomised controlled trial. *Lancet* 2004;363:1491–1502.

Mulè G, Nardi E, Andronico G, et al. Pulsatile and steady 24-h blood pressure components as determinants of left ventricular mass in young and middle-aged essential hypertensives. *J Human Hypertens* 2003;17:231–238.

Murabito JM, Evans JC, Lawson MG, et al. the ankle-brachial index in the elderly and risk of stroke, coronary disease, and death: The Framingham Study. *Arch Intern Med* 2003;163:1939–1942.

Murabito JM, Nam B-H, D'Agostino RB Sr, et al. Accuracy of offspring reports of parental cardiovascular disease history: The Framingham Offspring Study. *Ann Intern Med* 2004;140:434–440.

Narayan KMV, Boyle JP, Thompson TJ, et al. Lifetime risk for diabetes mellitus in the United States. *JAMA* 2003;290:1884–1890.

Neaton JD, Wentworth D. Serum cholesterol, blood pressure, cigarette smoking, and death from coronary heart disease: overall findings and differences by age for 316,099 white men. *Arch Intern Med* 1992;152:56–64.

Nienaber CA, Eagle KA. Aortic dissection: new frontiers in diagnosis and management. *Circulation* 2003;108:628–635, 772–778.

Njølstad I, Arnesen E. Preinfarction blood pressure and smoking are determinants for a fatal outcome of myocardial infarction. *Arch Intern Med* 1998;158:1326–1332.

Nürnberger J, Keflioglu-Scheiber A, Opazo Saez AM, et al. Augmentation index is associated with cardiovascular risk. *J Hypertens* 2002;20:2407–2414.

Obialo CI, Hewan-Lowe K, Fulong B. Nephrotic proteinuria as a result of essential hypertension. *Kidney Blood Press Res* 2002;25:250–254.

Obisesan TO, Vargas CM, Gillum RF. Geographic variation in stroke risk in the United States. *Stroke* 2000;31:19–25.

Oikarinen L, Nieminen MS, Viitasalo M, et al. QRS duration and QT interval predict mortality in hypertensive patients with left ventricular hypertrophy: The Losartan Intervention for Endpoint Reduction in Hypertension Study. *Hypertension* 2004;43:1029–1034.

Okin PM, Devereux RB, Jern S, et al. Regression of electrocardiographic left ventricular hypertrophy during antihypertensive treatment and the prediction of major cardiovascular events. *JAMA* 2004;292:2343–2349.

Olsen MH, Wachtell K, Bella JN, et al. Aortic valve sclerosis relates to cardiovascular events in patients with hypertension (A LIFE substudy). *Am J Cardiol* 2005;95:132–136.

O'Meara JG, Kardia SLR, Armon JJ, et al. Ethnic and sex differences in the prevalence, treatment, and control of dyslipidemia among hypertensive adults in the GENOA study. *Arch Intern Med* 2004;164:1313–1318.

O'Rourke MF, Safar ME. Relationship between aortic stiffening and microvascular disease in brain and kidney. *Hypertension* 2005;46. Available online at: http://www.hypertensionaha.org. Accessed May 23, 2005.

Pache M, Kube T, Wolf S, Kutschbach P. Do angiographic data support a detailed classification of hypertensive fundus changes? *J Human Hypertens* 2002;6:405–410.

Palacios C, Wigertz K, Martin BR, et al. Sodium retention in black and white female adolescents in response to salt intake. *J Clin Endocrin Metab* 2004;89:1858–1863.

Palatini P, Mormino P, Mos L, et al. Microalbuminuria, renal function and development of sustained hypertension: a longitudinal study in the early stage of hypertension. *J Hypertens* 2005;23:175–182.

Palombo C, Kozàkovà M, Magagna A, et al. Early impairment of coronary flow reserve and increase in minimum coronary resistance in borderline hypertensive patients. *J Hypertens* 2000;18:453–459.

Paran E, Galily Y, Abu-Rabia Y, Neuman L, Keynan A. Environmental and genetic factors of hypertension in a biracial Beduin population. *J Hum Hypertens* 1992;6:107–112.

Park Y-W, Zhu S, Palaniappan L, et al. The metabolic syndrome: prevalence and associated risk factor findings in the US population from the Third National Health and Nutrition Examination Survey, 1988–1994. *Arch Intern Med* 2003;163:427–436.

Parrinello G, Columba D, Bologna P, et al. Early carotid atherosclerosis and cardiac diastolic abnormalities in hypertensive subjects. *J Human Hypertens* 2004;18:201–205.

Perera GA. Hypertensive vascular disease. *J Chron Dis* 1955;1:33–42.

Pierini A, Bertinieri G, Pagnozzi G, et al. Effects of systemic hypertension on arterial dynamics and left ventricular compliance in patients 70 years of age. *Am J Cardiol* 2000;86:882–886.

Pocock SJ, McCormack V, Gueyffier F, et al. A score for predicting risk of death from cardiovascular disease in adults with raised blood pressure, based on individual patient data from randomized controlled trials. *BMJ* 2001;323:75–81.

Pratt JH, Ambrosius WT, Agarwal R, et al. Racial differences in the activity of amiloride-sensitive epithelial sodium channel. *Hypertension* 2002;40:903–908.

Price DA, Fisher NDL, Lansang MC, et al. Renal perfusion in blacks: alterations caused by insuppressibility of intrarenal renin with salt. *Hypertension* 2002;40:186–189.

Prinssen M, Verhoeven ELG, Buth J, et al. A randomized trial comparing conventional and endovascular repair of abdominal aortic aneurysms. *N Engl J Med* 2004;351:1607–1618.

Prospective Studies Collaboration. Age-specific relevance of usual blood pressure to vascular mortality: a meta-analysis of individual data for one million adults in 61 prospective studies. *Lancet* 2002;360:1903–1913.

Puisieux F, Bulckaen H, Fauchais AL, et al. Ambulatory blood pressure monitoring and postprandial hypotension in elderly persons with falls or syncopes. *J Gerontol* 2000;55A:M535-M540.

Qiu C, von Strauss E, Winblad B, Fratiglioni L. Decline in blood pressure over time and risk of dementia: a longitudinal study from the Kungsholmen project. *Stroke* 2004;35:1810–1815.

Qiu C, Winblad B, Viitanen M, Fratiglioni L. Pulse pressure and risk of Alzheimer disease in persons aged 75 years or older: a community-based, longitudinal study. *Stroke* 2003;34:594–599.

Querejeta R, Lopez B, Gonzalez A, et al. Increased collagen type I synthesis in patients with heart failure of hypertensive origin: relation to myocardial fibrosis. *Circulation* 2004;110:1263–1268.

Qureshi AI, Suri FK, Mohammad Y, et al. Isolated and borderline isolated systolic hypertension relative to long-term risk and type of stroke: a 20-year follow-up of the National Health and Nutrition Survey. *Stroke* 2002;33:2781–2788.

Räihä I, Luutonen S, Piha J, et al. Prevalence, predisposing factors, and prognostic importance of postural hypotension. *Arch Intern Med* 1995;155:930–935.

Ridker PM, Cannon CP, Morrow D, et al. C-reactive protein levels and outcomes after statin therapy. *N Engl J Med* 2005;352:20–28.

Rodin MB, Daviglus ML, Wong GC, et al. Middle age cardiovascular risk factors and abdominal aortic aneurysm in older age. *Hypertension* 2003;42:61–68.

Roger VL, Weston SA, Redfield MM, et al. Trends in heart failure incidence and survival in a community-based population. *JAMA* 2004;292:344–350.

Ronnback M, Fagerudd J, Forsblom C, et al. Altered age-related blood pressure pattern in type 1 diabetes. *Circulation* 2004;110:1076–1082.

Ross R. Atherosclerosis—An inflammatory disease. *N Engl J Med* 1999;340:115–126.

Rothwell PM, Coull AJ, Giles MF, et al. Change in stroke incidence, mortality, case-fatality, severity, and risk factors in Oxfordshire, UK from 1981 to 2004 (Oxford Vascular Study). *Lancet* 2004;363:1925–1933.

Rule AD, Larson TS, Bergstralh EJ, et al. Using serum creatinine to estimate glomerular filtration rate: accuracy in good health and in chronic kidney disease. *Ann Intern Med* 2004;141:929–937.

Rutter MK, Meigs JB, Sullivan LM, et al. C-reactive protein, the metabolic syndrome, and prediction of cardiovascular events in the Framingham Offspring Study. *Circulation* 2004;110:380–385.

Safar ME. Systolic hypertension in the elderly: arterial wall mechanical properties and the renin-angiotensin-aldosterone system. *J Hypertens* 2005;23:673–681.

Safar ME, Benetos A. Factors influencing arterial stiffness in systolic hypertension in the elderly: role of sodium and the renin-angiotensin system. *Am J Hypertens* 2003;16:249–258.

Safar ME, Smulyan H. Hypertension in women. *Am J Hypertens* 2004;17:82–87.

Salmasi A-M, Alimo A, Dancy M. Prevalence of unrecognized abnormal glucose tolerance in patients attending a hospital hypertension clinic. *Am J Hypertens* 2004;17:483–488.

Sarti C, Rastenyte D, Cepaitis Z, Tuomilehto J. International trends in mortality from stroke, 1968 to 1994. *Stroke* 2000;31:1588–1601.

Scherrer JF, Xian H, Bucholz KK, et al. A twin study of depression symptoms, hypertension, and heart disease in middle-aged men. *Psychosom Med* 2003;65:548–557.

Schieppati A, Remuzzi G. The future of renoprotection: frustration and promises. *Kidney Int* 2003;64:1947–1955.

Schillaci G, de Simone G, Reboldi G, et al. Change in cardiovascular risk profile by echocardiography in low- or medium-risk hypertension. *J Hypertens* 2002a;20:1519–1525.

Schillaci G, Vaudo G, Pasqualini L, et al. Left ventricular mass and systolic dysfunction in essential hypertension. *J Human Hypertens* 2002b;16:117–122.

Schlaich MP, Kaye DM, Lambert E, et al. Relation between cardiac sympathetic activity and hypertensive left ventricular hypertrophy. *Circulation* 2003;108:560–565.

Schmieder RE, Messerli FH. Hypertension and the heart. *J Hum Hypertens* 2000;14:597–604.

Segura J, Ruilope LM, Zanchetti A. On the importance of estimating renal function for cardiovascular risk assessment. *J Hypertens* 2004;22:1635–1639.

Selvin E, Erlinger TP. Prevalence of and risk factors for peripheral arterial disease in the United States: results from the National Health and Nutrition Examination Survey, 1999–2000. *Circulation* 2004;110:738–743.

Sever PS, Dahlöf B, Poulter NR, et al. Prevention of coronary and stroke events with atorvastatin in hypertensive patients who have average or lower-than-average cholesterol concentrations, in the Anglo-Scandinavian Cardiac Outcomes Trial—Lipid Lowering Arm (ASCOT-LLA): a multicentre randomised controlled trial. *Lancet* 2003;361:1149–1158.

SHEP Cooperative Research Group. Prevention of stroke by antihypertensive drug treatment in older persons with isolated systolic hypertension. *JAMA* 1991;265:3255–3264.

Shinn EH, Poston WSC, Kimball KT, et al. Blood pressure and symptoms of depression and anxiety: a prospective study. *Am J Hypertens* 2001;14:660–664.

Shlipak MG, Sarnak MJ, Katz R, et al. Cystatin c and the risk of death and cardiovascular events among elderly persons. *N Engl J Med* 2005;352:2049–2060.

Simon G, Nordgren D, Connelly S, Shultz PJ. Screening for abdominal aortic aneurysms in a hypertensive patient population. *Arch Intern Med* 1996;156:2081–2084.

Smith DE, Odel HM, Kernohan JW. Causes of death in hypertension. *Am J Med* 1950;9:516–527.

Smith WM. Treatment of mild hypertension. *Circ Res* 1977;40(Suppl 1):98–105.

Smoller JW, Pollack MH, Wassertheil-Smoller S, et al. Prevalence and correlates of panic attacks in postmenopausal women: results from an ancillary study to the Women's Health Initiative. *Arch Intern Med* 2003;163:2041–2050.

Song CK, Martinez JA, Kailasam MT, et al. Renal kallikrein excretion: role of ethnicity, gender, environment, and genetic risk of hypertension. *J Hum Hypertens* 2000;14:461–468.

Spence JD. Pseudo-hypertension in the elderly. *J Hum Hypertens* 1997;11:621–623.

Staessen JA, Fagard R, Thijs L, et al. Randomized double-blind comparison of placebo and active treatment for older patients with isolated systolic hypertension. *Lancet* 1997;350:757–764.

Staessen JA, Gasowski J, Wang JG, et al. Risks of untreated and treated isolated systolic hypertension in the elderly. *Lancet* 2000;355:865–872.

Starr JM, Inch S, Cross S, et al. Blood pressure and ageing. *BMJ* 1998;317:513–514.

Stevens LA, Levey AS. Clinical implications of estimating equations for glomerular filtration rate. *Ann Intern Med* 2004;141:959–961.

Stewart IMcDG. Headache and hypertension. *Lancet* 1953;1:1261–1266.

Strate M, Thygesen K, Ringsted C, et al. Prognosis in treated hypertension. *Acta Med Scand* 1986;219:153–159.

Stratton IM, Kohner EM, Aldington SJ, et al. Risk factors for incidence and progression of retinopathy in type II diabetes over 6 years from diagnosis. UKPDS 50. *Diabetologia* 2001;44:156–163.

Suthanthiran M, Li B, Song JO, et al. Transforming growth factor-$\beta_1$ hyperexpression in African-American hypertensives. *Proc Natl Acad Sci U S A* 2000;97:3479–3484.

Svetkey, LP. Management of Prehypertension. *Hypertension* 2005;45:1056–1061.

Swedko PJ, Clark HD, Paramsothy K, Akbari A. Serum creatinine is an inadequate screening test for renal failure in elderly patients. *Arch Intern Med* 2003;163:356–360.

Tedesco MA, Natale F, Di Salvo G, et al. Effects of coexisting hypertension and type II diabetes mellitus on arterial stiffness. *J Human Hypertens* 2004;18:469–473.

Thompson D, Edelsberg J, Colditz GA, et al. Lifetime health and economic consequences of obesity. *Arch Intern Med* 1999;159:2177–2183.

Toto RB. Hypertensive nephrosclerosis in African Americans. *Kidney Int* 2003;64:2331–2341.

Toto RD. Microalbuminuria: definition, detection, and clinical signficance. *J Clin Hypertens* 2004;6(Suppl 3):2–7.

Tsioufis C, Dimitriadis K, Antoniadis D, et al. Inter-relationships of microalbuminuria with the other surrogates of the atherosclerotic cardiovascular disease in hypertensive subjects. *Am J Hypertens* 2004;17:470–476.

Tuomilehto J, Linström J, Eriksson JG, et al. Prevention of type 2 diabetes mellitus by changes in lifestyle among subjects with impaired glucose tolerance. *N Engl J Med* 2001;344:1343–1350.

US Preventive Services Task Force. Screening for coronary heart disease: recommendation statement. *Ann Intern Med* 2004;140:569–572.

Vakili BA, Okin PM, Devereux RB. Prognostic implications of left ventricular hypertrophy. *Am Heart J* 2001;141:334-341.

Van De Water JM, Miller TW, Vogel RL, et al. Impedance cardiography: the next vital sign technology? *Chest* 2003;123:2028–2033.

Van der Vliet JA, Boll APM. Abdominal aortic aneurysm. *Lancet* 1997;349:863–866.

van Dijk EJ, Breteler MMB, Schmidt R, et al. The association between blood pressure, hypertension, and cerebral white matter lesions: Cardiovascular Determinants of Dementia study. *Hypertension* 2004;44:625–630.

Vasan RS, Benjamin EJ. Diastolic heart failure. *N Engl J Med* 2001;344:56–59.

Vasan RS, Beiser A, Seshadri S, et al. Residual lifetime risk for developing hypertension in middle-aged women and men: The Framingham Heart Study. *JAMA* 2002;287:1003–1010.

Vasan RS, Evans JC, Benjamin EJ, et al. Relations of serum aldosterone to cardiac structure: gender-related differences in the Framingham Heart Study. *Hypertension* 2004;43:957–962.

Vasan RS, Larson MG, Leip EP, et al. Impact of high-normal blood pressure on the risk of cardiovascular disease. *N Engl J Med* 2001a;345:1291–1297.

Vasan RS, Larson MG, Leip EP, et al. Assessment of frequency of progression of hypertension in non-hypertensive participants in the Framingham Heart Study: a cohort study. *Lancet* 2001b;358:1682–1686.

Vemmos KN, Spengos K, Tsivgoulis G, et al. Factors influencing acute blood pressure values in stroke subtypes. *J Human Hypertens* 2004;18:253–259.

Ventura HO, Taler SJ, Strobeck JE. Hypertension as a hemodynamic disease: the role of impedance cardiography in diagnostic, prognostic, and therapeutic decision making. *Am J Hypertens* 2005;18:26S–43S.

Verdecchia P, Angeli F, Gattobigio R, et al. Asymptomatic left ventricular systolic dysfunction in essential hypertension: prevalence, determinants and prognostic value. *Hypertension* 2005;45:412–418.

Verdecchia P, Angeli F, Reboldi G, et al. Improved cardiovascular risk stratification by a simple ECG index in hypertension. *Am J Hypertens* 2003a;16:646–652.

Verdecchia P, Reboldi GP, Gattobigio R, et al. Atrial fibrillation in hypertension: predictors and outcome. *Hypertension* 2003b;41:218–223.

Vermeer SE, Koudstaal PJ, Oudkerk M, et al. Prevalence and risk factors of silent brain infarcts in the population-based Rotterdam Scan Study. *Stroke* 2002;33:21–25.

Veterans Administration Cooperative Study Group on Antihypertensive Agents. Effects of treatment on morbidity in hypertension. *JAMA* 1967;202:116–122.

Veterans Administration Cooperative Study Group on Antihypertensive Agents. Effects of treatment on morbidity in hypertension. *JAMA* 1970;213:1143–1152.

Veterans Administration Cooperative Study Group on Antihypertensive Agents. Effects of treatment on morbidity in hypertension. III. Influence of age, diastolic pressure, and prior cardiovascular disease. *Circulation* 1972;45:991–1004.

von Birgelen C, Hartmann M, Mintz G, et al. Relationship between cardiovascular risk as predicted by established risk scores versus plaque progression as measured by serial intravascular ultrasound in left main coronary arteries. *Circulation* 2004;110:1579–1585.

Vos LE, Oren A, Uiterwaal C, et al. Adolescent blood pressure and blood pressure tracking into young adulthood are related to sublinical atherosclerosis: The Atherosclerosis Risk in Young Adults (ARYA) study. *Am J Hypertens* 2003;16:549–555.

Wachtell K, Rokkedal J, Bella JN, et al. Effect of electrocardiographic left ventricular hypertrophy on left ventricular systolic function in systemic hypertension. *Am J Cardiol* 2001;87:54–60.

Waddell TK, Dart AM, Gatzka CD, et al. Women exhibit a greater age-related increase in proximal aortic stiffness than men. *J Hypertens* 2001;19:2205–2212.

Waldstein SR, Giggey PP, Thayer JF, Zonderman AB. Non-linear relations of blood pressure to cognitive function: The Baltimore Longitudinal Study of Aging. *Hypertension* 2005;45:374–379.

Wallis EJ, Ramsay LE, Haq IU, et al. Coronary and cardiovascular risk estimation for primary prevention: validation of a new Sheffield table in the 1995 Scottish Health Survey population. *Br Med J* 2000;320:671–676.

Wang TJ, Levy D, Benjamin EJ, Vasan RS. The epidemiology of "asymptomatic" left ventricular systolic dysfunction: implications for screening. *Ann Intern Med* 2003; 138:907–916.

Warlow C, Sudlow C, Dennis M, et al. Stroke. *Lancet* 2003; 362:1211–1224.

Weaver FA, Kumar SR, Yellin AE, et al. Renal revascularization in Takayasu arteritis-induced renal artery stenosis. *J Vasc Surg* 2004;39:749–757.

Weiss A, Grossman E, Beloosesky Y, Grinblat J. Orthostatic hypotension in acute geriatric ward: is it a consistent finding? *Arch Intern Med* 2002;162:2369–2374.

Weiss JP, Blaivas JG. Nocturia. *J Urol* 2000;163:5–12.

Weiss NS. Relation of high blood pressure to headache, epistaxis, and selected other symptoms. *N Eng J Med* 1972;287:631–633.

Whelton PK, He J, Appel LJ, et al. Primary prevention of hypertension: clinical and public health advisory from the National High Blood Pressure Education Program. *JAMA* 2002;288:1882–1888.

Wilhelm FH, Gerlach AL, Roth WT. Slow recovery from voluntary hyperventilation in panic disorder. *Psychosom Med* 2001;63:638–649.

Williams B, Poulter NR, Brown MJ, et al. Guidelines for management of hypertension: report of the fourth working party of the British Hypertension Society, 2004—BHS IV. *J Human Hypertens* 2004;18:139–185.

Wilson PWF, Grundy SM. The metabolic syndrome: practical guide to origins and treatment: part I. *Circulation* 2003;108:1422–1425.

Wong TY, Mitchell P. Hypertensive retinopathy. *N Engl J Med* 2004;351:2310–2317.

Wong TY, Klein R, Sharrett AR, et al. Retinal arteriolar diameter and risk for hypertension. *Ann Intern Med* 2004;140:248–255.

Wong TY, Rosamond W, Chang PP, et al. Retinopathy and risk of congestive heart failure. *JAMA* 2005;293:63–69.

Woo D, Gebel J, Miller R, et al. Incidence rates of first-ever ischemic stroke subtypes among blacks. *Stroke* 1999; 30:2517–2522.

Yliharsila H, Eriksson J, Forsen T, et al. Self-perpetuating effects of birth size on blood pressure levels in elderly people. *Hypertension* 2003;41:446–450.

Young JH, Klag MJ, Muntner P, et al. Blood pressure and decline in kidney function: findings from the Systolic Hypertension in the Elderly Program (SHEP). *J Am Soc Nephrol* 2002;13:2776–2782.

Young-Xu Y, Ravid S. Optimal blood pressure control for the prevention of atrial fibrillation [Abstract]. *Circulation* 2004;110(Suppl 3):III-768.

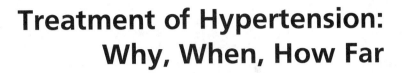

# Treatment of Hypertension: Why, When, How Far

In the preceding four chapters, the epidemiology, natural history, and pathophysiology of primary (essential) hypertension were reviewed. We will now turn to its treatment, examining the benefits and costs of therapy in this chapter and the use of nondrug and drug treatment in the two chapters that follow.

In this chapter, three main questions are addressed:

- First, what is the evidence that treatment is beneficial?
- Second, at what level of blood pressure (BP) should active drug therapy be started? Lifestyle modifications, which will be examined in the next chapter, can be justified for everyone, hypertensive or not.
- Third, what is the goal of therapy, and, further, are there different goals for different patients?

In order to answer these questions, in this chapter only data comparing active drug therapy against untreated or placebo-treated patients will be considered. In Chapter 7, data comparing one or another form of therapy will be examined.

## EVIDENCE FOR BENEFITS OF THERAPY

The evidence for benefits of therapy comes in part from epidemiologic and experimental evidence but mainly from the results of large-scale therapeutic trials.

### Epidemiologic Evidence

Epidemiologic evidence, covered in Chapter 1, provides a clear conclusion: The risks of cardiovascular morbidity and mortality rise progressively with increasing BP levels (Prospective Studies Collaboration, 2002).

### Interrupting the Progress of Hypertension

The 15- to 17-year longitudinal study of Welshmen by Miall and Chinn (1973) and the 24-year follow-up of American aviators by Oberman et al. (1967) showed that hypertension begets further hypertension. In both studies, the higher the BP, the greater was the rate of change of pressure, pointing to an obvious conclusion: Progressive rises in BP can be prevented by keeping the pressure down. This conclusion is further supported by the results of the major placebo-controlled trials of antihypertensive therapy: Whereas 10% to 17% of those on placebo progressed beyond the threshold of diastolic pressure above 110 mm Hg, only a small handful of those on drug treatment did so (see Chapter 4, Tables 4–3 and 4–4).

### Evidence from Natural Experiments in Humans

Vascular damage and the level of BP have been closely correlated in three situations: unilateral renal vascular disease, coarctation, and pulmonary hypertension. These three experiments of nature provide evidence that what is important is the level of the BP flowing through a vascular bed and not some other deleterious effect associated with systemic hypertension. Tissues with lower BP are protected; those with higher pressure are damaged.

- The kidney with renal artery stenosis is exposed to a lower pressure than is the contralateral kidney without stenosis. Arteriolar nephrosclerosis develops in the high-pressure nonstenotic kidney, occasionally to such a degree that hypertension can be relieved only by removal of the nonstenotic kidney, along with repair of the stenosis (Thal et al., 1963).
- The vessels exposed to the high pressure above the coarctation develop atherosclerosis to a much greater degree than do the vessels below the coarctation, where the pressure is low (Hollander et al., 1976).
- The low pressure within the pulmonary artery ordinarily protects these vessels from damage. When patients develop pulmonary hypertension secondary to mitral stenosis or certain types of congenital heart disease, both arteriosclerosis and arteriolar necrosis often develop within the pulmonary vessels (Heath & Edwards, 1958).

### Evidence from Animal Experiments

Just as hypertension accelerates and worsens atherosclerosis in humans, animals that are made hypertensive develop more atherosclerosis than do normotensive animals fed the same high-cholesterol diet (Chobanian, 1990). In animals, the lesions caused by hypertension, including accelerated atherosclerosis, can be prevented by lowering the pressure with antihypertensive agents (Chobanian et al., 1992).

### Evidence from Clinical Trials of Antihypertensive Therapy

The last piece of evidence—that there is benefit from lowering an elevated BP—is the most important. Over the past five decades, since oral antihypertensive therapy has become available, protection with antihypertensive therapy has been demonstrated at progressively lower levels of pressure and, more recently, even in the elderly. In multiple meta-analyses of all properly controlled trials (Blood Pressure Trialists, 2003; Psaty et al., 2003; Staessen et al., 2003), the conclusion reached earlier by Staessen et al. (2001) remains valid:

> . . . results of outcome trials for antihypertensive drugs can be explained by blood pressure differences between randomised groups. All antihypertensive drugs had similar long-term efficacy and safety. Our results show the desirability of lowering blood pressure as much as possible to achieve the greatest reduction in cardiovascular complications.

As will be noted, this wide umbrella covers disparate groups of patients who may differ in their responses to different drugs (Wong et al., 2003). However, the overall message is clear: The lower the blood pressure, the greater the protection.

### Problems in Applying Trial Results to Clinical Practice

Before examining the results of the multiple randomized, controlled trials (RCTs) and their meta-analyses that have been used to inform the guidelines for clinical practice, a few cautionary comments seem to be in order. Practitioners must be aware of the features, both good and bad, of both the performance and the presentation of clinical trials since they are the foundation of *evidence-based medicine,* the decision to use a therapy based on systematic analyses (usually meta-analyses) of unbiased scientific evidence. Though some object to the prior rigidity of evidence-based medicine (Swales, 1999), the concept has evolved to "emphasize the limitations of using evidence alone to make decisions, and the importance of the values and preference judgments that are implicit in every clinical management decision" (Guyatt et al., 2004).

The need for evidence-based medicine to improve upon the intuitive-based practice of the past has been nicely described by Califf and DeMets (2002):

> A practitioner's individual experience is simply not adequate to recognize treatment effects of the size usually seen in therapies to prevent future events in a chronic disease. . . . Although monitoring each individual patient closely for symptomatic and physiological improvements is critical in any clinical practice, it is not the best way to determine whether proposed treatments are effective (with the exception of suitable situations for the $n = 1$ trial), especially when the treatment is primarily given to alter the long-term course of a chronic disease. Furthermore, the experience with the last patient says little about what to expect in the next patient; rather, to detect modest treatment effects, large randomized trials are needed.

#### Problems with Trials

As noted, RCTs are required to assess reliably the modest effects of antihypertensive treatment on the major outcomes that are expected in typical hypertensive patients over the relatively short time, 3 to 5 years, wherein close observation remains possible (Collins & MacMahon, 2001). Vandenbroucke (2004) concluded that RCTs are needed because "observational studies about therapy will be credible only in exceptional circumstances."

As essential as they are, RCTs may be misleading, partly by their nature, partly because of human foibles (Rothwell, 2005). In particular, drug marketers' increasing financial sponsorship of clinical trials, although often essential for their performance (Bonaccorso & Smith, 2003), has been associated with selection of an inappropriate comparator (Carlberg et al., 2004), poorer quality of methods (Lexchin et al., 2003), selective reporting of outcomes (Chan et al., 2004), and more positive conclusions than seen in trials funded by nonprofit sources (Als-Nielsen et al., 2003).

Beyond these often subtle and unrecognized biases toward the financial sponsor, a number of other factors may either, on the one hand, exaggerate or, on the other, diminish the apparent benefits of therapy.

### Possible Underestimations of Benefit

Results of trials may underestimate the true benefits of antihypertensive therapy for a number of reasons, including the following.

#### Mislabeling of Patients

The ascertainment of hypertension for enrollment into trials is usually based on two or three sets of office-based BP measurements over 1 to 2 months. As amply noted in Chapter 2, such limited measurements are likely to capture a large number of transient or isolated clinic (white-coat) hypertensives, thereby diminishing the efficacy of therapy. All antihypertensive drugs lower BP more in relation to a higher starting BP, and most lower BP very little in the absence of persistent hypertension.

#### Intervention Too Late

Hypertension may produce damages well before patients have sufficiently high BP to be eligible for enrollment. Even if effectively treated, these damages may be irreversible, particularly if other risk factors are not also corrected.

#### Too Short Duration of Treatment

The duration of the trials is usually less than 5 years. However, the benefit of drugs may take much longer to become fully manifest, thereby minimizing the drugs' apparent efficacy.

#### Inadequate Therapy

The approximately 12/6 mm Hg overall decreases in BP accomplished in most clinical trials are likely too little to reduce the damages of hypertension maximally. The degree of damage clearly relates to the level of BP achieved during therapy and not to the pretreatment level (Adler et al., 2000). Because as many as 40% of patients in some trials did not reach the goal BP (Mancia & Grassi, 2002), the benefits may then be less than what could have been obtained by more intensive therapy.

#### Patients Lost to Follow-Up

In some trials, as many as 25% of patients are lost to follow-up before completion. In general, more high-risk patients are lost, weakening the evidence for benefit (Linjer & Hansson, 1997).

#### Switching of Patients

In all trials, a sizable number of patients initially randomized to placebo were switched to active therapy because their BP rose beyond the predetermined ceiling of presumed safety. As noted by Ramsay et al. (1996), "Treatment of these high-risk patients in the control groups will inevitably have reduced the cardiovascular disease event rates and led to underestimates of the absolute benefit."

#### Harm from Drugs

The drugs available and chosen for almost all the earlier trials in subjects younger than 60 years old were high doses of diuretics and adrenergic inhibitors, mostly nonselective β-blockers. As is noted in Chapter 7, multiple metabolic abnormalities, which particularly aggravate lipid and glucose-insulin levels, have been documented with these therapies. These drug-induced abnormalities, both from high doses of diuretics and β-blockers, may have blunted or reversed the improvement in coronary risk provided by reduction of the BP.

#### Noncompliance with Therapy

Patients assigned to active drug therapy may not have taken all of their medication and thereby would have had less benefit. Although pill counts are usually performed, no truly accurate assessment of compliance is available.

### Possible Overestimates of Benefit

On the other hand, antihypertensive therapy may be less effective than is seen in controlled trials because of poor external validity for application of the results to routine clinical practice (Rothwell, 2005). Data from clinical trials may overestimate the benefits of therapy as they are applied to the universe of hypertensives for the following reasons.

#### Inclusion of Inappropriate End Points

To maximize the impact of a therapy, multiple end points may be examined, some of questionable significance such as hospitalizations that occur at the subjective discretion of the investigator. Lauer and Topol (2003) argue that only all-cause mortality should be the primary end point since it is objective, unbiased, and clinically relevant. As they note: "Any end point that requires a measurement involving human judgment is inherently subject to bias."

#### Exclusion of High-Risk Patients

In many early RCTs, patients with various symptomatic cardiovascular diseases, target organ damage, or major risk factors were excluded, leaving a fairly healthy population who may respond better than the usual mix of patients.

### Better Compliance with Therapy

Patients enrolled in trials in which medications and all health care are free and follow-up is carefully monitored are more likely than patients in clinical practice to be compliant with therapy. Therefore, patients enrolled in trials may achieve greater benefit.

### Relative Versus Absolute Changes

In most reports of RCTs, the reductions in coronary heart disease (CHD) and stroke are relative—that is, they are the difference between the rates seen in treated versus untreated patients. However, as documented in Table 5–1, large relative differences may translate into small absolute differences. The 40% relative risk reduction by treatment of patients with diastolic ≤110 translates into only a 0.6% absolute risk reduction. The presentation of trial data as large relative reductions in risk is much more attractive than the usually much smaller absolute reductions (Steiner, 1999); however, the relative data may easily mislead the unwary into thinking that many more patients will be helped than is possible (Rothwell et al., 2005).

As shown in the far right column of Table 5–1, the measure *number needed to treat* (NNTs), calculated as the inverse of the absolute risk reduction, is recommended because it "conveys both statistical and clinical significance to the doctor" and "can be used to extrapolate published findings to a patient at an arbitrary specified baseline risk" (Cook & Sackett, 1995).

The need for using absolute risk, or number needed to treat, is well demonstrated in Figure 5–1 (Lever & Ramsay, 1995). Figure 5–1A shows the quite similar reductions in relative risk for stroke in six major trials in the elderly and in the earlier Medical Research Council trial of younger hypertensives. Figure 5–1B shows the same data in absolute terms, clearly portraying the progressively greater benefit of therapy with increasing pretherapy risk, as reflected in the rates in the placebo groups.

The use of NNTs based on absolute risk reduction is clearly more accurate than portrayal of relative risks. The NNT must be related to the duration of the trial. This is best done by using the *hazard difference,* expressed as mortality per unit of patient-time (Lubsen et al., 2000). However, in most recent reports, results are presented as *survival curves,* showing differences in outcomes that change over time, using the Kaplan-Meier lifetable methods for estimating the proportion of patients who experience an event by time since randomization (Pocock et al., 2001). When properly constructed, showing both the number of subjects remaining in the trial over time and a display of statistical uncertainty, such survival curves portray RCT results very well.

### Admixture of Drugs

In order to achieve the preset goal of therapy, e.g., BP below 140/90, most trials comparing a drug versus placebo (as examined in this chapter) or one drug versus another (as examined in Chapter 7) must add additional drugs to the study drug. In some trials, 80% or more of the patients end up

---

## TABLE 5–1

### Calculations of Relative and Absolute Risk Reduction and Numbers Needed to Be Treated for Patients with Hypertension

| Hypertension | Stroke in 5 Years | | Relative Risk Reduction, $(P_c - P_A)/P_c$ | Absolute Risk Reduction, $P_c - P_A$ | Number Needed to Treat, $1/(P_c - P_A)$ |
| --- | --- | --- | --- | --- | --- |
| | Control Group | Active Treatment Group | | | |
| Diastolic ≤115 mm Hg | | | | | |
| Event rate (*P*) | 0.20 | 0.12 | 0.40 | 0.08 | 13 |
| Total number of patients | 16,778 | 16,898 | | | |
| Diastolic ≤110 mm Hg | | | | | |
| Event rate (*P*) | 0.015 | 0.009 | 0.40 | 0.006 | 167 |
| Total number of patients | 15,165 | 15,238 | | | |

Modified from Cook RJ, Sackett DL. The number to treat: a clinically useful measure of treatment and effect. *BMJ* 1995;310:452–454. Based on the results of Collins R, Peto R, MacMahon S, et al. Blood pressure, stroke and coronary heart disease. Part 2: short-term reductions in blood pressure. *Lancet* 1990;335:827–838.

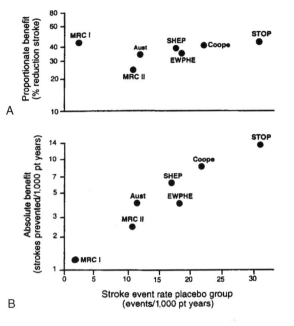

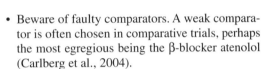

**FIGURE 5–1** ● Comparison of **(A)** proportionate (relative) and **(B)** absolute benefit from reduction in the incidence of stroke in six trials in the elderly and in one other [Medical Research Council I (MRC I)] having a similar design but in which the absolute stroke risk was much lower. Event rates are for fatal and nonfatal stroke combined. Aust, Australian study; EWPHE, European Working Party on High Blood Pressure in the Elderly trial; Coope, Coope and Warrender; SHEP, Systolic Hypertension in the Elderly Program; STOP, Swedish Trial in Old Patients with Hypertension. (Modified from Lever AF, Ramsay LE. Treatment of hypertension in the elderly. *J Hypertens* 1995;13:571–579.)

on two or more drugs. What is ascribed to only the study drug may represent the effect of many others (McAlister et al., 2003).

### Solutions to the Problems of Trials

Obviously those who perform and report RCTs must follow established guidelines such as CONSORT (Rennie, 2001) or those proposed by Rothwell (2005). However, clinicians themselves must be prepared to assess the validity of trial data since in the words of Montori et al. (2004):

> Science is often not objective. Emotional investment in particular ideas and personal interest in academic success may lead investigators to overemphasize the importance of their findings and the quality of their work. Even more serious conflicts arise when for-profit organizations, including pharmaceutical companies, provide funds for research and consulting, conduct data management and analyses, and write reports on behalf of the investigators.

Montori et al. (2004) provide this set of guides for clinicians to avoid being misled by biased presentation and interpretation of trial data:

- Read the Methods and Results sections. Remember that the Discussion section often offers inferences that differ from those a dispassionate reader would draw.
- Read abstracts and comments in objective secondary publications such as the *ACP Journal Club, Evidence-based Medicine, Up-To-Date, the Medical Letter,* etc.

- Beware of faulty comparators. A weak comparator is often chosen in comparative trials, perhaps the most egregious being the β-blocker atenolol (Carlberg et al., 2004).
- Beware of composite end points; as noted previously, all-cause mortality can hardly be fudged.
- Beware of small treatment effects, particularly when the data are reported as differences in relative risks. If the 95% confidence interval (CI) crosses the mid-line, beware.
- Beware of subgroup analyses. A number of provisos should be met to ensure that apparent differences in subgroup responses are real, particularly that only a small number of hypotheses were tested that were specified before the results became available (Freemantle, 2001).

Beyond these pitfalls to avoid in interpreting clinical trials is an increasing need for better and more practical clinical trials that are designed specifically to answer the questions faced by practitioners and their decision makers (Tunis et al., 2003). Most trials today are sponsored by pharmaceutical marketers whose primary interest, appropriately, is to document the superiority of their product. Funding from the National Institutes of Health and other nonprofit institutions is more likely to go for basic and focused clinical research, rather than to support the often very expensive, large clinical trials required to meet the needs of decision makers.

Meanwhile, students and practitioners need to take better advantage of available sources of evidence-based clinical information (Demaerschalk, 2004). The Cochrane Library is now the most prolific provider, but more and more sources are available, many at no cost.

## Problems with Meta-Analyses and Systematic Reviews

Meta-analyses and systematic reviews of multiple well-conducted RCTs are the highest level of evidence used by experts whether formulating practice guidelines, formulary composition, payment schedules, or textbook content (Thompson & Higgins, 2005). Unfortunately, biases may affect them as well. As Sterne et al. (2001) note:

> Studies that show a significant effect of treatment are more likely to be published, be published in English, be cited by other authors, and produce multiple publications than other studies. Such studies are therefore also more likely to be identified and included in systematic reviews, which may introduce bias. Low methodological quality of studies included in a systematic review is another important source of bias.
>
> All these biases are more likely to affect small studies than large ones. The smaller a study the larger the treatment effect necessary for the results to be significant. . . . Bias in a systematic review may therefore become evident through an association between the size of the treatment effect and study size—such associations may be examined both graphically [through funnel plots] and statistically.

Even under the best of conditions, meta-analyses and systematic reviews of RCTs may not be able to provide adequate information about long-term outcomes of such chronic diseases as hypertension since almost all RCTs are of relatively short-term duration.

## Problems with Guidelines

The most authoritative recommendations on how to best manage hypertension are the guidelines issued by national or international expert committees such as the U.S. Joint National Committee (Chobanian et al., 2003a; 2003b) or the World Health Organization/International Society of Hypertension (WHO/ISH Writing Group, 2003).

However, there are problems with current guidelines, including these:

- There are too many guidelines, often differing substantially (Fretheim et al., 2002).
- Guidelines are too long to be used when needed.
- The targets for therapy are too stringent and fail to take patients' beliefs and abilities into account (Campbell & Murchie, 2004).
- The participants in guideline committees may be too narrow in outlook, beholden to commercial interests, or not include the most critical observers (Alderman et al., 2002).

Numerous suggestions have been published on how to improve the preparation of guidelines including simplifying them (Avanzini et al., 2002), strengthening the quality of evidence (GRADE Working Group, 2004), and improving the process of reaching judgments (Raine et al., 2004).

Despite the problems with trials, meta-analyses, and guidelines, we must use them to determine the most effective way to manage hypertension. The following will examine the evidence that lowering blood pressure with drugs provides benefit, starting with the most severe degree of hypertension and ending with prehypertension.

## Trial Results

### Trials in Malignant Hypertension

The benefits of drug therapy in malignant hypertension were easy to demonstrate in view of its predictable, relatively brief, and almost uniformly fatal course in untreated patients. Starting in 1958, a number of studies appeared showing a significant effect of medical therapy in reducing mortality in malignant hypertension (see Chapter 8).

### Trials in Less Severe Hypertension

Demonstrating that therapy made a difference in nonmalignant, primary hypertension took a great deal longer. However, during the late 1950s and early 1960s, reports began to appear that suggested that therapy of nonmalignant hypertension was helpful (Hodge et al., 1961; Hood et al., 1963; Leishman, 1961). The first comparative, albeit small, study by Hamilton et al. (1964) showed a marked decrease in complications over a 2- to 6-year interval for 26 effectively treated patients as compared to 31 untreated patients.

#### Veterans Administration Cooperative Study

The first definitive proof of the protection provided by antihypertensive therapy in nonmalignant hypertension came from the Veterans Administration Cooperative Study, begun in 1963. The value of therapy in the 73 men with diastolic BPs of 115 to 129 mm Hg given hydrochlorothiazide, reserpine, and hydralazine versus the 70 men given placebo became obvious after less than 1.5 years, with a reduction in deaths from 4 to 0 and in major complications from 23 to 2 [Veterans Administration Cooperative Study Group (VA), 1967].

Along with the men with diastolic BPs of 115 to 129 mm Hg, another 380 with diastolic BPs between 90 and 114 mm Hg also were assigned randomly to either placebo or active therapy. It took a longer time—up to 5.5 years, with an average of 3.3 years—to demonstrate a statistically clear advantage of therapy in this group (VA, 1970). A total of 19 of the placebo group but only 8 of the treated group died of hypertensive complications, and serious morbidity occurred more often among the placebo group. Overall, major complications occurred in 29% of the placebo group and 12% of the treated group.

*Additional Randomized, Controlled Trials*

The promising results of the Veterans Administration study prompted the initiation of a number of additional controlled trials of therapy of hypertension. As previously emphasized, RCTs are required to assess reliably the modest effects of treatment on major outcomes that are expected in patients with mild to moderate hypertension over the relatively short duration of the observation. Fortunately, many more have now been completed, and a number of meta-analyses have been completed on the data

generated from the multiple RCTs performed over the past 40 years. Data from trials completed before 1995, primarily with diuretics and β-blockers are followed by those completed since 1995, primarily with angiotensin converting enzyme inhibitors (ACEIs), calcium channel blockers (CCBs), and angiotensin II-receptor blockers (ARBs).

### Trials Before 1995

The 21 trials listed in Table 5–2 included a total of 56,078 patients followed up for an average of 5 years (Psaty et al., 1997; 2003). In all these trials, the primary drugs were either β-blockers or diuretics; those trials done before the mid-1980s almost all used higher doses of diuretic. It should be noted that the entry BP criterion for all of the trials before the Systolic Hypertension in the Elderly Program-Pilot

## TABLE 5–2

### Randomized Placebo-Controlled Trials of Antihypertensive Drug Treatment Published Before 1995

| Trial (Reference) | Number of Patients | Entry BP mm Hg | Mean Age, Years | Duration, Years | Duration, Drugs |
|---|---|---|---|---|---|
| VA Coop I (1967) | 143 | 186/121 | 51 | 1.5 | D-high |
| VA Coop II (1970) | 380 | 163/104 | 51 | 3.3 | D-high |
| Carter (1970) | 97 | >160/110 | (60–79) | 4.0 | D-high |
| Barraclough et al. (1973) | 116 | –/109 | 56 | 2.0 | D-high |
| Hypertension-Stroke (1974) | 452 | 167/100 | 59 | 2.3 | D-high |
| USPHS (Smith, 1977) | 389 | 148/99 | 44 | 7.0 | D-high |
| VA-NHLBI (Perry et al., 1978) | 1,012 | –/93 | 38 | 1.5 | D-high |
| HDFP (1979) | 10,940 | 170/101 | 51 | 5.0 | D-high |
| Oslo (Hegeland, 1980) | 785 | 155/97 | 45 | 5.5 | D-high |
| Australian (Management Comm, 1980) | 3,427 | 165/101 | 50 | 4.0 | D-high |
| Kuramoto et al. (1981) | 91 | 168/86 | 76 | 4.0 | D-high |
| MRC-I (1985) | 17,354 | 161/98 | 52 | 5.0 | β-B/D-high |
| EWPHE (Amery et al., 1985) | 840 | 182/101 | 72 | 4.7 | D-low |
| HEP (Coope & Warrender, 1986) | 884 | 197/100 | 60 | 4.4 | β-B |
| SHEP-P (Perry et al., 1989) | 551 | 172/75 | 72 | 2.8 | D-low |
| SHEP (1991) | 4,736 | 170/77 | 72 | 4.5 | D-low |
| STOP-H (Dahlöf et al., 1991) | 1,627 | 195/102 | 76 | 2.0 | β-B |
| MRC-II (1992) | 4,396 | 185/91 | 70 | 5.8 | β-B/D-low |
| Dutch TIA (1993) | 1,473 | 157/91 | 52% >65 | 2.6 | β-B |
| PATS (1995) | 5,665 | 154/93 | 60 | 2.0 | D-high |
| TEST (Eriksson, 1995) | 720 | 161/89 | 70 | 2.6 | β-B |

β-B, beta-blocker; BP, blood pressure; D-high, diuretic dose ≥50 mg hydrochlorothiazide; D-low, diuretic dose <50 mg hydrochlorothiazide; EWPHE, European Working Party on Hypertension in the Elderly; HDFP, Hypertension Detection and Follow-up Program; MRC, Medical Research Council; NHLBI, National Heart, Lung, and Blood Institute; PATS, Post-Stroke Antihypertensive Treatment; SHEP, Systolic Hypertension in the Elderly Program; SHEP-P, SHEP Pilot Study; STOP-H, Swedish Trial in Old Patients with Hypertension; TEST, Tenormin after Stroke and TIA; USPHS, U.S. Public Health Service; VA, Veterans Administration.

Study (SHEP-P) in 1989 was the diastolic level, reflecting the greater emphasis placed, until recently, on diastolic rather than systolic BP as the major determinant of risk.

The trials published before 1985 mainly involved younger patients; those in the early 1990s enrolled elderly hypertensives with either combined hypertension or isolated systolic hypertension (ISH), who will be examined separately.

*Separation of the Data by Doses*

Psaty et al. (1997) separated the nine trials that involved high doses of diuretic (equivalent to 50 mg or more of hydrochlorothiazide) from the four that involved lower doses (equivalent to 12.5 mg to 25.0 mg hydrochlorothiazide) and the four that used a β-blocker as the primary drug (Figure 5–2). The Hypertension Detection and Follow-up Program study was considered separately, as it was not placebo controlled: Half of the patients were more intensively treated (stepped care); the other half were less intensively treated (referred care).

The separation of the data by doses clearly reveals the lack of protection from CHD by high doses of diuretic and β-blockers, whereas all therapies had a significant impact on stroke. The later four studies with low doses of diuretic showed excellent protection against CHD.

*Conclusion*

Based on these trials, primarily in middle-aged patients with combined systolic and diastolic hypertension, the evidence was clear: Reductions in BP of 10 to 12 mm Hg systolic and 5 to 6 mm Hg diastolic for a few years conferred relative reductions of 38% for stroke and 16% for CHD (Collins & MacMahon, 1994). The sizes of these reductions were consistent with those predicted from observational studies of the long-term relations between BP with risk of stroke and coronary disease (MacMahon et al., 1990). The relative reductions were similar in various subgroups of patients, seemingly independent of differences in the event rates in the placebo-treated controls.

### Placebo-Controlled Trials After 1995

After 1995, a new series of trials were completed and many more started to determine the effects of the newer antihypertensive agents—ACEIs, CCBs, and ARBs—and to broaden the patient population to those with associated conditions including coronary disease, diabetes, and renal insufficiency (Table 5–3). The most complete analyses of all of these more recent trials come from three sources. The first is the Blood Pressure Lowering Treatment Trialists' Collaboration (Blood Pressure Trialists, 2000; 2003).

To reduce random error and bias and to ensure comparability between various trials, in July 1995 the principal investigators from all the large-scale trials then in progress or in advanced stages of planning agreed to collaborate on prospective overviews in which treatment effects would be estimated from the combined results of individual studies not reported before July 1995 (World Health Organization, 1998). As will be described, separate overviews were planned for trials comparing active treatments against placebo, trials comparing more intensive with less intensive strategies (covered in the section Goal of Therapy, later in this chapter), and trials comparing different drug classes (covered in the first portion of Chapter 7). The trials had to have a minimum of 1,000 patient-years of follow-up, regardless of whether the intent

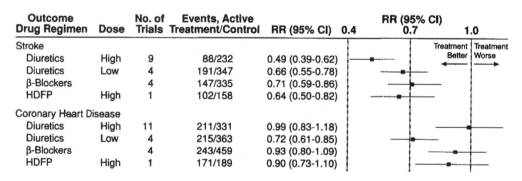

| Outcome Drug Regimen | Dose | No. of Trials | Events, Active Treatment/Control | RR (95% CI) | | |
|---|---|---|---|---|---|---|
| **Stroke** | | | | | | |
| Diuretics | High | 9 | 88/232 | 0.49 (0.39-0.62) | | |
| Diuretics | Low | 4 | 191/347 | 0.66 (0.55-0.78) | | |
| β-Blockers | | 4 | 147/335 | 0.71 (0.59-0.86) | | |
| HDFP | High | 1 | 102/158 | 0.64 (0.50-0.82) | | |
| **Coronary Heart Disease** | | | | | | |
| Diuretics | High | 11 | 211/331 | 0.99 (0.83-1.18) | | |
| Diuretics | Low | 4 | 215/363 | 0.72 (0.61-0.85) | | |
| β-Blockers | | 4 | 243/459 | 0.93 (0.80-1.09) | | |
| HDFP | High | 1 | 171/189 | 0.90 (0.73-1.10) | | |

*FIGURE 5–2* ● Meta-analysis of randomized, placebo-controlled clinical trials in hypertension according to first-line treatment strategy. For these comparisons, the numbers of participants randomized to active therapy and placebo were 7,758 and 12,075 for high-dose diuretic therapy; 4,305 and 5,116 for low-dose diuretic therapy; and 6,736 and 12,147 for β-blocker therapy. HDFP, Hypertension Detection and Follow-up Program; RR, relative risk; CI, confidence interval. (Adapted from Psaty BM, Smith NL, Siscovick DS, et al. Health outcomes associated with antihypertensive therapies used as first-line agents. *JAMA* 1997;277:739–745.)

## TABLE 5–3

### Randomized Placebo-Controlled Trials of Antihypertensive Drug Treatment Published After 1995

| Trial (Reference) | No. of Patients | Entry BP mm Hg | Mean Age, Years | Duration, Years | Primary Drugs |
|---|---|---|---|---|---|
| ACEI vs Placebo | | | | | |
| HOPE (Heart Outcomes, 2000a) | 9,297 | 139/79 | 66 | 5 | Ramipril |
| PART 2 (MacMahon et al., 2000) | 617 | 133/79 | 61 | 4 | Ramipril |
| OUIET (Cashin-Hemphill et al., 1999) | 1,750 | 123/74 | 58 | 2 | Quinapril |
| SCAT (Teo et al., 2000) | 460 | 130/78 | 61 | 5 | Enalapril |
| PROGRESS (2001) | 6,150 | 147/86 | 64 | 4 | Perindopril, Indapamide |
| CCB vs Placebo | | | | | |
| STONE (Gong, 1996) | 1,632 | 169/98 | 67 | 2 | Nifedipine |
| SYST-EUR (Staessen et al., 1997) | 4,695 | 174/86 | 70 | 2 | Nitrendipine |
| SYST-CHINA (Liu et al., 1998) | 2,394 | 170/86 | 67 | 3 | Nitrendipine |
| PREVENT (Pitt et al., 2000) | 825 | 129/79 | 57 | 3 | Amlodipine |
| IDNT (Lewis et al., 2001) | 1,136 | 159/97 | 59 | 3 | Amlodipine |
| ARB vs Placebo | | | | | |
| IDNT (Lewis et al., 2001) | 1,148 | 160/87 | 59 | 3 | Irbesartan |
| RENAAL (Brenner et al., 2001) | 1,513 | 152/82 | 60 | 4 | Losartan |
| SCOPE (Lithell et al., 2003) | 4,937 | 166/90 | 76 | 4 | Candesartan |

was to lower BP or whether the patients were selected on the basis of hypertension. The trialists obtained individual patient data from collaborating investigators and performed multiple analyses.

At the same time, Jan Staessen in Leuven, Belgium, and his coworkers have reported repeated meta-analyses of published data from RCTs that were available in 2001, 2003, and 2005 (Staessen et al., 2001; 2003; Wang et al., 2005). The Blood Pressure Trialists' meta-analysis covers 162,341 subjects in 29 RCTs; the Staessen group covered 149,407 subjects in 31 RCTs with almost complete overlap between the two groups.

Figure 5–3 is an interesting overview of data from the 31 RCTs included in Staessen et al.'s 2003 analysis, showing the relation between odds ratios for cardiovascular events and differences in systolic BP. The figure portrays data from 15 of the 21 placebo-controlled trials published before 1995 that are listed in Table 5–2, the others being too small or too short to be included. Most of the placebo-controlled trials published since 1995 are included. In addition, data from some of the comparative trials to be covered in Chapter 7 are

included since the purpose of the graph is to show the degree of protection with varying differences of systolic BP. In many of the comparative trials, higher systolic BP was seen with the "experimental" drug, with resultant increases in cardiovascular events, shown to the left of the dashed line.

The message of Figure 5–3 is clear: The degree of blood pressure reduction is the primary determinant of cardiovascular protection, not the type of drug that provided the reduction in BP.

The third meta-analysis is that of Psaty et al. (1997, 2003). Using somewhat different criteria for inclusion than the Trialists or Staessen et al., these investigators ended up with data from 41 trials encompassing 192,478 patients followed for an average of 3 to 4 years. Their comparisons of all active therapies versus placebo, shown in Table 5–4, agree with the other two analyses: Active therapy reduced all end points significantly better than placebo.

These three meta-analyses, though differing somewhat in methodology, provide a clear answer to the question as to whether treatment that lowers blood pressure is beneficial.

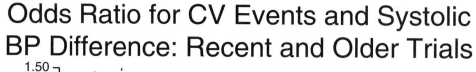

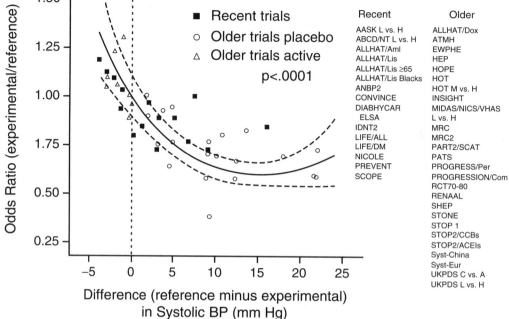

# Odds Ratio for CV Events and Systolic BP Difference: Recent and Older Trials

**FIGURE 5–3** ● Relationship between odds ratio for cardiovascular events and corresponding differences in systolic blood pressure in trials published before (*older*) and after (*recent*) 2000. The older trials included some comparing a drug against placebo, others comparing one drug against another, i.e., active. Odds ratios were calculated for experimental versus reference treatment. Blood pressure differences were obtained by subtracting achieved levels of experimental groups from those in reference groups. Negative values indicate tighter blood pressure on control than on reference treatment. The regression lines were plotted with 95% confidence interval and were weighted for the inverse of the variance of the individual odds ratios. (Modified from Staessen et al. Cardiovascular protection and blood pressure reduction: a quantitative overview updated until 1 March 2003. *J Hypertens* 2003;21:1055–1076.)

---

## TABLE 5–4

### Meta-analysis Comparing Any Antihypertensive Drug Treatment Versus No Treatment for Each Outcome

| Outcome | No. of Trials | Relative Risk (95% Confidence Interval) |
|---|---|---|
| Coronary heart disease | 24 | 0.86 (0.80–0.93) |
|  |  | 0.87 (0.80–0.94) |
| Stroke | 23 | 0.69 (0.64–0.74) |
|  |  | 0.68 (0.61–0.76) |
| Congestive heart failure | 7 | 0.54 (0.45–0.66) |
|  |  | 0.60 (0.49–0.74) |
| Major cardiovascular events | 28 | 0.78 (0.74–0.81) |
|  |  | 0.73 (0.62–0.87) |
| Cardiovascular mortality | 23 | 0.84 (0.78–0.90) |
|  |  | 0.84 (0.78–0.90) |
| Total mortality | 25 | 0.90 (0.85–0.95) |
|  |  | 0.90 (0.85–0.95) |

Data derived from Psaty BM, Lumly T, Furberg CD, et al. Health outcomes associated with various antihypertensive therapies used as first-line agents: a network meta-analysis. *JAMA* 2003;289:2534–2544.

### Active Drugs Versus Placebo

*Diuretics and β-Blockers*
Earlier trials documented the benefits of low-dose diuretic versus placebo (Figure 5–2). Starting with the first MRC trial (1985), β-blockers were introduced and compared exclusively against placebo in four trials. In all four of these trials, atenolol was the β-blocker chosen (Carlberg et al., 2004). As seen in Figure 5–4, atenolol was no better than placebo except against stroke. The stroke benefit arose primarily from the HEP trial (Coope & Warrender, 1986), wherein 60% of the patients also received a diuretic and achieved a greater fall in BP, averaging −18.0/−11.0 mm Hg, than in the other trials.

These and additional data on the lack of benefit with atenolol in comparative trials (to be described in Chapter 7) led Carlberg et al. (2004) to conclude that atenolol is not a suitable drug for hypertensive patients and challenge the use of atenolol as a reference drug in outcome trials in hypertension.

The status of other, more lipophilic β-blockers that more easily gain entry into the central nervous system for treatment of hypertension remains uncertain, despite their proven ability to prevent death after myocardial infarction and improve outcomes in congestive failure (see Chapter 7). Disturbing evidence about the potential hazards of β-blockers comes from an observational study that found a significant increase in myocardial infarctions among the 250 of 316 men who took a β-blocker over a 10-year interval (Dunder et al., 2003). The increased rate, 23% compared to 13.5% among those who did not take a β-blocker, was closely associated with a rise in blood glucose, now recognized to be a common accompaniment to β-blocker therapy.

*ACEIs, CCBs, and ARBs Versus Placebo*
In the 12 RCTs wherein one of the three newer classes has been compared to placebo, almost all three classes provide clear benefit with the exception of CCBs against heart failure (Blood Pressure Trialists, 2003) (Figure 5–5). The authors comment:

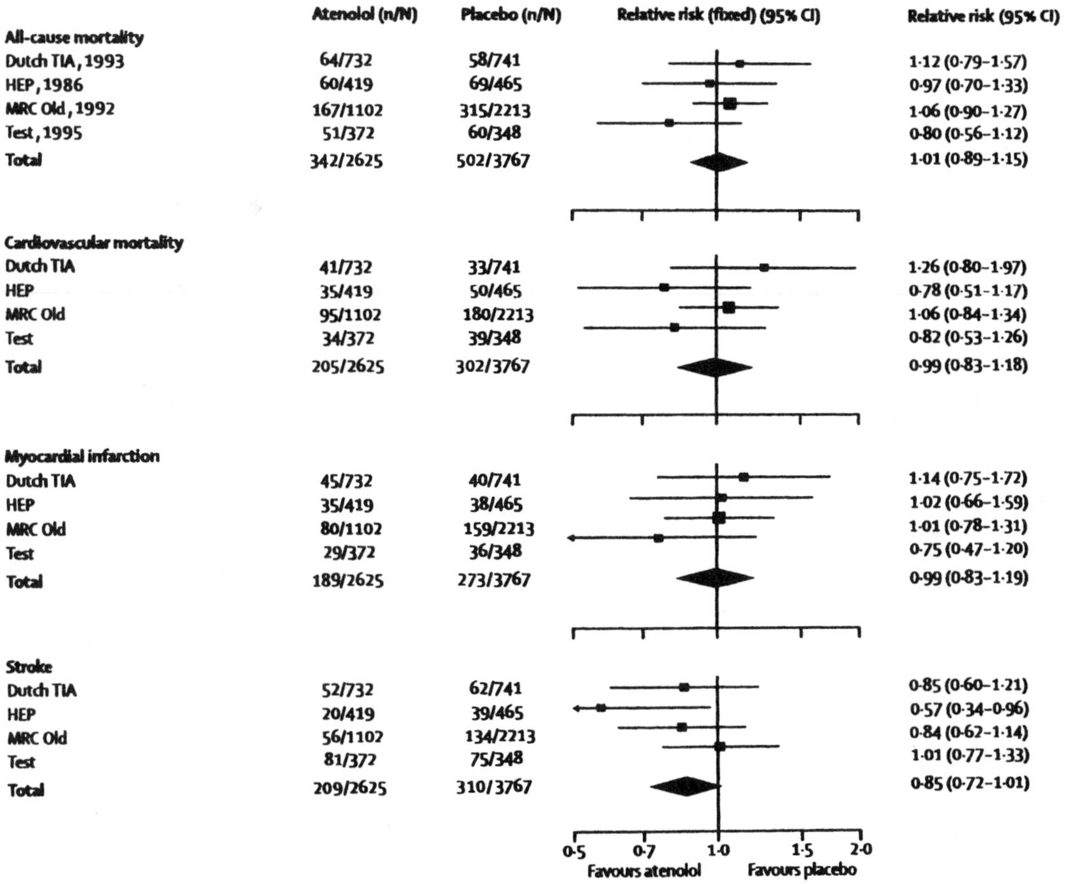

| | Atenolol (n/N) | Placebo (n/N) | Relative risk (fixed) (95% CI) | Relative risk (95% CI) |
|---|---|---|---|---|
| **All-cause mortality** | | | | |
| Dutch TIA, 1993 | 64/732 | 58/741 | | 1·12 (0·79–1·57) |
| HEP, 1986 | 60/419 | 69/465 | | 0·97 (0·70–1·33) |
| MRC Old, 1992 | 167/1102 | 315/2213 | | 1·06 (0·90–1·27) |
| Test, 1995 | 51/372 | 60/348 | | 0·80 (0·56–1·12) |
| **Total** | 342/2625 | 502/3767 | | 1·01 (0·89–1·15) |
| | | | | |
| **Cardiovascular mortality** | | | | |
| Dutch TIA | 41/732 | 33/741 | | 1·26 (0·80–1·97) |
| HEP | 35/419 | 50/465 | | 0·78 (0·51–1·17) |
| MRC Old | 95/1102 | 180/2213 | | 1·06 (0·84–1·34) |
| Test | 34/372 | 39/348 | | 0·82 (0·53–1·26) |
| **Total** | 205/2625 | 302/3767 | | 0·99 (0·83–1·18) |
| | | | | |
| **Myocardial infarction** | | | | |
| Dutch TIA | 45/732 | 40/741 | | 1·14 (0·75–1·72) |
| HEP | 35/419 | 38/465 | | 1·02 (0·66–1·59) |
| MRC Old | 80/1102 | 159/2213 | | 1·01 (0·78–1·31) |
| Test | 29/372 | 36/348 | | 0·75 (0·47–1·20) |
| **Total** | 189/2625 | 273/3767 | | 0·99 (0·83–1·19) |
| | | | | |
| **Stroke** | | | | |
| Dutch TIA | 52/732 | 62/741 | | 0·85 (0·60–1·21) |
| HEP | 20/419 | 39/465 | | 0·57 (0·34–0·96) |
| MRC Old | 56/1102 | 134/2213 | | 0·84 (0·62–1·14) |
| Test | 81/372 | 75/348 | | 1·01 (0·77–1·33) |
| **Total** | 209/2625 | 310/3767 | | 0·85 (0·72–1·01) |

0·5　0·7　1·0　1·5　2·0
Favours atenolol　　Favours placebo

**FIGURE 5–4** ● Outcome data for atenolol versus placebo or no treatment. *n*, number of patients with events. *N*, total number of patients. (Modified from Carlberg B, Samuelsson O, Lindholm LH. Atenolol in hypertension: is it a wise choice? *Lancet* 2004;364:1684–1689.)

| | Trials | Events/Participants | | Difference in BP (mean, mm Hg) | | Relative Risk (95%) |
|---|---|---|---|---|---|---|
| | | Drug | Placebo | | | |
| **Stroke** | | | | | | |
| ACEI vs Placebo | 5 | 473/9111 | 660/9118 | -5/-2 | | 0·72 (0·64–0·81) |
| CA vs Placebo | 4 | 76/3794 | 119/3688 | -8/-4 | | 0·62 (0·47–0·82) |
| ARB vs Placebo | 3 | 132/3461 | 141/2888 | -3/-2 | | 0·79 (0·63–0·99) |
| **Coronary Heart Disease** | | | | | | |
| ACEI vs Placebo | 5 | 667/9111 | 834/9118 | -5/-2 | | 0·80 (0·73–0·88) |
| CA vs Placebo | 4 | 125/3794 | 156/3688 | -8/-4 | | 0·78 (0·62–0·99) |
| ARB vs Placebo | 3 | 191/4183 | 177/3614 | -3/-2 | | 0·94 (0·77–1·14) |
| **Heart Failure** | | | | | | |
| ACEI vs Placebo | 5 | 219/8233 | 269/8246 | -5/-2 | | 0·82 (0·69–0·98) |
| CA vs Placebo | 3 | 104/3382 | 88/3274 | -8/-4 | | 1·21 (0·93–1·58) |
| ARB vs Placebo | 2 | 242/1655 | 240/1091 | -3/-2 | | 0·71 (0·60–0·83) |
| **Major Cardiovascular Events** | | | | | | |
| ACEI vs Placebo | 5 | 1283/9111 | 1648/9118 | -5/-2 | | 0·78 (0·73–0·83) |
| CA vs Placebo | 3 | 280/3382 | 337/3274 | -8/-4 | | 0·82 (0·71–0·95) |
| ARB vs Placebo | 3 | 755/3619 | 680/3111 | -3/-2 | | 0·96 (0·88–1·06) |
| **Cardiovascular Death** | | | | | | |
| ACEI vs Placebo | 5 | 488/9111 | 614/9118 | -5/-2 | | 0·80 (0·71–0·89) |
| CA vs Placebo | 4 | 107/3382 | 135/3274 | -8/-4 | | 0·78 (0·61–1·00) |
| ARB vs Placebo | 3 | 234/3359 | 198/2831 | -3/-2 | | 1·00 (0·83–1·20) |
| **Total Mortality** | | | | | | |
| ACEI vs Placebo | 5 | 839/9111 | 951/9118 | -5/-2 | | 0·88 (0·81–0·96) |
| CA vs Placebo | 4 | 239/3794 | 263/3688 | -8/-4 | | 0·89 (0·75–1·05) |
| ARB vs Placebo | 3 | 587/3787 | 514/3277 | -3/-2 | | 0·99 (0·89–1·11) |

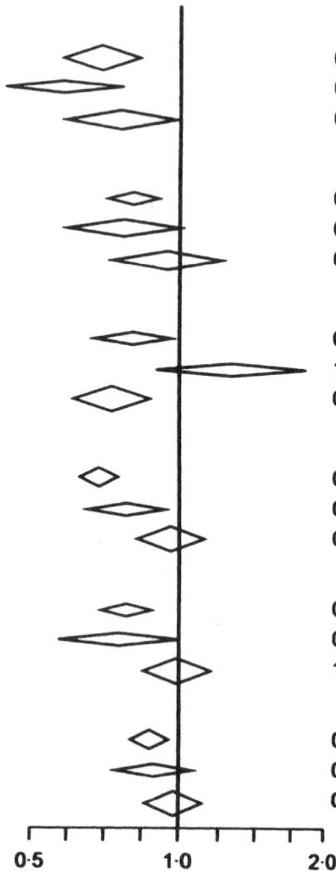

0·5                    1·0                    2·0

**FIGURE 5–5** ● Comparisons of the effects of therapy based on ACEI, angiotension converting enzyme inhibitor; CA, calcium antagonist; ARB, angiotensin II receptor blocker; all versus placebo, on cardiovascular events and mortality. (Modified from Blood Pressure Lowering Treatment Trialists' Collaboration. Effects of different blood-pressure-lowering regimens on major cardiovascular events: results of prospectively-designed overviews of randomised trials. *Lancet* 2003;362:1527–1535.)

Our results show that regimens based on ACE inhibitors or on diuretics or blockers are much more effective at preventing heart failure than are regimens based on calcium antagonists. Since the current analyses were restricted to cases of heart failure that resulted in death or admission to hospital, minor side-effects of calcium antagonists, such as peripheral oedema, are unlikely to be wholly responsible for this finding. The differences between these regimens are not easily accounted for by their comparative effects on blood pressure and are broadly consistent with results of trials of ACE inhibitors and calcium antagonists in patients with heart failure. . . . Unlike in earlier analyses, our results for coronary heart disease showed no trend towards a lesser effect of calcium antagonists compared with diuretics or blockers, or ACE inhibitors . . . questioning the validity of claims of large increases in coronary risk in hypertensive patients treated with calcium antagonists.

*An Issue About PROGRESS*
In Table 5–3, the PROGRESS trial (2001) is listed under "ACEI vs. Placebo," even though the effect of the ACEI alone was inconsequential (BP fell 5/3 mm Hg, strokes reduced by 5%). Only in those

given the ACEI with the addition of the diuretic indapamide was there a significant fall in BP (by 12/5 mm Hg) and reduction in stroke (by 43%) (Psaty et al., 2002). Unfortunately, the diuretic was not tested alone. However, in the original paper (PROGRESS Collaborative Group, 2001) and many subsequent ones about the data, the term "perindopril-based blood pressure-lowering regimen" is used, without mention that the addition of the diuretic provided the major benefit (Wennberg & Zimmermann, 2004). The investigators respond to this criticism simply by denying intent to deceive and calling attention to the major impact that their original observation has had on stroke management (MacMahon et al., 2004).

## Trial Results: Special Populations

### Trials in the Elderly with Isolated Systolic Hypertension

Although both the earlier and the later trials listed in Tables 5–2 and 5–3 include some elderly patients with ISH, defined in those trials as a systolic BP 160 mm Hg or higher, the fact that such patients make up the largest portion of hypertensive patients now, and to an even greater degree in the future, justifies a closer, separate look at the data on their therapy. Staessen et al. (2000) have provided a meta-analysis of these trials, which are listed in Table 5–5.

Figure 5–6 summarizes the data from all eight trials of the 15,693 elderly patients with ISH. The average BP at entry was 174/83 mm Hg and the mean fall in BP over the median 3.8-year follow-up was 10.4/4.1 mm Hg. Therapy significantly reduced all-cause and cardiovascular mortality, 13% and 18% respectively, but had an even greater impact on morbidity: Coronary events were reduced by 23% and strokes by 30%. As is noted in the next section on those older than 80 years in these trials, mortality is unlikely to be reduced greatly by any intervention in the elderly. However, as long as mortality is not increased, the ability of antihypertensive therapy to reduce disabling morbidities in the elderly is certainly adequate justification for its wider application.

In these trials, the absolute benefits of active therapy were greater in men, older patients, and those with prior cardiovascular complications, reflecting the higher initial risk status of such patients. To prevent one major cardiovascular event, the numbers of patients who needed to be treated for 5 years were 18 men versus 38 women; 19 patients 79 years or older versus 39 patients 60 to 69 years old; and 16 of those with prior cardiovascular complications versus 37 of

those without (Staessen et al., 2000). Moreover, in a 15-year follow-up of a portion of the participants in the SHEP trial, a persistent reduction in fatal plus nonfatal cardiovascular events was found among the original drug-treated group compared to the placebo group, 58% vs. 79%, despite the eventual use of antihypertensive therapy in 65% of the placebo group compared to 72% of the active group (Sutton-Tyrrell et al., 2003).

As impressive as these data are, they must be recognized as covering only the higher range (Stage 2) of ISH, i.e., systolics of 160 mm Hg or higher, which has uniformly been the criterion for entry into the trials shown in Table 5–5 and Figure 5–6. Most ISH is between 140 and 159 mm Hg and most premature cardiovascular events occur in patients in that range rather than in those with higher systolic BP (Chaudhry et al., 2004). As of now, there are no RCTs documenting the benefit for those with Stage 1 ISH.

### Trials in Those over Age 80

Attention must be given to patients over age 80, percentage-wise the fastest growing demographic group. To the results of a 1999 meta-analysis of seven RCTs including 1,670 patients over age 80 (Gueyffier et al., 1999), Bulpitt et al. (2003) have added data from an open-label study of drug therapy versus placebo in 1,283 patients, in the Hypertension in the Very Elderly Trial

## TABLE 5–5

### Randomized Placebo-Controlled Trials of Antihypertensive Drug Treatment in Elderly Patients with Isolated Systolic Hypertension Above 160 mm Hg[a]

| Trial (Reference) | Number of Patients | Entry BP mm Hg | Mean Age, Years | Duration, Years | Primary Drugs |
|---|---|---|---|---|---|
| EWPHE (Amery et al., 1985) | 172 | 178/92 | 73 | 4.3 | Diuretic |
| MRC-I (1985) | 428 | 174/92 | 62 | 5.2 | β-B/Diuretic |
| HEP (Coope & Warrender, 1986) | 349 | 191/85 | 70 | 3.6 | β-B |
| SHEP (1991) | 4,736 | 170/77 | 72 | 4.4 | Diuretic |
| STOP-H (Dahlöf et al., 1991) | 268 | 194/91 | 76 | 1.9 | β-B/Diuretic |
| MRC-II (1992) | 2,651 | 182/83 | 70 | 6.1 | β-B/Diuretic |
| Syst-Eur (Staessen et al., 1997) | 4,695 | 174/85 | 70 | 2.0 | CCB |
| Syst-China (Liu et al., 1998) | 2,394 | 170/86 | 67 | 3.0 | CCB |

β-B, beta-blocker; CCB, calcium channel blocker; EWPHE, European Working Party on Hypertension in the Elderly; MRC, Medical Research Council; SHEP, Systolic Hypertension in the Elderly Program; STOP-H, Swedish Trial in Old Patients with Hypertension; Syst-China, Systolic Hypertension in China trial; Syst-Eur, Systolic Hypertension in Europe trial.~

[a]Diagnosis of systolic hypertension based on systolic BP above 160, diastolic blood pressure below 95 mm Hg in all trials except SHEP, which required a diastolic blood pressure of ≤ 90 mm Hg.

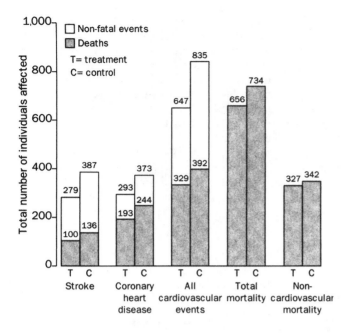

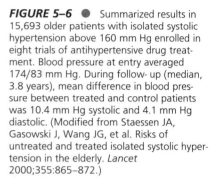

FIGURE 5–6 ● Summarized results in 15,693 older patients with isolated systolic hypertension above 160 mm Hg enrolled in eight trials of antihypertensive drug treatment. Blood pressure at entry averaged 174/83 mm Hg. During follow- up (median, 3.8 years), mean difference in blood pressure between treated and control patients was 10.4 mm Hg systolic and 4.1 mm Hg diastolic. (Modified from Staessen JA, Gasowski J, Wang JG, et al. Risks of untreated and treated isolated systolic hypertension in the elderly. *Lancet* 2000;355:865–872.)

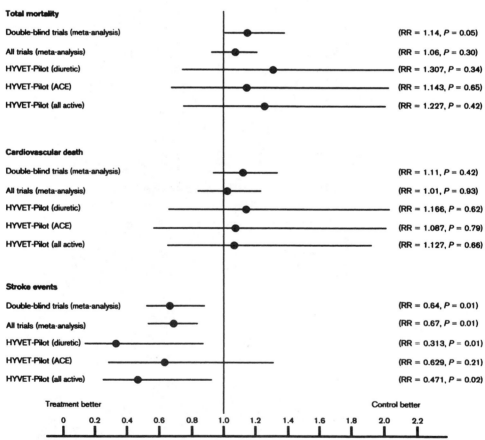

FIGURE 5–7 ● Comparison of Hypertension in the Very Elderly (HTVET-Pilot) results with those of the meta-analysis of Gueyffier et al. (1999). Point estimates of the relative hazard rates are given, together with the 95% confidence intervals. RR, relative risk; ACE, angiotensin-converting enzyme. (Modified from Bulpitt CJ, Beckett NS, Cooke J, et al. Results of the pilot study for the Hypertension in the Very Elderly Trial. *J Hypertens* 2003;21:2409.)

(HYVET) (Figure 5–7). In keeping with that found in Gueyffier et al.'s meta-analysis, the HYVET 1-year data show a reduction in strokes but a tendency toward an increase in mortality in those treated with antihypertensive drugs.

Despite, or perhaps because of, these disconcerting data, the larger controlled HYVET trial is now in progress. Meanwhile, caution is obviously advised in treating the very old.

### Trials in Younger Versus Older

Despite this disconcerting mortality trend in trials of the very elderly, older patients derive greater *absolute* benefit from any reduction in blood pressure than do younger patients and this reflects a greater fall in systolic BP. As shown by Wang et al. (2005), the relative slopes of decreasing events with therapy are similar in younger, older, and very old, but since the older start at higher degrees of risk, they achieve a greater absolute benefit (Figure 5–8). Wang et al. (2005) further show that the lowering of systolic pressure is the critical element of therapy, regardless of the magnitude of the fall in diastolic pressure.

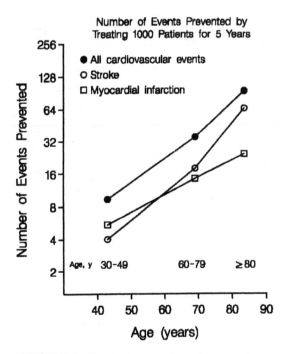

### FIGURE 5–8 ● Absolute benefits in the prevention of fatal and nonfatal cardiovascular events, stroke, and myocardial infarction in three age groups. Symbols represent the number of events that can be prevented by treating 1,000 patients for 5 years. (Modified from Wang J-G, Staessen JA, Franklin SS, et al. Systolic and diastolic blood pressure lowering as determinants of cardiovascular outcome on antihypertensive drug treatment. *Hypertension* 2005;45:907–913.)

### Trials in Women

In the various previously described trials, women achieve slightly less benefit from antihypertensive therapy than do men with similar levels of BP (Gueyffier et al., 1997). This reflects the lesser risk status for women than men, so that women achieve less absolute benefit. However, when women with equal degrees of risk as men are treated, they achieve virtually identical relative reductions in coronary disease and slightly greater protection against strokes (Gueyffier et al., 1997).

### Trials in Blacks

Blood pressure in Blacks responds less to renin-inhibiting drugs than it does in Whites, but there are no outcome data from RCTs against placebo to show a difference in Blacks' morbidity or mortality when treated for hypertension with any type of therapy (Brewster et al., 2004).

### Trials in Diabetic Patients

Two placebo-controlled trials have examined the effect of antihypertensive therapy on outcomes in hypertensive diabetic patients, the SHEP (Curb et al., 1996) and Syst-Eur (Tuomilehto et al., 1999) trials (Table 5–6). With considerable reductions in BP, significant decreases in cardiovascular events but not total mortality were seen. Of the remaining three trials, high-risk patients with diabetic nephropathy were studied in IDNT and RENAAL. The lesser degrees of protection likely reflect the small changes in BP. Nonetheless, the primary end point, a slowing of the fall in renal function, was observed in both trials. Further analyses of these and other trials in diabetic patients are available (Vijan & Hayward 2003; Zanchetti & Ruilope, 2002).

### Trials in Cardiac Patients

In addition to the documentation that coronary heart disease morbidity and mortality have been significantly prevented by low-dose diuretics, CCBs, ACEIs, and ARBs reviewed earlier in this chapter (see Figures 5–2 and 5–5, and Table 5–4), additional RCTs have examined the effect of antihypertensive agents in patients with preexisting coronary disease.

#### Angina and Coronary Disease

Nitrates, β-blockers, and CCBs had been used for many years on the basis of efficacy in reducing symptoms with little or no hard outcome data. More recently, trials of longer duration and with adequate power to provide hard outcome data have shown that the ACEIs ramipril (Heart Outcomes, 2000a) and perindopril (European Trial on Reduction, 2003) reduce major cardiovascular events, whereas the CCB nifedipine GITS had no effect on

## TABLE 5-6

### Outcomes in Placebo-controlled Trials in Diabetic Patients

| Trial | No. Pts. | Difference in BP | Duration (years) | Therapy | Relative Risks (95%) | | |
|-------|----------|------------------|------------------|---------|----------------------|---|---|
|       |          |                  |                  |         | CV Events Mortality | CV Mortality | Total |
| SHEP (Curb et al., 1996) | 583 | 10/2 | 5 | Chlorthalidone | .66 (.46–.94) | – | .74 (.46–1.18) |
| SYST-EUR (Tuomilehto et al., 1999) | 492 | 8/4 | 2 | Nitrendipine | .38 (.20–.81) | .30 (.11–.80) | .59 (.34–1.09) |
| MICRO-HOPE (Heart Outcomes, 2000b) | 3,577 | 2/1 | 4.5 | Ramipril | .77 (.64–.88) | .64 (.51–.80) | .77 (.63–.92) |
| IDNT (Lewis et al., 2001) | 1,148 | 4/3 | 2.6 | Irbesartan | 0.90 (.74–1.10) | 1.08 (.72–1.60) | .94 (.70–1.27) |
|  | 1,136 | 3/3 | 2.6 | Amlodipine | 1.0 (.83–1.21) | .79 (.51–1.22) | .90 (.68–1.18) |
| RENAAL (Brenner et al., 2001) | 1,513 | 2/1 | 3.4 | Losartan | .90 (.76–1.08) | 1.12 (.83–1.52) | 1.02 (.81–1.27) |

survival (Poole-Wilson et al., 2004). However, the CAMELOT trial (Nissen et al., 2004) showed that a CCB but not an ACEI further protected patients with coronary artery disease (CAD) even when they were normotensive.

### Congestive Heart Failure

In a similar manner, multiple trials, a few placebo-controlled, mostly of short duration, have shown reduction in hospitalizations and mortality in patients with chronic heart failure with diuretics, β-blockers, ACEIs, ARBs, aldosterone antagonists (Klein et al., 2003; Lee et al., 2004), and, in Blacks, a combination of hydralazine and nitrate (Taylor et al., 2004).

## Trials in Patients with Brain Disease

### Stroke

As noted earlier, a reduction in stroke events and mortality has been clearly documented in patients initially free of cerebrovascular disease. Equally impressive protection has been found in those with pre-existing disease (Lawes et al., 2004) (Figure 5–9). All classes of drugs save β-blockers have been effective. ARBs have been found to preserve cerebral blood flow in poststroke patients, which could add to their safety (Moriwaki et al., 2004). Whereas an ACEI alone did not reduce stroke recurrence, the addition of a diuretic did (PROGRESS, 2001), and Messerli et al. (2003) argue that diuretics confer specific protection against strokes.

Along with antihypertensive therapy, reduction of blood cholesterol with statins has provided another 21% reduction in stroke incidence in high-risk patients (Heart Protection Study, 2004) and a 27% reduction in hypertensives (Sever et al., 2003), an effect which is greater than expected from the fall in BP usually seen with statin therapy (Ferrier et al., 2002).

### Cognitive Function

In observational studies, antihypertensive therapy preserves cognitive function (Murray et al., 2002). The only specific drug that has been shown in an RCT to prevent dementia is the CCB nitrendipine in the Syst-Eur trial (Forette et al., 2002).

### Future Trials

The facts that there have been so many trials performed over the past 40 years and that many others are still in progress attest to the societal consequences of untreated hypertension and the financial gains for pharmaceutical companies that provide useful drugs. As many as we now have, we will have more.

A report by 36 experts in the hypertension arena provides a detailed description of what trials should be done next (NHLBI Working Group, 2005).

## An Overview of the Benefits of Therapy

Despite all of the preceding evidence that treatment of hypertension reduces cardiovascular disease, the

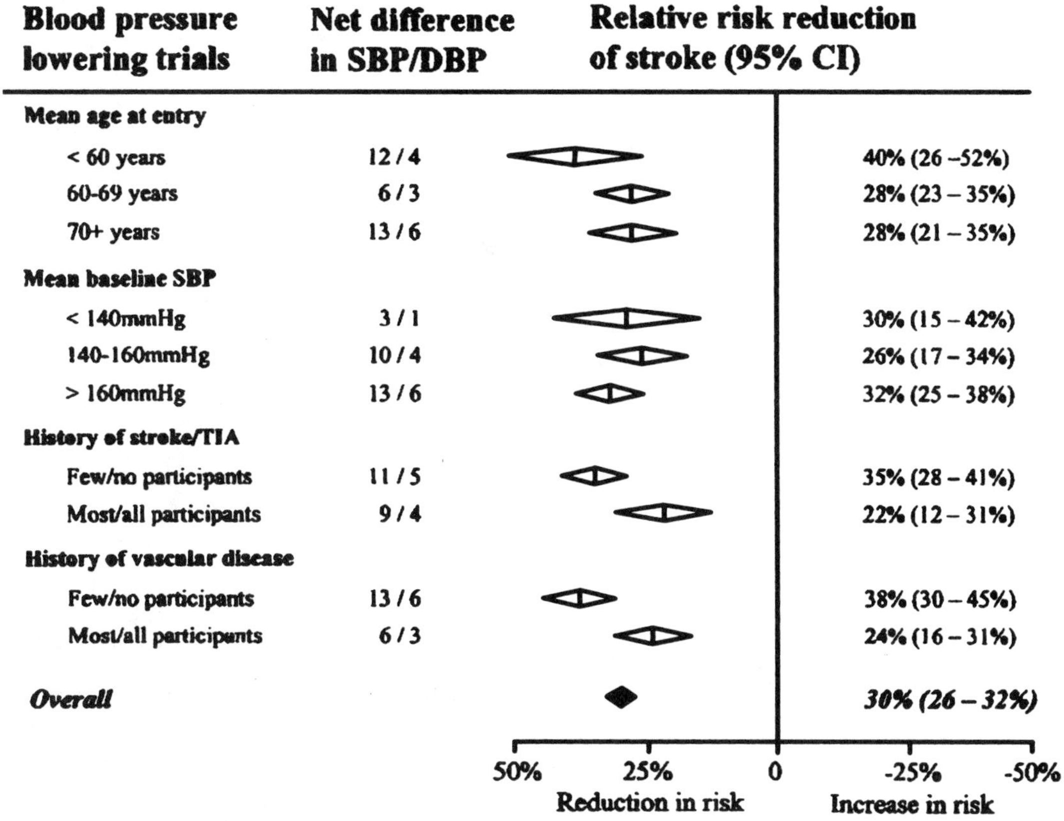

| Blood pressure lowering trials | Net difference in SBP/DBP | Relative risk reduction of stroke (95% CI) |
|---|---|---|
| **Mean age at entry** | | |
| < 60 years | 12 / 4 | 40% (26 –52%) |
| 60-69 years | 6 / 3 | 28% (23 – 35%) |
| 70+ years | 13 / 6 | 28% (21 – 35%) |
| **Mean baseline SBP** | | |
| < 140mmHg | 3 / 1 | 30% (15 – 42%) |
| 140-160mmHg | 10 / 4 | 26% (17 – 34%) |
| > 160mmHg | 13 / 6 | 32% (25 – 38%) |
| **History of stroke/TIA** | | |
| Few/no participants | 11 / 5 | 35% (28 – 41%) |
| Most/all participants | 9 / 4 | 22% (12 – 31%) |
| **History of vascular disease** | | |
| Few/no participants | 13 / 6 | 38% (30 – 45%) |
| Most/all participants | 6 / 3 | 24% (16 – 31%) |
| *Overall* | | *30% (26 – 32%)* |

**FIGURE 5–9** ● Results of over 40 randomized controlled trials comparing antihypertensive drugs with a placebo (or with no treatment) by subgroup for reduction of stroke. The *hollow diamonds* are centered on the pooled estimate of effect and represent 95% confidence interval. The *solid diamond* represents the pooled relative risk and 95% confidence interval for all contributing trials. (Modified from Lawes CMM, Bennett DA, Feigin VL, Rodgers A. Blood pressure and stroke: an overview of published reviews. *Stroke* 2004;35:776.)

overall role of antihypertensive therapy in the impressive falls in coronary and stroke mortality seen in most developed societies over the past 40 years turns out to be rather small. Recall from Chapter 1 that the best available evidence gives the treatment of hypertension only 3% and population-wide lowering of blood pressure 9.5% of the credit for the 62% decline in men and the 45% decline in women in coronary mortality in England and Wales between 1981 and 2000 (Unal et al., 2004).

The reasons for this limited role are multiple, including:

- Poor rates of adequate control of hypertension, in turn related to its basic nature and the inadequacies of current management.
- Inadequate attention to concomitant risk factors, leaving a large residual of risk even among those treated (Blacher et al., 2004).
- Too high levels of blood pressure both for initiation of therapy and for the goals of therapy

(Ivanovic et al., 2004), in accordance with the fact that risk increases above 115/75 mm Hg.

These issues and others are addressed in the remainder of this chapter and in Chapter 7, but first we will examine one of the more attractive aspects of treating hypertension, namely its cost effectiveness.

## Cost Effectiveness of Treating Hypertension

The treatment of hypertension is among the most cost-effective measures now available for preventing avoidable death. Using various mathematical modeling techniques and Markov decision analyses, most recent estimates find that treatment of hypertension provides additional quality-adjusted life-years (QALYs) for a far lower cost than treatment of dyslipidemia or diabetes. Marshall (2003) estimates that even intensive antihypertensive treatment with a diuretic, β-blocker, and ACEI would cost less than a third of statin therapy. Murray et al. (2003) estimate that, in addition to an overall reduction of dietary sodium, the treatment of hypertension is cost effective and could add 63 million QALYs per year worldwide.

Perhaps the most striking example of the cost-effectiveness of various therapies has been provided by the CDC Diabetes Cost-Effectiveness Group (2002), which estimate these costs of one QALY in type 2 diabetic patients: $41,384 for intensive glycemic control; $51,889 for reduction in serum cholesterol; and a positive + $1,959 for intensive control of hypertension. The reduction in cost reflects the decrease in money spent for care of the various complications provided by intensive control of hypertension.

These cost-effectiveness estimates often assume the use of the least expensive forms of therapy. With the current JNC-7 recommendations to start most patients with a low-dose diuretic and to use other medications as needed for various compelling indications, Fischer and Avorn (2004) project a savings of about $1.2 billion in the United States alone.

Such less expensive choices could obviously save the healthcare system money, but the seemingly insatiable desire of both practitioners and patients to mainly use those brand name products that are so heavily advertised on TV and in print will continue to inflate U.S. drug costs.

Although the use of a polypill containing a statin, three antihypertensives, aspirin, and folic acid to be given to everyone over age 55 and everyone with existing cardiovascular disease (Wald & Law, 2003) may seem far-fetched, the increasing need for inexpensive but effective preventive therapies may bring such a strategy to fruition (Jackson et al., 2005).

### Potential Constraints on Treatment of Hypertension

Such issues of cost-effectiveness may seem remote and almost irrelevant to those who care for hypertensive patients. However, there are three reasons for everyone to pay attention to such issues. First, there are unintended risks of continued growth of medical care under the assumption that more is better, particularly in an increasingly fatter and older population (Fisher & Welch, 1999). Second, financial constraints are being imposed everywhere on health care, so that the decision to treat hypertension may need to be based on cost effectiveness. Third, worldwide inequalities in health care are widening and availability of less costly but effective care is essential to overcome these inequalities (Gwatkin et al., 2004).

On the surface, the United States seems to be the exception, as healthcare spending will soon reach $2.2 trillion and, if current trends continue, will consume 25% of the gross national product by the year 2030 (Blumenthal, 2001). Even in the United States, however, the need to constrain the growth of the major federally financed Medicare and Medicaid programs is being recognized, particularly with the rapid growth in the number of people older than 65. And although the political will to provide universal healthcare coverage is not likely to develop in the near future, attention must be paid to the 45 million people in the United States who have no health insurance (Woolhandler & Himmelstein, 2002).

As these constraints increase, a collision may occur between the inherent desire to expand the number of hypertensive people under treatment and the societal need to limit healthcare expenditures. The late John Swales (2000), who served in the United Kingdom government for 3 years, wrote of this issue:

> The success of science has created painful dilemmas for health care across the world, whether funded through taxation or private insurance. A gap is opening up between aspiration and affordability. The treatment of hypertension provides an illuminating example of the problems this creates for clinical practice. These lead inevitably to social and political issues.
>
> The continuous gradient of risk associated with blood pressure implies that the benefits of reversing that risk will also be continuous. The lower the blood pressure level at which treatment is recommended, the smaller the probability of the individual benefiting and the greater the number of patients eligible for treatment. There is a continuous, inverse relationship between individual benefit and the total cost of health care. At some point a decision has to be made that the cost of treating a low level of risk is not justified. . . . The final decision concerning treatment clearly cannot be independent of the resources made available for treatment either by governments or private healthcare funders.
>
> Treatment of a hypertensive patient has to take place in the real world of constrained healthcare systems. . . . Excluding the social dimension can lead to serious errors and can weaken the case for more resources to be put into treating disorders such as hypertension. The cost of treating a large proportion of the population may be high, but the cost of not treating hypertension in terms of both hospital and social care is also high. The combined hospital and social care costs of treating stroke in England is four times the cost of managing hypertension, and there is actually a net return to society as a result of treating elderly hypertensives in terms of reduced indirect healthcare costs.

Constraints on the treatment of hypertension should be fairly easily resisted, because such treatment has been shown to be beneficial at costs that are low in comparison to most other therapies. As the demand for evidence-based medicine has grown, the treatment of hypertension stands as one of the prime examples wherein conclusive evidence is available for cost-effectiveness. At the same time, the critical decision as to when to institute therapy has been more rationally defined.

## WHEN SHOULD DRUG THERAPY BE STARTED?

Before addressing the question, "When should drug therapy be started?" one caveat must always be recalled: An initially elevated BP, above 140 mm Hg systolic or 90 mm Hg diastolic, must always be remeasured at least three times over at least 4 weeks to ensure that hypertension is present. Only if the level is very high (>180/110 mm Hg) or if symptomatic target organ damage is present should therapy be begun before the diagnosis is carefully established.

On the other hand, in view of the risks of even "high-normal" BP (Vasan et al., 2001), therapy in the future may be indicated for many more patients even without hypertension as currently defined.

### Problems with Past Guidelines

In the past, guidelines for the institution of therapy have been based solely on the level of BP, giving rise to major irrationalities and inconsistencies. As noted by Jackson et al. (1993),

> This has led to the situation in which a 60 year old woman with a diastolic BP of 100 mm Hg but no other risk factors (her absolute risk of cardiovascular disease is about 10% in 10 years) may meet the criteria for treatment, whereas a 70 year old man with multiple risk factors but a diastolic BP of 95 mm Hg (his absolute risk is about 50% in 10 years) may not. The treatment of these two patients would be expected to reduce the absolute risk in the 60-year-old woman by nearly 3% in 10 years (30% of 10%) but in the 70-year-old man by approximately 17% (30% of 50%).

### Guidelines Using Overall Risk

The situation has recently changed dramatically for the better with widespread acceptance of targeting treatment rationally on absolute cardiovascular risk rather than arbitrarily on certain levels of BP (Jackson et al., 2005). The change has been spurred on by numerous factors, including these:

- The repeated presentation of cardiovascular risk profiles covering the entire adult population from the phenomenally productive Framingham Heart Study (Kannel et al., 2004a; Lloyd-Jones et al., 2004). The Framingham bar graph surely is recognized everywhere (Figure 5–10).
- The presentation of relatively simple, easily used nomograms that translate the concept of risk

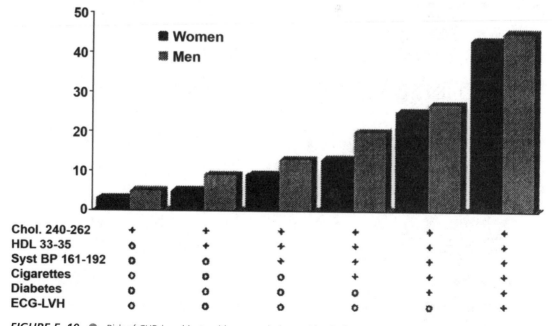

*FIGURE 5–10* ● Risk of CHD in subjects with serum cholesterol level of 240 to 262 mg/dL by level of other risk factors. Subjects were 42 to 43 years old in the Framingham Study. (Modified from Kannel WB, D'Agostino RB, Sullivan L, Wilson PWF. Concept and usefulness of cardiovascular risk profiles. *Am Heart J* 2004a;148:16.)

assessment into a practical method (Jackson, 2000; Jackson et al., 1993; Jackson et al., 2005; Pocock et al., 2001). Increasingly, computers are being used to make the individual patient's overall risk assessment and provide guidance on therapeutic choices.

- The recognition that blind adherence to levels of BP as the criterion for therapy provides many patients no benefit and may actually increase their risk (Hoes et al., 1995).
- The awareness that 90% or more of patients with coronary disease have multiple risk factors with hypertension being first or second in prevalence in various populations (Greenland et al., 2003; Khot et al., 2003).
- The recognition that blood pressure alone is variably related to coronary risk in different parts of the world (van den Hoogen et al., 2000). Addition of other risk factors strengthens the association.

### The New Zealand Recommendations

The New Zealand guidelines recommend that drug therapy be given for those with BP between 150/90 and 170/100 mm Hg if the predicted absolute 5-year risk of cardiovascular disease was 10% or higher from the Framingham data based on age, gender, levels of BP, ratio of total high-density lipoprotein cholesterol, smoking status, and presence of diabetes. The degree of risk can be easily determined

from their graphs, the one for men shown in Figure 5–11. The benefits of lowering BP by the usual 10 to 15 mm Hg systolic and 5 to 8 mm Hg diastolic has been shown for the various risk levels (Table 5–7).

### Problems with Current Assessments

As will be seen, different expert committees have issued national and international guidelines that differ in their modes of assessing risk and the level of risk they use as criteria for treatment. Jackson et al. (2005) summarize most of these risk prediction methods and suggest that the one chosen should be based on a population similar to which it is applied.

To improve the accuracy of risk assessments, addition of testing for microalbuminuria, carotid intima-media thickness by ultrasound, left ventricular mass index by echocardiography and C-reactive protein have been recommended (Viazzi et al., 2004). Only microalbuminuria has been added to recent guidelines; the others are considered too expensive for routine use.

### Current Guidelines

The guidelines from four expert committees published since 2003 have based the decision to start active drug therapy in those with BP of less than 140/90 mm Hg on the degree of overall cardiovascular risk (Table 5–8). The British guidelines (Williams et al., 2004a, 2004b) continue to be more

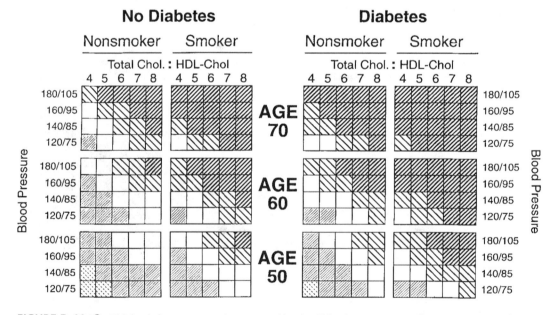

**FIGURE 5–11** ● Risk levels for men at varying ages and levels of blood pressure according to presence or absence of diabetes, smoking, and various levels of the ratio between total and high-density lipoprotein (HDL) cholesterol (chol). Risk of cardiovascular event in 5 years shown by *stippled squares,* 2.5% to 5.0%; *closely hatched squares,* 5% to 10%; *open squares,* 10% to 15%; *widely hatched squares,* 15% to 20%; and *medium hatched squares,* >20%. (Modified from Core Service Committee. *Guidelines for the management of mildly raised blood pressure in New Zealand.* Wellington, New Zealand: National Health Committee, 1995.)

## TABLE 5–7

### Expected Benefits of Treatment at Different Risk Levels

| 5-Year Cardiovascular Risk Level (Based on Framingham) | Cardiovascular Events Prevented/100 Treated for 5 Years[*] | Number Needed to Treat for 5 Years to Prevent 1 Event[*] |
|---|---|---|
| >30% | >10 | <10 |
| 25–30% | 9 | 11 |
| 20–25% | 7.5 | 13 |
| 15–20% | 6 | 16 |
| 10–15% | 5 | 25 |
| 5–10% | 2.5 | 40 |
| 2.5–5% | 1.25 | 80 |
| <2.5% | <0.8 | >120 |

[*]Based on a reduction of 10–15 mm Hg systolic or 5–8 mm Hg diastolic. Modified from Jackson R. Updated New Zealand cardiovascular disease risk-benefit prediction guide. *BMJ* 2000;320:710.

conservative, recommending drug treatment in those with BP between 140–159/90–99 only if there is target organ damage, cardiovascular complications, diabetes, or 10-year risk of cardiovascular disease >20%.

All four guidelines now agree that drug therapy should be started at 140/90 if risk factors or target organ damage is present, and all but the British recommend therapy for patients with diabetes or renal insufficiency at 130/80 (U.S., WHO/ISH) or 130/85 (European).

All but the U.S. JNC-7 continue to use overall risk assessment in determining the threshold to start therapy. The failure of JNC-7 to utilize even a crude profile is inexplicable, so, despite my American pride, the European approach will be detailed (Guidelines Committee, 2003).

As seen in Table 5–9, risk factors, target organ damage, and the presence of overt clinical disease are used to determine the overall degree of risk, using a stratification chart to classify risk from "average" to "very high" as seen in Table 5–10. In turn, the level of risk is used to decide upon the need to begin therapy or to continue to monitor (Figure 5–12).

As the ability to determine cardiovascular risk has become more reliable and accessible, all recommendations for initiation of therapy should be based on a quantitative assessment of risk (Jackson et al., 2005). In their latest review, the New Zealand group ends with this statement:

> A quantitative cardiovascular risk/benefit assessment should be a routine component of quality clinical practice in middle aged and older adults. It is timely for terms such as hypertension and hypercholesterolemia to be removed from our clinical vocabulary and the next generation of clinicians should treat risk not risk factors.

In clinical practice, most hypertensive people will have at least two risk factors, e.g., male gender, age above 55, abdominal obesity, dyslipidemia, etc. (Muntner et al., 2002). Therefore, few paragons of perfect health will be classified at "average" or "low" risk and most will be recommended to receive therapy at or above 140/90.

## TABLE 5–8

### Thresholds for Institution of Drug Therapy in Current Guidelines

| Level of Risk | US JNC-7 (Chobanian, 2003) | WHO-ISH (Writing Group, 2003) | British (Williams et al., 2004a, b) | European (Guidelines Committee, 2003) |
|---|---|---|---|---|
| No target organ damage or risk factors | ≥140/90 | ≥140/90 | ≥160/100 | ≥140/90 |
| With risk factors | ≥140/90 | ≥140/90 | ≥140/90 | |
| With target organ damage | ≥140/90 | ≥140/90 | ≥140/90 | |
| With diabetes or renal insufficiency | ≥130/80 | ≥130/80 | ≥140/90 | ≥130/85 |

JNC, Joint National Committee on Prevention, Detection, Evaluation, and Treatment of High Blood Pressure; WHO/ISH, World Health Organization/International Society of Hypertension.

## TABLE 5–9

### Factors Influencing Prognosis

**Risk Factors for Cardiovascular Disease Used for Stratification**

Levels of systolic and diastolic BP
Men >55 years
Women >65 years
Smoking
Dyslipidemia (total cholesterol >6.5 mmol/l, >250 mg/dl; or LDL-cholesterol >4.0 mmol/l, >144 mg/dl; or HDL-cholesterol M <1.0, W <1.2 mmol/l, M <40, W <48 mmg/dl)
Family history of premature cardiovascular disease (at age M <55 years, W <65 years)
Abdominal obesity (abdominal circumference M ≥102 cm, W ≥88 cm)
C-reactive protein ≥1 mg/dl
Diabetes mellitus (fasting plasma glucose 7.0 mmol/l, 126 mg/dl; postprandial plasma glucose >11.0 mmol/l, 198 mg/dl)

**Target Organ Damage (TOD)**

Left ventricular hypertrophy (electrocardiogram: Sokolow-Lyons >38 cm; Cornell >2,440 mm ms; echocardiogram LVMI M ≥125, W ≥110 g/m$^2$)
Ultrasound evidence of arterial wall thickening (carotid IMT ≥0.9 mm) or atherosclerotic plaque
Slight increase in serum creatinine (M 115–133, W 107–124 μmol/l; M 1.3–1.5, W 1.2–1.4 mg/dl)
Microalbuminuria (30–300 mg/24 h; albumin-creatinine ratio M ≥22, W ≥31 mg/g; M ≥2,5m W ≥ 3.5 mg/mmol)

**Associated Clinical Conditions (ACC)**

Cerebrovascular disease
   Ischemic stroke
   Cerebral hemorrhage
   Transient ischemic attack
Heart disease
   Myocardial infarction
   Angina
   Coronary revascularization
   Congestive heart failure
Renal disease
   Diabetic nephropathy
   Renal impairment (serum creatinine M >133, W >124 μmol/l; M >1.5, W >1.4 mg/dl)
   Proteinuria (>300 mg/24 h)
Peripheral vascular disease
Advanced retinopathy
   Hemorrhages or exudates
   Papilloedema

---

M, men; W, women; LDL, low-density lipoprotein; HDL, high-density lipoprotein; LVMI, left ventricular mass index; IMT, intima-media thickness.
Modified from Guidelines Committee. 2003 European Society of Hypertension-European Society of Cardiology guidelines for the management of arterial hypertension. *J Hypertens* 2003;21:1011–1053.

### Should the Threshold Be Lower?

As seen in Table 5–8, most current guidelines recommend antihypertensive drug therapy for patients with BP below the traditional definition of hypertension of 140/90 if they have a high overall risk status, in particular in patients with diabetes or renal insufficiency. Arguments have been made for a conservative approach to the use of active drug therapy for "mild," low-risk hypertensives. These concerns were delineated by Rose (1981), who wrote:

> In reality the care of the symptomless hypertensive person is preventive medicine, not therapeutics. . . . If a preventive measure exposes many people to a small risk, then the harm it does may readily outweigh the benefits, since these are received by relatively few. . . . We may thus be unable to identify that small level of harm to individuals from long-term intervention that would

## TABLE 5–10

### Stratification of Risk to Quantify Prognosis

| Other Risk Factors and Disease History | Blood Pressure (mm Hg) | | | | |
|---|---|---|---|---|---|
| | Normal SBP 120–129 or DBP 80–84 | High Normal SBP 130–139 or DBP 85–89 | Grade 1 SBP 140–159 or DBP 90–99 | Grade 2 SBP 160–179 or DBP 100–109 | Grade 3 SBP ≥ 180 or DBP ≥ 110 |
| No other risk factors | Average risk | Average risk | Low added risk | Moderate added risk | High added risk |
| 1–2 risk factors | Low added risk | Low added risk | Moderate added risk | Moderate added risk | Very high added risk |
| 3 or more risk factors or TOD or diabetes | Moderate added risk | High added risk | High added risk | High added risk | Very high added risk |
| ACC | High added risk | Very high added risk | Very high added risk | Very high added risk | Very high added risk |

ACC, associated clinical conditions; TOD, target organ damage; SBP, systolic blood pressure; DBP, diastolic blood pressure. Modified from Guidelines Committee. 2003 European Society of Hypertension-European Society of Cardiology guidelines for the management of arterial hypertension. *J Hypertens* 2003;21:1011–1053.

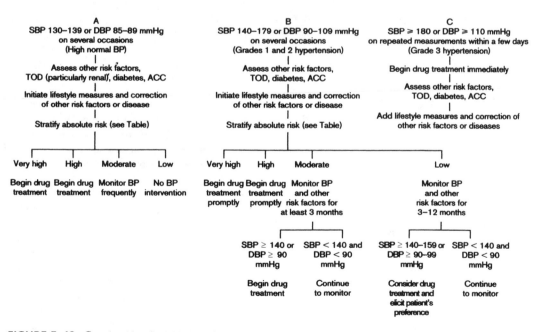

**FIGURE 5–12** ● Algorithm for initiation of antihypertensive treatment from the 2003 European Society of Hypertension-European Society of Cardiology guidelines. Decision based on initial blood pressure levels (A, B, C) and total risk level. BP, blood pressure; SBP, systolic blood pressure; DBP, diastolic blood pressure; TOD, target organ damage; ACC, associated clinical conditions. (Modified from Guidelines Committee. 2003 European Society of Hypertension-European Society of Cardiology guidelines for the management of arterial hypertension. *J Hypertens* 2003;21:1011–1053.)

be sufficient to make that line of prevention unprofitable or even harmful. Consequently we cannot accept long-term mass preventive medication.

Rose's comment was written at a time when adverse effects of antihypertensive drugs were fairly common and their ancillary benefits, as on endothelial function and arterial structure, had not been recognized. As easier to take and more effective drugs have become available, some have argued that they be given to people who are not yet hypertensive in an attempt to prevent both the onset of elevated BP and the vascular damage that may develop before the level goes beyond the 140/90 mm Hg threshold.

Stevo Julius (2000) in particular has argued that drug therapy should be started earlier despite the lack of evidence of benefit, a lack that is attributable to the absence of long-term trials in subjects with BP below 140/90 mm Hg. To provide such evidence, the TROPHY (Trial of Preventing Hypertension) trial was begun in 1999 using an angiotensin II receptor blocker in half of patients whose BP is between 130 and 139 mm Hg systolic and 85 and 89 mm Hg diastolic (Julius et al., 2004).

In support of this position is evidence from the Framingham study that those with such high-normal readings have a significantly increased risk of cardiovascular disease, 2.5 times higher in women and 1.6 times higher in men, compared to those with optimal BP (Vasan et al., 2001). Moreover, in a survey of a representative sample of English adults, 2,413 were found to have high-normal BP, i.e., 130–139/85–89 mm Hg (Yeo & Yeo, 2002). Among these 2,413 people, 12.9% had either overt cardiovascular disease, diabetes, or a 10-year risk of over 20% for cardiovascular event.

Additional aspects of Julius's argument include the unproved and unlikely ability of lifestyle modifications alone to prevent hypertension and the demonstration in spontaneously hypertensive rats that the use of ACEIs before the appearance of hypertension will markedly attenuate if not completely block the expected rise in BP (Harrap et al., 1990; Wu & Berecek, 1993).

## Thresholds for Higher Risk Patients

As seen in Table 5–8, all current guidelines save the British recommend lower thresholds for initiation of drug therapy in patients with diabetes or chronic renal disease (CRD). Such lower thresholds are given unequivocal support, not only in reports from expert committees such as JNC-7 (Chobanian et al., 2003a; 2003b) and the American Diabetes Association (2004) but also by virtually every author of papers addressing the issue over the past 5 years.

The increased risks of hypertensive cardiovascular and renal damage in both diabetic and CRD patients are certain, based on large amounts of observational data (Jafar et al., 2003; Vijan & Hayward, 2003) and experimental evidence (Bidani & Griffin, 2004). But the database for recommending considerably lower blood pressure levels for institution of drug therapy is small and unconvincing: Most of the data supporting the lower threshold that are repeatedly quoted do not, in fact, show what is claimed. In particular:

- For diabetes, the evidence comes from the UKPDS trial (1998) wherein better protection was seen at an achieved BP of 144/82 compared to 154/87 and from the HOT trial (Hansson et al., 1998) wherein better protection was seen at an achieved BP of 140/81 compared to 144/85 mm Hg.
- For CRD, the evidence comes largely from the MDRD trial, wherein better protection was seen *only in those CRD patients with proteinuria* >1.0 g/d but not in those with less proteinuria at an achieved BP of about 125/75 compared to 135/82 (Peterson et al., 1995). Additional studies, though not designed to address the issue of the threshold for therapy, but which provide data on the risk for progression of CRD by levels of achieved blood pressure, found protection below 130 mm Hg only in those with proteinuria greater than 1.0 g/d and no added protection from systolics as high as 160 down to <110 for those with less proteinuria (Jafar et al., 2003) (Figure 5–13).

Furthermore, in the African American Study of Kidney Disease and Hypertension (AASK), no additional benefit for slowing of progression of hypertensive nephrosclerosis was seen with an achieved BP of 128/78 than with an achieved BP of 141/85 (Wright et al., 2002).

The preceding is not intended to deny the value of starting higher-risk patients such as those with CRD or diabetes at lower levels of BP and pushing them to below that level with drug therapy. However, more widespread institution of therapy costs money and can induce side effects. We obviously need more data as noted in JNC-7, which observed that "available data are somewhat sparse to justify the lower target level of 130/80 mm Hg" (Chobanian et al., 2003b). As noted by Vijan and Hayward (2003) in their review of treatment of diabetic hypertensives:

> The current experimental evidence suggests that the diastolic blood pressure goal in patients with type 2 diabetes should be 80 mm Hg. . . .

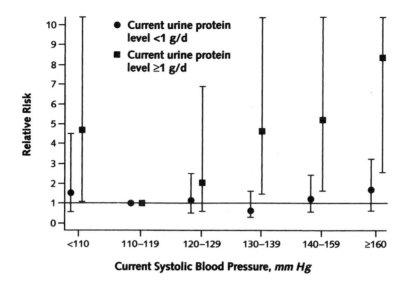

**FIGURE 5–13** ● The relative risk for CRD progression in patients with a current urine protein excretion of 1.0 g/d or greater represents 9,336 patients (223 events), and the relative risk for patients with a current urine excretion less than 1.0 g/d represents 13,274 patients (88 events). The reference group for each is defined at a systolic blood pressure of 110 to 119 mm Hg. Confidence intervals are truncated, as shown. (Modified from Jafar TH, Stark PC, Schmid CH, et al. Progression of chronic kidney disease: the role of blood pressure control, proteinuria, and angiotensin-converting enzyme inhibition: a patient-level meta-analysis. *Ann Intern Med* 2003;139:244–252.)

It may be reasonable to target systolic blood pressures at 135 mm Hg. We could find no evidence from randomized trials supporting the commonly recommended blood pressure goal of less than 130 mm Hg. Indeed, a less stringent goal of 140 mm Hg could be supported given the current evidence.

### Patients with Coronary Artery Disease

On the other hand, the use of a lower threshold even below those now recommended for patients with target organ damage (see Table 5–8) has been supported in an RCT, the CAMELOT study, of over 2,000 patients with preexisting CAD (Nissen et al., 2004). These patients were normotensive, average BP = 129/78. Most were receiving aspirin, β-blockers, a statin, and, for those 60% with prior hypertension, one or more antihypertensive drugs. They were randomly assigned to placebo, amlodipine, or enalapril. After a mean follow-up of 2.2 years, both drugs lowered blood pressure an average of 4.8/2.5 mm Hg. The number of cardiovascular events was significantly reduced (by 31%) but only in those who received the CCB.

As the authors conclude: "These results suggest that the optimal blood pressure range for patients with CAD may be substantially lower than indicated by current guidelines." Obviously, these results may not be applicable to lower-risk patients. Nonetheless, CAD is the most common cardiovascular complication in hypertensives so, even if applicable only to them, these findings deserve attention.

### Overall Management

The bottom line is this: Most hypertensives have fairly mild, asymptomatic hypertension, and the benefits of treatment—measured as the reduction in complications—progressively decline the milder the degree of hypertension. Many patients receive relatively little benefit yet are exposed both to adverse side effects and to the fairly large financial costs of therapy. On the other hand, those at higher degrees of risk likely achieve better protection when treated at lower levels of BP. Therefore, for maximal patient benefit, a management strategy based on overall risk is rational and appropriate. The situation would obviously change if and when the earlier use of antihypertensive drug therapy is shown to prevent the progression of BP and cardiovascular damage in those with BPs lower than the currently accepted lower threshold for institution of therapy.

Now that the rationale for the institution of therapy has been described, let us turn to the issue of how far to lower the pressure.

## GOAL OF THERAPY

Logically, the goal of therapy should be to lower BP below the threshold for starting therapy. Until recently, the general attitude was "the lower, the better." However, a number of factors have led to a more cautious approach, including the following:

- The progressively lower threshold for instituting therapy, previously as high as 160/110 mm Hg, now as low as 130/80 mm Hg for some patients.
- The inclusion of elderly patients with ISH and, by definition, low diastolic BP and the recognition that very low diastolic BP may be associated with increased risk whether occurring naturally or induced by therapy (Boutitie et al., 2002).
- Perhaps most important, concerns over the possible existence of a J-curve for both systolic and diastolic BP, i.e., a reduction in risk as BP is lowered down to some critical level but then an increased risk as the pressure is lowered further.

### Evidence for a J-Curve

An association between reduction of BP and ischemic injury was first suggested by Stewart (1979), who reported a fivefold increase in myocardial infarction among patients whose diastolic BP was reduced to less than 90 mm Hg (Korotkoff, phase 4). Stewart's report was largely neglected until Cruickshank et al. (1987) reported the same phenomenon.

A number of long-term studies in patients with diastolic hypertension have evaluated the incidence of cardiovascular complications according to the mean in-study diastolic BP. Rather than demonstrating a progressive benefit at lower pressures, many of these trials have shown a J-curve in which the risk of cardiac events declines as the diastolic pressure falls from more than 100 mm Hg to 85 mm Hg but then a rise in risk at diastolic pressures below 80 to 85 mg Hg (Farnett et al., 1991; Samuelsson et al., 1990). Kannel et al. (2004b) found an increased risk of cardiovascular disease with diastolic pressures below 80 only in those with elevated systolic BP above 140 mm Hg. On the other hand, in patients with isolated systolic hypertension with a diastolic pressure below 90, an increase in stroke has been retrospectively recognized in those whose diastolic pressures were reduced by therapy to below 65 mm Hg (Somes et al., 1999; Vokó et al., 1999). An even more obvious J-curve of myocardial infarction at lower diastolic BP was seen in the INVEST trial of 22,000 patients with hypertension and coronary disease treated with one of two antihypertensive regimens (Messerli et al., 2005). Compared to the MI rate at diastolic BP between 70 and 90, the rate was doubled at diastolic BP between 60 and 70 and quadrupled at diastolic BP <60.

In addition, apparent J-curves have been reported in the smokers enrolled in the HOT trial (Zanchetti et al., 2003), patients in the IDNT trial of diabetic nephropathy (Pohl et al., 2005), and elderly subjects followed for development of dementia (van Dijk et al., 2004).

### Evidence Against a J-Curve

Cruickshank's concept has not gone unchallenged. In particular, questions have been raised as to the exactness of the critical level at which the break in the curve appears and the relatively few events that make up the curves (Hansson, 2000). Moreover, a decrease in coronary events has been seen in patients with left ventricular dysfunction whose initially low pressures were reduced even further by ACEI therapy, well below the break of 85 to 90 mm Hg in the J-curve (Yusuf et al., 1992) as well as in the patients with CAD starting at a BP of 129/78 (Nissen et al., 2004) who were given a CCB. Fletcher and Bulpitt (1992), in their review of then-available evidence, concluded that "the J-curve is probably a consequence, not a cause of coronary heart disease."

The validity of this interpretation has been strongly supported by the meta-analysis of individual patient data from 40,233 subjects in seven RCTs (Boutitie et al., 2002). Their meticulous analysis is concluded thusly: "The increased risk for events observed in patients with low blood pressure was not related to antihypertensive treatment and was not specific to blood pressure-related events. Poor health conditions leading to low blood pressure and an increased risk for death probably explain the J-curve."

### Recommendations for the Goal of Therapy

The optimal goal of antihypertensive therapy in most patients with combined systolic and diastolic hypertension who were not at high risk is a BP of less than 140/90 mm Hg. The greatest benefit is likely derived from lowering the diastolic pressure to 80 to 85 mm Hg. Not only is there no proven benefit with more intensive control, but also there is added cost and probable increased side effects associated with more intensive antihypertensive therapy.

In elderly patients with ISH, the goal should be a systolic BP of 140 to 145 mm Hg, as that was the level reached in the RCTs wherein benefit was shown. Caution is advised if, inadvertently, diastolic pressures fall below 65 mm Hg. In such an event, less-than-ideal reductions in systolic levels need to be balanced against the potential of harm if diastolic levels fall below that level (Kaplan, 2001).

More intensive therapy to attain a systolic pressure below 140 and/or a diastolic pressure below 90 may be desirable in some groups, including the following:

- Black patients, who are at greater risk for hypertensive complications and who may continue to have progressive renal damage despite a diastolic pressure of 85 to 90 mm Hg.
- Patients with diabetes mellitus, in whom a BP of less than 140/80 mm Hg reduces the incidence of cardiovascular events (Hansson et al., 1998).
- Patients with slowly progressive CRD excreting more than 1 g of protein per day, in whom reducing the BP to 125/75 mm Hg may slow the rate of loss of renal function (Lazarus et al., 1997).
- Patients with coronary disease, if more evidence supports additional benefit of therapy down to a BP of 125/75 (Nissen et al., 2004).

## The Overriding Need: Adequate Therapy

Despite the concerns over a J-curve, we should not lose sight of the fact that the reason for the lesser protection found among most treated hypertensives reflects undertreatment, not overtreatment. Clearly, it is essential that all patients have their systolic BP brought down to 140 mm Hg and their diastolic BP to the 85- to 90-mm Hg range to provide the demonstrated benefits of therapy. The diastolic goal is usually reached, but the systolic is much more difficult to achieve (Mancia & Grassi, 2002).

## Importance of Population Strategies

Most of our current efforts are directed at the individual patient with existing hypertension. Clearly, we also need to advise the larger population to do those things that may protect against the development of hypertension, an approach directed toward "sick populations" rather than only sick individuals. At this time, such population strategies should not involve medications but rather should be based on lifestyle modifications. The next chapter describes these modifications.

## REFERENCES

Adler AI, Stratton IM, Neil HAW, et al. Association of systolic blood pressure with macrovascular and microvascular complications of type 2 diabetes (UKPDS 36). *BMJ* 2000;321:412–419.

Alderman MH, Furberg CD, Kostis JB, et al. Hypertension guidelines: criteria that might make them more clinically useful. *Am J Hypertens* 2002;15:917–923.

Als-Nielsen B, Chen W, Gluud C, Kjaergard LL. Association of funding and conclusions in randomized drug trials: a reflection of treatment effect or adverse effects? *JAMA* 2003;290:921–928.

American Diabetes Association. Hypertension management in adults with diabetes. *Diabetes Care* 2004;27(Suppl 1): S65–S82.

Amery A, Birkenhäger W, Brixko P, et al. Mortality and morbidity from the European Working Party on high blood pressure in the elderly trial. *Lancet* 1985;1:1350–1354.

Avanzini F, Corsetti A, Maglione T, et al. Simple, shared guidelines raise the quality of antihypertensive treatment in routine care. *Am Heart J* 2002;144:726–732.

Barraclough M, Joy MD, MacGregor GA, et al. Control of moderately raised blood pressure. *BMJ* 1973;3:434–436.

Bidani AK, Griffin KA. Pathophysiology of hypertensive renal damage: implications for therapy. *Hypertension* 2004;44:595–601.

Blacher J, Evans A, Arveiler D, et al. Residual coronary risk in men aged 50–59 years treated for hypertension and hyperlipidemia in the population: the PRIME study. *J Hypertens* 2004;22:415–423.

Blood Pressure Lowering Treatment Trialists' Collaboration. Effects of ACE inhibitors, calcium antagonists, and other blood-pressure-lowering drugs: results of prospectively designed overviews of randomised trials. *Lancet* 2000;355:1955–1964.

Blood Pressure Lowering Treatment Trialists' Collaboration. Effects of different blood-pressure-lowering regimens on major cardiovascular events: results of prospectively-designed overviews of randomised trials. *Lancet* 2003; 362:1527–1535.

Blumenthal D. Controlling health care expenditures. *N Engl J Med* 2001;344:766–769.

Bonaccorso S, Smith R. In praise of the "devil." *BMJ* 2003; 326:1220.

Boutitie F, Gueyffier F, Pocock S, et al. J-shaped relationship between blood pressure and mortality in hypertensive patients: new insights from a meta-analysis of individual-patient data. *Ann Intern Med* 2002;136:438–448.

Brenner BM, Cooper ME, de Zeeuw D, et al. Effects of losartan on renal and cardiovascular outcomes in patients with type 2 diabetes and nephropathy. *N Engl J Med* 2001; 345:861–869.

Brewster LM, van Montfrans GA, Kleijnen J. Systematic review: antihypertensive drug therapy in black patients. *Ann Intern Med* 2004;141:614–627.

Bulpitt CJ, Beckett NS, Cooke J, et al. Results of the pilot study for the Hypertension in the Very Elderly Trial. *J Hypertens* 2003;21:2409–2417.

Califf RM, DeMets DL. Principles from clinical trials relevant to clinical practice: part I. *Circulation* 2002; 106:1015–1021.

Campbell NC, Murchie P. Treating hypertension with guidelines in general practice: patients decide how low they can go, not targets. *BMJ* 2004;329:523–524.

Carlberg B, Samuelsson O, Lindholm LH. Atenolol in hypertension: is it a wise choice? *Lancet* 2004;364:1684–1689.

Carter AB. Hypotensive therapy in stroke survivors. *Lancet* 1970;1:485–489.

Cashin-Hemphill L, Holmvang G, Chan R, et al. Angiotensin converting enzyme inhibition as antiatherosclerotic therapy. *Am J Cardiol* 1999;83:43–47.

CDC Diabetes Cost-Effectiveness Group. Cost-effectiveness of intensive glycemic control, intensified hypertension control, and serum cholesterol level reduction for type 2 diabetes. *JAMA* 2002:287:2542–2551.

Chan A-W, Hróbjartsson A, Haahr MT, et al. Empirical evidence for selective reporting of outcomes in randomized trials: comparison of protocols to published articles. *JAMA* 2004;291:2457–2465.

Chaudhry SI, Krumholz HM, Foody JM. Systolic hypertension in older persons. *JAMA* 2004;292:1074–1080.

Chobanian AV. Adaptive and maladaptive responses of the arterial wall to hypertension. *Hypertension* 1990;15:666–674.

Chobanian AV, Bakris GL, Black HR, et al. The seventh report of the Joint National Committee on Prevention, Detection, Evaluation, and Treatment of High Blood Pressure: the JNC-7 report. *JAMA* 2003a;289:2560–2572.

Chobanian AV, Bakris GL, Black HR, et al. Seventh report of the Joint National Committee on Prevention, Detection, Evaluation, and Treatment of High Blood Pressure. *Hypertension* 2003b;42:1206–1252.

Chobanian AV, Haudenschild CC, Nickerson C, Hope S. Trandolapril inhibits atherosclerosis in the Watanabe heritable hyperlipidemic rabbit. *Hypertension* 1992;20:473–477.

Collins R, MacMahon S. Blood pressure, antihypertensive drug treatment and the risks of stroke and coronary heart disease. *Br Med Bull* 1994;50:272–298.

Collins R, MacMahon S. Reliable assessment of the effects of treatment on mortality and major morbidity. *Lancet* 2001;357:373–380.

Cook RJ, Sackett DL. The number needed to treat: a clinically useful measure of treatment effect. *BMJ* 1995;310:452–454.

Coope J, Warrender TS. Randomised trial of treatment of hypertension in elderly patients in primary care. *BMJ (Clin Res Ed)* 1986;294(6565):179.

Core Service Committee. *Guidelines for the management of mildly raised blood pressure in New Zealand.* Wellington, New Zealand: National Health Committee, 1995.

Cruickshank JM, Thorp JM, Zacharias FJ. Benefits and potential harm of lowering high blood pressure. *Lancet* 1987;1:581–584.

Curb JD, Pressel SL, Cutler JA, et al. Effect of diuretic-based antihypertensive treatment on cardiovascular disease risk in older diabetic patients with isolated systolic hypertension. *JAMA* 1996;276:1886–1892.

Dahlöf B, Lindholm LH, Hansson L, et al. Morbidity and mortality in the Swedish Trial in Old Patients with Hypertension (STOP-Hypertension). *Lancet* 1991;338:1281–1285.

Demaerschalk BM. Literature-searching strategies to improve the application of evidence-based clinical practice principles to stroke care. *Mayo Clin Proc* 2004;79:1321–1329.

Dunder K, Lind L, Zethelius B, et al. Increase in blood glucose concentration during antihypertensive treatment as a predictor of myocardial infarction: population based cohort study. *BMJ* 2003;326:681–685.

Dutch TIA Trial Study Group. Trial of secondary prevention with atenolol after transient ischemic attack or nondisabling ischemic stroke. *Stroke* 1993;24:543–548.

Eriksson S, Olofsson BO, Webster PO, for the TEST Study Group. Atenolol in secondary prevention after stroke. *Cerebrovasc Dis* 1995;5:21–25.

European Trial on Reduction of Cardiac Events with Perindopril in Stable Coronary Artery Disease Investigators. Efficacy of perindopril in reduction of cardiovascular events among patients with stable coronary artery disease: randomized, double-blind, placebo-controlled, multicentre trial (The EUROPA study). *Lancet* 2003;362:782–788.

Farnett L, Mulrow CD, Linn WD, et al. The J-curve phenomenon and the treatment of hypertension. *JAMA* 1991;265:489–495.

Ferrier KE, Muhlmann MH, Baguet J-P, et al. Intensive cholesterol reduction lowers blood pressure and large artery stiffness in isolated systolic hypertension. *J Am Coll Cardiol* 2002;39:1020–1025.

Fischer MA, Avorn J. Economic implications of evidence-based prescribing for hypertension: can better care cost less? *JAMA* 2004;291:1850–1856.

Fisher ES, Welch HG. Avoiding the unintended consequences of growth in medical care. *JAMA* 1999;281:446–453.

Fletcher AE, Bulpitt CJ. How far should blood pressure be lowered? *N Engl J Med* 1992;326:251–254.

Forette F, Seux M-L, Staessen JA, et al. The prevention of dementia with antihypertensive treatment: new evidence from the Systolic Hypertension in Europe (Syst-Eur) study. *Arch Intern Med* 2002;162:2046–2052.

Freemantle N. Interpreting the results of secondary end points and subgroup analyses in clinical trials: should we lock the crazy aunt in the attic? *BMJ* 2001;322:989–991.

Fretheim A, Williams JW Jr, Oxman AD, Herrin J. The relation between methods and recommendations in clinical practice guidelines for hypertension and hyperlipidemia. *J Fam Prac* 2002;51:963–968.

Gong L, Zhang W, Zhu Y, et al. Shanghai trial of nifedipine in the elderly (STONE). *J Hypertens* 1996;14:1237–1245.

GRADE Working Group. Grading quality of evidence and strength of recommendations. *BMJ* 2004;328:1490–1494.

Greenland P, Knoll MD, Stamler J, et al. Major risk factors as antecedents of fatal and non-fatal coronary heart disease events. *JAMA* 2003;290:891–897.

Gueyffier F, Boutitie F, Boissel J-P, et al. Effect of antihypertensive drug treatment on cardiovascular outcomes in women and men. *Ann Intern Med* 1997;126:761–767.

Gueyffier F, Bulpitt C, Boissel J-P, et al. Antihypertensive drugs in very old people. *Lancet* 1999;353:793–796.

Guidelines Committee. 2003 European Society of Hypertension-European Society of Cardiology guidelines for the management of arterial hypertension. *J Hypertens* 2003;21:1011–1053.

Guyatt G, Cook D, Haynes B. Evidence based medicine has come a long way: the second decade will be as exciting as the first. *BMJ* 2004;329:990–991.

Gwatkin DR, Bhuiya A, Victora CG. Making health systems more equitable. *Lancet* 2004;364:1273–1280.

Hamilton M, Thompson EN, Wisniewski TKM. The role of blood-pressure control in preventing complications of hypertension. *Lancet* 1964;1:235–238.

Hansson L. Antihypertensive treatment: does the J-curve exist? *Cardiovasc Drugs Ther* 2000;14:367–372.

Hansson L, Zanchetti A, Carruthers SG, et al. Effects of intensive blood-pressure lowering and low-dose aspirin in patients with hypertension. *Lancet* 1998;351:1755–1762.

Harrap SB, Van der Merwe WM, Griffin SA, et al. Brief angiotensin converting enzyme inhibitor treatment in young spontaneously hypertensive rats reduces blood pressure long term. *Hypertension* 1990;16:603–614.

Heart Outcomes Prevention Evaluation Study Investigators. Effects of an angiotensin-converting-enzyme inhibitor, ramipril, on cardiovascular events in high-risk patients. *N Engl J Med* 2000a;342:145–153.

Heart Outcomes Prevention Evaluation (HOPE) Study Investigators. Effects of ramipril on cardiovascular and microvascular outcomes in people with diabetes mellitus: results of the HOPE study and MICRO-HOPE substudy. *Lancet* 2000b;355:253–259.

Heart Protection Study Collaborative Group. Effects of cholesterol-lowering with simvastatin on stroke and other major vascular events in 20,536 people with cerebrovascular disease or other high-risk conditions. *Lancet* 2004;363: 757–767.

Heath D, Edwards JE. The pathology of hypertensive pulmonary vascular disease. *Circulation* 1958;18:533–547.

Hegeland A. Treatment of mild hypertension. *Am J Med* 1980;69:725–732.

Hodge JV, McQueen EG, Smirk H. Results of hypotensive therapy in arterial hypertension. *BMJ* 1961;1:1–7.

Hoes AW, Grobbee DE, Lubsen J. Does drug treatment improve survival? *J Hypertens* 1995;13:805–811.

Hollander W, Madoff I, Paddock J, Kirkpatrick B. Aggravation of atherosclerosis by hypertension in a subhuman primate model with coarctation of the aorta. *Circ Res* 1976;38(Suppl 2):631–672.

Hood D, Bjork S, Sannerstedt R, Angervall G. Analysis of mortality and survival in actively treated hypertensive disease. *Acta Med Scand* 1963;174:393–402.

Hypertension Detection and Follow-Up Program Cooperative Group. Five-year findings of the Hypertension Detection and Follow-Up Program. I. Reduction in mortality of persons with high blood pressure, including mild hypertension. *JAMA* 1979;242:2562–2571.

Hypertension-Stroke Cooperative Study Group. Effect of antihypertensive treatment on stroke recurrence. *JAMA* 1974;229:409–418.

Ivanovic B, Cumming ME, Pinkham CA. Relationships between treated hypertension and subsequent mortality in an insured population. *J Insur Med* 2004;36(1):16–26.

Jackson R. Updated New Zealand cardiovascular disease risk-benefit prediction guide. *BMJ* 2000;320:709–710.

Jackson R, Barham P, Biels J, et al. Management of raised blood pressure in New Zealand. *BMJ* 1993;307:107–110.

Jackson R, Lawes CMM, Bennett DA, et al. Treatment with drugs to lower blood pressure and blood cholesterol based on an individual's absolute cardiovascular risk. *Lancet* 2005;365:434–441.

Jafar TH, Stark PC, Schmid CH, et al. Progression of chronic kidney disease: the role of blood pressure control, proteinuria, and angiotensin-converting enzyme inhibition: a patient-level meta-analysis. *Ann Intern Med* 2003;139:244–252.

Julius S. Trials of antihypertensive treatment. *Am J Hypertens* 2000;13:11S–17S.

Julius S, Nesbitt S, Egan B, et al. Trial of preventing hypertension: design and 2-year progress report. *Hypertension* 2004;44:146–151.

Kannel WB, D'Agostino RB, Sullivan L, Wilson PWF. Concept and usefulness of cardiovascular risk profiles. *Am Heart J* 2004a;148:16–26.

Kannel WB, Wilson PWF, Nam B-H, D'Agostino RB. A likely explanation for the J-curve of blood pressure cardiovascular risk. *Am J Cardiol* 2004b;94:380–384.

Kaplan NM. Should new drugs be used without outcome data? *Arch Intern Med* 2001;161:511–512.

Khot UN, Khot MB, Bajzer CT, et al. Prevalence of conventional risk factors in patients with coronary heart disease. *JAMA* 2003;290:898–904.

Klein L, O'Connor CM, Gattis WA, et al. Pharmacologic therapy for patients with chronic heart failure and reduced systolic function: review of trials and practical considerations. *Am J Cardiol* 2003;91(Suppl):18F–40F.

Kuramoto K, Matsushita S, Kuwajima I, Murakami M. Prospective study on the treatment of mild hypertension in the aged. *Jpn Heart J* 1981;22:75–85.

Lauer MS, Topol EJ. Clinical trials: Multiple treatments, multiple end points, and multiple lessons. *JAMA* 2003; 289:2575–2577.

Lawes CMM, Bennett DA, Feigin VL, Rodgers A. Blood pressure and stroke: an overview of published reviews. *Stroke* 2004;35:776–785.

Lazarus JM, Bourgoignie JJ, Buckalew VM, et al. Achievement and safety of a low blood pressure goal in chronic renal disease. *Hypertension* 1997;29:641–650.

Lee VC, Rhew DC, Dylan M, et al. Meta-analysis: angiotensin-receptor blockers in chronic heart failure and high-risk acute myocardial infarction. *Ann Intern Med* 2004;141:693–704.

Leishman AWD. Hypertension—treated and untreated—a study of 400 cases. *BMJ* 1961;1:1–5.

Lever AF, Ramsay LE. Treatment of hypertension in the elderly. *J Hypertens* 1995;13:571–579.

Lewis EJ, Hunsicker LG, Clarke WR, et al. Renoprotective effect of the angiotensin-receptor antagonist irbesartan in patients with nephropathy due to type 2 diabetes. *N Engl J Med* 2001;345:851–860.

Lexchin J, Bero LA, Djulbegovic B, Clark O. Pharmaceutical industry sponsorship and research outcome and quality: systematic review. *BMJ* 2003;326:1167–1176.

Linjer E, Hansson L. Understatement of the true benefits of antihypertensive treatment. *J Hypertens* 1997;15:221–225.

Lithell H, Hansson L, Skoog I, et al. The Study of Cognition and Prognosis in the Elderly (SCOPE): principal results of a randomized double-blind interventional trial. *J Hypertens* 2003;21:875–886.

Liu L, Wang JG, Gong L, et al. Comparison of active treatment and placebo in older Chinese patients with isolated systolic hypertension. *J Hypertens* 1998;16:1823–1829.

Lloyd-Jones DM, Wilson PWF, Larson MG, et al. Framingham risk score and prediction of lifetime risk for coronary heart disease. *Am J Cardiol* 2004;94:20–24.

Lubsen J, Hoes A, Grobbee D. Implications of trial results: the potentially misleading notions of number needed to treat and average duration of life gained. *Lancet* 2000; 346:1757–1759.

MacMahon S, Neal B, Rodgers A, Chalmers J. Commentary: The PROGRESS trial three years later: time for more action, less distraction. *BMJ* 2004;329:970–971.

MacMahon S, Peto R, Cutler J, et al. Blood pressure, stroke, and coronary heart disease. Part 1: prolonged differences in blood pressure. *Lancet* 1990;335:765–774.

MacMahon S, Sharpe N, Gamble G, et al. Randomised, placebo-controlled trial of the angiotensin converting enzyme inhibitor, ramipril, in patients with coronary or other occlusive vascular disease. *J Am Coll Cardiol* 2000; 36:438–443.

Management Committee of the Australian National Blood Pressure Study. The Australian therapeutic trial in mild hypertension. *Lancet* 1980;1:1262–1267.

Mancia G, Grassi G. Systolic and diastolic blood pressure control in antihypertensive drug trials. *J Hypertens* 2002; 20:1461–1464.

Marshall T. Coronary heart disease prevention: insights from modelling incremental cost effectiveness. *BMJ* 2003;327:1264–1267.

McAlister FA, Straus SE, Sackett DL, Altman DG. Analysis and reporting of factorial trials: a systematic review. *JAMA* 2003;289:2545–2553.

Medical Research Council Working Party. MRC trial of treatment of mild hypertension. *BMJ* 1985;291:97–104.

Medical Research Council Working Party. Medical Research Council trial of treatment of hypertension in older adults. *BMJ* 1992;304:405–412.

Messerli FH, Grossman E, Lever AF. Do thiazide diuretics confer specific protection against strokes? *Arch Intern Med* 2003;163:2557–2560.

Messerli FH, Mancia G, Conti R, et al. J-curve in hypertension and coronary artery disease. *Am J Cardiol* 2005;95:160 (Letter to editor).

Miall WE, Chinn S. Blood pressure and ageing. *Clin Sci Mol Med* 1973;45(Suppl):23–33.

Montori VM, Jaeschke R, Schünemann HJ, et al. Users' guide to detecting misleading claims in clinical research reports. *BMJ* 2004;329:1093–1096.

Moriwaki H, Uno H, Nagakane Y, et al. Losartan, an angiotensin II (AT₁) receptor antagonists, preserves cerebral blood flow in hypertensive patients with a history of stroke. *J Human Hypertens* 2004;18:693–699.

Muntner P, He J, Roccella EJ, Whelton PK. The impact of JNC-VI guidelines on treatment recommendations in the U.S. population. *Hypertension* 2002;39:897–902.

Murray CJL, Lauer JA, Hutubessy RCW, et al. Effectiveness and costs of interventions to lower systolic blood pressure and cholesterol: a global and regional analysis on reduction of cardiovascular-disease risk. *Lancet* 2003; 361:717–725.

Murray MD, Lane KA, Gao S, et al. Preservation of cognitive function with antihypertensive medications: a longitudinal analysis of a community-based sample of African Americans. *Arch Intern Med* 2002;162:2090–2096.

NHLBI Working Group on Future Directions in Hypertension Treatment Trials. Major clinical trials of hypertension: what should be done next? *Hypertension* In press, 2005.

Nissen SE, Tuzcu EM, Libby P, et al. Effect of antihypertensive agents on cardiovascular events in patients with coronary disease and normal blood pressure. The CAMELOT Study: a randomized controlled trial. *JAMA* 2004;292:2217–2226.

Oberman A, Lane NE, Harlan WR, et al. Trends in systolic blood pressure in the thousand aviator cohort over a twenty-four-year period. *Circulation* 1967;36:812–822.

PATS Collaborating Group. Post-stroke antihypertensive treatment study: a preliminary result. *Chinese Med J* 1995;108:710–717.

Perry HM Jr, Goldman AI, Lavin MA, et al. Evaluation of drug treatment in mild hypertension. *Ann N Y Acad Sci* 1978;304:267–288.

Perry HM Jr, Smith WM, McDonald RH, et al. Morbidity and mortality in the Systolic Hypertension in the Elderly Program (SHEP) pilot study. *Stroke* 1989;20:4–13.

Peterson JC, Adler S, Burkart JM, et al. Blood pressure control, proteinuria, and the progression of renal disease in the modification of diet in renal disease study. *Ann Intern Med* 1995;123:754–762.

Pitt B, Byington R, Furberg C, et al. Effect of amlodipine on the progression of atherosclerosis and the occurrence of clinical events. *Circulation* 2000;102:1503–1510.

Pocock SJ, Clayton TC, Altman DG. Survival plots of time-to-event outcomes in clinical trials: good practice and pitfalls. *Lancet* 2002;359:1686–1689.

Pocock SJ, McCormack V, Gueyffier F, et al. A score for predicting risk of death from cardiovascular disease in adults with raised blood pressure, based on individual patient data from randomised controlled trials. *BMJ* 2001;323:75–81.

Pohl MA, Blumenthal S, Cordonnier DJ, et al. The independent and additive impact of blood pressure control and angiotensin II receptor blockade on renal outcomes in the Irbesartan Diabetic Nephropathy Trial (IDNT): clinical implications and limitations. *J Am Soc Nephrol* In press, 2005.

Poole-Wilson PA, Lubsen J, Kirwan B-A, et al. Effect of long-acting nifedipine on mortality and cardiovascular morbidity in patients with stable angina requiring treatment (ACTION trial): randomised controlled trial. *Lancet* 2004; 364:849–857.

PROGRESS Collaborative Group. Randomised trial of a perindopril-based blood-pressure-lowering regimen among 6,105 individuals with previous stroke or transient ischaemic attack. *Lancet* 2001;358:1033–1041.

Prospective Studies Collaboration. Age-specific relevance of usual blood pressure to vascular mortality: a meta-analysis of individual data for one million adults in 61 prospective studies. *Lancet* 2002;360:1903–1913.

Psaty BM, Lumly T, Furberg CD, et al. Health outcomes associated with various antihypertensive therapies used as first-line agents: a network meta-analysis. *JAMA* 2003; 289:2534–2544.

Psaty BM, Smith NL, Siscovick DS, et al. Health outcomes associated with antihypertensive therapies used as first-line agents. *JAMA* 1997;277:739–745.

Psaty BM, Weiss NS, Furberg CD. The PROGRESS trial: questions about the effectiveness of angiotensin converting enzyme inhibitors. *Am J Hypertens* 2002;15:472–474.

Raine R, Sanderson C, Hutchings A, et al. An experimental study of determinants of group judgments in clinical guideline development. *Lancet* 2004;364:429–437.

Ramsay LE, Hag IU, Yeo WW, Jackson PR. Interpretation of prospective trials in hypertension. *J Hypertens* 1996;14 (Suppl 5):S187–S194.

Rennie D. CONSORT revised: improving the reporting of randomized trials. *JAMA* 2001;285:2006–2007.

Rose G. Strategy of prevention. *BMJ* 1981;282:1847–1851.

Rothwell PM. External validity of randomised controlled trials: "to whom do the results of this trial apply?" *Lancet* 2005;365:82–93.

Rothwell PM, Mehta Z, Howard SC, et al. From subgroups to individuals: general principles and the example of carotid endarterectomy. Lancet 2005;365:256–265.

Samuelsson OG, Wilhelmesen LW, Pennert KM, et al. The J-shaped relation between coronary heart disease and achieved blood pressure level in treated hypertension. *J Hypertens* 1990;8:547–555.

Sever PS, Dahlöf B, Poulter NR, et al. Prevention of coronary and stroke events with atorvastatin in hypertensive patients who have average or lower-than-average cholesterol concentrations, in the Anglo-Scandinavian Cardiac Outcomes Trial—Lipid-Lowering Arm (ASCOT-LLA): a multicentre randomised controlled trial. *Lancet* 2003;361:1149–1158.

SHEP Cooperative Research Group. Prevention of stroke by antihypertensive drug treatment in older persons with isolated systolic hypertension. *JAMA* 1991;265:3255–3264.

Smith WM. Treatment of mild hypertension. *Hypertension* 1977;25(Suppl 1):I98–I105.

Somes GW, Pahor M, Shorr RI, et al. The role of diastolic blood pressure when treating isolated systolic hypertension. *Arch Intern Med* 1999;159:2004–2009.

Staessen JA, Fagard R, Thijs L, et al. Randomised double-blind comparison of placebo and active treatment for older patients with isolated systolic hypertension. *Lancet* 1997; 350:757–764.

Staessen JA, Gasowski J, Wang JG, et al. Risks of untreated and treated isolated systolic hypertension in the elderly. *Lancet* 2000;355:865–872.

Staessen JA, Wang J-G, Thijs L. Cardiovascular protection and blood pressure reduction. *Lancet* 2001;358:1305–1315.

Staessen JA, Wang J-G, Thijs L. Cardiovascular protection and blood pressure reduction: a quantitative overview updated until 1 March 2003. *J Hypertens* 2003;21:1055–1076.

Steiner JF. Talking about treatment: the language of populations and the language of individuals. *Ann Intern Med* 1999;130:618–622.

Sterne JAC, Egger M, Smith GD. Investigating and dealing with publication and other biases in meta-analysis. *BMJ* 2001;323:101–105.

Stewart IMG. Relation of reduction in pressure to first myocardial infarction in patients receiving treatment for severe hypertension. *Lancet* 1979;1:861–865.

Sutton-Tyrrell K, Wildman R, Newman A, Kuller LH. Extent of cardiovascular risk reduction associated with treatment of isolated systolic hypertension. *Arch Intern Med* 2003;163:2728–2731.

Swales JD. Evidence-based medicine and hypertension. *J Hypertens* 1999;17:1511–1516.

Swales JD. Hypertension in the political arena. *Hypertension* 2000;35:1179–1182.

Taylor AL, Ziesche S, Yancy C, et al. Combination of isosorbide dinitrate and hydralazine in blacks with heart failure. *N Engl J Med* 2004;351:2049–2057.

Teo K, Burton J, Buller C, et al. Long-term effects of cholesterol lowering and angiotensin-converting enzyme inhibition on coronary atherosclerosis. *Circulation* 2000;102:1748–1754.

Thal AP, Grage TB, Vernier RL. Function of the contralateral kidney in renal hypertension due to renal artery stenosis. *Circulation* 1963;27:36–43.

Thompson SG, Higgins JPT. Can meta-analysis help target interventions at individuals most likely to benefit? *Lancet* 2005;365:341–346.

Tunis SR, Stryer DB, Clancy CM. Practical clinical trials: increasing the value of clinical research for decision making in clinical and health policy. *JAMA* 2003;290:1624–1632.

Tuomilehto J, Rastenyte D, Birkenhäger WH, et al. Effects of calcium-channel blockade in older patients with diabetes and systolic hypertension. *N Engl J Med* 1999;340:677–684.

UKPDS Group. Tight blood pressure control and risk of macrovascular and microvascular complications in type 2 diabetes: UKPDS 38. *BMJ* 1998;317:703–713.

Unal B, Critchley JA, Capewell S. Explaining the decline in coronary heart disease mortality in England and Wales between 1981 and 2000. *Circulation* 2004;109:1101–1107.

van den Hoogen PCW, Feskens EJM, Nagelkerke NJD, et al. The relation between blood pressure and mortality due to coronary heart disease among men in different parts of the world. *N Engl J Med* 2000;342:1–8.

van Dijk EJ, Breteler MMB, Schmidt R, et al. The association between blood pressure, hypertension, and cerebral white matter lesions: Cardiovascular Determinants of Dementia study. *Hypertension* 2004;44:625–630.

Vandenbroucke JP. When are observational studies as credible as randomised trials? *Lancet* 2004;363:1728–1731.

Vasan RS, Larson MG, Leip EP, et al. Impact of high-normal blood pressure on the risk of cardiovascular disease. *N Engl J Med* 2001;345:1291–1297.

Veterans Administration Cooperative Study Group on Antihypertensive Agents. Effects of treatment on morbidity in hypertension. *JAMA* 1967;202:1028–1034.

Veterans Administration Cooperative Study Group on Antihypertensive Agents. Effects of treatment on morbidity in hypertension. *JAMA* 1970;213:1143–1152.

Viazzi F. Parodi D, Leoncini G, et al. Optimizing global risk evaluation in primary hypertension: the role of microalbuminuria and cardiovascular ultrasonography. *J Hypertens* 2004;22:907–913.

Vijan S, Hayward RA. Treatment of hypertension in type 2 diabetes mellitus: blood pressure goals, choice of agents, and setting priorities in diabetes care. *Ann Intern Med* 2003;138:593:602.

Vokó Z, Bots ML, Hofman A, et al. J-shaped relation between blood pressure and stroke in treated hypertensives. *Hypertension* 1999;34:1181–1185.

Wald NJ, Law MR. A strategy to reduce cardiovascular disease by more than 80%. *BMJ* 2003;326:1419–1424.

Wang J-G, Staessen JA, Franklin SS, et al. Systolic and diastolic blood pressure lowering as determinants of cardiovascular outcome on antihypertensive drug treatment. *Hypertension* 2005;45:907–913.

Wennberg R, Zimmermann C. The PROGRESS trial three years later: time for a balanced report of effectiveness. *BMJ* 2004;329:968–971.

WHO/ISH Writing Group. 2003 World Health Organization (WHO)/International Society of Hypertension (ISH) statement on management of hypertension. *J Hypertens* 2003;21:1983–1992.

Williams B, Poulter NR, Brown MJ, et al. British Hypertension Society guidelines for hypertension management 2004 (BHS-IV): summary. *BMJ* 2004a;328:634–640.

Williams B, Poulter NR, Brown MJ, et al. Guidelines for management of hypertension: report of the fourth working party of the British Hypertension Society, 2004—BHS IV. *J Human Hypertens* 2004b;18:139–185.

Wong ND, Thakral G, Franklin SS, et al. Preventing heart disease by controlling hypertension: impact of hypertensive subtype, stage, age, and sex. *Am Heart J* 2003; 145:888–895.

Woolhandler S, Himmelstein DU. National health insurance: liberal benefits, conservative spending. *Arch Intern Med* 2002;973–976.

World Health Organization. Protocol for prospective collaborative overviews of major randomized trials of blood-pressure-lowering treatments. *J Hypertens* 1998; 16:127–137.

Wright JT Jr, Bakris G, Greene T, et al. Effect on blood pressure lowering and antihypertensive drug class on progression of hypertensive kidney disease: results from the AASK trial. *JAMA* 2002;288:2421–2431.

Wu JN, Berecek KH. Prevention of genetic hypertension by early treatment of spontaneously hypertensive rats with the angiotensin converting enzyme inhibitor captopril. *Hypertension* 1993;22:139–146.

Yeo KR, Yeo WW. Should we treat high-normal blood pressure? *J Hypertens* 2002;20:2057–2062.

Yusuf S, Pepine CJ, Garces C, et al. Effect of enalapril on myocardial infarction and unstable angina in patients with low ejection fractions. *Lancet* 1992;340:1173–1178.

Zanchetti A, Ruilope LM. Antihypertensive treatment in patients with type-2 diabetes mellitus: what guidance from recent controlled randomized trials? *J Hypertens* 2002;20:2099–2110.

Zanchetti A, Hansson L, Clement D, et al. Benefits and risks of more intensive blood pressure lowering in hypertensive patients of the HOT study with different risk profiles: does a J-shaped curve exist in smokers? *J Hypertens* 2003;21:797–804.

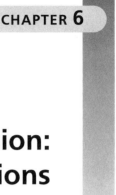

# CHAPTER 6

# Treatment of Hypertension: Lifestyle Modifications

With an appreciation of the benefits and costs of antihypertensive therapy, we now will consider the practical aspects of accomplishing a reduction in blood pressure (BP). In this chapter, *lifestyle modifications*—the term used rather than *nondrug therapies*—will be examined. At the end of this chapter, a number of miscellaneous therapies that are not lifestyle modifications are also covered. The next chapter covers the use of drugs.

Diet is the linchpin of lifestyle. Despite the advocacy of hundreds of diets, and with billions of dollars spent on the search for the ultimate weight loss program, the "ideal diet" for prevention of cardiovascular disease remains uncertain (Chahoud et al., 2004). However, those who consume less red meat, refined grains, and sweets and eat more fruits and vegetables, fish, and whole grains have fewer strokes (Fung et al., 2004). When extra olive oil and wine are added, i.e., the Mediterranean diet, life expectancy is prolonged (Trichopoulou et al., 2005).

These criteria are largely met by the Polymeal, described tongue-in-cheek by its proposers as "a more natural, safer, and probably tastier (than the Polypill) strategy to reduce cardiovascular disease by more than 75%" (Franco et al., 2004). The Polymeal is composed of these ingredients:

- Wine 150 mL/day
- Fish 114 g 4 times/week
- Dark chocolate 100 g/day
- Fruits and vegetables 400 g/day
- Garlic 2.7 g/day
- Almonds 68 g/day

This looks rather difficult, but recall how Atkins took over the world. Who can tell what will replace Atkins now that it is going out of style since it turns out to be no better than any other diet (Dansinger et al., 2005)?

## THE PLACE FOR LIFESTYLE MODIFICATIONS

Lifestyle modifications are recommended to help treat hypertension in all current guidelines by expert committees (Chobanian et al., 2003; Guidelines Committee, 2003; Williams et al., 2004; WHO/ISH Writing Group, 2003). As listed in Table 6–1, the recommendations are virtually identical except for a more liberal consumption of alcohol in the European and British guidelines and a more specific statement about increased fruits and vegetables and reduced fat, the DASH diet, recommended in the JNC-7 report (Chobanian et al., 2003).

### Potential for Prevention

Lifestyle modifications may also prevent hypertension (P. Whelton et al., 2002). The evidence for

## TABLE 6-1

### Lifestyle Modifications for Prevention and Treatment of Hypertension

Maintain normal body weight for adults (body mass index 18.5–24.9 kg/m$^2$)

Reduce dietary sodium intake to no more than 100 mmol per day (approximately 6 g of sodium chloride or 2.4 g of sodium per day)

Engage in regular aerobic physical activity, such as brisk walking, at least 30 minutes per day, most days of the week.

Limit alcohol consumption to no more than 1 oz (30 mL) of ethanol (e.g., 24 oz [720 mL] of beer, 10 oz [300 mL] of wine, or 2 oz [60 mL] of 100-proof whiskey) per day in most men and to no more than 0.5 oz (15 mL) ethanol per day in women and lighter-weight persons

Maintain adequate intake of dietary potassium (>90 mmol [3500 mg] per day)

Consume a diet that is rich in fruits and vegetables and in low-fat dairy products with a reduced content of saturated and total fat (Dietary Approaches to Stop Hypertension [DASH] eating plan)

their preventive potential remains fragmentary, and there is no proof that, individually or in combination, lifestyle modifications will reduce hypertension-induced morbidity and mortality. However, the evidence that such changes will lower BP and reduce other major cardiovascular risk factors is incontrovertible (Appel et al., 2003).

The benefits of a lifestyle that follows the features shown in Table 6–1 have been amply demonstrated in large populations observed over long periods. Examples include the 25% lower mortality rate in those Greek adults who closely adhere to a Mediterranean diet compared to those who do not (Trichopoulou et al., 2003) and the 50% lower mortality rate in European 70- to 90-year-olds who ate the Mediterranean diet, were physically active, drank alcohol in moderation, and did not smoke (Knoops et al., 2004). Another is the 7- to 10-year longer life expectancy for Seventh-Day Adventists who closely adhere to a healthy lifestyle (Fraser & Shavlik, 2001). The ways by which such lifestyle changes reduce mortality include a reduction in inflammatory markers, insulin resistance, and other components of the metabolic syndrome (Esposito et al., 2004b).

There is no doubt that the unhealthy lifestyle of people in most developed societies contributes to our high incidence of hypertension, diabetes, and cardiovascular disease. As noted in the JNC-7 report (Chobanian et al., 2003):

One hundred twenty two million Americans are overweight or obese. Mean sodium intake is approximately 4100 mg per day for men and 2750 mg per day for women, 75% of which comes from processed foods. Fewer than 20% of Americans engage in regular physical activity, and fewer than 25% consume five or more servings of fruits and vegetables daily.

Because the lifetime risk of developing hypertension is very high, a public health strategy that complements the hypertension treatment strategy is warranted. In order to prevent BP levels from rising, primary prevention measures should be introduced to reduce or minimize those causal factors in the population, particularly in individuals with prehypertension. A population approach that decreases the BP level in the general population by even modest amounts has the potential to substantially reduce morbidity and mortality or at least delay the onset of hypertension. . . .

Barriers to prevention include cultural norms: insufficient attention to health education by health care practitioners; lack of reimbursement for health education services; lack of access to places to engage in physical activity; larger servings of food in restaurants; lack of availability of healthy food choices in most schools, worksites, and restaurants; lack of exercise programs in schools; large amounts of sodium added to foods by the food industry and restaurants; and the higher cost of food products that are lower in sodium and calories. Overcoming the barriers will require a multipronged approach directed not only at high-risk populations but also to communities, schools, worksites, and the food industry.

Obviously, removal of these barriers will be difficult and will require major environmental changes, which demand a political advocacy and governmental financing that is sorely lacking. Meanwhile, more focused, smaller attempts have been made to document the ability of lifestyle changes to delay, if not prevent, the development of hypertension. As summarized in Table 6–2, three long-term, well-controlled preventive trials involving subjects with high-normal BP have shown that individual and combined lifestyle modifications lower BP and reduce the incidence of overt hypertension (Hypertension Prevention Trial, 1990; Stamler et al., 1989; Trials of Hypertension Prevention, 1992; 1997).

The effects of multiple lifestyle changes have also been examined in two groups of patients with somewhat higher blood pressures. The Trial of Nonpharmacologic Interventions in the Elderly (TONE) enrolled 975 men and women aged 60 to 80 years whose hypertension was controlled on one

## TABLE 6-2

### Trials of Lifestyle Modifications on the Incidence of Hypertension

| Trial (reference) | No. of subjects | Duration (yr) | Weight loss (kg) | Reduction of incidence (%) |
|---|---|---|---|---|
| Primary prevention trial (Stamler et al., 1989) | 201 | 5 | 2.7 | 54 |
| Hypertension Prevention Trial (Hypertension Prevention Trial Research Group, 1990) | 252 | 3 | 1.6 | 23 |
| Trials of hypertension prevention I (Trials of Hypertension Prevention Collaborative Research Group, 1992) | 564 | 1.5 | 3.9 | 51 |
| II (Trials of Hypertension Prevention Collaborative Research Group, 1997) | 595 | 4.0 | 1.9 | 21 |

antihypertensive drug (Whelton et al., 1998). They were randomly assigned to reduced sodium intake, weight loss, both of these, or no intervention (i.e., usual care). After 3 months, their antihypertensive drug was withdrawn. Over the ensuing 30 months, the proportion of patients who remained normotensive without antihypertensive drugs was only 16% in those on usual care, more than 35% in those on one of the two interventions, and 43.6% in those on both interventions (Figure 6–1). These impressive

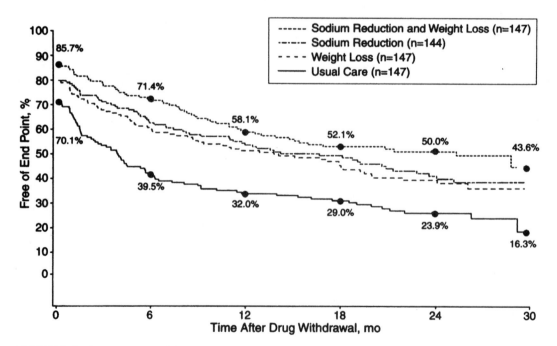

FIGURE 6–1 ● Percentages of the 144 participants assigned to reduced sodium intake, the 147 assigned to weight loss, the 147 assigned to reduced sodium intake and weight loss combined, and the 147 assigned to usual care (no lifestyle intervention) who remained free of cardiovascular events and high blood pressure and in whom no anti-hypertensive agent was prescribed during follow-up. (Modified from Whelton PK, Appel LJ, Espeland MA, et al. Sodium reduction and weight loss in the treatment of hypertension in older persons. *JAMA* 1998;279:839–846.)

effects were achieved with relatively small amounts of dietary sodium reduction (an average of 40 mmol per day) or weight reduction (an average of 4.7 kg).

Another trial involved 412 adults whose average age was 48 years and who had a BP between 120 and 159 mm Hg systolic and 80 to 95 mm Hg diastolic (Sacks et al., 2001). They were randomly given one of two already prepared diets, one typical of the U.S. diet (i.e., control), the other composed of more fruits, vegetables, and low-fat dairy foods [i.e., Dietary Approaches to Stop Hypertension (the DASH diet)]. In addition, they were randomly given one of three levels of sodium intake: high (150 mmol per day), intermediate (100 mmol per day), or low (50 mmol per day).

Each diet was consumed for 30 consecutive days, while weight was kept constant. Figure 6–2 graphically shows significant falls in systolic BP noted with the DASH diet at every level of sodium intake as compared to the control diet as well as significant falls in systolic BP with progressively lower sodium intakes on either diet. The effects were seen in normotensives and hypertensives, men and women, Blacks and non-Blacks, and were accompanied by falls in diastolic BP as well.

As impressive as these results are, they may not be applicable to the "real" world since they were obtained in a short study that was tightly controlled. A more realistic view of what can be expected comes from the PREMIER trial wherein participants were assigned to the DASH diet but prepared their own meals (Appel et al., 2003). Not surprisingly, at the end of 6 months, neither the extent of dietary change nor the reduction in blood pressure was as great as seen in the original DASH trial.

As Pickering (2004) notes:

> Given that healthcare practitioners have limited resources to improve hypertension control, it would seem appropriate to focus on the intervention that has the greatest chance of success; there can be little doubt that drug treatment wins hands down. This conclusion is not intended to negate the importance of lifestyle changes such as the DASH diet, and patients should certainly be encouraged to adopt them, but if behavioral medicine is to progress, practitioners need to find more cost-effective methods for instituting and maintaining behavior change. In the mean time, doctors are still going to need to take out the prescription pad.

## Protection Against Cardiovascular Disease

The larger issue of whether these lifestyle modifications will, in fact, reduce morbidity and mortality in hypertensive patients may never be settled. The difficulty of demonstrating such protection in the various therapeutic trials using much more potent antihypertensive drugs was described in Chapter 5. There is likely no way to document the efficacy of lifestyle modifications, which are less potent and

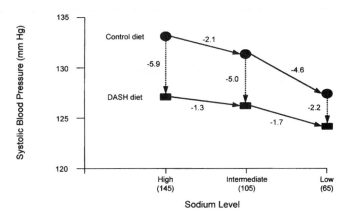

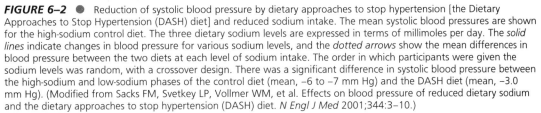

**FIGURE 6–2** ● Reduction of systolic blood pressure by dietary approaches to stop hypertension [the Dietary Approaches to Stop Hypertension (DASH) diet] and reduced sodium intake. The mean systolic blood pressures are shown for the high-sodium control diet. The three dietary sodium levels are expressed in terms of millimoles per day. The *solid lines* indicate changes in blood pressure for various sodium levels, and the *dotted arrows* show the mean differences in blood pressure between the two diets at each level of sodium intake. The order in which participants were given the sodium levels was random, with a crossover design. There was a significant difference in systolic blood pressure between the high-sodium and low-sodium phases of the control diet (mean, –6 to –7 mm Hg) and the DASH diet (mean, –3.0 mm Hg). (Modified from Sacks FM, Svetkey LP, Vollmer WM, et al. Effects on blood pressure of reduced dietary sodium and the dietary approaches to stop hypertension (DASH) diet. *N Engl J Med* 2001;344:3–10.)

more difficult to monitor than is drug treatment (Nicolson et al., 2004). Lifestyle modifications must be accepted on the evidence that they will lower the BP and other risk factors without risk and with a reasonable chance of adoption by most patients.

### The Problem of Individual Therapy

While there is no question that multiple lifestyle changes will lower blood pressure as amply demonstrated in controlled trials, there is another issue that must be recognized—practitioners dealing with individual patients may find much less benefit, despite their best efforts. Only minimal effects may be accomplished even with repeated counseling (Kastarinen et al., 2002) or other interventions (Little et al., 2004) as noted in the PREMIER trial (Appel et al., 2003).

The frustrations were described in a review of lifestyle interventions to prevent type 2 diabetes (Williamson et al., 2004):

> Although lifestyle interventions have great appeal, prescription medications are the intervention of choice in current practice. . . . Pharmaceutical interventions for chronic health conditions are appealing and straightforward. In contrast, even the most highly motivated physicians typically have minimal education or training in lifestyle intervention, and they usually have inadequate access in their practice to the resources needed to support lifestyle intervention. Well-intentional attempts by physicians to practice "lifestyle medicine" with scarce resources can lead to embittered rejection of health promotion.

Nonetheless, lifestyle changes of even a modest degree can reduce the incidence of hypertension (P. Whelton et al., 2002) and lower BPs that are high (Appel et al., 2003). Intensive patient education, motivation, and follow-up may be needed (Fleischmann et al., 2004) but relatively few U.S. practitioners provide such services (Mellen et al., 2004). The same techniques used to improve patient adherence to drug therapy, described in the next chapter, should help with lifestyle change as well. As difficult as it may be, the advice of JNC-7 (Chobanian et al., 2003) should be heeded:

> Adoption of healthy lifestyles by all persons is critical for the prevention of high BP and is an indispensable part of the management of those with hypertension. . . . Lifestyle modifications reduce BP, prevent or delay the incidence of hypertension, enhance antihypertensive drug efficacy, and decrease cardiovascular risk.

The effects of individual lifestyle modifications on hypertension will now be examined.

## AVOIDANCE OF TOBACCO

Smoking cessation is the most effective, immediate way to reduce cardiovascular risk (Doll et al., 2004). However, an effect on BP has not been generally thought to be involved in this risk reduction because chronic smokers as a group have a lower BP than do nonsmokers (Mikkelsen et al., 1997), likely because smokers weigh less than do nonsmokers. In fact, the role of a pressor effect of smoking has likely been missed because of the almost universal practice of having smokers abstain from smoking for some time before measuring their BP, usually because medical facilities are smoke-free. Thus, the significant, immediate, and repetitive pressor effect of smoking has been missed, because it lasts for only 15 to 30 minutes after each cigarette. Only with ambulatory BP monitoring has the major pressor effect of smoking been recognized (Oncken et al., 2001). The use of smokeless tobacco and cigars, if their smoke is inhaled, also may raise BP (Bolinder & de Faire, 1998). This pressor effect must be at least partly responsible for the major increase in strokes and coronary disease among smokers (Doll et al., 2004) as well as for their apparent resistance to antihypertensive therapy (Kawachi et al., 1994).

Thus, hypertensives who use tobacco must be repeatedly and unambiguously told to quit and given assistance in doing so (Lancaster et al., 2000). Nicotine patches may be effective and usually do not raise the BP (Tanus-Santos et al., 2001). Vigorous physical activity will help to prevent the usual gain in weight that occurs with smoking cessation (Chinn et al., 2005). If the patient continues to smoke, any antihypertensive drugs except nonselective β-blockers may attenuate the smoking-induced rise in BP (Pardell et al., 1998).

## WEIGHT REDUCTION

The nature of modern life, with more caloric intake, particularly from fast foods (Pereira et al., 2005), and less physical activity, engenders more obesity, which is now a worldwide epidemic (Eckel et al., 2004). Any degree of weight gain, even to a level that is not defined as overweight, is associated with an increasing incidence of hypertension and, even more strikingly, of type 2 diabetes. In a long-term follow-up of 85,000 nurses, the incidence of hypertension increased threefold and the incidence of diabetes more than sixfold at an initial BMI of 26 as compared to at an initial BMI of 21 (Willett et al., 1999).

Because the maintenance of significant weight loss is so difficult for most who are obese, physicians, patients, and society at large must do more to prevent weight gain, particularly among children (Ebbeling et al., 2002), in whom obesity and the metabolic syndrome are increasing so rapidly (Weiss et al., 2004). Effective health promotion in schools is an obvious way to slow the epidemic of childhood obesity (Hayman et al., 2004).

## Clinical Data

Short-term weight loss usually lowers BP, with an average fall of BP of 1.1/0.9 mm Hg for each kg of weight loss (Neter et al., 2003). The effects of long-term weight loss are less impressive. In studies with a 2-year or longer follow-up, a 10 kg weight loss was accompanied by a 6.0/4.6 mm Hg fall in BP (Aucott et al., 2005). Even less impressive falls in BP have accompanied the massive weight loss usually achieved by bariatric surgery, with better results by gastric bypass than gastroplasty (Livingston, 2005).

A persistent antihypertensive effect of long-term weight loss was seen in the Trials of Hypertension Prevention II study (Stevens et al., 2001), wherein 595 moderately obese subjects with high-normal BP were assigned to an intensive weight-loss program and compared to another 596 subjects who were simply observed. Over the 3-year follow-up, only 13% of the active participants were able to maintain a substantial weight loss of 4.5 kg or more, but, as shown in Figure 6–3, those subjects experienced a significant fall in BP and a 65% lower relative risk for the onset of hypertension as compared to the control group. Even those who did not sustain the weight loss (i.e., the relapse group) had a 25% lower risk for developing hypertension by the end of the 3 years.

## Mechanisms of Antihypertensive Effect

Weight loss likely lowers BP through multiple effects, including the following:

- Improvement in insulin sensitivity (Watkins et al., 2003)
- Decrease in sympathetic nervous system activity
- Decrease in renin-angiotensin-aldosterone activity (Engeli et al., 2005)
- Decrease in plasma leptin levels (Ogawa et al., 2000)
- Reduction of inflammatory cytokines (Ziccardi et al., 2002)
- Reversal of endothelial dysfunction (Perticone et al., 2001)
- Reduction in arterial stiffness (Wildman et al., 2005)

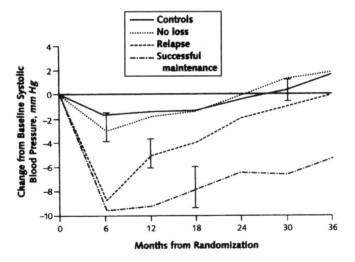

**FIGURE 6–3** ● Long-term changes in weight and systolic blood pressure. Data are adjusted for age, ethnicity, and gender, according to patterns of weight change. Usual-care controls were not assigned to intervention. Participants with successful maintenance of weight loss were defined as those who lost 4.5 kg or more at 6 months and maintained at least 4.5 kg of weight loss at 36 months. Participants with relapse were those who lost at least 4.5 kg at 6 months but whose weight loss at 36 months was less than 2.5 kg. Participants registered as having no weight loss had weight loss of 2.5 kg or less at 6 and 36 months. Error bars represent 95% confidence intervals. (Modified from Stevens VJ, Obarzanek E, Cook NR, et al. Long-term weight loss and changes in blood pressure: results of the Trials of Hypertension Prevention, phase II. *Ann Intern Med* 2001;134:1–11.)

## Recommendations

A structured, lower-calorie diet, along the lines of the Weight Watchers program (Tsai & Wadden, 2005), should be advised while avoiding "crash" diets and the latest fad of the moment. Although the low-carbohydrate, high-protein and fat diet that is currently popular seems inherently unhealthy, no short-term adverse effects on blood lipids, glucose, or insulin or changes in BP were found in a review of multiple studies (Bravata et al., 2003).

The ability to lose weight is greatly enhanced by an accompanying regularly performed program of physical activity (Jakicic et al., 1999), and both are strong and independent protectors against death (F. Hu et al., 2004). It takes a fairly vigorous exercise to overcome the decline in resting metabolic rate that occurs during dieting (Geliebter et al., 1997). An average of 80 minutes per day of moderate activity or 35 minutes per day of vigorous activity is needed to prevent weight gain after successful weight loss (Schoeller et al., 1997).

Among currently available drug therapies, orlistat does not raise BP (Aucott et al., 2005), but appetite suppressants such as sibutramine should be used only in concert with diet and exercise because, by themselves, they may raise BP (Arterburn et al., 2004). No effect on BP was seen with the cannabinoid-1 receptor blocker rimonabant despite a 10 kg weight loss (Van Gaal et al., 2005).

In view of the limited success of medical regimens in those with marked obesity (Norris et al., 2004), bariatric surgery is being increasingly performed with significant weight loss in more than 90% of patients but with only modest effects on BP (Sjöström et al., 2004).

## DIETARY SODIUM REDUCTION

Rigid restriction of dietary sodium intake was one of the first effective therapies for hypertension (Kempner, 1948). However, after thiazides were introduced during the late 1950s and their mode of action was shown to involve a mild state of sodium depletion, both physicians and patients eagerly adopted this form of therapy in place of dietary sodium reduction. In discarding rigid salt restriction, physicians disregarded the benefits of modest reduction both for its inherent antihypertensive effect and for its potential of reducing diuretic-induced potassium loss. Moreover, the amount of sodium chloride ingested by some patients—15 to 20 g per day—may completely overcome the antihypertensive effectiveness of diuretics (Winer, 1961).

## General Recommendations

Moderate sodium reduction to a level of 2.4 g per day (6 g NaCl per day, 100 mmol per day) for both prevention and treatment of hypertension has been included in all of the recent guidelines from expert committees (Chobanian et al., 2003; Guidelines Committee, 2003; Williams et al., 2004).

These recommendations are based on a large body of data from multiple clinical trials that have been repeatedly analyzed. In general, these analyses show a significant fall in blood pressure that is greater in hypertensives than in normotensives and correlated with the degree of sodium reduction (He & MacGregor, 2003) (Figure 6–4). This analysis was restricted to 26 trials that lasted 4 weeks or longer, but very similar results were found in an analysis of 40 trials that lasted only 2 weeks or longer (Geleijnse et al., 2003) (Table 6–3).

As noted in Table 6–3, both of these meta-analyses reported an average decrease in daily sodium excretion of over 75 mmol/day. However, the third meta-analysis, that of Hooper et al. (2002), was restricted to trials that lasted 6 months or longer, a few for 5 years. In these relatively few trials, the degree of sustained sodium reduction was obviously less and the degree of blood pressure reduction considerably less. In discussing their results, Hooper et al. (2002) comment:

> . . . most of the randomized controlled trials published have been of short duration and can show only that salt reduction is capable of reducing blood pressure but provide no useful information for primary care practice. . . . Is it realistic to ask people to alter their salt intake long term? Advice to reduce dietary salt is common in primary care and is a central part of the guidelines produced by the British Hypertension Society [Williams et al., 2004]. Despite a great deal of ongoing encouragement and support used in the trials included in this review, it seems that salt reduction attenuates over time. In routine primary care the intervention is likely to be less intense and therefore of more limited impact.

Despite this sobering conclusion, the same argument can be made about attempts to get obese people to lose weight or addicted smokers to quit: Most good advice is not readily accepted but the goals seem worth pursuing.

This likely inability to maintain enough dietary sodium reduction to achieve a meaningful effect on blood pressure over a longer period of time has led to a concerted effort to convince food processors to reduce the amount of sodium added to processed foods and drinks, the source of about three-fourths

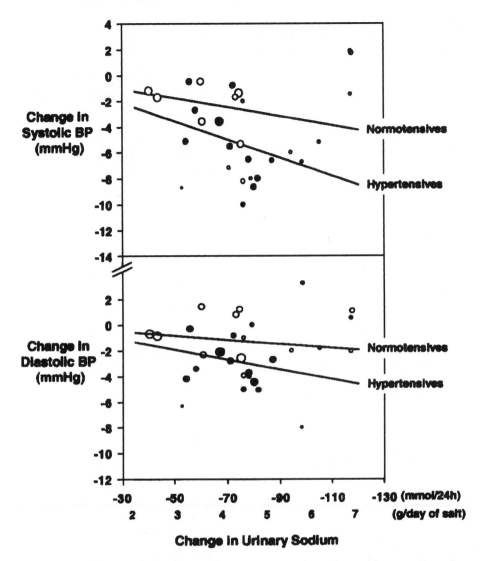

**FIGURE 6–4** ● Relationship between the net change in 24-hour urinary sodium excretion and blood pressure in a meta-analysis of 26 trials. *Open circles*, normotensive. *Solid circles*, hypertensives. The slope is weighted by the inverse of the variance of the net change in blood pressure. The size of the circle is proportional to the weight of the trial. (Modified from He FJ, MacGregor GA. How far should salt intake be reduced? *Hypertension* 2003;42:1093–1099.)

of current sodium consumption (P. Whelton et al., 2002). In the meantime, patients should be advised to read the label on processed products, avoiding those with more than 300 mg per portion. In addition, a number of websites provide advice and recipes for lower sodium diets. These include:

- http://www.saltfree.com
- http://www.geocities.com/NapaValley/7204/ DietingListservRecipeArchive/Indexes/ LowSodium.htm

- http://www.nhlbi.nih.gov/health/public/heart/ hbp/dash/
- http://www.megaheart.com/kit_recipes_index. html
- http://www.ianr.unl.edu/pubs/foods/g916.htm

### Additional Benefits of Sodium Reduction

In addition to lowering BP, other benefits have been observed with moderate sodium reduction, as summarized in Table 6–4.

## TABLE 6-3

### Meta-analyses of Trials of Dietary Sodium Reduction

| Reference | No. of Trials | Duration | Reduction in 24-hour Sodium Excretion | Reduction in Blood Pressure Normotensive syst/dias | Hypertensive syst/dias |
|-----------|---------------|----------|----------------------------------------|---------------------------------------------------|-------------------------|
| Geleijnse et al., 2003 | 40 | >2 wks | −77 mmol | −1.3/−1.1 | −5.2/−3.7 |
| He & MacGregor, 2003 | 26 | >4 wks | −78 mmol | −2.0/−1.0 | −5.0/−2.7 |
| Hooper et al., 2002 | 7 | 6–12 mo | −49 mmol | −2.5/−1.2 | |
| | 4 | 13–60 mo | −35 mmol | −1.1/−0.6 | |

### Enhancement of Efficacy of Antihypertensive Drugs

Moderate sodium reduction clearly increases the antihypertensive efficacy of all classes of antihypertensive drugs, with the possible exception of calcium channel blockers (Chrysant et al., 2000; Morgan et al., 1986). As is noted in Chapter 7, calcium channel blockers have an intrinsic natriuretic effect, which may explain the lesser potentiation with sodium reduction.

## TABLE 6-4

### Additional Benefits of Moderate Sodium Reduction

Enhancement of efficacy of antihypertensive drugs
(Chrysant et al., 2000)

Reduction of diuretic-induced potassium loss
(Crippa et al., 1996)

Regression of left ventricular hypertrophy
(Messerli et al., 1997)

Reduction in proteinuria (Weir, 2004)

Reduction in urine calcium excretion (Sakhaee et al., 1993)

Decrease in osteoporosis (Martini et al., 2000)

Decreased prevalence of stomach cancer
(Joossens et al., 1996)

Decreased mortality from stroke (Nagata et al., 2004)

Decreased prevalence of asthma (Peat, 1996)

Decreased prevalence of cataract (Cumming et al., 2000)

Protection against onset of hypertension
(P. Whelton et al., 2002)

### Protection from Diuretic-Induced Potassium Loss

High levels of dietary sodium make patients more vulnerable to the major side effect of diuretic therapy, potassium loss. The diuretic inhibits sodium reabsorption proximal to that part of the distal convoluted tubule where secretion of potassium is coupled with sodium reabsorption under the influence of aldosterone. When a diuretic is given daily while the patient ingests large amounts of sodium, the initial diuretic-induced sodium depletion shrinks plasma volume, activating renin release and secondarily increasing aldosterone secretion. As the diuretic continues to inhibit sodium reabsorption, more sodium is delivered to this distal site. The increased amounts of aldosterone act to increase sodium reabsorption, thereby increasing potassium secretion, and the potassium is swept into the urine.

With modest sodium reduction, less sodium is delivered to the distal exchange site, and therefore less potassium is swept into the urine. This modest restriction should not further activate the renin-angiotensin-aldosterone mechanism to cause more distal sodium-for-potassium exchange, because that usually occurs only with more rigid sodium restriction. This postulate was confirmed in a test of 12 hypertensive patients who were given one of three diuretics for 4-week intervals while ingesting a diet inclusive of either 72 or 195 mmol per day of sodium (Ram et al., 1981). While on the modestly restricted diet, total body potassium levels fell only half as much. Similar results have been observed with the diuretic indapamide (Crippa et al., 1996).

### Sodium Sensitivity and Cardiovascular Risk

As detailed in Chapter 3, varying degrees of BP sensitivity to varying levels of sodium intake have been documented in both normotensive and hypertensive people. By definition, those who are more sodium-sensitive have a greater fall in BP with dietary sodium reduction (Chrysant et al., 1997). Those who are more sodium-sensitive tend to have less of a nocturnal fall in BP (Suzuki et al., 2000), which may be involved in their amply documented increased risk for cardiovascular (Morimoto et al., 1997) and renal (Bihorac et al., 2000) target organ damage and mortality (Weinberger et al., 2001) as compared to sodium-resistant patients. These findings strengthen the need for sodium reduction to reduce the increased risks that accompany sodium sensitivity.

There seems to be no need to ascertain the individual patient's degree of sodium sensitivity before recommending moderate sodium reduction, particularly as testing may not be reliable or reproducible (Gerdts et al., 1999). Those who respond more to sodium reduction likely are more sodium-sensitive, but there is no harm and, as noted in Table 6–4, there are other potential benefits of moderate sodium reduction in all hypertensives. In view of the proved increased risk of cardiovascular and renal damage from higher sodium intake in hypertensives (du Cailar et al., 2002), all should be encouraged to reduce their levels to the 100 mmol per day goal.

### Additional Benefits

Of the additional benefits of moderate sodium reduction shown in Table 6–4, perhaps the most certain is the reduction in urinary calcium excretion, protecting against renal stones and osteoporosis, whereas the most exciting is the potential for prevention of hypertension, as suggested by the lower BP at age 15 of children who had been on a lower sodium intake as babies (Geleijnse et al., 1997).

### Mechanisms of Antihypertensive Effect

Despite considerable research, the mechanisms by which moderate sodium restriction lowers BP are not well characterized. After 6 months on a 120-mmol per day sodium diet, during which casual BP was reduced by 8/5 mm Hg, cardiac output was slightly reduced but peripheral resistance was not changed (Omvik & Myking, 1995). Others have noted improved large artery compliance (Gates et al., 2004), decreased plasma atrial natriuretic hormone levels (Jula et al., 1992), and improved β-adrenergic responsiveness (Feldman, 1992). The structure and function of the heart and kidneys may be improved after prolonged, moderate

sodium reduction: Left ventricular hypertrophy decreases (Messerli et al., 1997), and glomerular hyperfiltration and proteinuria are reduced (Weir et al., 1995).

The fall in BP tends to be greater in those with low plasma renin levels that rise little during sodium restriction (He et al., 1998). As noted in Chapter 3, the BP sensitivity to sodium tends to be enhanced in hypertensives, Blacks, and older people, all associated with lower renin, so that these patients tend to respond more to sodium reduction (Vollmer et al., 2001; Weinberger, 1996).

## A Dissenting View

However, there are dissenters to the value of such moderate sodium reduction. Their dissent is based on the possibility that such reduction will likely cause hazards that outweigh its benefits. These putative dangers include the following:

- *An increase in myocardial infarction* (Alderman et al., 1995). These data showed an increase in myocardial infarctions (but not strokes) in men (but not women) with the lowest urinary sodium excretion who were followed up for 3.8 years. These data have been faulted because of the small number of events (46 in 2,937 subjects), the failure to ascertain long-term sodium intake, and the likely presence of multiple confounding factors (Cook et al., 1995).
- *An increase in mortality* (Alderman et al., 1998). These data, based on a single-day dietary recall, showed an increased all-cause mortality the lower the sodium intake in a representative sample of 20,729 U.S. adults. These data also have been questioned mainly for the weakness of the measure of sodium intake, resulting in a level so low (30 mmol per day) as to be impossible to achieve in a free-living population; the presence of known and (likely) unknown confounding factors; and the inability to ascertain long-time sodium intake (de Wardener, 1999; Poulter, 1998). Moreover, when these same data were looked at separately for the 6,797 nonobese and the 2,688 obese subjects, highly significant direct associations between increased sodium intake and stroke, coronary heart disease, and cardiovascular and all-cause mortality were found among the obese subjects (He et al., 1999).

Methodologically stronger prospective data from Finland further document the positive correlation between higher sodium intake, ascertained from 24-hour urinary sodium excretion, and the risk of coronary heart disease in men, an association that was independent of other risk factors including BP and also primarily seen in those who were overweight (Tuomilehto et al., 2001).

• *Potentially harmful perturbations in various hormonal, lipid, and physiologic responses* (Graudal et al., 1998). These perturbations have usually been noted only when sodium intake has been severely restricted over short intervals. However, in 11 hypertensive patients given an 80 mmol per day sodium diet, sympathetic nervous system activation and rises in renin and angiotensin were observed (Grassi et al., 2002). Despite these changes, average blood pressure fell from 145/104 to 138/100.

## Conclusions

High sodium intake is harmful (Tuomilehto et al., 2001), and moderate sodium reduction is worthwhile and feasible (Jones, 2004). The reduction of BP possible with a universal reduction in sodium intake of 50 mmol per day down to the recommended level of 100 mmol per day has been estimated to translate into a 22% reduction of the incidence of stroke and a 16% reduction in the incidence of coronary disease (Law, 1997). Such estimates may be valid: Repeated surveys from 1966 to 1986 in Belgium showed a progressive decrease in average sodium intake from 203 to 144 mmol per day; these falls correlated closely with lesser rises in BP with increasing age and decreased stroke mortality in the population (Joossens & Kesteloot, 1991). Such population-wide reductions in sodium intake are likely to both improve health and reduce costs to society (Selmer et al., 2000). The real potential for benefit, with the remote possibility of harm, makes moderate sodium reduction a desirable goal both for the individual hypertensive patient and for the population at large.

## POTASSIUM SUPPLEMENTATION

Many of the benefits of reduced sodium intake could reflect an increased potassium intake, although in the TONE study the antihypertensive effects of the two were independent of each other (Appel et al., 2001). Intracellar potassium levels are lower in hypertensives, and, as the most abundant ion in the cell, it must be a fundamental factor in blood pressure control (Delgado, 2004).

### Clinical Data

He and Whelton (1999) identified 33 randomized, controlled trials of the effect of oral potassium supplementation on BP, 20 in hypertensives. A pooled analysis of the 33 trials found an overall reduction of 4.4/2.5 mm Hg (Figure 6–5). Greater effects were seen in the 28 trials wherein potassium excretion was increased by 20 mmol per day or more and in the 28 trials wherein no antihypertensive drugs were given. Overall, the response was greater in Blacks, the higher the baseline BP and the greater the sodium intake. Another analysis of 27 trials found that an average 44 mmol per day increase in potassium intake provided an average 3.5/2.5 mm Hg fall in BP among hypertensive subjects (Geleijnse et al., 2003).

The potassium supplement in almost all these trials was potassium chloride (KCl), in amounts from 48 to 120 mmol per day. Two randomized, controlled trials found a greater fall in BP after either potassium citrate (Overlack et al., 1995) or potassium bicarbonate (Morris et al., 1995) than equal amounts of KCl. In another trial, potassium citrate was equally as effective as KCl (He et al., 2005). Potassium citrate also prevented the caluresis and bone resorption caused by a high salt intake (Sellmeyer et al., 2002).

Considerable animal experimentation shows multiple mechanisms by which potassium may lower BP (Young & Ma, 1999).

### Protection Against Strokes

Increased potassium intake may protect against strokes. This was suggested by Acheson and Williams (1983) and supported by the finding that an increase in potassium intake of 10 mmol per day was associated with a 40% reduction in stroke mortality among 859 older people (Khaw & Barrett-Connor, 1987). Among men in the Framingham Heart Study, an increased intake of three servings per day of potassium-rich fruits and vegetables was associated with a 22% lesser risk for stroke over a 20-year follow-up (Gillman et al., 1995). In three even larger populations, increased dietary potassium intake was associated with fewer strokes (Ascherio et al., 1998; Bazzano et al., 2001; Fang et al., 2000) and lower all-cause mortality (Tunstall-Pedoe, 1999). These findings are supported by studies that demonstrate protection by high-potassium diets against vascular damage in the brain and kidneys of susceptible rats (Tobian, 1997) and various animal models (Young & Ma, 1999). In addition, KCl supplements diminish

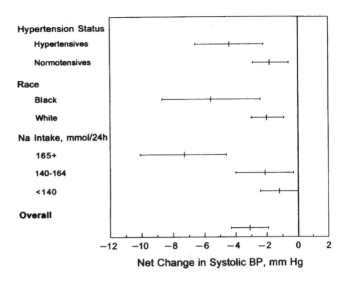

**FIGURE 6–5** ● Pooled net change in systolic BP by participants' characteristics in 33 randomized, controlled trials of potassium supplementation. Na, sodium. (Modified from Jiang H, Whelton PK. What is the role of dietary sodium and potassium in hypertension and target organ injury? *Am J Med Sci* 1999;317:152–159.)

platelet reactivity, a plausible path to stroke prevention (Kimura et al., 2004).

## Recommendations

Even though potassium supplements may lower the BP, they are too costly and potentially hazardous for routine use in the treatment of hypertension in normokalemic patients. They are indicated for diuretic-induced hypokalemia and, in the form of potassium-containing salt substitutes, will add little expense (Coca et al., 2005). For the larger population, a reduction of high-sodium, low-potassium processed foods with an increase of low-sodium, high-potassium natural foods is all that likely is needed to achieve the potential benefits. Fruits and beans provide the largest quantity of potassium per serving.

## CALCIUM SUPPLEMENTATION

There appears to be an inverse relation between dietary calcium intake and BP so that increased dairy consumption could help prevent hypertension as well as osteoporosis (Power et al., 1999). However, both dietary and nondietary calcium supplements have a minimal effect on BP, an effect too small to recommend their use to treat hypertension.

## Clinical Data

Griffith et al. (1999) performed a meta-analysis of 42 randomized, controlled trials of either dietary (dairy) or nondietary supplements of calcium. The pooled analysis found a reduction in BP of –1.44/0.84 mm Hg, with a trend toward larger effects with dietary supplements but with statistically significant heterogeneity of results across trials (Table 6–5). However, as Cappuccio (1999) noted, the dietary trials almost all included other ingredients that could have contributed to an antihypertensive effect. For example, in the DASH trial, calcium intake was increased by 800 mg, but fiber was increased by 240%, potassium by 150%, magnesium by 173%, and protein by 30%. Therefore, the possibility of a greater effect from dietary sources of calcium must be taken with a grain of salt.

Studies in addition to those in Griffith et al.'s (1999) analysis show a very limited effect of 1 to 2 g per day of calcium supplements on BP (Bostick et al., 2000; Reid et al., 2005). Similarly, no effect on BP was seen with 1,200 mg of calcium given to women whose habitual intake was low (Sacks et al., 1998).

## Recommendations

In the absence of data showing a significant effect of calcium supplementation on BP, this approach is not recommended for treatment of hypertension. Moreover, calcium supplements may increase further the hypercalciuria already present in many hypertensives and thereby lead to kidney stones and urinary tract infection (Curhan et al., 1997; Peleg et al., 1992). The best course is to ensure an adequate dietary calcium intake but not to give

## TABLE 6-5

**Summary Estimates Using Random Effects Model of Systolic and Diastolic Blood Pressure in 42 Randomized, Controlled Trials Comparing Calcium Supplementation with Placebo**

| Blood Pressure Type | Mean Change (mm Hg) in Blood Pressure (95% Confidence Interval) |
|---|---|
| All studies (*n* = 42) | |
|    Systolic blood pressure | −1.44 (−2.20, −0.68) |
|    Diastolic blood pressure | −0.84 (−1.44, −0.24) |
| Dietary (*n* = 9) and nondietary (*n* = 33) interventions | |
|    Systolic blood pressure | |
|      Dietary | −2.10 (−2.93, −1.26) |
|      Nondietary | −1.09 (−2.12, −0.06) |
|    Diastolic blood pressure | |
|      Dietary | −1.09 (−1.67, −0.52) |
|      Nondietary | −0.87 (−1.71, −0.03) |

Adapted from Griffith LE, Guyatt GH, Cook RJ, et al. The influence of dietary and nondietary calcium supplementation on blood pressure. *Am J Hypertens* 1999;12:84–92.

calcium supplements to either prevent or treat hypertension.

## MAGNESIUM SUPPLEMENTATION

The advice given for calcium supplements seems to be appropriate in regard to magnesium as well. Serum and intracellular magnesium levels are normal in most untreated hypertensives (Delva et al., 1996). However, low muscle magnesium concentration has been found in half of patients on chronic high-dose diuretic therapy (Drup et al., 1993), and magnesium deficiency usually is responsible when hypokalemia is not corrected by potassium repletion (Whang et al., 1992).

In a meta-analysis of 20 studies, 14 in hypertensives, involving 1,220 subjects, magnesium supplements provided only a 0.6/0.8 mm Hg average fall in blood pressure (Jee et al., 2002). Part of the impressive effects of the DASH diet may reflect its 173% higher magnesium content (Cappuccio, 1999). Therefore, rather than giving magnesium supplements, increasing dietary consumption with fresh fruits and vegetables seems preferable. Magnesium supplements should be given to patients found to be magnesium-deficient. For those patients, 15 mmol per day of magnesium may lower BP, enable potassium to be replenished, and improve glucose metabolism (Paolisso et al., 1992).

## INCREASED PHYSICAL ACTIVITY

At the same time as the evidence for protection from CVD and all-cause mortality by regular physical activity has become incontrovertible (Thompson et al., 2003), most people in all industrialized societies are becoming less physically active in their daily lives, spending more and more time in sedentary activities (Hancox et al., 2004). Not only will increased physical activity and higher levels of exercise capacity reduce mortality (Blair & Church, 2004), but they will likely prevent the development of hypertension. In a prospective 11-year follow-up of over 12,000 Finnish people, the incidence of hypertension was reduced by 28% in men and 35% in women who engaged in high levels of physical activity such as jogging or swimming (Barengo et al., 2005). In addition, regular physical activity during pregnancy reduced the incidence of preeclampsia (Saftlas et al., 2004).

### Clinical Data

Each episode of aerobic (dynamic) exercise is almost always accompanied by a lowering of BP. After each 30-minute period of aerobic exercise at 50% of maximal oxygen uptake, the BP remained lower for the rest of the 24-hour period, with an even greater reduction for the rest of the day after 30 minutes at

75% of maximal uptake (Quinn, 2000). A similar effect is seen in elderly hypertensives (Brandão Rondon et al., 2002) but their systolic BP may not be persistently reduced (Stewart et al., 2005).

Over longer intervals, regular aerobic exercise lowers BP which, in turn, reduces the incidence of stroke (Lee et al., 2003). In a meta-analysis of 54 randomized controlled trials with a total of 2,419 participants, those who performed aerobic exercise had an average 3.8/2.6 mm Hg fall in blood pressure compared to those who remained sedentary (S. Whelton et al., 2002). An even greater reduction, averaging 4.9/3.7 mm Hg, was seen in the hypertensive subjects and with longer intervals of exercise but not with higher intensity. Others have observed maximal effects with only moderate levels of aerobic exercise (Ishikawa-Takata et al., 2003). Although most studies involved aerobic exercise, progressive resistance (static) exercise (i.e., moving against resistance as with Nautilus-type equipment) also lowers BP (Cornelissen & Fagard, 2005) but may have adverse effects on arterial compliance (Miyachi et al., 2004).

Because the systolic BP rises during exercise and because the abrupt rise in BP after arising from sleep is associated with an increased incidence of cardiovascular events, concerns about exercise in the morning have been raised. However, even in patients with known coronary disease, no increase in events was noted with exercise performed in the morning versus the afternoon (Murray et al., 1993). On the other hand, strenuous physical exertion in patients who are habitually sedentary may precipitate an acute myocardial infarction, whereas habitual vigorous exercise reduces the risk of sudden death during exercise (Albert et al., 2000), so patients should always be advised to increase their level of activity slowly. With slowly increasing exercise, an exaggerated rise in BP, as can be seen during stress testing, can be moderated (Ketelhut et al., 2004).

Hypertensives may start with a reduced exercise capacity (Lim et al., 1996) and may experience additional difficulty if they take β-blockers, which blunt exercise-mediated increases in heart rate and cardiac output (Vanhees et al., 2000). Other antihypertensive agents should not interfere with exercise ability (Fahrenbach et al., 1995; Kaplan et al., 2005; Predel et al., 1996).

Concerns may arise about another activity that involves isometric exercise—sexual intercourse, which is accompanied by significant rises in pulse and BP (Nemec et al., 1976) (Table 6–6). The responses in ten healthy young men were essentially the same whether the man was on the top or on the bottom, despite the presumably greater isometric activity with the man-on-the-top position. Although actually quite rare even among patients with coronary disease, the triggering of myocardial infarction during sexual activity likely can be prevented by regular exercise (Muller et al., 1996). Moreover, erectile dysfunction may be overcome by a program of physical activity and weight loss in obese men (Esposito et al., 2004a).

## TABLE 6–6

### Blood Pressure and Pulse Responses During Sexual Intercourse in Ten Normal Men

|  | Rest | Intromission | Orgasm | 2 Min Later |
|---|---|---|---|---|
| Blood pressure (mm Hg) |  |  |  |  |
| Man on top | 112/66 | 148/79 | 163/81 | 118/69 |
| Man on bottom | 113/70 | 143/74 | 161/77 | 121/71 |
| Heart rate (bpm) |  |  |  |  |
| Man on top | 67 | 136 | 189 | 82 |
| Man on bottom | 65 | 125 | 183 | 77 |

*bpm*, beats per minute.

Adapted from Nemec ED, Mansfield L, Kennedy JW. Heart rate and blood pressure responses during sexual activity in normal males. *Am Heart J* 1976;92:274–277.

## Mechanisms of Antihypertensive Effect

Aerobic exercise lowers BP through multiple mechanisms, including the following:

- Increased endothelium-dependent vasodilation through increased production of nitric oxide (Goto et al., 2003)
- Reduced sympathetic nervous activity (Brownley et al., 2003)
- Reduced arterial stiffness (Boreham et al., 2004)
- Increased insulin sensitivity (Watkins et al., 2003)
- Reduced abdominal fat independent of weight loss (Wong et al., 2004)

## Recommendations

Without question, increased levels of physical activity either during ordinary life or with structured exercise will lower BP and prevent the onset of hypertension and diabetes, at least in part, through prevention of obesity (Hu et al., 2003). As little as 30 minutes of walking or its equivalent per day can have a major impact on cardiovascular morbidity (Manson et al., 2002) and mortality (Gregg et al., 2003) as well as slowing the decline in cognitive function in the elderly (Weuve et al., 2004).

Despite the obvious benefits, few physicians counsel their patients about exercise (Mellen et al., 2004), even though counseling has been shown to be effective in increasing patients' level of physical activity (Elley et al., 2003; Estabrooks et al., 2003). Perhaps of all attempts to modify lifestyle, this can have the greatest overall benefit.

## MODERATION OF ALCOHOL

A usual portion of alcohol-containing beverage, i.e., 12 oz of beer, 4 oz of wine, or 1.5 oz of whiskey, contains 10 to 12 ml of alcohol.

## Effects on Blood Pressure

Acutely, drinking 60 g of ethanol, the amount contained in five usual portions, induces an immediate fall in BP averaging 4/4 mm Hg followed, after 6 hours, by a rise averaging 7/4 mm Hg (Rosito et al., 1999). Among healthy normotensive men, daily drinking of 3.5 portions of either red wine or beer for 4 weeks raised daytime BP an average of 3/2 mm Hg (Zilkens et al., 2005). Chronically, the incidence of hypertension is increased among women who drink more than two portions a day (Thadhani et al., 2002) and among men who drink more than three per day (Fuchs et al., 2001). The BP rises during heavy binge drinking (Seppä & Sillanaukee, 1999), and, when heavy drinkers abstain, their BP usually goes down (Xin et al., 2001). An analysis of the relation between the risk of hypertension and the pattern of drinking found a slightly lower incidence among those who drank daily with meals but a 41% increased incidence in those who drank without food (Stranges et al., 2004).

## Beneficial Effects

Impressive evidence supports a protective effect of moderate, regular alcohol consumption of one-half to two portions per day on a host of cardiovascular and other diseases when compared to similar outcomes in nondrinkers or heavy drinkers. Protection has been seen against total mortality (Grønbæk et al., 2000), coronary disease mortality (Malinski et al., 2004), myocardial infarction (Mukamal et al., 2003), ischemic stroke (Djoussé et al., 2002), peripheral vascular disease (Djoussé et al., 2000), renal dysfunction (Schaeffner et al., 2005) incidence of type 2 diabetes (Koppes et al., 2005), osteoporosis (Rapuri et al., 2000), mild cognitive impairment (Anttila et al., 2004), and dementia (Truelsen et al., 2002).

Beneficial effects have been attributed to improvements in the lipid profile, in hemostatic factors, and in insulin sensitivity (Avogaro et al., 2002) and arterial stiffness (van den Elzen et al., 2005).

Wine may be more protective than beer or whiskey (Renaud et al., 2004), but wine drinkers tend to have a healthier lifestyle (Tjønneland et al., 1999), so this apparent benefit may be exaggerated. Although there is a common perception that red wine is more protective than white wine because of its increased levels of polyphenols, there is little evidence to support that conclusion (Vogel, 2003; Zilkens et al., 2005).

However, no mortality benefit is seen in young people and an increased prevalence of breast cancer has been seen in women who drink more than one portion per day (Smith-Warner et al., 1998) and of colon cancer in those who drink more than two portions per day (Cho et al., 2004). Drinking more than two portions per day increases risk for ischemic stroke (Mukamal et al., 2005).

## Recommendations

Beyond the obvious problems of increasing alcohol abuse, which could become more common with any increase in average consumption in the population at large (Colhoun et al., 1997), there seems to be no reason to advise patients, hypertensive or not, who drink in moderation to abstain from alcohol consumption. Whether those who do not drink should be advised of the many benefits observed with moderate drinking and thereby encouraged to begin drinking is a debatable issue. Some would encourage them to do so (Klatsky, 2003; Rimm, 2000); others would not (Goldberg et al., 2003), particularly those younger than 40 (White et al., 2002).

The following guidelines seem appropriate:

- Carefully assess alcohol intake, as some people drink well beyond moderate amounts without being aware of their excessive consumption or its deleterious effects.
- If intake is more than one portion per day in women or two per day in men, advise a reduction to that level.
- Strongly advise against binge drinking.
- Drink only with food intake.
- For most people who consume moderate amounts of alcohol, no change is needed.

## OTHER DIETARY FACTORS

The impressive results of the DASH diet (Figure 6–2) strongly support an antihypertensive effect of a diet low in saturated fat and high in fiber and minerals from fresh fruits and vegetables (Sacks et al., 2001). Moreover, among 1,710 middle-aged men followed up for 7 years, the rise in systolic BP was significantly less with diets higher in fruits and vegetables and lower in red meats (Miura et al., 2004).

Vegetarians tend to have low BP, but the reason for this is unknown. Compared to those eating a nonvegetarian diet, those consuming a vegetarian diet under controlled conditions in nine published studies had a lower blood pressure (Berkow & Barnard, 2005).

### Fiber Intake

One feature of a vegetarian diet is the increased amount of fiber. A meta-analysis of all 24 randomized, placebo-controlled clinical trials published from 1966 to 2003 of the effect on BP of supplements of dietary fiber averaging 11.5 g per day found an average fall of 1.1/1.3 mm Hg (Streppel et al., 2005). The effect was greater in older and hypertensive subjects. In a placebo-controlled trial among 110 untreated hypertensives, 8 g/d of water-soluble fiber from oat bran for 12 weeks was accompanied by a 2.0/1.0 mm Hg lower BP (He et al., 2004b). The benefits found in the DASH diet could reflect the increase in fiber from 9 to 31 g per day (Appel et al., 1997). Moreover, in the 12- to 14-year follow-up of the 75,000 women in the Nurses Health Study, the risk of stroke was significantly reduced by a higher intake of fruits and vegetables (Joshipura et al., 1999) and whole grain foods (Liu et al., 2000). In

addition, a pooled analysis of 10 prospective cohort studies found a decrease in the risk of coronary heart disease with increased consumption of dietary fiber (Pereira et al., 2004).

### Dietary Fat Intake

In keeping with the potential contribution of the low saturated fat content of the DASH diet, other smaller studies have shown a lowering of BP with a low-fat diet (Rantala et al., 1997; Straznicky et al., 1999).

The type of fat may also be important. As a component of the beneficial Mediterranean diet (Trichopoulou et al., 2003; 2005), olive oil may lower BP because of its high content of monounsaturated fatty acids or antioxidant polyphenols (Psaltopoulou et al., 2004). In a crossover trial of 13 hypertensives, 100 g/d of polyphenol-rich dark chocolate for 14 days was associated with a 5.1/1.8 mm Hg average fall in BP compared to the lack of effect of polyphenol-free white chocolate (Taubert et al., 2003).

### Lipid-Lowering Drugs

Beyond any antihypertensive effect, such lower-saturated-fat diets clearly protect against CVD (Mustad & Kris-Etherton, 2000). Both diet and lipid-lowering drugs, in particular statins, improve the endothelial dysfunction associated with dyslipidemia (Balk et al., 2004), which may contribute to both the lower BP (Ikeda et al., 2004) and the protection against atherosclerotic complications including stroke seen with statins (Collins et al., 2004; Sever et al., 2003).

### Fish Oil and Omega-3 Fatty Acids

Both increased fish consumption and fish oil supplements, i.e., omega-3 fatty acids, protect against coronary disease (Din et al., 2004; S. Whelton et al., 2004). The protective effect may involve a lowering of BP: In a total of 22 double-blind trials, an average daily supplement of 4.4 g/d of fish oil was associated with a 1.7/1.5 mm Hg lower BP, the effect being greater in older and hypertensive patients (Geleijnse et al., 2002).

### Protein Intake

Although high protein intake has been thought to be detrimental, in large part by placing an additional load on the kidney (Friedman, 2004), the INTER-SALT data showed a favorable effect: BPs averaged 3.0/2.5 mm Hg lower with a protein intake that was 30% higher than the mean as compared to an intake that was 30% lower than the mean (Stamler et al., 1996). Moreover, in a controlled study of 302 participants, 40 g per day of soybean protein for 8 weeks was associated with a significant fall in ambulatory 24-hour systolic and diastolic BP (He et al., 2004a). However, in the National Health and Nutrition Examination Survey III, increased dietary protein was positively associated with higher systolic BP (Hajjar et al., 2001).

## Antioxidants

Although the antihypertensive effect of a diet rich in fruits and vegetables has been related to the accompanying increase in antioxidant vitamins (John et al., 2002), supplements of Vitamin E have had no effect on BP (Palumbo et al., 2000) and may increase all-cause mortality (Miller et al., 2005). Vitamin C has given variable effects on BP (Svetkey & Loria, 2002).

## Caffeine

Acutely, 250 mg of caffeine, equivalent to three cups of coffee, raises blood pressure an average of 4/3 mm Hg (Hartley et al., 2004). The pressor effect may persist in regular caffeine consumers (Noordzij et al., 2005), but some develop tolerance (Lovallo et al., 2004). No increases in cardiovascular morbidity or mortality have been documented with chronic coffee drinking (Kleemola et al., 2000).

Acutely, three cups of black tea raised the BP in normotensives (Hodgson et al., 2005), but habitual consumption of more than 120 mL per day of green or oolong tea for at least a year was associated with a 46% reduction in the incidence of hypertension (Yang et al., 2004).

In summary, there seems no reason to restrict moderate amounts of caffeine-containing beverage (Myers, 2004).

## MISCELLANEOUS

A large number of complementary and alternative therapies are being used for hypertension among other indications, in part because of dissatisfaction with traditional medical practices (Adams et al., 2002). When such therapies are subjected to appropriately controlled study, they often are found to be ineffectual (Canter, 2003).

## Relaxation

In view of the evidence (more completely reviewed in Chapter 3) that stress-related anxiety and job strain may be involved in the development of hypertension (Esler & Parati, 2004), various stress-relieving techniques to lower BP have been used for many years (Jacobson, 1939). More recently, a variety of cognitive-behavioral therapies—including transcendental meditation, yoga, biofeedback, and psychotherapy—have been shown to reduce the BP of hypertensive patients at least transiently (Barnes et al., 2004; Linden et al., 2001). Although each therapy has its advocates, none has been shown conclusively to be either practical for the majority of hypertensives or effective in maintaining a significant long-term effect (Canter, 2003; Canter & Ernst, 2004).

If available and acceptable to the patient, one or another form of relaxation therapy may be tried, as such techniques may provide additional benefits in reducing coronary risk beyond any effect on BP. Patients should be forewarned that short-term effects may not be maintained, so continued surveillance is needed.

### Slow Breathing

Slow breathing guided by a device has been shown to reduce BP in hypertensives (Meles et al., 2004; Radaelli et al., 2004). Whether this provides more reduction in BP than other relaxation techniques is uncertain.

### Bed Rest and Sedatives

When patients, even those whose disease is difficult to control on an outpatient basis, are hospitalized, their BP frequently comes down, mainly because the sympathetic nervous system becomes less active (Nishimura et al., 1987). This fall in BP may largely reflect the removal of the white-coat effect, as little change has been noted by repeated ambulatory monitoring in hospitalized patients (Fotherby et al., 1995).

The BP usually falls considerably during sleep. However, there is no evidence that sedatives or tranquilizers lower BP (U.S. Public Health Service Cooperative Study, 1965). Monoamine oxidase inhibitors will lower the BP, but their use is limited by the potential for bad pressor reactions with tyramine-containing foods.

### Garlic and Herbal Remedies

*Garlic*, mainly as a deodorized powder, has been found to lower BP in a number of small, poorly controlled trials (Mashour et al., 1998).

*Herbal remedies* are being widely used for all sorts of unproved benefits, totally unsupervised in the United States because of congressional interference with the Food and Drug Administration's surveillance (Goldman, 2001). None has been shown to lower BP (with the obvious exceptions of *Rauwolfia* and *Veratrum*), and some, in fact, will raise BP, including *Ephedra* and licorice extract (De Smet, 2004).

## Other Modalities

*Ultraviolet irradiation* has been claimed to lower BP (Weber et al., 2004). In a controlled study, *acupuncture* was of no benefit (Robinson et al., 2004). *Pet owners* have demonstrated significantly lower systolic BPs and blood lipid levels than non-pet owners, effects not attributable to differences in obvious confounding factors (Anderson et al., 1992). They also have lesser BP rises in response to mental stress (Allen et al., 2001). *Melatonin,* 2.5 mg at bedtime for 3 weeks, was found to reduce nighttime BP by 6/4 mm Hg in a crossover trial in 16 hypertensives (Scheer et al., 2004). High intake of *folate* reduced the incidence of hypertension in the Nurses Health Study (Forman et al., 2005).

## Surgical Procedures

From approximately 1935 through the 1950s, surgical sympathectomy, along with a rigid low-salt diet, was about all that was available for treating hypertension. Sympathectomy was shown to be beneficial for those with severe disease (Thorpe et al., 1950). With current medical therapy, there is no place for sympathectomy.

*Neurovascular decompression* has been used to remove presumed vascular compression of the left ventrolateral medulla since Jannetta et al. (1985) claimed relief of hypertension in 32 of 42 hypertensives by the procedure when it was performed for unrelated cranial nerve dysfunctions. Although hypertension in a few patients with neurologic manifestations of compression of the lateral medulla has been helped by decompression (Salvi et al., 2000), the majority of published series claiming success have been poorly documented and the patients followed up for only a short time (Geiger et al., 1998). Nonetheless, considerable evidence points to heightened sympathetic nervous activity in hypertensives with medullary compression (Schobel et al., 2002; Smith et al., 2004). At the same time, carefully performed magnetic resonance imaging of the brainstem finds neurovascular contact in almost as many normotensives as hypertensives (Hohenbleicher et al., 2002; Thuerl et al., 2001; Žižka et al., 2004).

Patients should not be subjected to decompression in the absence of controlled outcome studies.

## CONCLUSIONS

Appropriate lifestyle modifications should be assiduously promoted in all patients. Those with mild hypertension may thereby be able to stay off drugs; those with more severe hypertension may need less medication. Hopefully, population-wide adoption of healthier lifestyles will reduce the incidence of hypertension. Meanwhile, most hypertensive patients will need antihypertensive drugs as described in the next chapter.

## REFERENCES

Acheson RM, Williams DRR. Does consumption of fruit and vegetables protect against stroke? *Lancet* 1983;1: 1191–1193.

Adams KE, Cohen MH, Eisenberg D, Jonsen AR. Ethical considerations of complementary and alternative medical therapies in conventional medical settings. *Ann Intern Med* 2002;137:660–664.

Albert CM, Mittleman MA, Chae CU, et al. Triggering of sudden death from cardiac disease by vigorous exertion. *N Engl J Med* 2000;343:1355–1361.

Alderman MH, Cohen H, Madhavan S. Dietary sodium intake and mortality: the National Health and Nutrition Examination Survey (NHANES I). *Lancet* 1998;351:781–785.

Alderman MH, Madhavan S, Cohen, et al. Low urinary sodium is associated with greater risk of myocardial infarction among treated hypertensive men. *Hypertension* 1995;25:1144–1152.

Allen K, Shykoff BE, Izzo JL Jr. Pet ownership, but not ACE inhibitor therapy, blunts home blood pressure responses to mental stress. *Hypertension* 2001;38:815–820.

Anderson WP, Reid CM, Jennings GL. Pet ownership and risk factors for cardiovascular disease. *Med J Aust* 1992; 157:298–301.

Anttila T, Helkala E-L, Viitanen M, et al. Alcohol drinking in middle age and subsequent risk of mild cognitive impairment and dementia in old age: a prospective population based study. *BMJ* 2004;329:539–544.

Appel LJ, Champagne CM, Harsha DW, et al. for the Writing Group of the PREMIER Collaborative Research Group. Effects of comprehensive lifestyle modification on blood pressure control: main results of the PREMIER clinical trial. *JAMA* 2003;289:2083–2093.

Appel LJ, Espeland MA, Easter L, et al. Effects of reduced sodium intake on hypertension control in older individuals: results from the Trial of Nonpharmacologic Interventions in the Elderly (TONE). *Arch Intern Med* 2001;161: 685–693.

Appel LJ, Moore TJ, Obarzanek E, et al. A clinical trial of the effects of dietary patterns on blood pressure. *N Engl J Med* 1997; 336:1117–1124.

Arterburn DE, Crane PK, Veenstra DL. The efficacy and safety of sibutramine for weight loss: a systematic review. *Arch Intern Med* 2004;164:994–1003.

Ascherio A, Rimm EB, Hernán MA, et al. Intake of potassium, magnesium, calcium, and fiber and risk of stroke among U.S. men. *Circulation* 1998;98:1198–1204.

Aucott L, Poobalan A, Smith WCS, et al. Effects of weight loss in overweight/obese individuals and long-term hypertension outcomes. *Hypertension* 2005;45:1035–1041.

Avogaro A, Watanabe RM, Gottardo L, et al. Glucose tolerance during moderate alcohol intake: insights on insulin action from glucose/lactate dynamics. *J Clin Endocrinol Metab* 2002;87:1233–1238.

Balk EM, Karas RH, Jordan HS, et al. Effects of statins on vascular structure and function: a systematic review. *Am J Med* 2004;117:775–790.

Barengo NC, Hu G, Kastarinen M, et al. Low physical activity as a predictor of antihypertensive drug treatment in 25–64-year-old populations in Eastern and south-western Finland. *J Hypertens* 2005;23:293–299.

Barnes VA, Treiber FA, Johnson MH. Impact of transcendental meditation on ambulatory blood pressure in African-American adolescents. *Am J Hypertens* 2004;17:366–369.

Bazzano LA, He J, Ogden LG, et al. Dietary potassium intake and risk of stroke in U.S. men and women: National Health and Nutrition Examination Survey I epidemiologic follow-up study. *Stroke* 2001;32:1473–1480.

Berkow SE, Barnard ND. Blood pressure regulation and vegetarian diets. *Nutr Rev* 2005;63:1–8.

Bihorac A, Tezcan H, Özener Ç, et al. Association between salt sensitivity and target organ damage in essential hypertension. *Am J Hypertens* 2000;13:864–872.

Blair SN, Church TS. The fitness, obesity, and health equation: is physical activity the common denominator? *JAMA* 2004;292:1232–1234.

Bolinder G, de Faire U. Ambulatory 24-h blood pressure monitoring in healthy, middle-aged smokeless tobacco users, smokers, and nontobacco users. *Am J Hypertens* 1998;11:1153–1163.

Boreham CA, Ferreira I, Twisk JW, et al. Cardiorespiratory fitness, physical activity, and arterial stiffness; the Northern Ireland Young Hearts Project. *Hypertension* 2004;44:721–726.

Bostick RM, Fosdick L, Grandits GA, et al. Effect of calcium supplementation on serum cholesterol and blood pressure. *Arch Fam Med* 2000;9:31–39.

Brandão Rondon MU, Alves MJ, Braga AM, et al. Postexercise blood pressure reduction in elderly hypertensive patients. *J Am Coll Cardiol* 2002;39:676–682.

Bravata DM, Sanders L, Huang J, et al. Efficacy and safety of low-carbohydrate diets: a systematic review. *JAMA* 2003;289:1837–1850.

Brownley KA, Hinderliter AL, West SG, et al. Sympathoadrenergic mechanisms in reduced hemodynamic stress responses after exercise. *Med Sci Sports Exerc* 2003;35:978–986.

Canter PH. The therapeutic effects of meditation. *BMJ* 2003;326:1049–1050.

Canter PH, Ernst E. Insufficient evidence to conclude whether or not transcendental meditation decreases blood pressure: results of a systematic review of randomized controlled trials. *J Hypertens* 2004;22:2049–2054.

Cappuccio FP. The "calcium antihypertension theory." *Am J Hypertens* 1999;12:93–95.

Chahoud G, Aude YW, Mehta JL. Dietary recommendations in the prevention and treatment of coronary heart disease: do we have the ideal diet yet? *Am J Cardiol* 2004;94:1260–1267.

Chinn S, Jarvis D, Melotti R, et al. Smoking cessation, lung function, and weight gain: a follow-up study. *Lancet* 2005; 365:1629–1635

Cho E, Smith-Warner SA, Ritz J, et al. Alcohol intake and colorectal cancer: a pooled analysis of 8 cohort studies. *Ann Intern Med* 2004;140:603–613.

Chobanian AV, Bakris GL, Black HR, et al. Seventh report of the Joint National Committee on Prevention, Detection, Evaluation, and Treatment of High Blood Pressure. *Hypertension* 2003;42:1206–1252.

Chrysant SG, Weder AB, McCarron DA, et al. Effects of isradipine or enalapril on blood pressure in salt-sensitive hypertensives during low and high dietary salt intake. *Am J Hypertens* 2000;13:1180–1188.

Chrysant SG, Weir MR, Weder AB, et al. There are no racial, age, sex, or weight differences in the effect of salt on blood pressure in salt-sensitive hypertensive patients. *Arch Intern Med* 1997;157:2489–2494.

Coca SG, Perazella MA, Buller GK. The cardiovascular implications of hypokalemia. *Am J Kidney Dis* 2005;45:233–247.

Colhoun H. Ben-Shlomo Y, Dong W, et al. Ecological analysis of collectivity of alcohol consumption in England: importance of average drinker. *BMJ* 1997;314:1164–1168.

Collins R, Armitage J, Parish S, et al. Effects of cholesterol-lowering with simvastatin on stroke and other major vascular events in 20,536 people with cerebrovascular disease or other high-risk conditions. Heart Protection Study Collaborative Group. *Lancet* 2004;363:757–767.

Cook NR, Cutler JA, Hennekens CH. An unexpected result for sodium—causal or casual? *Hypertension* 1995;25:1153–1154.

Cornelissen VA, Fagard RH. Effect of resistance training on resting blood pressure: a meta-analysis of randomized controlled trials. *J Hypertens* 2005;23:251–259.

Crippa G, Nuñez-Ruiz M, Sverzellati E, et al. Dietary sodium curtailment reduces indapamide kaliuretic effect and improves blood pressure control [Abstract]. *Am Soc Hypertens* 1996;9:145A.

Cumming RG, Mitchell P, Smith W. Dietary sodium intake and cataract: the Blue Mountains eye study. *Am J Epidemiol* 2000;151:624–626.

Curhan GC, Willett WC, Speizer FE, et al. Comparison of dietary calcium with supplemental calcium and other nutrients as factors affecting the risk for kidney stones in women. *Ann Intern Med* 1997;126:497–504.

Dansinger ML, Gleason JA, Griffith JL, et al. Comparison of the Atkins, Ornish, Weight Watchers, and Zone diets for weight loss and heart disease risk reduction: a randomized trial. *JAMA* 2005;293:43–53.

De Smet PAGM. Health risks of herbal remedies: an update. *Clin Pharmacol Ther* 2004;76:1–17.

de Wardener HE. Salt reduction and cardiovascular risk: the anatomy of a myth. *J Hum Hypertens* 1999;13:1–4.

Delgado MC. Potassium in hypertension. *Curr Hypertens Rep* 2004;6:31–35.

Delva PT, Pastori C, Degan M, et al. Intralymphocyte free magnesium in a group of subjects with essential hypertension. *Hypertension* 1996;28:433–439.

Din JN, Newby DE, Flapan AD. Omega 3 fatty acids and cardiovascular disease—fishing for a natural treatment. *BMJ* 2004;328:30–35.

Djoussé L, Ellison RC, Beiser A, et al. Alcohol consumption and risk of ischemic stroke: the Framingham Study. *Stroke* 2002;33:907–912.

Djoussé L, Levy D, Murabito JM, et al. Alcohol consumption and risk of intermittent claudication in the Framingham heart study. *Circulation* 2000;102:3092–3097.

Doll R, Peto R, Boreham J, Sutherland I. Mortality in relation to smoking: 50 years' observations on male British doctors. *BMJ* 2004;328:1519–1533.

Drup I, Skajaa K, Thybo NK. Oral magnesium supplementation restores the concentrations of magnesium, potassium and sodium-potassium pumps in skeletal muscle of patients receiving diuretic treatment. *J Int Med* 1993;233: 117–123.

du Cailar G, Ribstein J, Mimran A. Dietary sodium and target organ damage in essential hypertension. *Am J Hypertens* 2002;15:222–229.

Ebbeling CB, Pawlak DB, Ludwig DS. Childhood obesity: public-health crisis, common sense cure. *Lancet* 2002;360: 473–482.

Eckel RH, York DA, Rössner S, et al. Prevention Conference VII: obesity, a worldwide epidemic related to heart disease and stroke executive summary. *Circulation* 2004;110: 2968–2975.

Elley CR, Kerse N, Arroll B, Robinson E. Effectiveness of counselling patients on physical activity in general practice: cluster randomised controlled trial. *BMJ* 2003; 326:793–796.

Engeli S, Böhnke J, Gorzelniak K, et al. Weight loss and the renin-angiotensin-aldosterone system. *Hypertension* 2005; 45:356–362.

Esler M, Parati G. Is essential hypertension sometimes a psychosomatic disorder? *J Hypertens* 2004;22:873–876.

Esposito K, Giugliano F, Di Palo C, et al. Effect of lifestyle changes on erectile dysfunction in obese men: a randomized controlled trial. *JAMA* 2004a;291:2978–2984.

Esposito K, Marfella R, Ciotola M, et al. Effect of a Mediterranean-style diet on endothelial dysfunction and markers of vascular inflammation in the metabolic syndrome: a randomized trial. *JAMA* 2004b;292:1440–1446.

Estabrooks PA, Glasgow RE, Dzewaltowski DA. Physical activity promotion through primary care. *JAMA* 2003; 289:2913–2916.

Fahrenbach MC, Yurgalevitch SM, Zmuda JM, et al. Effect of doxazosin or atenolol on exercise performance in physically active, hypertensive men. *Am J Cardiol* 1995; 75:258–263.

Fang J, Madhavan S, Alderman MH. Dietary potassium intake and stroke mortality. *Stroke* 2000;31:1532–1537.

Feldman RD. A low-sodium diet corrects the defect in β-adrenergic response in older subjects. *Circulation* 1992; 85:612–618.

Fleischmann EH, Friedrich A, Danzer E, et al. Intensive training of patients with hypertension is effective in modifying lifestyle risk factors. *J Hum Hypertens* 2004; 18:127–131.

Forman JP, Rimm E, Stampfer M, Curhan G. Folate intake and the risk of incident hypertension in U.S. women. *JAMA* 2005;293:320–329.

Fotherby MD, Critchley D, Potter JF. Effect of hospitalization on conventional and 24-hour blood pressure. *Age Ageing* 1995;24:25–29.

Franco OH, Bonneux L, de Laet C, et al. The Polymeal: a more natural, safer, and probably tastier (than the Polypill) strategy to reduce cardiovascular disease by more than 75%. *BMJ* 2004;329:1147–1150.

Fraser GE, Shavlik DJ. Ten years of life: is it a matter of choice? *Arch Intern Med* 2001;161:1645–1652.

Friedman AN. High-protein diets: potential effects on the kidney in renal health and disease. *Am J Kidney Dis* 2004;44:950–962.

Fuchs FD, Chambless LE, Whelton PK, et al. Alcohol consumption and the incidence of hypertension: the Atherosclerosis Risk in Communities Study. *Hypertension* 2001;37:1242–1250.

Fung TT, Stampfer MJ, Manson JE, et al. Prospective study of major dietary patterns and stroke risk in women. *Stroke* 2004;35:2014–2019.

Gates PE, Tanaka H, Hiatt WR, Seals DR. Dietary sodium restriction rapidly improves large elastic artery compliance in older adults with systolic hypertension. *Hypertension* 2004;44:35–41.

Geiger H, Naraghi R, Schobel HP, et al. Decrease in blood pressure by ventrolateral medullary decompression in essential hypertension. *Lancet* 1998;352:446–449.

Geleijnse JM, Giltay EJ, Grobbee DE, et al. Blood pressure response to fish oil supplementation: metaregression analysis of randomized trials. *J Hypertens* 2002;20:1493–1499.

Geleijnse JM, Hofman A, Witteman JCM, et al. Long-term effects of neonatal sodium restriction on blood pressure. *Hypertension* 1997;29:913–917.

Geleijnse JM, Kok FJ, Grobbee DE. Blood pressure response to changes in sodium and potassium intake: a metaregression analysis of randomised trials. *J Hum Hypertens* 2003;17: 471–480.

Geliebter A, Maher MM, Gerace L, et al. Effects of strength or aerobic training on body composition, resting metabolic rate, and peak oxygen consumption in obese dieting subjects. *Am J Clin Nutr* 1997;66:557–563.

Gerdts E, Lund-Johansen P, Omvik P. Reproducibility of salt sensitivity testing using a dietary approach in essential hypertension. *J Hum Hypertens* 1999;13:375–384.

Gillman MW, Cupples A, Gagnon D, et al. Protective effect of fruits and vegetables on development of stroke in men. *JAMA* 1995;273:1113–1117.

Goldberg IJ. To drink or not to drink? *N Engl J Med* 2003; 348:163–164.

Goldman P. Herbal medicines today and the roots of modern pharmacology. *Ann Intern Med* 2001;135:594–600.

Goto C, Higashi Y, Kimura M, et al. Effect of different intensities of exercise on endothelium-dependent vasodilation in humans: role of endothelium-dependent nitric oxide and oxidative stress. *Circulation* 2003;108:530–535.

Grassi G, Dell'Oro R, Seravalle G, et al. Short- and long-term neuroadrenergic effects of moderate dietary sodium restriction in essential hypertension. *Circulation* 2002;106: 1957–1961.

Graudal N, Galløe A, Garred P. Effects of sodium restriction on blood pressure, renin, aldosterone, catecholamines, cholesterols, and triglyceride. *JAMA* 1998;279:1383–1391.

Gregg EW, Gerzoff RB, Caspersen CJ, et al. Relationship of walking to mortality among U.S. adults with diabetes. *Arch Intern Med* 2003;163:1440–1447.

Griffith LE, Guyatt GH, Cook RJ, et al. The influence of dietary and nondietary calcium supplementation on blood pressure. *Am J Hypertens* 1999;12:84–92.

Grønbæk M, Becker U, Johansen D, et al. Type of alcohol consumed and mortality from all causes, coronary heart disease, and cancer. *Ann Intern Med* 2000;133:411–419.

Guidelines Committee. 2003 European Society of Hypertension-European Society of Cardiology guidelines for the management of arterial hypertension. *J Hypertens* 2003;21:1011–1053.

Hajjar IM, Grim CE, George V, Kotchen TA. Impact of diet on blood pressure and age-related changes in blood pressure in the U.S. population. *Arch Intern Med* 2001; 161:589–593.

Hancox RJ, Milne BJ, Poulton R. Association between child and adolescent television viewing and adult health: a longitudinal birth cohort study. *Lancet* 2004;364: 257–262.

Hartley TR, Lovallo WR, Whitsett TL. Cardiovascular effects of caffeine in men and women. *Am J Cardiol* 2004; 93:1022–1026.

Hayman LL, Williams CL, Daniels SR, et al. Cardiovascular health promotion in the schools: a statement for health and education professionals and child health advocates from the Committee on Atherosclerosis, Hypertension, and Obesity in Youth (AHOY) of the Council on Cardiovascular Disease in the Young, American Heart Association. *Circulation* 2004;110:2266–2275.

He FJ, MacGregor GA. How far should salt intake be reduced? *Hypertension* 2003;42:1093–1099.

He FJ, Markandu ND, Coltart R, et al. Effect of short-term supplementation of potassium chloride and potassium citrate on blood pressure in hypertensives. *Hypertension* 2005; 45:571–574.

He FJ, Markandu ND, Sagnella GA, MacGregor GA. Importance of the renin system in determining blood pressure fall with salt restriction in black and white hypertensives. *Hypertension* 1998;32:820–824.

He J, Gu D, Duan X, Wu X, et al. Effect of soybean protein on blood pressure: a randomized controlled trial [Abstract]. *Circulation* 2004a;110(Suppl 3):III–778.

He J, Ogden LG, Vupputuri S, et al. Dietary sodium intake and subsequent risk of cardiovascular disease in overweight adults. *JAMA* 1999;282:2027–2034.

He J, Streiffer RH, Muntner P, et al. Effect of dietary fiber intake on blood pressure: a randomized, double-blind, placebo-controlled trial. *J Hypertens* 2004b;22:73–80.

He J, Whelton PK. What is the role of dietary sodium and potassium in hypertension and target organ injury? *Am J Med Sci* 1999;317:152–159.

Hodgson JM, Burke V, Puddey IB. Acute effects of tea on fasting and postprandial vascular function and blood pressure in humans. *J Hypertens* 2005;23:47–54.

Hohenbleicher H, Schmitz SA, Koennecke HC, et al. Neurovascular contact and blood pressure response in young, healthy, normotensive men. *Am J Hypertens* 2002;15(2 Pt 1): 119–124.

Hooper L, Bartlett C, Davey Smith G, Ebrahim S. Systematic review of long term effects of advice to reduce dietary salt in adults. *BMJ* 2002;325:628–632.

Hu FB, Li TY, Colditz GA, et al. Television watching and other sedentary behaviors in relation to risk of obesity and type 2 diabetes mellitus in women. *JAMA* 2003; 289:1785–1791.

Hu FB, Willett WC, Li T, et al. Adiposity as compared with physical activity in predicting mortality among women. *N Engl J Med* 2004;351:2694–2703.

Hu G, Barengo NC, Tuomilehto J, et al. Relationship of physical activity and body mass index to the risk of hypertension: a prospective study in Finland. *Hypertension* 2004;43:25–30.

Hypertension Prevention Trial Research Group. The Hypertension Prevention Trial: three-year effects of dietary changes on blood pressure. *Arch Intern Med* 1990; 150:153–162.

Ikeda T, Sakurai J, Nakayama D, et al. Pravastatin has an additional depressor effect in patients undergoing long-term treatment with antihypertensive drugs. *Am J Hypertens* 2004;17:502–506.

Ishikawa-Takata K, Ohta T, Tanaka H. How much exercise is required to reduce blood pressure in essential hypertensives: a dose-response study. *Am J Hypertens* 2003; 16:629–633.

Jacobson E. Variation of blood pressure with skeletal muscle tension and relaxation. *Ann Intern Med* 1939;12:1194–1212.

Jakicic JM, Winters C, Lang W, Wing RR. Effects of intermittent exercise and use of home exercise equipment on adherence, weight loss, and fitness in overweight women. *JAMA* 1999;282:1554–1560.

Jannetta PJ, Segal R, Wolfson SK. Neurogenic hypertension: etiology and surgical treatment. *Ann Surg* 1985;201: 391–398.

Jee SH, Miller ER 3rd, Guallar E, et al. The effect of magnesium supplementation on blood pressure: a meta-analysis of randomized clinical trials. *Am J Hypertens* 2002;15:691–696.

John JH, Ziebland S, Yudkin P, et al. Effects of fruit and vegetable consumption on plasma antioxidant concentrations and blood pressure: a randomised controlled trial. *Lancet* 2002;359:1969–1974.

Jones DW. Dietary sodium and blood pressure. *Hypertension* 2004;43:932–935.

Joossens JV, Hill MJ, Elliott P, et al. Dietary salt, nitrate and stomach cancer mortality in 24 countries. *Int J Epidemiol* 1996;25:494–504.

Joossens JV, Kesteloot H. Trends in systolic blood pressure, 24-hour sodium excretion, and stroke mortality in the elderly in Belgium. *Am J Med* 1991;90(Suppl 3A):5.

Joshipura KJ, Ascherio A, Manson JE, et al. Fruit and vegetable intake in relation to risk of ischemic stroke. *JAMA* 1999;282:1233–1239.

Jula A, Ronnemaa T, Tikkanen I, Karanko H. Responses of atrial natriuretic factor to long-term sodium restriction in mild to moderate hypertension. *J Intern Med* 1992;231: 521–529.

Kaplan NM, Gidding SS, Pickering TG, Wright JT. Task force 5: systemic hypertension. *JACC* 2005;45:1346–1348.

Kastarinen MJ, Puska PM, Korhonen MH, et al. Nonpharmacological treatment of hypertension in primary health care: a 2-year open randomized controlled trial of lifestyle intervention against hypertension in eastern Finland. *J Hypertens* 2002;20:2505–2512.

Kawachi I, Colditz GA, Stampfer MJ, et al. Smoking cessation and time course of decreased risks of coronary heart disease in middle-aged women. *Arch Intern Med* 1994; 154:169–175.

Kempner W. Treatment of hypertensive vascular disease with rice diet. *Am J Med* 1948;4:545–577.

Ketelhut RG, Franz IW, Scholze J. Regular exercise as an effective approach in antihypertensive therapy. *Med Sci Sports Exerc* 2004;36:4–8.

Khaw K-T, Barrett-Connor E. Dietary potassium and stroke-associated mortality: a 12-year prospective population study. *N Engl J Med* 1987;316:235–240.

Kimura M, Lu X, Skurnick J, et al. Potassium chloride supplementation diminishes platelet reactivity in humans. *Hypertension* 2004;44:969–973.

Klatsky AL. Drink to your health? *Sci Am.* 2003;288:74–81.

Kleemola P, Jousilahti P, Pietinen P, et al. Coffee consumption and the risk of coronary heart disease and death. *Arch Intern Med* 2000;160:3393–3400.

Knoops KTB, de Groot LCPGM, Kromhout D, et al. Mediterranean diet, lifestyle factors, and 10-year mortality in elderly European men and women: the HALE project. *JAMA* 2004;292:1433–1439.

Koppes LLJ, Dekker JM, Hendriks HFJ, et al. Moderate alcohol consumption lowers the risk of type 2 diabetes. *Diabetes Care* 2005;28:719–725.

Lancaster T, Stead L, Silagy C, Sowden A. Effectiveness of interventions to help people stop smoking: findings from the Cochrane Library. *BMJ* 2000;321:355–358.

Law MR. Epidemiologic evidence of salt and blood pressure. *Am J Hypertens* 1997;10:42S–45S.

Lee CD, Folsom AR, Blair SN. Physical activity and stroke risk: a meta-analysis. *Stroke* 2003;34:2475–2482.

Lim PO, MacFadyen RJ, Clarkson PBM, MacDonald TM. Impaired exercise tolerance in hypertensive patients. *Ann Intern Med* 1996;124:41–55.

Linden W, Lenz JW, Con AH. Individualized stress management for primary hypertension: a randomized trial. *Arch Intern Med* 2001;161:1071–1080.

Little P, Kelly J, Barnett J, et al. Randomized controlled factorial trial of dietary advice for patients with a single high blood pressure reading in primary care. *BMJ* 2004;328:1054–1058.

Liu S, Manson JE, Stampfer MJ, et al. Whole grain consumption and risk of ischemic stroke in women: a prospective study. *JAMA* 2000;284:1534–1540.

Livingston E. Treating obesity-related hypertension with surgery. *Am J Hypertens* 2005;18:443–445.

Lovallo WR, Wilson MF, Vincent AS, et al. Blood pressure response to caffeine shows incomplete tolerance after short-term regular consumption. *Hypertension* 2004;43:760–765.

Malinski MK, Sesso HD, Lopez-Jimenez F, et al. Alcohol consumption and cardiovascular disease mortality in hypertensive men. *Arch Intern Med* 2004;164:623–628.

Manson JE, Greenland P, LaCroix AZ, et al. Walking compared with vigorous exercise for the prevention of cardiovascular events in women. *N Engl J Med* 2002;347:716–725.

Martini LA, Cuppari L, Colugnati FAB, et al. High sodium chloride intake is associated with low bone density in calcium stone-forming patients. *Clin Nephrol* 2000; 54:85–93.

Mashour NH, Lin GI, Frishman WH. Herbal medicine for the treatment of cardiovascular disease. *Arch Intern Med* 1998;158:2225–2234.

Meles E, Giannattasio C, Failla M, et al. Nonpharmacologic treatment of hypertension by respiratory exercise in the home setting. *Am J Hypertens* 2004;17:370–374.

Mellen PB, Palla SL, Goff DC, Bonds DE. Prevalence of nutrition and exercise counseling for patients with hypertension: United States, 1999 to 2000. *J Gen Intern Med* 2004;19:917–924.

Messerli FH, Schmieder RE, Weir MR. Salt: a perpetrator of hypertensive target organ disease? *Arch Intern Med* 1997;157:2449–2452.

Mikkelsen KL, Wiinberg N, Hoegholm A, et al. Smoking related to 24-h ambulatory blood pressure and heart rate. *Am J Hypertens* 1997;10:483–491.

Miller ER III, Pastor-Barriuso R, Dalal D, et al. Meta-analysis. High-dosage vitamin E supplementation may increase all-cause mortality. *Ann Intern Med* 2005;142:37–46.

Miura K, Greenland P, Stamler J, et al. Relation of vegetable, fruit, and meat intake to 7-year blood pressure change in middle-aged men: the Chicago Western Electric study. *Am J Epidemiol* 2004;159:572–580.

Miyachi M, Kawano H, Sugawara J, et al. Unfavorable effects of resistance training on central arterial compliance; a randomized intervention study. *Circulation* 2004;110:2858–2863.

Morgan T, Anderson A, Wilson D, et al. Paradoxical effect of sodium restriction on blood pressure in people on slow-channel calcium blocking drugs. *Lancet* 1986;1:793.

Morimoto A, Uzu T, Fujii T, et al. Sodium sensitivity and cardiovascular events in patients with essential hypertension. *Lancet* 1997;350:1734–1737.

Morris RC Jr, O'Connor M, Forman A, et al. Supplemental dietary potassium with KHCO$_3$ but not KCI attenuates essential hypertension [Abstract]. *J Am Soc Nephrol* 1995;6(3):645.

Mukamal KJ, Ascherio A, Mittleman MA, et al. Alcohol and risk for ischemic stroke in men: the role of drinking patterns and usual beverage. *Ann Intern Med* 2005; 142:11–19.

Mukamal KJ, Conigrave KM, Mittleman MA, et al. Roles of drinking pattern and type of alcohol consumed in coronary heart disease in men. *N Engl J Med* 2003; 348:109–118.

Muller JE, Mittleman MA, Maclure M, et al. Triggering myocardial infarction by sexual activity. *JAMA* 1996;275: 1405–1409.

Murray PM, Herrington DM, Pettus CW, et al. Should patients with heart disease exercise in the morning or afternoon? *Arch Intern Med* 1993;153:833–836.

Mustad VA, Kris-Etherton PM. Beyond cholesterol lowering: deciphering the benefits of dietary intervention on cardiovascular diseases. *Curr Atherosclerosis Rep* 2000; 2:461–466.

Myers MG. Effect of caffeine on blood pressure beyond the laboratory. *Hypertension* 2004;43:724–725.

Nagata C, Takatsuka N, Shimizu N, Shimizu H. Sodium intake and risk of death from stroke in Japanese men and women. *Stroke* 2004;35:1543–1547.

Nemec ED, Mansfield L, Kennedy JW. Heart rate and blood pressure responses during sexual activity in normal males. *Am Heart J* 1976;92:274–277.

Neter JE, Stam BE, Kok FJ, et al. Influence of weight reduction on blood pressure: a meta-analysis of randomized controlled trials. *Hypertension* 2003;42:878–884.

Nicolson DJ, Dickinson HO, Campbell F, Mason JM. Lifestyle interventions or drugs for patients with essential hypertension: a systematic review. *J Hypertens* 2004;22:2043–2048.

Nishimura H, Nishioka A, Kubo S, et al. Multifactorial evaluation of blood pressure fall upon hospitalization in essential hypertensive patients. *Clin Sci* 1987;73:135–141.

Noordzij M, Uiterwaal CSPM, Arends LR, et al. Blood pressure response to chronic intake of coffee and caffeine: a meta-analysis of randomized controlled trials *J Hypertens* 2005;23:921–928.

Norris SL, Zhang X, Avenell A, et al. Efficacy of pharmacotherapy for weight loss in adults with type 2 diabetes mellitus: a meta-analysis. *Arch Intern Med* 2004;164: 1395–1404.

Ogawa Y, Aizawa-Abe M, Masuzaki H, et al. Role of leptin in blood pressure reduction during caloric restriction [Abstract]. *J Hypertens* 2000;18(Suppl 4):S15.

Omvik P, Myking OL. Unchanged central hemodynamics after six months of moderate sodium restriction with or without potassium supplement in essential hypertension. *Blood Pressure* 1995;4:32–41.

Oncken CA, White WB, Cooney JL, et al. Impact of smoking cessation on ambulatory blood pressure and heart rate in postmenopausal women. *Am J Hypertens* 2001;14:942–949.

Overlack A, Maus B, Ruppert M, et al. Kaliumcitrat versus kaliumchlorid bei essentieller hypertonie. Wirkung auf hämodynamische, hormonelle und metabolische parameter. *Dtsch Med Wochenschr* 1995;120:631–635.

Palumbo G, Avanzini F, Alli C, et al. Effects of vitamin E on clinic and ambulatory blood pressure in treated hypertensive patients. *Am J Hypertens* 2000;13:564–567.

Paolisso G, Di Maro G, Cozzolino D, et al. Chronic magnesium administration enhances oxidative glucose metabolism in thiazide treated hypertensive patients. *Am J Hypertens* 1992;5:681–686.

Pardell H, Tresserras R, Saltó E, et al. Management of the hypertensive patient who smokes. *Drugs* 1998;56:177–187.

Peat JK. Prevention of asthma. *Eur Resp J* 1996;9:1545–1555.

Peleg I, McGowan JE, McNagny SE. Dietary calcium supplementation increases the risk of urinary tract infection [Abstract]. *Clin Res* 1992;40:562A.

Pereira MA, Kartashov AI, Ebbeling CB, et al. Fast-food habits, weight gain, and insulin resistance (the CARDIA study): 15-year prospective analysis. *Lancet* 2005;365: 36–42.

Pereira MA, O'Reilly E, Augustsson K, et al. Dietary fiber and risk of coronary heart disease: a pooled analysis of cohort studies. *Arch Intern Med* 2004;164:370–376.

Perticone F, Ceravolo R, Candigliota M, et al. Obesity and body fat distribution induce endothelial dysfunction by oxidative stress. *Diabetes* 2001;50:159–165.

Pickering TG. Lifestyle modification: is it achievable and durable? *J Clin Hypertens* 2004;6:581–584.

Poulter NR. Dietary sodium intake and mortality: NHANES [Letter to the Editor]. *Lancet* 1998;352:987–988.

Power ML, Heaney RP, Kalkwarf HJ, et al. The role of calcium in health and disease. *Am J Obstet Gynecol* 1999; 181:1560–1569.

Predel HG, Schramm TH, Rohden C, et al. Effects of various antihypertensive treatment regimens in physically active patients with essential hypertension (EH) [Abstract]. *J Hypertens* 1996;14(Suppl 1):S230.

Psaltopoulou T, Naska A, Orfanos P, et al. Olive oil, the Mediterranean diet, and arterial blood pressure: the Greek European Prospective Investigation into Cancer and Nutrition (EPIC) study. *Am J Clin Nutr* 2004;80: 1012–1018.

Quinn TJ. Twenty-four hour, ambulatory blood pressure responses following acute exercise: impact of exercise intensity. *J Hum Hypertens* 2000;14:547–553.

Radaelli A, Raco R, Perfetti P, et al. Effects of slow, controlled breathing on baroreceptor control of heart rate and blood pressure in healthy men. *J Hypertens* 2004;22: 1361–1370.

Ram CVS, Garrett BN, Kaplan NM. Moderate sodium restriction and various diuretics in the treatment of hypertension. Effects of potassium wastage and blood pressure control. *Arch Intern Med* 1981;141:1015–1019.

Rantala M, Savolainen M, Kervinen K, Kesäniemi YA. Apolipoprotein E phenotype and diet-induced alteration of blood pressure. *Am J Clin Nutr* 1997;65:543–550.

Rapuri PB, Gallagher JC, Balhorn KE, Ryschon KL. Alcohol intake and bone metabolism in elderly women. *Am J Clin Nutr* 2000;72(5):1206–1213.

Reid IR, Horne A, Mason B, et al. Effects of calcium supplementation on body weight and blood pressure in normal older women–a randomized controlled trial. *J Clin Endocrinol Metab* 2005;10.1210:2004–2205.

Renaud SC, Guéguen R, Conard P, et al. Moderate wine drinkers have lower hypertension-related mortality: a prospective cohort study in French men. *Am J Clin Nutr* 2004;80:621–625.

Rimm E. Alcohol and cardiovascular disease. *Curr Atherosclerotic Rep* 2000;2:529–535.

Robinson RC, Wang Z, Victor RG, et al. Lack of effect of repetitive acupuncture on clinic and ambulatory blood pressure [Abstract]. *Am J Hypertens* 2004;17(5 pt 2):33A.

Rosito GA, Fuchs FD, Duncan BB. Dose-dependent biphasic effect of ethanol on 24-h blood pressure in normotensive subjects. *Am J Hypertens* 1999;12:236–240.

Sacks FM, Svetkey LP, Vollmer WM, et al. Effects on blood pressure of reduced dietary sodium and the dietary approaches to stop hypertension (DASH) diet. *N Engl J Med* 2001;344:3–10.

Sacks FM, Willett WC, Smith A, et al. Effect on blood pressure of potassium, calcium, and magnesium in women with low habitual intake. *Hypertension* 1998;31(Part 1):131–138.

Saftlas AF, Logsden-Sackett N, Wang W, et al. Work, leisuretime physical activity, and risk of preeclampsia and gestational hypertension. *Am J Epidemiol* 2004;160:758–765.

Sakhaee K, Harvey JA, Padalino PK, et al. The potential role of salt abuse on the risk for kidney stone formation. *J Urol* 1993;150:310–312.

Salvi F, Mascalchi M, Bortolotti C, et al. Hypertension, hyperekplexia, and pyramidal paresis due to vascular compression of the medulla. *Neurology* 2000;55:1381–1384.

Schaeffner ES, Kurth T, de Jong PE, et al. Alcohol consumption and the risk of renal dysfunction in apparently healthy men. *Arch Intern Med* 2005;165:1048–1053.

Scheer FA, Van Montfrans GA, van Someren EJ, et al. Daily nighttime melatonin reduces blood pressure in male patients with essential hypertension. *Hypertension* 2004;43: 192–197.

Schobel HP, Frank H, Naraghi R, et al. Hypertension in patients with neurovascular compression is associated with increased central sympathetic outflow. *J Am Soc Nephrol* 2002;13:35–41.

Schoeller DA, Shay K, Kushner RF. How much physical activity is needed to minimize weight gain in previously obese women? *Am J Clin Nutr* 1997;66:551–556.

Sellmeyer DE, Schloetter M, Sebastian A. Potassium citrate prevents increased urine calcium excretion and bone resorption induced by a high sodium chloride diet. *J Clin Endocrinol Metab* 2002;87:2008–2012.

Selmer RM, Kristiansen IS, Haglerød A, et al. Cost and health consequences of reducing the population intake of salt. *J Epidemiol Community Health* 2000;54:697–702.

Seppä K, Sillanaukee P. Binge drinking and ambulatory blood pressure. *Hypertension* 1999;33:79–82.

Sever PS, Dahlöf B, Poulter NR, et al. Prevention of coronary and stoke events with atorvastatin in hypertensive patients who have average or lower-than-average cholesterol concentrations, in the Anglo-Scandinavian cardiac outcomes trial—lipid lowering arm (ascot-lla): a multicentre randomized controlled trial. *Lancet* 2003;361:1149–1158.

Sjöström L, Lindroos A-K, Peltonen M, et al. Lifestyle diabetes, and cardiovascular risk factors 10 years after bariatric surgery. *N Engl J Med* 2004;351:2683–2693.

Smith PA, Meaney JF, Graham LN, et al. Relationship of neurovascular compression to central sympathetic discharge and essential hypertension. *J Am Coll Cardiol* 2004;43:1453–1458.

Smith-Warner SA, Spiegelman D, Yaun S-S, et al. Alcohol and breast cancer in women. *JAMA* 1998;279:535–540.

Stamler J, Elliott P, Kesteloot H, et al. Inverse relation of dietary protein markers with blood pressure. Findings for 10,020 men and women in the INTERSALT study. *Circulation* 1996;94:1629–1634.

Stamler R, Stamler J, Gosch FC, et al. Primary prevention of hypertension by nutritional-hygienic means. Final report of a randomized, controlled trial. *JAMA* 1989; 262:1801–1807.

Stevens VJ, Obarzanek E, Cook NR, et al. Long-term weight loss and changes in blood pressure: results of the Trials of Hypertension Prevention, Phase II. *Ann Intern Med* 2001;134:1–11.

Stewart KJ, Bacher AC, Turner KL, et al. Effect of exercise on blood pressure in older persons. *Arch Intern Med* 2005; 165:756–762.

Stranges S, Wu T, Dorn JM, et al. Relationship of alcohol drinking pattern to risk of hypertension: a population-based study. *Hypertension* 2004;44:813–819.

Straznicky NE, O'Callaghan CJ, Barrington VE, Louis WJ. Hypotensive effect of low-fat, high-carbohydrate diet can be independent of changes in plasma insulin concentrations. *Hypertension* 1999;34:580–585.

Streppel MT, Arends LR, van 't Veer P, et al. Dietary fiber and blood pressure: a meta-analysis of randomized placebo-controlled trials. *Arch Intern Med* 2005;165:150–156.

Suzuki M, Kimura Y, Tsushima M, Harano Y. Association of insulin resistance with salt sensitivity and nocturnal fall in blood pressure. *Hypertension* 2000;35:864–868.

Svetkey LP, Loria CM. Blood pressure effects of vitamin C: what's the key question? *Hypertension* 2002;40:789–791.

Tanus-Santos JE, Toledo JC, Cittadino M, et al. Cardiovascular effects of transdermal nicotine in mildly hypertensive smokers. *Am J Hypertens* 2001;14:610–614.

Taubert D, Berkels R, Roesen R, Klaus W. Chocolate and blood pressure in elderly individuals with isolated systolic hypertension. *JAMA* 2003;290:1029–1030.

Thadhani R, Camargo CA Jr, Stampfer MJ, et al. Prospective study of moderate alcohol consumption and risk of hypertension in young women. *Arch Intern Med* 2002;162:569–574.

Thompson PD, Buchner D, Pina IL, et al. Exercise and physical activity in the prevention and treatment of atherosclerotic cardiovascular disease: a statement from the Council on Clinical Cardiology (Subcommittee on Exercise, Rehabilitation, and Prevention) and the Council on Nutrition, Physical Activity, and Metabolism (Subcommittee on Physical Activity). *Circulation* 2003;107:3109–3116.

Thorpe JJ, Welch WJ, Poindexter CA. Bilateral thoracolumbar sympathectomy for hypertension. *Am J Med* 1950; 9:500–515.

Thuerl C, Rump LC, Otto M, et al. Neurovascular contact of the brainstem in hypertensive and normotensive subjects: MR findings and clinical significance. *AJNR Am J Neuroradiol* 2001;22:476–480.

Tjønneland A, Grønbæk M, Stripp C, Overvad K. Wine intake and diet in a random sample of 48,763 Danish men and women. *Am J Clin Nutr* 1999;69:49–54.

Tobian L. Dietary sodium chloride and potassium have effects on the pathophysiology of hypertension in humans and animals. *Am J Clin Nutr* 1997;65(Suppl):606S–611S.

Trials of Hypertension Prevention Collaborative Research Group. Effects of weight loss and sodium reduction intervention on blood pressure and hypertension incidence in overweight people with high-normal blood pressure. *Arch Intern Med* 1997;157:657–667.

Trials of Hypertension Prevention Collaborative Research Group. The effects of nonpharmacologic interventions on blood pressure of persons with high normal levels. Results of the Trials of Hypertension Prevention, Phase I. *JAMA* 1992;267:1213–1220.

Trichopoulou A, Costacou T, Bamia C, Trichopoulos D. Adherence to a Mediterranean diet and survival in a Greek population. *N Engl J Med* 2003;348:2599–2608.

Trichopoulou A, Orfanos P, Norat T, et al. Modified Mediterranean diet and survival: EPIC-elderly prospective cohort study. *BMJ* 2005;330:991–995.

Truelsen T, Thudium D, Grønbaek M. Amount and type of alcohol and risk of dementia: the Copenhagen City Heart Study. *Neurology* 2002;59:1313–1319.

Tsai AG, Wadden TA. Systematic review: an evaluation of major commercial weight loss programs in the United States. *Ann Intern Med* 2005;142:56–66.

Tunstall-Pedoe H. Does dietary potassium lower blood pressure and protect against coronary heart disease and death? Findings from the Scottish heart health study. *Semin Nephrol* 1999;19:500–502.

Tuomilehto J, Jousilahti P, Rastenyte D, et al. Urinary sodium excretion and cardiovascular mortality in Finland. *Lancet* 2001;357:848–851.

U.S. Public Health Service Cooperative Study. Evaluation of antihypertensive therapy. II. Double-blind controlled evaluation of mebutamate. *JAMA* 1965;193:103–105.

van den Elzen AP, Sierksma A, Oren A, et al. Alcohol intake and aortic stiffness in young men and women. *J Hypertens* 2005;23:731–735.

Van Gaal LF, Rissanen AM, Scheen AJ, et al. Effects of the cannabinoid-1 receptor blocker rimonabant on weight reduction and cardiovascular risk factors in overweight patients: 1-year experience from the RIO-Europe study. *Lancet* 2005;365:1389–1397.

Vanhees L, Defoor JGM, Schepers D, et al. Effect of bisoprolol and atenolol on endurance exercise capacity in healthy men. *J Hypertens* 2000;18:35–43.

Vogel RA. Vintners and vasodilators: are French red wines more cardioprotective? *J Am Coll Cardiol* 2003; 41:479–481.

Vollmer WM, Sacks FM, Ard J, et al. for the DASH-Sodium Trial Collaborative Research Group. Effects of diet and sodium intake on blood pressure: subgroup analysis of the DASH-sodium trial. *Ann Intern Med* 2001;135: 1019–1028.

Watkins LL, Sherwood A, Feinglos M, et al. Effects of exercise and weight loss on cardiac risk factors associated with syndrome X. *Arch Intern Med* 2003;163:1889–1895.

Weber KT, Rosenberg EW, Sayre RM. Suberythemal ultraviolet exposure and reduction in blood pressure. *Am J Med* 2004;117:281–282.

Wei M, Gibbons LW, Mitchell TL, et al. Alcohol intake and incidence of type 2 diabetes in men. *Diabetes Care* 2000;23:18–22.

Weinberger MH. Salt sensitivity of blood pressure in humans. *Hypertension* 1996;27:481–490.

Weinberger MH, Fineberg NS, Fineberg SE, Weinberger M. Salt sensitivity, pulse pressure and death in normal and hypertensive humans. *Hypertension* 2001:37:429–432.

Weir MR. Dietary salt, blood pressure, and microalbuminuria. *J Clin Hypertens* 2004;6(Suppl 3):23–26.

Weir MR, Dengel DR, Behrens MT, Goldbert AP. Salt-induced increases in systolic blood pressure affect renal hemodynamics and proteinuria. *Hypertension* 1995;25: 1339–1344.

Weiss R, Dziura J, Burgert TS, et al. Obesity and the metabolic syndrome in children and adolescents. *N Engl J Med* 2004;350:2362–2374.

Weuve J, Kang JH, Manson JE, et al. Physical activity, including walking, and cognitive function in older women. *JAMA* 2004;292:1454–1461.

Whang R, Whang DD, Ryan MP. Refractory potassium repletion. A consequence of magnesium deficiency. *Arch Intern Med* 1992;152:40–45.

Whelton PK, Appel LJ, Espeland MA, et al. Sodium reduction and weight loss in the treatment of hypertension in older persons. *JAMA* 1998;279:839–846.

Whelton PK, He J, Appel LJ, et al. Primary prevention of hypertension: clinical and public health advisory from the National High Blood Pressure Education Program. *JAMA* 2002;288:1882–1888.

Whelton SP, Chin A, Xin X, He J. Effect of aerobic exercise on blood pressure: a meta-analysis of randomized, controlled trials. *Ann Intern Med* 2002;136:493–503.

Whelton SP, He J, Whelton PK, Muntner P. Meta-analysis of observational studies on fish intake and coronary heart disease. *Am J Cardiol* 2004;93:1119–1123.

White IR, Altmann DR, Nanchahal K. Alcohol consumption and mortality: modelling risks for men and women at different ages. *BMJ* 2002;325:191–194.

WHO/ISH Writing Group. 2003 World Health Organization (WHO)/International Society of Hypertension (ISH) statement on management of hypertension. *J Hypertens* 2003;21:1983–1992.

Wildman RP, Farhat GN, Patel AS, et al. Weight change is associated with change in arterial stiffness among healthy, young adults. *Hypertension* 2005;45:187–192.

Willett WC, Dietz WH, Colditz GA. Guidelines for healthy weight. *N Engl J Med* 1999;341:427–434.

Williams B, Poulter NR, Brown MJ, et al. British Hypertension Society guidelines for hypertension management 2004 (BHS-IV): summary. *BMJ* 2004;328:634–640.

Williamson DF, Vinicor F, Bowman BA. Centers for Disease Control and Prevention Primary Prevention Working Group. Primary prevention of type 2 diabetes mellitus by lifestyle intervention: implications for health policy. *Ann Intern Med* 2004;140:951–957.

Winer BM. The antihypertensive mechanism of salt depletion induced by hydrochlorothiazide. *Circulation* 1961;24:788–796.

Wong SL, Katzmarzyk PT, Nichaman MZ, et al. Cardiorespiratory fitness is associated with lower abdominal fat independent of body mass index. *Med Sci Sports Exerc* 2004;36:286–291.

Xin X, Frontini MG, Ogden LG, et al. Effects of alcohol reduction on blood pressure: a meta-analysis of randomized controlled trials. *Hypertension* 2001;38:1112–1117.

Yang YC, Lu FH, Wu JS, et al. The protective effect of habitual tea consumption on hypertension. *Arch Intern Med* 2004;164:1534–1540.

Young DB, Ma G. Vascular protective effects of potassium. *Semin Nephrol* 1999;19:477–486.

Ziccardi P, Nappo F, Giugliano G, et al. Reduction of inflammatory cytokine concentrations and improvement of endothelial functions in obese women after weight loss over one year. *Circulation* 2002;105:804–809.

Zilkens RR, Burke V, Hodgson JM, et al. Both red wine and beer elevate blood pressure in normotensive men. *Hypertension* 2005;45:874–879.

Žižka J, Ceral J, Eliáš P, et al. Vascular compression of rostral medulla oblongata: prospective MR imaging study in hypertensive and normotensive subjects. *Radiology* 2004;230:65–69.

# Treatment of Hypertension: Drug Therapy

In the previous two chapters, I reviewed the evidence for the need for blood pressure (BP) reduction and the use of lifestyle modifications to lower the BP. This chapter begins with ways to improve on the currently inadequate control of the disease. Then each class of drugs currently available is covered. An analysis of initial drug choice and of the subsequent order of additional therapy follows; then comes considerations of the management of special populations and of hypertensives with various other conditions.

## BACKGROUND

Because the treatment of hypertension is the leading indication for the use of drugs in the United States (Woodwell & Cherry, 2004), new agents constantly are being introduced and heavily promoted. The choice of drugs is one of the factors that affects the efficacy of therapy, but choices are often based on promotional activities that may be biased (Blumenthal, 2004). In this chapter, I constantly attempt to maintain an objective view, both about the use of drugs overall and about the relative value of individual agents. Specific choices are often favored, in keeping with the recent guidelines from multiple expert committees in the United States (Chobanian et al., 2003a, 2003b), in the United Kingdom (Williams et al., 2004a, 2004b), Europe (Guidelines Committee, 2003), and international (Whitworth, 2003).

As we shall see, currently available antihypertensive drugs, used in concert with appropriate lifestyle modifications and self-monitoring, can control the BP in most hypertensives (Canzanello et al., 2005; Singer et al., 2004). Yet, in every survey, in only a minority of patients is the BP lower than 140/90 mm Hg (Hajjar & Kotchen, 2003), and those in most need of tight control such as stroke survivors are often even less well controlled (Amar et al., 2004). Therefore, before considering the drugs that are available and their indications, the issue of how to achieve better overall control of hypertension will be addressed.

## CURRENT STATE OF CONTROL OF HYPERTENSION

Inadequate rates of control have been reported in representative samples of the population from countries all over the world (Wolf-Maier et al., 2004), as well as from patients being seen in various healthcare settings, both subsidized (Borzecki et al., 2003; Spranger et al., 2004) and privately paid (Hajjar & Kotchen, 2003).

Particularly instructive are data from the participants in the longer than 50-year Framingham Heart Study, who are likely to be as aware of both the presence of hypertension and the need for its control as any group of people in the world. Among the entire 10,333 participants, of whom approximately 40% were hypertensive, the rate of use of antihypertensive medications increased from 2.3% to 24.6% in men and from 5.7% to 27.7% in women from 1950 to 1989 (Mosterd et al., 1999). These figures would translate into therapy being used by more than half of those with hypertension. As a consequence, the prevalence of BP higher than 160/100 mm Hg declined significantly. However, in the same group of hypertensives, the goal of therapy, a BP of less than 140/90 mm Hg, was reached by only 29% (Lloyd-Jones et al., 2000).

These figures are remarkably similar to those reported from the third survey of a representative sample of the entire U.S. population, the National Health and Nutrition Examination Survey (Hajjar & Kotchen, 2003). As bad as the results are, they are considerably better than found in other developed countries (Wolf-Maier et al., 2004).

## Reasons for Poor Control

Although practitioners are quick to blame patients as the main cause for poor control of their hypertension, all three players—physicians, patients, and therapies—are involved (Borzecki et al., 2005).

### Problems with Physicians

Many practitioners are either unaware of the need to more intensively treat hypertension, particularly isolated systolic hypertension in the elderly, or are unwilling to do so. Admittedly, systolic levels are more difficult to bring under control even under the best of circumstances, with fewer than half of patients enrolled in controlled trials having their systolics brought to 140 mm Hg or lower whereas 80% of diastolics were brought to 90 mm Hg or lower (Mancia & Grassi, 2002).

However, much of the problem in clinical practice is, as described by O'Connor (2003), "clinical inertia," the unwillingness to push therapy to the desired goal. This unwillingness may reflect inaccurate perceptions: that systolic elevations "aren't that bad"; that they can't be lowered without multiple medications and side effects; and that little benefit will accompany better control.

Moreover, many practitioners do not recognize their own shortcomings. They often underestimate the level of their patients' cardiovascular risk (Persson et al., 2004) and, even though they are unwilling to intensify therapy to the levels recommended in guidelines, they usually perceive their level of adherence to guidelines as being much better than it is (Steinman et al., 2004).

Hypertension "experts" (such as myself) have contributed to practitioners' problems by promoting conflicting positions, often at the same time: diuretics are bad—no, they are good; β-blockers are good—no, they are bad; CCBs are bad—no, they are good; and so on. On a higher level, the failure of national and international groups of experts to agree on such simple measures as the classification of hypertension and the goals of therapy adds to the confusion. And then the often subtle machinations of pharmaceutical marketers, particular in providing experts to tout somewhat hidden messages under the guise of Continuing Medical Education, must be playing a role in keeping practitioners from having a single, clear message of how best to manage hypertension.

In a capitalistic, competitive market system, multiple options will remain available, increasingly being touted directly to the public and profitably marketed to the profession. However, better directions are being provided by the National Institute for Clinical Excellence (NICE) in the United Kingdom, the Hypertension Education Program in Canada, and the National High Blood Pressure Education Program in the United States.

There is evidence that these efforts are helping. In Canada, use of diuretics rose and angiotensin-converting enzyme inhibitors (ACEIs) and angiotensin receptor blockers (ARBs) fell in the 4 months after widespread publicity about the Antihypertensive and Lipid-Lowering Treatment to Prevent Heart Attack Trial (ALLHAT) (Austin et al., 2004). In the U.S. Veterans Administration system, more diuretics and fewer CCBs are bring prescribed (Lopez et al., 2004). In a large U.S. health maintenance organization, more diuretics and fewer β-blockers are being used (Xie et al., 2005).

### Problems with Patients

As many as half of hypertensives prescribed a medication will not be taking it within a year (Borzecki et al., 2005). There are many reasons for poor adherence to antihypertensive therapy, including:

- Failure to identify and deal with patients' differing perceptions about their disease and beliefs about both the benefits and the problems of therapy (Ross et al., 2004). These may interfere with adherence, particularly among the poor and among recent immigrants who have different cultural attitudes and language barriers (Li et al., 2004).

- The largely asymptomatic nature of hypertension, making it difficult for patients to forego immediate pleasures (salt, calories, money, etc.) for distant, unrecognized benefits, even more so if therapy makes them feel worse.
- Competing problems such as poverty, psychological depression, and/or more immediately threatening diseases such as diabetes (Wang et al., 2002).
- Inability to access and maintain contact with a healthcare system that is affordable, available, and appropriate to their long-term needs, including 45 million people in the United States without health insurance.
- Real and imaginary concerns about the safety of lifelong medication. There likely never were many people willing to take whatever they were prescribed with full confidence in their physician, but there are even fewer today. The delayed recognition that an NSAID prescribed by thousands of physicians to millions of patients was responsible for heart attacks surely will further damage the patient-doctor relationship.

The patients' problems were nicely described in a *Lancet* editorial (Anonymous, 2004):

> Educating patients about the disease is a laudable undertaking. But a national health plan, affordable drugs, and evidence-based treatment regimens devised by knowledgeable clinicians who use their best judgment about the needs and wishes of individual patients would go much further to solve this public-health problem.

### Problems with the Therapy

As noted, hypertension has all the wrong characteristics to ensure adherence to therapy, but these are often compounded by problems of therapy, including:

- Difficulty in changing unhealthy lifestyles, in particular weight gain from too many calories and too little physical activity (see Chapter 6).
- The high cost of most new, trade-named medications.
- The prescription of two or more doses per day when long-acting, once-a-day options are available.
- Side effects of antihypertensive drugs, some not predicted such as impotence with diuretics.
- Even less obvious but perhaps more critical, the sympathetic nervous system may be chronically activated when the blood pressure is lowered (Fu et al., 2005).
- Interactions with other medications and substances: nonsteriodal antiinflammatory drugs (NSAIDs) being the most common, grapefruit juice likely the least recognized (Wilkinson et al.,

2005), and herbal remedies perhaps the most dangerous (Tannergren et al., 2004).
- Difficulty in assessment of adherence. Although there are multiple ways to assess the degree of patients' pill taking, none has been found to be particularly accurate. Just asking the patient in a nonthreatening way (e.g., "Patients often have difficulty in taking their pills. Have you missed taking any of yours?") is often productive (Fodor et al., 2005). More sophisticated techniques such as electronic medication monitors may be helpful in clinical practice (Burnier et al., 2001). Such monitors have shown that some patients omit drugs over weekends, increase doses before office visits, and often miss a dose (Steiner & Earnest, 2000).
- Variable responses to any dose of any medication. The starting and usual doses are determined by trials in only a limited number of usually uncomplicated patients. In practice, many patients respond more or less to any drug (Senn, 2004).

### Ways to Improve Adherence to Therapy

Many books and articles have suggested ways to keep more patients on effective therapy of hypertension, but the list of those that have been shown to work is relatively short. In truth, adequate studies are hard to do since it is difficult to separate effects and know which works, particularly since most people do better when they know they are being watched.

Recent reviews including Borzecki et al., 2005; Elwyn et al., 2003; Grol and Grimshaw, 2003; McDonald et al., 2002; and Schroeder et al., 2004, show these to improve adherence in most, but not in all, careful studies:

- Involving patients in making decisions about treatment.
- Involving patients by home blood pressure monitoring and using that data to adjust therapy (Canzanello et al., 2005).
- Simplifying the regimen to once-a-day dosing.
- Organizing health care so that patients have easy access to various providers, including nurses and physician assistants.
- Using motivational strategies, from financial rewards to simply providing feedback on performance.
- Sending reminders about appointments and continued adherence to therapy.

Patient education by itself does little (Hunt et al., 2004), but improvements in providing efficient care have a great potential. One clinical practice in Florida improved the level of control to below 130/85 in

53% of 469 hypertensive diabetic patients by involving nursing staff in case management, following evidence-based guidelines, and focusing the practice to the achievement of control (Wessell et al., 2003). Others have shown similar improvements, primarily by using ancillary personnel (Hill et al., 2003; New et al., 2003; Rudd et al., 2004), by following goal-oriented strategies (Singer et al., 2004), and by using home BP monitoring (Canzanello et al., 2005).

Beyond these more immediate measures, better organized and monitored health care as in the U.S. Veterans Administration system improves adherence (Furmaga et al., 2004). Even better would be the availability of nationwide, computerized, easily accessed medical records and the use of financial incentives to reward practitioners who improve the care and outcomes of their patients (Rundall et al., 2002).

I believe that if the amount of money now being spent on health care in the United States were applied in a more rational manner, as through a single-payer national health insurance plan (Woolhandler et al., 2003b), the care of hypertension and other chronic conditions would improve, but, absent the political will, the situation will apparently have to get a lot worse for the more affluent before it can get better for everyone else.

Until (or if) that time comes, application of the guidelines in Table 7–1 should certainly help even if their effectiveness has not been documented. A few of these deserve additional comment.

### Patient Involvement

Involvement of the patient is helpful, not only in making initial decisions, which are therefore more likely to be followed, but also in monitoring the course of the disease. Home BP readings should almost always be recommended, preferably for the patient to take, sometimes for other caregivers. As with diabetes, home monitoring should be used to adjust therapy, and some patients can be counseled to be able to make their own adjustments in doses of drugs, just as diabetics are encouraged to adjust their insulin doses. Remember, too, that the long-term benefits to therapy are more closely related to out-of-the-office measurements than office readings (Mancia & Parati, 2004). We need to use and trust home readings (Canzanello et al., 2005).

More details are provided in Chapter 2.

### Intensity of Therapy

The rapidity of reaching a goal is now in question since too fast a course may cause intolerable symptoms, but too slow may expose high-risk patients to immediate dangers. The greater exposure was graphically shown in the Valsartan Antihypertensive Long-term Use Evaluation (VALUE) trial wherein the quicker response over the first 3 to 6 months to the calcium channel blocker (CCB) amlodipine than to the adrenergic receptor blocker (ARB) valsartan provided greater protection against heart attacks and strokes (Julius et al., 2004c). The patients in VALUE were all at high risk for cardiovascular disease, so it still seems appropriate to "start low and go low" for most, particularly the elderly with systolic hypertension. For those with higher levels of blood pressure but, even more so, higher overall risk, a "higher and faster" approach should be used.

### Timing of Dosing

The time of day to take antihypertensive medications needs to be more carefully considered. Early morning has usually been recommended, but there are two potential problems: First, the pills may not exert a full 24-hour effect, as shown for atenolol (Neutel et al., 1990) and ramipril (Poirier et al., 2004); second, an even greater effect may be needed in the early morning, before the day's therapy has kicked in, to keep the pressure from surging in the immediate post-arising time, thereby contributing to the "morning surge" of cardiovascular catastrophes. In a study from Spain, the majority of hypertensives with well-controlled office readings had uncontrolled early morning readings (Redón et al., 2002).

The solution for the first problem is twofold: First, ensure full 24-hour control by having the patient measure early morning BP at home; second, choose intrinsically long-acting medications, e.g., metoprolol XL rather than atenolol, trandolapril rather than enalapril, amlodipine rather than felodipine, telmisartan rather than losartan.

The solution for the second problem seems as obvious but has never been definitely proven, i.e., take medications later in the day or even at bedtime. In the Heart Outcomes Prevention Evaluation (HOPE) trial (Heart Outcomes, 2000), the study medication, the ACEI ramipril, was taken at bedtime, purposely to prevent early morning events. The positive results were said not to reflect the 3/2 mm Hg lower average clinic blood pressure of those who took ramipril. However, the clinic pressures were taken hours after the morning surge so the possible benefit was undetectable. This belief is supported by a HOPE substudy wherein 38 participants had 24-hour ambulatory monitoring (Svensson et al., 2001). Among the 20 given bedtime ramipril, the midday pressures were the same as those in the 18 given placebo, but the overnight BPs were significantly lower (by 17/8 mm Hg) as were the 24-hour readings (by 10/4 mm Hg) in the ramipril group.

Another trial was specifically designed to test the use of bedtime versus early morning dosing. In the

## TABLE 7-1

### Guidelines to Improve Maintenance of Antihypertensive Therapy

Involve the patient in decision making to the extent desired.
    Assess attitudes and beliefs.
    Provide individual assessments of current risks and potential benefits of control.
    Inform the patient about the condition and its treatment.
    If patient agrees, involve family.
Articulate the goal of therapy: to reduce blood pressure to near normotension with few or no side effects.
Be alert for signs of inadequate intake of medications, e.g., absence of BP response or expected effects, e.g., bradycardia with β-blocker.
Recognize and manage depression.
Maintain contact with the patient.
    Encourage visits and calls to allied health personnel.
    Give feedback to the patient via home blood pressure readings.
    Make contact with patients who do not return.
Keep care inexpensive and simple.
    Do the least workup needed to rule out secondary causes.
    Obtain follow-up laboratory data only yearly unless indicated more often.
    Encourage lifestyle changes if needed.
    Use home blood pressure readings.
    Use once-daily doses of long-acting drugs.
    Use generic drugs and break larger doses of scored tablets in half.
    If appropriate, use combination tablets.
    Use calendar blister packs.
    Inspect all pill containers at each visit.
    If medications must be taken separately, provide clear, easily read instructions.
    Use clinical protocols monitored by nurses and assistants.
Prescribe according to pharmacologic principles.
    Add one drug at a time.
    Start with small doses, aiming for 5- to 10-mm Hg reductions at each step, unless more rapid response is indicated.
    Have medication taken immediately on awakening in the morning or after 4 a.m. if patient awakens to void. If morning surge of BP (above 160/100) persists, give all drugs at 6 p.m. or at bedtime, before using b.i.d. dosing.
Stop unsuccessful therapy and try a different approach.
Anticipate and address side effects.
    Adjust therapy to ameliorate side effects that do not spontaneously disappear.
Continue to add effective and tolerated drugs, stepwise, in sufficient doses to achieve the goal of therapy.
Provide feedback and validation of success.

Controlled Onset Verapamil Investigation of Cardiovascular End Points (CONVINCE) trial (Black et al., 2003), half of the 16,602 participants were given a bedtime dose of a specially formulated verapamil product (COER) that released the drug 4 to 8 hours after intake, doubling the likelihood that the early morning surge would be blunted. The other half were started on either hydrochlorothiazide (HCT) or atenolol to be taken each morning. Blood pressures, presumably taken sometime later in the day, were lowered equally for the evening verapamil groups (13.6/7.8 mm Hg) and the morning HCT or atenolol group (13.5/7.1 mm Hg). Although the sponsor of the trial withdrew its financial support before the trial could be completed, the data that were available showed no difference between the bedtime and morning dosing. It is doubly disturbing that a potentially useful trial for clinical medicine had an inherent flaw—the absence of early morning blood pressure measurements—and a socially irresponsible sponsor (Psaty & Rennie, 2003).

Additional studies have shown that a graded-release delivery system of diltiazem taken at bedtime lowers early morning BP better than a morning dose of amlodipine (Wright et al., 2004) or a bedtime dose of ramipril (White et al., 2004b). In addition, morning doses of the ARB candesartan were found to reduce early morning BP better than morning doses of the ACEI lisinopril in a crossover trial (Eguchi et al., 2003). None of these smaller trials were intended to reveal effects on cardiovascular events.

Therefore, "chronotherapeutics" sounds logical, but there are no data to either support or refute it. As Mosenkis and Townsend (2004) note:

> For now, the schedule of antihypertensive drug administration can be determined by other factors such as convenience, concurrence with the administration of other medications to foster adherence, and timing to minimize untoward effects of these medications. . . . If there are no other compelling timing considerations, one may choose nocturnal dosing (i.e., at bedtime for standard daily drugs and nighttime for extended-release preparations) so that their peak activities coincide with, and perhaps helps to blunt, the early morning BP increase.

### Dealing with Side Effects

Some medications are easier to take than others (Hollenberg et al., 2003), but some patients cannot seem to take any. Such patients with nonspecific intolerance to multiple antihypertensive drugs almost always have underlying psychiatric morbidity, often manifested as recurrent hyperventilation, panic attacks, generalized anxiety, or depression (Davies et al., 2003). As noted in Chapter 4, many people get anxious when their "silent killer" is diagnosed and even more when it cannot be easily controlled (Mena-Martin et al., 2003). Obviously, there are all grades of drug-related side effects. Fortunately, most currently available drugs do not interfere with cognitive performance (Muldoon et al., 2002) or other aspects of the quality of life. However, even such senses as smell and taste that seem unrelated to hypertension can be adversely affected by various antihypertensive drugs (Doty et al., 2003).

The astute clinician will remain open to all possibilities.

### Follow-up Visits

Achieving and maintaining target BP with the lowest possible dosage of medication requires ongoing patient follow-up and may involve multiple dosage adjustments. Most patients should be seen within 1 to 2 months after the initiation of therapy to determine the adequacy of BP control (preferably monitored by home readings), the degree of patient cooperation in taking pills, and the presence of adverse effects. Associated medical problems—including target organ damage, other major risk factors, and laboratory test abnormalities—also play a part in determining the frequency of patient follow-up. Once the BP is stabilized, follow-up at 3- to 6-month intervals (depending on the patient's status) is generally appropriate. In most patients, particularly the elderly and patients with orthostatic symptoms, monitoring should include BP measurement in the supine position and after standing for up to 5 minutes, to recognize postural hypotension.

Before considering the roles of individual drugs and the manner in which they are used in improving the overall management of hypertension, a detailed description of the various choices will be provided.

## SPECIFICS ABOUT ANTIHYPERTENSIVE DRUGS

The modern era of antihypertensive therapy began only slightly more than 40 years ago with the pioneering work of Ed Freis in the United States and Horace Smirk in New Zealand (Piepho & Beal, 2000). Since then, a large panoply of drugs have been developed, as listed in Table 7–2. We will consider the drugs in the order shown in Table 7–2. Some that are used extensively elsewhere but are not now available in the United States will also be covered, along with newer agents that are on the horizon.

In the year 2002 in the United States, the most commonly prescribed drugs were those used for the treatment of hypertension, totaling over 200 million prescriptions (Woodwell & Cherry, 2004). When the annual surveys of drug use are compared, diuretics have continued to be the most commonly prescribed, followed by ACEIs, $\beta$-blockers, and CCBs, with ARBs rising the fastest and $\alpha$-blockers continuing to fall. The initial rapid growth in the use of ARBs is almost certainly related to their intensive marketing; at least in the Netherlands, their increased use was not related to recognized indications (Greving et al., 2004). However, as will be noted, ARBs may be special so their continued growth clearly reflects more than marketing.

After a description of some of the basic pharmacology and clinical usefulness of each agent, we will consider the choice of first and second drugs, the selection of specific drugs for various types of hypertensive patients, the use of combinations,

## TABLE 7–2

## Antihypertensive Drugs Available in the United States (as of 2005)

| Diuretics | Adrenergic Inhibitors | | Vasodilators | |
|---|---|---|---|---|
| *Thiazides* | *Peripheral inhibitors* | *β-blockers* | *Direct* | *Angiotensin-converting enzyme inhibitors* |
| Chlorthalidone | Guanadrel | Acebutolol | Hydralazine | |
| Indapamide | Guanethidine | Atenolol | Minoxidil | |
| Metolazone | Reserpine | Betaxolol | *Calcium channel blockers* | Benazepril |
| Thiazides | *Central α₂-agonists* | Bisoprolol | | Captopril |
| *Loop diuretics* | Clonidine | Carteolol | Dihydropyridines | Enalapril |
| Bumetanide | Guanabenz | Metoprolol | Amlodipine | Fosinopril |
| Furosemide | Guanfacine | Nadolol | Felodipine | Lisinopril |
| Torsemide | Methyldopa | Penbutolol | Isradipine | Moexipril |
| *Aldosterone blockers* | *α₁-blockers* | Pindolol | Nicardipine | Quinapril |
| | Dozazosin | Propranolol | Nifedipine | Perindopril |
| Spironolactone | Prazosin | Timolol | Nisoldipine | Ramipril |
| Eplerenone | Terazosin | *Combined α-, β-blockers* | Diltiazem | Trandolapril |
| *Potassium sparers* | | | Verapamil | *Angiotensin-II receptor blockers* |
| Amiloride | | Carvediol | | Candesartan |
| Triamterene | | Labetalol | | Eprosartan |
| | | | | Irbesartan |
| | | | | Losartan |
| | | | | Telmisartan |
| | | | | Valsartan |

and conditions wherein special care is advised in the choice of drugs. The use of drugs in various secondary forms of hypertension (e.g., ACEIs in renovascular hypertension; spironolactone in primary aldosteronism) is considered in the respective chapters on these identifiable causes.

## DIURETICS

Among the first orally effective drugs to become available, diuretics are being used even more frequently because their effectiveness has been reiterated, and, with lower doses, their side effects minimized.

Diuretics differ in structure and major site of action within the nephron (Figure 7–1). The site of action determines their relative efficacy, as expressed in the maximal percentage of filtered sodium chloride excreted (Brater, 2000). Agents acting in the proximal tubule (site I) are seldom used to treat hypertension. Treatment is usually initiated with a thiazide-type diuretic (acting at site III, the distal

convoluted tubule). Chlorthalidone and indapamide are structurally different from, although still related to, the thiazides and will be covered with them. If renal function is significantly impaired (i.e., serum creatinine exceeding 1.5 mg per dL), a loop diuretic

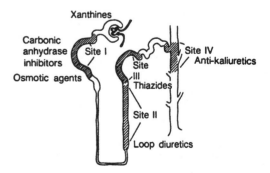

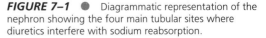

**FIGURE 7–1** ● Diagrammatic representation of the nephron showing the four main tubular sites where diuretics interfere with sodium reabsorption.

(acting at site II, the thick ascending limb of the loop of Henle) or metolazone likely will be needed. A potassium-sparing agent (acting at site IV) may be given with the diuretic to reduce the likelihood of hypokalemia. By themselves, potassium-sparing agents are relatively weak antihypertensives.

The specific agents now available in the United States are listed in Table 7–3. Aldosterone blockers, though potassium-sparers, are considered separately because of their additional effects.

## Thiazide Diuretics

### Mode of Action

The thiazide diuretics act by inhibiting sodium and chloride cotransport across the luminal membrane of the early segment of the distal convoluted tubule, where 5% to 8% of filtered sodium is normally reabsorbed (Puschett, 2000) (Figure 7–1, site III). Plasma and extracellular fluid volume are thereby shrunken, and cardiac output falls (Wilson & Freis, 1959).

## TABLE 7–3

### Diuretics and Potassium-Sparing Agents (U.S. Trade Names)

| Drug | Daily Dosage, MG | Duration of Action, H |
|---|---|---|
| Thiazides | | |
| Bendroflumethiazide (Naturetin) | 2.5–5.0 | 18 |
| Benzthiazide (Exna) | 12.5–50 | 12–18 |
| Chlorothiazide (Diuril) | 125–500 | 6–12 |
| Cyclothiazide (Anhydron) | 0.5–2.0 | 18–24 |
| Hydrochlorothiazide (Esidrix, | 12.5–50 | 12–18 |
| HydroDIURIL, Microzide) | 12.5–50 | 18–24 |
| Hydroflumethiazide (Saluron, Diucardin) | 2.5–5.0 | 24 |
| Methylclothiazide (Enduron, Aquatensen) | 1.0–4.0 | 24–48 |
| Polythiazide (Renese) | 1.0–4.0 | 24 |
| Trichlormethiazide (Metahydrin, Naqua) | 1.0–4.0 | 24 |
| Related sulfonamide compounds | | |
| Chlorthalidone (Hygroton, Thalitone) | 12.5–50 | 24–72 |
| Indapamide (Lozol) | 1.25–2.5 | 24 |
| Metolazone | | |
| Mykrox | 0.5–1.0 | 24 |
| Zaroxolyn | 2.5–10 | 24 |
| Quinethazone (Hydromox) | 25–100 | 18–24 |
| Loop Diuretics | | |
| Bumetanide (Bumex) | 0.5–5.0 | 4–6 |
| Ethacrynic acid (Edecrin)* | 25–100 | 12 |
| Furosemide (Lasix) | 20–480 | 4–6 |
| Torsemide (Demadex) | 5–40 | 12 |
| Potassium-sparing agents | | |
| Amiloride (Midamor) | 5–10 | 24 |
| Triamterene (Dyrenium) | 50–150 | 12 |
| Aldosterone blockers | | |
| Spironolactone (Aldactone) | 25–100 | 8–12 |
| Eplerenone (Inspra) | 50–100 | 12 |

*not being marketed in the United States

Humoral and intrarenal counterregulatory mechanisms rapidly reestablish the steady state so that sodium intake and excretion are balanced within 3 to 9 days in the presence of a decreased body fluid volume (Sica, 2004a). With chronic use, plasma volume returns partially toward normal, but, at the same time, peripheral resistance decreases (Conway & Lauwers, 1960; Zhu et al., 2005) (Figure 7–2).

### Determinants of Response

The degree of BP response to diuretics is predicated on their capacity to activate the counterregulatory defenses to a lower BP and a shrunken fluid volume—in particular, a reactive rise in renin and aldosterone levels. Those who start with low, suppressed plasma renin activity (PRA) and aldosterone levels and who are capable of mounting only a weak rise in these levels after diuretics are initiated have been shown to be more "diuretic-responsive" (Chapman et al., 2002a). This includes older, Black, and hypertensive people, all of whom frequently have lower renin levels (Kaplan, 1977). Those who respond less well, with a fall in mean BP of less than 10%, were found to have a greater degree of plasma volume depletion and greater stimulation of renin and aldosterone, contributing to a persistently high peripheral resistance (van Brummelen et al., 1980). Blockage of the reactive rise in renin-angiotensin-aldosterone, as with the addition of an ACEI or ARB, will potentiate the antihypertensive action (Ram, 2004).

Pharmacogenetic studies have related the responsiveness to thiazide diuretics to various polymorphisms of genes controlling the renin-angiotensin system (Frazier et al., 2004), the 11βHSD2 enzyme (Williams et al., 2005), and sodium channels (Maitland-van der Zee et al., 2004) that vary with both gender and ethnic background. Moreover, diuretic-treated carriers of a variant of the adducin gene, which is associated with increased renal sodium reabsorption, have been reported to have a lower risk of heart attack and stroke than seen in diuretic-treated patients who do not carry that variant or in those who are given other antihypertensive medications (Psaty et al., 2002). At the least, these studies foretell a probable application of pharmacogenetics to clinical practice in the near future.

### Thiazide-like Diuretics

Although commonly considered a thiazide, chlorthalidone is of a different chemical structure and milligram for milligram acts both stronger and longer than hydrochlorothiazide (HCTZ) (Carter et al., 2004a). Although HCTZ has become by far the most widely used diuretic to treat hypertension in the United States, chlorthalidone has been used in all trials conducted by the National Institutes of Health. When currently recommended lower doses, 12.5 to 25 mg a day, of the two agents were used in different trials, similar cardiovascular outcomes were found (Psaty et al., 2004). However, no direct comparisons between the two have been done and likely will not be done. Since HCTZ is the diuretic in most combination tablets, there is little reason not to use it, even though evidence-based purists might choose chlorthalidone (Choi et al., 2004; Kostis et al., 2005).

#### Indapamide

Indapamide (Lozol) is a chlorobenzene sulfonamide but has a methylindoline moiety, which may provide additional protective actions beyond its diuretic effect (Chillon & Baumbach, 2004). It is as effective in reducing the BP as are thiazides or CCBs (Emeriau et al., 2001); maintains a 24-hour effect; and, in appropriately low doses of 1.25 mg per day, rarely raises serum lipids (Hall et al., 1994) but, in larger doses, hyponatremia and hypokalemia may occur. With 1.5-mg doses, regression of left ventricular hypertrophy (LVH) was better (Gosse et al., 2000) and reduction in microalbuminuria equal to (Marre et al., 2004) that seen with enalapril, 20 mg per day. In a small group of patients with moderate renal insufficiency, indapamide preserved renal function better than did HCTZ (Madkour et al., 1995). On the background of an ACEI, indapamide provided a 43% reduction in recurrences of stroke (PROGRESS Collaborative Group, 2001).

#### Metolazone

Metolazone, a long-acting and more potent quinazoline thiazide derivative, maintains its effect in the presence of renal insufficiency (Paton & Kane, 1977). Small doses, 0.5 to 1.0 mg per day, of a new formulation (Mykrox) may be equal to ordinary long-acting thiazide diuretics (Miller et al., 1988); the agent is particularly useful in patients with renal insufficiency and resistant hypertension, but variable absorption may interfere with its efficacy.

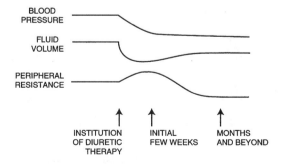

**FIGURE 7–2** ● Scheme of the hemodynamic changes responsible for the antihypertensive effects of diuretic therapy.

## Antihypertensive Efficacy

When used alone, thiazide diuretics provide efficacy similar to that of other classes of drugs (Psaty et al., 2003). Blacks and the elderly respond better to diuretics than do non-Blacks and younger patients (Brown et al., 2003), presumably because they have lower renin responsiveness. Diuretics may provide even better protection against strokes than would be expected from their antihypertensive efficacy (Messerli et al., 2003b).

Diuretics potentiate the effect of all other antihypertensive agents, including CCBs (Sica, 2004a). This potentiation depends on the contraction of fluid volume by the diuretic (Finnerty et al., 1970) and the prevention of fluid accumulation that frequently follows the use of nondiuretic antihypertensive drugs. Because of the altered pressure-natriuresis curve of primary hypertension (Saito & Kimura, 1996), whenever the BP is lowered, fluid retention is expected (Figure 7–3). The need for a diuretic may be lessened with ACEIs and ARBs, which inhibit the renin-aldosterone mechanism, and with CCBs, which have some intrinsic natriuretic activity, but potentiation persists with all classes.

## Duration of Action

The durations of action listed in Table 7–3 relate to the diuretic effect; the antihypertensive effect lasts beyond the diuretic effect. HCTZ once daily persistently reduced BP after 24 hours (Lacourcière & Provencher, 1989). HCTZ, 25 mg, at 7:00 a.m. for 4 weeks, converted hypertensives whose BP did not fall during the night, i.e., nondippers, into dippers, further documenting the duration of antihypertensive effect (Uzu & Kimura, 1999).

## Dosage

### Monotherapy

The recommended daily dose of thiazide diuretics has been progressively falling from as high as 200 mg HCTZ or equivalent doses of other thiazides in the early 1960s (Cranston et al., 1963) to as little as 6.25 to 12.5 mg today. In hypertensives with good renal function, most of the antihypertensive effect will be obtained from such small doses, with less hypokalemia and other side effects (Carlsen et al., 1990; Zimlichman et al., 2004). Flack and Cushman (1996) have summarized the evidence that 12.5 mg HCTZ lowers BP in most studies as effectively as 25- to 50-mg doses.

Even though most patients will have a good response to such small doses, some patients will require more, even up to 200 mg HCTZ per day (Freis et al., 1988). In another study, 12.5 mg HCTZ did not lower BP over a 4-week interval, but 25 mg did thereafter (Borghi et al., 1992). However, as shown by Carlsen et al. (1990), the full antihypertensive effect of low doses of diuretic may not become apparent in 4 weeks, so patience is advised when low doses are prescribed.

### Combination Therapy

Even more convincing data confirm a significant effect from small doses, even below 12.5 mg per day HCTZ, when diuretics are added to a variety of other drugs to enhance their antihypertensive efficacy. This was most clearly documented with the combination of 6.25 mg HCTZ plus the β-blocker bisoprolol (Frishman et al., 1994). Similar potentiation of ACEI efficacy with 6.25 mg HCTZ has been seen (Andrén et al., 1983).

Thiazides may also be coupled with loop diuretics in those with renal impairment, because

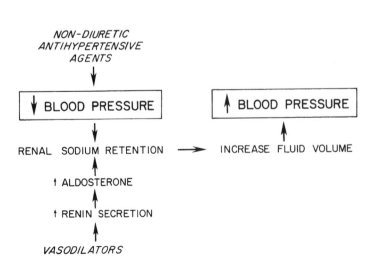

FIGURE 7–3 ● Manner by which nondiuretic antihypertensive agents may lose their effectiveness by reactive renal sodium retention.

they counter the distal nephron hypertrophy that occurs with loop diuretics alone (Brater, 2000).

## Conclusion

The overall evidence indicates that most hypertensives will respond over time to small doses of thiazide diuretic (i.e., 12.5 to 25 mg HCTZ) and that the relatively little additional effect that will be achieved by raising the daily dose beyond 25 mg per day comes at a high price in terms of side effects. In combinations, even 6.25 mg may be enough.

## Resistance to Diuretics

Resistance to the natriuretic and antihypertensive action of diuretics may occur for numerous reasons (Ellison, 1999):

- Excessive dietary sodium intake may overwhelm the diuretic's ability to maintain a shrunken fluid volume (Winer, 1961).
- For those with renal impairment (i.e., serum creatinine >1.5 mg per dL or creatinine clearance <30 mL per minute), thiazides likely will not work; because these drugs must be secreted into the renal tubules to work and because endogenous organic acids that build up in renal insufficiency compete with diuretics for transport into the proximal tubule, the renal response progressively falls with increasing renal damage (see Chapter 9).
- Food affects the absorption and bioavailability of different diuretics to variable degrees (Neuvonen & Kivistö, 1989), so the drugs should be taken in a uniform pattern in terms of the time of day and food ingestion.
- Nonsteroidal antiinflammatory drugs (NSAIDs) may blunt the effect of most diuretics. The problem may be even greater with selective COX-2 inhibitors (Cheng & Harris, 2004).

## Protection Against Cardiovascular Events

Diuretics in low doses protect against cardiovascular morbidity and mortality as well as any other class of drug (Psaty et al., 2003). In the review by the Blood Pressure Trialists (2003), diuretics were combined with β-blockers as "conventional therapy" but, in view of the inadequacy of β-blockers for primary protection, that is not appropriate. Diuretics stand on their own, as seen in the ALLHAT trial (ALLHAT Officers, 2002). Diuretic-based therapy lowered BP better than either ACEI- or CCC-based therapy, and a diuretic is recommended as the initial choice of therapy for most patients in the JNC-7 (Chobanian et al., 2003a, 2003b).

Diuretics may be particularly effective in prevention of strokes when compared to β-blockers and ACEIs (Messerli et al., 2003b). This issue will be addressed further in the section on ACEIs under "Other Uses: Cerebrovascular Diseases" (page 256).

## Side Effects

As shown in Figure 7–4, the likely pathogenesis for most of the more common complications related to diuretic use arises from the intrinsic activity of the drugs, and most complications are, therefore, related to the dose and duration of diuretic use. Logically, side effects occur with about the same frequency and severity with equipotent doses of all diuretics, and their occurrence will diminish with lower doses. In general, the longer the diuretic action, the more common the various complications: Hypokalemia was three times more common with the longer-acting chlorthalidone than with HCTZ in the Multiple Risk Factor Intervention Trial (Grimm et al., 1985).

*Hypokalemia*

As thiazides inhibit the coupled reabsorption of $Na^+/Cl^-$ in the early distal convoluted tubule, increased urinary $K^+$ loss may occur for multiple reasons: increased flow-dependent $K^+$ secretion in the distal nephron; volume contraction that activates release of both vasopressin and renin-aldosterone; and diuretic-induced hypochloremic metabolic alkalosis, which, in turn, redistributes $K^+$ into cells, leading to a further decrease in serum $K^+$ (Wilcox, 1999; Coca et al., 2005).

*Magnitude*

The degree of hypokalemia is dose dependent. With previously used, higher doses (50 to 100 mg HCTZ), the fall in serum potassium ranged from 0.1 to 1.4 mmol per L, averaging approximately 0.7 mmol per L (Grobbee & Hoes, 1995). With 25 mg HCTZ, the fall has ranged from 0.2 to 0.7 mmol per L, whereas with 12.5 mg HCTZ, no fall to as much as a 0.3-mm per L fall has been reported (Weir et al., 1996).

These falls translate to an incidence of hypokalemia (<3.5 mmol per L) of approximately 20% on higher doses (Widmer et al., 1995) and perhaps 5% to 10% on 12.5 to 25 mg per day of HCTZ or chlorthalidone (Franse et al., 2000a). Diuretic-induced hypokalemia will be accentuated by increased amounts of sodium intake (Ram et al., 1981) and in those with lower total body potassium stores, including many elderly patients (Flynn et al., 1989).

*Consequences*

The major potential risk of potassium depletion is to increase the incidence of stroke (Levine & Coull, 2002). This effect may be related to an increased platelet reactivity (Kimura et al., 2004). Muscle weakness, polyuria, and a propensity toward arrhythmias may appear with relatively mild hypokalemia. Patients on digitalis may develop toxicity, perhaps because both digitalis and hypokalemia inhibit the $Na^+/K^+$-adenosine

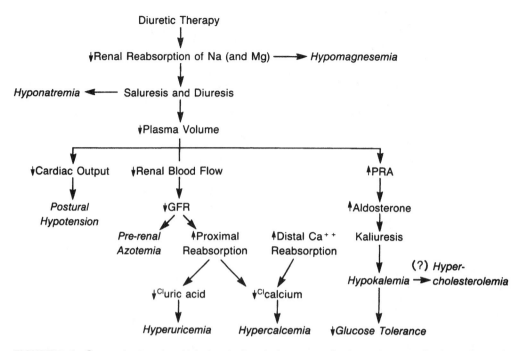

**FIGURE 7–4** ● Mechanisms by which chronic diuretic therapy may lead to various complications. The mechanism for hypercholesterolemia remains in question, although it is shown as arising via hypokalemia. Ca, calcium; Cl, chlorine; GFR, glomerular filtration rate; Na, sodium; Mg, magnesium; PRA, plasma renin activity.

triphosphatase ($Na^+/K^+$-ATPase) pump, the activity of which is essential to normal intracellular electrolyte balance and membrane potential (Nørgaard & Kjeldsen, 1991).

*Ventricular Arrhythmias and Sudden Death*
There appears to be a dose-dependent increase in sudden death with nonpotassium-sparing (naked) diuretics (Grobbee & Hoes, 1995). In two case-control studies, the risk of sudden death was nearly doubled in those on large doses of naked diuretics as compared to those on thiazide plus a potassium-sparing agent (Hoes et al., 1995; Siscovick et al., 1994). In the Systolic Hypertension in the Elderly Program (SHEP) trial, among those randomly allocated to 12.5 to 25 mg chlorthalidone, the 7.2% who developed hypokalemia had less than half the reduction in major cardiovascular events than those who remained normokalemic (Franse et al., 2000a). In the Studies of Left Ventricular Dysfunction (SOLVD) trial, use of a nonpotassium-sparing diuretic was associated with a 37% increased risk of arrhythmic death as compared to use of a potassium-sparing diuretic (HA Cooper et al., 1999).

*Effect on Blood Pressure*
Hypokalemia can set off various processes that can raise the BP (Coca et al., 2005), including a worsening of insulin resistance (Langford et al., 1990). Dietary potassium depletion has been found to

raise the BP (Krishna et al., 1989), whereas the correction of diuretic-induced hypokalemia lowered the mean BP by an average of 5.5 mm Hg in a group of 16 hypertensives on a constant dose of diuretic (Kaplan et al., 1985).

*Prevention of Diuretic-Induced Hypokalemia*
Prevention is preferable. By lowering dietary sodium, increasing dietary potassium, and using the least amount of diuretic needed, potassium depletion may be avoided. A lower dietary sodium intake (72 mmol per day) reduced diuretic-induced potassium loss by half of that observed on a higher sodium intake (195 mmol per day) (Ram et al., 1981). A potassium-sparing agent, β-blocker, or ACEI given with the diuretic will reduce the degree of potassium loss but may not prevent the development of hypokalemia (Sawyer & Gabriel, 1988). Aldosterone blockers may be even more efficient (Coca et al., 2005).

*Repletion of Diuretic-Induced Hypokalemia*
If prevention does not work, the potassium deficiency can be replaced with supplemental $K^+$, preferably given as the chloride; other anions (as found in most fruits rich in potassium) may not correct the alkalosis or the intracellular $K^+$ deficiency as well (Kopyt et al., 1985). However, potassium citrate (Sakhaee et al., 1991) or bicarbonate (Frassetto et al., 2000) will be more effective in reducing urinary calcium loss in patients with renal stones or

osteoporosis. The KCl may be given as a potassium-containing salt substitute; a number of these substitutes are available, and they are less expensive than potassium supplements.

If the patient is continued on the thiazide, 40 mmol per day of supplemental potassium or the addition of a potassium-sparing agent will usually overcome hypokalemia (Schnaper et al., 1989). Concomitant hypomagnesemia will also be corrected with the potassium sparer.

Caution is advised in giving potassium supplements to patients receiving ACEIs or ARBs whose aldosterone levels are suppressed and who may be unable to excrete extra potassium. The problem may be compounded in diabetics who may be unable to move potassium rapidly into cells and in those with renal insufficiency who may have a limited ability to excrete potassium.

### Hypomagnesemia

Some of the problems attributed to hypokalemia may be caused by hypomagnesemia instead, and potassium repletion may not be possible in the presence of magnesium depletion (Whang et al., 1985). Although loop diuretics tend to cause more urinary magnesium loss than do thiazides, hypomagnesemia and significant cellular depletion may occur with large doses of either (Dørup et al., 1993). However, conventional doses of diuretics rarely induce magnesium deficiency (Wilcox, 1999).

Clinical features include weakness, nausea, neuromuscular irritability, and the appearance of ventricular arrhythmias, which are resistant to treatment unless both hypomagnesemia and hypokalemia are corrected (Whang et al., 1985). Since, experimentally, magnesium inhibits norepinephrine release (Shimosawa et al., 2004), hypomagenesiumia may raise blood pressure.

Magnesium wastage is lessened by use of smaller doses of diuretics and concomitant use of a potassium-sparing agent (Schnaper et al., 1989). If repletion is needed, oral magnesium oxide, 200 to 400 mg per day (10 to 20 mmol), or potassium-magnesium citrate may be tolerated without gastrointestinal distress (Pak, 2000).

### Hyponatremia

By impairing the dilution of the tubular fluid, thiazides reduce the capacity for rapid and effective elimination of free water, and slight, asymptomatic falls in serum sodium concentration are common (Wilcox, 1999). Rarely, severe, symptomatic hyponatremia develops, usually soon after diuretics are started in elderly women who appear to have an expanded fluid volume from increased water intake in the face of a decreased ability to excrete free water (Sharabi et al., 2002).

### Hyperuricemia

Serum uric acid levels are high in as many as 30% of untreated hypertensives and may independently predict cardiovascular events (Franse et al., 2000b) and mortality (NisKanen et al., 2004). Moreover, Johnson and colleagues (2005) have provided evidence for a causal role of uric acid in the pathogenesis of hypertension. Thiazide therapy increases the incidence of hyperuricemia and may provoke gout, with an annual incidence of 4.9% at levels above 9 mg per dL (Campion et al., 1987). In a prospective 12-year follow-up of 47,150 men, both hypertension and diuretic use were independently associated with an increased incidence of gout (Choi et al., 2005).

With the possibility of a pathogenetic role of elevated uric acid, the prior neglect of hyperuricemia seems inappropriate. If therapy is given, the logical choice is probenecid to increase renal excretion of uric acid. The ARB losartan is uricosuric and may ameliorate diuretic-induced hyperuricemia.

### Calcium Metabolism Alterations

Renal calcium reabsorption also is increased with chronic thiazide therapy, and urinary calcium excretion is decreased by 40% to 50% (Friedman & Bushinsky, 1999). A slight rise in serum calcium (i.e., 0.1 to 0.2 mg per dL) is usual, and hypercalcemia is often provoked in patients with preexisting hyperparathyroidism or vitamin D-treated hypoparathyroidism. The fact that serum calcium levels do not continue to rise in the face of reduced calcium excretion likely reflects the combination of reduced intestinal absorption of calcium (Sakhaee et al., 1984) and retention of calcium in bone (Rejnmark et al., 2001). The former effect likely reflects a suppression of parathyroid hormone and vitamin D synthesis from the slight hypercalcemia and makes thiazide therapy a practical way to treat patients with renal stones caused by hypercalcemia from increased calcium absorption (Quereda et al., 1996). The retention of calcium in bone offers protection from osteoporosis and fractures (LaCroix et al., 2000).

### Hyperlipidemia

Kasiske et al. (1995) found that diuretics given in doses greater than the equivalent of 50 mg HCTZ induced these statistically significant increases (in millimoles per liter): total cholesterol, 0.12; low-density lipoprotein (LDL) cholesterol, 0.19; and triglycerides, 0.10. There was no significant change in high-density lipoprotein (HDL) cholesterol. In this analysis, cholesterol levels tended to decrease with time in both treated and untreated groups, whereas the effects of diuretics on triglycerides were seen only in short-term studies.

With currently used lower doses, thiazides induce minimal, if any, adverse changes in the lipid profile (Weir & Moser, 2000). It may still be useful to monitor lipid levels after a few months of thiazide use and, if elevated, to encourage a low-saturated-fat diet.

*Glucose Intolerance and Insulin Resistance*

Insulin resistance (Lithell, 1996), impairment of glucose tolerance, precipitation of overt diabetes (Samuelsson et al., 1996), and worsening of diabetic control (Goldner et al., 1960) have all been observed in patients taking larger doses of thiazides. Rarely, diuretics may precipitate hyperosmolar, nonketotic diabetic coma (Fonseca & Phear, 1982).

As with all the adverse effects of diuretics, the impairment of glucose utilization that connotes insulin resistance is seen more with high doses and less (or not at all) with therapeutically effective lower doses (equivalent to 12.5 mg HCTZ) (Harper et al., 1995). With currently used lower doses, no increase in the incidence of diabetes was noted in a prospective cohort study of 12,500 hypertensive subjects (Gress et al., 2000). However, the incidence of new-onset diabetes among the ALLHAT trial participants who took chlorthalidone (most at a dose of 25 mg, equivalent to 40 to 50 mg of HCTZ) was 11.5% compared to 8.3% in those who started with amlodipine and 7.6% in those who started with lisinopril (ALLHAT Officers, 2002). During the few years of the trial, no adverse consequences of this increase in diabetes was apparent, but the potential for future trouble should be recognized (Messerli et al., 2004). This is particularly true since patients with newly diagnosed diabetes have been reported to have a higher risk of heart attack (Dunder et al., 2003) and a higher mortality rate after a heart attack (Aguilar et al., 2004). Nonetheless, those patients given chlorthalidone in the SHEP trial, despite having an increased incidence of diabetes, compared to those given a placebo, did not have an increase in cardiovascular events even after an average of 14.3-year follow-up (Kostis et al., 2005).

It is likely that most of the increases in diabetes in diuretic-treated patients comes from the concomitant use of β-blockers, the "conventional" therapy of older trials.

*Erectile Dysfunction*

Impotence may be more common with diuretics than with other drugs. In the large, randomized Medical Research Council (MRC) trial, impotence was reported by 22.6% of the men on bendrofluazide, as compared to a rate of 10.1% among those on placebo, and 13.2% among those on propranolol [Medical Research Council Working Party (MRC), 1981]. In the Treatment of Mild Hypertension Study (TOMHS), the men randomized to chlorthalidone had a 17.1% incidence of erection problems through 24 months, as compared to an 8.1% incidence in those on placebo (Grimm et al., 1997). The problem is even greater in obese men but is lessened if they lose weight (Bursztyn, 2004).

*Other Side Effects*

Fever and chills, blood dyscrasias, cholecystitis, pancreatitis, necrotizing vasculitis, acute interstitial nephritis, and noncardiogenic pulmonary edema have been seen rarely. Excess volume depletion may induce prerenal azotemia and favor thrombosis (Lottermoser et al., 2000). Allergic skin rashes occur in 0.28% of patients, and approximately the same percentage develops photosensitivity (Diffey & Langtry, 1989). An increased relative risk of renal cell (and perhaps colon) cancer has been reported with diuretic therapy (Lip & Ferner, 1999), but the absolute risk is far below the proven benefits of these drugs.

## Conclusion

Diuretics can cause multiple metabolic perturbations that could reduce their ability to protect against progressive atherosclerosis as they lower BP. Clearly, these adverse effects are dose dependent and much less of a problem with appropriately lower doses (6.25 mg HCTZ in combination, 12.5 to 25 mg HCTZ alone), which will provide most, if not all, of their antihypertensive effects. Larger doses may be needed, but low doses should always be tried and, when they work, should be maintained for as long as the patient is being treated. When diuretics are withdrawn, the BP will usually promptly rise (Walma et al., 1997).

## Loop Diuretics

Loop diuretics primarily block chloride reabsorption by inhibition of the $Na^+/K^+/Cl^-$ cotransport system of the luminal membrane of the thick ascending limb of Henle's loop, the site where 35% to 45% of filtered sodium is reabsorbed (Figure 7–1). Therefore, the loop diuretics are more potent and have a more rapid onset of action than do the thiazides. However, they are no more effective in lowering BP or less likely to cause side effects if given in equipotent amounts. Their major use is in patients with renal insufficiency, in whom large enough doses can be given to achieve an effective luminal concentration (see Chapter 9). In addition, they may induce nitric-oxide mediated vasodilation (Costa et al., 2004).

## Furosemide

### Clinical Use

Although some report good antihypertensive effects from once-daily 40-mg doses of furosemide (van der Heijden et al., 1998), most find that even twice-daily furosemide is less effective than twice-daily HCTZ (Anderson et al., 1971; Holland et al., 1979) or once-daily chlorthalidone (Healy et al., 1970) while producing similar hyperuricemia and hypokalemia. The maintenance of a slightly shrunken body fluid volume, which is critical for an antihypertensive action from diuretic therapy, is not met by the short duration of furosemide action (<6 hours for an oral dose); during the remaining hours sodium is retained, so that net fluid balance over 24 hours is left unaltered (Wilcox et al., 1983). If furosemide is used twice daily, the first dose should be given early in the morning and the second in the midafternoon, both to provide diuretic action at the time of sodium intake and to avoid nocturia.

A long-held view that loop diuretics, unlike thiazides, do not increase renal reabsorption of lithium and therefore were preferable to prevent lithium toxicity appears not to be valid. In a study involving over 10,000 patients on lithium, the risk of hospitalization for lithium toxicity was increased 5.5-fold within the first 28 days of starting a loop diuretic (Juurlink et al., 2004b). Of further concern, new use of an ACEI increased the risk over sevenfold.

### Side Effects

Loop diuretics may cause fewer metabolic problems than do longer-acting agents, because of their shorter duration of action (Reyes & Taylor, 1999). With similar durations of action, the side effects are similar. Pancreatitis (Stenvinkel & Alvestrand, 1988) and allergic reactions (Sullivan, 1991) are two more of the thiazide-associated problems also seen with furosemide. In an experimental model, large doses of furosemide worsened the course of heart failure, presumably by reducing intracellular magnesium and calcium (Weber, 2004).

## Bumetanide

Bumetanide, although 40 times more potent and two times more bioavailable than furosemide on a weight basis, is identical in its actions when given in an equivalent dose (Brater et al., 1983).

## Torsemide

Torsemide differs from the other diuretics in that it is mainly eliminated by hepatic metabolism, with only 20% being excreted unchanged in the urine (Brater, 1993). Therefore, it has a more prolonged duration of action, as long as 12 hours.

In small doses of 2.5 to 5 mg, torsemide may lower BP in uncomplicated hypertension, whereas larger doses are needed for chronic edematous states or with renal insufficiency (Dunn et al., 1995). In patients with chronic renal disease, 40 mg of torsemide once a day provided equal natriuresic and hypertensive effect as 40 mg of furosemide twice a day (Vasavada et al., 2003).

## Ethacrynic Acid

Although structurally different from furosemide, ethacrynic acid also works primarily in the ascending limb of Henle's loop and has an equal potency. It is used much less than furosemide, mainly because of its greater propensity to cause permanent hearing loss. Since it does not contain a sulfonamide moiety, its main use has been in patients with sulfonamide sensitivity. However, the oral form of the drug is no longer being manufactured (Wall et al., 2003). A slowly increasing dose of furosemide may be tolerated in patients unable to take sulfa-containing diuretics (Earl et al., 2003).

## Potassium-Sparing Agents

Amiloride and triamterene act directly to inhibit sodium reabsorption by the epithelial sodium channels in the renal distal tubule, decreasing the net negative potential in the tubular lumen and thereby reducing potassium and hydrogen secretion and excretion, independent of aldosterone. Since neither are potent natriuretics, they are almost exclusively used in combination with thiazides to counter the $K^+$-wasting effect of the diuretic. Presumably by preventing hypokalemia, the use of $K^+$-sparing diuretics reduced the risk of death compared to the use of non-$K^+$-sparing diuretics in a large study of patients with systolic dysfunction (Domanski et al., 2003).

## Amiloride

Beyond experimental use in studies of sodium channels, most is used clinically with a thiazide diuretic as Moduretic containing 50 mg of HCTZ and 5 mg of amiloride. The drug has been used as medical therapy for hyperaldosteronism in patients intolerant to aldosterone blockers and in patients with mutations of the genes regulating sodium channels that lead to the full-blown Liddle's syndrome (see Chapter 13) or to a less severe prototype from the T594M polymorphism (Baker et al., 2002).

### Side Effects

Nausea, flatulence, and skin rash have been the most frequent side effects and hyperkalemia the most serious. Moreover, a number of cases of hyponatremia in elderly patients have been reported after its use in combination with HCTZ (Mathew et al., 1990).

### Triamterene

For many years, a combination of HCTZ (25 mg) and triamterene (50 mg), marketed as Dyazide, was the most widely prescribed antihypertensive drug in the United States. A more bioavailable tablet formulation of HCTZ and triamterene (Maxzide) has been marketed and shown to have equal antihypertensive efficacy (Casner & Dillon, 1990).

*Side Effects*

Triamterene may be excreted into the urine and may find its way into renal stones (Sörgel et al., 1985). Because triamterene is a folic acid antagonist, it should not be used during pregnancy (Hernández-Díaz et al., 2000).

### Aldosterone Blockers

The first of these agents, spironolactone, has long been available in the United States but little used until publication of the Randomized Evaluation Study (RALES) in 1999 (Pitt et al., 1999). This study showed a 30% decrease in mortality in patients with severe heart failure given 25 mg of spironolactone in addition to their other medications (Pitt et al., 1999). Since then, a large body of experimental and clinical evidence has revealed a multiorgan profibrotic effect of aldosterone so that blocking the hormone has assumed an important place in clinical medicine. At the same time, the marketing of a more specific aldosterone blocker, eplerenone, has stimulated the use of these agents.

### Mode of Action

The primary mineralocorticoid aldosterone causes hypertension when present in large excess, the syndrome of primary aldosteronism covered in Chapter 13. As noted in Chapter 3, even "normal" amounts of aldosterone in the presence of the relatively high sodium intake of most people in modern societies are now known to activate mineralocorticoid receptors in multiple organs including the brain, heart, kidney, and blood vessels (Rocha & Funder, 2002). In turn, vasculitis and fibrosis are induced, independent of the traditional renal sodium-retaining effect of the hormone.

On the foundation of considerable experimental evidence wherein blocking the mineralocorticoid receptor prevented all of the tissue damage, the RALES trial demonstrated that the addition of the aldosterone blocker spironolactone to therapy which included inhibitors of the renin-angiotensin system further reduced mortality in severe heart failure (Pitt et al., 1999), likely by reducing cardiac fibrosis (Zannad et al., 2000).

Subsequently, a more selective aldosterone receptor blocker, eplerenone, was marketed on the basis of its virtual equivalence to spironolactone in blocking the mineralocorticoid receptor but its much lesser blockade of androgen and progesterone receptors (Funder, 2002). In 2003, the addition of eplerenone was shown to reduce morbidity and mortality among patients with acute myocardial infarction complicated by left ventricular dysfunction in the Eplerenone Post-Acute Myocardial Infarction Heart Failure Efficacy and Survival Study (EPHESUS) (Pitt et al., 2003).

The antihypertensive effect of eplerenone appears to occur largely independent of its effect on epithelial electrolyte and fluid transport (Levy et al., 2004).

In both the RALES and EPHESUS trials, the aldosterone blocker provided additional benefit to patients receiving full doses of blockers of the renin-angiotensin system, ACEIs or ARBs. It is now known that aldosterone synthesis is not completely suppressed with these agents, breaking through to maintain the pretreatment aldosterone levels even if angiotensin II levels remain suppressed (Sato & Saruta, 2003). Such a breakthrough was not seen in the Valsartan Heart Failure Trial (Cohn et al., 2003), but the role of breakthrough has been documented in trials of hypertension therapy wherein addition of an aldosterone blocker to ACEIs or ARBs provided additional benefit (Black, 2004).

### Antihypertensive Efficacy

Spironolactone has been used alone to treat hypertension for many years, particularly in France (Jeunemaitre et al., 1988), but its major use in the United States has been as a $K^+$-sparer in combination with a thiazide diuretic (as in Aldactazide), providing an effect equivalent to 32 mmol of KCl (Toner et al., 1991). More recently, it has been found to effectively control patients with refractory hypertension when added in doses of 1 mg/kg per day (Ouzan et al., 2002). As expected, the drug lowers blood pressure more in patients with low plasma renin and higher aldosterone levels (Lim et al., 1999) and it has been the primary drug for hyperaldosteronism due to bilateral adrenal hyperplasia (Lim et al., 2001).

Eplerenone alone has been found to have an antihypertensive effect equivalent to ACEIs and CCBs, working well in Blacks and the elderly (Weinberger, 2004). It has also been shown to provide additional effect when added to an ACEI or ARB (Black, 2004). It improves diastolic function (Grandi et al., 2002) and reduces proteinuria in patients with diabetic nephropathy (Sato et al., 2003).

### Other Uses

In view of the strong experimental evidence and increasing clinical experience that aldosterone blockers provide major protection against damage to the heart, brain, kidneys, and blood vessels, the enthusiasm expressed by Pitt (2004) and Struthers and MacDonald (2004) may certainly be warranted. As the latter investigators state:

> Aldosterone interacts with mineralocorticoid receptors to promote endothelial dysfunction, facilitate thrombosis, reduce vascular compliance, impair baroreceptor function, and cause myocardial and vascular fibrosis. Although angiotensin II has been considered the major mediator of cardiovascular damage, increasing evidence suggests that aldosterone may mediate and exacerbate the damaging effects of angiotensin II. While angiotensin-converting enzyme (ACE) inhibitors and angiotensin II receptor blockers reduce plasma aldosterone levels initially, aldosterone rebound, or "escape" may occur during long-term therapy. Therefore, aldosterone blockage is required to reduce the risk of progressive target organ damage in patients with hypertension and heart failure. This may be achieved nonselectively with spironolactone or with the use of the selective aldosterone blocker eplerenone.

### Side Effects

The less specific spironolactone induces gynecomastia in about 10% of patients and occasional menstrual irregularities and impotence (Gumieniak & Williams, 2004). The more specific eplerenone induced gynecomastia in fewer than 1% of men and less of the other endocrine side effects, as well.

Hyperkalemia may occur with either agent but is uncommon in the absence of renal insufficiency, concomitant β-blocker, ACEI, or ARB therapy, or the use of potassium supplements (Gumieniak & Williams, 2004; Tamirisa et al., 2004). However, with the much greater use of spironolactone in patients with heart failure also being treated with ACEIs after publication of the RALES trial in 1999, the rate of hospitalization for hyperkalemia in a Toronto hospital rose from 2.4 per 1,000 patients in 1994 to 11.0 per 1,000 in 2001 and mortality rose from 0.3 to 2.0 per 1,000 (Juurlink et al., 2004a). Others have reported similar experiences (Svensson et al., 2003; Tamirisa et al., 2004), so care is obviously needed in combining an aldosterone blocker with a β-blocker, ACEI, or ARB.

## ADRENERGIC-INHIBITING DRUGS

Of the adrenergic-inhibiting agents currently used to treat hypertension, some act centrally on $\alpha_2$-receptors to inhibit sympathetic nerve activity, some inhibit postganglionic sympathetic neurons, and some block the $\alpha$- or $\beta$-adrenoreceptors on target organs (Figure 7–5). Agents that act by blocking ganglia are no longer used.

### Central α-Agonists

Central α agents stimulate central $\alpha_{2a}$-adrenergic receptors that are involved in depressor sympathoinhibitory mechanisms (van Zwieten, 1999b) (Figure 7–6). Some are selective, whereas clonidine also acts on central imidazoline receptors. These drugs have well-defined effects, including:

- A marked decline in sympathetic activity reflected in lower levels of norepinephrine.
- A reduction of the ability of the baroreceptor reflex to compensate for a decrease in BP, accounting for the relative bradycardia and enhanced hypotensive action noted on standing.
- A modest decrease in both peripheral resistance and cardiac output.
- A fall in plasma renin levels.

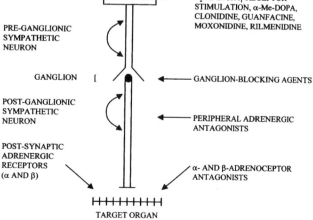

**FIGURE 7–5** ● Drug targets in the sympathetic nervous system. Virtually all structures, neurons, and receptors of the sympathetic nervous system can be influenced more or less selectively by antihypertensive drugs. α-Me-DOPA, α-Methyl-dioxyphenylalanine. (Modified from van Zwieten PA. Beneficial interactions between pharmacological, pathophysiological and hypertension research. *J Hypertens* 1999a;17:1787–1797.)

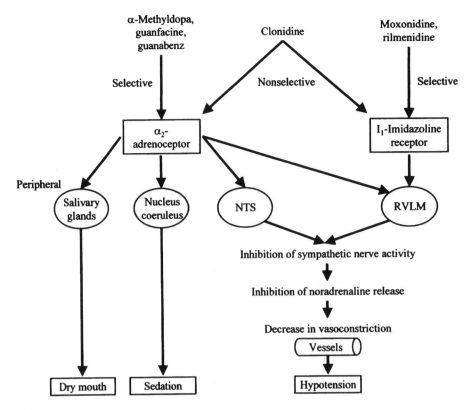

**FIGURE 7-6** ● Central antihypertensive mechanisms of various types of centrally acting antihypertensive drugs. Note the different targets of $\alpha_2$-adrenoceptor agonists and $I_1$-imidazoline stimulants. The adverse reactions, dry mouth and sedation, are mediated by $\alpha_2$-adrenoceptors but not by $I_1$-imidazoline receptors. NTS, nucleus tractus solitarii; RVLM, rostral ventrolateral medulla. (Modified from van Zwieten PA. The renaissance of centrally acting antihypertensive drugs. *J Hypertens* 1999b;17(Suppl 3):S15–S21.)

- Maintenance of renal blood flow despite a fall in BP.
- In addition to fluid retention, common side effects reflect their central site of action: sedation, decreased alertness, and a dry mouth.

When central $\alpha$-agonists are abruptly stopped, a rapid rebound and, rarely, an overshoot of the BP may be experienced with or without accompanying features of excess sympathetic nervous activity. This discontinuation syndrome likely represents a sudden surge of catecholamine release, freed from the prior state of inhibition.

## Methyldopa

From the early 1960s to the late 1970s, when β-blockers became available, methyldopa (Aldomet) was the second most popular drug (after diuretics) used to treat hypertension.

### Mode of Action

Methyldopa is the $\alpha$-methylated derivative of dopa, the natural precursor of dopamine and norepinephrine. Its mode of action involves the formation of methylnorepinephrine, which acts as a potent agonist at $\alpha$-adrenergic receptors within the central nervous system (CNS) (van Zwieten, 1999b).

### Antihypertensive Efficacy

Blood pressure is lowered maximally approximately 4 hours after an oral dose of methyldopa, and some effect persists for up to 24 hours. For most patients, therapy should be started with 250 mg two times per day, and the daily dosage can be increased to a maximum of 3.0 g on a twice-per-day schedule. In patients with renal insufficiency, the dosage should be halved.

### Side Effects

In addition to the anticipated sedative effects, postural hypotension, and fluid retention, an impairment of reticuloendothelial function (Kelton, 1985) and a variety of autoimmune side effects, including fever and liver dysfunction, are peculiar to methyldopa. Liver dysfunction usually disappears when the drug is stopped, but at least 83 cases of serious hepatotoxicity were reported by 1975 (Rodman et al., 1976), with diffuse parenchymal injury similar to autoimmune chronic active hepatitis (Lee, 1995).

An impairment of psychometric performance (Johnson et al., 1990) and a selective loss of upper airway motor activity (Lahive et al., 1988) may not be obvious until the drug is stopped. Overall, in large surveys, the number and range of the adverse reactions to methyldopa are impressive (Webster & Koch, 1996). In view of its unique and potentially serious side effects, other central α-agonists should be used in place of methyldopa. In the United States, it remains a favored drug only for the treatment of hypertension during pregnancy (see Chapter 11).

### Guanabenz

Guanabenz, an aminoguanidine, works like clonidine and methyldopa and causes similar side effects; unlike these other agents, it offers the advantages of not causing reactive fluid retention, so it has been approved for initial use as monotherapy. Its use is usually associated with slight lowering of serum cholesterol, and it can be safely used in diabetics (Gutin & Tuck, 1988) and asthmatics (Deitch et al., 1984).

Therapy should begin with 4 mg twice per day, with increments up to a total of 64 mg per day.

The side effects mimic those seen with other central $\alpha_2$-agonists; sedation and dry mouth are the most prominent, being seen in 20% to 30% of patients. A withdrawal syndrome may occur if the drug is stopped abruptly (Ram et al., 1979).

### Guanfacine

Another selective central $\alpha_2$-agonist, guanfacine appears to enter the brain more slowly and to maintain its antihypertensive effect longer then guanabenz (Sorkin & Heel, 1986). These differences translate into a once-per-day dosage and perhaps fewer CNS side effects (Lewin et al., 1990). Withdrawal symptoms are less common than with clonidine (Wilson et al., 1986). These characteristics make it the most attractive of this group of centrally acting $\alpha_2$-agonists.

### Clonidine

#### Mode of Action

Clonidine acts centrally on both $\alpha_2$-receptors and imidazoline receptors (Figure 7–6). It is readily absorbed, and plasma levels peak within an hour; the plasma half-life is 6 to 13 hours. When taken orally, the BP begins to fall within 30 minutes, with the greatest effect occurring between 2 and 4 hours. The duration of effect is from 8 to 12 hours.

#### Antihypertensive Efficacy

The starting dose may be as little as 0.075 mg twice daily (Clobass Study Group, 1990), with a maximum of 1.2 mg per day. Repeated hourly doses of 0.1 to 0.2 mg have been used to lower markedly elevated BP (Houston, 1986). Clonidine has been used to prevent the reflex sympathetic overactivity that follows direct vasodilator therapy and to serve as a screening test for pheochromocytoma (see Chapter 12).

A transdermal preparation that delivers clonidine continuously over a 7-day interval is effective and causes milder side effects than oral therapy (Giugliano et al., 1998), but it may cause considerable skin irritation and side effects similar to those seen with the oral drug (Langley & Heel, 1988), including rebound hypertension when discontinued (Metz et al., 1987). It is available in doses of 0.1, 0.2, and 0.3 mg per day.

#### Side Effects

Clonidine and methyldopa share the two most common side effects, sedation and dry mouth, although these effects are more common with clonidine (Webster & Koch, 1996). Clonidine does not share the autoimmune hepatic and hematologic derangements induced by methyldopa. Depression of sinus and atrioventricular (AV) nodal function may be common, and a few cases of severe bradycardia have been reported (Byrd et al., 1988). Large overdoses will lead to hypertension, presumably by stimulation of peripheral α receptors, causing vasoconstriction (Hunyor et al., 1975).

#### Rebound and Discontinuation Syndromes

If any antihypertensive therapy is inadvertently stopped abruptly, various discontinuation syndromes may occur: (a) a rapid asymptomatic return of the BP to pretreatment levels, which occurs in the majority of patients; (b) a rebound of the BP plus symptoms and signs of sympathetic overactivity; and (c) an overshoot of the BP above pretreatment levels.

A discontinuation syndrome has been reported most frequently with clonidine (Neusy & Lowenstein, 1989), likely reflecting a rapid return of catecholamine secretion that had been suppressed during therapy. Those who had been on a combination of a central adrenergic inhibitor, e.g., clonidine, and a β-blocker may be particularly susceptible if the central inhibitor is withdrawn while the β-blocker is continued (Lilja et al., 1982). This leads to a sudden surge in plasma catecholamines in a situation in which peripheral α-receptors are left unopposed to induce vasoconstriction because the β-receptors are blocked and cannot mediate vasodilation.

If a discontinuation syndrome appears, clonidine should be restarted, and the symptoms will likely recede rapidly. If needed, labetalol will effectively lower a markedly elevated BP (Mehta & Lopez, 1987).

## Other Uses

Clonidine has been reported to be useful in numerous conditions that may accompany hypertension, including:

- Restless legs syndrome (Wagner et al., 1996)
- Opiate withdrawal (Bond, 1986)
- Menopausal hot flashes (Pandya et al., 2000)
- Diarrhea due to diabetic neuropathy (Fedorak et al., 1985) or ulcerative colitis (Lechin et al., 1985)
- Sympathetic nervous hyperactivity in patients with alcoholic cirrhosis (Esler et al., 1992)
- Congestive heart failure (CHF) (Gavras et al., 1999)
- Perioperative protection for patients at high risk of coronary events (Wallace et al,. 2004)

### Imidazoline Receptor Agonists

Not available in the United States but used elsewhere, monoxidine and rilmenidine are two centrally acting drugs that have as their primary site of action the imidazoline receptor located in the rostral ventrolateral medulla oblongata, wherein $\alpha_2$-receptors are less abundant (Figure 7–6) (van Zwieten, 1999b). They effectively reduce sympathetic activity (Esler et al., 2004) and may diminish insulin resistance so they are being used for patients with the metabolic syndrome (Sharma et al., 2004), with less of the sedation and dry mouth seen with clonidine and selective $\alpha_2$-agonists.

### Peripheral Adrenergic Inhibitors

Of these, only reserpine continues to be used.

### Reserpine

First reported to be effective in the 1940s (Bhatia, 1942), reserpine became popular in the 1960s but has been used less and less for various reasons:

- An inexpensive generic drug, reserpine has no constituency pushing for its use.
- Reserpine has become old hat; the advent of every new "miracle" antihypertensive makes it look more and more outdated.
- The scare of cancer tainted reserpine, although the claims have been refuted (Horwitz & Feinstein, 1985).
- Reserpine is associated with a lurking specter of insidious depression.

#### Mode of Action

Reserpine, one of the many alkaloids of the Indian snakeroot *Rauwolfia serpentine,* is absorbed readily from the gut, is taken up rapidly by lipid-containing tissue, and binds to sites involved with storage of biogenic amines. Its effects start slowly and persist, so only one dose per day is needed.

Reserpine blocks the transport of norepinephrine into its storage granules so that less of the neurotransmitter is available when the adrenergic nerves are stimulated. The resultant decrease in sympathetic tone results in a decrease in peripheral vascular resistance. Catecholamines also are depleted in the brain, which may account for the sedative and depressant effects of the drug, and in the myocardium, which may decrease cardiac output and induce a slight bradycardia (Cohen et al., 1968).

#### Antihypertensive Efficacy

By itself, reserpine has limited antihypertensive potency, resulting in an average decrease of only 3/5 mm Hg; when combined with a thiazide, the reduction averaged 14/11 mm Hg (VA Cooperative Study, 1962). It works as well as other drugs (Krönig et al., 1997) and induces significant regression of LVH (Horn et al., 1997). With a diuretic, as little as 0.05 mg once daily will provide most of the antihypertensive effect of 0.25 mg and is associated with less lethargy and impotence (Participating VA Medical Centers, 1982).

#### Side Effects

Side effects, which are relatively infrequent at appropriately low doses (Prisant et al., 1991), include nasal stuffiness, increased gastric acid secretion, which rarely may activate an ulcer, and CNS depression, which may simply tranquilize an apprehensive patient and is rarely severe enough to lead to serious depression

### Guanethidine

Guanethidine at one time was frequently used for moderate hypertension because it requires only one dose per day and has a steep dose-response relationship, thus producing an effect in almost every patient. As other effective drugs with fewer side effects became available, the use of guanethidine rapidly diminished.

#### Mode of Action

Guanethidine is taken into the adrenergic nerves by an active transport mechanism. Once inside the adrenergic nerves, guanethidine initially blocks the exit of norepinephrine; it then causes an active release of norepinephrine from its storage granules, depleting the reserve pool of the neurotransmitter and decreasing the amount released when the nerve is stimulated, thereby reducing peripheral resistance. The BP is reduced somewhat in the supine position but much more so when the patient is upright, because the normal vasoconstrictive response to posture is blunted (Goldberg & Raftery, 1976). The amount required to lower standing BP to an acceptable and tolerable level varies from 25 to 300 mg daily.

### Side Effects

Most of the complications are in keeping with the known effects of guanethidine: postural hypotension, fluid retention, diarrhea, and failure of ejaculation. The appearance of minimal postural hypotension is an indication that the therapeutic end point has been reached.

### Guanadrel Sulfate

A close relative of guanethidine, guanadrel sulfate has almost all the attributes of that drug with a shorter onset and offset of action, which diminish the frequency of side effects and make it more tolerable (Owens & Dunn, 1988).

### α-Adrenergic Receptor Blockers

Selective $\alpha_1$-blockers have had a relatively small share of the overall market for antihypertensive drugs in the United States and as a consequence of the ALLHAT trial (ALLHAT Officers, 2000), their use in the United States is now almost exclusively for relief of prostatism. Nonetheless, the availability of more of these drugs, the increasing awareness of their special ability to improve lipid levels (Hirano et al., 2001) and insulin sensitivity, and their unique ability to quickly relieve the symptoms of benign prostatic hypertrophy (Schwinn et al., 2004) support their more widespread use.

### Mode of Action

The nonselective α-blockers phenoxybenzamine and phentolamine are used almost exclusively in the medical management of pheochromocytoma, because they are only minimally effective in primary hypertension (see Chapter 12).

After recognition of the two major subtypes of α-receptors—the $\alpha_1$ postsynaptic and the $\alpha_2$ presynaptic—prazosin was recognized to act as a competitive antagonist of postsynaptic $\alpha_1$-receptors, an effect shared by doxazosin and terazosin (Figure 7–7). These agents block the activation of postsynaptic $\alpha_1$-receptors by circulating or by neurally released catecholamines, an activation that normally induces vasoconstriction. Peripheral resistance falls without major changes in cardiac output.

The presynaptic $\alpha_2$-receptors remain open, capable of binding neurotransmitter and thereby inhibiting the release of additional norepinephrine through a direct negative-feedback mechanism. This inhibition of norepinephrine release explains the lesser frequency of tachycardia, increased cardiac output, and rise in renin levels that characterize the response to drugs that block both the presynaptic $\alpha_2$-receptor and the postsynaptic $\alpha_1$-receptor (e.g., phentolamine). Despite this selective blockade, neurally

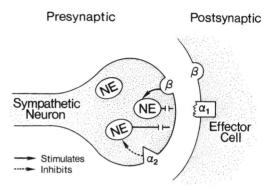

**FIGURE 7–7** ● Schematic view of the action of selective postsynaptic $\alpha_1$-blockers. By blocking the $\alpha_1$-adrenergic receptor on the vascular smooth muscle, catecholamine-induced vasoconstriction is inhibited. The $\alpha_2$-adrenergic receptor on the neuronal membrane is not blocked; therefore, inhibition of additional norepinephrine (NE) release by the short feedback mechanism is maintained.

mediated responses to stress and exercise are unaffected, and the baroreceptor reflex remains active.

Accompanying these desirable attributes may be other actions that lessen the usefulness of α-adrenergic blockers: They relax the venous bed as well and, at least initially, may affect the visceral vascular bed more than the peripheral vascular bed, and the subsequent pooling of blood in the viscera may explain the propensity to first-dose hypotension seen with the fast-acting prazosin (Saxena & Bolt, 1986). Volume retention is common, perhaps because renin and aldosterone levels are less suppressed than they are with other adrenergic-inhibiting drugs (Webb et al., 1987).

A quinazoline derivative, prazosin is rapidly absorbed, reaching maximal blood levels at 2 hours and having a plasma half-life of approximately 3 hours. Terazosin and doxazosin are less lipid-soluble and have half or less of the affinity for $\alpha_1$-receptors as compared with prazosin. Therefore, they induce a slower and less profound initial fall in BP, particularly after standing, than does prazosin. This translates into a lesser propensity for hypotensive symptoms (Achari et al., 2000) and a longer duration of action for the second-generation $\alpha_1$-blockers.

Tamsulosin produces a lesser blockade of the $\alpha_1$-receptors on blood vessels than in the prostate (Harada et al., 2000). It is not approved for treatment of hypertension.

### Antihypertensive Efficacy

The antihypertensive efficacy of doxazosin and terazosin is equivalent to that of diuretics, β-blockers,

ACEIs, and CCBs (Achari et al., 2000). The drugs work equally well in Black and in non-Black patients (Batey et al., 1989) and in the elderly (Cheung et al., 1989) and can be effectively combined with a diuretic, β-blockers, or CCBs. In the presence of renal failure, the hypotensive action is enhanced, so lower doses should be used. The addition of doxazosin has been shown to control hypertension effectively in patients resistant to two or more other agents (Black et al., 2000).

The initial dose should be 1 mg, slowly titrated upward to achieve the desired fall in BP, with a total daily dose of up to 20 mg sometimes required. α-blockers can be given at bedtime to provide a greater nocturnal fall in BP in patients who fail to have a normal dipping of BP during the night (Kario et al., 2000) and a maximal effect on the early morning surge in BP that is involved in the increased incidence of cardiovascular events at that time (Pickering et al., 1994). No tachyphylaxis to the antihypertensive action has been seen after 3 years of doxazosin use (Talseth et al., 1991). However, if reactive fluid retention occurs, the BP may rise, only to fall again with the addition of a small dose of diuretic.

### Other Uses

#### Genitourinary Function

Doxazosin, tamsulosin, and terazosin have been found to provide excellent relief from the obstructive symptoms of benign prostatic hypertrophy (BPH) (Schwinn et al., 2004). The combination of doxazosin and the 5α-reductace inhibitor finasteride slowed the clinical progression of BPH better than either drug alone (McConnell et al., 2003). In those who are also hypertensive, the expected fall in BP is noted; in those who are normotensive, little effect on BP is seen (Lepor et al., 1997).

In the TOMHS trial, which involved a representative from each of the five major classes of antihypertensives, only doxazosin reduced the incidence of impotence below that seen with placebo (Grimm et al., 1997).

#### Metabolic Effects

$\alpha_1$-blockers have been repeatedly found to improve both the lipid profile (Kasiske et al., 1995) and insulin sensitivity (Lithell, 1996). The mechanisms responsible for these generally favorable effects may include a decrease in fractional catabolic rate of HDL cholesterol (Sheu et al., 1990), an increase in lipoprotein lipase and lecithin-cholesterol acyltransferase activity (Rabkin, 1993), and an inhibition of LDL oxidation (Kinoshita et al., 2001).

### The ALLHAT Experience

Despite these generally attractive features, the termination of the doxazosin arm of the ALLHAT (ALLHAT Officers, 2000) has been used as an argument to restrict the use of α-blockers (Stafford et al., 2004). However, the design of the study and the interpretation of the results have exaggerated the patative dangers of α-blockers (Davis et al., 2004).

In ALLHAT, more than 90% of the participants were on various antihypertensive drugs at the time of enrollment (Grimm et al., 2001). Their previous drugs were stopped abruptly or after one period of partial withdrawal, and they were started on their randomly allocated study drug (α-blocker, ACEI, CCB, or diuretic) as monotherapy. These enrollees were, overall, a high-risk population: significantly hypertensive, elderly, and with a high proportion of diabetics, dyslipidemics, Blacks, and patients having had prior cardiovascular events. It is not very surprising, then, that some of these subjects switched from a diuretic with or without ACEI therapy to a low dose of an α-blocker would develop CHF as compared to those assigned to a diuretic.

At the same time, neither cardiovascular nor all-cause mortality was increased in the doxazosin group, suggesting that the twofold increased numbers of heart failure likely were not of severe degree. Moreover, the diagnosis of CHF was based on clinical grounds and was much more commonly observed in the ALLHAT than in other randomized, controlled trials (RCTs) with equally severe hypertension (Brown, 2001).

I believe that the doxazosin arm of ALLHAT could have been continued in the absence of any increase in mortality. Nonetheless, the ALLHAT experience clearly indicates the need to use a diuretic with an α-blocker for the treatment of hypertension, particularly in those with LVH or other risk factors for CHF. α-blockers remain useful as add-on therapy in patients with resistant hypertension (Black et al., 2000). They remain the preferred initial therapy for many hypertensive patients with benign prostatic hypertrophy.

### Side Effects

Side effects include headache, drowsiness, fatigue, and weakness—likely nonspecific effects of a lowering of the BP. Rather surprisingly, dizziness and asthma, the most common side effects seen in men given terazosin for benign prostatic hypertrophy, were not related to changes in BP (Lepor et al., 2000). For most patients, the side effects diminish with continued therapy. Rarely, a first-dose response of postural hypotension developing in 30 to 90 minutes is seen, particularly in volume-depleted patients given the shorter-acting prazosin (Stokes et al., 1977). The problem generally can be avoided by initiating therapy with a small dose and ensuring that the patient is not volume-depleted as a result of diuretic therapy. Urinary incontinence in women may be caused by α-blockers (Marshall & Beevers, 1996). Even massive overdoses do little harm if the patient remains supine (Lip & Ferner, 1995a).

## β-Adrenergic Receptor Blockers

For many years, β-adrenergic blocking agents were the second most popular antihypertensive drugs after diuretics. Although they are no more effective than other antihypertensive agents and may, on occasion, induce serious side effects, they offer the special advantage of relieving a number of concomitant diseases. In view of their proven ability to provide secondary cardioprotection after an acute myocardial infarction (MI), it was hoped that they would provide special primary protection against initial coronary events as well. This hope remains unfulfilled. To the contrary, β-blockers have failed to reduce either heart attacks or strokes, and in the words of Messerli et al. (2003a): "The time has come to admit that beta-blockers should no longer be considered appropriate first-line therapy in uncomplicated hypertension." This is particularly true for the most popular, atenolol (Carlberg et al., 2004).

Nonetheless, the proven benefits of β-blockers in patients with either coronary disease (particularly after an acute MI) or CHF ensure that these drugs will continue to be widely used (Estep et al., 2004).

### Mode of Action

These agents are chemically similar to β-agonists and to each other (Figure 7–8). The competitive inhibition of β-blockers on β-adrenergic receptors produces numerous effects on functions that regulate the BP, including a reduction in cardiac output, a diminution of renin release, perhaps a decrease in central sympathetic nervous outflow, a presynaptic

blockade that inhibits catecholamine release, and a probable decrease in peripheral vascular resistance. The hemodynamic effects appear to change over time. Cardiac output usually falls acutely (except with high-ISA pindolol) and remains lower chronically; peripheral resistance, on the other hand, usually rises acutely but falls toward, if not to, normal with time (Man in't Veld et al., 1988).

### *Pharmacologic Differences*

Since the introduction of propranolol in 1964 (Black et al., 1964), a number of similar drugs have been synthesized, approximately 20 being marketed throughout the world, 12 in the United States. The various β-blockers can be conveniently classified by their relative selectivity for the $\beta_1$-receptors (primarily in the heart) and presence of intrinsic sympathomimetic activity (ISA), also referred to as *partial agonist activity* and their *lipid solubility* (Figure 7–9) (Table 7–4). In addition, some agents (labetalol, carvedilol) have both α- and β-blocking effects, and they are considered separately.

*Lipid Solubility*

Those that are more lipid-soluble (lipophilic) tend to be taken up and metabolized extensively by the liver. As an example, with oral propranolol and metoprolol, up to 70% is removed on the first pass of portal blood through the liver. The bioavailability of these β-blockers is, therefore, less after oral than after intravenous administration.

Those such as nadolol, which is much less lipid-soluble (lipophobic), escape hepatic metabolism and are mainly excreted by the kidneys, unchanged. As a result, its plasma half-life and duration of action is much longer.

*$\beta_1$-Receptor Cardioselectivity*

All currently available β-blockers antagonize cardiac $\beta_1$-receptors competitively, but they vary in their degree of $\beta_2$-receptor blockade in extracardiac tissues. The assumption that an agent with relative cardioselectivity is automatically less likely to cause side effects must be tempered by these considerations:

- No β-blocker is purely cardioselective, particularly in large doses.
- No tissue contains exclusively only one subgroup of receptors: The heart has both, with $\beta_1$ predominating; bronchioles have both, with $\beta_2$ predominating.
- When high endogenous catechol levels are needed, as during an attack of asthma, even minimal degrees of $\beta_2$-blockade from a cardioselective drug such as bisoprolol may cause trouble (Haffner et al., 1992).

Nonetheless, $\beta_1$-receptor cardioselective agents have some advantages. For instance, they have been

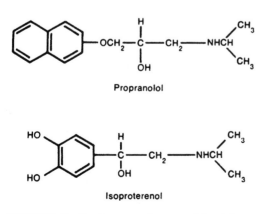

**FIGURE 7–8** ● Structure of propranolol and the β-agonist isoproterenol.

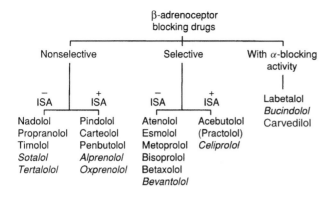

**FIGURE 7–9** ● Classification of β-adrenoreceptor blockers based on cardioselectivity and intrinsic sympathomimetic activity. Drugs not approved for use in the United States for the treatment of hypertension are in italics. ISA, intrinsic sympathomimetic activity.

shown to disturb lipid and carbohydrate metabolism less than do nonselective agents (Dujovne et al., 1993), and they can be safely used in patients with mild to moderate reactive airway disease (Salpeter et al., 2002).

On the other hand, in the presence of certain concomitant diseases, such as migraine and tremor, a nonselective $\beta_2$-antagonist effect may be preferable. Also, $\beta_2$-receptors are involved in stress-induced hypokalemia, so nonselective agents will block this fall in plasma potassium more than selective ones will (Brown et al., 1983). This could have clinical relevance, as stress-induced hypokalemia could cause sudden death.

## TABLE 7–4

### Pharmacologic Properties of Some β-Blockers

| Drug | U.S. Trade Name | $\beta_1$-Selectivity | Intrinsic Sympathomimetic Activity | $\alpha$-Blockage | Lipid Solubility | Usual Daily Dosage (Frequency) |
|---|---|---|---|---|---|---|
| Acebutolol | Sectral | + | + | – | + | 200–1200 mg (1) |
| Atenolol | Tenormin | ++ | – | – | – | 25–100 mg (2) |
| Betaxolol | Kerlone | ++ | – | – | – | 5–40 mg (1) |
| Bisoprolol | Zebeta | +++ | – | – | + | 2.5–20 mg (1) |
| Bucindolol | | – | – | – | + | 50–200 mg |
| Carteolol | Cartrol | – | + | – | – | 2.5–10 mg (1) |
| Carvedilol | Coreg | – | – | + | +++ | 12.5–50 mg (2) |
| Celiprolol | Selectol | ++ | + | – | – | 200–400 mg (1) |
| Esmolol | Brevibloc | ++ | – | – | – | 25–300 µg/kg/min iv |
| Labetalol | Normodyne, Trandate | – | – | + | ++ | 200–1200 mg (2) |
| Metoprolol | Lopressor, Toprol XL | ++ | – | – | ++ | 50–200 mg (2, 1) |
| Nadolol | Corgard | – | – | – | – | 20–240 mg (1) |
| Nebivolol | | ++ | – | – | ++ | 5–10 mg (1) |
| Penbutolol | Levatol | – | + | – | +++ | 10–20 mg (1) |
| Pindolol | Visken | – | +++ | – | ++ | 10–60 (2) |
| Propranolol | Inderal, LA | – | – | – | +++ | 40–240 mg (2, 1) |
| Timolol | Blocadren | – | – | – | ++ | 10–40 mg (2) |

+, ++, and +++ signs indicate the magnitude of the effect on various properties; – sign indicates no effect.

*Intrinsic Sympathomimetic Activity*

Of the β-blockers now available in the United States, pindolol and, to a lesser degree, acebutolol have ISA, implying that even in concentrations that fully occupy the β-receptors, the biologic effect is less than that seen with a full agonist. When background sympathetic activity is low, the partial agonist acts as an agonist; when background activity is high, the partial agonist acts as an antagonist (Cruickshank, 1990).

The presence of ISA may be clinically reflected in various beneficial features: less bradycardia, less bronchospasm, less decrease in peripheral blood flow, and less derangement of blood lipids.

## Antihypertensive Efficacy

In the usual doses prescribed (Table 7–4), various β-blockers have equal antihypertensive efficacy (Wilcox, 1978). However, they may not all provide full 24-hour lowering of the BP, which may be particularly critical in protecting against early morning cardiovascular catastrophes. Metoprolol blunted this rapid early morning rise, but atenolol and pindolol did not (Raftery & Carrageta, 1985). Neutel et al. (1990) found a similar lack of 24-hour effect with once-daily atenolol but a sustained effect with acebutolol. This less than 24-hour efficacy of atenolol may be responsible, along with its lesser penetration into the brain, for the higher stroke and mortality rates seen with atenolol in multiple trials comparing it to other antihypertensive drugs (Carlberg et al., 2004).

The blood pressure responds less to β-blockers in Blacks than in Whites (Brewster et al., 2004). The elderly seem to have an equal blood pressure response as younger patients, but cardiovascular events in the elderly have not been reduced with their use (Messerli et al., 2003a). Two polymorphisms of the β-receptor genes have been associated with a greater antihypertensive response to a β-blocker (Filigheddu et al., 2004; Sofowora et al., 2003).

## Other Uses

*Coexisting Coronary Disease*

The antianginal and antiarrhythmic effects of β-blockers make them especially useful in hypertensive patients with coexisting coronary disease (Goldstein, 1996). They are recommended as the first therapy for chronic angina (Snow et al., 2004). Their use is particularly important for those with coronary artery disease (CAD) who are about to undergo surgery, either cardiac or noncardiac (Lindenauer et al., 2004).

Equally strong evidence supports the routine use of β-blockers after an acute MI (Freemantle et al., 1999), including patients with conditions often

considered contraindications to β-blockade, such as diabetes, heart failure, and older age (Gottlieb et al., 1998).

*Congestive Heart Failure*

β-blockers have now been documented to be of value, first in those with idiopathic dilated cardiomyopathy, later in those with ischemic and other forms of systolic dysfunction, extending to the elderly with severe chronic heart failure (Tandon et al., 2004). As of now, excellent results have been reported with long-acting metoprolol, bisoprolol, and the α-β-blocker carvedilol (Gheorghiade et al., 2003).

β-blocker therapy in CHF can induce hypotension, dizziness, and bradycardia, but the overall risks are small and far outweighed by the benefits (Ko et al., 2004).

*Hypertrophic Cardiomyopathy*

β-blockers are also useful in patients with hypertrophic cardiomyopathy, particularly for those with obstruction (Spirito et al., 1997).

*Patients Needing Direct Vasodilator Therapy*

When used alone, direct vasodilators such as hydralazine set off reflex sympathetic stimulation of the heart. The simultaneous use of β-blockers prevents this undesired increase in cardiac output, which not only bothers the patient but also dampens the antihypertensive effect of the vasodilator.

*Marked Anxiety and Stress*

The somatic manifestations of anxiety—tremor, sweating, and tachycardia—can be reduced with β-blockers, which has been found useful for violin players, surgeons, race car drivers, and sufferers from phobias and panic attacks (Fogari et al., 1992). Propanolol given to patients with severe burns reversed muscle-protein catabolism (Herndon et al., 2001).

## Side Effects

These have been reported to be more common in patients receiving β-blockers:

- Fatigue (Ko et al., 2002)
- Diminished exercise ability (Vanhees et al., 2000)
- Weight gain (Sharma et al., 2001)
- Worsening of insulin sensitivity (Jacob et al., 1998)
- New onset of diabetes (Gress et al., 2000)
- Rise in serum triglycerides, fall in HDL-cholesterol (Kasiske et al., 1995)
- Slight rise in serum potassium (Traub et al., 1980)
- Increased rate of suicide (Sørensen et al., 2001)
- Worsening of psoriasis (Savola et al., 1987)

Two additional groups of patients may experience special problems: insulin-taking diabetics who are prone to hypoglycemia and coronary patients. As for diabetics, the responses to hypoglycemia—both the symptoms and the counterregulatory hormonal changes that raise the blood sugar level—are largely mediated by epinephrine, particularly in those who are insulin-dependent because they usually are also deficient in glucagon. If these patients become hypoglycemic, the β-blockade of epinephrine responses delays the return of the blood sugar. The only symptom of hypoglycemia may be sweating, which may be enhanced by the presence of a β-blocker (Molnar et al., 1974).

Patients with coronary disease who discontinued chronic β-blocker therapy may experience a discontinuation syndrome of increasing angina, infarction, or sudden death (Psaty et al., 1990). These ischemic episodes likely reflect the phenomenon of supersensitivity: An increased number of β-receptors appear in response to the functional blockade of receptors by the β-blocker; when the β-blocker is discontinued and no longer occupies the receptors, the increased number of receptors are suddenly exposed to endogenous catecholamines, resulting in a greater α-agonist response for a given level of catechols. Hypertensives, with a high frequency of underlying coronary atherosclerosis, may be particularly susceptible to this type of withdrawal syndrome; thus, when the drugs are discontinued, their dosage should be cut by half every 2 or 3 days, and the drugs should be stopped after the third reduction.

In addition, patients with genetic long QT syndrome may experience a spectrum of cardiac events from syncope to sudden death (Priori et al., 2004). These side effects have *not* been consistently or significantly found to be more common with β-blocker use:

- Depression (Ko et al., 2002)
- Sexual dysfunction (Ko et al., 2002)
- Cognitive loss (Pérez-Stable et al., 2000)
- Worsening of peripheral vascular disease (Radack & Deck, 1991)
- Worsening of mild to moderate reactive airway disease or obstructive lung disease (Prichard & Vallance, 2004). In fact, in a cohort of 1,966 patients with chronic obstructive pulmonary disease, the use of β-blocker monotherapy was associated with a lower mortality rate than seen with other antihypertensive drugs (Au et al., 2004).

Moveover, on the positive side, β-blockers may reduce urine calcium excretion (Lind et al., 1994) and thereby decrease the risk of fractures (Schlienger et al., 2004).

## Vasodilating β-Blockers

In this category, I have included one old drug (labetalol) whose vasodilatory properties come from its high level of α-blockade, one newer drug (carvedilol) with a little α-blocking activity but primarily a direct vasodilatory action mediated by nitric oxide (NO) generation, and two as yet unapproved drugs (celiprolol and nebivolol) that are highly selective β$_1$-blockers that also work by generating NO. From the wealth of papers in the hypertension research literature, nebivolol seems most likely to be the first antihypertensive drug to be marketed as an endogenous NO generator as opposed to drugs such as nitrates which provide exogenous NO.

### Labetalol

#### Mode of Action
Labetalol is a nonselective β$_1$- and β$_2$-receptor blocker combined with α-blocking action in a 4-to-1 ratio. The hemodynamic consequences of a combined α- and β-blockade are a fall in BP, mainly via a fall in systemic vascular resistance, with little effect on cardiac output. The lack of reflex tachycardia is a consequence of β-blockade. Plasma renin activity decreases acutely and then rises, whereas norepinephrine levels increase (Weidmann et al., 1978). An apparent increased urinary excretion of catecholamines has been found to be a chemical interference and not a true increase in excretion. As a result, diagnostic confusion may arise if workup for pheochromocytoma is done with nonspecific catechol measurements while the patient is on labetalol (see Chapter 12).

#### Antihypertensive Efficacy
Labetalol is an effective antihypertensive when given twice daily, maintaining good 24-hour control and blunting the early morning surges in pressure (Ruilope, 1994). The usual starting doses are 100 mg b.i.d. The maximal daily dose is 1,200 mg.

#### Other Uses
Labetalol has been used both orally and intravenously to treat hypertensive emergencies, including postoperative hypertension (Lebel et al., 1985) and acute aortic dissection (Grubb et al., 1987). It has been successfully used to treat hypertension during pregnancy (Pickles et al., 1992).

#### Side Effects
Symptomatic orthostatic hypotension is the most common side effect, seen most often during initial therapy with larger doses. A variety of other side effects have been seen, including intense scalp itching, ejaculatory failure (Goa et al., 1989), and bronchospasm (George et al., 1985). An increased titer of antinuclear and antimitochondrial antibodies develops in some patients; although a systemic lupus syndrome has not been reported, lichenoid skin eruptions have been (Goa et al., 1989).

Perhaps the most serious side effect of labetalol is hepatotoxicity: At least three deaths have been reported (Clark et al., 1990). As a result, a warning has been added to its label in the United States, stating, "Hepatic injury may be slowly progressive despite minimal symptomatology. Appropriate laboratory testing should be done at the first symptom or sign of liver dysfunction."

In keeping with its α-blocking effect, labetalol (Lardinois & Neuman, 1988) has less adverse effect on lipids as do β-blockers.

## Carvedilol

This "third" generation nonselective β-blocker with only one-tenth as much α-blocking activity has been used mainly for treatment of heart failure. It is approved for hypertension but in a twice-a-day dosage, which has reduced its use.

*Mode of Action*

Beyond its slight α-blocking effect, carvedilol vasodilates by increasing generation of endogenous NO from endothelial cells (Kalinowski et al., 2003). It also exerts antioxidant and antiproliferative effects. As with labetalol, blood pressure falls without a fall in cardiac output but rather a decrease in peripheral resistance (Dupont et al., 1987).

*Antihypertensive Efficacy*

In doses starting at 6.25 mg twice a day and proceeding up to 25 mg bid, carvedilol is equal to 50 up to 200 mg of metoprolol bid (Bakris et al., 2004b).

*Other Uses*

Carvedilol has been extensively tested against metoprolol and found to provide additional survival benefit in patients with varying grades of CHF (Poole-Wilson et al., 2003), even in those with low systolic pressure, (Rouleau et al., 2004) while better preserving renal function (Di Lenarda et al., 2004b).

*Side Effects*

Unlike traditional β-blockers, carvedilol does not worsen insulin sensitivity or have as much of an adverse effect on lipids (Bakris et al., 2004b).

## Celiprolol

This selective β$_1$-blocker has vasodilating properties similar to carvedilol and nebivolol (Liao et al., 2004).

## Nebivolol

Like celiprolol, this drug has been studied for a long time but is receiving a great amount of attention lately, both in its mode of action (Ignarro, 2004), its antihypertensive efficacy (Zanchetti, 2004), and its ancillary properties (Galderisi et al., 2004; McEniery et al., 2004). It is the most selective β$_1$-blocker of this family of drugs and exerts its effect by generating and releasing NO while having a complimentary antioxidant effect (Ignarro, 2004).

## DIRECT VASODILATORS

In this category, I have added nitrates to those agents which vasodilate by entering vascular smooth muscle cells. This is in contrast to those that vasodilate in other ways—by inhibiting hormonal vasoconstrictor mechanisms (e.g., ACEIs), by preventing calcium entry into the cells that initiate constriction (e.g., CCBs), or by blocking α-receptor-mediated vasoconstriction (e.g., α$_1$-blockers). The various vasodilators differ considerably in their power, mode of action, and relative activities on arteries and veins (Table 7–5). The intravenous direct vasodilators are covered in Chapter 8.

The use of hydralazine and the only currently available long-acting nitrates, isosorbide mono- and di-nitrate, may both increase as a consequence of the favorable results of the African-American Heart Failure Trial (A-HeFT) (Taylor et al., 2004). When added to full standard therapy for severe CHF, this combination reduced mortality by 43% in the 518 patients given the active drug compared to the 532 given placebo.

The explanation for the results provided by Hare (2004) is the ability of isosorbide dinitrate to stimulate nitric oxide (NO) signaling and of hydralazine to inhibit the enzymatic formation of reactive oxygen species that would disrupt NO signaling, thereby restoring what Hare labels "nitroso-redox balance."

Whether these results in a purely Black population will apply to other ethnic groups in heart failure or in any ethnic group with hypertension or other vascular diseases remains to be seen. Endothelial

## TABLE 7–5

### Vasodilator Drugs Used to Treat Hypertension

| Drug | Relative Action on Arteries (A) or Veins (V) |
|---|---|
| Direct | |
|   Hydralazine | A >> V |
|   Minoxidil | A >> V |
|   Nitroprusside | A + V |
|   Diazoxide | A > V |
|   Nitroglycerin | V > A |
| Calcium channel blockers | A >> V |
| ACE inhibitors | A > V |
| α-blockers | A + V |

>, greater than; >>, much greater than; +, equal or both

cells from healthy Blacks have been found to have diminished bioavailability of NO as a result of increased oxidative stress (Kalinowski et al., 2004), so these results may apply only to Blacks with high levels of oxidative stress.

## Hydralazine

Hydralazine was introduced in the early 1950s (Freis et al., 1953) but was little used because of its activation of the sympathetic nervous system. Its use increased in the 1970s when the rationale for triple therapy—a diuretic, an adrenergic inhibitor, and a direct vasodilator—was demonstrated (Zacest et al., 1972). However, its use receded again with the advent of the newer vasodilating drugs.

### Mode of Action

Hydralazine acts directly to relax the smooth muscle in the walls of peripheral arterioles, the resistance vessels more so than the capacitance vessels, thereby decreasing peripheral resistance and BP (Saxena & Bolt, 1986).

For many years, hydralazine has been known to serve as an antioxidant, inhibiting vascular production of reactive oxygen species, and thereby preventing the development of tolerance to exogenous nitrates, which serve as a source of nitric oxide (Münzel et al., 1996). In the more recent past, endogenous NO has been shown to serve as the locally produced endothelial relaxing factor in large capacitance vasculature but to be carried by

S-nitroso-hemoglobin into the microcirculation where it regulates arteriolar blood flow (Singel & Stamler, 2004). Therefore, hydralazine may induce arteriolar vasodilation by preventing oxidation of NO and thereby lower blood pressure.

Coincidental to the peripheral vasodilation, the heart rate, stroke volume, and cardiac output rise, reflecting a baroreceptor-mediated reflex increase in sympathetic discharge (Lin et al., 1983) and direct stimulation of the heart (Khatri et al., 1977). In addition, the sympathetic overactivity and the fall in BP increase renin release, further counteracting the vasodilator's effect and likely adding to the reactive sodium retention that accompanies the fall in BP (Figure 7–10). Therefore, it has usually been given along with a β-blocker and a diuretic in the treatment of more severe hypertension.

### Antihypertensive Efficacy

Hydralazine should usually be started at 25 mg two times per day. The maximal dose should probably be limited to 200 mg per day to lessen the likelihood of a lupuslike syndrome and because higher doses seldom provide additional benefit.

The inactivation of hydralazine involves acetylation in the liver by the enzyme N-acetyltransferase. The level of this enzyme activity is genetically determined, and rapid acetylators require larger doses than do slow acetylators to achieve an equivalent effect (Ramsay et al., 1984). Perry (1973) showed that patients who develop a lupuslike toxicity tend

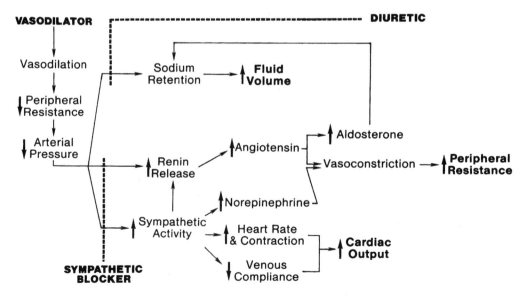

FIGURE 7–10  ●  Primary and secondary effects of vasodilator therapy in essential hypertension and the manner by which diuretic and β-adrenergic blocker therapy can overcome the undesirable secondary effects. (Modified from Koch-Weser J. Vasodilator drugs in the treatment of hypertension. *Arch Intern Med* 1974;133:1017–1027.)

to be slow acetylators and thus are exposed to the drug longer.

### Side Effects

Three kinds of side effects are seen: those due to reflex sympathetic activation, those due to a lupuslike reaction, and those due to nonspecific problems. Headaches, flushing, and tachycardia should be anticipated and prevented by concomitant use of adrenergic inhibitors. The drug should be given with caution to patients with CAD and should be avoided in patients with a dissecting aortic aneurysm or recent cerebral hemorrhage, in view of its propensity to increase cardiac output and cerebral blood flow (CBF) (Schroeder & Sillesen, 1987).

The lupuslike reaction has been described by Perry (1973), who reviewed his experience with 371 patients given the drug for as long as 20 years. An early, febrile reaction resembling serum sickness was seen in 11 patients; late toxicity developed in 44 (with serious symptoms in 14), resembling systemic lupus erythematosus or rheumatoid arthritis. These symptoms almost invariably went away when therapy was stopped or the dosage was lowered.

The lupuslike syndrome is clearly dose-dependent. In a prospective study of 281 patients, the syndrome did not occur in those taking 50 mg daily, whereas it occurred in 5.4% taking 100 mg daily and in 10.4% taking 200 mg daily (Cameron & Ramsay, 1984). A smaller number of patients develop a vasculitis primarily affecting the skin or kidneys (Short & Lockwood, 1995).

Other side effects of hydralazine include anorexia, nausea, vomiting, and diarrhea; less common effects are paresthesias, tremor, and muscle cramps. An additional potential disadvantage of hydralazine and other direct vasodilators is their failure when given alone to regress LVH, presumably because of their marked stimulation of sympathetic nervous activity (Leenen et al., 1987).

## Minoxidil

More potent than hydralazine, minoxidil has become a mainstay in the therapy of severe hypertension associated with renal insufficiency (see Chapter 9). Its propensity to grow hair precludes its use in many women, but this effect has led to its use as a topical ointment for male-pattern baldness.

### Mode of Action

Minoxidil induces smooth muscle relaxation by opening cardiovascular ATP-sensitive potassium channels, a mechanism apparently unique among vasodilators currently available in the United States but similar to the mode of action of various potassium channel openers (e.g., nicorandil) (Ito et al., 2004b).

Because minoxidil is both more potent and longer lasting than hydralazine, it turns on the various reactions to direct arteriolar vasodilation to an even greater degree. Therefore, large doses of potent loop diuretics and adrenergic blockers will be needed in most patients (see Figure 7–10).

### Antihypertensive Efficacy

When used with diuretics and adrenergic inhibitors, minoxidil controls hypertension in more than 75% of patients whose disease was previously resistant to multiple drugs (Sica, 2004b). It can be given once daily in a range of 2.5 to 80 mg.

### Side Effects

The most common side effect, seen in nearly 80% of patients, is hirsutism, beginning with fairly fine hair on the face and then with coarse hair increasing everywhere. It is apparently related to the vasodilation produced by the drug and not to hormonal effects. The hair gradually disappears when the drug is stopped (Kidwai & George, 1992).

Beyond generalized volume expansion, pericardial effusions appear in approximately 3% of patients who receive minoxidil (Martin et al., 1980).

## Nitrates

Nitrates, both nitroglycerin (Kawakami et al., 1995) and oral isosorbide nitrate (Stokes et al., 2003), by their vasodilating properties as exogenous endothelium-derived relaxing factor (NO), can also be used as antihypertensives. Stokes et al. (2005) found isosorbide mononitrate to lower systolic BP to a much greater degree than diastolic BP in 16 elderly patients with resistant systolic hypertension. The pulse pressure fell by 13% and the augmentation index, a measure of pulse wave reflection, fell by 25%.

Tolerance did not seem to develop. Despite the attractiveness of this approach for treatment of systolic hypertension, the lack of a commercial sponsor for testing a generic drug in a large clinical trial makes it unlikely that a nitrate will be approved as an antihypertensive drug. The benefits of combined hydralazine and isosorbide dinitrate in Blacks with CHF (Taylor et al., 2004) may change the situation.

## CALCIUM CHANNEL BLOCKERS

Calcium channel blockers were introduced as antianginal agents in the 1970s and as antihypertensives in the 1980s. Their use grew rapidly so that they became the second most popular group of drugs used by U.S. practitioners for the treatment of hypertension in the early 2000s.

## Mode of Action

Three types of CCBs are now available. Another, mibefradil, was marketed but withdrawn. Those now available interact with the same calcium channel: the L-type voltage-gated plasma membrane channel. They have major differences in their structure and cardiovascular effects (Eisenberg et al., 2004) (Table 7–6).

*Diltiazem,* a benzothiazepine, and *verapamil,* a phenylalkylamine, the currently available nondihydropyridine (nonDHP), are rate slowing: At equivalent concentrations, they induce vasodilation, depress cardiac contractility, and inhibit atrioventricular (AV) conduction.

*Dihydropyridines* (DHP) are predominantly vasodilators. The first generation, exemplified by nifedipine, had modest effects on cardiac contractility. The second generation, such as amlodipine, felodipine, and nicardipine, has more effect on vascular dilation than on myocardial contractility or cardiac conduction. A number of other dihydropyridines are not yet approved in the United States but are being used elsewhere; these include azelnidipine, benidipine, efonidipine, lacidipine, lercanidipine, manidipine, and nitrendipine. Although the major differences are between non-DHP and the DHP-CCBs, there are enough differences between the multiple DHP-CCBs so that "caution should be exercised in assuming that all dihydropyridine CCBs licensed for once-daily administration are equivalent

in their durations of action and overall antihypertensive efficacy" (Meredith & Elliott, 2004).

### Sympathetic Activation

One pharmacologic feature that may explain some of the initial side effects of CCBs and has been incriminated as a possible contributor to adverse cardiovascular effects of short-acting agents (Psaty et al., 1995) is their activation of the sympathetic nervous system. Such activation is a transient phenomenon that is seen with acute BP reduction even with central sympathetic-inhibitory drugs such as clonidine (Wallin & Frisk-Holmberg, 1981) and that may be affected by the lipophilicity of the agent and the age of the patient. Those agents that are more lipophilic and thereby gain entry into the brain where they may depress the vasomotor center, such as nifedipine or lercanidipine, have a lesser degree of sympathetic activation. On the other hand, long-acting nifedipine for 4 weeks activated sympathetic activity in younger (average age 45) hypertensives who had minimal falls in BP (1/1 mm Hg) compared to older (average age 67) hypertensives who experienced no sympathetic activation but had a significant (10/7 mm Hg) fall in BP (Ruzicka et al., 2004).

Two studies in subjects whose average age was 57 provide further evidence of initial but not chronic effects of CCBs on sympathetic activity. Grassi et al. (2003) found marked increases in heart rate, plasma norepinephrine, and muscle sympathetic nerve traffic on the first day of intake of two long-acting DHP-CCBs, felodipine and lercanidipine, which lowered BP equally. After 8 weeks of daily

## TABLE 7–6

### Cardiovascular Profile of Calcium Channel Blockers

|                                    | Nidefipine | Amlodipine | Diltiazem        | Verapamil       |
|------------------------------------|:----------:|:----------:|:----------------:|:---------------:|
| Heart rate                         | ↑          | ↑/0        | ↓                | ↓               |
| Sinoatrial node conduction         | 0          | 0          | ↓↓               | ↓               |
| Atrioventricular node conduction   | 0          | 0          | ↓                | ↓               |
| Myocardial contractility           | ↓/0        | ↓/0        | ↓                | ↓↓              |
| Neurohormonal activation           | ↑          | ↑/0        | ↑                | ↑               |
| Vascular dilatation                | ↑↑         | ↑↑         | ↑                | ↑               |
| Coronary flow                      | ↑          | ↑          | ↑                | ↑               |

↓ = decrease; 0 = no change; ↑ = increase
Adapted from Eisenberg MJ, et al. Calcium channel blockers: an update. *Am J Med* 2004;116:35–43.

therapy, which continued to provide similar BP reductions, the heart rate, plasma norepinephrine, and muscle nerve traffic were markedly attenuated, virtually back to baseline in the lercanidipine group but not quite with the felodipine.

The validity of these observations was confirmed in a comparative study of long-acting formulations of two DHP-CCBs, amlodipine and nifedipine, and a nonDHP-CCB, verapamil, given to hypertensives for 8 weeks (Binggeli et al., 2002). All three led to similar falls in BP and there were no significant differences in muscle sympathetic nerve traffic from baseline between the three drugs. However, with more marked reductions in BP over 8 weeks, amlodipine induced a persistent increase in plasma norepinephrine levels (Karas et al., 2005).

The bottom line is that sympathetic activation is seen with CCBs as it is with all drugs when they lower BP but is usually minimized during chronic therapy, with the degree of initial activation and subsequent return affected by the age of the patient and the nature of the CCB.

### Duration of Action

One of the major differences between older and newer CCBs is their duration of action. As shown in Table 7–7, some of these, such as the formulation of verapamil that affords 24-hour effectiveness, are provided by special delivery systems; others, such

as amlodipine, have intrinsically long durations of action. The slow onset and long duration of action of amlodipine provide continued effects even if daily doses are missed (Elliott et al., 2002).

As has become increasingly obvious in the recent past, short-acting agents may induce abrupt falls in BP, which may incite coronary ischemia (Psaty et al., 1995). Such effects are not seen with long-acting agents, which lower the BP gradually and smoothly (Eisenberg et al., 2004).

### Antihypertensive Efficacy

The currently available CCBs seem comparable in their antihypertensive potency, although no direct comparisons have been made among all of them. The relative effectiveness in protecting against major cardiovascular events of various types of CCBs—short- and long-acting, DHP and nonDHP—has been tested in 12 randomized controlled trials against three of the other major classes of antihypertensives: diuretics or β-blockers or ACEIs (Eisenberg et al., 2004). As seen in Table 7–8, various types of CCBs have proven to be equally effective as other classes in overall protection against all major cardiovascular events. However, they have provided *less* protection against heart failure but *more* protection against stroke than other classes (Angeli et al., 2004).

---

## TABLE 7-7

### Calcium Channel Blockers Approved for Use in the Treatment of Hypertension in the United States

| Drug | Form and Dose | Time to Peak Effect (hrs) | Elimination Half-Life (hrs) |
|------|---------------|---------------------------|-----------------------------|
| Amlodipine | Tablet; 2.5–10 mg | 6–12 | 30–50 |
| Diltiazem[a] | Immediate-release tablet; dose varies | 0.5–1.5 | 2–5 |
| | Sustained-release tablet; 180–480 mg | 6–11 | 2–5 |
| Felodipine | Sustained-release tablet; 2.5–10 mg | 2.5–5 | 11–16 |
| Isradipine | Tablet; 2.5–10 mg | 1.5 | 8–12 |
| Nicardipine[a] | Immediate-release tablet; 20–40 mg | 0.5–2.0 | 8 |
| | Sustained-release tablet; 60–120 mg | ? | 8 |
| Nifedipine | Immediate-release capsule; dose varies | 0.5 | 2 |
| | Sustained-release tablet; 30–120 mg | 6 | 7 |
| Nisoldipine | Sustained-release tablet; 20–40 mg | 6–12 | 7–12 |
| Verapamil[a] | Immediate-release tablet; dose varies | 0.5–1.0 | 4.5–12 |
| | Sustained-release tablet; 120–480 mg | 4–6 | 4.5–12 |

[a] Also available in an intravenous formation, with a time to peak effect ranging from 5 to 15 minutes after administration.

## TABLE 7-8

### Major Cardiovascular Events with CCBs Versus Other Antihypertensive Drugs

| CCB Formulation | Number of Trials | Major Cardiovascular Events[a] No. Events/No. Patients (%) | | Relative Risk (95% CI) |
|---|---|---|---|---|
| | | CCBs | Others | |
| Short acting | 7 | 1,222/9351 (13.1) | 1,768/11,691 (15.1) | 1.09 (1.00–1.18) |
| Long acting | 5 | 2,567/31,934 (8.0) | 3,546/38,278 (9.3) | 1.01 (0.96–1.07) |
| Nondihydropyridine | 4 | 1,359/25,625 (5.3) | 1,365/25,848 (5.3) | 1.00 (0.93–1.09) |
| Dihydropyridine | 8 | 2,430/15,630 (15.5) | 3,949/24,121 (16.4) | 1.05 (0.99–1.11) |

[a]Major cardiovascular events included myocardial infarction, heart failure, stroke, and cardiovascular mortality, except in ALLHAT, where composite coronary heart disease included death from coronary heart disease, nonfatal myocardial infarction, coronary revascularization procedures, and angina requiring hospitalization, and in INVEST, where the primary outcome was cardiovascular mortality.
Composed from Eisenberg MJ, Brox A, Bestawros AN. Calcium channel blockers: an update. *Am J Med* 2004;116:35–43.

## Determinants of Efficacy

### Age

An apparently greater antihypertensive effectiveness of CCBs in the elderly (Lacourcière et al., 1995) may reflect the characteristically higher systolic BP levels of the elderly and the more pronounced efficacy of CCBs as the level of BP increases (Donnelly et al., 1988). In addition, elderly patients may be more responsive because of pharmacokinetic changes that increase the bioavailability of various CCBs, providing more active drug at any given dose than in younger patients (Lernfelt et al., 1998).

### Race

In Blacks, the repsonse of the blood pressure to monotherapy with CCBs is better than to ACEIs, ARBs, or β-blockers and equal to the response to diuretics (Brewster et al., 2004).

### Additive Effect of Diuretic or Low-Sodium Intake

A decrease in the antihypertensive efficacy of CCBs has been claimed under two conditions: dietary sodium restriction (Valdés et al., 1982) and concomitant diuretic therapy (Magagna et al., 1986).

Numerous studies have examined these relationships. In general, the findings support the view that dietary sodium restriction may reduce (but not abolish) the antihypertensive effect of CCBs, whereas high-sodium intake may enhance (or not diminish) their efficacy (Luft et al., 1991; Nicholson et al., 1987). The explanation may be simple: CCBs have a mild natriuretic effect (Krekels et al., 1997); this effect would be more obvious in the presence of a higher sodium diet so that the BP would fall

more. With a low-sodium intake, this natriuretic effect would not be as pronounced, so the BP would diminish less. This explanation fits with the observation that the fall in BP with a CCB is greater in more sodium-sensitive patients (Damasceno et al., 1999).

On the other hand, most well-controlled studies have shown an additional antihypertensive effect when diuretics are combined with CCBs (Stergiou et al., 1997). The combination of a diuretic with a CCB has been shown to provide additive effects equal to those seen when a diuretic is added to a β-blocker (Thulin et al., 1991) or to an ACEI (Elliott et al., 1990).

## Potential for Good or Bad Renal Effects

The mild natriuretic action of CCBs likely reflects their unique ability, unlike other vasodilators, to maintain or increase effective renal blood flow, glomerular fitration rate (GFR), and renal vascular resistance, which has been attributed to their selective vasodilative action on the renal afferent arterioles (Delles et al., 2003). On the surface, this preferential vasodilation of afferent arterioles with increases in GFR, renal blood flow, and natriuresis appears to favor the use of CCBs as a way of maintaining good renal function. However, a large body of experimental data suggests that increased renal plasma flow and GFR may accelerate the progression of glomerulosclerosis by increasing intraglomerular pressure (Griffin et al., 1995).

In hypertensive patients with renal damage, as manifested by proteinuria, DHP-CCBs do not reduce proteinuria, whereas verapamil and diltiazem do about as well as ACEIs (Bakris et al., 2004c). In the African-American Study of Kidney Disease and Hypertension, amlodipine did not slow the rate of decline of renal function in hypertensive Blacks with renal insufficiency and heavy proteinuria as well as did the ACEI ramipril (Agodoa et al., 2001). Therefore, CCBs should be only added to an ACEI or ARB if needed to control hypertension in patients with renal insufficiency.

Moreover, as shown in the RENAAL trial, the addition of a DHP-CCB should not diminish the benefits of an ACEI or ARB on the slowing of progression of nephropathy (Bakris et al., 2003). However, verapamil did no better than placebo in preventing the onset of microalbuminuria in type 2 diabetes (Ruggenenti et al., 2004), so CCBs should not be used in an attempt to prevent nephropathy.

## Other Uses

### Cardiac Diseases

#### Coronary Artery Disease
Although usually considered as second or third choice for chronic stable angina, the use of CCBs will likely be more highly regarded for patients with CAD in view of the results of the Comparison of Amlodipine vs Enalapril to Limit Occurrences of Thrombosis (CAMELOT) trial (Nissen et al., 2004). In this trial of 1,991 patients with angiographically proven CAD and normal blood pressure (often provided by other antihypertensive drugs), the addition of amlodipine, 10 mg, provided a 31% reduction in cardiovascular events and less progression of coronary atherosclerosis than seen in the placebo-treated patients. Moreover, amlodipine was considerably better than enalapril, 20 mg, despite the equal additional blood pressure reduction with the CCB and ACEI.

DHP-CCBs are effective for relief of chronic stable angina (Poole-Wilson et al., 2004) and vasospastic angina (Ito et al., 2004a). NonDHP-CCBs are used for supraventricular tachyarrhythmias and hypertrophic obstructive cardiomyopathy (Roberts & Sigwart, 2001). Calcium channel blockers are not generally used immediately postmyocardial infarction, although diltiazem was safe and reduced nonfatal cardiac events (Boden et al., 2000).

#### Congestive Heart Failure
The incidence of heart failure has been usually found to be increased in hypertensives given CCBs in large RCTs whether DHP (ALLHAT Officers, 2002; Julius et al., 2004b) or nonDHP (Black et al., 2003).

In patients with CHF, CCBs, particularly nonDHPs, are generally avoided but if there is a need for a CCB, amlodipine has been found to be safe (Packer et al., 1996).

#### Left Ventricular Hypertrophy
Left ventricular hypertrophy is not in itself a disease, but it is common in hypertensives, whether treated or not (Mancia et al., 2002), is associated with an increased risk of cardiovascular events (Okin et al., 2004), and, if regressed, this risk is significantly reduced (Devereux et al., 2004b; Verdecchia et al., 2003). Calcium channel blockers reduce LVH, as well as other major classes of antihypertensive drugs (Klingbeil et al., 2003) (Figure 7–11).

#### Arrhythmias
Verapamil and, to a lesser degree, diltiazem have been widely used to treat supraventricular tachyarrhythmias, particularly reentrant AV nodal tachycardia and atrial fibrillation (Abernethy & Schwartz, 1999).

#### Valvular Diseases
In asymptomatic patients with chronic aortic regurgitation, long-term use of nifedipine has delayed the need for operation (Levine & Gaasch, 1996). In patients with mild to moderate aortic stenosis, an ACEI, ramipril 7.5 mg b.i.d. was well tolerated over 8 weeks even though conventional wisdom has been that any vasodilator would worsen the course of aortic stenosis (O'Brien et al., 2004).

#### Cerebrovascular Diseases
##### Stroke
The use of CCBs provided a 38% reduction in stroke incidence when compared to placebo in four RCTs and a 12% further reduction when compared to ACEI-based therapy in five RCTs (Blood Pressure Trialists, 2003). Using more liberal criteria for inclusion of trials, Angeli et al. (2004) found a 10% lower incidence of stroke with CCBs than with other antihypertensive drugs in 13 comparative trials. According to Angeli et al. (2004), the added protection provided by CCB-based therapy "appeared unrelated to the degree of systolic blood pressure reduction."

The DHP-CCB nimodipine has been approved for relief of vasospasm after subarachnoid hemorrhage (Feigen et al., 1998). For secondary prevention of stroke recurrence, there are no RCTs examining the benefit of CCBs. The consensus is that tight control of blood pressure, however achieved, is the primary need (Pedelty & Gorelick, 2004).

#### Dementia
The only prospective RCT examining the ability to prevent dementia remains the Systolic Hypertension in Europe (Syst-Eur) trial which reported a 55% reduction in dementia with therapy based on the DHP-CCB nitrendipine (Forette et al., 2002).

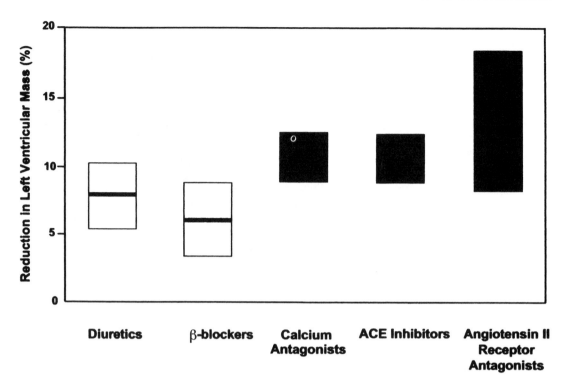

**FIGURE 7–11** ● Change in left ventricular mass index (as percentage from baseline) with antihypertensive treatment by drug class. Mean values and 95% confidence intervals, adjusted for change in diastolic blood pressure and treatment duration, are given. ACE, angiotensin-converting enzyme. (Modified from Klingbeil AU et al. A meta-analysis of the effects of treatment on left ventricular mass in essential hypertension. *Am J Med* 2003;115:41–46.)

## Other Conditions

Some improvement has been reported with the use of CCBs in these conditions:

- Peripheral vascular disease (Bagger et al., 1997)
- Primary pulmonary hypertension (Rubin, 1997)
- Raynaud's phenomenon (Wigley, 2002)
- Preterm labor (Lockwood, 1997)

## Side Effects

Serious consequences of the use of short-acting CCBs were reported in retrospective observational studies involving diltiazem, nifedipine, and verapamil (Pahor et al., 1996a, 1996b; Psaty et al., 1995). The subsequent results from multiple prospective RCTs comparing CCBs against placebo and other classes of antihypertensive drugs clearly show that the observational studies were largely invalid with the possible exception of an increased risk with short-acting CCBs (Table 7–8 and Figure 7–16, page 266). Observational studies are confounded by inclusion of high-risk patients among those given CCBs (Leader et al., 2001). As noted earlier, none of these claims has been documented with the use of long-acting CCBs, which

induce distinctly different hemodynamic and hormonal responses than do the short-acting agents (Meredith & Elliott, 2004).

### More Common

Relatively mild but sometimes bothersome side effects will preclude the use of these drugs in perhaps 10% of patients. Most side effects—headaches, flushing, local ankle edema—are related to the vasodilation for which the drugs are given. With slow-release and longer-acting formulations, vasodilative side effects are reduced. The side effects of the three major classes of CCBs differ considerably (Table 7–9).

### Verapamil

Constipation is the most common side effect, and AV block is the most serious one. To avoid conduction problems, the drug should generally be avoided in patients with sick sinus syndrome, second- or third-degree AV block, or CHF.

### Diltiazem

The incidence of both gastrointestinal symptoms and conduction problems is lower with diltiazem, but this drug is best avoided in patients with the

> **TABLE 7–9**
>
> **Relative Frequency of Side Effects of Calcium Channel Blockers**

| Effect | Verapamil | Diltiazem | Dihydropyridines |
|---|---|---|---|
| *Cardiovascular system* | | | |
|    Hypotension | + | + | ++ |
|    Flush | + | – | ++ |
|    Headache | + | + | ++ |
|    Ankle edema | + | + | ++ |
|    Palpitation | – | – | + |
|    Conduction disturbances | ++ | + | – |
|    Bradycardia | ++ | + | – |
| *Gastrointestinal tract* | | | |
|    Nausea | + | + | + |
|    Constipation | ++ | (+) | – |

+, increase; –, no effect.

underlying conduction disturbances noted previously for verapamil (Abernethy & Schwartz, 1999).

### Dihydropyridines

Vasodilative side effects are more common with the dihydropyridines but less so with the second generation of slower-release and longer-acting preparations. On the other hand, dependent edema remains a relatively common problem, related to localized vasodilation and not generalized fluid retention and not prevented or relieved by diuretics (van der Heijden et al., 2004). If the pedal edema is bothersome, either a nonDHP-CCB should be substituted (Weir et al., 2001) or the DHP-CCB combined with an ACEI to reduce the edema (Gradman et al., 1997).

### Other Side Effects

Gingival hyperplasia is most common with dihydropyridines (Missouris et al., 2000). Eye pain, possibly due to ocular vasodilation, has been noted with nifedipine (Coulter, 1988). A wide spectrum of adverse cutaneous reactions, some quite serious, has been reported to occur rarely with various CCBs (Orme & da Costa, 1997). Impotence seems rare, but 31 patients have been reported to develop gynecomastia (Tanner & Bosco, 1988).

No adverse effects on glucose, insulin, or lipids have been seen and fewer cases of new onset diabetes developed in the INVEST trials among those given verapamil than those given atenolol (Pepine et al., 2003). Overdoses usually are manifested by hypotension and conduction disturbances and can usually be overcome with parenteral calcium and sympathomimetics (Abernethy & Schwartz, 1999).

### Drug Interactions

A problem noted with most other classes of antihypertensive drugs—interference from NSAIDs—is usually not seen with CCBs (Celis et al., 2001). Another interaction has been noted with the dihydropyridines felodipine and nifedipine but not with amlodipine (Vincent et al., 2000): an increased plasma level and duration of action when taken along with grapefruit juice (Bailey et al., 2000) which prevents the usual inactivation of the CCB in the gut (Wilkinson, 2005). Most other drug interactions with CCBs are of little consequence except the possible major cost savings represented by the lower doses of cyclosporine needed with concomitant CCB therapy (Valantine et al., 1992).

### Perspective on Use

Calcium channel blockers have been found to reduce the risk of coronary disease equally, stroke more, but heart failure less than other antihypertensive therapies while having similar effects on overall mortality (Blood Pressure Lowering, 2003). They work well and are usually well tolerated across the entire spectrum of hypertensives. They have some particular niches: the elderly, coexisting angina, and cyclosporine or NSAID use. If chosen, an inherently long-acting, second-generation dihydropyridine seems the best choice, because it will maintain better BP control in the critical early morning hours and on through the next day if the patient misses a daily dose (Meredith & Elliott, 2004). Rate-slowing CCBs, verapamil or diltiazem, may be preferable in certain circumstances.

The phenomenal growth over the past 20 years of the use of CCBs for the treatment of hypertension may have been slowed by the previous observational reports of problems with short-acting formulations. However, impressively consistent and strong data from prospective RCTs have confirmed both the efficacy and safety of currently available long-acting CCBs. Even more may be marketed in the United States as they are elsewhere. The use of these agents will continue to increase.

## ANGIOTENSIN-CONVERTING ENZYME INHIBITORS

There are four ways to reduce the activity of the renin-angiotensin system in humans (Figure 7–12). The first way, the use of β-blockers to reduce renin release from the juxtaglomerular cells, has been covered. The second way, the direct inhibition of the activity of renin, is being actively investigated with a variety of renin inhibitors. The third way is to inhibit the activity of the angiotensin-converting enzyme (ACE) which converts the inactive decapeptide angiotensin I (AI) to the potent hormone angiotensin II (AII); i.e., ACEIs. The fourth way is to use a competitive antagonist that attaches to the AII receptors and blocks the attachment of the native hormone, i.e., angiotensin receptor blockers

(ARBs). Multiple ARBs are now available and are challenging ACEIs.

This section examines the use of ACEIs. Thereafter, the use of ARBs will be described.

### Mode of Action

Peptides from the venom of the Brazilian viper *Bothrops jararaca* were discovered to potentiate the effects of bradykinin by inhibiting its degradation (Ferreira, 1965). Soon thereafter, Ng and Vane (1967) recognized that the same enzyme from the carboxypeptidase family could be responsible for both the conversion of AI to AII and the degradation of bradykinin. The nature of this ACE was identified by Erdös and coworkers in 1970 (Yang et al., 1970). Biochemists at the Squibb laboratories identified the first inhibitor for the ACE enzyme, teprotide or SQ20881 (Ondetti et al., 1971), which was shown to lower BP when given intravenously (Gavras et al., 1974). The Squibb group then identified the active site on the ACE and developed the first orally effective ACEI, captopril (Ondetti et al., 1977).

Three chemically different classes of ACEIs have been developed, classified by the ligand of the zinc ion of ACE: sulfhydryl, carboxyl, and phosphoryl (Table 7–10). Their different structures influence their tissue distribution and routes of elimination (Brown & Vaughan, 1998), differences that could alter their effects on various organ functions beyond their shared ability to lower the BP by blocking the circulating renin-angiotensin mechanism. Differences in tissue penetration of the ACEIs may result in different clinical effects (Anderson et al., 2000), but these have not yet been proved (Re, 2004).

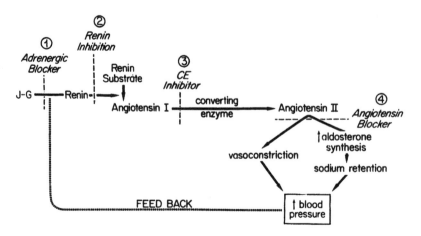

**FIGURE 7–12** ● The renin-angiotensin system and four sites where its activity may be inhibited. CE, converting enzyme; J-G, juxtaglomerular.

## TABLE 7–10

### Characteristics of Angiotensin-Converting Enzyme Inhibitors

| Drug | U.S. Trade Name | Zinc Ligand | Prodrug | Rate of Elimination | Duration of Action, h | Dose Range, mg |
|------|-----------------|-------------|---------|---------------------|------------------------|----------------|
| Benazepril | Lotensin | Carboxyl | Yes | Renal | 24 | 5–40 |
| Captopril | Capoten | Sulfhydryl | No | Renal | 6–12 | 25–150 |
| Enalapril | Vasotec | Carboxyl | Yes | Renal | 18–24 | 5–40 |
| Fosinopril | Monopril | Phosphoryl | Yes | Renal-hepatic | 24 | 10–40 |
| Imidapril | – | Carboxyl | Yes | Renal | 24+ | 5–10 |
| Lisinopril | Prinivil, Zestril | Carboxyl | No | Renal | 24 | 5–40 |
| Moexipril | Univasc | Carboxyl | Yes | Renal | 12–18 | 7.5–30 |
| Perindopril | Aceon | Carboxyl | Yes | Renal | 24 | 4–16 |
| Quinapril | Accupril | Carboxyl | Yes | Renal | 24 | 5–80 |
| Ramipril | Altase | Carboxyl | Yes | Renal | 24 | 1.25–20 |
| Spirapril | – | Carboxyl | Yes | Hepatic | 24 | 12.5–50 |
| Trandolapril | Mavik | Carboxyl | Yes | Renal | 24+ | 1–8 |

### Pharmacokinetics

As seen in Table 7–10, most ACEIs are prodrugs, esters of the active compounds that are more lipid-soluble, so that they are more quickly and completely absorbed. Although there are large differences in bioavailability, these seem to make little difference in the clinical effects, likely because of the variable degrees of binding to ACE, tissue penetration, and elimination that contribute to the overall effects (Komajda & Wimart, 2000).

Most ACEIs, except fosinopril and spirapril, are eliminated through the kidneys, having undergone variable degrees of metabolism. Fosinopril has a balanced route of elimination, with increasingly more of the drug removed through the liver as renal function decreases (Hui et al., 1991).

### Pharmacodynamics

As seen in Figure 7–12, the most obvious manner by which ACEIs lower the BP is to reduce the circulating levels of AII markedly, thereby removing the direct vasoconstriction induced by this peptide. However, with usual doses of ACEIs, plasma angiotensin II levels begin to "escape" after a few hours, in part because of the release of more renin, freed from its feedback suppression (Azizi & Ménard, 2004).

Although the presence of the complete renin-angiotensin system within various tissues, including vessel walls, heart, and brain, is certain, the role of these tissue renin-angiotensin systems in pathophysiology remains uncertain, as does the contribution of inhibition of tissue ACE to the antihypertensive effects of ACEIs (Re, 2004).

Moreover, nonclassical pathways may be involved in the elaboration of AII, involving either nonrenin effects on angiotensinogen or nonACE effects on AI (Figure 7–13). Because ACEIs block only AII production via the classical pathway, there could then be additional effects of ARBs. On the other hand, some of the effects of ACEIs may be mediated via their inhibition of the breakdown of bradykinin (Erdös et al., 1999), with an additional contribution from kinin stimulation of nitric oxide production (Burnier & Brunner, 2000). Nonsteroidal antiinflammatory drugs clearly reduce the antihypertensive effect of ACEIs, likely by inhibiting vasodilatory prostaglandin production (Polónia et al., 1995).

Regardless of the contributions of various other mechanisms beyond the reduction in AII levels, the lower AII levels certainly play a major role. In addition to the relief of vasoconstriction, multiple other effects likely contribute to their antihypertensive effect:

- A decrease in aldosterone secretion that may not be persistent (Sato & Saruta, 2003).
- An increase in bradykinin, which in turn increases release of tissue plasminogen activator (Labinjoh et al., 2001).
- An increase in the activity of the $11\beta$-hydroxysteroid dehydrogenase-2 enzyme, which could

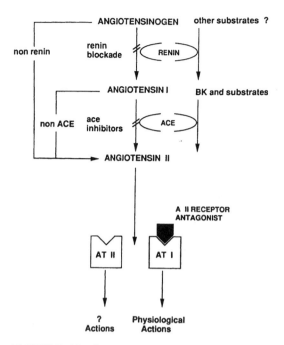

**FIGURE 7–13** ● Theoretic biochemical and physiologic consequences of blocking the renin-angiotensin system at different steps in the pathway. ACE, angiotensin-converting enzyme; AT, angiotensin; BK, bradykinin. (Modified from Johnston CI, Burrell LM. Evolution of blockade of the renin-angiotensin system. *J Hum Hypertens* 1995;9:375–380.)

increase renal sodium excretion by protecting the nonselective mineralocorticoid receptor from cortisol (Ricketts & Stewart, 1999).

- Blunting of the expected increase in sympathetic nervous system activity typically seen after vasodilation (Lyons et al., 1997). As a result, heart rate is not increased and cardiac output does not rise, as is seen with direct vasodilators such as hydralazine.
- Suppression of endogenous endothelin secretion (Brunner & Kukovetz, 1996).
- Improvement in endothelial dysfunction (Ghiadoni et al., 2003).
- Reduction in oxidative stress by reducing production of reactive oxygen species (Hamilton et al., 2004) and inflammatory factors (Sattler et al., 2005).
- Stimulation of endothelial progenitor cells (Bahlmann et al., 2005).

As a consequence of these multiple effects, ACE inhibition results in a dampening of arterial wave reflections and increased aortic distensibility (London et al., 1996). These hemodynamic improvements contribute to the reversal of hypertrophy both in the heart and vasculature. As will be noted, ACEIs lower the BP in a manner that tends to protect the function of two vital organs—the heart and the kidneys. In addition, ACEIs have reduced the incidence of new-onset diabetes in patients enrolled in multiple RCTs to a greater degree than any other antihypertensive drug (Opie & Schall, 2004).

Angiotensin-converting enzyme inhibitors are also venodilators (Zarnke & Feldman, 1996), which may be responsible for their ability to reduce the accumulation of ankle edema seen with CCBs when the two agents are combined (Gradman et al., 1997).

## Antihypertensive Efficacy

A rather remarkable turnabout has occurred since 1979 when captopril was approved only for use in patients with severe hypertension unresponsive to other agents. Angiotensin-converting enzyme inhibitors are now included among the drugs recommended for initial monotherapy of patients with a variety of comorbid conditions accompanying hypertension by all expert guidelines (Chobanian et al., 2003a; 2003b; Guidelines Committee, 2003; Williams, 2004). This turnabout reflects the use of smaller doses, the recognition of equal efficacy but apparently fewer side effects than are seen with other classes, and the provision of some special advantages not provided by other drugs now available.

### Monotherapy

An immediate fall in BP occurs in approximately 70% of patients given captopril, and the decrease is sometimes rather precipitous (Postma et al., 1992). Such a dramatic fall is more likely in those with high renin levels, particularly if they are volume-depleted by prior dietary sodium restriction or diuretic therapy.

Black hypertensives, with lower renin levels as a group, have been found to respond less well to ACEIs than do White hypertensives (Brewster et al., 2004). Younger patients tend to respond better than elderly patients (Morgan et al., 2001).

As expected, patients with high-renin forms of hypertension (e.g., renovascular hypertension) may respond particularly well to ACEIs, but the removal of AII's support of perfusion to the ischemic kidney may precipitously reduce renal function, particularly in those with bilateral stenoses (Hricik et al., 1983) (see Chapter 10). If such patients are excluded, ACEIs are usually effective and well tolerated in patients with renal insufficiency. Renal function may worsen if the BP is reduced too much (Toto et al., 1991) or in the presence of heart failure (Kalra et al., 1999). However, an initial decline of 25% to 30% in renal function after starting ACEI therapy in patients with mild to moderate renal insufficiency was found to be associated with *better* long-term renoprotection (Apperloo et al., 1997), presumably reflecting a beneficial dilation of efferent arterioles, which reduces intraglomerular pressure and filtration (Bakris & Weir, 2000).

Sublingual captopril is effective in lowering severe hypertension (Angeli et al., 1991) but is just as likely as sublingual nifedipine to lower the BP too much too quickly, so it too should be used rarely, if ever, for this purpose (see Chapter 8).

### Combination Therapy

The addition of a diuretic, even in as low a dose as 6.25 mg HCTZ, will enhance the efficacy of an ACEI (Cheng & Frishman, 1998), normalizing the BP of another 20% to 25% of patients with mild to moderate hypertension more effectively than would raising the dose of the ACEI (Townsend & Holland, 1990). The marked additive effect of a diuretic likely reflects the ACEI blunting of the reactive rise of AII that usually occurs with diuretic use and that opposes the antihypertensive effect of the diuretic. Combinations of an ACEI and a CCB provide additive effects (de Leeuw et al., 1997) and likely reduce the prevalence of pedal edema seen with CCBs alone (Gradman et al., 1997). The combination of an ACEI and an ARB is being increasingly used to reduce proteinuria to a greater degree than seen with either agent alone (Azizi & Ménard, 2004). The dual blockade may provide greater benefit than doubling the dose of the ACEI (Kincaid-Smith et al., 2004).

### Effectiveness in Reducing Morbidity and Mortality

In multiple RCTs in comparison to placebo, ACEIs reduced stroke by 28%, CHD by 20%, CHF by 18%, and cardiovascular mortality by 12% (Blood Pressure Trialists, 2003) (Figure 7–16, page 266). In comparison to diuretics ± β-blocker therapy, ACEIs were slightly less effective against strokes but equal against the other end points, whereas against CCBs, ACEIs were better against CHF but less effective against stroke. In two recent trials, an ACEI was less effective than a diuretic in ALLHAT (ALLHAT Officers, 2002) but more effective than a diuretic in the males enrolled in the Second Australian National Blood Pressure Study (ANBP2) trial (Wing et al., 2003). These differences were likely related to the different characteristics of the patients in the two trials.

As will be noted, ACEIs are particularly effective for cardio- and renoprotection.

## Other Uses

### Heart Diseases

#### Coronary Artery Disease

Although not antianginal, ACEIs have been recommended for all patients with known coronary disease, whether hypertensive or not (White, 2003). The evidence is derived from two large RCTs, the Heart Outcomes Prevention Evaluation (HOPE) and European Trial on Reduction of Cardiac Events with Perindopril (EUROPA) trials. Both involved adding an ACEI, ramipril in HOPE, perindopril in EUROPA (Fox, 2003), or a placebo to other therapies in patients with known CAD. In both, significant reductions in subsequent cardiovascular events were seen although the absolute reductions in both were quite small (Badrinath, 2002). Moreover, the benefits may have largely been related to lower blood pressure in the ACEI-added groups (Svensson et al., 2001), although investigators from both trials believe the positive results reflect intrinsic benefits of ACE inhibition and not lower BP (Remme, 2004; Sleight et al., 2001).

However, in two more recently completed trials, an ACEI did not offer as much protection as a CCB in high-risk patients with CAD (Nissen et al., 2004) or any more protection than placebo in lower-risk CAD patients (PEACE Investigators, 2004). In the CAMELOT trial, 20 mg per day of enalapril protected CAD patients less well than amlodipine 10 mg per day (Nissen et al., 2004). In the Prevention of Events with Angiotensin-converting enzyme Inhibition (PEACE) trial, 8,290 patients with stable CAD and normal left ventricular function while on "standard therapy" were randomly given either trandolapril 4 mg per day or placebo (PEACE Investigators, 2004). After a median follow-up of 4.8 years, the incidences of cardiovascular death, myocardial infarction, and coronary revascularization were 21.7% for the ACEI group and 22.5% for the placebo group.

#### Postmyocardial Infarction

ACEIs reduce subsequent mortality after an acute MI, ramipril perhaps better than other ACEIs (Pilote et al., 2004), but there are no head-to-head comparisons to be sure. In one comparison between the ACEI captopril and the ARB losartan in postMI patients, the ACEI was marginally better (Dickstein & Kjekshus, 2002).

#### Congestive Heart Failure

ACEIs are now the primary treatment of CHF due to systolic dysfunction even in the face of perceived contraindications to their use (Ahmed et al., 2005). Usually a shorter-acting one such as captopril is started in a low dose to minimize hypotension and azotemia. If tolerated, the dose is gradually increased to at least 40 mg of a once-daily ACEI such as quinapril. Most experts recommend larger doses to maximize benefits.

### Cerebrovascular Diseases

Angiotensin-converting enzyme inhibitors compared to placebo reduced strokes by an average 28% in the five trials included in the Blood Pressure Trialists analysis (2003). However, ACEIs were less effective in comparison to both diuretic ± β-blocker or CCB-based therapies, by 9% and 12% respectively, whereas ARBs have reduced strokes by 21% in four placebo-controlled RCTs.

Fournier and colleagues (2004) have presented a provocative but reasonable explanation for the observed better cerebroprotection by diuretics and ARBs than by ACEIs (and β-blockers). Their argument is based on the hypothesis of Brown and Brown (1986) that "angiotensin II could protect against stroke by causing vasoconstriction of the proximal cerebral arteries thereby preventing Charcot-Bouchard aneurysms from rupturing" (Fournier et al., 2004). This 1986 hypothesis presaged the identification of two major angiotensin II receptors, $AT_1$ and $AT_2$, both restrained by ACEIs which lower circulating angiotensin II, whereas only the $AT_1$ receptor is blocked by the ARBs, leaving the $AT_2$ receptor even more stimulated by higher levels of circulating angiotensin II. Stimulation of $AT_1$ receptors evokes vasoconstriction and vascular damage (Ryan et al., 2004). Stimulation of $AT_2$ receptors, at least experimentally, evokes a number of helpful effects including vasodilation, antiinflammation, and regeneration of neuronal tissues (Thöne-Reineke et al., 2004). Further support for a protective effect against stroke by $AT_2$ stimulation are data from an animal model showing a protective effect on ischemic brain lesions, at least partly through an increase of cerebral blood flow and a decrease in superoxide formulation (Iwai et al., 2004).

Whether or not these conjectures are valid, they support the clinical evidence: ACEIs (and β-blockers) prevent strokes less well than ARBs (and diuretics and CCBs). Further support for this construct is the inadequacy of ACEI alone to prevent recurrent strokes except with the addition of a diuretic in the Perindopril Protection Against Recurrent Stroke Study (PROGRESS) trial (PROGRESS Collaborative Group, 2001).

### Renal Diseases

Angiotensin-converting enzyme inhibitors preferentially dilate the renal efferent arteriole, reducing intraglomerular pressure and restraining glomerulosclerosis, podocyte damage, and proteinuria.

Their antiproteinuric effect may involve a number of additional mechanisms (Lassila et al., 2004). The clinical consequences have been profound: a significant slowing of the progress of renal damage in those with nephropathy (Thurman & Schrier, 2003) but an even more potentially helpful prevention of the development of nephropathy (Ruggenenti et al., 2004).

In Ruggenenti et al.'s study, 1,204 type 2 diabetic patients free of albuminuria were assigned either the ACEI trandolapril alone, the nonDHP-CCB verapamil alone, the two together, or placebo for at least 3 years. In those on the ACEI alone, microalbuminuria developed in 6.0%; on the CCB alone, 11.9%; on the combination, 5.7%; and on the placebo, 10%. The obvious conclusion is that the ACEI works, the CCB adds nothing.

Angiotensin-converting enzyme inhibitors have been extensively studied in type 1 diabetic and nondiabetic nephropathies and found to be protective against progression (Thurman & Schrier, 2003). ARBs have been shown to be protective in type 2 diabetic nephropathy (Brenner et al., 2001; Lewis et al., 2001). In the only currently available head-to-head comparison, the ACEI enalapril was equal to the ARB telmisartan in type 2 diabetic nephropathy (Barnett et al., 2004).

More and more, a combination of an ACEI and an ARB is being used to minimize proteinuria. Whether the combination protects renal function or lowers BP better than full doses of one or the other remains to be seen (Doulton et al., 2005).

### Other Uses

Angiotensin-converting enzyme inhibitors have been found to ameliorate altitude polycythemia with its attendant proteinuria (Plata et al., 2002), maintain muscle strength in older hypertensive women (Onder et al., 2002), diminish hypertriglyceridemia in nephrotic patients (Ruggenenti et al., 2003), and ameliorate migraine (Schrader et al., 2001). All of this good is only partly countered by an increased sensitivity to pain (Guasti et al., 2002).

### Side Effects

With large doses of captopril in patients with severe hypertension, many of whom also had renal insufficiency, a high incidence of side effects was initially reported. As smaller doses have been used in patients with normal renal function, the incidence of side effects has fallen significantly. For example, the incidence of neutropenia was 7.2% in patients with collagen vascular disease and impaired renal function and 0.4% in patients with renal insufficiency from other causes but only 0.02%

in patients with normal renal function (Warner & Rush, 1988).

The recognized side effects of ACEIs logically can be divided into three types: (a) those anticipated from their specific pharmacologic actions, (b) those probably related to their chemical structure, and (c) nonspecific effects, as seen with any drug that lowers the BP.

### Effects Anticipated from Pharmacologic Actions

*First-Dose Hypotension*
An immediate fall in mean arterial BP of more than 30% was seen in 3.3% of 240 hypertensive patients given 25 mg captopril (Postma et al., 1992). The likelihood of such an abrupt fall is less with other ACEIs, which are prodrugs and have a slower onset of action (Table 7–10).

*Hyperkalemia*
Hyperkalemia occurs in about 10% of patients taking an ACEI (Palmer, 2004). The reasons are

## TABLE 7–11

**Risk Factors for Hyperkalemia with the Use of Drugs That Interfere with the Renin-Angiotensin-Aldosterone System**

Chronic kidney disease, particularly with GFR < 30

Bilateral renal artery stenosis

Diabetes mellitus

Volume depletion

Advanced age

Drugs used concomitantly that interfere in renal potassium excretion

    Nonsteroidal antiinflammatory drugs

    β-blockers

    Calcineurin inhibitors: cyclosporine, tacrolimus

    Heparin

    Ketoconazole

    Potassium-sparing diuretics: spironolactone, eplerenone, amiloride, triamterine

    Trimethoprim

    Pentamidine

Potassium supplements, including salt substitutes and certain herbs

Modified from Palmer BF. Managing hyperkalemia caused by inhibitors of the renin-angiotensin-aldosterone system. *N Engl J Med* 2004;351:585–592.

multiple (Table 7–11), mostly reflecting diminished renal perfusion, decreased aldosterone, and reduced renal tubular function (Palmer, 2004). If recognized, the problem can usually be managed by deleting drugs that further increase potassium load or interfere with its excretion.

*Hypoglycemia*
Perhaps as a reflection of increased insulin sensitivity, ACEI use has been accompanied by hypoglycemia both in insulin-dependent and noninsulin-dependent diabetics (Herings et al., 1995).

*Interference with Erythropoietin*
Angiotensin II enhances erythrocytosis and ACEIs may interefere with the action of erythropoieten in correcting the anemia of CRD patients but also reduce secondary erythrocytosis as after transplantation (Fakhouri et al., 2004).

*Deterioration of Renal Function*
Most reports of acute loss of renal function involved patients with CHF, volume depletion, or renal artery stenoses, either bilaterally or to a solitary kidney (Table 7–11).Within 6 months, 0.2% of 18,977 patients given lisinopril had more than a doubling of serum creatinine but none developed renal failure (Thorp et al., 2005). However, acute increases of serum creatinine of up to 30% that stabilize within the first 2 months of ACEI therapy are associated with *better* long-term renoprotection (Bakris & Weir, 2000), and so such rises should not lead to withdrawal of ACEI therapy.

*Pregnancy*
Angiotensin-converting enzyme inhibitors are contraindicated during the second and third trimesters of pregnancy, because they cause fetal injury and death (Shotan et al., 1994). No definite evidence of ACEI fetal damage has been noted among 48 infants born to mothers who took an ACEI during the first trimester (Feldkamp et al., 1997).

*Cough and Bronchospasm*
A dry, hacking, nonproductive, and sometimes intolerable cough is the most frequent side effect of ACEI therapy; bronchospasm may be the second most frequent. In a controlled cohort study of 1,013 patients on an ACEI and 1,017 on lipid-lowering drugs, cough developed in 12.3% and bronchospasm in 5.5% of patients on an ACEI versus 2.7% and 2.3%, respectively, in those on the lipid-lowering drugs (Wood, 1995). The incidence may differ between ACEIs. In a crossover trial, cough occured less than half as often with imidapril as with enalapril (Saruta et al., 1999).

An increase in bradykinin has been assumed to be the mechanism for the cough (Yeo et al., 1995), and a genetic polymorphism of the bradykinin $\beta_2$-receptor has been found in a higher proportion of patients who have an ACEI-related cough (Mukae et al., 2000).

Cough is more common in older patients, women, and Blacks (Morimoto et al., 2004) and was reported in almost half of Chinese patients (Woo & Nicholls, 1995). It usually goes away in a few weeks after the drug is withdrawn and usually recurs with reexposure to an ACEI. Although the cough may be effectively treated with inhaled sodium cromoglycate (Hargreaves & Benson, 1995) or aspirin (Tenenbaum et al., 2000), the easiest way to resolve the problem is to replace the ACEI with an ARB.

*Angioedema*

Angioedema occurs in 0.1% to 0.2% of patients given an ACEI, usually within hours but sometimes after prolonged use (Cicardi et al., 2004). Recurrent episodes, some with visceral involvement, may not be attributed to ACEI use until years after they are begun. Fatal airway obstruction has been reported so that it is mandatory that patients with angioedema on an ACEI never be given an ACEI again. Switching to an ARB may or may not be associated with recurrence and should be done very cautiously if at all (Sica & Black, 2002).

### Effects Related to Chemical Structure

Effects related to chemical structure may be more common with captopril than with the nonsulfhydryl ACEIs, because most are also seen with other sulfhydryl-containing drugs such as penicillamine (Hammarström et al., 1991). Most, but not all, patients who experience one of these reactions while on captopril can be safely crossed over to another ACEI (Jackson et al., 1988).

*Taste Disturbance*

Although usually of little consequence and self-limited with continued drug intake, taste disturbance may be so bad as to interfere with nutrition. It appears to be related to the binding of zinc by the ACEI (Abu-Hamdan et al., 1988).

*Rash*

The rash is usually a nonallergic, pruritic, maculopapular eruption that appears during the first few weeks of therapy and may disappear despite continuation of the ACEI. Serious skin reactions including Schönlein-Henoch purpura have been reported (Gonçalves et al., 1998).

*Leukopenia*

Leukopenia probably occurs exclusively in patients with renal insufficiency (Cooper, 1983), particularly those with underlying immunosuppression either from a disease or from a drug.

*Nonspecific Side Effects*

Angiotensin-converting enzyme activity is present in intestinal brush border, and adverse gastrointestinal effects have been reported with ACEI use (Edwards et al., 1992). Other rare effects include pancreatitis (Roush et al., 1991) and cholestatic jaundice (Nissan et al., 1996).

Angiotensin-converting enzyme inhibitors have no major effects on cognitive function (Ebert & Kirch, 1999) and are "lipid-neutral" (Kasiske et al., 1995), escaping some of the common side effects of other drugs. Headache, dizziness, fatigue, diarrhea, and nausea are listed in reviews but are seldom problems. Sudden withdrawal does not usually lead to a rebound (Vlasses et al., 1981). Overdose causes hypotension that should be easily managed with fluids and, if needed, dopamine (Lip & Ferner, 1995).

### Perspective on Use

Captopril, when first introduced for use in severe hypertensives and in high doses, earned a bad reputation that was quickly overcome. As appropriately lower doses were used and found to be as effective as other drugs, often with fewer side effects, captopril and then enalapril became increasingly popular. Over the past few years, many more ACEIs have been marketed, most with the added advantage of longer duration of action, allowing for once-daily dosing.

As ACEIs have been used in various situations, three places have been recognized wherein they provide special benefits beyond those provided by other agents: relief of acute and chronic heart failure, prevention of remodeling and progressive ventricular dysfunction after MI, and slowing of glomerular sclerosis in diabetic and other nephropathies. Beyond these specific indications, the evidence from the HOPE and EUROPA trials led to the recommendation that an ACEI be given to all patients with CHD, whether hypertensive or not (White, 2003) but that recommendation should now be reconsidered on the basis of the CAMELOT and PEACE trials. Moreover, they (along with ARBs) are more likely to prevent the onset of diabetes than any antihypertensive agent (Opie & Schall, 2004).

Even as ACEIs have become increasingly popular, their popularity has been threatened by the introduction of ARBs, agents that act at a more distal site of the renin-angiotensin system (Figure 7–13).

### ANGIOTENSIN II-RECEPTOR BLOCKERS

Even before ACEIs were available, a peptidic antagonist of AII receptors, saralasin, was shown to lower BP (Brunner et al., 1973). However, its use was limited by the need for intravenous administration and its pressor effect in low-renin patients resulting from its partial agonist effects (Case et al., 1976). Subsequently, the AII receptor was found to have at least two major subtypes, with the type 1 ($AT_1$) receptor mediating most of the physiologic roles of AII. The signaling mechanisms and functions of these receptor subtypes are different, and they may exert opposite effects on cell growth and BP regulation (Nickenig, 2004) (Figure 7–14). Agents that selectively block the $AT_1$-receptor have been synthesized and marketed for the treatment of hypertension. Losartan was the first, and now six more have been approved for use in the United States (Table 7–12).

## Mode of Action

Angiotensin II-receptor blockers displace AII from its specific $AT_1$-receptor, antagonizing all of its known effects and resulting in a dose-dependent fall in peripheral resistance and little change in heart rate or cardiac output (Burnier, 2001). As a consequence of the competitive displacement, circulating levels of AII increase while at the same time the blockade of the renin-angiotensin mechanism is more complete, including any AII that is generated through pathways that do not involve ACE (Figure 7–13). No obvious good or bad effects of the increased AII levels have been proven but, in experimental animals, chronic stimulation of $AT_2$

receptors exerts a hypertrophic and antiangiogenic influence that, if seen in humans, could lead to cardiac hypertrophy, vascular fibrosis, and a decrease in neovascularization in hypoxic tissues (Levy, 2004). On the other hand, chronic stimulation of $AT_2$ receptors has been found in experimental models to provide neuroprotection (Thöne-Reineke et al., 2004).

More may be involved in the action of ARBs than blocking the $AT_1$ receptor. β-adrenergic blockers have been shown to cross react with ARBs at their respective receptors, individually inhibiting the major functional and physiological effects of the other (Barki-Harrington et al., 2003). The investigators conclude: "A single receptor antagonist effectively blocks downstream signaling and trafficking of both receptors simultaneously." They advance their experimental data as support for the additive effect of β-blockers and ARBs in the treatment of heart failure.

### Differences Between ARBs and ACEIs

Since their introduction, the major obvious difference between ARBs and ACEIs has been thought to be the absence of an increase in kinin levels with the ARB, increases that may be responsible for some of the beneficial effects of ACEIs and likely

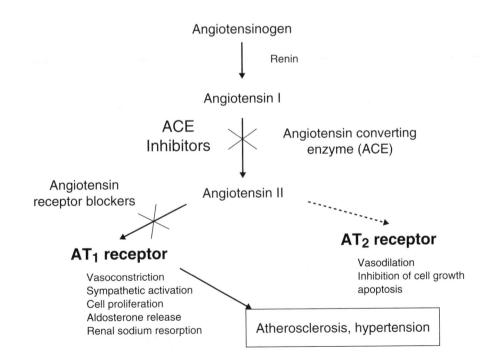

**FIGURE 7–14** ● The renin-angiotensin system with the major effects of stimulation at $AT_1$ and $AT_2$ receptors and the sites of action of ACEIs and ARBs. (Modified from Nickenig G. Should angiotensin II receptor blockers and statins be combined? *Circulation* 2004;110:1013–1020.)

## TABLE 7–12

### Angiotensin II-Receptor Blockers

| Drug | Trade Name | Half-Life (h) | Active Metabolite | Daily Dosage (mg) |
|------|-----------|---------------|-------------------|-------------------|
| Candesartan | Atacand (Astra) | 3–11 | Yes | 8–32 in 1 dose |
| Eprosartan | Tevetan (Smith Kline) | 5–7 | No | 400–800 in 1–2 doses |
| Irbesartan | Avapro (BMS, Sanofi) | 11–15 | No | 150–300 in 1 dose |
| Losartan | Cozaar (Merck) | 2 (6–9) | Yes | 50–100 in 1–2 doses |
| Olmesartan | Benicar (Sankyo) | 13 | Yes | 20–40 in 1 dose |
| Telmisartan | Micardis (BI) | 24 | No | 40–80 in 1 dose |
| Valsartan | Diovan (Novartis) | 9 | No | 80–320 in 1 dose |

even more of their side effects. However, Campbell et al. (2005) have found twofold increases in blood levels of bradykinin after 4 weeks use of losartan 50 mg a day and slightly smaller increases with eprosartan 600 mg a day. These increases are similar to those seen with ACEIs, but they did not find increases in blood kallidin levels, which are seen with ACEIs. They believe the absence of this rise is responsible for the lesser incidence of angioedema with ARBs.

Direct comparisons between the two types of drugs show few differences in antihypertensive efficacy and long-term renoprotection (Barnett et al., 2004). Although cough is not provoked by ARBs (Tanser et al., 2000), angioedema has been seen (Sica & Black, 2002) and ageusia reported with losartan (Schlienger et al., 1996). The ARB valsartan improved some cognitive functions in elderly hypertensives whereas enalapril did not (Fogari et al., 2004b).

As evidence of differences between the two classes, Stergiou et al. (2004) found at least 10/5 mm Hg difference in the response to 80 mg telmisartan or 20 mg lisinopril each given for 5 weeks in 28% of 32 hypertensives in a crossover trial.

As seen with ACEIs, ARBs have been found to improve endothelial dysfunction and correct the altered structure of resistance arteries in patients with hypertension (Schiffrin et al., 2000). Major antiinflammatory effects of various ARBs have been reported in experimental models (Ando et al., 2004), human cells (Dandona et al., 2003), and hypertensive patients (Koh et al., 2003). These effects include suppression of reactive oxygen species and a variety of inflammatory cytokines (Fliser et al., 2004). These effects have been translated into attenuation of nitrate tolerance (Hirai et al., 2003) and stabilization of atherosclerotic plaques (Cipollone et al., 2004).

### Differences Between ARBs

To gain position in a crowded market of ARBs (and ACEIs), pharmaceutical marketers have expended a lot of effort and money to provide a special niche for their product. Most of these studies show little difference in efficacy with comparable doses but a definitely longer duration of action for those with a longer half-life(!). It comes as no surprise that telmisartan acts longer than losartan (Neutel et al., 2004) or valsartan (White et al., 2004a).

On the other hand, some ARBs may be different in other respects:

- Losartan has a uricosuric effect (Würzner et al., 2001)
- Valsartan enhances insulin sensitivity in the skeletal muscles of diabetic mice (Shiuchi et al., 2004)
- Telmisartan and, to a lesser extent, irbesartan but not the other ARBs act as partial peroxisome proliferator-activated receptor-γ (PPARγ) agonists (Benson et al., 2004; Schupp et al., 2004). Both groups of investigators found similar effects on adipocyte differentiation and PPARγ target gene expression. Benson et al. (2004) also found that telmisartan reduced glucose, insulin, and triglyceride levels in rats fed a high-fat, high-carbohydrate diet. These results suggest "a potential mechanism for insulin-sensitizing/antidiabetic effects" (Schupp et al., 2004) and "unique opportunities for the prevention and treatment of diabetes and cardiovascular disease in high-risk

populations" (Benson et al., 2004). Obviously, clinical proof of these exciting potentials is eagerly awaited.

## Antihypertensive Efficacy

In the recommended doses (Table 7–12), all seven currently available ARBs have comparable antihypertensive efficacy, and all are potentiated by addition of a diuretic (Conlin et al., 2000). The dose-response curve is fairly flat for all, although increasing doses of candesartan show an increasing effect (Lacourcière & Asmar, 1999).

As noted, a single daily dose of 50 mg losartan does not provide as complete 24-hour efficacy as do single daily doses of the other ARBs (Fogari et al., 2000). However, either the 100-mg dose or the combination of losartan with HCTZ does provide full 24-hour efficacy (Weber et al., 1995).

Angiotensin II-receptor blockers may be combined with other agents for additive effects. Multiple studies have shown additive effects when submaximal doses of an ARB are added to submaximal doses of an ACEI, but the only convincing evidence now available for additive effects of presumably maximal doses of an ARB and an ACEI is in reduction of proteinuria (Nakao et al., 2003). Whereas the combination of high doses of ACEIs and ARBs to provide "complete" inhibition of the renin-angiotensin-aldosterone system may be useful, Ménard and Azizi (2004) warn: "Environmental aggression, such as acute dehydration, regional or general anaesthesia, onset or aggravation of CHF or dysrhythmia, may suddenly transform 'healthy' treated subjects into high-risk subjects, if RAS and aldosterone blockade are not rapidly ceased and/or if sodium repletion is not performed."

## Other Uses

### Renal Diseases

Angiotensin II-receptor blockers have been shown to be renoprotective in three placebo-controlled trials in type II diabetics with nephropathy (Brenner et al., 2001; Lewis et al., 2001; Parving et al., 2001), two using irbesartan, the third losartan, all three showing 20% to 30% reductions in progression of renal damage. However, ARBs did not reduce mortality in those trials, unlike the 21% reduction in mortality in the 36 trials comparing ACEIs to placebo in patients with diabetic nephropathy (Strippoli et al., 2004).

### Effects on Morbidity and Mortality

In the four trials available in early 2003, ARBs reduced stroke by 21%, heart failure by 16%, but had no significant effect on coronary disease or mortality, either cardiovascular or all-cause (Blood Pressure Trialists, 2003).

Subsequently, many more trials using ARBs have been published, particularly in patients with nephropathy or heart failure. As will be reviewed under "Other Uses," these trials have in general been positive, showing benefits from ARBs. However, as noted by Verma and Strauss (2004), ARB's record against preventing myocardial infarction has been negative, with more MIs seen with ARBs than with placebo or other antihypertensive drugs:

- In VALUE, valsartan was associated with 19% more MIs than amlodipine (Julius et al., 2004b).
- In CHARM-alternative, candesartan was associated with 36% more MIs than a placebo (Granger et al., 2003).
- In SCOPE, candesartan was associated with 10% more MIs than placebo (Lithell et al., 2003).
- In IDNT, irbesartan was associated with 36% more MIs than amlodipine (Lewis et al., 2001).
- Verma and Strauss's claim has been said to be based on incomplete data and incorrect (Lewis, 2005; McMurray, 2005). Direct comparisons between ARBs and ACEIs are obviously needed (Opie, 2005).

### Cardiac Diseases

In their 2003 meta-analysis, the Blood Pressure Trialists reported that ARB-based therapy reduced heart failure by 16% but coronary heart disease and cardiovascular mortality by only 4% in four RCTs—the SCOPE (Lithell et al., 2003), IDNT (Lewis et al., 2001), RENAAL (Brenner et al., 2001), and LIFE (Dahlöf et al., 2002). Of the trials, LIFE has been extensively touted in multiple publications of subgroup analyses as evidence that the ARB losartan was better than the β-blocker atenolol among hypertensives with LVH in multiple ways: regression of LVH, cardiovascular morbidity and mortality in the entire 9,193 patients (Dahlöf et al., 2002), as well as in the 1,195 diabetic subjects (Lindholm et al., 2002); in the 6,886 participants without clinically evident vascular disease (Devereux et al., 2003); and in the 1,325 with isolated systolic hypertension (Kjeldsen et al., 2002). Moreover, sudden cardiac death was also separately reported to have been reduced more by the ARB than the β-blocker (Lindholm et al., 2003a) as was echocardiographically defined LVH in the 960 participants who had that procedure (Devereux et al., 2004a) as well as stroke (Kizer et al., 2005).

These multiple publications (and the many more likely to come) had the expected effect: ARBs in general and losartan in particular were hailed as "a promise fulfilled" (Brunner & Gavras, 2002) and proof that ARBs have "come of age" (Sica & Weber, 2002). Others have pointed out that atenolol is an ineffective drug (but a good one to compare against) (Carlberg et al., 2004), that almost 80% of patients who remained on therapy in the LIFE trial were also taking a diuretic, and that 25% of patients were off the study drugs by the end of the study. Nonetheless, the study deserves credit for putting losartan "on the map" even if subsequent data suggest that other ARBs may be preferable.

In smaller studies, losartan but not atenolol has been shown to reduce myocardial fibrosis (Ciulla et al., 2004), valsartan to regress LVH better than amlodipine (Yasunari et al., 2004), but candesartan to regress LVH no better than enalapril (Cuspidi et al., 2002).

## Heart Failure

Angiotensin II-receptor blockers have been extensively studied in patients with chronic heart failure and found to be equally effective as ACEIs. In a meta-analysis of 24 trials involving 38,080 patients, Lee et al. (2004) reported these findings:

- Angiotensin II-receptor blockers as compared to placebo provided a 17% decrease in all-cause mortality and a 36% decrease in heart failure hospitalizations.
- ARBs as compared to ACEIs did not differ in either end point. However, in the OPTIMAL trial most end points showed a trend in favor of captopril over losartan, with cardiovascular death significantly lower in the captopril group (Dickstein et al., 2002).
- Angiotensin II-receptor blockers combined with ACEIs did not further reduce all-cause mortality but reduced heart failure hospitalizations by 23%.

## Post-Myocardial Infarction

Lee et al. (2004) examined the two trials in high-risk post-MI patients—OPTIMAL, comparing losartan to captopril (Dickstein et al., 2002) and VALIANT, comparing valsartan to captopril and the two together (Pfeffer et al., 2003). No differences in all-cause mortality or heart failure hospitalizations were found.

In a review of these data on the use of ARBs in CHF and postMI, McMurray et al. (2004) conclude:

We believe that the available trial data provide clear evidence that certain ARBs, when used at the clinically effective dose (titration of either valsartan to 160 mg twice daily or candesartan to 32 mg daily) can reduce cardiovascular morbidity and mortality. . . . in CHF, ARBs provide a clear advance, offering an additional

opportunity to further reduce cardiovascular morbidity and mortality when used concomitantly with both a β-blocker and ACE inhibitor. In AMI complicated by LVSD, acute heart failure, or both, the combination of an ARB with a proven dose of an ACE inhibitor does not result in incremental clinical benefits, although a proven dose of a proven ARB is as effective as an ACE inhibitor.

These conclusions must be contrasted with the claim that ARBs have not been effective in preventing acute MIs (Verma & Strauss, 2004).

## Side Effects

In virtually every trial of ARBs given to hypertensive patients, ARBs have been better tolerated than other classes of antihypertensives, usually causing no more symptoms than placebo with no increase in cough as seen with ACEIs although angioedema may still occur (Mancia et al., 2003). Such tolerability is likely responsible for the higher maintenance of therapy with ARBs than with other antihypertensives (Conlin et al., 2001).

In trials of patients with CHF and postMI, more problems arose as would be expected in such hemodynamically unstable patients. As McMurray et al. (2004) observe: "A consistent finding from all the major trials is that effective doses of these ARBs lead to hypotension and increases in creatinine and potassium."

Beyond these expected side effects, along with fetal toxicity (Chen et al., 2004), no major surprises have surfaced. A minor surprise is the rare occurrence of a rash and even rarer acute nephritis with candesartan reported from Australia (Morton et al., 2004).

## Perspective on Use

Angiotensin II-receptor blockers have rapidly taken their place as excellent drugs for the treatment of hypertension, proteinuric renal diseases, and heart failure, in general equal to but no better than the effects of ACEIs except, as noted earlier, for the potential for better neuroprotection. Their major current advantage is their better tolerability over other classes, in particular the absence of the cough seen in about 10% of ACEI users.

Since generic ACEIs are (or should be) less expensive than trade-named ARBs, the argument could easily be made to use ACEIs wherever a renin-angiotensin inhibitor is indicated and switch to an ARB if a cough develops, since the ACEI cough is only an irritant, not a danger. This approach may be even more appropriate in view of the putative inability of ARBs to reduce heart attacks in high-risk patients.

On the other hand, the combination of an ACEI and an ARB has been quickly adopted by nephrologists for use in proteinuria patients, and the combination may prove better in other patients as well.

Whereas Wald and Law (2003) have recommended the incorporation of an ACEI in their polypill, Nickenig (2004) suggests the combination of an ARB with a statin, providing preliminary evidence of synergism between the two. Since a combination of a CCB and a statin has been approved, other superpills may be on their way.

Meanwhile, as always happens in clinical medicine, something even better may be on the horizon.

## DRUGS UNDER INVESTIGATION

### Renin Inhibitors

Long under study, orally effective inhibitors of the action of renin to cleave the decapeptide AI from angiotensinogen are now being tested in hypertensive patients. The first of these, aliskiren, seems both effective and safe (Gradman et al., 2005; Stanton et al., 2003). Such agents are attractive not only because they can inhibit the production of AI and AII, but also because they prevent the reactive rise in renin release that follows the use of ACEIs and ARBs. Whether any will become available for clinical use remains to be seen.

### *Renin-Angiotensin Vaccine*

Although immunogenic, an angiotensin I vaccine had no antihypertensive effect (Brown et al., 2004).

### Vasopeptidase Inhibitors

The most exciting new class of drugs recently examined are vasopeptidase inhibitors, single molecules that simultaneously inhibit ACE and the neutral endopeptidase (NEP), which normally degrades a number of endogenous natriuretic peptides so that decreases in AII and increases in bradykinin are combined with increases in natriuretic peptides (Burnett, 1999). The most widely studied of these agents is omapatrilat (Vanlev) (Kostis et al., 2004).

The obvious attraction of the combined ACE and NEP inhibitors is the ability to have effects on both high and low renin states while providing a natriuresis without activating the renin system as do traditional diuretics. Clinical studies in patients with hypertension or heart failure were encouraging (Mitchell et al., 2002).

However, not surprisingly, the high levels of bradykinin induced by these agents led to a disturbing incidence of severe angioedema, so that the expected approval of omapatrilat was rejected in 2002 (Pickering, 2002). It is unlikely that vasopeptidease inhibitors will see the light of clinical use.

**Endothelin Antagonists**

Although able to inhibit endothelin-induced vasoconstriction experimentally (Gössl et al., 2004), the currently available endothelin antagonists are only weak antihypertensives (Kirchengast & Luz, 2005). The orally active antagonist, darusentan, did not improve symptoms or outcomes in patients with chronic CHF receiving an ACEI, β-blocker, or aldosterone antagonist (Anand et al., 2004).

### Possible Drugs for the Far Future

- Stimulants of calcitonin gene-related peptide synthesis (Deng et al., 2004)
- Inhibitors of endogenous cannabinoids breakdown (Batkai et al., 2004)
- Breaker of advanced glycation end product cross links (Bakris et al., 2004a)
- Targeted inhibitors of the brain renin-angiotensin system (Fournie-Zaluski et al., 2004)
- Inhibitors of angiotensin-converting enzyme 2 (Huentelman et al., 2004)
- Gene therapy (Tang et al., 2004)

### Conclusion

A number of different drugs are under investigation. Time—and, in the United States, the U.S. Food and Drug Administration—will tell which of them will become available for clinical use. More drugs will be available, probably in rate-controlled forms, so that a single capsule or a patch may provide smooth control over many days. In the meantime, proper use of what is available will control BP in virtually every hypertensive patient, and whether new drugs will necessarily improve our ability to do so is questionable. As Pickering (2002) notes:

> We have witnessed the introduction of two completely new classes of antihypertensive drugs, the ACE inhibitors and the angiotensin receptor blockers, and the annual expenditure on antihypertensive drugs has increased dramatically, but there is not a shred of evidence that there has been any meaningful improvement in the rate of blood pressure control, which remains 27%–29%. In contrast to this dismal state of affairs, two recent studies, the Antihypertensive and Lipid-Lowering Treatment to Prevent Heart Attack Trial (ALLHAT) (ALLHAT Officers, 2002) and the Controlled Onset Verapamil Investigation of Cardiovascular End Points (CONVINCE) (Black et al., 2003), both treating hypertensive patients who were at somewhat increased

risk, have reported that simply following a predetermined protocol, and using conventional and readily available drugs, could increase the control rate more than 65%.

## GENERAL GUIDELINES FOR DRUG CHOICES

An attempt will be made to put our current knowledge about the drugs available to treat hypertension into a useful clinical context, proceeding to considerations of the appropriate choices for multiple types of hypertensive patients.

### Comparisons Between Drugs: Efficacy

The individual practitioner's choice of drug is often based on perceived differences in efficacy in lowering BP and the likelihood of side effects. In fact, overall antihypertensive efficacy varies little between the various available drugs; to gain U.S. Food and Drug Administration approval for marketing in the United States, the drug must have been shown to be effective in reducing the BP in a large portion of the 1,500 or more patients given the drug during its clinical investigation. Moreover, the dose and formulation of drug are chosen so as not to lower the BP too much or too fast, to avoid hypotensive side effects. Virtually all oral drugs are designed to do the same thing: lower the BP at least 10% in the majority of patients with mild to moderate hypertension.

Not only must each new drug be shown to be effective in large numbers of hypertensive patients, but the drug also must have been tested against currently available agents to show at least equal efficacy. When comparisons between various drugs are made, they almost always come out close to one another. The best such comparison was performed in the TOMHS study (Neaton et al., 1993) with random allocation of five drugs (chlorthalidone, acebutolol, doxazosin, amlodipine, and enalapril), each given to almost 200 mild hypertensives, while another group took a placebo, and all patients remained on a nutritional-hygienic program. The overall antihypertensive efficacy of the five drugs over 4 years was virtually equal (Neaton et al., 1993).

Despite the fairly equal overall efficacy of various antihypertensive drugs, individual patients may vary considerably in their response to different drugs, often for no obvious reason (Senn, 2004). However, some of this variability can be accounted for by patient characteristics, including age and race. This was seen in a VA cooperative 1-year trial in which 1,292 men were randomly given one of six drugs from each major class: Overall, and in the Black patients, the CCB was most effective, but the

ACEI was best in younger Whites, and the β-blocker was best in older Whites (Materson et al., 1993, 1995). Similarly, in a randomized crossover trial of elderly patients with isolated systolic hypertension given a representative of four major classes—ACEI, β-blocker, CCB, and diuretic—each for 1 month, the diuretics and CCB were more effective than the β-blocker or ACEI (Morgan et al., 2001). In similarly designed trials of younger patients with combined systolic and diastolic hypertension, the ACEI and β-blocker were more effective than the CCB or diuretic (Deary et al., 2002; Dickerson et al., 1999). These different effects, which are at least partly related to the level of renin-angiotensin activity, resulted in the AB/CD concept (Figure 7–15). This concept is now incorporated in the guidelines of the British Hypertension Society (Williams et al., 2004a) to be more fully covered later in this chapter.

### Individual Trials of Efficacy

Because individual patients do vary in their response, individual patient randomized clinical trials, referred to as "n of 1" (Jaeschke & Guyatt, 1990), have been proposed to ascertain the best drug for each patient. The idea is simple: The patient undergoes successive treatment periods, each providing an active drug and a matched placebo assigned at random, with both the patient and the physician blinded to the choice, which is made by the pharmacist. The process can go on as long as needed until an effective and well-tolerated agent is found for each individual patient, using home BP monitoring (Chatellier et al., 1995).

Although the concept is simple, I doubt whether many practitioners (or their patients) will go to that much trouble. Fortunately, the physician can make a fairly exact ascertainment, if not of the best drug, certainly of an effective and well-tolerated one. This simply requires an open mind, a willingness to try one drug after another (each chosen from the major classes of available antihypertensive agents) with careful monitoring of the patient (preferably by using home BP readings), and a thorough ascertainment of side effects.

### Comparisons Between Drugs: Reductions in Morbidity and Mortality

The critical issue is not efficacy in lowering BP but rather effectiveness in reducing morbidity and mortality. As detailed in Chapter 5, all major classes of antihypertensive drugs except α-blockers have been shown to reduce mortality and morbidity in large RCTs, and there are few differences between them (Blood Pressure Lowering, 2003; Psaty et al., 2003; Staessen et al., 2003).

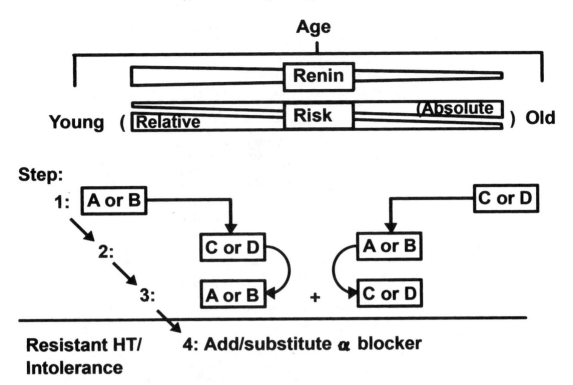

**FIGURE 7–15** ● Steps one and two are monotherapy, with the order influenced by the patient's renin status. This is partly determined by the patient's age and ethnic group, permitting initial selection of treatment without actual renin measurements. Steps three and four are combination treatment. Progress to each step is indicated by failure to meet the treatment target. A, ACEI; B, β-blocker; C, CCB; D, diuretic. (Modified from Dickerson JEC, et al. Optimisation of antihypertensive treatment by crossover rotation of four major classes. *Lancet* 1999;353:2008–2013.

In all of the 18 RCTs completed before 1995, diuretics or β-blockers were used (Psaty et al., 1997). Both classes reduced the incidence of stroke and heart failure, but only low doses of diuretic significantly reduced CHD. Over the past few years, the relative impotence of β-blockers, in particular atenolol, in reducing coronary disease has relegated them only to patients with a compelling indication for β-blocker.

In the 29 RCTs completed between 1995 and 2003, ACEIs or CCBs were compared either against placebo or against a diuretic with or without a β-blocker or against one another (Blood Pressure Lowering, 2003). As seen in Figure 7–16, one conclusion from these more recent trials seems obvious: Neither ACEI-based nor CCB-based therapies are better than are therapies based on diuretics with or without a β-blocker. Calcium channel blocker therapy did protect better against stroke and less well against CHF, but ACEIs and CCBs provided identical effects on overall morbidity and mortality. Only one comparison against an ARB was available, the LIFE trial comparing losartan against the weak sister atenolol.

In one sense, the issue of determining which one drug is best is irrelevant. As the need to achieve lower goals of therapy has become obvious, the need to use more than one drug in the majority of hypertensives has also become obvious. Therefore, the best combination of agents, almost always to include a low dose of diuretic, will be a more pertinent object of trials in the future.

**Comparisons Between Drugs: Adverse Effects**

As to the issue of differences in adverse effects among different agents, two points are obvious: First, no drug that causes dangerous adverse effects beyond a rare idiosyncratic reaction when given in usual doses will remain on the market, even if it slips by the approval process, as witnessed by the CCB mibefradil. Second, drugs that cause frequent bothersome although not dangerous adverse effects, such as guanethidine, will likely no longer be used now that so many other choices are available.

The various antihypertensive agents vary significantly, both in the frequency of adverse effects

| | Trials | Events/participants 1st listed | Events/participants 2nd listed | Difference in BP* (mean, mm Hg) | | Relative risk (95% CI) | p |
|---|---|---|---|---|---|---|---|
| **Stroke** | | | | | | | |
| ACEI vs D/BB | 5 | 984/20 195 | 1178/26 358 | +2/0 | | 1·09 (1·00–1·18) | 0·13 |
| CA vs D/BB | 9 | 999/31 031 | 1358/37 418 | +1/0 | | 0·93 (0·86–1·00) | 0·67 |
| ACEI vs CA | 5 | 701/12 562 | 622/12 541 | +1/+1 | | 1·12 (1·01–1·25) | 0·20 |
| **Coronary heart disease** | | | | | | | |
| ACEI vs D/BB | 5 | 1172/20 195 | 1658/26 358 | +2/0 | | 0·98 (0·91–1·05) | 0·21 |
| CA vs D/BB | 9 | 1394/31 031 | 1840/37 418 | +1/0 | | 1·01 (0·94–1·08) | 0·48 |
| ACEI vs CA | 5 | 907/12 562 | 948/12 541 | +1/+1 | | 0·96 (0·88–1·04) | 0·01 |
| **Heart failure** | | | | | | | |
| ACEI vs D/BB | 3 | 547/12 498 | 809/18 652 | +2/0 | | 1·07 (0·96–1·19) | 0·43 |
| CA vs D/BB | 7 | 732/23 425 | 850/29 734 | +1/0 | | 1·33 (1·21–1·47) | 0·92 |
| ACEI vs CA | 4 | 502/10 357 | 609/10 345 | +1/+1 | | 0·82 (0·73–0·92) | 0·75 |
| **Major cardiovascular events** | | | | | | | |
| ACEI vs D/BB | 6 | 2581/20 631 | 3450/26 799 | +2/0 | | 1·02 (0·98–1·07) | 0·31 |
| CA vs D/BB | 9 | 2998/31 031 | 3839/37 418 | +1/0 | | 1·04 (1·00,1·09) | 0·92 |
| ACEI vs CA | 5 | 1953/12 562 | 2011/12 541 | +1/+1 | | 0·97 (0·92–1·03) | 0·22 |
| **Cardiovascular death** | | | | | | | |
| ACEI vs D/BB | 6 | 1061/20 631 | 1440/26 799 | +2/0 | | 1·03 (0·95–1·11) | 0·36 |
| CA vs D/BB | 9 | 1237/31 031 | 1584/37 418 | +1/0 | | 1·05 (0·97–1·13) | 0·33 |
| ACEI vs CA | 5 | 870/12 562 | 840/12 541 | +1/+1 | | 1·03 (0·94–1·13) | 0·56) |
| **Total mortality** | | | | | | | |
| ACEI vs D/BB | 6 | 2176/20 631 | 3067/26 799 | +2/0 | | 1·00 (0·95–1·05) | 0·76 |
| CA vs D/BB | 9 | 2527/31 031 | 3437/37 418 | +1/0 | | 0·99 (0·95–1·04) | 0·71 |
| ACEI vs CA26 | 6 | 1763/12 998 | 1683/12 758 | +1/+1 | | 1·04 (0·98–1·10) | 0·68 |

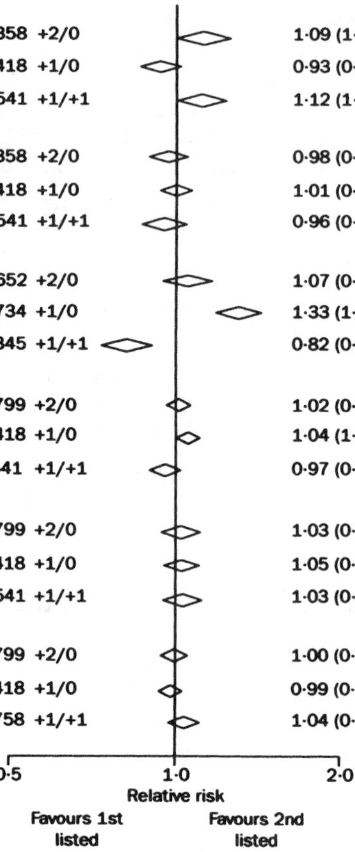

```
          0·5              1·0              2·0
                      Relative risk

        Favours 1st           Favours 2nd
          listed                 listed
```

**FIGURE 7–16** ● ACEI, ACE inhibitor; CA, calcium antagonist; C/BB, diuretic or β-blocker. p values from $|^2$ test for homogeneity. *Overall mean blood pressure difference (systolic/diastolic) during follow-up in the group assigned the first-listed treatment compared with the group assigned second-listed treatment, calculated by weighting the difference observed in each contributing trial by the number of individuals in the trial. Positive values indicate a higher mean follow-up blood pressure in the first-listed group. (Modified from Blood Pressure Lowering Trialists, *Lancet* 2003;362:1527–1536.)

and, to an even greater degree, in their nature. The only currently available comparisons of a representative drug from all major classes given as monotherapy to sizable numbers of patients are TOMHS (Neaton et al., 1993) and the VA Cooperative Study (Materson et al., 1993, 1995). Side effects differed between the drugs, but no one drug was markedly more or less acceptable than the others were. The differences may include sexual dysfunction. Impotence was twice as common in men in the TOMHS study given the diuretic chlorthalidone than in those given a placebo, whereas less impotence was seen among those given the α-blocker doxazosin (Grimm et al., 1997).

Angiotensin II-receptor blockers were not available when these trials were done. Clearly, they win first prize for tolerability, often with no more

immediate side effects than placebo (Mancia et al., 2003).

### Quality of Life

Over the past 25 years, a number of studies have examined the side effects of antihypertensive agents on quality of life (QOL) using various questionnaires and scales (Testa, 2000). The results show that, although 10% to 20% of patients will experience bothersome adverse effects from virtually any and every antihypertensive drug (ARBs not included), the overall impact of therapies on QOL over 2 to 6 months of observation is positive (Weir et al., 1996; Wiklund et al., 1999).

The most important component of QOL is cognitive function. The only currently available evidence for the ability to delay dementia remains the

Syst-Eur trial, which found that CCB-based therapy reduced the incidence by 55% over a mean follow-up of 3.9 years (Forette et al., 2002).

### Apparent Intolerance to All Drugs

Some patients have adverse effects from every drug they take, often bringing to the office a long list of what they have been unable to tolerate. In a few, this may reflect successful reduction in BP below the threshold of cerebral autoregulation by usual doses of drugs so that the patient appears to be intolerant to all medications. Some of these highly susceptible patients can be treated with very small doses of an appropriate agent, because they may be to the far left of the curve of responsiveness. More likely, such patients have psychiatric morbidity that sometimes can respond to behavioral cognitive therapy or antidepressants (Davies et al., 2003).

### Serious Side Effects

In addition to these QOL issues, more serious problems have been blamed on various classes of antihypertensive drugs. Virtually all these claims have come from noncontrolled, often retrospective, observational case-control studies, and most of them have been subsequently proven to be wrong (Kizer & Kimmel, 2001).

### Cancer from Reserpine, Calcium Channel Blockers, and Diuretics

The first and perhaps most egregious claim was that the use of reserpine was associated with a twofold to fourfold increased risk of breast cancer in women, a claim made in three simultaneously published papers from outstanding investigators (Armstrong et al., 1974; Boston Collaborative, 1974; Heinonen et al., 1974). As subsequently shown by Feinstein (1988), these studies were all contaminated by the bias of excluding women at high risk for cancer from the control groups. Multiple subsequently published prospective studies showed no association (Mayes et al., 1988).

More recently, Pahor et al. (1996a, 1996c) reported a twofold greater risk for cancer in elderly patients taking short-acting CCBs as compared to users of β-blockers. Unfortunately, they made no ascertainment of drug use after the original observation that the subjects had the respective drugs in their possession, so that the actual intake of drugs is totally unknown. Multiple subsequent reports of much larger populations in which drug use was appropriately ascertained have found no increase in cancer among users of CCBs (Kizer & Kimmel, 2001). Moreover, in the massive placebo-controlled Syst-Eur trial in the elderly, the incidence of cancer

was 31% less in those taking the CCB than in those on placebo (Staessen et al., 1997).

On the other hand, there may be an association between diuretic use and cancers arising in renal cells (Grossman et al., 2001) or colon (Tenenbaum et al., 2001). The association with renal cell cancers has been repeatedly observed and could reflect conversion of thiazides to mutagenic nitroso derivatives in the stomach. As noted by Hamet (1996), these claims must all be balanced against the multiple observations that the rates of cancer are increased among untreated hypertensives as well as obese patients (Yuan et al., 1998). Even if the association is true, the incidence is nonetheless so low as to be far overshadowed by the known benefits of diuretic therapy (Lip & Ferner, 1999).

### Coronary Disease from Calcium Channel Blockers and β-Blockers

Psaty et al. (1995) reported a 60% increase in the risk of acute MI among patients taking short-acting CCBs. This report coincided with republication of a metaanalysis of the adverse effects of high doses of short-acting CCBs in the immediate postMI period (Furberg et al., 1995). The two publications received tremendous press coverage claiming that CCBs could endanger more than 6 million hypertensives in the United States alone, leading to major disruptions in the management of patients with both angina and hypertension who were receiving these agents.

Psaty et al. (1995) and Furberg et al. (1995) strongly suggested that their claims against short-acting CCBs (which had never been approved for the treatment of hypertension) also carried over to the longer-acting agents (which are approved for the treatment of hypertension). In view of the significant differences in the hemodynamic and hormonal responses to short-acting versus long-acting CCBs, the faults of the former should not be assumed to apply to the latter. In fact, the multiple RCTs comparing long-acting CCBs against placebo show a decrease in coronary morbidity and mortality in the CCB users whereas comparisons between CCBs and other drugs show no differences (Blood Pressure Trialists, 2003).

Despite such repeated failures of observational studies to prove causality, they continue to appear in mainstream journals. A recent example is the claim that women who were supposedly taking a CCB and a diuretic at baseline experienced a higher rate of cardiovascular mortality than did those taking a β-blocker and diuretic (Wassertheil-Smoller et al., 2004). Again, there were no ascertainment of actual drug intake, monitoring of blood pressure, or certainty of end points. In the presence of such strong data from RCTs, the continued publication of what is almost hearsay evidence seems counterproductive.

## Dose-Response Relationships

### Need to Avoid Overdosing

Beyond the individual variabilities in response to drugs, there is a more generalized problem with the use of antihypertensive agents: They often are prescribed in doses that are too high. The problem of overdosing has been obvious with virtually every new drug introduced, wherein the initial recommended doses have been gradually reduced because, after widespread clinical experience, they proved to be too high (Johnston, 1994). Whereas 100 to 200 mg HCTZ was initially used, 12.5 mg is now recognized as enough for many patients. The initial recommended daily dose of captopril was up to 600 mg; now 50 to 100 mg is usually prescribed.

The problem arises in the preapproval testing of new drugs, as described by Herxheimer (1991):

> For a new drug to penetrate the market quickly, it should be rapidly effective in a high proportion of patients and simple to use. To achieve this, the dosage of the first prescription is therefore commonly set at about the ED90 level—i.e., the dose which the early clinical (phase II) studies have shown to be effective in 90% of the target population, provided that the unwanted effects at this dose are considered acceptable. In 25% of patients a smaller, perhaps much smaller, dose (the ED25) will be effective. The patients in this quartile are the most sensitive to the drug and are liable to receive far more than they need if they are given the ED90. They are also likely to be more sensitive to the dose-related side effects of the drug.

The obvious solution to this problem is for practitioners to start patients with doses that will not be fully effective and to titrate the dose gradually to the desired response. As Herxheimer (1991) notes:

> The disadvantage from the marketing standpoint is that for the majority of patients the dose must be titrated. That is time-consuming for doctors and patients and more difficult to explain to them. A drug requiring dose titration cannot be presented as the quick fix, the instant good news that marketing departments love.

### Need to Lower the Pressure Gradually

While it may be true that more rapid reduction in BP is needed to protect high-risk hypertensives as seen in the VALUE trial (Julius et al., 2004b), the "quick fix" is inappropriate for most patients, who are at low to moderate risk. In a large trial with an ACEI,

slower dose escalation (every 6 weeks) was shown to provide higher BP control rates and fewer serious adverse events than more rapid escalation (every 2 weeks) (Flack et al., 2000). These results are in keeping with what is known about the autoregulation of cerebral and coronary blood flow (Strandgaard & Haunsø, 1987) supporting the need for a slow and gradual fall in BP to maintain blood flow to vital organs. Normally, CBF remains relatively constant at approximately 50 mL per minute/100 g of brain (Strandgaard & Paulson, 1996). When the systemic BP falls, the vessels dilate; when the BP rises, the vessels constrict. The limits of cerebral autoregulation in normal people are between mean arterial BPs of about 60 and 120 mm Hg (e.g., 80/50 to 160/100 mm Hg).

In hypertensives without neurologic deficits, the CBF is not different from that found in normotensives (Eames et al., 2003; Traon et al., 2002). This constancy of the CBF reflects a shift in the range of autoregulation to the right to a range of mean BP from approximately 100 to 180 mm Hg (e.g., 130/85 to 240/150). As seen in Figure 7–17, this shift maintains a normal CBF despite the higher BP, but makes the hypertensive vulnerable to cerebral ischemia when the BP falls to a level that is well tolerated by normotensives.

Note that the lower limit of autoregulation capable of preserving CBF in hypertensive patients shown in Figure 7–17 is at a mean BP of nearly 110 mm Hg. Thus, acutely lowering the BP from 160/100 mm Hg (mean, 127 mm Hg) to 140/85 mm Hg (mean, 102 mm Hg) may induce cerebral hypoperfusion, although hypotension in the usual sense has not been induced. This likely explains why many patients experience manifestations of cerebral hypoperfusion (weakness, easy fatigability, and postural dizziness) at the start of antihypertensive therapy, even though BP levels do not seem inordinately low.

Fortunately, with slow and effective control of the BP by medication, the curve drifts back toward normal, explaining the eventual ability of hypertensive patients to tolerate falls in BP to levels that initially produced symptoms of cerebral ischemia. In a study of elderly hypertensives treated for 6 months, reduction of systolic BP to less than 140 mm Hg with various drugs resulted in increases in cerebral blood flow velocity and carotid distensibility, decreases in cerebrovascular resistance, and unimpaired cerebral autoregularion (Lipsitz et al., 2005).

### Need for 24-Hour Coverage

As noted in Chapter 2, self-recorded measurements and ambulatory automatic BP monitoring are being increasingly used to ensure the 24-hour duration of action of antihypertensive agents. This is particularly critical with the increasing use of once-a-day

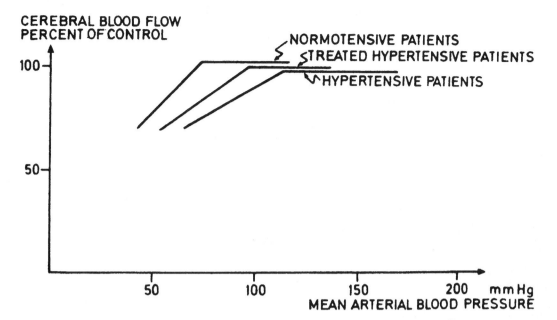

**FIGURE 7–17** ● Autoregulation of cerebral blood flow. Mean cerebral blood flow autoregulation curves from normotensive, severely hypertensive, and effectively treated hypertensive patients are shown. (Modified from Strandgaard S, Haunsø S. Why does antihypertensive treatment prevent stroke but not myocardial infarction? *Lancet* 1987;2:658–661.)

medications that often do not provide 24-hour efficacy (Lacourcière et al., 2000). Therefore, the patient is exposed to the full impact of the early morning, abrupt rise in BP that is almost certainly involved in the increased incidence of various cardiovascular events immediately after arising (Munger & Kenney, 2000).

Although ambulatory automatic BP monitoring is not available for most patients, self-recorded measurements with inexpensive semiautomatic devices should be possible for most, thereby ensuring the adequacy of control throughout the waking hours—particularly the early morning hours. As noted earlier, this may require taking medications in the evening or bedtime rather than the usually recommended early morning.

### Value of Greater than 24-Hour Efficacy

Drugs that continue to work beyond 24 hours are even more attractive to prevent loss of control in the considerable number who skip a dose at least once weekly, as documented in 30% or more of patients with hypertension (Rudd, 1995). Among those currently available drugs that will maintain good efficacy on a missed day are the CCB amlodipine (Elliott et al., 2002), the ACEIs perindopril (Tan & Leenen, 1999), trandolapril (Meredith, 1996), and the ARB telmisartan (Lacourcière et al., 2004). In the study shown in Figure 7–18, once-daily enalapril did not have sustained efficacy in the initial 24 hours and provided almost no effect in the second 24

hours, whereas trandolapril maintained full efficacy throughout the day of intake and most of its effect on the next day as well, when no drug was taken.

## CHOICE OF DRUGS: FIRST, SECOND, AND BEYOND

Now that the effectiveness and safety of various antihypertensive agents have been compared and important pharmacologic considerations have been emphasized, we will turn to the practical issue of which of the many drugs now available (Table 7–13) should be the first, second, or subsequent choices in individual patients. As noted previously, major changes in these choices have occurred.

Before proceeding into the specifics, we need to recall the overriding issue: to lower the BP to reduce cardiovascular risk maximally without decreasing (and perhaps even improving) the enjoyment of life. The preferred qualities of the drugs are fairly obvious, but none now available (or likely to become available) meets all the criteria for perfection. Nonetheless, currently available choices come close and, used adroitly, can protect almost all patients without much bother.

One impediment is threatening to interfere with clinicians' ability to use the therapy of their choice: restrictive formularies that often provide only the least expensive drugs even if they are not the most appropriate for patients' needs. Moreover, with a plethora of healthcare organizations, multiple

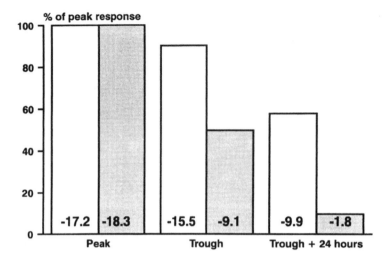

**FIGURE 7–18** ● Systolic BP responses to enalapril (*shaded bars*) and trandolapril (*open bars*) at steady state and 24 hours after a missed dose. (Modified from Meredith PA. Implications of the links between hypertension and myocardial infarction for choice of drug therapy in patients with hypertension. *Am Heart J* 1996b;132:222–228.)

formularies may compound the problems, irritating physicians who must receive authorization before using a nonformulary drug and confusing patients with frequent switches in their medication. Care must be taken to ensure that formularies provide long-acting, once-a-day preparations of at least one member of each major class of antihypertensive, thereby allowing improvement of patient care and reduction of costs.

## Choice of First Drug

As more patients with less severe hypertension are being treated with drugs, the choices of therapy, particularly for the first drug, should be made with care. The first drug chosen may be taken for 10, 20, 30, or 40 years. Therefore, adverse effects that may not be obvious must be considered. The issue was portrayed in a one-year comparison between diuretic/β-blocker therapy versus ARB/CCB therapy (Lindholm et al., 2003). Although hypertension was well controlled with both, more abnormalities in lipids and glucose/insulin developed in those on the diuretic/β-blocker. I attribute most of the metabolic mischief to the β-blocker, but, one way or the other, the choice of drugs is important.

### Comparative Trials

As previously noted, multiple RCTs have compared the long-term ability of four classes of antihypertensive drugs—diuretics, ACEIs, ARBs, and CCBs—to protect patients from overall and cardiovascular morbidity and mortality, the only meaningful criterion (Figure 7–16). Additional trials, most comparing two or more drugs against one another, are in progress and one, the Anglo-Scandinavian Cardiac Outcomes Trial (ASCOT), has been completed. Those who believe that clinical decisions must be

evidence-based argue that those drugs that have been tested and found to reduce cardiovascular morbidity and mortality should be chosen (Antman & Ferguson, 2003).

### Expert Committee Recommendations

The position taken in the JNC-7 (Chobanian et al., 2003a; 2003b), as seen in Figure 7–19, is that if there are no specific indications for another type of drug, a diuretic should be chosen because numerous RCTs have shown a reduction in morbidity and mortality with diuretic-based therapy. As will be noted, JNC-7 recommends two-drug combinations for those with stage 2 hypertension, above 160 systolic or 100 diastolic. Some believe that low-dose combinations are the best initial and subsequent choice for almost all hypertensives, thereby increasing efficiency and reducing side effects (Law et al., 2003).

The other recent expert guidelines take different approaches:

- The WHO/ISH (2003) recommends a low-dose diuretic unless compelling indications for other drugs are present (Whitworth, 2003).
- The European Hypertension Society-European Society of Cardiology recommend any of the five major classes (Guidelines Committee, 2003).
- The British Hypertension Society recommends the choice be based on age and race, the AB/CD algorithm (see Figure 7–15).
- Of interest, the British National Institute for Clinical Excellence (NICE) (2004) recommends a thiazide diuretic for all patients.
- The Canadian Hypertension Education Program recommends any one of the five drug classes but "initial therapy should include thiazide diuretics" (Khan et al., 2004).

## TABLE 7–13

### Oral Antihypertensive Drugs Available in the United States

| Drug | Trade Name | Usual Dose Range, Total mg per Day (frequency per day)[a] | Selected Side Effects and Comments[b] |
|---|---|---|---|
| *Diuretics* (partial list) | | | |
| Chlorthalidone[c] | Hygroton | 12.5–50(1) | High doses: ↑ cholesterol, ↑glucose, ↓ |
| Hydrochlorothiazide[c] | Hydrodiuril, Microzide, Esidrix | 12.5–50(1) | potassium, ↑uric acid, ↑calcium, ↓ magnesium |
| Indapamide[c] | Lozol | 1.25–2.5(1) | (Less ↓ cholesterol) |
| Metolazone | Mykrox | 0.5–1.0(1) | Rare: blood dyscrasias, photosensitivity, pancreatitis |
| | Zaroxolyn | 2.5–10(1) | |
| *Loop Diuretics* | | | No hypercalcemia |
| Bumetanide[c] | Bumex | 0.5–4(2–3) | (Short duration of action) |
| Ethacrynic acid | Edecrin | 25–100(2–3) | (Only nonsulfonamide diuretic) |
| Furosemide[c] | Lasix | 20–240(2–3) | (Short duration of action) |
| Torsemide | Demadex | 2.5–100(2) | |
| *Potassium-sparing agents* | | | Hyperkalemia |
| Amiloride[c] | Midamor | 5–10(1) | |
| Triamterene[c] | Dyrenium | 25–100(1) | |
| *Aldosterone blockers* | | | |
| Eplerenone | Inspra | 50–100(1) | |
| Spironolactone | Aldactone | 25–100(1) | (Gynecomastia) |
| **Adrenergic inhibitors** | | | |
| *Peripheral-acting* | | | |
| Guanadrel[c] | Hylorel | 10–75(2) | (Postural hypotension, diarrhea) |
| Guanethidine | Ismelin | 10–150(1) | (Same as above) |
| Reserpine[c] | Serpasil | 0.05–0.25(1) | (Nasal congestion, sedation, depression) |
| *Centrally acting α-agonists* | | | Sedation, dry mouth, withdrawal hypertension |
| Clonidine[c] | Catapres | 0.2–1.2(2–3) | (More withdrawal) |
| Guanabenz[c] | Wytensin | 8–32(2) | (Less withdrawal) |
| Guanfacine[c] | Tenex | 1–3(1) | |
| Methyldopa[c] | Aldomet | 500–3000(2) | (Autoimmune disorders) |
| *α-Blockers* | | | *Postural hypotension* |
| Doxazosin | Cardura | 1–16(1) | |
| Prazosin[c] | Minipress | 2–30(2–3) | |
| Terazosin | Hytrin | 1–20(1) | |
| *β-Blockers* | | | Bronchospasm, fatigue, bradycardia, heart failure, masking of insulin-induced hypoglycemia; decreased exercise tolerance, hypertriglyceridemia |
| Acebutolol | Sectral | 20–1200(1) | |
| Atenolol[c] | Tenormin | 25–100(1–2) | |
| Betaxolol | Kerlone | 5–40(1) | |
| Bisoprolol | Zebeta | 2.5–20(1) | |

*(continued)*

## TABLE 7–13 (Continued)

### Oral Antihypertensive Drugs Available in the United States

| Drug | Trade Name | Usual Dose Range, Total mg per Day (frequency per day)[a] | Selected Side Effects and Comments[b] |
|------|-----------|-------------------------------|-------------------------------|
| Metoprolol[c] | Lopressor, Toprol XL | 50–200(2,1) | |
| Nadolol[c] | Corgard | 20–240(1) | |
| Penbutolol[c] | Levatol | 10–20(1) | |
| Pindolol[c] | Visken | 10–60(2) | |
| Propranolol[c] | Inderal, Inderal LA | 40–240(2,1) | |
| Timolol[c] | Blocadren | 10–40(2) | |
| *Combined α- and β-blockers* | | | Postural hypotension, bronchospasm |
| Carvedilol | Coreg | 12.5–50(2) | |
| Labetalol[c] | Normodyne, Trandate | 200–1200(2) | |
| **Direct vasodilators** | | | Headaches, fluid retention, tachycardia |
| Hydralazine[c] | Apresoline | 50–300(2) | (Lupus syndrome) |
| Minoxidil[c] | Loniten | 5–100(1) | (Hirsutism) |
| **Calcium channel blockers** | | | |
| *Nondihydropyridines* | | | Conduction defects |
| Diltiazem | Cardizem SR Cardizem CD, | 120–480(2) | (Nausea, headache) |
| | Dilacor XL, Tiazac | 120–480(1) | |
| Verapamil | Isoptin SR, Calan SR | 90–480(2) | (Constipation) |
| | Verelan, Covera HS | 120–480(1) | |
| *Dihydropyridines* | | | |
| Amlodipine | Norvasc | 2.5–10(1) | Ankle edema, flushing, headache, gingival hyperplasia |
| Felodipine | Plendil | 2.5–20(1) | |
| Isradipine | DynaCirc, DynaCirc CR | 5–20(2, 1) | |
| Nicardipine | Cardene SR | 60–120(2) | |
| Nifedipine | Procardia XL, Adalat CC | 30–120(1) | |
| Nisoldipine | Sular | 20–40(1) | |
| **Angiotensin-converting enzyme inhibitors** | | | Common: cough |
| Benazepril[c] | Lotensin | 5–40(1) | Rare: angioedema, hyperkalemia, rash, loss of taste, leucopenia, fetal toxicity |
| Captopril[c] | Capoten | 25–150(2–3) | |
| Enalapril | Vasotec | 5–40(2) | |
| Fosinopril | Monopril | 10–40(1) | |
| Lisinopril[c] | Prinivil, Zestril | 5–40(1) | |
| Moexipril | Univasc | 7.5–30(2) | |
| Perindopril | Aceon | 4–16(1) | |
| Quinapril | Accupril | 5–80(1) | |
| Ramipril | Altace | 1.25–20(1) | |
| Trandolapril | Mavik | 1–4(1) | |

(continued)

## TABLE 7–13 (Continued)

### Oral Antihypertensive Drugs Available in the United States

| Drug | Trade Name | Usual Dose Range, Total mg per Day (frequency per day)[a] | Selected Side Effects and Comments[b] |
|---|---|---|---|
| *Angiotensin II-receptor blockers* | | | Angioedema, hyperkalemia, fetal toxicity |
| Candesartan | Atacand | 8–32(1) | |
| Eprosartan | Teveten | 400–800(1) | |
| Irbesartan | Avapro | 150–300(1) | |
| Losartan | Cozaar | 50–100(1–2) | |
| Olmesartan | Benicar | 20–40(1) | |
| Telmisartan | Micardis | 40–80(1) | |
| Valsartan | Diovan | 80–320(1) | |

[a] These dosages may vary from those listed in the *Physicians' Desk Reference*, which may be consulted for additional information. The listing of side effects is not all-inclusive, and clinicians are urged to refer to the package insert for more detailed listing.
[b] Parentheses are individual drug effects. All others are class effects.
[c] Generic available.

Obviously, disagreements persist, but low-dose diuretics are included in all.

### Once-Daily Therapy

One point agreed upon by all expert guidelines is the need for long-acting, once-a-day therapy. As noted in Table 7–13, either inherently or artificially long-acting choices are available in every category. Some may work to reduce the early morning surge of BP if taken in the evening or at bedtime. That requires home BP monitoring which, hopefully, will be done by more and more patients.

### Compelling Indications

Another point of agreement is the need for certain drugs for those compelling indications that have shown to respond better to them. Table 7–14 is the listing shown in JNC-7. A more liberal listing is shown in Table 7–15 with a number of combinations matched to choices that seem logical but that have not been tested in RCTs.

### Other Factors

#### Characteristics of the Patient

Individual patient's characteristics may affect the likelihood of a good response to various classes of drugs. As shown in crossover rotations of the four major classes (Deary et al., 2002; Morgan et al., 2001), younger, White patients will usually respond better to either an ACEI/ARB or a β-blocker, perhaps because they tend to have higher renin levels, whereas older and Black patients will respond better to diuretics and CCBs, perhaps because they have lower renin levels and their hypertension is more "volume-mediated" (Laragh, 2001). These differences apply to monotherapy; with a low dose of a diuretic as part of the regimen, responses to all other agents are largely equalized. Moreover, for the individual patient, any drug may work well or poorly, and there is no set formula that can be used to predict certain success without side effects (Senn, 2004).

#### Plasma Renin Levels

As noted, the differences in BP response between younger versus older and Blacks versus non-Blacks could reflect differences in the activity of the renin-angiotensin system, as measured by plasma renin activity (PRA) or direct renin assays.

Laragh and co-workers, as far back as 1972 (Bühler et al., 1972), have used the level of PRA to guide the choice of initial therapy. As attractive as the concept is, in practice it often does not work: Donnelly et al. (1992) found that pretreatment PRA accounted for considerably less than 10% of the variability in response to treatment.

#### Characteristics of the Drug

The five major classes differ in their characteristics that play a role in their advantages and disadvantages (Table 7–16). Some agents—such as the

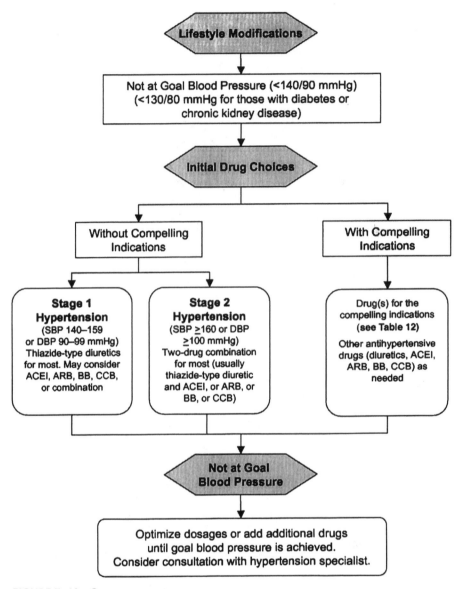

**FIGURE 7–19** ● The JNC-7 algorithm. BP, blood pressure; ACE, angiotensin-converting enzyme; ARB, angiotenin-receptor blocker; CCB, calcium channel blocker. (From Chobanian et al. The Seventh Report of the Joint National Committee on Prevention, Detection, Evaluation, and Treatment of High Blood Pressure: The JNC 7 report. *JAMA* 2003a;289:2560–2572.)

direct-acting smooth-muscle vasodilators, central $\alpha_2$-agonists, and peripheral-acting adrenergic antagonists—are not well suited for initial monotherapy because they produce annoying adverse effects in a large number of patients. However, as repeatedly documented, if they effectively lower BP, all drugs provide protection from cardiovascular events.

### Cost of the Drug

Three issues need to be considered: (a) the overall cost of antihypertensive therapy; (b) the overall

cost-effectiveness of antihypertensive therapy; and (c) the relative cost-effectiveness of specific antihypertensive drugs.

First, the treatment of hypertension in the United States in 1998 was estimated to cost $22.8 billion, whereas the cost of treatment of hypertension-induced or related complications was estimated to cost $86.1 billion (Hodgson & Cai, 2001). It seems obvious that with more treatment the number of complications would be reduced and money would be saved.

## TABLE 7-14

### Clinical Trial and Guideline Basis for Compelling Indications for Individual Drug Classes

| Compelling Indication | Recommended Drugs | | | | | |
|---|---|---|---|---|---|---|
| | Diuretic | βB | ACEI | ARB | CCB | Aldo Ant |
| Heart failure | • | • | • | • | • | • |
| Postmyocardial infarction | | • | • | | | • |
| High coronary disease risk | • | • | • | | • | |
| Diabetes | • | • | • | • | • | |
| Chronic kidney disease | | | • | • | | |
| Recurrent stroke prevention | • | | • | | | |

*βB*, beta-blocker; *ACEI*, angiotensin-converting enzyme inhibitor; *ARB*, angiotensin receptor blocker; *CCB*, calcium channel blocker; *Aldo Ant*, aldosterone antagonist.

Modified from Chobanian AV, et al. Seventh report of the Joint National Committee on Prevention, Detection, Evaluation, and Treatment of High Blood Pressure. *Hypertension* 2003b;42:1206–1252.

Second, multiple analyses have documented the positive cost-effectiveness of antihypertensive therapy, particularly in comparison to other therapies. These include:

- An analysis of worldwide cost effectiveness of interventions to reduce cardiovascular risk found that, beyond a population-wide reduction in sodium intake, treatment of all people in Europe with a systolic BP above 140 mm Hg would add 82,000,000 quality-adjusted life years (QALYs) at a cost of $454 per QALY (Murray et al., 2003).
- For low-risk hypertensives, the cost of one QALY ranged between $1,600 and $5,000; for the high-risk hypertensives, the cost per QALY was as little as $50 to $500 (Montgomery et al., 2003).
- For patients at 10% coronary risk over 5 years, the cost of preventing one coronary event was estimated to be $5,000 for aspirin, $20,000 for antihypertensive therapy, $100,000 for clopidrogel, and $110,000 for simvastatin (Marshall, 2003).
- For type 2 hypertensive diabetics, the cost per QALY was estimated to be $41,000 for intensive glycemic control, $52,000 for reduction of serum cholesterol, and –$2,000 (money saved) for intensive hypertension control (CDC Diabetes Cost-Effectiveness Group, 2002).

Third, there are differences in cost effectiveness of specific antihypertensive drugs. These differences mainly revolve around availability of lower-cost generics versus higher-cost trade-name drugs. For instance, in the state of Pennsylvania in 2001, if a diuretic costing $5.33 per month was substituted for a CCB costing $33.39 per month in all the prescriptions written for elderly hypertensives covered by Medicare, over $16.5 million would have been saved (Fischer & Avorn, 2004). The authors project a nationwide savings of $1.2 billion if JNC guidelines were followed.

There is more to the cost of the drug than the cost of the tablet: If a less expensive choice causes problems that need to be treated (diabetes from a β-blocker), the cost is considerably more; if a more expensive choice relieves problems that need to be treated (nephropathy with an ACEI), the cost is considerably less. Regardless, cost must be considered as more people, particularly the elderly poor, need more drugs for longer times.

Absent from many arguments about cost in the United States is the less expensive and more effective control of hypertension that could be possible under a national healthcare system (Woolhandler et al., 2003b) that would remove the extra 20% burden from heathcare administration (Woolhandler et al., 2003a).

### Combinations as Initial Therapy

Another possible way to reduce the costs of antihypertensive care is to use those combination tablets that cost less than their separate ingredients.

As JNC-7 and all other guidelines recognize, most patients will end up on two or more drugs to achieve adequate control. Therefore, the idea of

## TABLE 7–15

### Considerations for Individualizing Antihypertensive Drug Therapy[a]

| May Have Favorable Effects on Comorbid Conditions | | May Have Unfavorable Effects on Comorbid Conditions[b] | |
|---|---|---|---|
| Condition | Drug | Condition | Drug |
| Angina | β-blockers, CCB | Bronchospasic disease | β-blockers |
| Atrial tachycardia and fibrillation | β-blockers CCB (non-DHP) | 2° or 3° heart block | β-blockers CCB (non-DHP) |
| Cough from ACEI | ARB | Depression | Central α-agonists |
| Cyclosporine-induced hypertension | CCB | | Reserpine[c] |
| | | Dyslipidemia | β-blockers (non-ISA) |
| Diabetes mellitus, particularly with proteinuria | ACEI, ARB, low-dose diuretics, CCBs, β-blockers | | Diuretics (high-dose) |
| | | Gout | Diuretics |
| Dyslipidemia | α-blockers | Heart failure | CCB[b] |
| Essential tremor | β-blockers (non-CS) | Hyperkalemia | ACEI, ARB |
| Heart failure | ACEI, ARB, Carvedilol, β-blockers, diuretics | Liver disease | Labetalol Methyldopa[c] |
| Hyperthyroidism | β-blockers | Peripheral vascular disease | β-blockers[b] |
| Migraine | β-blockers (non-CS) | | |
| Osteoporosis | CCB, Thiazides | Pregnancy | ACEI[c] ARB[c] |
| Preoperative hypertension | β-blockers | | |
| Prostatism | α-blockers | Renal insufficiency | Potassium-sparing agents, aldosterone blockers[b] |
| Renal insufficiency | ACEI, ARB | Renovascular disease, bilateral | ACEI ARB |
| Systolic hypertension in elderly | Diuretics, CCB | Type I and II diabetes | β-blockers High-dose diuretics |

[a] Conditions and drugs are listed in alphabetical order. See also Figure 7–20.
[b] These drugs may be used with special monitoring, unless contraindicated.
[c] Contraindicated.
  ACEI, angiotensin-converting enzyme inhibitor; ARB, angiotensin II receptor blocker; CCB, calcium channel blocker; DHP, dihydropyridine; non-CS, non-cardioselective; non-ISA, non–intrinsic sympathomimetic activity.

starting with two drugs is gaining currency, in the JNC-7 for all with BP above 160/100. In JNC-7 and the Canadian guidelines, a low-dose diuretic is suggested as one of the two.

A number of combination tablets are available (Table 7–17). In keeping with the JNC-7 recommendation, almost all ACEIs, ARBs, and β-blockers are marketed in the United States with low doses of a diuretic in most. Calcium channel blockers are not because of the incorrect perception that adding a diuretic would be of no benefit.

The recently completed ASCOT showed superiority of an ACEI/CCB combination over a diuretic/β-blocker combination (www.Ascotstudy.org).

### Choice of Second Drug

If a moderate dose of the first choice is well tolerated and effective but not enough to bring the BP down to the desired level, a second drug can be added, and thereby control will likely be better achieved than by increasing the dose of the first drug (Elliott et al., 1999). A logical overall algorithm by the choice of second drug based upon the compelling indications is shown in Figure 7–20.

Particularly among nephrologists, an increasingly popular combination is an ACEI and an ARB, which has been found to reduce proteinuria better than the individual drugs (Nakao et al., 2003). No

## Characteristics of Major Classes of Antihypertensive Drugs

| Consideration | Diuretics | α-Blockers | β-Blockers | ACE Inhibitors; All Blockers | CCBs |
|---|---|---|---|---|---|
| Hemodynamic effect | Initial volume shrinkage; peripheral vasodilation | Peripheral vasodilation | Initially reduce cardiac output | Peripheral vasodilation | Peripheral vasodilation |
| Side effects | | | | | |
| Overt | Weakness, palpitations | Postural dizziness | Bronchospasm; fatigue; prolong hypoglycemia | Cough; angioedema | Flushing; local edema; constipation (verapamil) |
| Hidden | Hypokalemia; hypercholesterolemia; glucose intolerance; hyperuricemia | | Glucose intolerance; hypertriglyceridemia; decrease HDL cholesterol | Fetal toxicity | AV conduction (verapamil, diltiazem) |
| Contraindications | Pre-existing volume contraction | Orthostatic hypotension | Asthma; heartblock | Pregnancy | PostMI (dihydropyridines) |
| Cautions | Diabetes mellitus; gout; digitalis toxicity | Congestive heart failure | Peripheral vascular disease; insulin-dependent diabetes; allergy; coronary spasm | Renal insufficiency; renovascular disease | Heart failure |
| Special advantages | Effective in Blacks and elderly; enhance effectiveness of all other agents | No decrease in cardiac output; no alteration in blood lipids; no sedation; relieves symptoms of prostatic hypertrophy | Reduce recurrences of coronary disease; reduce manifestations of anxiety; coexisting angina, CHF, migraine, tremor | No CNS side effects; treat CHF; postMI, reduce coronary disease and CHF; renal protection | Effective in Blacks and elderly; no CNS side effects; coronary vasodilation |

## TABLE 7–17

## Combination Drugs for Hypertension

| Drug | Trade Name |
| --- | --- |
| *Diuretics and potassium-sparers* | |
| Amiloride 5 mg/hydrochlorothiazide 50 mg | Moduretic |
| Spironolactone 25 or 50 mg/hydrochlorothiazide 25 or 50 mg | Aldactazide |
| Triamterene 37.5, 50 or 75 mg/hydrochlorothiazide 25 or 50 mg | Dyazide, Maxide |
| *β-Blockers and diuretics* | |
| Atenolol 50 or 100 mg/chlorthalidone 25 mg | Tenoretic |
| Bisoprolol 2.5, 5 or 10 mg/hydrochlorothiazide 6.25 mg | Ziac[a] |
| Metoprolol 50 or 100 mg/hydrochlorothiazide 25 or 50 mg | Lopressor HCT |
| Nadolol 40 or 80 mg/bendroflumethiazide 5 mg | Corzide |
| Propranolol 40 or 80 mg/hydrochlorothiazide 25 mg | Inderide |
| Propranolol (extended release) 80, 120 or 160 mg/hydrochlorothiazide 50 mg | Inderide LA |
| Timolol 10 mg/hydrochlorothiazide 25 mg | Timolide |
| *ACE inhibitors and diuretics* | |
| Benazepril 5, 10 or 20 mg/hydrochlorothiazide 6.25, 12.5 or 25 mg | Lotensin HCT |
| Captopril 25 or 50 mg/hydrochlorothiazide 15 or 25 mg | Capozide[a] |
| Enalapril 5 or 10 mg/hydrochlorothiazide 12.5 or 25 mg | Vaseretic |
| Fosinopril 10 or 20 mg/hydrochlorothiazide 12.5 mg | Monopril HCT |
| Lisinopril 10 or 20 mg/hydrochlorothiazide 12.5 or 25 mg | Prinzide; Zestoretic |
| Moexipril 7.5 or 15 mg/hydrochlorothiazide 12.5 mg | Uniretic |
| Quinipril 10 or 20 mg/hydrochlorothiazide 12.5 mg | Accuretic |
| *Angiotensin II-receptor antagonists and diuretics* | |
| Candesartan 16 or 32 mg/hydrochlorothiazide 12.5 or 25 mg | Atacand HCT |
| Irbesartan 150 or 300 mg/hydrochlorothiazide 12.5 or 25 mg | Avalide |
| Losartan 50 or 100 mg/hydrochlorothiazide 12.5 or 25 mg | Hyzaar |
| Valsartan 80 or 160 mg/hydrochlorothiazide 12.5 or 25 mg | Diovan HCT |
| *CCBs and ACE inhibitors* | |
| Amlodipine 2.5 or 5 mg/benazepril 10 or 20 mg | Lotrel |
| Diltiazem 180 mg/enalapril 5 mg | Teczem |
| Felodipine 2.5 or 5 mg/enalapril 5 mg | Lexxel |
| Verapamil (extended release) 180 or 240 mg/trandolapril 1, 2 or 4 mg | Tarka |
| *Other combinations* | |
| Clonidine 0.1, 0.2 or 0.3 mg/chlorthalidone 15 mg | Combipres |
| Hydralazine 25, 50 or 100 mg/hydrochlorothiazide 25 or 50 mg | Apresazide |
| Methyldopa 250 or 500 mg/hydrochlorothiazide 15, 25, 30 or 50 mg | Aldoril |
| Reserpine 0.10 mg/hydralazine 25 mg/hydrochlorothiazide 15 mg | Ser-ap-es |
| Reserpine 0.125 mg/hydrochlorothiazide 25 or 50 mg | Hydropres |

[a] Approved for initial therapy.

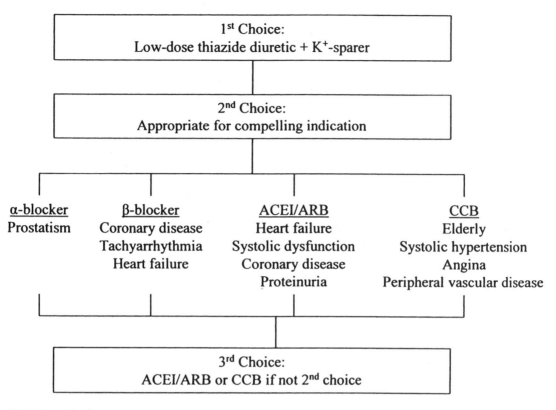

**FIGURE 7–20** ● A treatment algorithm based on JNC-7.

cardiovascular outcome data as yet attest to the greater benefit of the ACEI plus ARB combination.

## Choice of Third or Fourth Drug

Various combinations usually work. The key, as with two drugs, is to combine agents with different mechanisms of action. The most rational is a diuretic, an ACEI, and a CCB.

Few patients should need more than three drugs, particularly if the various reasons for resistance to therapy are considered. For those who do, the JNC-7 recommends considering consultation with a hypertension specialist (Chobanian et al., 2003a; 2003b).

## Resistant Hypertension

### Causes

The reasons for a poor response are numerous (Table 7–18); the most likely is volume overload (Graves, 2000). In one series of 91 patients whose BPs remained above 140/90 mm Hg despite use of three antihypertensive agents, the mechanisms were a suboptimal drug regimen (mainly inadequate diuretic) in 43%, intolerance to medications in 22%, noncompliance in 10%, and secondary

hypertension in 11% (Yakovlevitch & Black, 1991). Similar findings were noted among 141 patients seen more recently (Gang et al., 2005). Patients who are elderly, uninformed about the goal of therapy, on multiple drugs, or having drug side effects are more likely to be uncontrolled (Knight et al., 2001) as are diabetics (Singer et al., 2002). In a disadvantaged minority population, uncontrolled hypertension is most closely related to limited access to care, noncompliance with therapy, and alcohol-related problems (Shea et al., 1992).

*Pseudoresistance*

Before starting workup for identifiable causes and altering drug therapy, BPs should be checked out of the office setting, because as many as a third (Brown et al., 2001) to a half (Redon et al., 1998) of resistant patients turn out to have controlled hypertension by out-of-office measurements.

*Nonadherence to Therapy*

Patients often do not take their medications because they cannot afford them and because they have no access to consistent and continuous primary care. As noted earlier in this chapter, there are ways to simplify the regimen and improve access. Recall as well the evidence that patients may appear to be resistant only because their physicians simply do not keep increasing patient therapy (Amar et al., 2003).

## TABLE 7-18

## Causes of Inadequate Responsiveness to Therapy

Pseudoresistance
  White coat or office elevations
  Pseudohypertension in the elderly
Nonadherence to therapy
  Side effects or costs of medication
  Lack of consistent and continuous primary care
  Inconvenient and chaotic dosing schedules
  Instructions not understood
  Organic brain syndrome (e.g., memory deficit)
Drug-related causes
  Doses too low
  Inappropriate combinations
  Rapid inactivation (e.g., hydralazine)
  Drug actions and interactions
    NSAIDS
    Sympathomimetics
      Nasal decongestants
      Appetite suppressants
      Cocaine and other street drugs
      Caffeine
    Oral contraceptives
    Adrenal steroids
    Licorice (as may be found in chewing tobacco)
    Cyclosporine, tacrolimus
    Erythropoietin
Associated conditions
  Smoking
  Increased obesity
  Sleep apnea
  Insulin resistance or hyperinsulinemia
  Ethanol intake more than 1 ounce a day
  Anxiety-induced hyperventilation or panic attacks
  Chronic pain
  Intense vasoconstriction (Raynaud phenomenon, arteritis)
Identifiable causes of hypertension
Volume overload
  Excess sodium intake
  Progressive renal damage (nephrosclerosis)
  Fluid retention from reduction of blood pressure
  Inadequate diuretic therapy

### Drug-related Causes

In a survey of 1,377 hypertensives over 9 months, 75% had some potential interaction with their antihypertensive drugs and in 35% the interaction was considered highly significant (Carter et al., 2004b).

The most common of these in the United States is likely the interference with the antihypertensive effect of virtually all agents save CCB by nonsteroidal antiinflammatory drugs (NSAIDs). All of them can interfere, particularly the COX-2 specific rofecoxib (Vioxx) (Solomon et al., 2004), which has been removed from the U.S. market. The estimated cost in money and lives from using NSAIDs for osteoarthritis is staggering (Grover et al., 2005), and it is likely that their use in hypertensives will continue to fall. Large doses of aspirin also pose a problem but 80 mg a day does not (Zanchetti et al., 2002).

A number of other drug interactions may be seen, mostly reducing the effectiveness of one or both participants. Some interactions increase the duration or degree of action, e.g., large amounts of grapefruit juice and Seville oranges (Lilja et al., 2004) inhibit the activity of the cytochrome P450 isoenzyme CYP3A4 which is involved in the metabolism of many drugs and can raise the blood levels of some statins, CCBs, and immune-suppressive drugs (Wilkinson, 2005).

The mechanism of most serious interactions involves administration of a drug known to cause an interaction and therefore avoidable (Juurlink et al., 2003). In these days of increasing use of herbal remedies, which in the United States are totally unregulated because of Senator Hatch's bill prohibiting FDA surveillance of these agents, a number of herb-drug interactions are seen (Fugh-Berman, 2000). More about such interactions, which can raise BP, is provided in Chapter 15.

### Associated Conditions

Nicotine transiently raises blood pressure, but the effect is often not recognized because the blood pressure is almost ways taken in a no-smoking environment. The combination of abdominal and generalized obesity, insulin resistance, and sleep apnea is an increasingly common cause of resistant hypertension (Logan et al., 2001).

### Identifiable Causes of Hypertension

Identifiable causes of hypertension are covered in Chapters 9 through 15. Recently, a much higher prevalence of primary aldosteronism than previously recognized has been reported and the presence of a low plasma renin level in a resistant hypertensive can be the tip-off for the condition (Eide et al., 2004).

*Volume Overload*

As seen in Table 7–18, there are multiple reasons for volume overload and they are often allowed to persist because of inadequate diuretic.

### Treatment

The need for adequate diuretic is obvious. The need for blockade of high or even "normal" levels of aldosterone, whether or not associated with autonomous hypersecretion, has become increasingly documented by impressive relief of resistance with even low doses of spironolactone (Nishizaka et al., 2003; Ouzan et al., 2002).

A careful search of the cause(s) and appropriate antihypertensive therapy almost always can correct resistance. If not, consultation with a hypertension specialist should be utilized.

### Reduction or Discontinuation of Therapy

Once a good response has occurred and has been maintained for a year or longer, medications may be reduced or discontinued. In a review of all published series of planned withdrawal, 42% of selected patients with mild hypertension were found to remain normotensive for 12 months or longer off medication (Nelson et al., 2001). However, in a closely monitored group of over 6,200 hypertensives who had been successfully controlled, only 18% were able to remain normotensive after stopping therapy (Nelson et al., 2003). The characteristics that make withdrawal more likely to be successful were lower levels of BP before and after therapy; fewer and lower doses of medication needed to control hypertension; and patient's willingness to follow lifestyle modifications.

Whether it is worth the trouble to stop successful drug therapy completely is questionable. The more sensible approach in well-controlled patients would be first to decrease the dose of whatever is being used. If this succeeds, withdrawal may be attempted with continued close surveillance of the BP.

## SPECIAL CONSIDERATIONS IN THE CHOICE OF THERAPY

Children are covered in Chapter 16; women who are pregnant or on hormones are covered in Chapter 11.

### Women

In an analysis by Gueyffier et al. (1997) women were found to derive less relative benefit from therapy because they start with lower risk for cardiovascular disease. In absolute terms, their response was identical to that of men. Moreover, in the Second Australian National Blood Pressure Study, women randomly assigned to ACEI derived equal reduction in the hazard ratio for cardiovascular events or mortality than those assigned to a diuretic whereas the men on an ACEI had a 17% reduction in hazard compared to those on a diuretic despite equal and substantial reductions in BP in both women and men (Wing et al., 2003).

### Blacks and Other Ethnic Groups

As noted in Chapter 4, Black hypertensives have many distinguishing characteristics, some of which could affect their responses to antihypertensive therapy. However, when they achieve adequate control, Blacks usually respond as Whites do and experience similar reductions in the incidences of cardiovascular disease as Whites (Brewster et al., 2004). However, in the LIFE trial, the small number of Blacks (*n* = 533) did not receive the cardiovascular protection from an ARB as did the larger number of Whites (*n* = 8,660) despite equal reductions in BP (Julius et al., 2004a).

Blacks respond less well to monotherapy with renin-suppressing drugs, i.e., β-blockers, ACEIs and ARBs, perhaps because they tend to have lower renin levels, and equally as well to diuretics and CCBs (Brewster et al., 2004). In this systematic review of 30 trials involving 20,006 Black hypertensives, the mean falls in blood pressure (mm Hg) with the different agents were:

- Diuretics . . . 11.8/8.1
- CCBs . . . 12.1/9.4
- β-blockers . . . 3.5/5.4
- ACEIs . . . 7.0/3.8
- ARBs . . . 3.6/2.1

Nonetheless, Blacks should not be denied β-blockers, ARBs, or ACEIs if special indications for their use are present. Moreover, their response to these drugs is equalized by addition of a diuretic (Libhaber et al., 2004).

There is no good evidence that Hispanics, Asians, or other ethnic groups differ from Whites in their responses to various antihypertensive agents. As noted, both Blacks and Asians have a higher incidence of ACEI-induced cough.

### Elderly Patients

The majority of people over age 65 have hypertension; in most, the hypertension is predominantly or purely systolic from arterial stiffness. As described in Chapter 4, the risks for such patients are significant. As detailed in Chapter 5, the benefits of treating hypertension in the elderly have been well documented. Now that such evidence is available, many more elderly hypertensives should be brought into active therapy with assurance that debilitating morbidities will be reduced (Staessen et al., 2004), likely including dementia (Williams, 2004). At present, only a small minority of elderly patients with systolic hypertension are being adequately treated (Chobanian et al., 2003b).

Recall the evidence described in Chapter 2 showing that white-coat hypertension is even more common in the elderly than in younger patients (Pickering, 2004). Therefore, before making the diagnosis, out-of-the-office readings should be obtained, if possible.

Regardless of age, as long as the patient appears to have a reasonable life expectancy, active therapy is appropriate for all who have a systolic level above 160 mm Hg, with or without an elevated diastolic pressure. No RCTs have involved elderly with systolic BP between 140 and 160 so the decision to treat should be based on overall risk. Those at high risk (e.g., diabetics or smokers) should be started on therapy at systolic levels above 140 mm Hg.

Table 7–19 lists factors often present in the elderly that may complicate their therapy. Because the elderly may have sluggish baroreceptor and sympathetic nervous responsiveness, as well as impaired cerebral autoregulation, therapy should be gentle and gradual, avoiding drugs that are likely to cause postural hypotension.

Even more caution is advised with the very elderly. The relatively small amount of data from RCTs in those over age 80 indicate a statistically significant 30% to 50% reduction in stroke with antihypertensive therapy but a consistently though statistically insignificant 6% to 23% *increase* in total mortality among those treated (Bulpitt et al., 2003). The ongoing Hypertension in the Very Elderly Trial (HYVET) will hopefully provide more definitive evidence.

### Lifestyle Modifications

Before we rush into drug therapy, the multiple benefits of nondrug therapies that were described in Chapter 6 need to be reaffirmed. The ability of lifestyle changes to lower BP in the elderly has been well documented (Moore et al., 2001; Whelton et al., 1998). In particular, dietary sodium should be moderately restricted down to 100 to 120 mmol per day, because the pressor effect of sodium excess and the antihypertensive efficacy of sodium restriction progressively increase with age (Geleijnse et al., 1994; Weinberger & Fineberg, 1991). However, the elderly may have at least two additional hurdles to overcome in achieving this goal: First, their taste sensitivity may be lessened, so they may ingest more sodium to compensate; and second, they may depend more on processed, prepackaged foods that are high in sodium rather than fresh foods that are low in sodium.

### Drug Treatment

If lifestyle changes are not enough, drug therapy should be started following the principles listed

---

## TABLE 7–19

### Factors That Might Contribute to Complications from Pharmacologic Treatment of Hypertension in the Elderly

| Factors | Potential Complications |
|---|---|
| Diminished baroreceptor activity | Orthostatic hypotension |
| Impaired cerebral autoregulation | Cerebral ischemia with small falls in systolic pressure |
| Decreased intravascular volume | Orthostatic hypotension<br>Volume depletion, hyponatremia |
| Sensitivity to hypokalemia | Arrhythmia, muscular weakness |
| Decreased renal and hepatic function | Drug accumulation |
| Polypharmacy | Drug interaction |
| CNS changes | Depression, confusion |

## TABLE 7–20

### Guidelines in Treating Hypertension in the Elderly

1. Check for postural and postprandial hypotension before starting
2. Choose drugs that will help other concomitant conditions
   a. For uncomplicated patients, a thiazide diuretic + $K^+$ sparer
   b. If a second agent is needed, a CCB
   c. β-blockers are not appropriate unless an indication is present, e.g., coronary disease
3. Start with small doses, titrating gradually
4. Use longer acting, once daily formulations
5. Avoid drug interactions, particularly from over-the-counter medications, e.g., NSAIDs
6. Look for subtle drug-induced adverse effects, e.g., weakness, dizziness, depression, confusion
7. Monitor home blood pressures to avoid over and under treatment
8. Aim for the goal of SBP = 140–145, DBP = 80–85

---

in Table 7–20. Some of these deserve additional comment.

*Postural Hypotension*

Defined as a fall in BP of either 20 mm Hg systolic or 10 mm Hg diastolic upon unsupported standing from the supine position, postural or orthostatic hypotension is found in 10% to 30% of ambulatory hypertensives over age 60 and in 50% of those in a geriatric ward (Weiss et al., 2004). It is often associated with postprandial hypotension induced by splanchnic pooling; it is more common in diabetics and is a marker of increased mortality. As noted in Figure 7–21 (Tonkin, 1995), numerous causes may be responsible, including arterial stiffness (Boddaert et al., 2004) and baroreceptor insensitivity (Wilson, 2004). Postural hypotension is often found with supine hypertension (Goldstein et al., 2003) and is a component of more severe syndromes of autonomic failure (Ketch et al., 2002).

Postural hypotension must be recognized before antihypertensive therapy is begun to avoid traumatic falls when the BP is lowered further. Fortunately, the physical therapies listed in Figure 7–21 can usually manage the problem, but various medications have been tried with limited success, including the sympathomimetic midodrine (Schrage et al., 2004) and β-blockers, which provide some degree of peripheral vasoconstriction (Cleophas et al., 2002).

*Choice of Drugs for the Elderly*

The initial choice of drug therapy for elderly with isolated systolic hypertension should be a low-dose diuretic or a dihydropyridine CCB. This recommendation is based on the cardiovascular protection found in the RCTs in which these drugs were used (Staessen et al., 2000). Stokes (2004) has advocated the use of extended-release isosorbide mononitrate, which he finds to lower the elevated systolic pressure but not the already low diastolic pressure. In older patients with combined systolic and diastolic hypertension, therapy based on an ACEI or ARB has been shown to be effective (Lithell et al., 2003).

Therapy should begin with small doses and then should be slowly increased: Start low and go slow. Small doses may be fully effective. Even more so than in younger patients, the elderly do better with long-acting (once-daily), smoothly working agents since they may have trouble following complicated dosage schedules, reading the labels, and opening bottles with safety caps. Fortunately, when therapy is carefully provided, no loss of cognitive function is seen and dementia may be prevented, as seen in the Syst-Eur trial with therapy based on the CCB nitrendipine (Forette et al., 2002).

Home BP recording may be particularly useful, first in overcoming the white-coat effect, which is quantitatively greater in the elderly, and, second, in ensuring that therapy is enough but not too much. The white-coat effect may obscure considerable overtreatment.

*Goal of Therapy*

As I have written elsewhere (Kaplan, 2000):

> The question of how much should blood pressure be lowered is perhaps the most disturbing in view of evidence that serious consequences are seen with low diastolic blood pressures. These low pressures may occur naturally, as part of the atherosclerotic process (Staessen et al., 2000), or as part of antihypertensive therapy. In the Rotterdam

| CAUSAL FACTOR | PATHOPHYSIOLOGY | THERAPY |
|---|---|---|
| Rapid rising | Pooling of blood in lower body | Slow rising, particularly from sleep |
| Vasodilation | Venous pooling<br>Splanchnic pooling<br>Sympatholytic drugs | Supportive panty hose<br>Avoid large meals<br>Avoid such agents |
| Volume depletion | Low cardiac output<br>- diuretic<br>- very low sodium intake | Maintain intravascular volume by avoiding over-diuresis and sleeping with head of bed elevated |
| Baroreflex dysfunction | Loss of normal vasoconstriction by sympathetic stimulation | Drinking 16 oz water before arising<br>Various drugs:<br>- sympathomimetics<br>- volume expanders<br>Isometric exercise |
| Cerebrovascular disease | Low cerebral perfusion | Avoid overtreatment of hypertension<br>Correct dyslipidemia<br>Stop smoking |

FIGURE 7–21  ● Summary of the pathophysiologic events that occur during the development of symptoms of postural hypotension (*middle column*) and the interaction of exacerbating factors (*left column*) and remedial measures (*right column*) with these events.

Study involving 2,351 elderly hypertensives, the risk of stroke was significantly higher in those given antihypertensive drugs whose diastolic blood pressure was <65 mm Hg compared with those who had a diastolic pressure between 65 and 74 mm Hg (Vokó et al., 1999). In the recent reanalysis of data from the SHEP, those who experienced a cardiovascular event while on antihypertensive drug therapy had lower diastolic levels than those who did not have an event (Somes et al., 1999). Overall, a further decrease of 5 mm Hg in a diastolic blood pressure (which initially averaged 77 mm Hg) among those who were treated resulted in statistically significant 11% to 14% increases in stroke and cardiovascular events.

Thus there may very well be a J-curve of increasing cardiovascular disease when the diastolic pressure is lowered below the level needed to maintain perfusion to vital organs. . . . Therefore, caution is advised in treating those with

[isolated systolic hypertension], who obviously start with already low diastolic blood pressures.

On the other hand, no J-curve for systolic BP has been documented. However, in the RCTs of treatment of the elderly, the final average treated systolic pressures were between 140 and 150 mm Hg, so the goal for systolic BP remains uncertain (Pickering, 2004).

## The Metabolic Syndrome and Obesity

The five primary features of the Metabolic Syndrome, as described in Chapter 3, include hypertension. With the marked increase in obesity worldwide, the syndrome will increase in prevalence, reaching down into childhood (Hedley et al., 2004). In managing the hypertension, care must be taken not to worsen the other components of the syndrome.

## Lifestyle Modifications

The major focus must be prevention of obesity. Failing that, weight loss and increased physical activity will slow the onset of diabetes (Knowler et al., 2002; Tuomilehto et al., 2001) likely by improving insulin sensitivity (Rhéaume et al., 2002). A Mediterranean-style diet, even with little weight loss, reduced the prevalence of the syndrome by more than half (Esposito et al., 2004). If all else fails, gastric bypass will usually work (Sugerman et al., 2003).

## Antihypertensive Drug Therapy

High doses of diuretics and, even more, β-blockers should be avoided in those who are prone to develop or who have the Metabolic Syndrome, as noted earlier in this chapter. The incidence of new-onset diabetes in multiple RCTs has been reduced significantly with therapy based on ACEIs, ARBs, and CCBs compared to therapy based on diuretics, β-blockers, or their combination (Messerli et al., 2004). Which among the three safer classes to choose is uncertain although many prefer ACEIs or ARBs because they more favorably reduce insulin resistance (Furuhashi et al., 2004; Prasad & Quyyumi, 2004).

## Insulin Sensitizers and Other Drugs

Thiazolidinediones are the most effective insulin sensitizers (Yki-Järvinen, 2004) and lower the blood pressure by about 4 mm Hg (Raji et al., 2003).

Metformin reduced the appearance of diabetes in the Diabetes Prevention Program (Knowler et al., 2002) and acarbose improved multiple features of the Metabolic Syndrome (Chiasson et al., 2003).

## Diabetes

When diabetes develops, the scenario becomes much more ominous with a much higher likelihood of hypertension and more than a doubling of cardiovascular events (Fox et al., 2004) through the interaction of multiple mechanisms (Lim et al., 2004) (Figure 7–22).

## Lifestyle Modifications

The same principles apply as with the Metabolic Syndrome: Weight loss and physical activity are critical, even if minimal in degree (Gregg et al., 2003; Gregg et al., 2004). The 40% reduction in mortality among those diabetics who simply walked 2 hours or more per week reported by Gregg et al. (2003) is truly remarkable and likely could be reduced even more with more strenuous walking (Tanasescu et al., 2003).

## Antihypertensive Drug Therapy

Therapy should be started at levels of BP above 130/80 and intensified enough to keep the BP below 130/80. Such therapy will save the patient misery and the healthcare system money, even better than will glycemic or lipid control (CDC Diabetes Cost-Effectiveness Group, 2002).

Despite only a limited database to determine the best BP for diabetics (Snow et al., 2003), lower

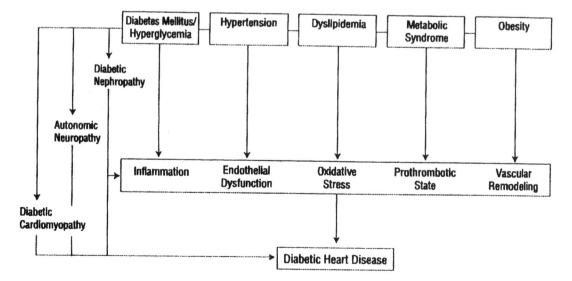

**FIGURE 7–22** ● Multiple paths that lead to the major complications of diabetes. (Modified from Lim et al. Diabetes mellitus, the renin-angiotensin-aldosterone system, and the heart. *Arch Intern Med* 2004;164:1737–1748.)

levels of BP increasingly seem better (Lüscher et al., 2003), particularly in those with existing vascular or renal disease (Mehler et al., 2003).

The best drugs to achieve control are, in order, ACEIs, ARBs, diuretics, and CCBs (Vijan & Hayward, 2003). A combination of an ACEI with a nonDHP-CCB provided better BP control than the ACEI alone (Ruilope et al., 2004). An ACEI, trandolapril, alone reduced the onset of microalbuminuria by 40%, equal to the effect of the ACEI plus a nonDHP-CCB, verapamil (Ruggenenti et al., 2004). Chapter 9 details management of diabetic nephropathy.

Whichever drug is chosen as first, almost all diabetic hypertensives will need between two and four drugs to accomplish the goal of 130/80, and that often will include a CCB (Grossman & Messerli, 2004). If that goal can even be approximated, marked protection against most diabetic complications will be provided (Gæde et al., 2003).

### Lipid-Lowering Therapy

A strong argument has been made for routine use of a statin in all diabetics regardless of lipid levels (Colhoun et al., 2004). In their study of 2,838 type 2 diabetics, those given atovastatin 10 mg a day had a 37% reduction in major cardiovascular risk compared to those given placebo, and the protection was almost the same in those without elevated lipids as in those with dyslipidemia (Colhoun et al., 2004).

### Other Drugs

The same benefits of thiazolidinediones (Sarafidis et al., 2004) and metformin (Manzella et al., 2004) have been seen in diabetes as with the Metabolic Syndrome.

### Conclusion

The bottom line is that everything possible to tightly control hypertension, hyperglycemia, and dyslipidemia should be provided. Unfortunately, in the United States, the costs of the multiple drugs usually needed are not covered by insurance whereas the much greater costs of end-stage renal disease and congestive heart failure often are covered. Perhaps a national healthcare system would provide the preventive care that would cost far less than what we spend today on caring for the complications of diabetes.

## Dyslipidemia

What is true for diabetic hypertensives is likely true for nondiabetic hypertensives: Statins will reduce morbidity and mortality regardless of the lipid profile. The clearest affirmation of this belief comes from the Anglo-Scandinavian Cardiac Outcomes Trial—Lipid Lowering Arm (ASCOT-LLA) (Sever et al., 2003). In this trial, half of 19,342 high-risk hypertensives were randomly assigned to placebo or atorvastatin 10 mg a day. The lipid-lowering arm of the trial was prematurely stopped after a median of 3.3 years in view of a 36% reduction in fatal and nonfatal coronary events and a 27% reduction in strokes in those on the statin, whose average total serum cholesterol fell by 1.1 mmol/L (44 mg/dL). These benefits were seen in those with or without baseline hypercholesterolemia.

Impressive protection from strokes has been noted in other statin trials, averaging 21% in 12 trials involving 85,039 patients whose LDL-cholesterol was reduced an average of 1 mmol/L (Collins et al., 2004).

### Mechanisms

The mechanisms for protection against heart attack and stroke likely reflect more than the reduction in lipid levels. Blood pressure is lowered and large artery stiffness is reduced by statins (Ferrier et al., 2002). When combined with an ACEI, a statin improved endothelial function and fibrinolysis potential while reducing markers of oxidative stress and inflammation (Koh et al., 2004). When combined with a CCB, a statin improved arterial compliance (Leibovitz et al., 2003) and fibrinolytic balance (Fogari et al., 2004a).

### Current Recommendations

In view of the large and consistent evidence that statin therapy is useful in medium- and high-risk people (which would include virtually all hypertensives), the National Cholesterol Education Program Adult Treatment Panel III (ATP III) has modified its recommendations thusly (Grundy et al., 2004):

- Lifestyle changes remain essential for all.
- In high-risk patients, including all diabetics, the goal is an LDL-cholesterol below 100 mg/dL.
- In very high-risk patients, the goal is an LDL-cholesterol below 70 mg/dL.
- In high-risk patients with high triglycerides or low HDL-cholesterol, adding a fibrate or nicotinic acid should be considered.
- In moderately high-risk or high-risk patients, at least a 30% to 40% reduction in LDL-cholesterol should be achieved.

## Patients with Existing Cardiovascular or Renal Disease

### Left Ventricular Hypertrophy

Whether detected by electrocardigraphy or more sensitive echocardiography, LVH is a significant risk factor. There is now convincing evidence that the risks are reduced by regression of LVH (Devereux et al., 2004a; Okin et al., 2004; Verdecchia et al., 2003).

Any drug that reduces BP will regress LVH except for naked direct vasodilators. Better and equal results have been seen with ACEIs, ARBs, and CCBs. Less regression has been seen with diuretics and β-blockers (Klingbeil et al., 2003).

## Coronary Disease

### Chronic Stable Angina

β-blockers, ACEIs, CCBs, and nitrates are usually recommended in that order along with aspirin and a statin (Snow et al., 2004). The CAMELOT trial (Nissen et al., 2004) suggests that DHP-CCBs may be listed before ACEIs (at least before once a day enalapril). Concerns about an increase in myocardial infarctions with ARBs (Verma & Strauss, 2004) hopefully will be settled by comparative trials.

### Postmyocardial Infarction

Angiotensin-converting enzyme inhibitors, β-blockers, and aldosterone-blockers are recommended (Chobanian et al., 2003a). Despite acceptance by experts on the equivalence of ARBs with ACEIs (Lee et al., 2004; McMurray et al., 2004), the limited amount of data on ARB use recommends caution.

## Congestive Heart Failure

JNC-7 lists diuretics, β-blockers, ACEIs, ARBs, and aldosterone blockers as "compelling" for CHF related to systolic dysfunction (Chobanian et al., 2003a; 2003b).

Diastolic heart failure with preserved left ventricular systolic function is common, particularly in Blacks who have a worse prognosis than Whites (East et al., 2004). Therapy is less well established but should be directed at diastolic relaxation, regression of left ventricular hypertrophy, and avoidance of both tachycardia and volume contraction (Krishnan et al., 2003). Rate-slowing nonDHP-CCBs and ACEIs seem to be appropriate, but no outcome data are now available.

## Cerebrovascular Disease

### Carotid Stenosis

Increased cartotid intima-media thickness (IMT) is a risk factor for stroke as is the presence of carotid atherosclerosis (Kitamura et al., 2004). Reduction of blood pressure and lipid levels with a combination of a statin and an ACEI limited the progression of asymptomatic carotid atherosclerosis (Zanchetti et al., 2004).

High-grade stenoses may be relieved by either protected carotid-artery stenting or endarterectomy (Yadav et al., 2004). A few such patients develop a post-endarterectomy reperfusion syndrome (Karapanayiotides et al., 2005).

### Acute Ischemic Stroke

Unlike other hypertensive emergencies, elevated BP in the setting of an acute ischemic stroke is best left untreated unless the level is so high as to pose a danger to other organs (Goldstein, 2004). Table 7–21 is taken from the latest guidelines of the Stroke Council of the American Stroke Association (Adams et al., 2005).

The basis for such caution is the almost consistent finding that the prognosis is worse when BP is lowered. The paradox is explained by two features of cerebral ischemia: First, a loss of cerebral autoregulation so that perfusion is reduced when pressure is lowered; and second, the presence of a penumbra of reduced blood flow around the infarcted area that is potentially salvageable but which could be further damaged by a further fall in perfusion (Goldstein, 2004).

As seen in Table 7–21, the exception to the nontreatment rule is the need to gently lower BP to below 185/110 if the patient is a candidate for thrombolytic therapy. Those with lower BP have a higher rate of vessel recanalization (Mattle et al., 2005).

One large exploratory trial provides the first convincing evidence that the recommendations in Table 7–21 may be too conservative. In the Acute Candesartan Cilexetil Therapy in Stroke Survivors (AC-CESS) trial, half of 342 patients with acute ischemic stroke and BP above 200 mm Hg systolic or 110 mm Hg diastolic within the first 6 to 24 hours were given a placebo, the other half the ARB candesartan, started at 4 mg and increased up to 16 mg if BP remained above 160/100 (Schrader et al., 2003). The aim was a 10% to 15% reduction in the average initial BP of 197/102 within 24 hours. Surprisingly, the subsequent BP levels over the next 7 days with placebo and ARB were identical. After 7 days, both groups were given the ARB for 12 months. There were no differences in outcome, either neurological or cardiovascular at 3 months, but a significant (52%) reduction in 12-month mortality and vascular event in those given the ARB during the first 7 days.

As Goldstein (2004) concludes: "Further studies will be required to determine the optimal management of blood pressure and the use of antihypertensives in this patient population."

### Acute Hemorrhagic Stroke

Unlike ischemic strokes, hypertension in the setting of hemorrhagic strokes is definitely considered in need of reduction, usually by parenteral antihypertensives (see Chapter 8). In a series from Japan, hematoma enlargements were more frequent with target systolic BPs of 160 mm Hg compared to target BPs below 150 mm Hg (Ohwaki et al., 2004).

### Chronic Stroke or TIA Survivors

Virtually in every study of *primary* prevention in hypertensives, strokes have been reduced more than

## TABLE 7–21

## Management of Hypertension in Acute Ischemic Stroke

| Clincial Situation | Recommendation |
| --- | --- |
| Systolic BP <220 mm Hg; diastolic BP <120 mm Hg | Observe BP unless there is other end organ involvement, such as aortic dissection, renal failure, or acute myocardial infarction that would mandate emergent treatment. |
| Systolic BP >220 mm Hg or diastolic BP 121–140 mm Hg | Labetalol 10–20 mg IV over 1–2 min. May repeat or double every 10 min to a maximum dose of 300 mg OR nicardipine 5 mg per hour IV infusion as initial dose; titrate to desired effect by increasing by 2.5 mg per hour every 5 min to maximum of 15 mg/h (target 10%–15% reduction). |
| Diastolic BP >140 mm Hg | Sodium nitroprusside 0.5 µg/kg per min IV with continuous BP monitoring (target 10%–15% reduction) |
| Patient otherwise candidate for intravenous rt-PA | If systolic BP >185 mm Hg or diastolic >110 mm Hg, intravenous labetalol, 10–20 mg over 1–2 min, or 1–2 inches of nitropaste; if BP is not reduced and maintained at desired levels (<185 mm Hg systolic BP and <110 mm Hg diastolic BP), do not administer rt-PA. |

BP, blood pressure. Adapted from Goldstein LB. Blood pressure management in patients with acute ischemic stroke. *Hypertension* 2004;43:137–141 and Adams H, Adams R, Del Zoppo G, Goldstein LB. Guidelines for the early management of patients with ischemic stroke. *Stroke* 2005;36:916–921.

coronary events. In a meta-analysis of more than 40 RCTs of hypertensive patients whose average age was 70 years, a 10 mm Hg reduction in systolic BP was associated with a one-third reduction in the risk of stroke (Lawes et al., 2004). Although some find evidence that CCBs are best (Angeli et al., 2004), others find ARBs to provide additional benefit (Papademetriou et al., 2004). Lawes et al. (2004) conclude: "The benefits from stroke [prevention] appear similar between agents . . . with evidence of greater benefit with a larger BP reduction."

Additional proven benefit has been shown for statins (Amarenco et al., 2004) and aspirin perhaps better taken at bedtime to provide maximal antithrombotic effect in the early morning when more strokes occur (Kriszbacher et al., 2004).

The available evidence for *secondary* prevention in stroke or TIA survivors is much more limited but also strongly recommends reduction of both blood pressure and lipids. The largest trial in stroke survivors is the Perindopril Protection Against Recurrent Stroke Study (PROGRESS) trial, which showed a significant (43%) reduction in stroke recurrence by the combination of the diuretic indapamide and the ACEI perindopril (PROGRESS Collaborative Group, 2001).

In a systemic review, Rashid et al. (2003) identified seven RCTs including PROGRESS and concluded that lowering BP with a variety of antihypertensive agents reduced stroke by 24% and total vascular events by 21% but with no impact on vascular or all-cause mortality. They found the reduction in stroke recurrence to be related to the degree of reduction of systolic BP.

The neurologist Keith Muir (2004) believes that all stroke and TIA survivors should be given antihypertensive and lipid-lowering therapies "irrespective of starting levels of blood pressure." His argument seems well founded.

### Peripheral Vascular Disease

Because ACEIs (or, if not tolerated, ARBs) and CCBs have been shown to normalize endothelial dysfunction and vascular remodeling in arteries from hypertensive patients (Park & Schiffrin, 2000), they are the logical choices in patients with concomitant peripheral vascular disease.

### Renal Disease

Because there are so many facets to hypertension in renal disease, Chapter 9 covers that combination in depth. Two points seem worth mentioning here: First, the presence of renal dysfunction can complicate the treatment of hypertension (Palmer, 2002). Second, microalbuminuria is known to be a serious risk factor and should be looked for in every new hypertensive; if present, reduction in the level of proteinuria may serve as a useful marker of successful therapy (Ibsen et al., 2005).

### Sexual Dysfunction

Hypertension and its treatment are widely believed to be commonly associated and causally connected to sexual dysfunction. Almost nothing is known about sexual dysfunction in women, but over the past few years, since Viagra has been marketed, more and more data address the issue of sexual dysfunction in men, with the easiest measured indicator, erectile dysfunction (ED), providing the hardest evidence. In a word, the evidence is soft.

### Incidence

Despite statements such as "erectile dysfuction is one of the major obstacles for noncompliance in antihypertensive treatment" (Della Chiesa et al., 2003), most data do not firmly indicate a hard relation between ED and hypertension beyond what is expected in elderly men with an increased number of comorbid conditions. In a survey of 29,228 health professionals older than 50 years, 33% reported ED in the prior 3 months (Bacon et al., 2003). Along with a large number of other factors that were adjusted for age (the strongest association) and other known variables, hypertension had an increased relative risk of 20%, as compared to diabetes, which had a 50% increase, smoking with 30%, being married with 30%, watching television more than 20 hours per week with 20%, and a BMI of over 28.7 with 20%. The only lower associations were with physical activity and consumption of up to 30 grams of alcohol per day (1 usual sized drink = 12 grams). The intake of antidepressants increased the relative risk (RR) of ED by 70% and β-blockers by 20%, but diuretics decreased the RR an insignificant 10%.

Looked at in a different way, of 272,325 ED patients, 41.6% were hypertensive, 42.4% dyslipidemic, 20.2% diabetic, and 11.1% depressed (Seftel et al., 2004). Thus, there is no question that a lot of ED patients are hypertensive but only a modest amount of data that hypertension is an independent predictor of ED (Russell et al., 2004).

### Mechanisms

There are a number of logical reasons why ED and hypertension may intercouple, including:

- The typical fall in plasma testosterone with age (Araujo et al., 2004) which may be weakly accentuated by hypertension (Fogari et al., 2002),
- A higher association with sleep apnea (Russell et al., 2004),
- More extensive atherosclerotic stiffness of the pudendal vessels and endothelial dysfunction (Kaiser et al., 2004),
- Adverse effects of diuretics as noted in the TOMHS trial (Grimm et al., 1997) and likely, most importantly,

- The psychological distress of having an incurable, lifelong disease which is widely said to cause impotence.

Regardless of why, men with ED may have more angiographic coronary disease so that "if you can't get an erection, your heart may be heading in the wrong direction" (Chawla, 2004).

### Treatment

If an antihypertensive drug is thought to induce ED (perhaps by further lowering arterial pressure into the pudendal vessels), that drug should be stopped and another from a different class given in small dose to gradually lower BP.

If androgen deficiency is proven, a difficult task (McLachlan & Allan, 2004), androgen replacement can be considered but better by an endocrinologist.

If no reversible cause is found, a phosphodiesterase-5 inhibitor (PDI) can almost always be safely given (Pickering et al., 2004) with an expectation of return of erectile function in 50% to 70% of cases (Kloner, 2004). Caution is needed if nitrates of α-blockers are being used. If the patient fails to respond to PDI, extreme psychological distress may develop (Tomlinson & Wright, 2004).

### Competitive Athletes

One group of patients who should not lack androgens are those who engage in competitive athletics. Not unexpectedly, "white-coat" hypertension may be noted during their precompetition physical exam so that out-of-office BP readings may be indicated. After a limited workup that may be extended to include an echocardiogram, those with persistent, stage 1 hypertension need not be limited in their training or competition (Kaplan et al., 2005). Those with stage 2 hypertension likely should be limited, at least until lifestyle changes (including cessation of androgens, sympathomimetics, growth hormones, etc.) and medication has brought the BP under control. Resistance training should be restricted in those who are not well controlled (Miyachi et al., 2004). The only drugs that may limit physical performance are β-blockers (Vanhees et al., 2000).

### Hypertensive Pilots

The U.S. Federal Aviation Administration has changed the regulations considerably as to the limits of BP and the types of antihypertensive medications that can be taken by people who wish to be certified as pilots (www.faa.gov/avr/aam/game/version_2/03amemanual/PROTOCOLS/Hypertension.htm). Most antihypertensive drugs can be used, with the exceptions of those that act centrally, such as reserpine, guanethidine, guanadrel, methyldopa, and guanabenz.

## Hypertension with Anesthesia and Surgery

Although there is little evidence that poorly controlled hypertension poses a threat and should delay elective surgery (Casadei & Abuzeid, 2005), if possible, blood pressure should be well controlled before elective surgery. A preoperative history of hypertension (>180/110) increased the risk of perioperative mortality (Fleisher, 2002), and the prior administration of antihypertensive therapy reduced that risk (Bach, 1998). In randomized trials, preoperative administration of atenolol (Mangano et al., 1996), bisoprolol (Poldermans et al., 1999), or clonidine (Wallace et al., 2004) provided a reduction in fatal and nonfatal cardiac events in higher-risk patients. In lower-risk patients with stage 1 hypertension, there is no conclusive evidence of greater risk or of the need for additional BP lowering (Eagle et al., 2002).

Whatever drugs hypertensive patients are taking before surgery should be continued until the time of surgery, using parenteral or transdermal forms. When any antihypertensive drug is stopped before surgery, severe hypertension may develop in the postoperative period, particularly with agents such as oral clonidine that have a propensity to rebound hypertension. The exception may be ARBs. In a small group of patients, hypotensive episodes occurred more frequently after anesthetic induction in those receiving an ARB than in those receiving β-blockers, CCBs, or ACEIs (Brabant et al., 1999). Subsequently, these same investigators reported a high incidence of severe hypotension in patients on an ARB undergoing general anesthesia and recommend that it be stopped the day before surgery (Bertrand et al., 2001). Those on a CCB may experience an increase in surgical bleeding (Zuccalá et al., 1997).

If hypertension needs to be treated during surgery, intravenous labetalol, nitroprusside, nicardipine, or esmolol can be used (See Chapter 8).

For those in need of postoperative BP reduction, successful use of parenteral forms of various agents has been reported, including the short-acting β-blocker esmolol, labetalol, nicardipine, or enalaprilat. Sublingual nifedipine is inappropriate, because it does not allow for the control provided by parenteral agents.

Postoperatively, significant lowering of BP may occur as a nonspecific response to surgery and may persist for months (Volini & Flaxman, 1939). Do not be deceived by what appears to be an improvement in the patient's hypertension: Anticipate a gradual return to preoperative levels.

Special problems in postoperative patients after coronary bypass surgery, trauma, and burns are covered in Chapter 15. Anesthetic considerations in patients with pheochromocytoma are covered in Chapter 12.

## Paroxysmal Hypertension and Hypovolemia

Cohn (1966) reported on a group of patients who were severely hypertensive and rapidly went into peripheral vascular collapse when treated with antihypertensive agents. These patients were hypovolemic, and their initial hypertension was at least partly a reflection of compensatory sympathetic nervous system overactivity and an activated renin-angiotensin system. When their compensatory support was removed by treatment, profound hypotension quickly followed. Similar patients have been observed to have a fall in BP as their shrunken fluid volume is replaced, quieting their activated sympathetic nervous and renin-angiotensin systems (Bissler et al., 1991).

## CONCLUSION

The large numbers of drugs now available can be used to treat virtually every hypertensive patient successfully under most any circumstance. Perhaps of even greater eventual value will be the treatment of prehypertensives to prevent the onset of hypertension, only now being examined (Julius et al., 2004c). Lifestyle modifications should always be the first attempt, but, failing that, drug therapy may be indicated in the future. Meanwhile, even those at highest risk—the few who develop a hypertensive emergency—can be effectively treated, as is described in the next chapter.

## REFERENCES

Abernethy DR, Schwartz JB. Calcium-antagonist drugs. *N Engl J Med* 1999;341:1447–1457.

Abu-Hamdan DK, Desai H, Sondheimer J, et al. Taste acuity and zinc metabolism in captopril-treated hypertensive male patients. *Am J Hypertens* 1988;1:303S–308S.

Achari R, Hosmane B, Bonacci E, O'Dea R. The relationship between terazosin dose and blood pressure response in hypertensive patients. *J Clin Pharmacol* 2000;40:1166–1172.

Adams H, Adams R, Del Zoppo G, Goldstein LB. Guidelines for the early management of patients with ischemic stroke: 2005 guidelines update; a scientific statement from the Stroke Council of the American Heart Association/American Stroke Association. *Stroke* 2005;36:916–921.

Agodoa LY, Appel L, Bakris GL, et al. Effect of ramipril vs amlodipine on renal outcomes in hypertensive nephrosclerosis. *JAMA* 2001;285:2719–2728.

Aguilar D, Solomon SD, Kober L, et al. Newly diagnosed and previously known diabetes mellitus and 1-year outcomes of acute myocardial infarction: the VALsartan In Acute myocardial iNfarcTion (VALIANT) trial. *Circulation* 2004;110:1572–1578.

Ahmed A, Centor RM, Weaver MT, Perry GJ. A propensity score analysis of the impact of angiotensin–converting enzyme inhibitors on long-term survival of older adults with heart failure and perceived contraindications. *Am Heart J* 2005;149:737–743.

ALLHAT Officers and Coordinators for the ALLHAT Collaborative Research Group. Major cardiovascular events in hypertensive patients randomized to doxazosin vs chlorthalidone. *JAMA* 2000;283:1967–1975.

ALLHAT Officers and Coordinators for the ALLHAT Collaborative Research Group. The Antihypertensive and Lipid-Lowering Treatment to Prevent Heart Attack Trial. Major outcomes in high-risk hypertensive patients randomized to angiotensin-converting enzyme inhibitor or calcium channel blocker vs diuretic: the Antihypertensive and Lipid-Lowering Treatment to Prevent Heart Attack Trial (ALLHAT). *JAMA* 2002;288: 2981–2997.

Amar J, Cambou JP, Touze E, et al. Comparison of hypertension management after stroke and myocardial infarction: results from ECLAT1—a French nationwide study. *Stroke* 2004;35:1579–1583.

Amar J, Chamontin B, Genes N, et al. Why is hypertension so frequently uncontrolled in secondary prevention? *J Hypertens* 2003;21:1199–1205.

Amarenco P, Labreuche J, Lavallee P, Touboul PJ. Statins in stroke prevention and carotid atherosclerosis: systematic review and up-to-date meta-analysis. *Stroke* 2004;35: 2902–2909.

Anand I, McMurray J, Cohn JN, et al. Long-term effects of darusentan on left-ventricular remodelling and clinical outcomes in the EndothelinA Receptor Antagonist Trial in Heart Failure (EARTH): randomised, double-blind, placebo-controlled trial. *Lancet* 2004;364:347–354.

Anderson J, Godfrey BE, Hill DM, et al. A comparison of the effects of hydrochlorothiazide and of furosemide in the treatment of hypertensive patients. *QJM* 1971;40:541–560.

Anderson TJ, Elstein E, Haber H, Charbonneau F. Comparative study of ACE-inhibition, angiotensin II antagonism, and calcium channel blockade on flow-mediated vasodilation in patients with coronary disease (BANFF study). *J Am Coll Cardiol* 2000;35:60–66.

Ando H, Zhou J, Macova M, et al. Angiotensin II AT1 receptor blockade reverses pathological hypertrophy and inflammation in brain microvessels of spontaneously hypertensive rats. *Stroke* 2004;35:1726–1731.

Andrén L, Weiner L, Svensson A, Hansson L. Enalapril with either a "very low" or "low" dose of hydrochlorothiazide is equally effective in essential hypertension. *J Hypertens* 1983;1:384–386.

Angeli F, Verdecchia P, Reboldi GP, et al. Calcium channel blockade to prevent stroke in hypertension: a meta-analysis of 13 studies with 103,793 subjects. *Am J Hypertens* 2004;17:817–822.

Angeli P, Chiesa M, Caregaro L, et al. Comparison of sublingual captopril and nifedipine in immediate treatment of hypertensive emergencies. *Arch Intern Med* 1991; 151: 678–682.

Anonymous. Educating, with evidence. *Lancet* 2004;363: 1485.

Antihypertensive and Lipid-Lowering Treatment to Prevent Heart Attack Trial Collaborative Research Group. Diuretic versus alpha-blocker as first-step antihypertensive therapy: final results from the Antihypertensive and Lipid-Lowering Treatment to Prevent Heart Attack Trial (ALLHAT). *Hypertension* 2003;42:239–246.

Antman EM, Ferguson JJ. Should evidence-based proof of efficacy as defined for a specific therapeutic agent be extrapolated to encompass a therapeutic class of agents? *Circulation* 2003;108:2604–2607.

Apperloo AJ, de Zeeuw D, de Jong PE. A short-term antihypertensive treatment-induced fall in glomerular filtration rate predicts long-term stability of renal function. *Kidney Int* 1997;51:793–797.

Araujo AB, O'Donnell AB, Brambilla DJ, et al. Prevalence and incidence of androgen deficiency in middle-aged and older men: estimates from the Massachusetts Male Aging Study. *J Clin Endocrinol Metab* 2004;89:5920–5926.

Armstrong B, Stevens N, Doll R. Retrospective study of the association between use of rauwolfia derivatives and breast cancer in English women. *Lancet* 1974;21:672–675.

Au DH, Bryson CL, Fan VS, Beta-blockers as single-agent therapy for hypertension and the risk of mortality among patients with chronic obstructive pulmonary disease. *Am J Med* 2004;117:925–931.

Austin PC, Mamdani MM, Tu K, Zwarenstein M. Changes in prescribing patterns following publication of the ALLHAT trial. *JAMA* 2004;291:44–45.

Azizi M, Ménard J. Combined blockade of the renin-angiotensin system with angiotensin-converting enzyme inhibitors and angiotensin II type 1 receptor antagonists. *Circulation* 2004;109:2492–2499.

Bach DS. Management of specific medical conditions in the perioperative period. *Prog Cardiovasc Dis* 1998;40: 469–476.

Bacon CG, Mittleman MA, Kawachi I, et al. Sexual function in men older than 50 years of age: results from the health professionals follow-up study. *Ann Intern Med* 2003;139: 161–168.

Badrinath P. Preventing stroke with ramipril. Results should have been presented in ways that help practicing clinicians. *BMJ* 2002;325:439.

Bagger JP, Helligsoe P, Randsback F, et al. Effect of verapamil in intermittent claudication. *Circulation* 1997;95: 411–414.

Bahlmann FH, de Groot K, Mueller O, et al. Stimulation of endothelial progenitor cells: a new putative therapeutic effect of angiotensin II receptor antagonists. *Hypertension* 2005;45:526–529.

Bailey DG, Dresser GK, Kreeft JH, et al. Grapefruit-felodipine interaction. *Clin Pharmacol Ther* 2000;68:468–477.

Baker EH, Duggal A, Dong Y, et al. Amiloride, a specific drug for hypertension in black people with T594M variant? *Hypertension* 2002;40:13–17.

Bakris GL, Bank A, Kass DA, et al. Advanced glycation end-product cross-link breakers. *Am J Hypertens* 2004a; 17(Suppl):23S-30S.

Bakris GL, Fonseca V, Katholi RE, et al. Metabolic effects of carvedilol vs metoprolol in patients with type 2 diabetes mellitus and hypertension: a randomized controlled trial. *JAMA* 2004b;292:2227–2236.

Bakris GL, Weir MR, Secic M, et al. Differential effects of calcium antagonist subclasses on markers of nephropathy progression. *Kidney Int* 2004c;65:1991–2002.

Bakris GL, Weir MR, Shanifar S, et al. Effects of blood pressure level on progression of diabetic nephropathy: results from the RENAAL study. *Arch Intern Med* 2003;163: 1555–1565.

Bakris GL, Weir MR. Angiotensin-converting enzyme inhibitor-associated elevations in serum creatinine: is this a cause for concern? *Arch Intern Med* 2000;160:685–693.

Barki-Harrington L, Luttrell LM, Rockman HA. Dual inhibition of beta-adrenergic and angiotensin II receptors by a single antagonist: a functional role for receptor-receptor interaction *in vivo*. *Circulation* 2003;108:1611–1618.

Barnett AH, Bain SC, Bouter P, et al. Angiotensin-receptor blockade versus converting-enzyme inhibition in type 2 diabetes and nephropathy. *N Engl J Med* 2004;351:1952–1961.

Batey DM, Nicolich MJ, Lasser VI, et al. Prazosin versus hydrochlorothiazide as initial antihypertensive therapy in black versus white patients. *Am J Med* 1989;86:74–78.

Batkai S, Pacher P, Osei-Hyiaman D, et al. Endocannabinoids acting at cannabinoid-1 receptors regulate cardiovascular function in hypertension. *Circulation* 2004;110:996–2002.

Benson SC, Pershadsingh HA, Ho CI, et al. Identification of telmisartan as a unique angiotensin II receptor antagonist with selective PPARgamma-modulating activity. *Hypertension* 2004;43:993–1002.

Bertrand M, Godet G, Meersschaert K, et al. Should the angiotensin II antagonists be discontinued before surgery? *Anesth Analg* 2001;92:26–30.

Bhatia BB. On the use of rauwolfia serpentina in high blood pressure. *J Ind Med Assoc* 1942;11:262–265.

Binggeli C, Corti R, Sudano I, et al. Effects of chronic calcium channel blockade on sympathetic nerve activity in hypertension. *Hypertension* 2002;39:892–896.

Bissler JJ, Welch TR, Loggie JM. Paradoxical hypertension in hypovolemic children. *Pediatr Emerg Care* 1991;7:350–352.

Black HR. Evolving role of aldosterone blockers alone and in combination with angiotensin-converting enzyme inhibitors or angiotensin II receptor blockers in hypertension management: a review of mechanistic and clinical data. *Am Heart J* 2004;147:564–572.

Black HR, Elliott WJ, Grandits G, et al. Principal results of the Controlled Onset Verapamil Investigation of Cardiovascular End Points (CONVINCE) trial. *JAMA* 2003;289:2073–2082.

Black HR, Sollins JS, Garofalo JL. The addition of doxazosin to the therapeutic regimen of hypertensive patients inadequately controlled with other antihypertensive medications. *Am J Hypertens* 2000;13:468–474.

Black JW, Crowther AF, Shanks RG, et al. A new adrenergic beta-receptor antagonist. *Lancet* 1964;2:1080–1081.

Blood Pressure Lowering Treatment Trialists' Collaboration. Effects of different blood-pressure-lowering regimens on major cardiovascular events: results of prospectively designed overviews of randomised trials. *Lancet* 2003;362:1527–1535.

Blumenthal D. Doctors and drug companies. *N Engl J Med* 2004;351:1885–1890.

Boddaert J, Tamim H, Verny M, Belmin J. Arterial stiffness is associated with orthostatic hypotension in elderly subjects with history of falls. *J Am Geriatr Soc* 2004;52:568–572.

Boden WE, van Gilst WH, Scheldewaert RG, et al. Diltiazem in acute myocardial infarction treated with thrombolytic agents. *Lancet* 2000;355:1751–1756.

Bond WS. Psychiatric indications for clonidine. *J Clin Psychopharmacol* 1986;6:81–87.

Borghi C, Boschi S, Costa FV, et al. Effects of different dosages of hydrochlorothiazide on blood pressure and the renin-angiotensin-aldosterone system in mild to moderate essential hypertension. *Curr Ther Res* 1992;51:859–869.

Borzecki AM, Oliveria SA, Berlowitz DR. Barriers to hypertension control. *Am Heart J* 2005;149:785–794.

Borzecki AM, Wong AT, Hickey EC, et al. Hypertension control: how well are we doing? *Arch Intern Med* 2003;163:2705–2711.

Boston Collaborative Drug Surveillance Program. Reserpine and breast cancer. *Lancet* 1974;2:669–671.

Brabant SM, Bertrand M, Eyraud D, et al. The hemodynamic effects of anesthetic induction in vascular surgical patients chronically treated with angiotensin II receptor antagonists. *Anesth Analg* 1999;88:1388–1392.

Brater DC, Chennavasin P, Day B, et al. Bumetanide and furosemide. *Clin Pharm Ther* 1983;34:207–213.

Brater DC. Pharmacokinetics and pharmacodynamics of torasemide in health and disease. *J Cardiovasc Pharmacol* 1993;22(Suppl 3):S24–S31.

Brater DC. Pharmacology of diuretics. *Am J Med Sci* 2000;319:38–50.

Brenner BM, Cooper ME, de Zeeuw D, et al. Effects of losartan on renal and cardiovascular outcomes in patients with type 2 diabetes and nephropathy. *N Engl J Med* 2001;345:861–869.

Brewster LM, van Montfrans GA, Kleijnen J. Systematic review: antihypertensive drug therapy in black patients. *Ann Intern Med* 2004;141:614–627.

Brown MA, Buddle ML, Martin A. Is resistant hypertension really resistant? *Am J Hypertens* 2001;14:1263–1269.

Brown MJ. Blood pressure lowering treatment. *Lancet* 2001;357:715–716.

Brown MJ, Brown DC, Murphy MB. Hypokalemia from beta-receptor stimulation by circulating epinephrine. *N Engl J Med* 1983;309:1414–1419.

Brown MJ, Brown J. Does angiotensin-II protect against strokes? *Lancet* 1986;2:427–429.

Brown MJ, Coltart J, Gunewardena K, et al. Randomized double-blind placebo-controlled study of an angiotensin immunotherapeutic vaccine (PMD3117) in hypertensive subjects. *Clin Sci (Lond)* 2004;107:167–173.

Brown MJ, Cruickshank JK, Dominiczak AF, et al. Better blood pressure control: how to combine drugs. *J Hum Hypertens* 2003;17:81–86.

Brown NJ, Vaughan DE. Angiotensin-converting enzyme inhibitors. *Circulation* 1998;97:1411–1420.

Brunner F, Kukovetz WR. Postischemic antiarrhythmic effects of angiotensin-converting enzyme inhibitors. *Circulation* 1996;94:1752–1761.

Brunner HR, Gavras H. Angiotensin blockade for hypertension: a promise fulfilled. *Lancet* 2002;359:990–992.

Brunner HR, Gavras H, Laragh JH, Keenan R. Angiotensin-II blockade in man by Sar$^1$-Ala$^8$-angiotensin II for understanding and treatment of high blood pressure. *Lancet* 1973;2:1045–1048.

Bühler FR, Laragh JH, Baer L, et al. Propranolol inhibition of renin secretion. *N Engl J Med* 1972;287:1209–1214.

Bulpitt CJ, Beckett NS, Cooke J, et al. Results of the pilot study for the Hypertension in the Very Elderly Trial. *J Hypertens* 2003;21:2409–2417.

Burnett JC Jr. Vasopeptidase inhibition: a new concept in blood pressure management. *J Hypertens* 1999;17 (Suppl 1):S37–S43.

Burnier M. Angiotensin II type 1 receptor blockers. *Circulation* 2001;103:904–912.

Burnier M, Brunner HR. Angiotensin II receptor antagonists. *Lancet* 2000;355:637–645.

Burnier M, Schneider MP, Chioléro A, et al. Electronic compliance monitoring in resistant hypertension: the basis for rational therapeutic decisions. *J Hypertens* 2001;19:335–341.

Bursztyn M. Erectile dysfunction in obese men. *JAMA* 2004;292:2466.

Byrd BF III, Collins HW, Primm RK. Risk factors for severe bradycardia during oral clonidine therapy for hypertension. *Arch Intern Med* 1988;148:729–733.

Cameron HA, Ramsay LE. The lupus syndrome induced by hydralazine. *BMJ* 1984;289:410–412.

Campbell DJ, Krum H, Esler MD. Losartan increases bradykinin levels in hypertensive humans. *Circulation* 2005;111:315–320.

Campion EW, Glynn RJ, DeLabry LO. Asymptomatic hyperuricemia. *Am J Med* 1987;82:421–426.

Canzanello VJ, Jensen PL, Schwartz LL, et al. Improved blood pressure control with a physician-nurse team and home blood pressure measurement. *Mayo Clin Proc* 2005; 80:31–36.

Carlberg B, Samuelsson O, Lindholm LH. Atenolol in hypertension: is it a wise choice? *Lancet* 2004;364:1684–1689.

Carlsen JE, Køber L, Torp-Pedersen C, Johansen P. Relation between dose of bendrofluazide, antihypertensive effect, and adverse biochemical effects. *BMJ* 1990;300: 974–978.

Carter BL, Ernst ME, Cohen JD. Hydrochlorothiazide versus chlorthalidone: evidence supporting their interchangeability. *Hypertension* 2004a;43:4–9.

Carter BL, Lund BC, Hayase N, Chrischilles E. A longitudinal analysis of antihypertensive drug interactions in a Medicaid population. *Am J Hypertens* 2004b;17:421–427.

Casadei B, Abuzeid H. Is there a strong rationale for deferring elective surgery in patients with poorly controlled hypertension? *J Hypertens* 2005;23:19–22.

Case DB, Wallace JM, Keim Hj, et al. Usefulness and limitations of saralasin, a partial competitive agonist of angiotensin II for evaluating the renin and sodium factors in hypertensive patients. *Am J Med* 1976;60:824–836.

Casner PR, Dillon KR. A comparison of the antihypertensive effectiveness of two triamterene/hydrochlorothiazide combinations: Maxzide versus Dyazide. *J Clin Pharmacol* 1990;30:714–719.

CDC Diabetes Cost-Effectiveness Group. Cost-effectiveness of intensive glycemic control, intensified hypertension control, and serum cholesterol level reduction for type 2 diabetes. *JAMA* 2002;287:2542–2551.

Celis H, Thijs L, Staessen JA, et al. Interaction between nonsteroidal anti-inflammatory drug intake and calcium-channel blocker-based antihypertensive treatment in the Syst-Eur trial. *J Hum Hypertens* 2001;15:613–618.

Chapman AB, Schwartz GL, Boerwinkle E, Turner ST. Predictors of antihypertensive response to a standard dose of hydrochlorothiazide for essential hypertension. *Kidney Int* 2002a;61:1047–1055.

Chapman MD, Hanrahan R, McEwen J, Marley JE. Hyponatraemia and hypokalaemia due to indapamide. *Med J Aust* 2002b;176:219–221.

Chatellier G, Day M, Bobrie G, Menard J. Feasibility study of N-of-1 trials with blood pressure self-monitoring in hypertension. *Hypertension* 1995;25:294–301.

Chawla R. Erectile dysfunction may be an early sign of heart disease, suggests new research. *BMJ* 2004;329:1366.

Chen Y, Lasaitiene D, Gabrielsson BG, et al. Neonatal losartan treatment suppresses renal expression of molecules involved in cell-cell and cell-matrix interactions. *J Am Soc Nephrol* 2004;15:1232–1243.

Cheng A, Frishman WH. Use of angiotensin-converting enzyme inhibitors as monotherapy and in combination with diuretics and calcium channel blockers. *J Clin Pharmacol* 1998;38:477–491.

Cheng HF, Harris RC. Cyclooxygenases, the kidney, and hypertension. *Hypertension* 2004;43:525–530.

Cheung DG, Hoffman CA, Ricci ST, Weber MA. Mild hypertension in the elderly. *Am J Med* 1989;86:87–90.

Chiasson JL, Josse RG, Gomis R, et al. Acarbose treatment and the risk of cardiovascular disease and hypertension in patients with impaired glucose tolerance: the STOP-NIDDM trial. *JAMA* 2003;290:486–494.

Chillon JM, Baumbach GL. Effects of indapamide, a thiazide-like diuretic, on structure of cerebral arterioles in hypertensive rats. *Hypertension* 2004;43:1092–1097.

Chobanian AV, Bakris GL, Black HR, et al. The Seventh Report of the Joint National Committee on Prevention, Detection, Evaluation, and Treatment of High Blood Pressure: the JNC-7 report. *JAMA* 2003a;289:2560–2572.

Chobanian AV, Bakris GL, Black HR, et al. Seventh report of the Joint National Committee on Prevention, Detection, Evaluation, and Treatment of High Blood Pressure. *Hypertension* 2003b;42:1206–1252.

Choi HK, Atkinson K, Karlson EW, Curhan G. Obesity, weight change, hypertension, diuretic use, and risk of gout in men: The Health Professionals Follow-up Study. *Arch Intern Med* 2005;165:742–748.

Choi KL, Chua D, Elliott WJ. Chlorthalidone vs other low-dose diuretics. *JAMA* 2004;292:1816–1817.

Cicardi M, Zingale LC, Bergamaschini L, Agostoni A. Angioedema associated with angiotensin-converting enzyme inhibitor use: outcome after switching to a different treatment. *Arch Intern Med* 2004;164:910–913.

Cipollone F, Fazia M, Iezzi A, et al. Blockade of the angiotensin II type 1 receptor stabilizes atherosclerotic plaques in humans by inhibiting prostaglandin E2-dependent matrix metalloproteinase activity. *Circulation* 2004;09:1482–1488.

Ciulla MM, Paliotti R, Esposito A, et al. Different effects of antihypertensive therapies based on losartan or atenolol on ultrasound and biochemical markers of myocardial fibrosis: results of a randomized trial. *Circulation* 2004;110: 552–557.

Clark JA, Zimmerman HJ, Tanner LA. Labetalol hepatotoxicity. *Ann Intern Med* 1990;113:210–213.

Cleophas TJ, Grabowsky I, Niemeyer MG, et al. Paradoxical pressor effects of beta-blockers in standing elderly patients with mild hypertension: a beneficial side effect. *Circulation* 2002;105:1669–1671.

Clobass Study Group. Low-dose clonidine administration in the treatment of mild or moderate essential hypertension. *J Hypertens* 1990;8:539–546.

Coca SG, Perazella MA, Buller GK. The cardiovascular implications of hypokalemia. *Am J Kidney Dis* 2005;45:233–247.

Cohen SI, Young MW, Lau SH, et al. Effects of reserpine therapy on cardiac output and atrioventricular conduction during rest and controlled heart rates in patients with essential hypertension. *Circulation* 1968;37:738–745.

Cohn JN. Paroxysmal hypertension and hypovolemia. *N Engl J Med* 1966;275:643–646.

Cohn JN, Anand IS, Latini R, et al. Sustained reduction of aldosterone in response to the angiotensin receptor blocker valsartan in patients with chronic heart failure: results from the Valsartan Heart Failure Trial. *Circulation* 2003; 108:1306–1309.

Colhoun HM, Betteridge DJ, Durrington PN, et al. Primary prevention of cardiovascular disease with atorvastatin in type 2 diabetes in the Collaborative Atorvastatin Diabetes Study (CARDS): multicentre randomised placebo-controlled trial. *Lancet* 2004;364:685–696.

Collins R, Armitage J, Parish S, et al. Effects of cholesterol-lowering with simvastatin on stroke and other major vascular events in 20,536 people with cerebrovascular disease or other high-risk conditions. *Lancet* 2004;363: 757–767.

Conlin PR, Gerth WC, Fox J, et al. Four-year persistence patterns among patients initiating therapy with the angiotensin II receptor antagonist losartan versus other antihypertensive drug classes. *Clin Ther* 2001;23: 1999–2010.

Conlin PR, Spence JD, Williams B, et al. Angiotensin II antagonists for hypertension: are there differences in efficacy? *Am J Hypertens* 2000;13:418–426.

Conway J, Lauwers P. Hemodynamic and hypotensive effects of long-term therapy with chlorothiazide. *Circulation* 1960;21:21–26.

Cooper HA, Dries DL, Davis CE, et al. Diuretics and risk of arrhythmic death in patients with left ventricular dysfunction. *Circulation* 1999;100:1311–1315.

Cooper RA. Captopril-associated neutropenia. Who is at risk? *Arch Intern Med* 1983;143:659–660.

Costa MA, Loria A, Elesgaray R, et al. Role of nitric oxide pathway in hypotensive and renal effects of furosemide during extracellular volume expansion. *J Hypertens* 2004; 22:1561–1569.

Coulter DM. Eye pain with nifedipine and disturbance of taste with captopril. *BMJ* 1988;296:1086–1088.

Cranston WI, Juel-Jensen BE, Semmence AM, et al. Effects of oral diuretics on raised arterial pressure. *Lancet* 1963; 2:966–970.

Cruickshank JM. Measurement and cardiovascular relevance of partial agonist activity (PAA) involving $\beta_1$- and $\beta_2$-adrenoceptors. *Pharmacol Ther* 1990;46:199–242.

Cuspidi C, Meani S, Fusi V, et al. Home blood pressure measurement and its relationship with blood pressure control in a large selected hypertensive population. *J Hum Hypertens* 2004;18:725–731.

Cuspidi C, Muiesan ML, Valagussa L, et al. Comparative effects of candesartan and enalapril on left ventricular hypertrophy in patients with essential hypertension: the Candesartan Assessment in the Treatment of Cardiac Hypertrophy (CATCH) study. *J Hypertens* 2002;20:2293–2300.

Dahlöf B, Devereux RB, Kjeldsen SE, et al. Cardiovascular morbidity and mortality in the Losartan Intervention For Endpoint reduction in hypertension study (LIFE): a randomised trial against atenolol. *Lancet* 2002;359:995–1003.

Damasceno A, Santos A, Pestana M, et al. Acute hypotensive, natriuretic, and hormonal effects of nifedipine in salt-sensitive and salt-resistant black normotensive and hypertensive subjects. *J Cardiovasc Pharmacol* 1999;34: 346–353.

Dandona P, Kumar V, Aljada A, et al. Angiotensin II receptor blocker valsartan suppresses reactive oxygen species generation in leukocytes, nuclear factor-kappa B, in mononuclear cells of normal subjects: evidence of an antiinflammatory action. *J Clin Endocrinol Metab* 2003; 88:4496–4501.

Davies SJ, Jackson PR, Ramsay LE, Ghahramani P. Drug intolerance due to nonspecific adverse effects related to psychiatric morbidity in hypertensive patients. *Arch Intern Med* 2003;163:592–600.

Davis BR, Furberg CD, Wright JT Jr, et al. ALLHAT: setting the record straight. *Ann Intern Med* 2004;141:39–46.

de Leeuw PW, Notter T, Zilles P. Comparison of different fixed antihypertensive combination drugs. *J Hypertens* 1997; 15:87–91.

Deary AJ, Schumann AL, Murfet H, et al. Double-blind, placebo-controlled crossover comparison of five classes of antihypertensive drugs. *J Hypertens* 2002;20:771–777.

Deitch MW, Littman GS, Pascucci VL. Antihypertensive therapy with guanabenz in patients with chronic obstructive pulmonary diseases. *J Cardiovasc Pharmacol* 1984;6: S818–S822.

Della Chiesa A, Pfiffner D, Meier B, Hess OM. Sexual activity in hypertensive men. *J Hum Hypertens* 2003;17: 515–521.

Delles C, Klingbeil AU, Schneider MP, et al. Direct comparison of the effects of valsartan and amlodipine on renal hemodynamics in human essential hypertension. *Am J Hypertens* 2003;16:1030–1035.

Deng PY, Ye F, Cai WJ, et al. Stimulation of calcitonin gene-related peptide synthesis and release: mechanisms for a novel antihypertensive drug, rutaecarpine. *J Hypertens* 2004; 22:1819–1829.

Devereux RB, Dahlöf B, Gerdts E, et al. Regression of hypertensive left ventricular hypertrophy by losartan compared with atenolol: the Losartan Intervention for Endpoint Reduction in Hypertension (LIFE) trial. *Circulation* 2004a; 110:1456–1462.

Devereux RB, Dahlöf B, Kjeldsen SE, et al. Effects of losartan or atenolol in hypertensive patients without clinically evident vascular disease: a substudy of the LIFE randomized trial. *Ann Intern Med* 2003;139:169–177.

Devereux RB, Wachtell K, Gerdts E, et al. Prognostic significance of left ventricular mass change during treatment of hypertension. *JAMA* 2004b;292:2350–2356.

Di Lenarda A, Charlesworth A, Gleland JG, et al. Carvedilol better preserves renal function in heart failure than metoprolol: a potential link to its beneficial effect on prognosis in COMET? [Abstract] *Circulation* 2004;110 (Suppl 3): III–431.

Dickerson JE, Hingorani AD, Ashby MJ, et al. Optimisation of antihypertensive treatment by crossover rotation of four major classes. *Lancet* 1999;353:2008–2013.

Dickstein K, Kjekshus J. Effects of losartan and captopril on mortality and morbidity in high-risk patients after acute myocardial infarction: the OPTIMAAL randomised trial. Optimal Trial in Myocardial Infarction with Angiotensin II Antagonist Losartan. *Lancet* 2002;360: 752–760.

Diffey BL, Langtry J. Phototoxic potential of thiazide diuretics in normal subjects. *Arch Dermatol* 1989;125:1354–1358.

Domanski M, Norman J, Pitt B, et al. Diuretic use, progressive heart failure, and death in patients in the Studies Of Left Ventricular Dysfunction (SOLVD). *J Am Coll Cardiol* 2003;42:705–708.

Donnelly R, Elliott HL, Meredith PA, et al. Nifedipine: individual responses and concentration-effect relationships. *Hypertension* 1988;12:443–449.

Donnelly R, Elliott HL, Meredith PA. Antihypertensive drugs: individualized and clinical relevance of kinetic dynamic relationships. *Pharmacol Ther* 1992;53:67–79.

Dørup I, Skajaa K, Thybo NK. Oral magnesium supplementation restores the concentrations of magnesium, potassium, and sodium-potassium pumps in skeletal muscle of patients receiving diuretic treatment. *J Intern Med* 1993; 233:117–123.

Doty RL, Philip S, Reddy K, Kerr KL. Influences of antihypertensive and antihyperlipidemic drugs on the senses of taste and smell: a review. *J Hypertens* 2003;21:1805–1813.

Doulton TW, He FJ, MacGregor GA. Systematic review of combined angiotensin-converting enzyme inhibition and angiotensin receptor blockade in hypertension. *Hypertension* 2005;45:880–886.

Dujovne CA, Eff J, Ferraro L, et al. Comparative effects of atenolol versus celiprolol on serum lipids and blood pressure in hyperlipidemic and hypertensive subjects. *Am J Cardiol* 1993;72:1131–1136.

Dunder K, Lind L, Zethelius B, et al. Increase in blood glucose concentration during antihypertensive treatment as a predictor of myocardial infarction: population based cohort study. *BMJ* 2003;326:681.

Dunn CJ, Fitton A, Brogden RN. Torasemide. *Drugs* 1995; 49:121–142.

Dupont AG, Van der Niepen P, Taeymans Y, et al. Effect of carvedilol on ambulatory blood pressure, renal hemodynamics, and cardiac function in essential hypertension. *J Cardiovasc Pharmacol* 1987;10(Suppl 11):S130–S136.

Dykman D, Simon EE, Avioli LV. Hyperuricemia and uric acid nephropathy. *Arch Intern Med* 1987;147:1341–1345.

Eagle KA, Berger PB, Calkins H, et al. ACC/AHA guideline update for perioperative cardiovascular evaluation for non-cardiac surgery—executive summary a report of the American College of Cardiology/American Heart Association Task Force on Practice Guidelines (Committee to Update the 1996 Guidelines on Perioperative Cardiovascular Evaluation for Noncardiac Surgery). *Circulation* 2002;105:1257–1267.

Eames PJ, Blake MJ, Panerai RB, Potter JF. Cerebral autoregulation indices are unimpaired by hypertension in middle aged and older people. *Am J Hypertens* 2003; 16:746–753.

Earl G, Davenport J, Narula J. Furosemide challenge in patients with heart failure and adverse reactions to sulfa-containing diuretics. *Ann Intern Med* 2003;138:358–359.

East MA, Peterson ED, Shaw LK, et al. Racial differences in the outcomes of patients with diastolic heart failure. *Am Heart J* 2004;148:151–156.

Ebert U, Kirch W. Effects of captopril and enalapril on electroencephalogram and cognitive performance in healthy volunteers. *Eur J Clin Pharmacol* 1999;55:255–257.

Edwards IR, Coulter DM, Macintosh D. Intestinal effects of captopril. *Br Med J* 1992;304:359–360.

Eguchi K, Kario K, Shimada K. Comparison of candesartan with lisinopril on ambulatory blood pressure and morning surge in patients with systemic hypertension. *Am J Cardiol* 2003;92:621–624.

Eide IK, Torjesen PA, Drolsum A, et al. Low-renin status in therapy-resistant hypertension: a clue to efficient treatment. *J Hypertens* 2004;22:2217–2226.

Eisenberg MJ, Brox A, Bestawros AN. Calcium channel blockers: an update. *Am J Med* 2004;116:35–43.

Elliott HL, Elawad M, Wilkinson R, Singh SP. Persistence of antihypertensive efficacy after missed doses: comparison of amlodipine and nifedipine gastrointestinal therapeutic system. *J Hypertens* 2002;20:333–338.

Elliott WJ, Montoro R, Smith D, et al. Comparison of two strategies for intensifying antihypertensive treatment. *Am J Hypertens* 1999;12:691–696.

Elliott WJ, Polascik TB, Murphy MB. Equivalent antihypertensive effects of combination therapy using diuretic + calcium antagonist compared with diuretic + ACE inhibitor. *J Hum Hypertens* 1990;4:717–723.

Ellison DH. Diuretic resistance: physiology and therapeutics. *Semin Nephrol* 1999;19:581–597.

Elwyn G, Edwards A, Britten N. What information do patients need about medicines? "Doing prescribing": how doctors can be more effective. *BMJ* 2003;327:864–867.

Emeriau JP, Knauf H, Pujadas JO, et al. A comparison of indapamide SR 1.5 mg with both amlodipine 5 mg and hydrochlorothiazide 25 mg in elderly hypertensive patients. *J Hypertens* 2001;19:343–350.

Erdös EG, Deddish PA, Marcic BM. Potentiation of bradykinin actions by ACE inhibitors. *Trends Endocrinol Metab* 1999;10:223–229.

Esler M, Dudley F, Jennings G, et al. Increased sympathetic nervous activity and the effects of its inhibition with clonidine in alcoholic cirrhosis. *Ann Intern Med* 1992;116:446–455.

Esler M, Lux A, Jennings G, et al. Rilmenidine sympatholytic activity preserves mental stress, orthostatic sympathetic responses and adrenaline secretion. *J Hypertens* 2004;22:1529–1534.

Esposito K, Marfella R, Ciotola M, et al. Effect of a Mediterranean-style diet on endothelial dysfunction and markers of vascular inflammation in the metabolic syndrome: a randomized trial. *JAMA* 2004;292:1440–1446.

Estep JD, Mehta SK, Uddin F, et al. ®-blocker therapy in patients with heart failure in the urban setting: moving beyond clinical trials. *Am Heart J* 2004;148:958–963.

Fakhouri F, Grunfeld JP, Hermine O, Delarue R. Angiotensin-converting enzyme inhibitors for secondary erythrocytosis. *Ann Intern Med* 2004;140:492–493.

Fedorak RN, Field M, Chang EB. Treatment of diabetic diarrhea with clonidine. *Ann Intern Med* 1985;102:197–199.

Feigin VL, Rinkel GJ, Algra A, et al. Calcium antagonists in patients with aneurysmal subarachnoid hemorrhage. *Neurology* 1998;50:876–883.

Feinstein AR. Scientific standards in epidemiologic studies of the menace of daily life. *Science* 1988;242:1257–1263.

Feldkamp M, Jones KL, Ornoy A, et al. Postmarketing surveillance for angiotensin-converting enzyme inhibitor use during the first trimester of pregnancy. *Morb Mortal Wkly Rep* 1997;46:240–242.

Ferreira SH. A bradykinin-potentiating factor (BPF) present in the venom of Bothrops jararaca. *Br J Pharmacol* 1965; 24:163–169.

Ferrier KE, Muhlmann MH, Baguet JP, et al. Intensive cholesterol reduction lowers blood pressure and large artery stiffness in isolated systolic hypertension. *J Am Coll Cardiol* 2002;39:1020–1025.

Filigheddu F, Reid JE, Troffa C, et al. Genetic polymorphisms of the beta-adrenergic system: association with essential hypertension and response to beta-blockade. *Pharmacogenomics J* 2004;4:154–160.

Finnerty FA Jr, Davidov M, Mroczek WJ, Gavrilovich L. Influence of extracellular fluid volume on response to antihypertensive drugs. *Circ Res* 1970;26(Suppl 1):71–80.

Fischer MA, Avorn J. Economic implications of evidence-based prescribing for hypertension: can better care cost less? *JAMA* 2004;291:1850–1856.

Flack JM, Cushman WC. Evidence for the efficacy of low-dose diuretic monotherapy. *Am J Med* 1996;101:53S–60S.

Flack JM, Yunis C, Preisser J, et al. The rapidity of drug dose escalation influences blood pressure response and adverse effects burden in patients with hypertension. *Arch Intern Med* 2000;160:1842–1847.

Fleisher LA. Preoperative evaluation of the patient with hypertension. *JAMA* 2002;287:2043–2046.

Fliser D, Buchholz K, Haller H. Antiinflammatory effects of angiotensin II subtype 1 receptor blockade in hypertensive patients with microinflammation. *Circulation* 2004;110:1103–1107.

Flynn MA, Nolph GB, Baker AS, et al. Total body potassium in aging humans: a longitudinal study. *Am J Clin Nutr* 1989;50:713–717.

Fodor GJ, Kotrec M, Bacskai K, et al. Is interview a reliable method to verify the compliance with antihypertensive therapy? An international central-European study. *J Hypertens* 2005;23:1261–1266.

Fogari R, Derosa G, Lazzari P, et al. Effect of amlodipine-atorvastatin combination on fibrinolysis in hypertensive hypercholesterolemic patients with insulin resistance. *Am J Hypertens* 2004a;17:823–827.

Fogari R, Mugellini A, Zoppi A, et al. A double-blind, crossover study of the antihypertensive efficacy of angiotensin II-receptor antagonists and their activation of the renin- angiotensin system. *Curr Ther Res* 2000;61:669–679.

Fogari R, Mugellini A, Zoppi A, et al. Effects of valsartan compared with enalapril on blood pressure and cognitive function in elderly patients with essential hypertension. *Eur J Clin Pharmacol* 2004b;59:863–868.

Fogari R, Zoppi A, Preti P, et al. Sexual activity and plasma testosterone levels in hypertensive males. *Am J Hypertens* 2002;15:217–221.

Fogari R, Zoppi A, Tettamanti F, et al. Effects of nifedipine and indomethacin on cough induced by angiotensin-converting enzyme inhibitors. *J Cardiovasc Pharmacol* 1992;19: 670–673.

Fonseca V, Phear DN. Hyperosmolar non-ketotic diabetic syndrome precipitated by treatment with diuretics. *BMJ* 1982;284:36–37.

Forette F, Seux ML, Staessen JA, et al. The prevention of dementia with antihypertensive treatment: new evidence from the Systolic Hypertension in Europe (Syst-Eur) study. *Arch Intern Med* 2002;162:2046–2052.

Fournier A, Messerli FH, Achard JM, Fernandez L. Cerebroprotection mediated by angiotensin II: a hypothesis supported by recent randomized clinical trials. *J Am Coll Cardiol* 2004;43:1343–1347.

Fournie-Zaluski MC, Fassot C, Valentin B, et al. Brain renin-angiotensin system blockade by systemically active aminopeptidase A inhibitors: a potential treatment of salt-dependent hypertension. *Proc Natl Acad Sci USA* 2004; 101:7775–7780.

Fox CS, Coady S, Sorlie PD, et al. Trends in cardiovascular complications of diabetes. *JAMA* 2004;292:2495–2499.

Fox KM. Efficacy of perindopril in reduction of cardiovascular events among patients with stable coronary artery disease: randomised, double-blind, placebo-controlled, multicentre trial (the EUROPA study). *Lancet* 2003; 362: 782–788.

Franse LV, Pahor M, Di Bari M, et al. Hypokalemia associated with diuretic use and cardiovascular events in the Systolic Hypertension in the Elderly Program. *Hypertension* 2000a;35:1025–1030.

Franse LV, Pahor M, Di Bari M, et al. Serum uric acid, diuretic treatment and risk of cardiovascular events in the Systolic Hypertension in the Elderly Program (SHEP). *J Hypertens* 2000b;18:1149–1154.

Frassetto LA, Nash E, Morris RC Jr, Sebastian A. Comparative effects of potassium chloride and bicarbonate on thiazide-induced reduction in urinary calcium excretion. *Kidney Int* 2000;58:748–752.

Frazier L, Turner ST, Schwartz GL, et al. Multilocus effects of the renin-angiotensin-aldosterone system genes on blood pressure response to a thiazide diuretic. *Pharmacogenomics J* 2004;4:17–23.

Freemantle N, Cleland J, Young P, et al. β blockade after myocardial infarction. *BMJ* 1999;318:1730–1737.

Freis ED, Reda DJ, Materson BJ. Volume (weight) loss and blood pressure response following thiazide diuretics. *Hypertension* 1988;12:244–250.

Freis ED, Rose JC, Higgins TF, et al. The hemodynamic effects of hypotensive drugs in man. IV. 1-hydrazinophthalazine. *Circulation* 1953;8:199.

Friedman PA, Bushinsky DA. Diuretic effects on calcium metabolism. *Semin Nephrol* 1999;19:551–556.

Frishman WH, Bryzinski BS, Coulson LR, et al. A multifactorial trial design to assess combination therapy in hypertension. *Arch Intern Med* 1994;154:1461–1468.

Fu Q, Zhang R, Witkowski S, et al. Persistent sympathetic activation during chronic antihypertensive therapy: a potential mechanism for hypertension morbidity or treatment failure? *Hypertension* 2005;45:513–521.

Fugh-Berman A. Herb-drug interactions. *Lancet* 2000;355: 134–138.

Funder JW. New biology of aldosterone, and experimental studies on the selective aldosterone blocker eplerenone. *Am Heart J* 2002;144(5 Suppl):S8–S11.

Furberg CD, Psaty BM, Meyer JV. Nifedipine. Dose-related increase in mortality in patients with coronary heart disease. *Circulation* 1995;92:1326–1331.

Furmaga EM, Cunningham FE, Cushman WC, et al. Treatment and control of hypertension in the Veterans Health Administration [Abstract]. *Am J Hypertens* 2004;17:107A.

Furuhashi M, Ura N, Takizawa H, et al. Blockade of the renin-angiotensin system decreases adipocyte size with improvement in insulin sensitivity. *J Hypertens* 2004;22: 1977–1982.

Gæde P, Vedel P, Larsen N, et al. Multifactorial intervention and cardiovascular disease in patients with type 2 diabetes. *N Engl J Med* 2003;348:383–393.

Garg JP, Elliott WJ, Folker A, et al. Resistant hypertension revisited: a comparison of two university-based cohorts. *Am J Hypertens* 2005;18:619–626.

Gavras H, Brunner HR, Laragh JH, et al. An angiotensin converting-enzyme inhibitor to identify and treat vasoconstrictor and volume factors in hypertensive patients. *N Engl J Med* 1974;291:817–821.

Gavras I, Manolis AJ, Gavras H. The economics of therapeutic advances. *Arch Intern Med* 1999;159:2634–2636.

Geleijnse JM, Witteman JC, Bak AA, et al. Reduction in blood pressure with a low sodium, high potassium, high magnesium salt in older subjects with mild to moderate hypertension. *BMJ* 1994;309:436–440.

George RB, Light RW, Hudson LD, et al. Comparison of the effects of labetalol and hydrochlorothiazide on the ventilatory function of hypertensive patients with asthma and propranolol sensitivity. *Chest* 1985;88:814–818.

Gheorghiade M, Colucci WS, Swedberg K. Beta-blockers in chronic heart failure. *Circulation* 2003;107:1570–1575.

Ghiadoni L, Magagna A, Versari D, et al. Different effect of antihypertensive drugs on conduit artery endothelial function. *Hypertension* 2003;41:1281–1286.

Giugliano D, Acampora R, Marfella R, et al. Hemodynamic and metabolic effects of transdermal clonidine in patients with hypertension and noninsulin-dependent diabetes mellitus. *Am J Hypertens* 1998;11:184–189.

Goa KL, Benfield P, Sorkin EM. Labetalol. *Drugs* 1989;37: 583–627.

Goldberg AD, Raftery EB. Patterns of blood-pressure during chronic administration of postganglionic sympathetic blocking drugs for hypertension. *Lancet* 1976;2:1052–1054.

Goldner MG, Zarowitz H, Akgun S. Hyperglycemia and glycosuria due to thiazide derivatives administered in diabetes mellitus. *Med Intel* 1960;262:403–405.

Goldstein DS, Pechnik S, Holmes C, et al. Association between supine hypertension and orthostatic hypotension in autonomic failure. *Hypertension* 2003;42:136–142.

Goldstein LB. Blood pressure management in patients with acute ischemic stroke. *Hypertension* 2004;43:137–141.

Goldstein S. Beta-blockers in hypertensive and coronary heart disease. *Arch Intern Med* 1996;156;1267–1276.

Gonçalves R, Pinto HC, Serejo F, Ramalho F. Adult Schönlein-Henoch purpura after enalapril. *J Intern Med* 1998; 244:356.

Gosse P, Sheridan DJ, Zannad F, et al. Regression of left ventricular hypertrophy in hypertensive patients treated with indapamide SR 1.5 mg versus enalapril 20 mg. *J Hypertens* 2000;18:1465–1475.

Gössl M, Mitchell A, Lerman A, et al. Endothelin-B-receptor-selective antagonist inhibits endothelin-1 induced potentiation on the vasoconstriction to noradrenaline and angiotensin II. *J Hypertens* 2004;22:1909–1916.

Gottlieb SS, McCarter RJ, Vogel RA. Effect of beta-blockade on mortality among high-risk and low-risk patients after myocardial infarction. *N Engl J Med* 1998;339: 489–497.

Gradman AH, Cutler NR, Davis PJ, et al. Combined enalapril and felodipine extended release (ER) for systemic hypertension. *Am J Cardiol* 1997;79:431–435.

Gradman AH, Schmieder RE, Lins RL, et al. Aliskiren, a novel orally effective renin inhibitor, provides dose-dependent antihypertensive efficacy and placebo-like tolerability in hypertensive patients. *Circulation* 2005;111:1012–1018.

Grandi AM, Imperiale D, Santillo R, et al. Aldosterone antagonist improves diastolic function in essential hypertension. *Hypertension* 2002;40:647–652.

Granger CB, McMurray JJ, Yusuf S, et al. Effects of candesartan in patients with chronic heart failure and reduced left-ventricular systolic function intolerant to angiotensin-converting-enzyme inhibitors: the CHARM-Alternative trial. *Lancet* 2003;362:772–776.

Grassi G, Seravalle G, Turri C, et al. Short- versus long-term effects of different dihydropyridines on sympathetic and baroreflex function in hypertension. *Hypertension* 2003; 41:558–562.

Graves JW. Management of difficult to control hypertension. *Mayo Clin Proc* 2000;75:278–284.

Gregg EW, Gerzoff RB, Caspersen CJ, et al. Relationship of walking to mortality among U.S. adults with diabetes. *Arch Intern Med* 2003;163:1440–1447.

Gregg EW, Gerzoff RB, Thompson TJ, Williamson DF. Trying to lose weight, losing weight, and 9-year mortality in overweight U.S. adults with diabetes. *Diabetes Care* 2004;27:657–662.

Gress TW, Nieto FJ, Shahar E, et al. Hypertension and antihypertensive therapy as risk factors for type 2 diabetes mellitus. *N Engl J Med* 2000;342:905–912.

Greving JP, Denig P, van der Veen WJ, et al. Does comorbidity explain trends in prescribing of newer antihypertensive agents? *J Hypertens* 2004;22:2209–2215.

Griffin KA, Picken MM, Bidani AK. Deleterious effects of calcium channel blockade on pressure transmission and glomerular injury in rat remnant kidneys. *J Clin Invest* 1995;96:793–800.

Grimm RH Jr, Cohen JD, Smith WM, et al. Hypertension management in the Multiple Risk Factor Intervention Trial (MRFIT). *Arch Intern Med* 1985;145:1191–1199.

Grimm RH Jr, Grandits GA, Prineas RJ, et al. Long-term effects on sexual function of five antihypertensive drugs and nutritional hygienic treatment of hypertensive men and women. *Hypertension* 1997;29:8–14.

Grimm RH Jr, Margolis KL, Papademetriou V, et al. Baseline characteristics of participants in the Antihypertensive and Lipid Lowering Treatment to Prevent Heart Attack Trial (ALLHAT). *Hypertension* 2001;37:19–27.

Grobbee DE, Hoes AW. Nonpotassium-sparing diuretics and risk of sudden cardiac death. *J Hypertens* 1995;13: 1539–1545.

Grol R, Grimshaw J. From best evidence to best practice: effective implementation of change in patients' care. *Lancet* 2003;362:1225–1230.

Grossman E, Messerli FH. Are calcium antagonists beneficial in diabetic patients with hypertension? *Am J Med* 2004;116:44–49.

Grossman E, Messerli FH, Goldbourt U. Antihypertensive therapy and the risk of malignancies. *Eur Heart J* 2001;22: 1343–1352.

Grover SA, Coupal L, Zowall H. Treating osteoarthritis with cyclooxygenase-2-specific inhibitors: what are the benefits of avoiding blood pressure destabilization? *Hypertension* 2005;45:92–97.

Grubb BP, Sirio C, Zelis R. Intravenous labetalol in acute aortic dissection. *JAMA* 1987;258:78–79.

Grundy SM, Cleeman JI, Merz CN, et al. Implications of recent clinical trials for the National Cholesterol Education Program Adult Treatment Panel III guidelines. *Circulation* 2004;110:227–239.

Guasti L, Zanotta D, Diolisi A, et al. Changes in pain perception during treatment with Angiotensin-converting enzyme-inhibitors and angiotensin II type 1 receptor blockade. *J Hypertens* 2002;20:485–491.

Gueyffier F, Boulitie F, Boissel JP, et al. Effect of antihypertensive drug treatment on cardiovascular outcomes in women and men. *Ann Intern Med* 1997;126:761–767.

Guidelines Committee. 2003 European Society of Hypertension-European Society of Cardiology guidelines for the management of arterial hypertension. *J Hypertens* 2003; 21:1011–1053.

Gumieniak O, Williams GH. Mineralocorticoid receptor antagonists and hypertension: is there a rationale? *Curr Hypertens Rep* 2004;6:279–287.

Gutin M, Tuck ML. Metabolic control during guanabenz antihypertensive therapy in diabetic patients with hypertension. *Curr Ther Res* 1988;43:774–785.

Haffner CA, Horton RC, Lewis HM, et al. A metabolic assessment of the beta$_1$ selectivity of bisoprolol. *J Hum Hypertens* 1992;6:397–400.

Hajjar I, Kotchen TA. Trends in prevalence, awareness, treatment, and control of hypertension in the United States, 1988–2000. *JAMA* 2003;290:199–206.

Hall WD, Weber MA, Ferdinand K, et al. Lower dose diuretic therapy in the treatment of patients with mild to moderate hypertension. *J Hum Hypertens* 1994;8:571–575.

Hamet P. Cancer and hypertension. *Hypertension* 1996;28: 321–324.

Hamilton CA, Miller WH, Al-Benna S, et al. Strategies to reduce oxidative stress in cardiovascular disease. *Clin Sci (Lond)* 2004;106:219–234.

Hammarström L, Smith CI, Berg U. Captopril-induced IgA deficiency. *Lancet* 1991;337:436.

Harada K, Kawaguchi A, Ohmori M, Fujimura A. Antagonistic activity of tamsulosin against human vascular $\alpha_1$-adrenergic receptors. *Clin Pharmacol Ther* 2000;67:405–412.

Hare JM. Nitroso-redox balance in the cardiovascular system. *N Engl J Med* 2004;351:2112–2114.

Hargreaves MR, Benson MK. Inhaled sodium cromoglycate in angiotensin-converting enzyme inhibitor cough. *Lancet* 1995;345:13–16.

Harper R, Ennis CN, Heaney AP, et al. A comparison of the effects of low- and conventional-dose thiazide diuretic on insulin action in hypertensive patients with NIDDM. *Diabetologia* 1995;38:853–859.

Healy JJ, McKenna TJ, Canning B, et al. Body composition changes in hypertensive subjects on long-term diuretic therapy. *BMJ* 1970;1:716–719.

Heart Outcomes Prevention Evaluation (HOPE) Study Investigators. Effects of an angiotensin-converting-enzyme inhibitor, ramipril, on cardiovascular events in high-risk patients. *N Engl J Med* 2000;342:145–153.

Hedley AA, Ogden CL, Johnson CL, et al. Prevalence of overweight and obesity among U.S. children, adolescents, and adults, 1999–2002. *JAMA* 2004;291:2847–2850.

Heinonen OP, Shapiro S, Tuomenen L, Turunen MI. Reserpine use in relation to breast cancer. *Lancet* 1974;2:674–677.

Herings RM, de Boer A, Stricker BH, Leufkens HG. Hypoglycemia associated with use of inhibitors of Angiotensin-converting enzyme. *Lancet* 1995;345:1194–1198.

Hernández-Díaz S, Werler MM, Walker AM, Mitchell AA. Folic acid antagonists during pregnancy and the risk of birth defects. *N Engl J Med* 2000;343:1608–1614.

Herndon DN, Hart DW, Wolf SE, et al. Reversal of catabolism by beta-blockade after severe burns. *N Engl J Med* 2001;345:1223–1229.

Herxheimer A. How much drug in the tablet? *Lancet* 1991; 337:346–348.

Hill MN, Han HR, Dennison CR, et al. Hypertension care and control in underserved urban African American men:

behavioral and physiologic outcomes at 36 months. *Am J Hypertens* 2003;16:906–913.

Hirai N, Kawano H, Yasue H, et al. Attenuation of nitrate tolerance and oxidative stress by an angiotensin II receptor blocker in patients with coronary spastic angina. *Circulation* 2003;108:1446–1450.

Hirano T, Yoshino G, Kashiwazaki K, Adachi M. Doxazosin reduces prevalence of small dense low density lipoprotein and remnant-like particle cholesterol levels in nondiabetic and diabetic hypertensive patients. *Am J Hypertens* 2001;14:908–913.

Hodgson TA, Cai L. Medical care expenditures for hypertension, its complications, and its comorbidities. *Med Care* 2001;39:599–615.

Hoes AW, Grobbee DE, Lubsen J, et al. Diuretics, beta-blockers, and the risk for sudden cardiac death in hypertensive patients. *Ann Intern Med* 1995;123:481–487.

Holland OB, Gomez-Sanchez CE, Kuhnert LV, et al. Antihypertensive comparison of furosemide with hydrochlorothiazide for black patients. *Arch Intern Med* 1979;139:1014–1021.

Hollenberg NK, Williams GH, Anderson R, et al. Symptoms and the distress they cause: comparison of an aldosterone antagonist and a calcium channel blocking agent in patients with systolic hypertension. *Arch Intern Med* 2003;163:1543–1548.

Horn HJ, Detmar K, Pittrow DB, et al. Impact of a low-dose reserpine/thiazide combination on left ventricular hypertrophy assessed with magnetic resonance tomography and echocardiography. *Clin Drug Invest* 1997;14:109–116.

Horwitz RI, Feinstein AR. Exclusion bias and the false relationship of reserpine and breast cancer. *Arch Intern Med* 1985;145:1873–1875.

Houston MC. Treatment of hypertensive emergencies and urgencies with oral clonidine loading and titration. *Arch Intern Med* 1986;146:586–589.

Hricik DE, Browning PJ, Kopelman R, et al. Captopril-induced functional renal insufficiency in patients with bilateral renal-artery stenoses or renal-artery stenosis in a solitary kidney. *N Engl J Med* 1983;308:373–376.

Huentelman MJ, Zubcevic J, Hernandez Prada JA, et al. Structure-based discovery of a novel angiotensin-converting enzyme 2 inhibitor. *Hypertension* 2004;44:903–906.

Hui KK, Duchin KL, Kripalani KJ, et al. Pharmacokinetics of fosinopril in patients with various degrees of renal function. *Clin Pharmacol Ther* 1991;49:457–467.

Hunt JS, Siemienczuk J, Touchette D, Payne N. Impact of educational mailing on the blood pressure of primary care patients with mild hypertension. *J Gen Intern Med* 2004;19:925–930.

Hunt SA, Baker DW, Chin MH, et al. ACC/AHA guidelines for the evaluation and management of chronic heart failure in the adult: executive summary. *Circulation* 2001;104:2996–3007.

Hunyor SN, Bradstock K, Somerville PJ, Lucas N. Clonidine overdose. *BMJ* 1975;4:23.

Ibsen H, Olsen MH, Wachtell K, et al. Reduction in albuminuria translates to reduction in cardiovascular events in hypertensive patients: a LIFE study. *Hypertension* 2005;45:198–202.

Ignarro LJ. Experimental evidences of nitric oxide-dependent vasodilatory activity of nebivolol, a third-generation beta-blocker. *Blood Press Suppl* 2004;1:2–16.

Ito A, Fukumoto Y, Shimokawa H. Changing characteristics of patients with vasospastic angina in the era of new calcium channel blockers. *J Cardiovasc Pharmacol* 2004a;44:480–485.

Ito I, Hayashi Y, Kawai Y, et al. Prophylactic effect of intravenous nicorandil on perioperative myocardial damage in patients undergoing off-pump coronary artery bypass surgery. *J Cardiovasc Pharmacol* 2004b;44:501–506.

Iwai M, Liu HW, Chen R, et al. Possible inhibition of focal cerebral ischemia by angiotensin II type 2 receptor stimulation. *Circulation* 2004;110:843–848.

Jackson B, McGrath BP, Maher D, et al. Lack of cross sensitivity between captopril and enalapril. *Aust N Z J Med* 1988;18:21–27.

Jacob S, Rett K, Henriksen EJ. Antihypertensive therapy and insulin sensitivity: do we have to redefine the role of β-blocking agents? *Am J Hypertens* 1998;11:1258–1265.

Jaeschke R, Guyatt GH. Randomized trials in the study of antihypertensive drugs. *Am J Hypertens* 1990;3:811–814.

Jeunemaitre X, Kreft-Jais C, Chatellier G, et al. Long-term experience of spironolactone in essential hypertension. *Kidney Int* 1988;34:S14–S17.

Johnson B, Hoch K, Errichetti A, Johnson J. Effects of methyldopa on psychometric performance. *J Clin Pharmacol* 1990;30:1102–1105.

Johnson RJ, Feig DI, Herrera-Acosta J, Kang DH. Resurrection of uric acid as a causal risk factor in essential hypertension. *Hypertension* 2005;45:18–20.

Johnston GD. Selecting appropriate antihypertensive drug dosages. *Drugs* 1994;47:567–575.

Julius S, Alderman MH, Beevers G, et al. Cardiovascular risk reduction in hypertensive black patients with left ventricular hypertrophy: the LIFE study. *J Am Coll Cardiol* 2004a;43:1047–1055.

Julius S, Kjeldsen SE, Weber M, et al. Outcomes in hypertensive patients at high cardiovascular risk treated with regimens based on valsartan or amlodipine: the VALUE randomised trial. *Lancet* 2004b;363:2022–2031.

Julius S, Nesbitt S, Egan B, et al. Trial of preventing hypertension: design and 2-year progress report. *Hypertension* 2004c;44:146–151.

Juurlink DN, Mamdani M, Kopp A, et al. Drug-drug interactions among elderly patients hospitalized for drug toxicity. *JAMA* 2003;289:1652–1658.

Juurlink DN, Mamdani MM, Lee DS, et al. Rates of hyperkalemia after publication of the Randomized Aldactone Evaluation Study. *N Engl J Med* 2004a;351:543–551.

Juurlink DN, Mamdani MM, Kopp A, et al. Drug-induced lithium toxicity in the elderly: a population-based study. *J Am Geriatr Soc* 2004b;52:794–798.

Kaiser DR, Billups K, Mason C, et al. Impaired brachial artery endothelium-dependent and -independent vasodilation in men with erectile dysfunction and no other clinical cardiovascular disease. *J Am Coll Cardiol* 2004;43:179–184.

Kalinowski L, Dobrucki I, Malinski T. Race-specific differences in endothelial function: predisposition of African Americans to vascular disease. *Circulation* 2004;109:2511–2517.

Kalinowski L, Dobrucki LW, Szczepanska-Konkel M, et al. Third-generation beta-blockers stimulate nitric oxide release from endothelial cells through ATP efflux: a novel mechanism for antihypertensive action. *Circulation* 2003;107:2747–2752.

Kalra PA, Kumwenda M, MacDowall P, Roland MO. Questionnaire study and audit of use of Angiotensin-converting enzyme inhibitor and monitoring in general practice. *BMJ* 1999;318:234–237.

Kaplan NM. New issues in the treatment of isolated systolic hypertension. *Circulation* 2000;102:1079–1081.

Kaplan NM. Renin profiles. The unfulfilled promises. *JAMA* 1977;238:611–613.

Kaplan NM, Carnegie A, Raskin P, et al. Potassium supplementation in hypertensive patients with diuretic-induced hypokalemia. *N Engl J Med* 1985;312:746–749.

Kaplan NM, Gidding SS, Pickering TG, Wright JT Jr. Task Force 5: systemic hypertension. *J Am Coll Cardiol* 2005;45:1346–1348.

Karapanayiotides T, Muili R, Devuyst G, et al. Postcarotid endarterectomy hyperperfusion or reperfusion syndrome. *Stroke* 2005;36:21–26.

Karas M, Lacourcière Y, LeBlanc AR, et al. Effect of the renin-angiotensin system or calcium channel blockade on the circadian variation of heart rate variability, blood pressure and circulating catecholamines in hypertensive patients. *J Hypertens* 2005;23:1251–1260.

Kario K, Schwartz JE, Pickering TG. Changes of nocturnal blood pressure dipping status in hypertensives by nighttime dosing of α-adrenergic blocker, doxazosin: results from the HALT study. *Hypertension* 2000;35:787–794.

Kasiske BL, Ma JZ, Kalil RS, Louis TA. Effects of antihypertensive therapy on serum lipids. *Ann Intern Med* 1995;122:133–141.

Kawakami H, Sumimoto T, Hamada M, et al. Acute effect of glyceryl trinitrate on systolic blood pressure and other hemodynamic variables. *Angiology* 1995;46:151–156.

Kelton JG. Impaired reticuloendothelial function in patients treated with methyldopa. *N Engl J Med* 1985;313:596–600.

Ketch T, Biaggioni I, Robertson R, Robertson D. Four faces of baroreflex failure: hypertensive crisis, volatile hypertension, orthostatic tachycardia, and malignant vagotonia. *Circulation* 2002;105:2518–2523.

Khan NA, McAlister FA, Campbell NR, et al. The 2004 Canadian recommendations for the management of hypertension: Part II—Therapy. *Can J Cardiol* 2004;20: 41–54.

Khatri I, Uemura N, Notargiacomo A, Freis ED. Direct and reflex cardiostimulating effects of hydralazine. *Am J Cardiol* 1977;40:38–42.

Kidwai BJ, George M. Hair loss with minoxidil withdrawal. *Lancet* 1992;340:609–610.

Kimura M, Lu X, Skurnick J, et al. Potassium chloride supplementation diminishes platelet reactivity in humans. *Hypertension* 2004;44:969–973.

Kincaid-Smith P, Fairley KF, Packham D. Dual blockade of the renin-angiotensin system compared with a 50% increase in the dose of angiotensin-converting enzyme inhibitor: effects on proteinuria and blood pressure. *Nephrol Dial Transplant* 2004;19:2272–2274.

Kinoshita M, Shimazu N, Fujita M, et al. Doxazosin, and α$_1$-adrenergic antihypertensive agent, decreases serum oxidized LDL. *Am J Hypertens* 2001;14:267–270.

Kirchengast M, Luz M. Endothelin receptor antagonists: clinical realities and future directions. *J Cardiovasc Pharmacol* 2005;45:182–191.

Kitamura A, Iso H, Imano H, et al. Carotid intima-media thickness and plaque characteristics as a risk factor for stroke in Japanese elderly men. *Stroke* 2004;35:2788–2794.

Kizer JR, Dahlöf B, Kjeldsen SE, et al. Stroke reduction in hypertensive adults with cardiac hypertrophy randomized to losartan versus atenolol: the Losartan Intervention for Endpoint Reduction in Hypertension Study. *Hypertension* 2005;45:46–52.

Kizer JR, Kimmel SE. Epidemiologic review of the calcium channel blocker drugs. *Arch Intern Med* 2001;161:1145–1158.

Kjeldsen SE, Dahlöf B, Devereux RB, et al. Effects of losartan on cardiovascular morbidity and mortality in patients with isolated systolic hypertension and left ventricular hypertrophy: a Losartan Intervention for Endpoint Reduction (LIFE) substudy. *JAMA* 2002;288:1491–1498.

Klingbeil AU, Schneider M, Martus P, et al. A meta-analysis of the effects of treatment on left ventricular mass in essential hypertension. *Am J Med* 2003;115:41–46.

Kloner RA. Cardiovascular effects of the 3 phosphodiesterase-5 inhibitors approved for the treatment of erectile dysfunction. *Circulation* 2004;110:3149–3155.

Knight EL, Bohn RL, Wang PS, et al. Predictors of uncontrolled hypertension in ambulatory patients. *Hypertension* 2001;38:809–814.

Knowler WC, Barrett-Connor E, Fowler SE, et al. Reduction in the incidence of type 2 diabetes with lifestyle intervention or metformin. *N Engl J Med* 2002;346:393–403.

Ko DT, Hebert PR, Coffey CS, et al. Beta-blocker therapy and symptoms of depression, fatigue, and sexual dysfunction. *JAMA* 2002;288:351–357.

Ko DT, Hebert PR, Coffey CS, et al. Adverse effects of beta-blocker therapy for patients with heart failure: a quantitative overview of randomized trials. *Arch Intern Med* 2004;164:1389–1394.

Koh KK, Ahn JY, Han SH, et al. Pleiotropic effects of angiotensin II receptor blocker in hypertensive patients. *J Am Coll Cardiol* 2003;42:905–910.

Koh KK, Son JW, Ahn JY, et al. Simvastatin combined with ramipril treatment in hypercholesterolemic patients. *Hypertension* 2004;44:180–185.

Komajda M, Wimart MC. Angiotensin-converting enzyme inhibition: from viper to patient. *Heart* 2000;84(Suppl 1): i11–i14, discussion i50.

Kopyt N, Dalal F, Narins RG. Renal retention of potassium in fruit. *N Engl J Med* 1985;313:582–583.

Kostis JB, Packer M, Black HR, et al. Omapatrilat and enalapril in patients with hypertension: the Omapatrilat Cardiovascular Treatment vs. Enalapril (OCTAVE) trial. *Am J Hypertens* 2004;17:103–111.

Kostis JB, Wilson AC, Freudenberger RS, et al. Long-term effect of diuretic-based therapy on fatal outcomes in subjects with isolated systolic hypertension with and without diabetes. *Am J Cardiol* 2005;95:29–35.

Krekels MM, Gaillard CA, Viergever PP, et al. Natriuretic effect of nitrendipine is preceded by transient systemic and renal hemodynamic effects. *Cardiovasc Drugs Ther* 1997;11:33–38.

Krishna GG, Miller E, Kapor S. Increased blood pressure during potassium depletion in normotensive men. *N Engl J Med* 1989;320:1177–1182.

Krishnan P, Ventura HO, Uber PA, et al. Treatment of hypertension for patients with diastolic dysfunction. *Curr Opin Cardiol* 2003;18:272–277.

Kriszbacher I, Koppan M, Bodis J. Aspirin for stroke prevention taken in the evening? *Stroke* 2004;35:2760–2761.

Krönig B, Pittrow DB, Kirch W, et al. Different concepts in first-line treatment of essential hypertension. Comparison of a low-dose reserpine-thiazide combination with nitrendipine monotherapy. *Hypertension* 1997;29:651–658.

Labinjoh C, Newby DE, Pellegrini MP, et al. Potentiation of bradykinin-induced tissue plasminogen activator release by angiotensin-converting enzyme inhibition. *J Am Coll Cardiol* 2001;38:1402–1408.

Lacourcière Y, Asmar R. A comparison of the efficacy and duration of action of candesartan cilexetil and losartan as assessed by clinic and ambulatory blood pressure after a missed dose, in truly hypertensive patients. *Am J Hypertens* 1999;12:1181–1187.

Lacourcière Y, Krzesinski JM, White WB, et al. Sustained antihypertensive activity of telmisartan compared with valsartan. *Blood Press Monit* 2004;9:203–210.

Lacourcière Y, Poirier L, Lefebvre J, et al. Antihypertensive effects of amlodipine and hydrochlorothiazide in elderly patients with ambulatory hypertension. *Am J Hypertens* 1995;8:1154–1159.

Lacourcière Y, Poirier L, Lefebvre J. A comparative review of the efficacy of antihypertensive agents on 24 h ambulatory blood pressure. *Can J Cardiol* 2000;16:1155–1166.

Lacourcière Y, Provencher P. Comparative effects of zofenopril and hydrochlorothiazide on office and ambulatory blood pressures in mild to moderate essential hypertension. *Br J Clin Pharmacol* 1989;27:371–376.

LaCroix AZ, Ott SM, Ichikawa L, et al. Low-dose hydrochlorothiazide and preservation of bone mineral density in older adults. *Ann Intern Med* 2000;133:516–526.

Lahive KC, Weiss JW, Weinberger SE. α-methyldopa selectively reduces alae nasi activity. *Clin Sci* 1988;74:547–551.

Langford HG, Blaufox MD, Borhani NO, et al. Is thiazide-produced uric acid elevation harmful? Analysis of data from the hypertension detection and follow-up program. *Arch Intern Med* 1987;147:644–649.

Langford HG, Cutter G, Oberman A, et al. The effect of thiazide therapy on glucose, insulin, and cholesterol metabolism and of glucose on potassium. *J Hum Hypertens* 1990;4:491–500.

Langley MS, Heel RC. Transdermal clonidine. *Drugs* 1988;35:123–142.

Laragh J. Laragh's lessons in pathophysiology and clinical pearls for treating hypertension. Lesson I. A brief history of hypertension research: renin is twice rejected. *Am J Hypertens* 2001;14:186–194.

Lardinois CK, Neuman SL. The effects of antihypertensive agents on serum lipids and lipoproteins. *Arch Intern Med* 1988;148:1280–1288.

Lassila M, Cooper ME, Jandeleit-Dahm K. Antiproteinuric effect of RAS blockade: new mechanisms. *Curr Hypertens Rep* 2004;6:383–392.

Law MR, Wald NJ, Morris JK, Jordan RE. Value of low dose combination treatment with blood pressure lowering drugs: analysis of 354 randomised trials. *BMJ* 2003;326:1427.

Lawes CM, Bennett DA, Feigin VL, Rodgers A. Blood pressure and stroke: an overview of published reviews. *Stroke* 2004;35:776–785.

Leader S, Mallick R, Roht L. Using medication history to measure confounding by indication in assessing calcium channel blockers and other antihypertensive therapy. *J Hum Hypertens* 2001;15:153–159.

Lebel M, Langlois S, Belleau LJ, Grose JH. Labetalol infusion in hypertensive emergencies. *Clin Pharmacol Ther* 1985;37:614–618.

Lechin F, van der Dijs B, Insausti CL, et al. Treatment of ulcerative colitis with clonidine. *J Clin Pharmacol* 1985;25:219–226.

Lee VC, Rhew DC, Dylan M, et al. Meta-analysis: angiotensin-receptor blockers in chronic heart failure and high-risk acute myocardial infarction. *Ann Intern Med* 2004;141:693–704.

Lee W. Drug-induced hepatotoxicity. *N Engl J Med* 1995;17:1118–1127.

Leenen FH, Smith DL, Farkas RM, et al. Vasodilators and regression of left ventricular hypertrophy. *Am J Med* 1987;82:969–978.

Leibovitz E, Beniashvili M, Zimlichman R, et al. Treatment with amlodipine and atorvastatin have additive effect in improvement of arterial compliance in hypertensive hyperlipidemic patients. *Am J Hypertens* 2003;16:715–718.

Lepor H, Jones K, Williford W. The mechanism of adverse events associated with terazosin. *J Urol* 2000;163:1134–1137.

Lepor H, Kaplan SA, Klimberg I, Mobley DF. Doxazosin for benign prostatic hyperplasia. *J Urol* 1997;157:524–530.

Lernfelt B, Landahl S, Johansson P, et al. Haemodynamic and renal effects of felodipine in young and elderly patients. *Eur J Clin Pharmacol* 1998;54:595–601.

Levine HJ, Gaasch WH. Vasoactive drugs in chronic regurgitant lesions of the mitral and aortic valves. *J Am Coll Cardiol* 1996;28:1083–1091.

Levine SR, Coull BM. Potassium depletion as a risk factor for stroke: will a banana a day keep your stroke away? *Neurology* 2002;59:302–303.

Levy BI. Can angiotensin II type 2 receptors have deleterious effects in cardiovascular disease? Implications for therapeutic blockade of the renin-angiotensin system. *Circulation* 2004;109:8–13.

Levy DG, Rocha R, Funder JW. Distinguishing the antihypertensive and electrolyte effects of eplerenone. *J Clin Endocrinol Metab* 2004;89:2736–2740.

Lewin A, Alderman MH, Mathur P. Antihypertensive efficacy of guanfacine and prazosin in patients with mild to moderate essential hypertension. *J Clin Pharmacol* 1990;30:1081–1087.

Lewis EJ. Angiotensin receptor blockers and myocardial infarction: results reflect different cardiovascular states in patients with types 1 and 2 diabetes [Letter to the Editor]. *BMJ* 2005;330:1269–1270.

Lewis EJ, Hunsicker LG, Clarke WR, et al. Renoprotective effect of the angiotensin-receptor antagonist irbesartan in patients with nephropathy due to type 2 diabetes. *N Engl J Med* 2001;345:851–860.

Li W-W, Stewart AL, Stotts N, Froelicher ES. Cultural factors of Chinese immigrants as predictors of hypertensive medication compliance [Abstract]. *Circulation* 2004;110:III-393.

Liao Y, Asakura M, Takashima S, et al. Celiprolol, a vasodilatory beta-blocker, inhibits pressure overload-induced cardiac hypertrophy and prevents the transition to heart failure via nitric oxide-dependent mechanisms in mice. *Circulation* 2004;110:692–699.

Libhaber EN, Libhaber CD, Candy GP, et al. Effect of slow-release indapamide and perindopril compared with amlodipine on 24-hour blood pressure and left ventricular mass in hypertensive patients of African ancestry. *Am J Hypertens* 2004;17:428–432.

Lilja JJ, Juntti-Patinen L, Neuvonen PJ. Orange juice substantially reduces the bioavailability of the beta-adrenergic-blocking agent celiprolol. *Clin Pharmacol Ther* 2004;75:184–190.

Lilja M, Jounela AJ, Juustila HJ, Paalzow L. Abrupt and gradual change from clonidine to beta-blockers in hypertension. *Acta Med Scand* 1982;211:374–380.

Lim HS, MacFadyen RJ, Lip GY. Diabetes mellitus, the renin-angiotensin-aldosterone system, and the heart. *Arch Intern Med* 2004;164:1737–1748.

Lim PO, Jung RT, MacDonald TM. Raised aldosterone to renin ratio predicts antihypertensive efficacy of spironolactone. *Br J Clin Pharmacol* 1999;48:756–760.

Lim PO, Young WF, MacDonald TM. A review of the medical treatment of primary aldosteronism. *J Hypertens* 2001;19:353–361.

Lin MS, McNay JL, Shepherd AM, et al. Increased plasma norepinephrine accompanies persistent tachycardia after hydralazine. *Hypertension* 1983;5:257–263.

Lind L, Hänni A, Hvarfner A, et al. Influences of different antihypertensive treatments on indices of systemic mineral metabolism. *Am J Hypertens* 1994;7:302–307.

Lindenauer PK, Fitzgerald J, Hoople N, Benjamin EM. The potential preventability of postoperative myocardial infarction: underuse of perioperative beta-adrenergic blockade. *Arch Intern Med* 2004;164:762–766.

Lindholm LH, Dahlöf B, Edelman JM, et al. Effect of losartan on sudden cardiac death in people with diabetes: data from the LIFE study. *Lancet* 2003a;362:619–620.

Lindholm LH, Ibsen H, Dahlöf B, et al. Cardiovascular morbidity and mortality in patients with diabetes in the Losartan Intervention For Endpoint reduction in hypertension study (LIFE): a randomised trial against atenolol. *Lancet* 2002;359:1004–1010.

Lindholm LH, Persson M, Alaupovic P, et al. Metabolic outcome during 1 year in newly detected hypertensives: results of the Antihypertensive Treatment and Lipid Profile in a North of Sweden Efficacy Evaluation (ALPINE study). *J Hypertens* 2003b;21:1563–1574.

Lip GYH, Ferner RE. Diuretic therapy for hypertension: a cancer risk? *J Hum Hypertens* 1999;13:421–423.

Lip GYH, Ferner RE. Poisoning with anti-hypertensive drugs. *J Hum Hypertens* 1995a;9:523–526.

Lip GY, Ferner RE. Poisoning with anti-hypertensive drugs: angiotensin-converting enzyme inhibitors. *J Hum Hypertens* 1995b;9:711–715.

Lipsitz LA, Gagnon M, Vyas M, et al. Antihypertensive therapy increases cerebral blood flow and carotid distensibility in hypertensive elderly subjects. *Hypertension* 2005;45:216–221.

Lithell H, Hansson L, Skoog I, et al. The Study on Cognition and Prognosis in the Elderly (SCOPE): Principal results of a randomized double-blind intervention trial. *J Hypertens* 2003;21:875–886.

Lithell HO. Hyperinsulinemia, insulin resistance, and the treatment of hypertension. *Am J Hypertens* 1996;9:150S-154S.

Lloyd-Jones DM, Evans JC, Larson MG, et al. Differential control of systolic and diastolic blood pressure. *Hypertension* 2000;36:594–599.

Lockwood CJ. Calcium-channel blockers in the management of preterm labour. *Lancet* 1997;350:1339–1340.

Logan AG, Perlikowski SM, Mente A, et al. High prevalence of unrecognized sleep apnoea in drug-resistant hypertension. *J Hypertens* 2001;19:2271–2277.

London GM, Pannier B, Vicaut E, et al. Antihypertensive effects and arterial haemodynamic alterations during Angiotensin-converting enzyme inhibition. *J Hypertens* 1996;14:1139–1146.

Lopez J, Meier J, Cunningham F, Siegel D. Antihypertensive medication in VA: a national analysis of medication use patterns for 2000–2002. *Am J Hypertens* 2004;17:1095–1099.

Lottermoser K, Hertfelder HJ, Vetter H, Düsing R. Fibrinolytic function in diuretic-induced volume depletion. *Am J Hypertens* 2000;13:359–363.

Luft FC, Fineberg NS, Weinberger MH. Long-term effect of nifedipine and hydrochlorothiazide on blood pressure and sodium homeostasis at varying levels of salt intake in mildly hypertensive patients. *Am J Hypertens* 1991;4: 752–760.

Lüscher TF, Creager MA, Beckman JA, Cosentino F. Diabetes and vascular disease: pathophysiology, clinical consequences, and medical therapy: part II. *Circulation* 2003; 108:1655–1661.

Lyons D, Roy S, O'Byrne S, Swift CG. ACE inhibition: postsynaptic adrenergic sympatholytic action in men. *Circulation* 1997;96:911–915.

Madkour H, Gadallah M, Riveline B, et al. Comparison between the effects of indapamide and hydrochlorothiazide on creatinine clearance in patients with impaired renal function and hypertension. *Am J Nephrol* 1995;15: 251–255.

Magagna A, Abdel-Haq B, Pedrinelli R, Salvetti A. Does chlorthalidone increase the hypotensive effect of nifedipine? *J Hypertens* 1986;4:S519-S521.

Maitland-van der Zee A-H, Turner ST, Chapman AB, et al. Multifocus approach to the pharmacogenetics of thiazide diuretics [Abstract]. *Circulation* 2004;110:III-428.

Man in't Veld AJ, Van den Meiracker AH, Schalekamp MA. Do beta-blockers really increase peripheral vascular resistance? *Am J Hypertens* 1988;1:91–96.

Mancia G, Carugo S, Grassi G, et al. Prevalence of left ventricular hypertrophy in hypertensive patients without and with blood pressure control: data from the PAMELA population. *Hypertension* 2002;39:744–749.

Mancia G, Grassi G. Systolic and diastolic blood pressure control in antihypertensive drug trials. *J Hypertens* 2002; 20:1461–1464.

Mancia G, Parati G. Office compared with ambulatory blood pressure in assessing response to antihypertensive treatment: a meta-analysis. *J Hypertens* 2004;22:435–445.

Mancia G, Seravalle G, Grassi G. Tolerability and treatment compliance with angiotensin II receptor antagonists. *Am J Hypertens* 2003;16:1066–1073.

Mangano DT, Layug EL, Wallace A, et al. Effect of atenolol on mortality and cardiovascular morbidity after noncardiac surgery. *N Engl J Med* 1996;335:1713–1720.

Manzella D, Grella R, Esposito K, et al. Blood pressure and cardiac autonomic nervous system in obese type 2 diabetic patients: effect of metformin administration. *Am J Hypertens* 2004;17:223–227.

Marre M, Puig JG, Kokot F, et al. Equivalence of indapamide SR and enalapril on microalbuminuria reduction in hypertensive patients with type 2 diabetes: the NESTOR Study. *J Hypertens* 2004;22:1613–1622.

Marshall HJ, Beevers DG. α-adrenoceptor blocking drugs and female urinary incontinence. *Br J Clin Pharmacol* 1996; 42:507–509.

Marshall T. Coronary heart disease prevention: insights from modelling incremental cost effectiveness. *BMJ* 2003; 327:1264.

Martin WB, Spodick DH, Zins GR. Pericardial disorders occurring during open-label study of 1,869 severely hypertensive patients treated with minoxidil. *J Cardiovasc Pharmacol* 1980;2:S217–S227.

Materson BJ, Reda DJ, Cushman WC, et al. Single-drug therapy for hypertension in men. *N Engl J Med* 1993; 328:914–921.

Materson BJ, Reda DJ, Cushman WC. Department of Veterans Affairs single-drug therapy of hypertension study. *Am J Hypertens* 1995;8:189–192.

Mathew TH, Boyd IW, Rohan AP. Hyponatraemia due to the combination of hydrochlorothiazide and amiloride (Moduretic). *Med J Aust* 1990;152:308–309.

Mattle HP, Kappeler L, Arnold M, et al. Blood pressure and vessel recanalization in the first hours after ischemic stroke. *Stroke* 2005;36:264–269.

Mayes LC, Horwitz R, Feinstein AR. A collection of 56 topics with contradictory results in case-control research. *Int J Epidemiol* 1988;17:680–685.

McConnell JD, Roehrborn CG, Bautista OM, et al. The long-term effect of doxazosin, finasteride, and combination therapy on the clinical progression of benign prostatic hyperplasia. *N Engl J Med* 2003;349:2387–2398.

McDonald HP, Garg AX, Haynes RB. Interventions to enhance patient adherence to medication prescriptions: scientific review. *JAMA* 2002;288:2868–2879.

McEniery CM, Schmitt M, Qasem A, et al. Nebivolol increases arterial distensibility *in vivo. Hypertension* 2004; 44:305–310.

McLachlan RI, Allan CA. Defining the prevalence and incidence of androgen deficiency in aging men: where are the goal posts? *J Clin Endocrinol Metab* 2004;89:5916–5919.

McMurray J. Angiotensin receptor blockers and myocardial infarction: analysis of evidence is incomplete and inaccurate [Letter to the Editor]. *BMJ* 2005;330:1269.

McMurray JJ, Pfeffer MA, Swedberg K, Dzau VJ. Which inhibitor of the renin-angiotensin system should be used in chronic heart failure and acute myocardial infarction? *Circulation* 2004;110:3281–3288.

Medical Research Council Working Party on Mild Hypertension. Adverse reactions to bendrofluazide and propranolol for the treatment of mild hypertension. *Lancet* 1981; 2:539–543.

Mehler PS, Coll JR, Estacio R, et al. Intensive blood pressure control reduces the risk of cardiovascular events in patients with peripheral arterial disease and type 2 diabetes. *Circulation* 2003;107:753–756.

Mehta JL, Lopez LM. Rebound hypertension following abrupt cessation of clonidine and metoprolol. *Arch Intern Med* 1987;147:389–390.

Mena-Martin FJ, Martin-Escudero JC, Simal-Blanco F, et al. Health-related quality of life of subjects with known and unknown hypertension: results from the population-based Hortega study. *J Hypertens* 2003;21:1283–1289.

Ménard J, Azizi M. Renin-angiotensin system blockade: to what extent? *J Hypertens* 2004;22:459–462.

Meredith PA, Elliott HL. Dihydropyridine calcium channel blockers: basic pharmacological similarities but fundamental therapeutic differences. *J Hypertens* 2004;22:1641–1648.

Meredith PA. Implications of the links between hypertension and myocardial infarction for choice of drug therapy in patients with hypertension. *Am Heart J* 1996;132: 222–228.

Messerli FH, Beevers DG, Franklin SS, Pickering TG. Beta-blockers in hypertension—the emperor has no clothes: an open letter to present and prospective drafters of new guidelines for the treatment of hypertension. *Am J Hypertens* 2003a;16:870–873.

Messerli FH, Grossman E, Leonetti G. Antihypertensive therapy and new onset diabetes. *J Hypertens* 2004;22: 1845–1847.

Messerli FH, Grossman E, Lever AF. Do thiazide diuretics confer specific protection against strokes? *Arch Intern Med* 2003b;163:2557–2560.

Metz S, Klein C, Morton N. Rebound hypertension after discontinuation of transdermal clonidine therapy. *Am J Med* 1987;82:17–19.

Miller RP, Woodworth JR, Graves DA, et al. Comparison of three formulations of metolazone. *Curr Ther Res* 1988; 43:1133–1142.

Missouris GG, Kalaitzidis RG, Cappuccio FP, et al. Gingival hyperplasia caused by calcium channel blockers. *J Hum Hypertens* 2000;14:155–156.

Mitchell GF, Izzo JL Jr, Lacourcière Y, et al. Omapatrilat reduces pulse pressure and proximal aortic stiffness in patients with systolic hypertension: results of the conduit hemodynamics of omapatrilat international research study. *Circulation* 2002;105:2955–2961.

Miyachi M, Kawano H, Sugawara J, et al. Unfavorable effects of resistance training on central arterial compliance: a randomized intervention study. *Circulation* 2004;110: 2858–2863.

Molnar GW, Read RC, Wright FE. Propranolol enhancement of hypoglycemic sweating. *Clin Pharmacol Ther* 1974;15:490–496.

Montgomery AA, Fahey T, Ben-Shlomo Y, Harding J. The influence of absolute cardiovascular risk, patient utilities, and costs on the decision to treat hypertension: a Markov decision analysis. *J Hypertens* 2003;21:1753–1759.

Moore TJ, Conlin PR, Ard J, Svetkey LP. The DASH diet is effective treatment for stage 1 isolated systolic hypertension. *Hypertension* 2001;38:155–158.

Morgan TO, Anderson AIE, MacInnis RJ. ACE inhibitors, beta-blockers, calcium blockers, and diuretics for the control of systolic hypertension. *Am J Hypertens* 2001;14: 241–247.

Morimoto T, Gandhi TK, Fiskio JM, et al. Development and validation of a clinical prediction rule for angiotensin-converting enzyme inhibitor-induced cough. *J Gen Intern Med* 2004;19:684–691.

Morton A, Muir J, Lim D. Rash and acute nephritic syndrome due to candesartan. *BMJ* 2004;328:25.

Mosenkis A, Townsend RR. What time of day should I take my antihypertensive medications? *J Clin Hypertens* 2004; 6:593–594.

Mosterd A, D'Agostino RB, Silbershatz H, et al. Trends in the prevalence of hypertension, antihypertensive therapy, and left ventricular hypertrophy from 1950 to 1989. *N Engl J Med* 1999;340:1221–1227.

Muir KW. Secondary prevention for stroke and transient ischaemic attacks. *BMJ* 2004;328:297–298.

Mukae S, Aoki S, Itoh S, et al. Bradykinin B$_2$ receptor gene polymorphism is associated with angiotensin-converting enzyme inhibitor-related cough. *Hypertension* 2000;36: 127–131.

Muldoon MF, Waldstein SR, Ryan CM, et al. Effects of six anti-hypertensive medications on cognitive performance. *J Hypertens* 2002;20:1643–1652.

Munger MA, Kenney JK. A chronobiologic approach to the pharmacotherapy of hypertension and angina. *Ann Pharmacother* 2000;34:1313–1319.

Münzel T, Kurz S, Rajagopalan S, et al. Hydralazine prevents nitroglycerin tolerance by inhibiting activation of a membrane-bound NADH oxidase. A new action for an old drug. *J Clin Invest* 1996;98:1465–1470.

Murray CJ, Lauer JA, Hutubessy RC, et al. Effectiveness and costs of interventions to lower systolic blood pressure and cholesterol: a global and regional analysis on reduction of cardiovascular-disease risk. *Lancet* 2003;361:717–725.

Nakao N, Yoshimura A, Morita H, et al. Combination treatment of angiotensin-II receptor blocker and angiotensin-converting-enzyme inhibitor in non-diabetic renal disease (COOPERATE): a randomised controlled trial. *Lancet* 2003; 361:117–124.

National Institute for Clinical Excellence. Hypertension—management of hypertension in adults in primary care: clinical guidelines 18 August 2004.

Neaton JD, Grimm RH Jr, Prineas RJ, et al. Treatment of mild hypertension study (TOMHS). *JAMA* 1993;270:713–724.

Nelson MR, Reid CM, Krum H, et al. Short-term predictors of maintenance of normotension after withdrawal of antihypertensive drugs in the second Australian National Blood Pressure Study (ANBP2). *Am J Hypertens* 2003; 16:39–45.

Nelson M, Reid C, Krum H, McNeil J. A systematic review of predictors of maintenance of normotension after withdrawal of antihypertensive drugs. *Am J Hypertens* 2001;14:98–105.

Neusy AJ, Lowenstein J. Blood pressure and blood pressure variability following withdrawal of propranolol and clonidine. *J Clin Pharmacol* 1989;29:18–24.

Neutel JM, Chrysant SG, Littlejohn TW. Telmisartan 40 or 80 mg/HCT 12.5 mg fixed dose combinations provide superior BP reductions compared to losartan 50 mg/HCT 12.5 mg fixed dose combinations during the last 6 hours of the dosing interval: an ABPM comparison [Abstract]. *Am J Hypertens* 2004;17:118A.

Neutel JM, Schnaper H, Cheung DG, et al. Antihypertensive effects of β-blockers administered once daily. *Am Heart J* 1990;120:166–171.

Neuvonen PJ, Kivistö KT. The clinical significance of food-drug interactions. *Med J Aust* 1989;150:36–40.

New JP, Mason JM, Freemantle N, et al. Specialist nurse-led intervention to treat and control hypertension and hyperlipidemia in diabetes (SPLINT): a randomized controlled trial. *Diabetes Care* 2003;26:2250–2255.

Ng KFF, Vane JR. Conversion of angiotensin I to angiotensin II. *Nature* 1967;216:762–766.

Nicholson JP, Resnick LM, Laragh JH. The antihypertensive effect of verapamil at extremes of dietary sodium intake. *Ann Intern Med* 1987;107:329–324.

Nickenig G. Should angiotensin II receptor blockers and statins be combined? *Circulation* 2004;110:1013–1020.

Nishizaka MK, Zaman MA, Calhoun DA. Efficacy of low-dose spironolactone in subjects with resistant hypertension. *Am J Hypertens* 2003;16:925–930.

Niskanen LK, Laaksonen De, Nyyssönen K, et al. Uric acid level as a risk factor for cardiovascular and all-cause mortality in middle-aged men: a prospective cohort study. *Arch Intern Med* 2004;164:1546–1551.

Nissan A, Spira RM, Seror D, Ackerman Z. Captopril-associated "Pseudocholangitis." *Arch Surg* 1996;131:670–671.

Nissen SE, Tuzcu EM, Libby P, et al. Effect of antihypertensive agents on cardiovascular events in patients with coronary disease and normal blood pressure. the CAMELOT study: a randomized controlled trial. *JAMA* 2004;292: 2217–2225.

Nørgaard A, Kjeldsen K. Interrelation of hypokalaemia and potassium depletion and its implications. *Clin Sci* 1991; 81:449–455.

O'Brien KD, Zhao XQ, Shavelle DM, et al. Hemodynamic effects of the angiotensin-converting enzyme inhibitor, ramipril, in patients with mild to moderate aortic stenosis and preserved left ventricular function. *J Investig Med* 2004;52:185–191.

O'Connor PJ. Overcome clinical inertia to control systolic blood pressure. *Arch Intern Med* 2003;163:2677–2678.

Ohwaki K, Yano E, Nagashima H, et al. Blood pressure management in acute intracerebral hemorrhage: relationship between elevated blood pressure and hematoma enlargement. *Stroke* 2004;35:1364–1367.

Okin PM, Devereux RB, Jern S, et al. Regression of electrocardiographic left ventricular hypertrophy during antihypertensive treatment and the prediction of major cardiovascular events. *JAMA* 2004;292:2343–2349.

Onder G, Penninx BW, Balkrishnan R, et al. Relation between use of angiotensin-converting enzyme inhibitors and muscle strength and physical function in older women: an observational study. *Lancet* 2002;359:926–930.

Ondetti MA, Rubin B, Cushman DW. Design of specific inhibitors of angiotensin-converting enzyme. *Science* 1977; 196:441–444.

Ondetti MA, Williams NJ, Sabo EF, et al. Angiotensin-converting enzyme inhibitors from the venom of Bothrops jararaca. *Biochemistry* 1971;10:4033–4039.

Opie LH. Angiotensin receptor blockers and myocardial infarction: direct comparative studies are needed [Letter to the Editor]. *BMJ* 2005;330:1270.

Opie LH, Schall R. Old antihypertensives and new diabetes. *J Hypertens* 2004;22:1453–1458.

Orme S, da Costa D. Drug points: generalised pruritus associated with amlodipine. *Br Med J* 1997;315:463.

Ouzan J, Pérault C, Lincoff AM, et al. The role of spironolactone in the treatment of patients with refractory hypertension. *Am J Hypertens* 2002;15:333–339.

Owens SD, Dunn MI. Efficacy and safety of guanadrel in elderly hypertensive patients. *Arch Intern Med* 1988; 148:1514–1518.

Packer M, O'Connor CM, Ghali JK, et al. Effect of amlodipine on morbidity and mortality in severe chronic heart failure. *N Engl J Med* 1996;335:1107–1114.

Pahor M, Guralnik JM, Ferrucci L, et al. Calcium-channel blockade and incidence of cancer in aged populations. *Lancet* 1996a;348:493–497.

Pahor M, Guralnik JM, Salive ME, et al. Do calcium channel blockers increase the risk of cancer? *Am J Hypertens* 1996b;9:694–699.

Pahor M, Guralnik JM, Salive ME, et al. Do calcium channel blockers increase the risk of cancer? *Am J Hypertens* 1996c;9:694–699.

Pak CYC. Correction of thiazide-induced hypomagnesemia by potassium-magnesium citrate from review of prior trials. *Clin Nephrol* 2000;54:271–275.

Palmer BF. Renal dysfunction complicating the treatment of hypertension. *N Engl J Med* 2002;347:1256–1261.

Palmer BF. Managing hyperkalemia caused by inhibitors of the renin-angiotensin-aldosterone system. *N Engl J Med* 2004;351:585–592.

Pandya KJ, Raubertas RF, Flynn PJ, et al. Oral clonidine in postmenopausal patients with breast cancer experiencing tamoxifen-induced hot flashes. *Ann Intern Med* 2000;132: 788–793.

Papademetriou V, Farsang C, Elmfeldt D, et al. Stroke prevention with the angiotensin II type 1-receptor blocker candesartan in elderly patients with isolated systolic hypertension: the Study on Cognition and Prognosis in the Elderly (SCOPE). *J Am Coll Cardiol* 2004;44:1175–1180.

Park JB, Schiffrin EL. Effects of antihypertensive therapy on hypertensive vascular disease. *Curr Hypertens Rep* 2000;2:280–288.

Participating VA Medical Centers. Low doses v standard dose of reserpine. *JAMA* 1982;248:2471–2477.

Parving H-H, Lehnert H, Bröchner-Mortensen J, et al. The effect of irbesartan on the development of diabetic nephropathy in patients with type 2 diabetes. *N Engl J Med* 2001; 345:870–878.

Paton RR, Kane RE. Long-term diuretic therapy with metolazone of renal failure and the nephrotic syndrome. *J Clin Pharm* 1977;17:243–251.

PEACE Trial Investigators. Angiotensin-converting-enzyme inhibition in stable coronary artery disease. *N Engl J Med* 2004;351:2058–2068.

Pedelty L, Gorelick PB. Chronic management of blood pressure after stroke. *Hypertension* 2004;44:1–5.

Pepine CJ, Handberg EM, Cooper-DeHoff RM, et al. A calcium antagonist vs a non-calcium antagonist hypertension treatment strategy for patients with coronary artery disease. The International Verapamil-Trandolapril Study (INVEST): a randomized controlled trial. *JAMA* 2003;290: 2805–2816.

Pérez-Stable E, Halliday R, Gardiner PS, et al. The effects of propranolol on cognitive function and quality of life. *Am J Med* 2000;108:359–365.

Perry HM Jr. Late toxicity to hydralazine resembling systemic lupus erythematosus or rheumatoid arthritis. *Am J Med* 1973;54:58–72.

Persson M, Carlberg B, Tavelin B, Lindholm LH. Doctors' estimation of cardiovascular risk and willingness to give drug treatment in hypertension: fair risk assessment but defensive treatment policy. *J Hypertens* 2004;22:65–71.

Pfeffer MA, McMurray JJ, Velazquez EJ, et al. Valsartan, captopril, or both in myocardial infarction complicated by heart failure, left ventricular dysfunction, or both. *N Engl J Med* 2003;349:1893–1906.

Pickering TG. Effects of stress and behavioral interventions in hypertension: the rise and fall of omapatrilat. *J Clin Hypertens* 2002;4:371–373.

Pickering TG. Treatment of hypertension in the elderly. *J Clin Hypertens* 2004;6(10 Suppl 2):18–23.

Pickering TG, Levenstein M, Walmsley P. Nighttime dosing of doxazosin has peak effect on morning ambulatory blood pressure. *Am J Hypertens* 1994;7:844–847.

Pickering TG, Shepherd AMM, Puddey I, et al. Sildenafil citrate for erectile dysfunction in men receiving multiple antihypertensive agents. *Am J Hypertens* 2004;17:1135–1142.

Pickles CJ, Pipkin FB, Symonds EM. A randomised placebo controlled trial of labetalol in the treatment of mild to moderate pregnancy induced hypertension. *Br J Obstet Gynaecol* 1992;99:964–968.

Piepho RW, Beal J. An overview of antihypertensive therapy in the 20th century. *J Clin Pharmacol* 2000;40:967–977.

Pilote L, Abrahamowicz M, Rodrigues E, et al. Mortality rates in elderly patients who take different angiotensin-converting enzyme inhibitors after acute myocardial infarction: a class effect? *Ann Intern Med* 2004;141:102–112.

Pitt B. A new HOPE for aldosterone blockade? *Circulation* 2004;110:1714–1716.

Pitt B, Remme W, Zannad F, et al. Eplerenone, a selective aldosterone blocker, in patients with left ventricular dysfunction after myocardial infarction. *N Engl J Med* 2003;348:1309–1321.

Pitt B, Zannad F, Remme WJ, et al. The effect of spironolactone of morbidity and mortality in patients with severe heart failure. *N Engl J Med* 1999;341:709–717.

Plata R, Cornejo A, Arratia C, et al. Angiotensin-converting-enzyme inhibition therapy in altitude polycythaemia: a prospective randomised trial. *Lancet* 2002;359:663–666.

Poirier L, de Champlain J, Larochelle P, et al. A comparison of the efficacy and duration of action of telmisartan, amlodipine and ramipril in patients with confirmed ambulatory hypertension. *Blood Press Monit* 2004;9:231–236.

Poldermans D, Boersma E, Bax JJ, et al. The effect of bisoprolol on perioperative mortality and myocardial infarction in high-risk patients undergoing vascular surgery. *N Engl J Med* 1999;341:1789–1794.

Polónia J, Boaventura I, Gama G, et al. Influence of nonsteroidal anti-inflammatory drugs on renal function and h24 ambulatory blood pressure-reducing effects of enalapril and nifedipine gastrointestinal therapeutic system in hypertensive patients. *J Hypertens* 1995;13:924–931.

Poole-Wilson PA, Lubsen J, Kirwan BA, et al. Effect of long-acting nifedipine on mortality and cardiovascular morbidity in patients with stable angina requiring treatment (ACTION trial): randomised controlled trial. *Lancet* 2004;364:849–857.

Poole-Wilson PA, Swedberg K, Cleland JG, et al. Comparison of carvedilol and metoprolol on clinical outcomes in patients with chronic heart failure in the Carvedilol Or Metoprolol European Trial (COMET): randomised controlled trial. *Lancet* 2003;362:7–13.

Postma CT, Dennesen PJW, de Boo T, Thien T. First dose hypotension after captopril; can it be predicted? *J Hum Hypertens* 1992;6:204–209.

Prasad A, Quyyumi AA. Renin-angiotensin system and angiotensin receptor blockers in the metabolic syndrome. *Circulation* 2004;110:1507–1512.

Prichard BN, Vallance P. ESH/ESC guidelines. *J Hypertens* 2004;22:859–861.

Priori SG, Napolitano C, Schwartz PJ, et al. Association of long QT syndrome loci and cardiac events among patients treated with beta-blockers. *JAMA* 2004;292: 1341–1344.

Prisant LM, Spruill WJ, Fincham JE, et al. Depression associated with antihypertensive drugs. *J Fam Pract* 1991;33:481–485.

PROGRESS Collaborative Group. Randomised trial of a perindopril-based blood-pressure-lowering regimen among 6105 individuals with previous stroke or transient ischaemic attack. *Lancet* 2001;358:1033–1041.

Psaty BM, Heckbert SR, Koepsell TD, et al. The risk of myocardial infarction associated with antihypertensive drug therapies. *JAMA* 1995;274:620–625.

Psaty BM, Koepsell TD, Wagner EH, et al. The relative risk of incident coronary heart disease associated with recently stopping the use of beta-blockers. *JAMA* 1990;263: 1653–1657.

Psaty BM, Lumley T, Furberg CD, et al. Health outcomes associated with various antihypertensive therapies used as first-line agents: a network meta-analysis. *JAMA* 2003; 289:2534–2544.

Psaty BM, Lumley T, Furberg CD. Meta-analysis of health outcomes of chlorthalidone-based vs nonchlorthalidone-based low-dose diuretic therapies. *JAMA* 2004;292:43–44.

Psaty BM, Rennie D. Stopping medical research to save money: a broken pact with researchers and patients. *JAMA* 2003;289:2128–2131.

Psaty BM, Smith NL, Heckbert SR, et al. Diuretic therapy, the alpha-adducin gene variant, and the risk of myocardial infarction or stroke in persons with treated hypertension. *JAMA* 2002;287:1680–1689.

Psaty BM, Smith NL, Siscovick DS, et al. Health outcomes associated with antihypertensive therapies used as first-line agents. *JAMA* 1997;277:739–745.

Puschett JB. Diuretics and the therapy of hypertension. *Am J Med Sci* 2000;319:1–9.

Quereda C, Orte L, Sabater J, et al. Urinary calcium excretion in treated and untreated essential hypertension. *J Am Soc Nephrol* 1996;7:1058–1065.

Rabkin SW. Mechanisms of action of adrenergic receptor blockers on lipids during antihypertensive drug treatment. *J Clin Pharmacol* 1993;33:286–291.

Radack K, Deck C. Beta-adrenergic blocker therapy does not worsen intermittent claudication in subjects with peripheral arterial disease. *Arch Intern Med* 1991;151:1769–1776.

Raftery EB, Carrageta MO. Hypertension and beta-blockers. Are they all the same? *Int J Cardiol* 1985;7:337–346.

Raji A, Seely EW, Bekins SA, et al. Rosiglitazone improves insulin sensitivity and lowers blood pressure in hypertensive patients. *Diabetes Care* 2003;26:172–178.

Ram CVS. Antihypertensive efficacy of angiotensin receptor blockers in combination with hydrochlorothiazide: a review of the factorial-design studies. *J Clin Hypertens* 2004;6:569–577.

Ram CVS, Garrett BN, Kaplan NM. Moderate sodium restriction and various diuretics in the treatment of hypertension. *Arch Intern Med* 1981;141:1014–1019.

Ram CVS, Holland OB, Fairchild C, Gomez-Sanchez CE. Withdrawal syndrome following cessation of guanabenz therapy. *J Clin Pharmacol* 1979;19:148–150.

Ramsay LE, Silas JH, Ollerenshaw JD, et al. Should the acetylator phenotype be determined when prescribing hydralazine for hypertension? *Eur J Clin Pharmacol* 1984;26:39–42.

Rashid P, Leonardi-Bee J, Bath P. Blood pressure reduction and secondary prevention of stroke and other vascular events: a systematic review. *Stroke* 2003;34:2741–2748.

Re RN. Tissue renin angiotensin systems. *Med Clin NA* 2004;88:19–38.

Redon J, Campos C, Narciso ML, et al. Prognostic value of ambulatory blood pressure monitoring in refractory hypertension. *Hypertension* 1998;31:712–718.

Rédon J, Roca-Cusachs A, Mora-Maciá J. Uncontrolled early morning blood pressure in medicated patients: the ACAMPA study. Analysis of the Control of Blood Pressure using Ambulatory Blood Pressure Monitoring. *Blood Press Monit* 2002;7:111–116.

Rejnmark L, Vestergaard P, Heickendorff L, et al. Effect of thiazide- and loop-diuretics, alone or in combination, on calcitropic hormones and biochemical bone markers. *J Intern Med* 2001;250:144–153.

Remme WJ. Prevention of cardiovascular events by perindopril in patients with stable coronary disease does not depend on blood pressure and its reduction: results from the EUROPA study [Abstract]. *Circulation* 2004;110:III–628.

Reyes AJ, Taylor SH. Diuretics in cardiovascular therapy. *Cardiovasc Drugs Ther* 1999;13:371–398.

Rhéaume C, Waib PH, Lacourcière Y, et al. Effects of mild exercise on insulin sensitivity in hypertensive subjects. *Hypertension* 2002;39:989–995.

Ricketts ML, Stewart PM. Regulation of 11beta-hydroxysteroid dehydrogenase type 2 by diuretics and the renin-angiotensin-aldosterone axis. *Clin Sci* 1999;96:669–675.

Roberts R, Sigwart U. New concepts in hypertrophic cardiomyopathies, part II. *Circulation* 2001;104:2249–2252.

Rocha R, Funder JW. The pathophysiology of aldosterone in the cardiovascular system. *Ann N Y Acad Sci* 2002;970:89–100.

Rodman JS, Deutsch DJ, Gutman SI. Methyldopa hepatitis. *Am J Med* 1976;60:941–948.

Ross S, Walker A, MacLeod MJ. Patient compliance in hypertension: role of illness perceptions and treatment beliefs. *J Hum Hypertens* 2004;18:607–613.

Rouleau JL, Roecker EB, Tendera M, et al. Influence of pretreatment systolic blood pressure on the effect of carvedilol in patients with severe chronic heart failure: the Carvedilol Prospective Randomized Cumulative Survival (COPERNICUS) study. *J Am Coll Cardiol* 2004;43:1423–1439.

Roush MK, McNutt RA, Gray TF. The adverse effect dilemma. *Ann Intern Med* 1991;114:298–299.

Rubin LJ. Primary pulmonary hypertension. *N Engl J Med* 1997;336:111–117.

Rudd P, Miller NH, Kaufman J, et al. Nurse management for hypertension. A systems approach. *Am J Hypertens* 2004;17:921–927.

Rudd P. Clinicians and patients with hypertension. *Am Heart J* 1995;130:572–578.

Ruggenenti P, Fassi A, Ilieva AP, et al. Preventing microalbuminuria in type 2 diabetes. *N Engl J Med* 2004;351:1941–1951.

Ruggenenti P, Mise N, Pisoni R, et al. Diverse effects of increasing lisinopril doses on lipid abnormalities in chronic nephropathies. *Circulation* 2003;107:586–592.

Ruilope LM. Comparison of a new vasodilating beta-blocker, carvedilol, with atenolol in the treatment of mild to moderate essential hypertension. *Am J Hypertens* 1994;7: 129–136.

Ruilope LM, Usan L, Segura J, Bakris GL. Intervention at lower blood pressure levels to achieve target goals in type 2 diabetes: PRADID (PResion Arterial en DIabeticos tipo Dos) study. *J Hypertens* 2004;22:217–222.

Rundall TG, Shortell SM, Wang MC, et al. As good as it gets? Chronic care management in nine leading U.S. physician organisations. *BMJ* 2002;325:958–961.

Russell ST, Khandheria BK, Nehra A. Erectile dysfunction and cardiovascular disease. *Mayo Clin Proc* 2004;79:782–794.

Ruzicka M, Coletta E, Floras J, Leenen FH. Effects of low-dose nifedipine GITS on sympathetic activity in young and older patients with hypertension. *J Hypertens* 2004;22:1039–1044.

Ryan MJ, Didion SP, Mathur S, et al. Angiotensin II-induced vascular dysfunction is mediated by the AT1A receptor in mice. *Hypertension* 2004;43:1074–1079.

Saito F, Kimura G. Antihypertensive mechanism of diuretics based on pressure-natriuresis relationship. *Hypertension* 1996;27:914–918.

Sakhaee K, Alpern R, Jacobson HR, Pak CYC. Contrasting effects of various potassium salts on renal citrate excretion. *J Clin Endocrinol Metab* 1991;72:396–400.

Sakhaee K, Nicar MJ, Glass K, et al. Reduction in intestinal calcium absorption by hydrochlorothiazide in postmenopausal osteoporosis. *J Clin Endocrinol Metab* 1984;59:1037–1043.

Salpeter SR, Ormiston TM, Salpeter EE. Cardioselective beta-blockers in patients with reactive airway disease: a meta-analysis. *Ann Intern Med* 2002;137:715–725.

Samuelsson O, Pennert K, Andersson O, et al. Diabetes mellitus and raised serum triglyceride concentration in treated hypertension—are they of prognostic importance? *BMJ* 1996;313:660–663.

Sarafidis PA, Lasaridis AN, Nilsson PM, et al. Ambulatory blood pressure reduction after rosiglitazone treatment in patients with type 2 diabetes and hypertension correlates with insulin sensitivity increase. *J Hypertens* 2004;22:1769–1777.

Saruta T, Arakawa K, Iimura O, et al. Difference in the incidence of cough induced by angiotensin converting enzyme inhibitors: a comparative study using imidapril hydrochloride and enalapril maleate. *Hypertension Res* 1999;22:197–202.

Sato A, Hayashi K, Naruse M, Saruta T. Effectiveness of aldosterone blockade in patients with diabetic nephropathy. *Hypertension* 2003;41:64–68.

Sato A, Saruta T. Aldosterone breakthrough during angiotensin-converting enzyme inhibitor therapy. *Am J Hypertens* 2003;16:781–788.

Sattler KJE, Woodrum JE, Galili O, et al. Concurrent treatment with renin-angiotensin system blockers and acetylsalicylic acid reduces nuclear factor κB activation and C-reactive protein expression in human carotid artery plaques. *Stroke* 2005;36:14–20.

Savola J, Vehviäinen O, Väätäinen NJ. Psoriasis as a side effect of beta blockers. *BMJ* 1987;295:637.

Sawyer N, Gabriel R. Progressive hypokalaemia in elderly patients taking three thiazide potassium-sparing diuretic combinations for thirty-six months. *Postgrad Med J* 1988;64:434–437.

Saxena PR, Bolt GR. Haemodynamic profiles of vasodilators in experimental hypertension. *Trends Pharmacol Sci* 1986;7:501–506.

Schiffrin EL, Park JB, Intengan HD, Touyz RM. Correction of arterial structure and endothelial dysfunction in human essential hypertension by the angiotensin receptor antagonist losartan. *Circulation* 2000;101:1653–1659.

Schlienger RG, Kraenzlin ME, Jick SS, Meier CR. Use of beta-blockers and risk of fractures. *JAMA* 2004;292: 1326–1332.

Schlienger RG, Saxer M, Haefeli W. Reversible ageusia associated with losartan. *Lancet* 1996;347:471–472.

Schnaper HW, Freis ED, Friedman RG, et al. Potassium restoration in hypertensive patients made hypokalemic by hydrochlorothiazide. *Arch Intern Med* 1989;149:2677–2681.

Schrader H, Stovner LJ, Helde G, et al. Prophylactic treatment of migraine with Angiotensin-converting enzyme inhibitor (lisinopril). *BMJ* 2001;322:19–22.

Schrader J, Luders S, Kulschewski A, et al. The ACCESS Study: evaluation of acute candesartan cilexetil therapy in stroke survivors. *Stroke* 2003;34:1699–1703.

Schrage WG, Eisenbach JH, Dinenno FA, et al. Effects of midodrine on exercise-induced hypotension and blood pressure recovery in autonomic failure. *J Appl Physiol* 2004; 97:1978–1984.

Schroeder K, Fahey T, Ebrahim S. How can we improve adherence to blood pressure-lowering medication in ambulatory care? Systematic review of randomized controlled trials. *Arch Intern Med* 2004;164:722–732.

Schroeder T, Sillesen H. Dihydralazine induces marked cerebral vasodilation in man. *Eur J Clin Invest* 1987;17: 214–217.

Schupp M, Janke J, Clasen R, et al. Angiotensin type 1 receptor blockers induce peroxisome proliferator-activated receptor-gamma activity. *Circulation* 2004;109:2054–2057.

Schwinn DA, Price DT, Narayan P. Alpha1-adrenoceptor subtype selectivity and lower urinary tract symptoms. *Mayo Clin Proc* 2004;79:1423–1434.

Seftel AD, Sun P, Swindle R. The prevalence of hypertension, hyperlipidemia, diabetes mellitus and depression in men with erectile dysfunction. *J Urol* 2004;171:2341–2345.

Senn S. Individual response to treatment: is it a valid assumption? *BMJ* 2004;329:966–968.

Sever PS, Dahlöf B, Poulter NR, et al. Prevention of coronary and stroke events with atorvastatin in hypertensive patients who have average or lower-than-average cholesterol concentrations, in the Anglo-Scandinavian Cardiac Outcomes Trial—Lipid Lowering Arm (ASCOT-LLA): a multicentre randomised controlled trial. *Lancet* 2003;361:1149–1158.

Sharabi Y, Illan R, Kamari Y, et al. Diuretic induced hyponatraemia in elderly hypertensive women. *J Hum Hypertens* 2002;16:631–635.

Sharma AM, Pischon T, Hardt S, et al. Hypothesis: beta-adrenergic receptor blockers and weight gain: a systematic analysis. *Hypertension* 2001;37:250–254.

Sharma AM, Wagner T, Marsalek P. Moxonidine in the treatment of overweight and obese patients with the metabolic syndrome: a postmarketing surveillance study. *J Hum Hypertens* 2004;18:669–675.

Shea S, Misra D, Ehrlich MH, et al. Predisposing factors for severe, uncontrolled hypertension in an inner-city minority population. *N Engl J Med* 1992;327:776–781.

Sheu WH-H, Swislocki ALM, Hoffman BB, et al. Effect of prazosin treatment on HDL kinetics in patients with hypertension. *Am J Hypertens* 1990;3:761–768.

Shimosawa T, Takano K, Ando K, Fujita T. Magnesium inhibits norepinephrine release by blocking N-type calcium channels at peripheral sympathetic nerve endings. *Hypertension* 2004;44:897–902.

Shiuchi T, Iwai M, Li HS, et al. Angiotensin II type-1 receptor blocker valsartan enhances insulin sensitivity in skeletal muscles of diabetic mice. *Hypertension* 2004;43: 1003–1010.

Short AK, Lockwood CM. Antigen specificity in hydralazine associated ANCA positive systemic vasculitis. *QJM* 1995; 88:774–783.

Shotan A, Widerhorn J, Hurst A, Elkayam U. Risks of angiotensin-converting enzyme inhibition during pregnancy. *Am J Med* 1994;96:451–456.

Sica DA. Current concepts of pharmacotherapy in hypertension. Thiazide-type diuretics: ongoing considerations on mechanism of action. *J Clin Hypertens* 2004a;6:661–664.

Sica DA. Minoxidil: an underused vasodilator for resistant or severe hypertension. *J Clin Hypertens* 2004b;6:283–287.

Sica DA, Black HR. Current concepts of pharmacotherapy in hypertension. ACE inhibitor-related angioedema: Can angiotensin-receptor blockers be safely used? *J Clin Hypertens* 2002;4:375–380.

Sica DA, Weber M. The Losartan Intervention for Endpoint Reduction (LIFE) trial—have angiotensin-receptor blockers come of age? *J Clin Hypertens* 2002;4:301–305.

Singel DJ, Stamler JS. Blood traffic control. *Nature* 2004; 430:297.

Singer GM, Izhar M, Black HR. Goal-oriented hypertension management: translating clinical trials to practice. *Hypertension* 2002;40:464–469.

Singer GM, Izhar M, Black HR. Guidelines for hypertension: are quality-assurance measures on target? *Hypertension* 2004;43:198–202.

Siscovick DS, Raghunathan TE, Wicklund KG, et al. Diuretic therapy for hypertension and the risk of primary cardiac arrest. *N Engl J Med* 1994;330:1852–1857.

Sleight P, Yusuf S, Pogue J, et al. Blood-pressure reduction and cardiovascular risk in HOPE study. *Lancet* 2001; 358:2130–2131.

Snow V, Barry P, Fihn SD, et al. Primary care management of chronic stable angina and asymptomatic suspected or known coronary artery disease: a clinical practice guideline from the American College of Physicians. *Ann Intern Med* 2004;141:562–567.

Snow V, Weiss KB, Mottur-Pilson C. The evidence base for tight blood pressure control in the management of type 2 diabetes mellitus. *Ann Intern Med* 2003;138: 587–592.

Sofowora GG, Dishy V, Muszkat M, et al. A common beta1-adrenergic receptor polymorphism (Arg389Gly) affects blood pressure response to beta-blockade. *Clin Pharmacol Ther* 2003;73:366–371.

Solomon DH, Schneeweiss S, Levin R, Avorn J. Relationship between COX-2 specific inhibitors and hypertension. *Hypertension* 2004;44:140–145.

Somes GW, Pahor M, Shorr RI, et al. The role of diastolic blood pressure when treating isolated systolic hypertension. *Arch Intern Med* 1999;159:2004–2009.

Sørensen HT, Mellemkjær L, Olsen JH. Risk of suicide in users of beta-adrenoceptor blockers, calcium channel blockers and Angiotensin-converting enzyme inhibitors. *Br J Clin Pharmacol* 2001;52:313–318.

Sörgel F, Ettinger B, Benet LZ. The true composition of kidney stones passed during triamterene therapy. *J Urol* 1985;134:871–873.

Sorkin EM, Heel RC. Guanfacine. *Drugs* 1986;31:301–336.

Spirito P, Seidman CE, McKenna WJ, Maron BJ. The management of hypertrophic cardiomyopathy. *N Engl J Med* 1997;336:774–785.

Spranger CB, Ries AJ, Berge CA, et al. Identifying gaps between guidelines and clinical practice in the evaluation and treatment of patients with hypertension. *Am J Med* 2004;117:14–18.

Staessen JA, Fagard R, Thijs L, et al. Randomised double-blind comparison of placebo and active treatment for older patients with isolated systolic hypertension. *Lancet* 1997; 350:757–764.

Staessen JA, Gasowski J, Wang JG, et al. Risks of untreated and treated isolated systolic hypertension in the elderly. *Lancet* 2000;355:865–872.

Staessen JA, Thijisq L, Fagard R, et al. Effects of immediate versus delayed antihypertensive therapy on outcome in the Systolic Hypertension in Europe Trial. *J Hypertens* 2004; 22:847–857.

Staessen JA, Wang J-G, Thijs L. Cardiovascular protection and blood pressure reduction: a quantitative overview updated until 1 March 2003. *J Hypertens* 2003;21:1055–1076.

Stafford RS, Furberg CD, Finkelstein SN, et al. Impact of clinical trial results on national trends in alpha-blocker prescribing, 1996–2002. *JAMA* 2004;291:54–62.

Stanton A, Jensen C, Nussberger J, O'Brien E. Blood pressure lowering in essential hypertension with an oral renin inhibitor, aliskiren. *Hypertension* 2003;42:1137–1143.

Steiner JF, Earnest MA. The language of medication-taking. *Ann Intern Med* 2000;132:926–930.

Steinman MA, Fischer MA, Shlipak MG, et al. Clinician awareness of adherence to hypertension guidelines. *Am J Med* 2004;117:747–754.

Stenvinkel P, Alvestrand A. Loop diuretic-induced pancreatitis with rechallenge in a patient with malignant hypertension and renal insufficiency. *Acta Med Scand* 1988; 224:89–91.

Stergiou GS, Efstathiou SP, Roussias LG, Mountokalakis TD. Comparison of intraindividual blood pressure responses to ACE inhibition and angiotensin blockade [Abstract]. *Am J Hypertens* 2004;17:123A.

Stergiou GS, Malakos JS, Achimastos AD, Mountokalakis TD. Additive hypotensive effect of a dihydropyridine calcium antagonist to that produced by a thiazide diuretic. *J Cardiovasc Pharmacol* 1997;29:412–416.

Stokes GS. Systolic hypertension in the elderly: pushing the frontiers of therapy—a suggested new approach. *J Clin Hypertens* 2004;6:192–197.

Stokes GS, Barin ES, Gilfillan KL. Effects of isosorbide mononitrate and AII inhibition on pulse wave reflection in hypertension. *Hypertension* 2003;41:297–301.

Stokes GS, Bune AJ, Huon N, Barin ES. Long-term effectiveness of extended-release nitrate for the treatment of systolic hypertension. *Hypertension* 2005;45:380.

Stokes GS, Graham RM, Gain JM, Davis PR. Influence of dosage and dietary sodium on the first-dose effects of prazosin. *Br Med J* 1977;1:1507–1508.

Strandgaard S, Haunsø S. Why does antihypertensive treatment prevent stroke but not myocardial infarction? *Lancet* 1987;2:658–661.

Strandgaard S, Paulson OB. Antihypertensive drugs and cerebral circulation. *Eur J Clin Invest* 1996;26:625–630.

Strippoli GF, Craig M, Deeks JJ, et al. Effects of Angiotensin-converting enzyme inhibitors and angiotensin II receptor antagonists on mortality and renal outcomes in diabetic nephropathy: systematic review. *BMJ* 2004;329:828.

Struthers AD, MacDonald TM. Review of aldosterone- and angiotensin II-induced target organ damage and prevention. *Cardiovasc Res* 2004;61:663–670.

Sugerman HJ, Wolfe LG, Sica DA, Clore JN. Diabetes and hypertension in severe obesity and effects of gastric bypass-induced weight loss. *Ann Surg* 2003;237:751–756.

Sullivan TJ. Cross-reactions among furosemide, hydrochlorothiazide, and sulfonamides. *JAMA* 1991;265: 120–121.

Svensson M, Gustafsson F, Galatius S, et al. Hyperkalaemia and impaired renal function in patients taking spironolactone for congestive heart failure: retrospective study. *BMJ* 2003;327:1141–1142.

Svensson P, de Faire U, Sleight P, et al. Comparative effects of ramipril on ambulatory and office blood pressures: a HOPE substudy. *Hypertension* 2001;38:E28–E32.

Talseth T, Westlie L, Daae L. Doxazosin and atenolol as monotherapy in mild and moderate hypertension. *Am Heart J* 1991;121:280–285.

Tamirisa KP, Aaronson KD, Koelling TM. Spironolactone-induced renal insufficiency and hyperkalemia in patients with heart failure. *Am Heart J* 2004;148:1–8.

Tan KW, Leenen FHH. Persistence of antihypertensive effect after missed dose of perindopril. *Br J Clin Pharmacol* 1999;48:628–630.

Tanasescu M, Leitzmann MF, Rimm EB, Hu FB. Physical activity in relation to cardiovascular disease and total mortality among men with type 2 diabetes. *Circulation* 2003; 107:2435–2439.

Tandon P, McAlister FA, Tsuyuki RT, et al. The use of beta-blockers in a tertiary care heart failure clinic: dosing, tolerance, and outcomes. *Arch Intern Med* 2004;164: 769–774.

Tang YL, Tang Y, Zhang YC, et al. Protection from ischemic heart injury by a vigilant heme oxygenase-1 plasmid system. *Hypertension* 2004;43:746–751.

Tanner LA, Bosco LA. Gynecomastia associated with calcium channel blocker therapy. *Arch Intern Med* 1988;148: 379–380.

Tannergren C, Engman H, Knutson L, et al. St John's wort decreases the bioavailability of R- and S-verapamil through induction of the first-pass metabolism. *Clin Pharmacol Ther* 2004;75:298–309.

Tanser PH, Campbell LM, Carranza J, et al. Candesartan cilexetil is not associated with cough in hypertensive patients with enalapril-induced cough. *Am J Hypertens* 2000; 13:214–218.

Taylor AL, Ziesche S, Yancy C, et al. Combination of isosorbide dinitrate and hydralazine in blacks with heart failure. *N Engl J Med* 2004;351:2049–2057.

Tenenbaum A, Grossman E, Shemesh J, et al. Intermediate but not low doses of aspirin can suppress angiotensin-converting enzyme inhibitor-induced cough. *Am J Hypertens* 2000;13:776–782.

Tenenbaum A, Motro M, Jones M, et al. Is diuretic therapy associated with an increased risk of colon cancer? *Am J Med* 2001;110:143–145.

Teo K, Yusuf S, Sleight P, et al. Rationale, design, and baseline characteristics of 2 large, simple, randomized trials evaluating telmisartan, ramipril, and their combination in high-risk patients: the Ongoing Telmisartan Alone and in Combination with Ramipril Global Endpoint Trial/Telmisartan Randomized Assessment Study in ACE Intolerant Subjects with Cardiovascular Disease (ONTARGET/TRANSCEND) trials. *Am Heart J* 2004;148:52–61.

Testa MA. Methods and applications of quality-of-life measurement during antihypertensive therapy. *Curr Hypertens Rep* 2000;2:530–537.

Thöne-Reineke C, Zimmermann M, Neumann C, et al. Are angiotensin receptor blockers neuroprotective? *Curr Hypertens Rep* 2004;6:257–266.

Thorp ML, Ditmer DG, Nash MK, et al. A study of the prevalence of significant increases in serum creatinine following angiotensin-converting enzyme inhibitor administration. *J Hum Hypertens* 2005;19:389–392.

Thulin T, Hedneer T, Gustafsson S, Olsson S-O. Diltiazem compared with metoprolol as add-on-therapies to diuretics in hypertension. *J Human Hypertens* 1991;5:107–114.

Thurman JM, Schrier RW. Comparative effects of angiotensin-converting enzyme inhibitors and angiotensin receptor blockers on blood pressure and the kidney. *Am J Med* 2003;114:588–598.

Tomlinson J, Wright D. Impact of erectile dysfunction and its subsequent treatment with sildenafil: qualitative study. *BMJ* 2004;328:1037–1040.

Toner JM, Brawn LA, Yeo WW, Ramsay LE. Adequacy of twice daily dosing with potassium chloride and spironolactone in thiazide treated hypertensive patients. *Br J Clin Pharmacol* 1991;31:457–461.

Tonkin AL. Postural hypotension. *Med J Aust* 1995;162: 436–438.

Toto RD, Mitchell HC, Lee H-C, et al. Reversible renal insufficiency due to Angiotensin-converting enzyme inhibitors in hypertensive nephrosclerosis. *Ann Intern Med* 1991;115:513–519.

Townsend RR, Holland OB. Combination of converting enzyme inhibitor with diuretic for the treatment of hypertension. *Arch Intern Med* 1990;150:1174–1183.

Traon AP, Costes-Salon MC, Galinier M, et al. Dynamics of cerebral blood flow autoregulation in hypertensive patients. *J Neurol Sci* 2002;195:139–144.

Traub YM, Rabinov M, Rosenfeld JB, Treuherz S. Elevation of serum potassium during beta blockade. *Clin Pharmacol Ther* 1980;28:764–768.

Tuomilehto J, Lindstrom J, Eriksson JG, et al. Prevention of type 2 diabetes mellitus by changes in lifestyle among subjects with impaired glucose tolerance. *N Engl J Med* 2001;344:1343–1350.

U.S. Department of Transportation. *Guide for Aviation Medical Examiners*. Washington, DC: Federal Aviation Administration, October 1999;95–98.

Uzu T, Kimura G. Diuretics shift circadian rhythm of blood pressure from nondipper to dipper in essential hypertension. *Circulation* 1999;100:1635–1638.

Valantine H, Keogh A, McIntosh N, et al. Cost containment: coadministration of diltiazem with cyclosporine after heart transplantation. *J Heart Lung Transplant* 1992;11:1–8.

Valdés G, Soto ME, Croxatto HR, et al. Effects of nifedipine during low, normal and high intakes of sodium in patients with essential hypertension. *Clin Sci* 1982;63:447S–450S.

van Brummelen P, Man in't Veld AJ, Schalekamp MA. Hemodynamic changes during long-term thiazide treatment of essential hypertension in responders and nonresponders. *Clin Pharmacol Ther* 1980;27:328–336.

van der Heijden AG, Huysmans FT, van Hamersvelt HW. Foot volume increase on nifedipine is not prevented by pretreatment with diuretics. *J Hypertens* 2004;22:425–430.

van der Heijden M, Donders SH, Cleophas TJ, et al. A randomized, placebo-controlled study of loop diuretics in patients with essential hypertension. *J Clin Pharmacol* 1998;38:630–635.

van Zwieten PA. Beneficial interactions between pharmacological, pathophysiological and hypertension research. *J Hypertens* 1999a;17:1787–1797.

van Zwieten PA. The renaissance of centrally acting antihypertensive drugs. *J Hypertens* 1999b;17(Suppl 3):S15–S21.

Vanhees L, Defoor JG, Schepers D, et al. Effect of bisoprolol and atenolol on endurance exercise capacity in healthy men. *J Hypertens* 2000;18:35–43.

Vasavada N, Saha C, Agarwal R. A double-blind randomized crossover trial of two loop diuretics in chronic kidney disease. *Kidney Int* 2003;64:632–640.

Verdecchia P, Angeli F, Borgioni C, et al. Changes in cardiovascular risk by reduction of left ventricular mass in hypertension: a meta-analysis. *Am J Hypertens* 2003;16:895–899.

Verma S, Strauss M. Angiotensin receptor blockers and myocardial infarction. *BMJ* 2004;329:1248–1249.

Veterans Administration Cooperative Study on Antihypertensive Agents. Double blind control study of antihypertensive agents, II: further report on the comparative effectiveness of reserpine, reserpine and hydralazine, and three ganglion blocking agents, chlorisondamine, mecamylamine, and pentolinium tartrate. *Arch Intern Med* 1962;110:222–229.

Vijan S, Hayward RA. Treatment of hypertension in type 2 diabetes mellitus: blood pressure goals, choice of agents, and setting priorities in diabetes care. *Ann Intern Med* 2003;138:593–602.

Vincent J, Harris SI, Foulds G, et al. Lack of effect of grapefruit juice on the pharmacokinetics and pharmacodynamics of amlodipine. *Br J Clin Pharmacol* 2000;50:455–463.

Vlasses PH, Koffer H, Ferguson RK, Green PJ, McElwain GE. Captopril withdrawal after chronic therapy. *Clin Exp Hypertens* 1981;3:929–937.

Vokó Z, Bots ML, Hofman A, et al. J-shaped relation between blood pressure and stroke in treated hypertensives. *Hypertension* 1999;34:1181–1185.

Volini IF, Flaxman N. The effect of nonspecific operations on essential hypertension. *JAMA* 1939;112:2126–2128.

Wagner ML, Walters AS, Coleman RG, et al. Randomized, double-blind, placebo-controlled study of clonidine in restless legs syndrome. *Sleep* 1996;19:52–58.

Wald NJ, Law MR. A strategy to reduce cardiovascular disease by more than 80%. *BMJ* 2003;326:1419.

Wall GC, Bigner D, Craig S. Ethacrynic acid and the sulfa-sensitive patient. *Arch Intern Med* 2003;163:116–117.

Wallace AW, Galindez D, Salahieh A, et al. Effect of clonidine on cardiovascular morbidity and mortality after noncardiac surgery. *Anesthesiology* 2004;101:284–293.

Wallin BG, Frisk-Holmberg M. The antihypertensive mechanism of clonidine in man. Evidence against a generalized reduction of sympathetic activity. *Hypertension* 1981;3:340–346.

Walma EP, Hoes AW, van Dooren C, et al. Withdrawal of long term diuretic medication in elderly patients. *BMJ* 1997;315:464–468.

Wang PS, Bohn RL, Knight E, et al. Noncompliance with antihypertensive medications: the impact of depressive symptoms and psychosocial factors. *J Gen Intern Med* 2002;17:504–511.

Warner NJ, Rush JE. Safety profiles of the angiotensin-converting enzyme inhibitors. *Drugs* 1988;35:89–97.

Wassertheil-Smoller S, Psaty B, Greenland P, et al. Association between cardiovascular outcomes and antihypertensive drug threatment in older women. *JAMA* 2004;292:2849–2859.

Webb DJ, Fulton JD, Leckie BJ, et al. The effect of chronic prazosin therapy on the response of the renin-angiotensin system in patients with essential hypertension. *J Hum Hypertens* 1987;1:194–200.

Weber KT. Furosemide in the long-term management of heart failure: the good, the bad, and the uncertain. *J Am Coll Cardiol* 2004;44:1308–1310.

Weber MA, Byyny RL, Pratt H, et al. Blood pressure effects of the angiotensin II receptor blocker, losartan. *Arch Intern Med* 1995;155:405–411.

Webster J, Koch H-F. Aspects of tolerability of centrally acting antihypertensive drugs. *J Cardiovasc Pharmacol* 1996;27:S49–S54.

Weidmann P, de Chätel R, Ziegler WH, et al. Alpha and beta adrenergic blockade with orally administered labetalol in hypertension. *Am J Cardiol* 1978;41:570–576.

Weinberger MH. The use of selective aldosterone antagonists. *Curr Hypertens Rep* 2004;6:342–345.

Weinberger MH, Fineberg NS. Sodium and volume sensitivity of blood pressure. *Hypertension* 1991;18:67–71.

Weir MR, Moser M. Diuretics and beta-blockers: is there a risk for dyslipidemia? *Am Heart J* 2000;139:174–184.

Weir MR, Prisant LM, Papademetriou V, et al. Antihypertensive therapy and quality of life. *Am J Hypertens* 1996;9:854–859.

Weir MR, Rosenberger C, Fink JC. Pilot study to evaluate a water displacement technique to compare effects of diuretics and ACE inhibitors to alleviate lower extremity edema due to dihydropyridine calcium antagonists. *Am J Hypertens* 2001;14:963–968.

Weiss A, Chagnac A, Beloosesky Y, et al. Orthostatic hypotension in the elderly: are the diagnostic criteria adequate? *J Hum Hypertens* 2004;18:301–305.

Wessell AM, Ornstein SM, Nietert PJ, et al. Achieving blood pressure control in patients with diabetes: a case study in primary care. *Top Health Inf Manage* 2003;24:3–7.

Whang R, Flink EB, Dyckner T, et al. Magnesium depletion as a cause of refractory potassium repletion. *Arch Intern Med* 1985;145:1686–1689.

Whelton PK, Appel LJ, Espeland MA, et al. Sodium reduction and weight loss in the treatment of hypertension in older persons. *JAMA* 1998;279:839–846.

White HD. Should all patients with coronary disease receive angiotensin-converting-enzyme inhibitors? *Lancet* 2003; 362:755–757.

White WB, Lacourciere Y, Davidai G. Effects of the angiotensin II receptor blockers telmisartan versus valsartan on the circadian variation of blood pressure: impact on the early morning period. *Am J Hypertens* 2004a;17:347–353.

White WB, Lacourciere Y, Gana T, et al. Effects of graded-release diltiazem versus ramipril, dosed at bedtime, on early morning blood pressure, heart rate, and the rate-pressure product. *Am Heart J* 2004b;148:628–634.

Whitworth JA. 2003 World Health Organization (WHO)/International Society of Hypertension (ISH) statement on management of hypertension. *J Hypertens* 2003;21:1983–1992.

Widmer P, Maibach R, Knzi UP, et al. Diuretic-related hypokalaemia. *Eur J Clin Pharmacol* 1995;49:31–36.

Wigley FM. Raynaud's Phenomenon. *N Engl J Med* 2002; 347:1001–1008.

Wiklund I, Halling K, Ryden-Bergsten T, et al. What is the effect of lowering the blood pressure on quality of life? *Arch Mal Couer Vaiss* 1999;92:1079–1082.

Wilcox CS. Metabolic and adverse effects of diuretics. *Semin Nephrol* 1999;19:557–568.

Wilcox CS, Mitch WE, Kelly RA, et al. Response of the kidney to furosemide. I. Effects of salt intake and renal compensation. *J Lab Clin Med* 1983;102:450–458.

Wilcox RG. Randomised study of six beta-blockers and a thiazide diuretic in essential hypertension. *BMJ* 1978;2: 383–385.

Wilkinson GR. Drug metabolism and variability among patients in drug response. *N Engl J Med* 2005;352:2211–2221.

Williams B. Protection against stroke and dementia: an update on the latest clinical trial evidence. *Curr Hypertens Rep* 2004;6:307–313.

Williams B, Poulter NR, Brown MJ, et al. British Hypertension Society guidelines for hypertension management 2004 (BHS-IV): summary. *BMJ* 2004a;328:634–640.

Williams B, Poulter NR, Brown MJ, et al. Guidelines for management of hypertension: report of the fourth working party of the British Hypertension Society, 2004-BHS IV. *J Hum Hypertens* 2004b;18:139–185.

Williams TA, Mulatero P, Filigheddu F, et al. Role of HSD11B2 polymorphisms in essential hypertension and the diuretic response to thiazides. *Kidney Int* 2005;67:631–637.

Wilson IM, Freis ED. Relationship between plasma and extracellular fluid volume depletion and the antihypertensive effect of chlorothiazide. *Circulation* 1959;20:1028–1036.

Wilson JF. Frailty—and its dangerous effects—might be preventable. *Ann Intern Med* 2004;141:489–492.

Wilson MF, Haring O, Lewin A, et al. Comparison of guanfacine versus clonidine for efficacy, safety and occurrence of withdrawal syndrome in step-2 treatment of mild to moderate essential hypertension. *Am J Cardiol* 1986;57: 43E–49E.

Winer BM. The antihypertensive mechanisms of salt depletion induced by hydrochlorothiazide. *Circulation* 1961;24: 788–796.

Wing LM, Reid CM, Ryan P, et al. A comparison of outcomes with angiotensin-converting-enzyme inhibitors and diuretics for hypertension in the elderly. *N Engl J Med* 2003;348:583–592.

Wolf-Maier K, Cooper RS, Kramer H, et al. Hypertension treatment and control in five European countries, Canada, and the United States. *Hypertension* 2004;43:10–17.

Woo KS, Nicholls MG. High prevalence of persistent cough with Angiotensin-converting enzyme inhibitors in Chinese. *Br J Clin Pharmacol* 1995;40:141–144.

Wood R. Bronchospasm and cough as adverse reactions to the ACE inhibitors captopril, enalapril and lisinopril. *Br J Clin Pharmacol* 1995;39:264–270.

Woodwell DA, Cherry DK. National Ambulatory Medical Care Survey: 2002 summary. *Adv Data* 2004;346:1–44.

Woolhandler S, Campbell T, Himmelstein DU. Costs of health care administration in the United States and Canada. *N Engl J Med* 2003a;349:768–775.

Woolhandler S, Himmelstein DU, Angell M, Young QD. Proposal of the Physicians' Working Group for Single-Payer National Health Insurance. *JAMA* 2003b;290:798–805.

Wright JT Jr, Sica DA, Gana TJ, et al. Antihypertensive efficacy of night-time graded-release diltiazem versus morning amlodipine in African Americans. *Am J Hypertens* 2004;17:734–742.

Würzner G, Gerster J-C, Chiolero A, et al. Comparative effects of losartan and irbesartan on serum uric acid in hypertensive patients with hyperuricaemia and gout. *J Hypertens* 2001;19:1855–1860.

Xie F, Petitti DB, Chen W. Prescribing patterns for antihypertensive drugs after the Antihypertensive and Lipid-Lowering Treatment to Prevent Heart Attack Trial: report of experience in a health maintenance organization. *Am J Hypertens* 2005;18:464–469.

Yadav JS, Wholey MH, Kuntz RE, et al. Protected carotid-artery stenting versus endarterectomy in high-risk patients. *N Engl J Med* 2004;351:1493–1501.

Yakovlevitch M, Black HR. Resistant hypertension in a tertiary care clinic. *Arch Intern Med* 1991;151:1786–1792.

Yang HYT, Erdös EG, Levin YA. Dipeptidyl carboxypeptidase that converts angiotensin I and inactivates bradykinin. *Biochem Biophys Acta* 1970;214:374–376.

Yasunari K, Maeda K, Watanabe T, et al. Comparative effects of valsartan versus amlodipine on left ventricular mass and reactive oxygen species formation by monocytes in hypertensive patients with left ventricular hypertrophy. *J Am Coll Cardiol* 2004;43:2116–2123.

Yeo WW, Chadwick IG, Kraskiewics M, et al. Resolution of ACE inhibitor cough. *Br J Clin Pharmacol* 1995;40: 423–429.

Yki-Järvinen H. Thiazolidinediones. *N Engl J Med* 2004; 351:1106–1118.

Yuan J-M, Castelao JE, Gago-Dominguez M, et al. Hypertension, obesity and their medications in relation to renal cell carcinoma. *Br J Cancer* 1998;77:1508–1513.

Zacest R, Gilmore E, Koch-Weser J. Treatment of essential hypertension with combined vasodilation and beta-adrenergic blockade. *N Engl J Med* 1972;286:617–622.

Zanchetti A. Clinical pharmacodynamics of nebivolol: new evidence of nitric oxide-mediated vasodilating activity and peculiar haemodynamic properties in hypertensive patients. *Blood Press Suppl* 2004;1:17–32.

Zanchetti A, Crepaldi G, Bond MG, et al. Different effects of antihypertensive regimens based on fosinopril or hydrochlorothiazide with or without lipid lowering by pravastatin on progression of asymptomatic carotid atherosclerosis: principal results of PHYLLIS—a randomized double-blind trial. *Stroke* 2004;35:2807–2812.

Zanchetti A, Hansson L, Leonetti G, et al. Low-dose aspirin does not interfere with the blood pressure-lowering effects of antihypertensive therapy. *J Hypertens* 2002;20:1015–1022.

Zannad F, Alla F, Dousset B, et al. Limitation of excessive extracellular matrix turnover may contribute to survival benefit of spironolactone therapy in patients with congestive heart failure: insights from the randomized aldactone evaluation study (RALES). Rales Investigators. *Circulation* 2000;102:2700–2706.

Zarnke KB, Feldman RD. Direct Angiotensin-converting enzyme inhibitor-mediated venodilation. *Clin Pharmacol Ther* 1996;59:559–568.

Zhu Z, Zhu S, Liu D, et al. Thiazide-like diuretics attenuate agonist-induced vasoconstriction by calcium desensitization linked to rho kinase. *Hypertension* 2005;45:233–239.

Zimlichman R, Shargorodsky M, Wainstein J. Prolonged treatment of hypertensive patients with low dose HCTZ improves arterial elasticity but not if they have NIDDM or IFG. Treatment with full dose HCTZ (25 mg/d) aggravates metabolic parameters and arterial stiffness [Abstract]. *Am J Hypertens* 2004;17:138A.

Zuccalá G, Pahor M, Landi F, et al. Use of calcium antagonists and need for perioperative transfusion in older patients with hip fracture. *BMJ* 1997;314:643–644.

# Hypertensive Crises

Although only a small spot in the large panorama of hypertension, hypertensive crises represent, on one hand, the most immediate danger to those afflicted and, on the other, the most dramatic proof of the lifesaving potential of antihypertensive therapy. Such crises are less likely now to be the end result of chronic hypertension but may be seen at any age, representing the manifestations of suddenly developing hypertension from such diverse causes as substance abuse, immunosuppressive drugs, and human immunodeficiency virus infection (Vaughn & Delanty, 2000).

## DEFINITIONS

A *hypertensive emergency* is a situation that requires immediate reduction in blood pressure (BP) with parenteral agents because of acute or progressing target organ damage (Table 8–1).

A *hypertensive urgency* is a situation with markedly elevated BP but without severe symptoms or progressive target organ damage, wherein the BP should be reduced within hours, often with oral agents. Some of the circumstances listed in Table 8–1 may be urgencies rather than emergencies if of lesser severity, including some patients with accelerated-malignant hypertension, perioperative or rebound hypertension, less severe body

burn, or epistaxis. The distinction between an emergency and an urgency is often ambiguous.

*Accelerated-malignant hypertension* represents markedly elevated BP with papilledema (grade 4 Keith-Wagener retinopathy) and/or hemorrhages and exudates (grade 3 Keith-Wagener retinopathy). The clinical features and prognosis are similar with grade 3 or grade 4 retinopathy (Ahmed et al., 1986).

*Hypertensive encephalopathy* is a sudden, marked elevation of BP with severe headache and altered mental status, reversible by reduction of BP. Encephalopathy is more common in previously normotensive individuals whose pressures rise suddenly, such as during pregnancy with eclampsia; the accelerated-malignant course often appears without encephalopathy in individuals with more chronic hypertension whose pressures progressively rise.

## ACCELERATED-MALIGNANT HYPERTENSION

### Mechanisms

When BP reaches some critical level—in experimental animals at a mean arterial pressure of 150 mm Hg—lesions appear in arterial walls, and the syndrome of accelerated-malignant hypertension begins (Figure 8–1). This may be provoked by one or more vasoactive factors, but the accelerated-malignant phase is likely to be a nonspecific consequence of very high BP (Beilin & Goldby, 1977). Any form of hypertension may progress to the accelerated-malignant phase, some without activation of the renin-angiotensin system or other known humoral mechanisms (Gavras et al., 1975).

## TABLE 8-1

### Hypertensive Emergencies

Accelerated-malignant hypertension with papilledema

Cerebrovascular conditions

    Hypertensive encephalopathy

    Atherothrombotic brain infarction with severe hypertension

    Intracerebral hemorrhage

    Subarachnoid hemorrhage

    Head trauma

Cardiac conditions

    Acute aortic dissection

    Acute left ventricular failure

    Acute or impending myocardial infarction

    After coronary bypass surgery

Renal conditions

    Acute glomerulonephritis

    Renovascular hypertension

    Renal crises from collagen-vascular diseases

    Severe hypertension after kidney transplantation

Excess circulating catecholamines

    Pheochromocytoma crisis

    Food or drug interactions with monoamine oxidase inhibitors

    Sympathomimetic drug use (cocaine)

    Rebound hypertension after sudden cessation of antihypertensive drugs

    Automatic hyperreflexia after spinal cord injury

Eclampsia

Surgical conditions

    Severe hypertension in patients requiring immediate surgery

    Postoperative hypertension

    Postoperative bleeding from vascular suture lines

Severe body burns

Severe epistaxis

Thrombotic thrombocytopenic purpura

### Structural Changes

In animal models, the level of the arterial pressure correlates closely with the development of fibrinoid necrosis, the experimental hallmark of accelerated-malignant hypertension (Byrom, 1974). In humans, fibrinoid necrosis is rare, perhaps because those who die from an acute attack have not had time to develop the lesion, and those who live with therapy are able to repair it. The typical lesions, best seen in the kidney, are hyperplastic arteriosclerosis and accelerated glomerular obsolescence (Kitiyakara & Guzman, 1998).

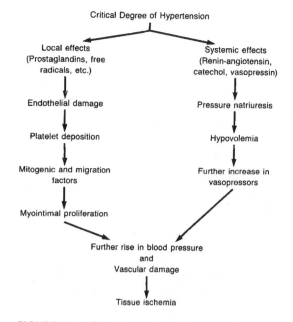

FIGURE 8–1 ● Scheme for initiation and progression of accelerated-malignant hypertension.

### Humoral Factors

There is support, however, for the involvement of factors besides the level of the BP in setting off the accelerated-malignant phase (Kincaid-Smith, 1991). As shown on the right side of Figure 8–1, in both rats (Gross et al., 1975) and dogs (Dzau et al., 1981) with unilateral renal artery stenosis, the accelerated-malignant phase was preceded by natriuresis that markedly activated the renin-angiotensin system. The progression was delayed by giving saline loads after the natriuresis.

Whether these animal models involving a major insult to renal blood flow are applicable to most human accelerated-malignant hypertension is uncertain; however, renal artery stenosis is a common cause of accelerated-malignant hypertension in humans, found in 20% to 35% of patients with this form of hypertension (Davis et al., 1979; Webster et al., 1993).

Evidence for the pathway shown on the left side of Figure 8–1 includes the presence of circulating endothelial and platelet microparticles in patients with severe uncontrolled hypertension (Preston et al., 2003) and markers of endothelial dysfunction and platelet activation in patients with malignant hypertension (Lip et al., 2001).

### Clinical Features

Accelerated-malignant hypertension may be accompanied by various symptoms and signs (Table 8–2).

## TABLE 8–2

### Clinical Characteristics of Accelerated–Malignant Hypertension

Blood pressure: usually >140 mm Hg diastolic

Funduscopic findings: hemorrhages, exudates, papilledema

Neurologic status: headache, confusion, somnolence, stupor, vision loss, focal deficits, seizures, coma

Renal status: oliguria, azotemia

Gastrointestinal status: nausea, vomiting

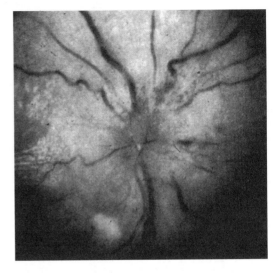

**FIGURE 8–2** ● Funduscopic photography showing typical features of accelerated-malignant hypertension.

However, it is not uncommon to see patients, particularly young Black men, who deny any prior symptoms when seen in the end stages of the hypertensive process, with their kidneys destroyed, heart failing, and brain function markedly impaired. Even in the elderly, hypertension may initially present in the accelerated-malignant phase (Lip et al., 2000).

Less common clinical presentations include:

- Fibrinoid necrosis within abdominal arteries producing major gastrointestinal tract infarction with an acute abdomen (Padfield, 1975).
- Acute pancreatitis (Mathur & Warren, 1989).
- Rapidly progressive necrotizing vasculitis as a feature of lupus (Mitchell, 1994) or polyarteritis nodosa (Blaustein et al., 2004).

### Funduscopic Findings

The effects of the markedly elevated BP are displayed in the optic fundi (Figure 8–2). Acute changes may include arteriolar spasm, either segmental or diffuse; retinal edema, with a sheen or ripples; retinal hemorrhages, either superficial and flame-shaped or deep and dot-shaped; retinal exudates, either hard and waxy from resorption of edema or with a raw cotton appearance from ischemia; and papilledema and engorged retinal veins.

Similar retinopathy with hemorrhages and even papilledema rarely occurs in severe anemia, collagen diseases, and subacute bacterial endocarditis. Some patients have pseudopapilledema associated with congenital anomalies, hyaline bodies (drusen) in the disc, or severe farsightedness. Fluorescein fundus photography will distinguish between the true and the pseudo states. In addition, benign intracranial hypertension may produce real papilledema but is usually a minimally symptomatic and self-limited process (Jain & Rosner, 1992).

### Evaluation

In addition to an adequate history and physical examination, a few laboratory tests should be done immediately to assess the patient's status (Table 8–3).

### Laboratory Findings

#### Hematology and Urine Analysis

Microangiopathic hemolytic anemia with red cell fragmentation and intravascular coagulation may occur in accelerated-malignant hypertension, possibly originating from the fibrinoid necrotic arterial lesions (van den Born et al., 2005).

The urine contains protein and red cells. In a few patients, acute oliguric renal failure may be the presenting manifestation (Lip et al., 1997).

#### Blood Chemistry

Various features of renal insufficiency may be present. Approximately half of patients have hypokalemia, reflecting secondary aldosteronism from increased renin secretion induced by intrarenal ischemia (Kawazoe et al., 1987). Hyponatremia is usual and can be extreme (Trivelli et al., 2005), in contrast to the hypernatremia found in primary aldosteronism.

#### Cardiography

The electrocardiogram usually displays evidence of left ventricular hypertrophy, strain, and lateral ischemia. Echocardiography may show significant left ventricular hypertrophy, systolic dysfunction and dilated left atria (Nadar et al., 2005).

### Evaluation for Identifiable Causes

Once causes for the presenting picture other than severe hypertension are excluded and necessary

## TABLE 8-3

### Initial Evaluation of Patients with a Hypertensive Emergency

History
   Prior diagnosis and treatment of hypertension
   Intake of pressor agents: street drugs, sympathomimetics
   Symptoms of cerebral, cardiac, and visual dysfunction
Physical examination
   Blood pressure
   Funduscopy
   Neurologic status
   Cardiopulmonary status
   Body fluid volume assessment
   Peripheral pulses
Laboratory evaluation
   Hematocrit and blood smear
   Urine analysis
   Automated chemistry: creatinine, glucose, electrolytes
   Plasma renin activity and aldosterone (if primary aldosteronism is suspected)
   Plasma renin activity before and 1 h after 25 mg captopril (if renovascular hypertension is suspected)
   Spot urine or plasma for metanephrine (if pheochromocytoma is suspected)
Chest radiograph (if heart failure or aortic dissection is suspected)
Electrocardiogram

immediate therapy is provided, an appropriate evaluation for identifiable causes of the hypertension should be performed as quickly as possible. It is preferable to obtain necessary blood and urine samples for required laboratory studies before institution of therapies that may markedly complicate subsequent evaluation. None of these procedures should delay effective therapy.

*Renovascular Hypertension*
Renovascular hypertension is by far the most likely secondary cause and, unfortunately, the one that may be least obvious by history, physical examination, and routine laboratory tests. It should be particularly looked for in older patients with extensive atherosclerosis (see Chapter 10).

A single-dose captopril challenge test, measuring plasma renin activity before and 1 hour after administration of 25 mg captopril, can be performed when the patient presents, because the captopril

will almost certainly lower the BP during the subsequent hour, protecting the patient while helping to rule out—or in—renovascular hypertension.

*Pheochromocytoma*
If there are suggestive symptoms, blood for a plasma metanephrine assay should be collected.

*Primary Aldosteronism*
If significant hypokalemia is noted on the initial blood test, a plasma renin and aldosterone level should be obtained. In most cases of primary aldosteronism presenting with malignant hypertension, plasma renin activity has initially been elevated, later being suppressed as the intrarenal necrotizing process subsides (Suzuki et al., 2002).

## Prognosis

If untreated, most patients with accelerated-malignant hypertension will die within 6 months. The 1-year survival rate was only 10% to 20% without therapy (Dustan et al., 1958). With current therapy, 5-year survival rates of greater than 70% are usual (Lip et al., 2000; Webster et al., 1993), clearly showing the major protection provided by antihypertensive therapy.

### Renal Function and Prognosis

Many patients when first seen with accelerated-malignant hypertension have significant renal damage, which markedly worsens their prognosis (van den Born et al., 2005). In one series of 100 consecutive patients with malignant hypertension (Bing et al., 1986), the 5-year survival rate of those without renal impairment (serum creatinine <1.5 mg/dL) was 96%, no different from that of the general population. However, among those with renal impairment, 5-year survival fell to 65%. When vigorous antihypertensive therapy is begun, renal function often worsens transiently, but in nearly half of those with initial renal insufficiency, function remains invariant or improves (Lip et al., 1997). Of 54 patients with malignant hypertension requiring dialysis, 12 recovered sufficient renal function to allow withdrawal of dialysis (James et al., 1995).

### Causes of Death

Therapy used over the past 50 years has dramatically reduced immediate deaths from acute renal failure, hemorrhagic strokes, and congestive heart failure. With longer survival, death from an acute myocardial infarction (MI) is more likely (Webster et al., 1993), but death from renal failure is still common in those who present with an elevated serum creatinine (Lip et al., 2000).

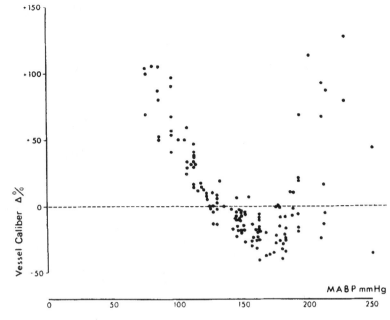

**FIGURE 8–3** ● Observed change in the caliber of pial arterioles with a caliber of less than 50 mm in eight cats, calculated as a percentage of change from the caliber at a mean arterial blood pressure (MABP) of 135 mm Hg. The blood pressure was raised by intravenous infusion of angiotensin II. (Reprinted from MacKenzie ET, Strandgaard S, Graham DI, et al. Effects of acutely induced hypertension in cats on pial arteriolar caliber, local cerebral blood flow, and the blood-brain barrier. *Circ Res* 1976;39:33, with permission.)

## HYPERTENSIVE ENCEPHALOPATHY

With or without the structural defects of accelerated-malignant hypertension, progressively higher BP can lead to hypertensive encephalopathy.

## Pathophysiology

### Breakthrough Vasodilation

With changes in BP, cerebral vessels dilate or constrict to maintain a relatively constant level of cerebral blood flow (CBF), the process of autoregulation that is regulated by sympathetic nervous activity (Tuor, 1992). Figure 8–3 shows direct measurements taken in cats, with progressive vasodilation as pressures are lowered and progressive vasoconstriction as pressures rise (MacKenzie et al., 1976). Note, however, that when mean arterial pressures reach a critical level, approximately 180 mm Hg, the previously constricted vessels, unable to withstand such high pressures, are stretched and dilated—first in areas with less muscular tone, producing irregular sausage-string patterns, and later diffusely, producing generalized vasodilation. This vasodilation allows a breakthrough of CBF, which hyperperfuses the brain under high pressure, with leakage of fluid into the perivascular tissue, leading to cerebral edema and the clinical syndrome of hypertensive encephalopathy (Strandgaard & Paulson, 1989).

Breakthrough vasodilation has also been demonstrated in humans (Strandgaard et al., 1973). Figure 8–4 shows curves of autoregulation constructed by measuring CBF repetitively while arterial BP was lowered by vasodilators or raised by vasoconstrictors. Cerebral blood flow is constant between mean arterial pressures of 60 and 120 mm Hg in normotensive subjects. However, when pressure was raised beyond the limit of autoregulation, breakthrough hyperperfusion occurred.

Pressures such as these are handled without obvious trouble in chronic hypertensives, whose blood

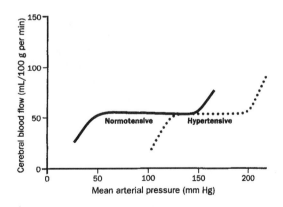

**FIGURE 8–4** ● Idealized curves of cerebral blood flow at varying levels of systemic blood pressure in normotensive and hypertensive subjects. Rightward shift in autoregulation is shown with chronic hypertension. (Adapted from Strandgaard S, Olesen J, Skinhøj E, Lassen NA. Autoregulation of brain circulation in severe arterial hypertension. *BMJ* 1973;1:507–510.)

vessels adapt to the chronically elevated BP with structural thickening, presumably mediated by sympathetic nerves (Tuor, 1992). Thereby the entire curve of autoregulation is shifted to the right (Figure 8–4). Even with this shift, breakthrough will occur if mean arterial pressures are markedly raised to levels beyond 180 mm Hg.

These findings explain a number of clinical observations. Previously normotensive people who suddenly become hypertensive may develop encephalopathy at relatively low levels of hypertension, which are nonetheless beyond their upper limit of autoregulation. These include children with acute glomerulonephritis and young women with eclampsia. On the other hand, chronically hypertensive patients less commonly develop encephalopathy and only at much higher pressures.

In regard to the lower portion of the curve, when the BP is lowered by antihypertensive drugs too quickly, chronic hypertensives often are unable to tolerate the reduction without experiencing cerebral hypoperfusion, manifested by weakness and dizziness. These symptoms may appear at levels of BP that are still well within the normal range of autoregulation and well tolerated by normotensives. The reason is that the entire curve of autoregulation shifts, so that the lower end also is moved, with a fall-off of CBF at levels of 100 to 120 mm Hg mean arterial pressure (Figure 8–4). Moreover, chronic hypertensives may lose their ability to autoregulate, increasing their risk of cerebral ischemia when BP is lowered acutely (Jansen et al., 1987).

As detailed in Chapter 7, if the BP is lowered gradually, the curve can shift back toward normal so that greater reductions in pressure can eventually be tolerated. However, maneuvers that increase CBF further and thereby increase intracranial pressure, such as $CO_2$ inhalation or cerebral vasodilators (e.g., hydralazine and nitroprusside), may be harmful in patients with encephalopathy.

### Central Nervous System Changes

Encephalopathic patients have many of the same laboratory findings seen in patients with malignant hypertension, but they have more central nervous system manifestations. The cerebrospinal fluid rarely shows pleocytosis (McDonald et al., 1993) but is usually under increased pressure. Computed tomography or magnetic resonance imaging shows a characteristic posterior leukoencephalopathy predominantly affecting the parietooccipital white matter, often the cerebellum and brainstem (Karampekios et al., 2004), and occasionally other areas as well (Vaughan & Delanty, 2000).

## Differential Diagnosis

There are clinical situations in which the BP is elevated and the patient has findings that suggest hypertension-induced target organ damage wherein the findings are unrelated to the elevated BP. Table 8–4 lists conditions that may mimic a hypertensive emergency. A less aggressive approach to lowering of the BP is indicated in such patients. Particular caution is warranted after a stroke, when a rapid decrease in BP may shunt blood away from the ischemic area and extend the lesion (Adams et al., 2005).

In addition to the two specific presentations of accelerated-malignant hypertension and hypertensive encephalopathy, hypertension may be life threatening when it accompanies other acute conditions wherein a markedly elevated BP contributes to the ongoing tissue damage (Table 8–1). The role of hypertension in most of these conditions is covered in Chapter 4, and some of the other specific circumstances (e.g., pheochromocytoma crises and eclampsia) are covered in their respective chapters.

## THERAPY FOR HYPERTENSIVE EMERGENCIES

The majority of patients with the conditions shown in Table 8–1 require immediate reduction in BP. In those patients with hypertensive encephalopathy, if

### TABLE 8–4

### Conditions That May Mimic a Hypertensive Emergency

Acute left ventricular failure

Uremia, particularly with volume overload

Cerebrovascular accident

Subarachnoid hemorrhage

Brain tumor

Head injury

Epilepsy (postictal)

Collagen diseases, particularly systemic lupus, with cerebral vasculitis

Encephalitis

Drug ingestion: sympathomimetics (e.g., cocaine)

Acute intermittent porphyria

Hypercalcemia

Acute anxiety with hyperventilation syndrome or panic attack the pressure is not reduced, cerebral edema will worsen, and the lack of autoregulation in ischemic brain tissue may result in further increases in the volume of the ischemic tissue, which may cause either acute herniation or more gradual compression of normal brain.

On the other hand, the shift to the right of the curve of cerebral autoregulation in most patients who develop encephalopathy exposes them to the hazards of a fall in CBF when systemic pressure is lowered abruptly by more than approximately 25%, even though these levels are not truly hypotensive (Immick et al., 2004; Strandgaard & Paulson, 1996) (Figure 8–4).

## Initiating Therapy

With encephalopathy or evidence of progressive myocardial ischemia, no more than a very few minutes should be taken to admit a patient to an intensive care unit, set up intravenous access, and begin frequent monitoring of the BP, usually with automatic syphygmomanometry. The initial blood and urine samples should be obtained, and antihypertensive therapy should begin immediately thereafter.

## Monitoring Therapy

Abrupt falls in pressure should be avoided, and the goal of immediate therapy should be to lower the diastolic pressure only to approximately 110 mm Hg. The reductions may need to be even less if signs of tissue ischemia develop as the pressure is lowered. Most of the catastrophes seen with treatment of hypertensive emergencies were related to overly aggressive reduction of the BP (Jansen et al., 1987).

Particular care should be taken in elderly patients and in patients with known cerebrovascular disease, who are even more vulnerable to sudden falls in systemic BP (Fischberg et al., 2000). In patients with recent ischemic stroke, the American Stroke Association recommends cautious reduction of BP by 10% to 15% if systolic levels are above 220 mm Hg or diastolic above 120 mm Hg (Adams et al., 2005).

If the neurologic status worsens as treatment proceeds, urgent computed tomography of the brain should be obtained and, if potentially life-threatening cerebral edema is identified, osmotic diuresis with mannitol, often plus intravenous furosemide, can be effective (Brott & Bogousslavsky, 2000). It may be possible to monitor intracranial pressure and cerebral autoregulation noninvasively (Schmidt et al, 2003).

## Parenteral Drugs

Table 8–5 lists the choices of parenteral therapy now available. All are capable of inducing hypotension, a risk that mandates careful monitoring of BP. They are covered in the order shown in Table 8–5.

### Diuretics

A potent diuretic, usually furosemide, is often initially given intravenously. In one controlled trial involving 64 patients with hypertensive encephalopathy and diastolic pressure above 135 mm Hg, 40 mg intravenous furosemide alone brought the pressure down from an average of 225/144 to 166/102 mm Hg over 5 hours in 12 patients (McNair et al., 1986). The remaining 52 patients still had a diastolic pressure higher than 125 mm Hg 1 hour after the furosemide; they were given additional therapy.

Even if not given initially, a diuretic will likely be needed after other antihypertensives are used, because reactive renal sodium retention usually accompanies a fall in pressure and may blunt the efficacy of nondiuretic agents. On the other hand, if the patient is volume-depleted from pressure-induced natriuresis and prior nausea and vomiting, additional diuresis could be dangerous. In a few documented instances, volume expansion with intravenous saline has been shown to lower the BP (Baer et al., 1977; Kincaid-Smith, 1973).

### Nitroprusside

The BP always falls when nitroprusside is given, although it occasionally takes much more than the usual starting dose of 0.25 µg/kg per minute for a response. The antihypertensive effect disappears within minutes after the drug is stopped. Obviously, the drug should be used only with constant monitoring of the BP, preferably with a computer-controlled device (Chitwood et al., 1992).

The nitric oxide that is part of the nitroprusside structure induces immediate arteriolar and venous dilation with no effects on the autonomic or central nervous system (Mansoor & Frishman, 2002). Nitroprusside is metabolized to cyanide by sulfhydryl groups in red cells, and the cyanide is rapidly metabolized to thiocyanate in the liver (Schulz, 1984). If high levels of thiocyanate (>10 mg/dL) remain for days, toxicity may be manifested as fatigue, nausea, disorientation, and psychosis. If cyanide toxicity is suspected because of metabolic acidosis and venous hyperoxemia, nitroprusside should be discontinued, and 4 to 6 mg of 3% sodium nitrite given intravenously over 2 to 4 minutes, followed by an infusion of 50 mL of 25% sodium thiosulfate

## TABLE 8–5

### Parenteral Drugs for Treatment of Hypertensive Emergency

| Drug[a] | Dose | Onset of Action | Duration of Action | Adverse Effects[b] | Special Indications |
|---|---|---|---|---|---|
| **DIURETICS** | | | | | |
| Furosemide | 20–40 mg in 1–2 min, repeated and higher doses with renal insufficiency | 5–15 min | 2–3 h | Volume depletion, hypokalemia | Usually needed to maintain efficacy of other drugs |
| **VASODILATORS** | | | | | |
| Nitroprusside (Nipride, Nitropress) | 0.25–10.00 µg/kg per min as i.v. infusion | Immediate | 1–2 min | Nausea, vomiting, muscle twitching, sweating, thiocyanate and cyanide intoxication | Most hypertensive emergencies; caution with high intracranial pressure or azotemia |
| Nitroglycerin (Nitro-bid IV) | 5–100 µg per min as i.v. infusion | 2–5 min | 5–10 min | Headache, vomiting, methemoglobinemia, tolerance with prolonged use | Coronary ischemia |
| Fenoldopam (Corlopam) | 0.1–0.6 µg/kg per min as i.v. infusion | 4–5 min | 10–15 min | Reflex tachycardia, increased intraocular pressure, headache | Renal insufficiency, after surgery |
| Nicardipine[c] (Cardene IV) | 5–15 mg per h as i.v. | 5–10 min | 1–4 h | Headache, nausea, flushing, tachycardia, local phlebitis | Most hypertensive emergencies; caution with acute heart failure |
| Hydralazine (Apresoline) | 5–20 mg as i.v. 10–40 mg IM | 10–20 min 20–30 min | 1–4 h 4–6 h | Tachycardia, flushing, headache, vomiting, aggravation of angina | Eclampsia; caution with high intracranial pressure |
| Enalaprilat (Vasotec IV) | 1.25–5 mg every 6 h | 15 min | 6 h | Precipitous fall in pressure in high-renin states; response variable | Acute left ventricular failure |
| **ADRENERGIC INHIBITORS** | | | | | |
| Phentolamine | 5–15 mg as i.v | 1–2 min | 3–10 min | Tachycardia, flushing, headache | Catecholamine excess |
| Esmolol (Brevibloc) | 200–500 µg/kg per min for 4 min, then 50–300 µg/kg per min as i.v. | 1–2 min | 10–20 min | Hypotension, nausea | Aortic dissection, after operation |
| Labetalol (Normodyne, Trandate) | 20–80 mg as i.v. bolus every 10 min or 2 mg per min as i.v. infusion | 5–10 min | 3–6 h | Vomiting, scalp tingling, burning in throat, dizziness, nausea, heart block, orthostatic hypotension | Most hypertensive emergencies except acute heart failure |

[a]In order of rapidity of action. [b]Hypotension may occur with any. [c]Intravenous formulations of other calcium channel blockers are also available.

(Gifford, 1991). Cyanide toxicity has been prevented by concomitant administration of hydroxocobalamin (Zerbe & Wagner, 1993).

### Nitroglycerin

Intravenous nitroglycerin is often chosen for patients with myocardial ischemia since it dilates coronary vessels and decreases myocardial wall tension and oxygen consumption (Mansoor & Frishman, 2002). Like nitroprusside, it causes cerebral vasodilation and can increase intracranial pressure (Dahl et al., 1989). Methemoglobin is formed during the administration of all organic nitrates, but its mean concentration in patients receiving nitroglycerin for 48 hours or longer averaged only 1.5%, with no clinical symptoms (Kaplan et al., 1985).

### Fenoldopam

Fenoldopam, a peripheral dopamine-I agonist, unlike other parenteral antihypertensive agents, maintains or increases renal perfusion while it lowers BP (Murphy et al., 2001). It maintains most of its efficacy for 48 hours of constant rate infusion without rebound hypertension when discontinued. Although theoretically attractive in maintaining renal perfusion, it was no better than nitroprusside when compared in a sequential study of 43 patients with hypertensive emergencies (Devlin et al., 2004).

### Nicardipine and Other Calcium Channel Blockers

When given by continuous infusion, the intravenous formulations of various dihydropyridine calcium channel blockers (CCBs) produce a steady, progressive fall in BP with little change in heart rate and a small increase in cardiac output (Mansoor & Frishman, 2002). Nicardipine has been found to provide responses virtually equal to those seen with nitroprusside, with few side effects (Neutel et al., 1994). Other intravenous CCBs also are effective, including verapamil (Brush et al., 1989). Nimodipine, with an apparently greater selectivity for cerebral vessels, has been approved for use in relieving the vasospasm that accompanies subarachnoid hemorrhage (Wong & Haley, 1990) but was detrimental in patients after ischemic stroke (Fogelholm et al., 2004).

### Hydralazine

The direct vasodilator hydralazine can be given by repeated intramuscular injections as well as intravenously with a fairly slow onset and prolonged duration of action, allowing for less intensive monitoring. Significant compensatory increases in cardiac output preclude its use as a sole agent except in young patients, as with preeclampsia, who can handle the increased cardiac work without the likelihood that coronary ischemia will be induced. Hydralazine's primary use is for severe hypertension during pregnancy, as noted in Chapter 11.

### Enalaprilat

Enalaprilat, the intravenous preparation of the active, free form of the prodrug enalapril, may be used for treatment of hypertensive emergencies wherein angiotensin-converting enzyme (ACE) inhibition is thought to offer special advantages, such as in severe congestive heart failure (CHF) (Varriale et al., 1993). An initial dose of 0.625 mg is as effective as larger doses and may be less likely to induce severe hypotension in those with high renin-angiotensin levels (Hirschl et al., 1997). Angiotensin-converting enzyme inhibitors (ACEI) and angiotensin II-receptor blockers (ARBs) may maintain cerebral regulation, resetting the autoregulatory curve to a lower pressure level and thereby could be safer than direct vasodilators (Strandgaard, 2004).

### Phentolamine

The α-blocker phentolamine is specifically indicated for pheochromocytoma or tyramine-induced catecholamine crisis.

### Esmolol

Esmolol, a relatively cardioselective β-blocker, is rapidly metabolized by blood esterases and has a short (approximately 9-minute) half-life and total duration of action (approximately 30 minutes). Its effects begin almost immediately, and it has found particular use during anesthesia to prevent postintubation hemodynamic perturbations (Oxorn et al., 1990).

### Labetalol

The combined α- and β-blocker labetalol has been found to be both safe and effective when given intravenously either by repeated bolus (Huey et al., 1988) or by continuous infusion (Leslie et al., 1987). It starts acting within 5 minutes, and its effects last for 3 to 6 hours. Labetalol can likely be used in almost any situation requiring parenteral antihypertensive therapy, except when left ventricular dysfunction could be worsened by the predominant β-blockade. Caution is needed to avoid postural hypotension if patients are allowed out of bed. Nausea, itching, tingling of the skin, and β-blocker side effects may be noted.

### Criteria for Drug Selection

Because no clinical comparisons are available of the eventual outcome after the use of various agents, the choice of therapy is based on rapidity of action, ease of administration, and propensity for side effects. Although nitroprusside has been most widely used and most authors continue to cite it as the preferred choice for most hypertensive emergencies, nitroprusside's propensity to increase intracranial pressure and the need for constant monitoring support the wider use of other effective parenteral agents such as labetalol, nicardipine, and fenoldopam.

The management of hypertensive emergencies in a number of special circumstances is considered in other chapters of this book: renal insufficiency, Chapter 9; eclampsia, Chapter 11; pheochromocytoma, Chapter 12; drug abuse, Chapter 15; and, in children and adolescents, Chapter 16.

## THERAPY FOR HYPERTENSIVE URGENCIES

Hypertensive urgencies, including some cases of accelerated-malignant hypertension or perioperative or rebound hypertension, can usually be managed with oral therapy. The management of the overwhelming majority of patients who are found to have a very high BP but who are asymptomatic and in little danger of rapidly progressive target organ damage, referred to as *uncontrolled severe hypertension* rather than a *hypertensive urgency,* is considered at the end of this chapter.

In particular, patients in a surgical recovery room or a nursing home whose BP is found to be above some arbitrary danger level such as 180/110 mm Hg should not automatically be given sublingual nifedipine or any other antihypertensive drug. This practice has been widespread. In a 2-month survey

in three hospitals, 3.4% of all patients had been given sublingual nifedipine: 63% of the orders were given over the telephone for arbitrary and asymptomatic BP elevations and 98% with no bedside evaluation (Rehman et al., 1996).

Rather than such inappropriate prescribing, the proximate causes for abrupt increases in BP should be identified and managed (e.g., hypoxia, pain, or volume overload in the postoperative patient; a distended bladder, disturbed sleep, or arthritic pain in the nursing home patient). Only if the BP remains above 180/110 mm Hg after 15 to 30 minutes may there be a need for additional antihypertensive therapy but not for rapid and precipitous reduction of BP as may be induced by sublingual nifedipine. If such rises in BP are frequent, appropriate increases in long-term therapy may be indicated.

### Choice of Oral Agents

Virtually every available antihypertensive drug with a fairly short onset of action has been shown to be effective in patients with uncontrolled, severe hypertension. None is clearly better than the rest, and a combination will often be needed for long-term control. Those most widely used are listed in Table 8–6; complete information about them is provided in Chapter 7.

### *Nifedipine*

The rapidly acting formulation of the CCB nifedipine has been widely used for the treatment of hypertensive urgencies (Grossman et al., 1996). Liquid nifedipine in a capsule will usually lower

## TABLE 8–6

### Oral Drugs for Hypertensive Urgencies

| Drug | Class | Dose | Onset | Duration (h) |
|------|-------|------|-------|--------------|
| Captopril (Capoten) | Angiotensin-converting enzyme inhibitor | 6.5–50.0 mg | 15 min | 4–6 |
| Clonidine (Catapres) | Central α-agonist | 0.2 mg initially, then 0.1 mg per h, up to 0.8 mg total | 0.5–2.0 h | 6–8 |
| Furosemide (Lasix) | Diuretic | 20–40 mg | 0.5–1.0 h | 6–8 |
| Labetalol (Normodyne, Trandate) | α- and β-blocker | 100–200 mg | 0.5–2.0 h | 8–12 |
| Nifedipine (Procardia, Adalat) | Calcium channel blocker | 5–10 mg | 5–15 min | 3–5 |
| Propranolol (Inderal) | β-blocker | 20–40 mg | 15–30 min | 3–6 |

BP after a single 5- or 10-mg oral dose (Maharaj & van der Byl, 1992). The drug is effective even more quickly when the capsule is chewed and the contents are swallowed than when it is squirted under the tongue (van Harten et al., 1987).

As might be expected with any drug that induces such a significant and rapid fall in BP, with no way to titrate or overcome the response, occasional symptomatic hypotension can occur, resulting in severe cerebral or cardiac ischemia (Grossman et al., 1996). Grossman et al. (1996), therefore, recommended that the use of short-acting nifedipine be abandoned. However, if taken in the unbroken capsule, it seems no more likely to cause a precipitous fall in BP than other short-acting agents (e.g., captopril). Certainly, there is no place for such short-acting formulations in the chronic treatment of hypertension, but if the BP needs to be lowered over a few hours, short-acting nifedipine is an acceptable choice. Other slower and, therefore, possibly safer oral CCB formulations such as short-acting diltiazem, felodipine, or verapamil can be used (Shayne & Pitts, 2003).

### Captopril

Captopril is the fastest acting of the oral ACEIs now available, and it can also be used sublingually in patients who cannot swallow (Angeli et al., 1991). As noted earlier in this chapter, an ACEI may be particularly attractive because it shifts the entire curve of cerebral autoregulation to the left, so CBF should be well maintained as the systemic BP falls (Barry, 1989).

Abrupt and marked first-dose hypotension after an ACEI has been observed rarely, usually in patients with an activated renin-angiotensin system (Postma et al., 1992). Caution is advised in patients who have significant renal insufficiency or who are volume-depleted. Despite the small potential for hypotension, oral captopril may be the safest of nonparenteral agents for urgent hypertension.

### Clonidine

Clonidine, a central α-agonist, has been widely used in repeated hourly doses to safely and effectively reduce very high BP (Jaker et al., 1989). Significant sedation is the major side effect that contraindicates its use in patients with central nervous system involvement. Because it has a greater proclivity than other drugs to cause rebound hypertension if it is suddenly discontinued, it should not be used by patients who have demonstrated poor compliance with therapy. Despite its past popularity, clonidine seems to be a most unattractive drug for such patients.

### Labetalol

The α- and β-blocker labetalol has been given in hourly oral doses ranging from 100 to 200 mg. It has reduced elevated pressures as effectively as repeated doses of oral nifedipine; it works somewhat more slowly and, perhaps, more safely (McDonald et al., 1993).

### Diuretics

Diuretics, specifically furosemide or bumetanide, often are needed in patients with hypertensive urgencies, both to lower the BP by getting rid of excess volume and to prevent the loss of potency from nondiuretic antihypertensives because of their tendency to cause fluid retention as they lower blood pressure. However, volume depletion may be overdone, particularly in patients who start off with a shrunken fluid volume. Thereby renin secretion may be further increased, producing more intensive vasoconstriction and worsening the hypertension.

## Management After Acute Therapy

After the patient is out of danger, a careful search should continue for possible identifiable causes, as delineated earlier in this chapter in the section "Evaluation." Identifiable causes, in particular renovascular hypertension, are much more likely in patients with severe hypertension.

After control of the acute presentation, most patients will likely require multiple drug therapy, and chronic treatment should likely begin with a diuretic and an appropriate second agent. The guidelines delineated in Chapter 7 should be followed to ensure adherence to effective therapy.

## UNCONTROLLED SEVERE HYPERTENSION

Most patients who are diagnosed and treated as a hypertensive urgency are not in the immediate danger of uncontrolled hypertension that this diagnosis connotes. They are simply patients with very high BP, often as a consequence of discontinuing prior therapy, but in no distress. They may need nothing more than observation for a few minutes for the BP to come down to levels not deemed to require immediate therapy (Lima et al., 1997). As shown in Figure 8–5, if BP remains higher than 180/120 mm Hg, such patients should be started on appropriate oral therapy, perhaps with a combination of medications; if prior therapy was successful and well tolerated, that regimen could be restarted; if prior therapy was unsuccessful or not well tolerated, appropriate changes should be

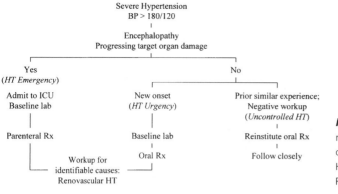

**FIGURE 8–5** ● Pathways for management of patients with severe hypertension, defined as BP in excess of 180/120 mm Hg. HT, hypertension; ICU, intensive care unit; Rx, therapy.

made. If this is the first instance of severe hypertension, a workup for possible identifiable causes should be performed.

Logically, shorter-acting formulations of whatever class of drug that seems appropriate for long-term therapy should be used (Table 8–6). Thus, if a diuretic and an ACEI are to be used chronically, an oral dose of furosemide and captopril could be given acutely.

Although most such patients could be safely started on one or more oral drugs and sent home to return in 24 or 48 hours for confirmation of their responsiveness, it seems preferable to observe them for a few hours after administration of antihypertensive therapy to ensure responsiveness. Once BP is down to a safer level, i.e., below 170/110, chronic therapy should be started.

We will now leave the realm of primary hypertension and look in depth at the various secondary forms of hypertension, starting with the most common: renal parenchymal disease.

## REFERENCES

Adams H, Adams R, Del Zoppo G, Goldstein LB. Guidelines for the early management of patients with ischemic stroke. 2005 Guideline Update: a scientific statement from the Stroke Council of the American Heart Association/American Stroke Association. *Stroke* 2005; 36:916–921.

Ahmed MEK, Walker JM, Beevers DG, Beevers M. Lack of difference between malignant and accelerated hypertension. *BMJ* 1986;292:235–237.

Angeli P, Chiesa M, Caregaro L, et al. Comparison of sublingual captopril and nifedipine in immediate treatment of hypertensive emergencies a randomized, single-blind clinical trial. *Arch Intern Med* 1991;151:678–682.

Baer L, Parra-Carrillo JZ, Radichevich I, Williams GS. Detection of renovascular hypertension with angiotensin II blockade. *Ann Intern Med* 1977;86:257–260.

Barry DI. Cerebrovascular aspects of antihypertensive treatment. *Am J Cardiol* 1989;63:14C–18C.

Beilin LJ, Goldby FS. High arterial pressure versus humoral factors in the pathogenesis of the vascular lesions of malignant hypertension. The case of pressure alone. *Clin Sci Mol Med* 1977;52:111–117.

Bing BF, Heagerty AM, Russell GI, et al. Prognosis in malignant hypertension. *J Hypertens* 1986;4(Suppl 6):42–44.

Blaustein DA, Kumbar L, Srivastava M, Avram MM. Polyarteritis nodosa presenting as isolated malignant hypertension. *Am J Hypertens* 2004;17:380–381.

Brott T, Bogousslavsky J. Treatment of acute ischemic stroke. *N Engl J Med* 2000;343:710–722.

Brush JE Jr, Udelson JE, Bacharach SL, et al. Comparative effects of verapamil and nitroprusside on left ventricular function in patients with hypertension. *J Am Coll Cardiol* 1989;14:515–522.

Byrom FB. The evolution of acute hypertensive arterial disease. *Prog Cardiovasc Dis* 1974;17:31–37.

Chitwood WR Jr, Cosgrove DM III, Lust RM, and the Titrator Multicenter Study Group. Multicenter trial of automated nitroprusside infusion for postoperative hypertension. *Ann Thorac Surg* 1992;54:517–522.

Dahl A, Russell D, Nyberg-Hansen R, Rootwelt K. Effect of nitroglycerin on cerebral circulation measured by transcranial Doppler and SPECT. *Stroke* 1989;20: 1733–1736.

Davis BA, Crook JE, Vestal RE, Oates JA. Prevalence of renovascular hypertension in patients with grade III or IV hypertensive retinopathy. *N Engl J Med* 1979;301: 1273–1276.

Devlin JW, Seta ML, Kanji S, Somerville AL. Fenoldopam versus nitroprusside for the treatment of hypertensive emergency. *Ann Pharmacother* 2004;38:755–759.

Dustan HP, Schneckloth RE, Corcoran AC, Page IH. The effectiveness of long-term treatment of malignant hypertension. *Circulation* 1958;18:644–651.

Dzau VJ, Siwek LG, Rosen S, et al. Sequential renal hemodynamics in experimental benign and malignant hypertension. *Hypertension* 1981;3(Suppl 1):63–68.

Fischberg GM, Lozano E, Rajamani K, et al. Stroke precipitated by moderate blood pressure reduction. *J Emerg Med* 2000;19:339–346.

Fogelholm R, Palomaki H, Erila T, et al. Blood pressure, nimodipine, and outcome of ischemic stroke. *Acta Neurol Scand* 2004;109:200–204.

Gavras H, Brunner HR, Laragh JH, et al. Malignant hypertension resulting from deoxycorticosterone acetate and salt excess. *Circ Res* 1975;36:300–310.

Gifford RW Jr. Management of hypertensive crises. *JAMA* 1991;266:829–835.

Gross F, Dietz R, Mast GJ, Szokol M. Salt loss as a possible mechanism eliciting an acute malignant phase in renal hypertensive rats. *Clin Exp Pharmacol Physiol* 1975;2: 323–333.

Grossman E, Messerli FH, Grodzicki T, Kowey P. Should a moratorium be placed on sublingual nifedipine capsules given for hypertensive emergencies and pseudoemergencies? *JAMA* 1996;276:1328–1331.

Hirschl MM, Binder M, Bur A, et al. Impact of the renin-angiotensin-aldosterone system on blood pressure response to intravenous enalaprilat in patients with hypertensive crises. *J Hum Hypertens* 1997;11:177–183.

Huey J, Thomas JP, Hendricks DR, et al. Clinical evaluation of intravenous labetalol for the treatment of hypertensive urgency. *Am J Hypertens* 1988;1:284S–289S.

Immick RV, van den Born B-JH, van Montfrans GA, et al. Impaired cerebral autoregulation in patients with malignant hypertension. *Circ* 2004;110:2241–2245.

Jain N, Rosner F. Idiopathic intracranial hypertension: report of seven cases. *Am J Med* 1992;93:391–395.

Jaker M, Atkin S, Soto M, et al. Oral nifedipine vs oral clonidine in the treatment of urgent hypertension. *Arch Intern Med* 1989;149:260–265.

James SH, Meyers AM, Milne FJ, Reinach SG. Partial recovery of renal function in black patients with apparent end-stage renal failure due to primary malignant hypertension. *Nephron* 1995;71:29–34.

Jansen PAF, Schulte BPM, Gribnau FWJ. Cerebral ischaemia and stroke as side effects of antihypertensive treatment; special danger in the elderly. A review of the cases reported in the literature. *Neth J Med* 1987;30:193–201.

Kaplan KJ, Taber M, Teagarden JR, et al. Association of methemoglobinemia and intravenous nitroglycerin administration. *Am J Cardiol* 1985;55:181–183.

Karampekios SK, Contopoulou E, Basta M, et al. Hypertensive encephalopathy with predominant brain stem involvement: MRI findings. *J Hum Hypertens* 2004;18: 133–134.

Kawazoe N, Eto T, Abe I, et al. Pathophysiology in malignant hypertension: with special reference to the renin-angiotensin system. *Clin Cardiol* 1987;19:513–518.

Kincaid-Smith P. Malignant hypertension. *J Hypertens* 1991;9:893–899.

Kincaid-Smith P. Management of severe hypertension. *Am J Cardiol* 1973;32:575–581.

Kitiyakara C, Guzman NJ. Malignant hypertension and hypertensive emergencies. *J Am Soc Nephrol* 1998;9: 133–142.

Leslie JB, Kalayjian RW, Sirgo MA, et al. Intravenous labetalol for treatment of postoperative hypertension. *Anesthesiology* 1987;67:413–416.

Lima E Jr, Zytynski LA, Camargo RF, et al. Placebo effects in hypertensive urgency. [Abstract] *Am J Hypertens* 1997; 10 (Suppl 1): 113A.

Lip GYH, Beevers M, Beevers DG. Does renal function improve after diagnosis of malignant phase hypertension? *J Hypertens* 1997;15:1309–1315.

Lip GYH, Beevers M, Beevers DG. Do patients with *de novo* hypertension differ from patients with previously known hypertension when malignant phase hypertension occurs? *Am J Hypertens* 2000;13:934–939.

Lip GY, Edmunds E, Hee FL, et al. A cross-sectional, diurnal, and follow-up study of platelet activation and endothelial dysfunction in malignant phase hypertension. *Am J Hypertens* 2001;14:823–828.

MacKenzie ET, Strandgaard S, Graham DI, et al. Effects of acutely induced hypertension in cats on pial arteriolar caliber, local cerebral blood flow, and the blood-brain barrier. *Circ Res* 1976;39:33–41.

Maharaj B, van der Byl K. A comparison of the acute hypotensive effects of two different doses of nifedipine. *Am Heart J* 1992;124:720–725.

Mansoor GA, Frishman WH. Comprehensive management of hypertensive emergencies and urgencies. *Heart Dis* 2002;4:358–371.

Mathur R, Warren JP. Malignant hypertension presenting as acute pancreatitis. *J Hum Hypertens* 1989;3:479–480.

McDonald AJ, Yealy DM, Jacobson S. Oral labetalol versus oral nifedipine in hypertensive urgencies in the ED. *Am J Emerg Med* 1993;11:460–463.

McNair A, Krogsgaard AR, Hilden T, Nielsen PE. Severe hypertension with cerebral symptoms treated with furosemide, fractionated diazoxide or dihydralazine. Danish Multicenter Study. *Acta Med Scand* 1986;220:15–23.

Mitchell I. Cerebral lupus. *Lancet* 1994;343:579–582.

Murphy MB, Murray C, Shorten GD. Fenoldopam: a selective peripheral dopamine-receptor agonist for the treatment of severe hypertension. *N Engl J Med* 2001;345:1548–1557.

Nadar S, Beevers DG, Lip GYH. Echocardiographic changes in patients with malignant phase hypertension: The West Birmingham Malignant Hypertension Register. *J Human Hypertens* 2005;19:69–75.

Neutel JM, Smith DHG, Wallin D, et al. A comparison of intravenous nicardipine and sodium nitroprusside in the immediate treatment of severe hypertension. *Am J Hypertens* 1994;7:623–628.

Oxorn D, Knox JWD, Hill J. Bolus doses of esmolol for the prevention of perioperative hypertension and tachycardia. *Can J Anaesth* 1990;37:206–209.

Padfield PL. Malignant hypertension presenting with an acute abdomen. *BMJ* 1975;3:353–354.

Postma CT, Dennesen PJW, de Boo T, Thien T. First dose hypotension after captopril: can it be predicted? A study of 240 patients. *J Hum Hypertens* 1992;6:205–209.

Preston RA, Jy W, Jimenez JJ, et al. Effects of severe hypertension on endothelial and platelet microparticles. *Hypertension* 2003;41:211–217.

Rehman F, Mansoor GA, White WB. "Inappropriate" physician habits in prescribing oral nifedipine capsules in hospitalized patients. *Am J Hypertens* 1996;9:1035–1039.

Schmidt B, Czosnyka M, Raabe A, et al. Adaptive noninvasive assessment of intracranial pressure and cerebral autoregulation. *Stroke* 2003;34:84–89.

Schulz V. Clinical pharmacokinetics of nitroprusside, cyanide, thiosulphate and thiocyanate. *Clin Pharmacokinet* 1984; 9:239–251.

Shapiro LM, Beevers DG. Malignant hypertension: cardiac structure and function at presentation and during therapy. *Br Heart J* 1983;49:477–484.

Shayne PH, Pitts SR. Severely increased blood pressure in the emergency department. *Ann Emerg Med* 2003;41: 513–529.

Strandgaard S. The management of elevated blood pressure in acute stroke: preferential use of angiotensin II receptor antagonists? *J Hypertens* 2004;22:877–878.

Strandgaard S, Olesen J, Skinhøj E, Lassen NA. Autoregulation of brain circulation in severe arterial hypertension. *BMJ* 1973;1:507–510.

Strandgaard S, Paulson OB. Antihypertensive drugs and cerebral circulation. *Eur J Clin Invest* 1996;26:625–630.

Strandgaard S, Paulson OB. Cerebral blood flow and its pathophysiology in hypertension. *Am J Hypertens* 1989;2: 486–492.

Suzuki H, Asano K, Eiro M, et al. Recovery from renal failure in malignant hypertension associated with primary aldosteronism: effect of an ACE inhibitor. *Q J Med* 2002; 95:128–130.

Trivelli A, Ghiggeri GM, Canepa A, et al. Hyponatremic-hypertensive syndrome with extensive and reversible renal defects. *Ped Nephrol* 2005;20:101–104.

Tuor UI. Acute hypertension and sympathetic stimulation: local heterogeneous changes in cerebral blood flow. *Am J Physiol* 1992;263:H511–H518.

van den Born BJH, Honnebier UPF, Koopmans RP, van Montfrans GA. Microangiographic hemolysis and renal failure in malignant hypertension. *Hypertension* 2005; 45:246–251.

van Harten J, Burggraaf K, Danhof M, et al. Negligible sublingual absorption of nifedipine. *Lancet* 1987;2:1363–1365.

Varriale P, David W, Chryssos BE. Hemodynamic response to intravenous enalaprit in patients with severe congestive heart failure and mitral regurgitation. *Clin Cardiol* 1993;16: 235–238.

Vaughan CJ, Delanty N. Hypertensive emergencies. *Lancet* 2000;356:411–417.

Webster J, Petrie JC, Jeffers TA, Lovell HG. Accelerated hypertension—patterns of mortality and clinical factors affecting outcome in treated patients. *QJM* 1993;86: 485–493.

Wong MCW, Haley EC Jr. Calcium antagonists: stroke therapy coming of age. *Stroke* 1990;21:494–501.

Zerbe NF, Wagner BKJ. Use of vitamin B12 in the treatment and prevention of nitroprusside-induced cyanide toxicity. *Crit Care Med* 1993;21:465–467.

# CHAPTER 9

# Renal Parenchymal Hypertension

T he kidney is important in most forms of hypertension, either as victim or culprit. As described in Chapter 3, a defect in renal function is almost certainly involved in the pathogenesis of primary hypertension, and renal damage often develops during its course. Clinically, there is often a vicious circle: Hypertension causes renal damage, which causes more hypertension. Moreover, even before hypertension appears, the earliest discernable degree of renal damage—very low levels of microalbuminuria—increases the risk of cardiovascular morbidity and mortality (Ritz, 2005).

As noted in Chapter 1, chronic renal disease (CRD) is the most common of the identifiable causes of hypertension. In the United States, an estimated 11% of the adult population—19.2 million people—have CRD defined as persistent microalbuminuria or a glomerular filtration rate (GFR) below 60 mL/min/1.73m$^2$, and most of them are hypertensive (Coresh et al., 2003). Parenthetically, these estimates are more than twice those based on serum creatinine levels in the same population (Coresh et al., 2001).

The prevalence of CRD increases progressively with increasing levels of BP (Hsu et al., 2005). In the 40,514 high-risk hypertensives enrolled in the Antihypertensive and Lipid-Lowering Treatment to Prevent Heart Attack Trial (ALLHAT), 57% had mild CRD (GFR 60 to 89) and 17.2% had moderate CRD (GFR 30 to 59) (Rahman et al., 2004). Not surprisingly, hypertension is second only to diabetes among the causes of end-stage renal disease (ESRD) (Jones et al., 2005; U.S. Renal Data System, 2003). Moreover, although progression into ESRD may appear to be the primary problem with CRD, increased cardiovascular morbidity and mortality are much more common outcomes, as seen both in trials involving high-risk patients (Mann et al., 2001) and in community-based studies (Go et al., 2004; Weiner et al., 2004). Therefore, the presence of CRD is considered to be a major risk factor for the development of cardiovascular disease (Sarnak et al., 2003).

For multiple reasons, CRD and ESRD will become even more common and use an increasing share of health care expenditures. In the United States, projections from 2000 to the year 2010 indicate almost a doubling of the numbers with over 650,000 patients with ESRD being treated with dialysis and transplants (Levey et al., 2003). By the year 2030, the current projection is more than 2 million ESRD patients (Szczech & Lazar, 2004). The reasons for these marked increases in renal disease are multiple, including the risk factors for the initiation and progression of CRD shown in Table 9–1. Of these, the major roles will be played by the increasing age of the population, the progressive rise in obesity and consequent diabetes mellitus (Fox et al., 2004), and the growing proportion of Hispanics and Blacks, both more susceptible to renal disease (Hsu et al., 2003). Moreover, the incidence of ESRD is growing faster than the prevalence of CRD, largely because of more liberal criteria for entry into ESRD treatment programs (Hsu et al., 2004).

## TABLE 9-1

### Risk Factors for Chronic Kidney Disease and Progression

| Level of Risk | Risk Factors |
| --- | --- |
| Susceptibility factors | Older age, family history of chronic kidney disease, reduction in kidney mass, low birthweight, U.S. racial or ethnic minority status, low income or education |
| Initiation factors | Diabetes, high blood pressure, autoimmune diseases, systemic infections, urinary tract infections, urinary stones, lower urinary tract obstruction, drug toxicity |
| Progression factors | Higher level of proteinuria, higher blood pressure, poor glycemic control in diabetes, smoking |
| End-stage factors | Late referral, lower dialysis dose, nonpermanent vascular access, anemia, low serum albumin level |

Modified from Levey AS, Coresh J, Balk E, et al. National Kidney Foundation practice guidelines for chronic kidney disease: evaluation, classification, and stratification. *Ann Intern Med* 2003;139:137–147.

As noted in Chapter 4, primary hypertension may be less common a cause of progressive renal disease than was previously thought (Kincaid-Smith, 2004). However, over an average 13-year follow-up, CRD, defined as a GFR <60, developed in 14.6% of a closely followed group of 281 hypertensive patients with initially normal GFR (Segura et al., 2004). This percentage is similar to the reported prevalence of microalbuminuria in nondiabetic patients with primary hypertension (de Jong & Brenner, 2004). Moreover, hypertension, if not as often the primary cause for progressive renal disease, almost always develops in the course of all other causes and speeds their progression (Ruggenenti et al., 2000).

As bad as this scenario looks, there is a countervailing, brighter aspect: The control of hypertension undoubtedly can slow, if not stop, the progression of renal damage (Jafar et al., 2003). Therefore, the identification and control of hypertension is the most practical way to slow the onslaught of renal disease (National Kidney Foundation K/DOQI Clinical Practice Guidelines, 2004).

We will now examine specific varieties of renal disease and how they relate to hypertension, starting from acute renal insults and progressing eventually to posttransplantation. Renovascular hypertension is covered in the next chapter. It should always be kept in mind as a potentially curable form of ESRD (Safian & Textor, 2001).

Before proceeding, a word about the measurement of renal function is needed. In the past, the level of serum creatinine has been most widely used, but GFR has long been recognized to be a more accurate assessor (Stevens & Levey, 2004). Glomerular filtration rate is cumbersome to measure, but formulas to calculate GFR from serum creatinine with the patient's age, weight, gender, and race are available. The best of these, the abbreviated Modification of Diet in Renal Disease (MDRD) equation, has been repeatedly found to give an accurate estimate in patients with significant renal damage. However, it underestimates GFR in people with fairly good renal function such as renal donors (Rule et al., 2004). Less error has been reported with computerized networks trained to generate accurate output from input variables (Marshall et al., 2005). Meanwhile, the calculated GFR from the MDRD equation should be provided whenever a serum creatinine is measured. If not provided by the laboratory, the GFR calculation can be provided instantly by accessing these websites: http://www.HDCN.com or http://www.NKF.org.

## ACUTE RENAL DISEASE

A rapid decline in renal function may appear from various causes: prerenal (e.g., volume depletion), intrinsic (e.g., glomerulonephritis), or postrenal (e.g., obstructive uropathy). Nonsteriodal antiinflammatory drugs (NSAIDs) are among the most common causes of acute renal failure, particularly in patients whose already reduced renal perfusion depends on prostaglandin-mediated vasodilation (Huerta et al., 2005). Hypertension is rarely a problem because most of these patients are also volume contracted from prior therapy with diuretics and angiotensin-converting enzyme inhibitor (ACEI) or angiotensin receptor blocker (ARB) therapy (Braden et al., 2004).

### Acute Glomerulonephritis

The classic presentation of acute glomerulonephritis is a child with recent streptococcal pharyngitis or impetigo who suddenly passes dark urine and develops facial edema. The renal injury represents the trapping of antibody-antigen complexes within the glomerular capillaries. Although the syndrome has become less common, it still occurs, sometimes in adults past middle age. Typically, in the acute phase, patients are hypertensive, and there is a close temporal relation between oliguria, edema, and hypertension. On occasion, hypertension of a severe, even malignant, nature may be the overriding feature.

The hypertension should be treated by salt and water restriction and, in mild cases, diuretics and other oral antihypertensives. In keeping with an apparent role of renin, ACEI therapy has been effective (Jardine, 1995). In the classic disease, the patient is free of edema and hypertension within days, of proteinuria within weeks, and of hematuria within months. Hypertension was found in only 3 of 88 children followed up for 10 to 17 years (Popovic-Rolovic et al., 1991).

More common than poststreptococcal glomerulonephritis are a variety of primary renal diseases (e.g., IgA nephropathy) and systemic diseases (e.g., systemic lupus erythematosus) (Chadban & Atkins, 2005). These may present with acute renal crises marked by hypertension (Madaio & Harrington, 2001) that may be effectively treated with an ACEI (Steen & Medsger, 2000).

## Urinary Tract Obstruction and Reflux

Vesicoureteric reflux is seen in 1% to 2% of children and can lead to hypertension, renal scarring, and ESRD (Fanos & Cataldi, 2004). Among 157 hypertensives in India over age 18, vesicourteral reflux was found in 30 (19.1%) without overt evidence of renal parenchymal damage (Barai et al., 2004).

Hypertension may develop after unilateral (Berka et al., 1994) or bilateral (Jones et al., 1987) obstruction to the ureters or the urethra (Robinson et al., 1992). Obstruction in rats is associated with activation of renin and suppression of kallikrein (El-Dahr et al., 1992). In most patients, the hypertension is fairly mild, but significant hypertension and severe renal insufficiency may occur with hydronephrosis from prostatic obstruction (Rule et al., 2005). Catheter drainage of the residual urine may lead to rapid resolution of the hypertension and circulatory overload (Ghose & Harindra, 1989).

## Other Causes of Acute Renal Disease

Other causes of acute renal disease include:

- Bilateral renal artery occlusion, either by emboli or thromboses.
- Removal of angiotensin II support of blood flow with ACEI therapy in the presence of bilateral renal artery disease (Safian & Textor, 2001).
- Trauma to the kidney (Watts & Hoffbrand, 1987).
- Cholesterol emboli, which may shower the kidney after radiologic or surgical procedures, producing

rapidly worsening renal function and hypertension (Vidt, 1997).

- Extracorporeal shock wave lithotripsy for kidney stones, which may be followed by a rise in BP that lasts at least 6 months in 20% to 30% of patients (Hammond et al., 1993). The incidence of persistent hypertension seems quite small (Lingeman et al., 1995), but long-time follow-up is appropriate.

### Renal Donors

Removal of half of a living donor's renal mass could be looked upon as an acute injury, but in normal humans, the removal of a kidney does not result in hypertension, likely because of downward adjustments in glomerular hemodynamics to maintain normal fluid volume (Guidi et al., 2001). However, the possibility of subsequent damage to the remaining kidney has been raised, since removal of one kidney could lead to hyperperfusion and progressive glomerulosclerosis in the other.

No increase in the prevalence of hypertension was found in a meta-analysis of 48 studies with 2,988 patients who had had a unilateral nephrectomy and were carefully followed for a mean follow-up of 10.6 years (range, 2 to 50 years) (Kasiske et al., 1995). Among 148 living donors who were hypertensive before nephrectomy, no adverse effects on either BP or renal function were seen over a 1-year follow-up (Textor et al., 2004). However, 20 of 73 patients who had unilateral nephrectomy for various renal diseases developed proteinuria and CRD (Praga et al., 2000).

As summarized by Gridelli and Remuzzi (2000), "To date, the development of proteinuria in kidney donors has not been correlated with the development of hypertension or with the interval since nephrectomy; moreover, donors in whom proteinuria developed have not had progressive proteinuria or renal failure."

## NONDIABETIC CHRONIC RENAL DISEASE

Of the various discernable primary causes of ESRD among patients starting dialysis in the United States, diabetic nephropathy is the most common, comprising about 40%, followed by vascular diseases, including hypertensive nephrosclerosis (20%), primary glomerular disease (18%), tubulointerstitial diseases (7%), and cystic diseases (5%) (Levey et at., 2003).

The prevalence of hypertension and the responses to antihypertensive therapy differ among the various causes of renal damage: Chronic pyelonephritis may be less commonly associated with hypertension (Goodship et al., 2000); polycystic diseases may be more commonly associated, even before significant renal dysfunction develops (Tee et al., 2004). Patients with these various causes of CRD may start at either end of the spectrum: Hypertension without overt renal damage on the one end and severe renal insufficiency without hypertension on the other. Eventually, however, both groups move toward the middle—renal insufficiency with hypertension—so that hypertension is found in approximately 85% of patients with CRD of diverse causes (Levey et al., 2003) and is closely related to the progression of nephropathy (Hsu et al., 2005). Renal insufficiency as a consequence of primary hypertension is described in Chapter 4. This section examines the development of hypertension as a secondary process in the presence of primary renal disease. Diabetic nephropathy is covered later in this chapter.

Patients whose underlying problem is bilateral renovascular disease may present with refractory hypertension and renal insufficiency (Safian & Textor, 2001). The recognition of the renovascular etiology of these patients' condition is critical, because revascularization may relieve their hypertension and improve their renal function. More about this important group of patients with ischemic nephropathy is provided in the next chapter, as well as hypertension associated with renal tumors.

## Significance

Hypertension is associated with a more rapid progression of renal damage, regardless of the underlying cause. This was demonstrated in the Modification of Diet in Renal Disease (MDRD) study, involving 585 patients with a GFR between 25 and 55 mL per minute and 255 patients with a GFR between 13 and 24 mL per minute (Lazarus et al., 1997). Among those with proteinuria of more than 1 g per day at baseline, the rate of decline in GFR was significantly less over a mean follow-up of 2.2 years in both groups whose BPs remained an average of 5 mm Hg lower as a result of more intensive therapy. After a longer follow-up, those assigned to the lower BP target (mean BP less than 92 mm Hg) had a 32% lower hazard ratio for progressing into ESRD than did those assigned to the usual BP target (mean less than 107 mm Hg) (Sarnak et al., 2005).

As noted in Chapter 4, Blacks develop ESRD at a higher rate, almost fourfold higher than Whites in the large Multiple Risk Factor Intervention Trial population (Klag et al., 1997). Most of their higher risk is derived from their higher prevalence of hypertension (Hsu et al., 2003) and, perhaps, a genetic susceptibility to renal dysfunction when hypertensive (Bochud et al., 2005). Together, these are major contributors to the excess mortality of U.S. Blacks (Young & Gaston, 2000).

In addition to its role in advancing renal damage, hypertension may be the most common risk factor for the many-fold increased risk for cardiovascular diseases seen in patients with renal insufficiency (Weiner et al., 2004).

In patients with CRD, ambulatory blood pressure monitoring, which often identifies a loss of nocturnal dipping, is better than office readings in predicting progression of renal damage and mortality (Mentari & Rahman, 2004). Home monitoring is also more accurate than office readings (Andersen et al., 2005).

## Mechanisms

Hypertension develops and progresses in patients with renal diseases for multiple reasons (Table 9–2). Most of these funnel into a common path: impaired renal autoregulation that normally attenuates the transmission of elevated systemic pressure to the glomeruli (Bidani & Griffin, 2004) because

## TABLE 9–2

### Features Associated with High Blood Pressure in Chronic Kidney Disease

Pre-existing essential hypertension

Extracellular fluid volume expansion

Renin-angiotensin aldosterone system stimulation

Increased sympathetic activity

Endogenous digitalis-like factors

Prostaglandins/bradykinins

Alteration in endothelium-derived factors (nitric oxide/endothelin)

Increased body weight

Insulin resistance

Erythropoietin administration

Parathyroid hormone secretion/increased intracellular calcium/hypercalcemia

Renal vascular disease and renal arterial stenosis

Chronic allograft dysfunction

Cadaver allografts, especially from a donor with a family history of hypertension

Cyclosporine, tacrolimus, other immunosuppresive and corticosteroid therapy

Modified from Levey AS, Coresh J, Bolton K, et al. Clinical practice guidelines for chronic kidney disease. *Am J Kidney Dis* 2002;39:S112–S119.

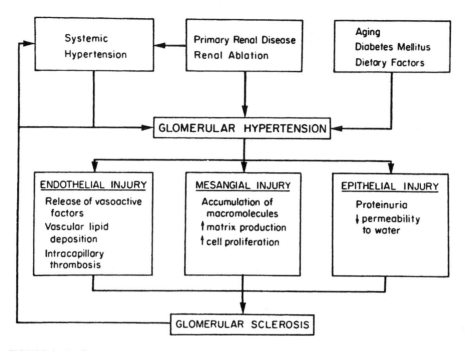

**FIGURE 9–1** ● Pivotal role in glomerular hypertension in the initiation and progression of structural injury. (Modified from Anderson S, Brenner BM. Progressive renal disease: a disorder of adaptation. *QJM* 1989;70:185–189.)

afferent arteriolar resistance fails to increase adequately. The resultant glomerular hypertension damages glomerular cells and leads to progressive sclerosis, setting off a vicious cycle (Anderson & Brenner, 1989) (Figure 9–1).

Of the contributing or aggravating factors listed in Table 9–2, volume expansion from impaired natriuresis has traditionally been given primacy. However, in view of the increased peripheral vascular resistance typically seen in these patients, both an activated renin-angiotensin-aldosterone mechanism (Hollenberg, 2004) and an overactive sympathetic nervous system (Augustyniak et al., 2002; Campese, 2000; Neumann et al., 2004) have received increasing attention.

### Proteinuria

The degree of proteinuria serves as a strong predictor of the rate of progression to ESRD (Zhang et al., 2005). Increased protein trafficking through the glomerular capillaries directly damages podocytes and tubular interstitium (Schieppati & Remuzzi, 2003). The role of heavy proteinuria in progression of renal damage was documented in a meta-analysis of data from 11 randomized controlled trials involving 1,860 patients (Jafar et al., 2003). As seen in Figure 9–2, proteinuria above 1 g per day was associated with a higher relative risk for progression at all levels of systolic blood pressure above 120 mm Hg. The greater the proteinuria, the more the progression. In one trial of patients with nondiabetic CRD, progression of renal damage occurred in one-third of those with proteinuria in the highest tertile (>3.8 g/day) but in only 1 of the 67 in the lowest tertile (<1.9 g/day) (Ruggenenti et al., 1996). Moreover, the degree of change in proteinuria was closely related to the rate of progression of hypertensive renal damage in the African American Kidney Disease and Hypertension (AASK) trial (Lea et al., 2005).

### Management

#### Intensity of Therapy

Reduction of BP and proteinuria has been clearly shown to slow the rate of progression of nondiabetic CRD (Jafar et al., 2003). However, as seen in Figure 9–2, only those with proteinuria above 1 g per day have been shown to benefit from more intensive lowering of BP. This was found in the MDRD study (Lazarus et al., 1997) and reconfirmed in the AASK study (Wright et al., 2002) and in the REIN-2 study (Ruggenenti et al., 2005). In the AASK study, no additional slowing of the progression of CRD was found in those given more therapy to provide an average BP of 128/78 compared to

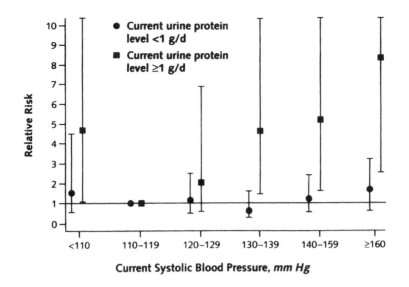

**FIGURE 9–2** ● The relative risk for progression of renal disease in patients with proteinuria either below or above 1 g per day by levels of systolic blood pressure. The reference group (*RR*=1) is a systolic pressure of 110–119 mm Hg. (Modified from Jafar TH, Stark PC, Schmid CH, et al., Progression of chronic kidney disease; the role of blood pressure control, proteinuria, and angiotensin-converting enzyme inhibition: a patient-level meta-analysis. *Ann Intern Med* 2003;139:244–252.)

those given less therapy who ended up with an average BP of 141/85. Therefore, the widely held view, as in JNC-7 (Chobanian et al., 2003), that all patients with CRD should be treated to below 130/80 may be appropriate but remains unproven.

Nonetheless, the overall benefits of lowering BP and proteinuria are undeniable. Many patients who progress into ESRD have not been adequately treated (Levey et al., 2003). Despite the absence of evidence that additional benefit is provided by more intensive therapy in those with proteinuria <1 g per day, there is also no evidence that those more intensively treated have worse outcomes. Moreover, these data apply only to progression of renal disease whereas cardiovascular diseases, the most common cause of death in CRD patients, have been clearly shown to be reduced by further lowering of BP (Chobanian et al., 2003).

## Mode of Therapy

An overall plan of treatment based on that recommended by Schieppati and Remuzzi (2003) is shown in Figure 9–3. The primacy of ACEIs and/or ARBs is accepted by most authorities, but the supporting evidence is slim (Bidani & Griffin, 2004), and some believe it is the lowered BP and not the agent that lowers the BP that matters (Locatelli et al., 2005).

### Dietary Sodium Reduction

The algorithm shown in Figure 9–3 starts with dietary sodium reduction. Patients with CRD may have a narrow range of sodium excretory capacity: If their dietary salt is markedly reduced, they may not be able to conserve sodium and will become volume depleted; if given modest salt loads, they may be unable to excrete enough sodium to prevent volume expansion and hypertension.

Sodium reduction to the range of 1 to 2 g per day (sodium, 44 to 88 mEq per day) is both feasible and often necessary to control the hypertension in these patients (De Nicola et al., 2004). The importance of dietary sodium restriction in proteinuric patients goes beyond the ability to enhance the antihypertensive effect of all drugs (save CCBs). If dietary sodium intake is as high as 200 mmol per day, the antiproteinuric efficacy of both ACEIs (Heeg et al., 1989) and nondihydropyridine CCBs (Bakris & Smith, 1996) may be inhibited, presumably reflecting hyperfiltration induced by the high sodium intake (Weir & Fink, 2005).

### Angiotensin-Converting Enzyme Inhibitors

Angiotensin-converting enzyme inhibitors are recommended for initial antihypertensive drug therapy by most authorities. The evidence favoring the special benefits of ACEIs in patients with nondiabetic CRD is impressive: In the 11 RCTs analyzed

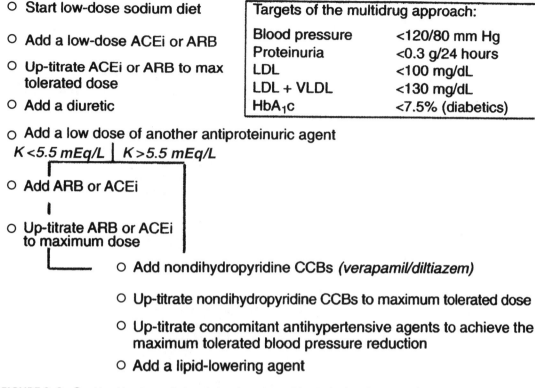

○ Start low-dose sodium diet

○ Add a low-dose ACEi or ARB

○ Up-titrate ACEi or ARB to max tolerated dose

○ Add a diuretic

| Targets of the multidrug approach: | |
|---|---|
| Blood pressure | <120/80 mm Hg |
| Proteinuria | <0.3 g/24 hours |
| LDL | <100 mg/dL |
| LDL + VLDL | <130 mg/dL |
| $HbA_1c$ | <7.5% (diabetics) |

○ Add a low dose of another antiproteinuric agent

*K <5.5 mEq/L* | *K >5.5 mEq/L*

○ Add ARB or ACEi

○ Up-titrate ARB or ACEi to maximum dose

○ Add nondihydropyridine CCBs *(verapamil/diltiazem)*

○ Up-titrate nondihydropyridine CCBs to maximum tolerated dose

○ Up-titrate concomitant antihypertensive agents to achieve the maximum tolerated blood pressure reduction

○ Add a lipid-lowering agent

**FIGURE 9–3** ● Algorithm for remission of chronic nephropathies. In the box the targets for remission are shown. ACEi, angiotensin-converting enzyme inhibitor; ARB, angiotensin II receptor blocker; CCB, calcium channel blocker; LDL, low-density lipoprotein; VLDL, very low-density lipoprotein; $HbA1_c$, hemoglobin A1$_c$. (Adapted from Schieppati A, Remuzzi G. The future of renoprotection: frustration and promises. *Kidney Int* 2003;64:1947–1955.)

by Jafar et al. (2003), the use of an ACEI was associated with a 33% decrease in risk of progression after adjustments for reduction of both blood pressure and proteinuria. In eight RCTs including 142 patients with advanced polycystic kidney disease, ACEIs were effective in reducing proteinuria (Jafar et al., 2005).

Such better effects of ACEIs likely reflect their greater ability to reduce intraglomerular pressure by their preferential dilation of efferent arterioles (Figure 9–4) (Tolins & Raij, 1991). The reduction in intraglomerular pressure protects the glomeruli from progressive sclerosis and reduces the escape of protein into the tubule. At the same time, GFR is reduced and serum creatinine increased, usually to only a small degree. This expected, initial slight lowering of GFR is not a cause for stopping the use of an ACEI and is, in fact, followed by even greater renal protection (Bakris et al., 2000).

If the serum creatinine rises or GFR falls more than 30% of the pre-ACEI level, the ACEI should be stopped and other possible contributing causes identified and corrected, including volume contraction, concomitant use of NSAIDs, or most dramatically, the presence of bilateral renovascular hypertension.

Another reflection of the ACEI-induced inhibition of the renin-angiotensin-aldosterone system is a rise in serum potassium, usually less than 0.5 mEq/L. However, if hyperkalemia above 5.5 mEq/L develops, the dose of ACEI may need to be reduced or the drug discontinued. Obviously, blood chemistries should be monitored within a few days of starting ACEI therapy in patients with CRD, as a rapid and sustained rise in serum creatinine may occur with unrecognized bilateral renovascular disease, or significant hyperkalemia may develop.

***Angiotensin Receptor Blockers***

As seen in Figure 9–3, an ARB may be added in those without hyperkalemia. *Angiotensin receptor blockers* have been shown to be protective in diabetic nephropathy, but there are as yet no RCTs with ARB-based therapy in nondiabetic CRD. There is, however, increasingly convincing evidence of additional reductions of proteinuria when ARBs are added to ACEIs (Andersen & Mogensen, 2004; Campbell et al., 2003; Nakao et al., 2003). Certainly, an ARB should be substituted in those who develop an ACEI-induced cough. As with ACEIs, larger doses of ARBs may further reduce

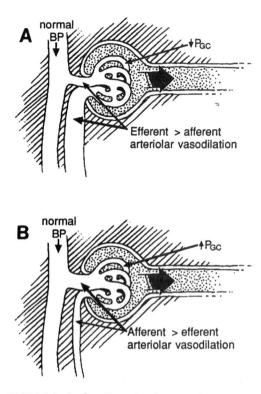

**FIGURE 9–4** ● Effect of antihypertensive treatment on glomerular hemodynamics as determined by micro-puncture studies in rats. (**A**) Angiotensin-converting enzyme inhibition results in normalization of BP associated with vasodilatation, predominantly of the efferent arteriole, resulting in normalization of intraglomerular capillary pressure ($P_{GC}$). (**B**) With calcium channel blockers, reduction of BP is offset by afferent arteriolar vasodilatation, and therefore, $P_{GC}$ remains elevated. (Modified from Tolins JP, Raij L. Antihypertensive therapy and the progression of chronic renal disease. Are there renoprotective drugs? *Semin Nephrol* 1991;11:538–548.)

proteinuria even if BP does not fall further (Laverman et al., 2005).

### Diuretics

All diuretics must gain entry to the tubular fluid and have access to the luminal side of the nephron to work. They reach the tubular fluid by secretion across the proximal tubule by way of organic acid or base secretory pathways. Patients with CRD thus are resistant to acidic diuretics such as thiazides and the loop diuretics, both because of their reduced renal blood flow and because of the accumulation of organic acid end products of metabolism that compete for the secretory pump. To effect diuresis, enough of the diuretic must be given to deliver adequate amounts of the agent to the tubular sites of action. This translates into a "sequential doubling of single doses until a ceiling dose is reached" (Brater, 1988). Once the ceiling dose is reached, that dose should be given as often as needed as a maintenance dose.

As Brater (1988) points out, thiazides would probably work in many CRD patients if given in high enough doses; "however, such a strategy is still not worth pursuing [because of] the low intrinsic efficacy of these drugs compared to loop diuretics." On the other hand, in severely resistant patients, combining a loop diuretic with a thiazide may effect a response when neither is effective alone (Knauf & Mutschler, 1995).

In those with a serum creatinine above 1.5 mg/dL, metolazone may work as well as loop diuretics, with the added benefit of providing a full 24-hour effect with once-a-day dosing (Bennett & Porter, 1973).

Caution should be exercised to avoid excessive diuresis with such potent diuretics, on the one hand, and interference with diuretic action by NSAIDs, on the other. COX-2 inhibitors are likely just as nephrotoxic and interfere as much with sodium excretion as do the older NSAIDs (Braden et al., 2004). Spironolactone, eplerenone, triamterene, and amiloride should be avoided in most patients with severe CRD, because they may induce hyperkalemia. On the other hand, the favorable effects of low doses of spironolactone in heart failure patients and the likely pathogenetic role of aldosterone in renal injury (Hollenberg, 2004) may lead to a greater use of aldosterone antagonists in CRD patients in the future (Bianchi et al., 2005; Nitta et al., 2004).

### Calcium Channel Blockers

In Figure 9–3, nondihydropyridine calcium channel blockers (nonDHP-CCBs) are recommended as third or fourth choices. The advocacy of nonDHP-CCBs is largely based on their greater antiproteinuric effect than seen with DHP-CCBs (Bakris et al., 2004). This difference is attributed by Bakris et al. to a greater effect of nonDHP-CCBs on efferent arteriolar vasodilation than seen with DHP-CCBs in experimental models (Griffin et al., 1999). In addition, nonDHP-CCBs have been found to reduce glomerular permeability (Russo et al., 2002).

These differences in antiproteinuric effects, though in themselves a cause for concern, have not been shown to eventuate in differences in renal protection between DHP-CCBs and nonDHP-CCBs. However, additional concern arose from the AASK trial, wherein those with proteinuria greater than 300 mg per day had a faster decline in GFR if started in the DHP-CCB amlodipine than if started on the ACEI ramipril (Agodoa et al., 2001). It should be noted, however, that in the majority of these patients with CRD from hypertensive nephrosclerosis wherein proteinuria was less than 300 mg per day, GFR was better preserved in those on amlodipine and both progression to ESRD and mortality were lower in those in the lower BP group who were on amlodipine (Contreras et al., 2005). However, in the Ramipril Efficacy in Nephropathy (REIN) trial, the addition of the DHP-CCB felodipine did not improve renoprotection when added to an ACEI even though BP was reduced more (Ruggenenti et al., 2005).

In conclusion, nonDHP-CCBs may be preferable to DHP-CCBs, but either type of CCB can safely be used *when added to an ACEI* in patients with nondiabetic CRD.

### Minoxidil

Those with refractory hypertension and renal insufficiency may be successfully treated with minoxidil (Toto et al., 1995). As noted in Chapter 7, minoxidil is a potent vasodilator and must be given with an adrenergic blocker (usually a β-blocker) to prevent reflex cardiac stimulation and with a loop diuretic to prevent fluid retention. The drug need be given in only a single daily dose.

## Restriction of Dietary Protein

A protein-restricted diet has been recommended for predialysis patients (Walser et al., 1999), and an analysis of multiple randomized trials has shown a delay in ESRD or death (Fouque et al., 2000), but individualized decisions seem appropriate in view of the malnutrition often seen with CRD (Levey et al., 2003).

## Correction of Anemia

Anemia is a risk factor for progression of CRD (Rossing et al., 2004), and treatment with erythropoeitin may improve morbidity (Jones et al., 2004), but proper controlled trials are only now underway to document this effect.

## Lipid-Lowering Agents

In view of the common presence of dyslipidemia in CRD patients and the high rate of atherosclerotic vascular disease they suffer, the use of lipid-lowering agents seems appropriate (Levey et al., 2003). Pooled data from three randomized, placebo-controlled trials involving 4,491 patients with GFR between 30 and 60 showed a 23% reduction in myocardial infarction (MI), coronary death, and revascularization with pravastatin (Tonelli et al., 2004). Atorvastatin has also been shown to reduce proteinuria and slow the progression of CRD (Bianchi et al., 2003).

## Dose Modification of Other Drugs

The presence of CRD can influence the dosing of a variety of drugs, in particular those with considerable renal clearance (Table 9–3) (Kappel & Calissi, 2002).

## TABLE 9–3

### Dose Modification for Patients with Renal Insufficiency

| Drugs Requiring Dose Modification | | Drugs Not Requiring Dose Modification |
|---|---|---|
| *All antibiotics* | EXCEPT | Cloxacillin, clindamycin, metronidazole, macrolides |
| **Antihypertensives** | | **Antihypertensives** |
| Atenolol, nadolol, angiotensin-converting-enzyme inhibitors | | Calcium channel blockers, minoxidil, angiotensin receptor blockers, clonidine, α-blockers |
| **Other cardiac medications** | | **Other cardiac medications** |
| Digoxin, sotalol | | Amiodarone, nitrates |
| **Diuretics** | | **Narcotics** |
| AVOID potassium-sparing diuretics in patients with creatinine clearance <30 mL/min | | Fentanyl hydromorphone, morphine |
| **Lipid-lowering agents** | | **Psychotropics** |
| HMG-CoA reductase inhibitors, benafibrate, clofibrate, fenofibrate | | Tricyclic antidepressants, nefazodone, other selective serotonin reuptake inhibitors |
| **Narcotics** | | **Hypoglycemia medications** |
| Codeine, meperidine | | Repaglinide, rosiglitazone |
| **Psychotropics** | | **Miscellaneous** |
| Lithium, chloral hydrate, gabapentin, trazodone, paroxetine, primidone, topiramate, vigabatrin | | Proton pump inhibitors |
| **Hypoglycemia medications** | | |
| Acarbose, chlorpropamide, glyburide, gliclazide, metformin, insulin | | |
| **Miscellaneous** | | |
| Allopurinol, colchicine, histamine$_2$ receptor antagonists, diclofenac, ketorolac, terbutaline | | |

Modified from Kappel J, Calissi P. Nephrology: 3. Safe drug prescribing for patients with renal insufficiency. *CMAJ* 2002;166:473–477.

## DIABETIC NEPHROPATHY

Now the most common cause of ESRD leading to dialysis, diabetic nephropathy will become even more common for two main reasons: first, the current epidemic of obesity which induces type 2 diabetes at an early age; second, diabetics are living long enough to develop nephropathy.

Fortunately, tight control of hyperglycemia (Writing Team, 2003) and hypertension (Bakris et al., 2003) can slow the progression, and intensive multifactorial interventions may prevent the development of nephropathy (Gæde et al., 2004; McCullough et al., 2004).

### Pathology and Clinical Features

As delineated by Kimmelstiel and Wilson (1936), renal disease occurs among diabetics with a high incidence and with a particular glomerular pathology—nodular intercapillary glomerulosclerosis. The clinical description has been improved very little since their original paper (Kimmelstiel & Wilson, 1936):

> The clinical picture appears . . . to be almost as characteristic as the histological one: the patients are relatively old; hypertension is present, usually of the benign type, and the kidneys frequently show signs of decompensation; there is a history of diabetes, usually of long standing; the presenting symptoms may be those of edema of the nephrotic type, renal decompensation or heart failure; the urine contains large amounts of albumin and there is usually impairment of concentrating power with or without nitrogen retention.

The pathologic specificity of the nodular glomerular lesion for diabetes has been upheld, although diffuse glomerulosclerosis may be just as common (White & Bilous, 2000). Before overt glomerulosclerosis appears, basement membrane thickening, mesangial expansion, and podocyte loss are noted, usually associated with microalbuminuria (Adler, 2004). The clinical description should be altered to include younger patients who have been diabetic for more than 15 years, to involve hypertension in approximately 50% to 60% of patients, and to almost always be accompanied by retinal capillary microaneurysms. In the absence of retinopathy, nearly 30% of proteinuric type 2 diabetics will have renal disease unrelated to diabetes (Christensen et al., 2000).

### Course

Progression of nephropathy in type 2 diabetics is associated with higher baseline levels of albuminuria, hemoglobin $A_{1c}$, and systolic BP, along with lower GFR and hemoglobin (Rossing et al., 2004).

Persistent microalbuminuria, as the first manifestation of diabetic nephropathy, has been observed in about one third of newly diagnosed type 1 diabetics within 20 years (Hovind et al., 2004) and in about one quarter of newly diagnosed type 2 diabetics within 10 years (Adler et al., 2003). The difference in time of onset may largely reflect the long asymptomatic background of type 2 compared to the usual abrupt onset of type 1. Rather surprisingly, regression of microalbuminuria has been observed in a significant percentage of type 1 diabetics, generally associated with lower levels of blood pressure and glycemia (Hovind et al., 2004; Perkins et al., 2003).

Although there are differences between type 1 and type 2 diabetes in the mechanisms and courses of nephropathy, the course of type 2 diabetes will be emphasized, particularly because such a clear description of its progression has been presented (Nelson et al., 1996).

Nelson et al. (1996) studied renal function every 6 to 12 months over 4 years in 194 Pima Indians who were selected as representative of different stages in the development of diabetic nephropathy: from normal glucose tolerance to overt diabetes; from normal albumin excretion to macroalbuminuria. As shown in Figure 9–5, the major findings generally were as follows: Glomerular hyperfiltration is present from the onset until macroalbuminuria appears. Thereafter, GFR declines rapidly because of a progressive loss of intrinsic ultrafiltration capacity. Although the rather abrupt fall in GFR that occurs after approximately 15 years was not prevented by control of BP, higher baseline pressures predicted increasing urinary albumin excretion, which in turn mediated a fall in GFR.

### Mechanisms

The critical role of glomerular hypertension as reflected by the hyperfiltration seen in Figure 9–5 has been strongly supported by the ability of antihypertensive therapy to prevent the progression of nephropathy (Bakris et al., 2003). In addition to multiple clinical studies, the role is supported by the observation that nodular glomerulosclerosis developed in only the nonobstructed kidney of a diabetic patient with unilateral renal artery stenosis (Berkman & Rifkin, 1973). Moreover, normal kidneys transplanted into diabetic patients develop typical diabetic lesions (Mauer et al., 1983), denying an essential role for genetic factors.

The progression from glomerular hypertension to overt nephropathy has been portrayed by Adler (2004):

> Mesangial expansion is the defining lesion in diabetic nephropathy. . . . The mesangial

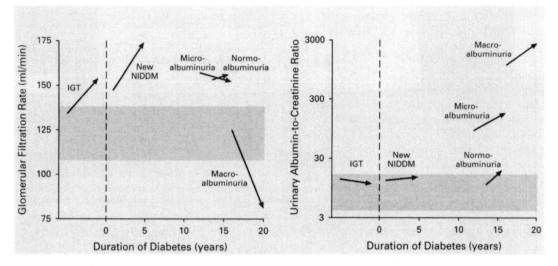

**FIGURE 9–5** ● Changes in the mean glomerular filtration rate and median urinary albumin (mg/L) to creatinine (g/L) ratio from baseline to the end of follow-up in subjects with impaired glucose tolerance (IGT); newly diagnosed noninsulin-dependent diabetes mellitus (New NIDDM); NIDDM and normal urinary albumin excretion (normoalbuminuria); NIDDM and microalbuminuria ; and NIDDM and macroalbuminuria. *Arrows* connect the value of the baseline examination with the value at the end of follow-up; *dashed lines* indicate the time of diagnosis; *shaded areas* indicate the twenty-fifth and seventy-fifth percentiles of values in subjects with normal glucose tolerance. (Modified from Nelson RG, Bennet PH, Beck GH, et al. Development and progression of renal disease in Pima Indians with non-insulin-dependent diabetes mellitus. *N Engl J Med* 1996;334:1636–1642.)

expansion encroaches on capillary lumena and results in slow progression toward end-stage renal disease. But the diabetic lesion also involves podocyte injury mediated by signal transduction change, cytoskeletal change, alterations in the podocyte slit pore membrane, detachment from the GBM, and apoptosis, all of which contribute to the development of proteinuria. In turn, proteinuria accelerates progression by its effects on tubulointerstitial fibrosis and atrophy, the final common pathway of progressive renal insufficiency. Adding insult to injury are the arterial and arteriolar sclerotic lesions, which superimpose ischemia on each of the other three renal regions.

Dr. Adler identifies angiotensin II as the primary mediator of this progression. She states that:

angiotensin II interacts on the cell membrane with its receptor(s), and then triggers the elaboration of signaling molecules, the activation of transcription factors, and the up-regulation of gene expression, ultimately inducing the fibrosis, cell growth, and even the inflammation that characterize the renal damage in diabetic nephropathy. . . . Angiotensin II interacts with many other growth factors and cytokines that also are activated in diabetic nephropathy and that simultaneously utilize the same and parallel signaling pathways, all factors or systems contributing to the histologic picture and functional decline of the diabetic kidney. (Figure 9–6)

**FIGURE 9–6** ● Schema outlining potential interactions between metabolic and hemodynamic factors in the pathogenesis of diabetic nephropathy. PKC, protein kinase C; TGF-β, transforming growth factor-β; VEGF, vascular endothelial growth factor. (Modified from Cooper ME. Pathogenesis, prevention, and treatment of diabetic nephropathy. *Lancet* 1998;352:213–219.)

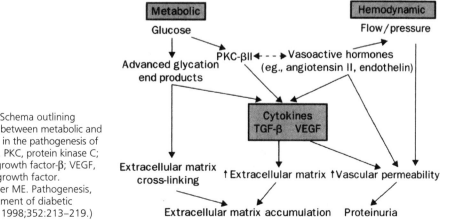

## Albuminuria

Microalbuminuria, defined as a urine albumin level between 30 and 300 mg per day, is the usual earliest manifestation of nephropathy. The presence of an even minimally elevated albumin-creatinine ratio in morning first-voided samples beyond 30 µg/mg creatinine is an early indicator of the risk of nephropathy (American Diabetes Association, 2004).

In addition to its role in nephropathy, proteinuria is associated with a two- to threefold increase in the risk for cardiovascular mortality over a 12-year follow-up in type 2 diabetics as compared to that seen in those without proteinuria (Valmadrid et al., 2000). Moreover, a reduction in albuminuria with therapy is associated with a reduction in cardiovascular risk (Atkins et al., 2005; de Zeeuw et al., 2004).

## Hypertension

As reviewed by Mogensen (1999), the associations between hypertension and both increasing albuminuria and falling GFR have been recognized for more than 30 years and repeatedly confirmed. An increase in nocturnal systolic blood pressure has been found to precede the development of microalbuminuria (Lurbe et al., 2002).

## Renin-Angiotensin

The progressive glomerulosclerosis would be expected to knock out the juxtaglomerular cells that secrete renin and, in some diabetics, a state of *hyporeninemic hypoaldosteronism* appears, usually manifested by hyperkalemia (Perez et al., 1977). However, serum total and prorenin levels are often increased before the onset of microalbuminuria, serving as a potential marker for the development of nephropathy (Deinum et al., 1999). Moreover, the intrarenal renin-angiotensin system is activated in both type 1 (Hollenberg et al., 2003) and type 2 (Mezzano et al., 2003) diabetics. These findings suggest autonomy of the intrarenal renin system and set the stage for the major benefits of ACEIs and ARBs seen in diabetic nephropathy. Moreover, elevated plasma aldosterone levels have been noted in type 1 diabetics (Hollenberg et al., 2004), presumably reflecting an activated systemic renin-angiotensin system as well.

## Management

An overall plan for management of diabetic nephropathy is shown in Table 9–4. The plan is similar to the algorithm for management of hypertension in nondiabetic CRD, but there are differences. The management of hypertension in diabetics without nephropathy is covered in Chapter 7.

## TABLE 9-4

### Measures to Prevent Progression of Overt Nephropathy in Patients with Type 2 Diabetes

Achieve glycemic control as reflected by a normal glycosylated hemoglobin concentration

Maintain blood pressure in the mid-normal range (below 130/80 mm Hg), preferably with the use of angiotensin-converting enzyme inhibitors or angiotensin II-receptor blockers

Reduce the level of proteinuria to <0.3 g per day

Stop smoking

Restrict dietary protein intake to approximately 0.8 g per kg of body weight per day, preferably by reducing the intake of animal proteins

Control dyslipidemia

## Glycemic Control

The first step is control of hyperglycemia, shown conclusively to slow the progress of nephropathy in the long-term follow-up study of 1,349 type 1 diabetic patients in the Diabetes Control and Complications Trial (Writing Team, 2003) and in less structured studies of type 2 diabetics (Levin et al., 2000).

## Antihypertensive Therapy

Evidence has been available since 1976 that reduction of elevated BP will slow the progression of diabetic nephropathy (Mogensen, 1976). The evidence accumulated from multiple subsequent trials has made two certain conclusions: First, the degree of BP reduction needed to protect against progression is much lower than the previously accepted goal of 140/90 mm Hg and, second, multiple drugs will usually be needed to achieve the necessary goal (National Kidney Foundation K/DOQI Clinical Practice Guidelines, 2004). The evidence is nicely portrayed in Figure 9–7 (Bakris et al., 2000) showing that the rate of progression of nephropathy was directly related to the level of BP achieved in these six trials of patients with diabetic nephropathy and the three trials in nondiabetic renal disease. It required on average more than two, sometimes four or more, drugs to achieve the lower targets of therapy. More so than with nondiabetic CRD, considerable evidence supports a goal of therapy to below 130/80 in diabetic CRD (Bakris et al., 2003; Gæde et al., 2004; Ruilope et al., 2001; Schrier et al., 2002). In the Irbesartan Diabetic Nephropathy Trial (IDNT), progressive lowering of systolic BP down to 120 mm Hg was associated with increased renal and patients' survival,

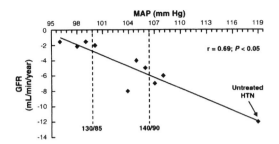

**FIGURE 9–7** ● Relationship between achieved blood pressure control and declines in GFR in six clinical trials of diabetic and three trials of nondiabetic renal disease. HTN, hypertension; MAP, mean arterial pressure. (Modified from Bakris GL, Williams M, Dworkin L, et al. Preserving renal function in adults with hypertension and diabetes: a consensus approach. *Am J Kidney Dis* 2000;36:646–661.)

whereas with systolic BP below 120 mm Hg, all-cause mortality increased (Pohl et al., 2005).

### Choices of Drugs

#### ACEIs and ARBs

Although the renoprotection provided in the original trials by Mogensen (1976) and Parving et al. (1983) used diuretics, β-blockers, and direct vasodilators—the major drugs available in the 1970s—more recent trials have almost all used ACEIs or ARBs as the primary drug (Deferrari et al., 2004; Strippoli et al., 2004). As reviewed earlier in this chapter, ACEIs and ARBs theoretically should reduce intraglomerular pressure better than do other drugs (Lassila et al., 2004) and, practically, they do. The evidence, starting with overt nephropathy in hypertensive type 1 diabetics, has now progressed to encompass normotensive type 1 diabetics either with microalbuminuria (ACE Inhibitors in Diabetic Nephropathy Trialist Group, 2001) or with normoalbuminuria (Kvetny et al., 2001).

In type 2 diabetics, similar renal protection has been found in those who are normotensive with either an ACEI (Ravid et al., 1998) or an ARB (Zandbergen et al., 2003). Larger controlled trials with ARBs have shown impressive renal protection in those with microalbuminuria (Parving et al., 2001) or macroalbuminuria (Brenner et al., 2001; Lewis et al., 2001).

Unfortunately, there have been no major trials of ACEIs in type 2 diabetics and only one direct comparison between an ACEI and an ARB in diabetic nephropathy. In that trial of 250 type 2 diabetics with early nephropathy (mean GFR = 93), the fall in GFR after 5 years averaged 17.9 with the ARB telmisartan 80 mg per day, and 14.9 with the ACEI enalapril 20 mg per day (Barnett et al., 2004). This statistically insignificant difference was interpreted as showing that telmisartan is not inferior to enalapril in providing long-term renoprotection in persons with type 2 diabetes.

The equality of renoprotection with the two classes has been well documented in 36 RCTs comparing an ACEI against placebo and in four RCTs comparing an ARB against placebo (Strippoli et al., 2004). However, this systematic review included only three trials with only 206 patients wherein an ACEI was compared directly against an ARB, providing inconclusive evidence of superiority of one or the other as to renal protection, However, the trial reported at a later time by Barnett et al. (2004) comparing telmisartan to enalapril does support equal renoprotective effects of the two classes.

On the other hand, when all-cause mortality (not reported by Barnett et al., 2004) was examined by Strippoli et al. (2004), the two classes differed significantly: ACEIs were associated with a significant 21% reduction, ARBs with an insignificant 1% reduction. Obviously, more direct comparisons between ACEIs and ARBs examining both renoprotection and mortality are needed.

In the meantime, increasingly strong evidence supports the combination of an ACEI and an ARB (Anderson & Mogensen, 2004; McCall, 2004). Beyond the clinical evidence, Adler (2004) notes that: "depending on ACE inhibition to block angiotensin II synthesis in the kidney will miss up to 30% of the total angiotensin II that is synthesized by other pathways. Thus, to block the effects of that angiotensin II that evades ACE inhibition, it becomes necessary to block the receptor directly."

For now, the wisest course would be to start with an ACEI, substitute an ARB if a cough develops, and combine the two if proteinuria persists despite large doses of the ACEI. The combination of an ACEI and an ARB may be appropriate for most proteinuric patients.

Meanwhile, uncertainty remains over the maximal doses of ACEIs and ARBs needed for full renoprotection (Weinberg et al., 2003). In one trial, 300 mg of the ARB irbesartan provided additional benefit over 150 mg (Parving et al., 2001). In a rat model of CRD, a 10-fold higher dose of an ARB was more renoprotective than the usual dose (Fujihara et al., 2005).

#### Additional Drugs

More than one drug will usually be needed and the second one should almost always be a diuretic (Mogensen et al., 2003), as volume expansion is usual with any degree of renal insufficiency. The third one could be a β-blocker, as atenolol was somewhat more effective than captopril in protecting the type 2 diabetics in the U.K. Prospective Diabetes Study (1998). On the other hand, a CCB may be needed to achieve BP control. As noted previously in this chapter, evidence of lesser decreases in proteinuria with DHP-CCBs than seen with nonDHP-CCBs (Bakris et al., 2004) have prompted the recommendation that only nonDHP-CCBs be used as add-on therapy in patients with diabetic nephropathy (Remuzzi et al., 2002). However, DHP-CCBs have provided equal renal protection as ACEIs in long-term comparisons (Schrier et al., 2002; Tarnow et al., 2000). Moreover, even though ARB-based therapy provided better renal protection than DHP-CCB-based therapy in the IDNT trial, the two were equal in prevention of cardiovascular outcomes (Berl et al., 2003). It should be further noted that over half of the ARB-based group in the RENAAL trial received a DHP-CCB with no apparent loss of renal protection (Brenner et al., 2001). Therefore, while a nonDHP-CCB may be theoretically preferable, a DHP-CCB will likely do as well when added to maximal ACEI or ARB.

Other choices for third or fourth add-ons include α-blockers, which have many attractive features and were as effective as ACEIs in reducing proteinuria (Rachmani et al., 1998). Although aldosterone antagonists are usually avoided in CRD because of the threat of hyperkalemia, particularly on top of an ACEI or ARB, aldosterone escape has been noted in 40% of ACEI-treated patients with diabetic nephropathy (Sato et al., 2003). Therefore, cautious use of an aldosterone antagonist may be appropriate in resistant patients (Sato et al., 2005).

### Other Therapies

Although the evidence is not conclusive, a *low-protein diet* should be helpful (Mogensen, 1999). *Moderate sodium restriction* is clearly necessary (MacGregor, 2001), particularly as these patients tend to be very sensitive to the pressor effect of sodium (Imanishi et al., 2001). *Control of dyslipidemia* may also lower BP, reduce proteinuria, slow the decline in GFR (Bianchi et al., 2003), and reduce cardiovascular events (Tonelli et al., 2004). As an aid to achieve control of hyperglycemia, a *thiazolidinedione* may also lower BP (Parulkar et al., 2001).

Gæde et al. (2004) have provided a striking demonstration of the ability of a multifaceted approach involving tight control of hypertension, hyperglycemia, and dyslipidemia, along with aspirin and an ACEI, to reduce the progression of nephropathy as well as retinopathy and autonomic neuropathy in patients with type 2 diabetes and microalbuminuria. Despite the costs and problems of such intensive therapy, the benefits are surely worth the expense and effort.

# CHRONIC DIALYSIS

Hypertension is common in patients entering dialysis and is a risk for premature mortality, mostly due to cardiovascular disease (CVD) (Agarwal, 2005; Kiss et al., 2005). Despite the obvious connection between persistent hypertension and poor outcome, the majority of chronic dialysis patients remain hypertensive—in spite of widespread use of various antihypertensive medications (Agarwal et al., 2003). As will be noted, the current inadequacy of blood pressure control almost certainly reflects the persistence of volume overload (Scribner, 1999). While emphasizing the critical role of volume expansion, Khosla and Johnson (2004) recognize a number of other possible contributions to the hypertension (Table 9–5).

As important as control of hypertension is after start of dialysis, the key to improved dialysis outcomes is improved predialysis care (Pereira, 2000), in particular the adequacy of control of hypertension (Fernández Lucas, 2003).

## Patterns of Blood Pressure

Most patients have systolic hypertension and a wide pulse pressure as a consequence of atherosclerotic arterial stiffness (Locatelli et al., 2004). The BP of patients on chronic dialysis may vary considerably with the timing of dialysis. Ambulatory BP monitoring reveals a frequent white-coat effect before dialysis, higher readings on the day after dialysis, and a blunting of nocturnal dipping (Mitra et al., 1999). The absence of a nocturnal fall in BP is a potent indicator of mortality (Amar et al., 2000). Mitra et al. (1999) recommend the 20-minute postdialysis reading as most representative of interdialytic BP.

## Management of Hypertension

As summarized by Locatelli et al. (2004):

> The principles of hypertension treatment in dialysis are an achievement of dry body weight, proper dialysis prescription with respect to dialysis time and intra-dialytic sodium balance, and dietary sodium and water restriction. Pharmacological treatment should only be the second option, after the adequate and complete application of all other means.

As little as a 2.5-kg weight gain between dialysis sessions is associated with a significant rise in BP, and there is a significant correlation between BP and interdialytic weight gain in hypertensive patients (Rahman et al., 2000). Despite the use of multiple

**TABLE 9–5**

## Mechanisms of Hypertension in the Hemodialysis Patient

Pre-existing hypertension
ECV expansion
    Inability to excrete sodium
    Blood volume-related vasoactive substances
    Dietary salt noncompliance
Renal-dependent mechanisms
    Dysregulation of renin-angiotensin system
    Sympathetic hyperactivity
    Loss of inherent renal vasodilatory factors
Vascular mechanisms
    Elevated calcium/phosphate product
    Secondary hyperparathyroidism
    Vascular calcification and stiffening
Medications and toxins
    Sympathomimetics
    Erythropoietin
    Cigarette smoking
    Lead exposure
Circulating factors
    Endogenous inhibitors of nitric oxide system
    Endogenous inhibitors of vascular $Na^+$, $K^+$-ATPase
    Parathyroid hormone
    "Uremic toxins"
Hemodialysis prescription
    Dialysate $Na^+$ and $K^+$ concentrations
    Shorter dialysis sessions
    Overestimation of dry weight
    Impaired sleep; sleep apnea

Modified from Khosla UM, Johnson RJ. Hypertension in the hemodialysis patient and the "lag phenomenon": insights into pathophysiology and clinical management. *Am J Kidney Dis* 2004;43:739–751.

antihypertensive drugs, control of BP may not be possible if dry weight is not achieved by ultrafiltration and dietary sodium restriction as emphasized by the late Belding Scribner (1999). Even after the achievement of dry weight, there may be a long "lag" time before blood pressure remains normal without antihypertensive drugs (Khosla & Johnson, 2004). Measurement of B-type natriuretic peptide (BNP) may be an effective way to estimate volume load (Dastoor et al., 2005).

### Choices of Antihypertensive Drugs

Before dry weight can control hypertension or if this ideal cannot be achieved, antihypertensive drugs may be needed. As noted by Locatelli et al. (2004): "No comparative pharmacological trials have specifically addressed the issue of hypertension control in dialysis patients." Nonetheless, there are some data supporting the use of an ACEI (Efrati et al., 2002; Li et al., 2003) or an ARB (Suzuki et al., 2004) in chronic dialysis patients, to maintain residual renal function and prolong survival. If these agents are used, careful monitoring of serum potassium is critical since hyperkalemia is a serious threat (Knoll et al., 2002).

Calcium channel blockers are widely used in ESRD patients, and their use was associated with a 21% lower risk of mortality in a large cohort (Kestenbaum et al., 2002). Similar reductions in mortality have been associated with β-blockers (Foley et al., 2002), but, as with other drugs, the data are purely observational and may be related to effects on coexisting conditions.

### Hypotension

Hypotension during dialysis can arise from multiple causes (Table 9–6) and may be a major problem, especially in debilitated patients (Port et al., 1999). In such cases, the extracellular volume (ECV) becomes even more difficult to control, and a constant state of ECV excess may be necessary to avoid severe episodes of hypotension during dialysis.

**TABLE 9–6**

## Causes of Dialysis-Related Hypotension

Excessive ultrafiltration
Decrease of plasma osmolality
Dialysate problems: temperature, bioincompatibility
Hyperinsulinemia from dialysate-induced hyperglycemia
Reflex sympathetic inhibition
Autonomic neuropathy
Bleeding
Electrolyte abnormalities (hypokalemia, hyperkalemia, hypocalcemia)
Sepsis
Heart disease (ischemia, arrhythmias, pericardial effusion with cardiac tamponade)
Restoration of nitric oxide by removal of endogenous inhibitors

## Other Risk Factors

In view of the high level of cardiovascular risk in most of these patients, full attention to other risk factors should be provided, even though they do not fully explain the high prevalence of coronary disease (Cheung et al., 2000), which may be explained by other manifestations of ESRD (McClellan & Chertow, 2005). An apparent paradox of an increased mortality in dialysis patients with lower cholesterol levels has been explained by the association of low cholesterol with inflammation and malnutrition (Liu et al., 2004). A similar scenario may explain the "reverse" association between lower BP and higher mortality (Kalantar-Zadeh et al., 2004).

## HYPERTENSION AFTER KIDNEY TRANSPLANTATION

Hypertension has been recognized as a major complication, one that may, if uncontrolled, quickly destroy the transplant or add to the risk of accelerated atherosclerosis (Kasiske et al., 2004). The majority of transplant recipients are hypertensive, and the higher the level of BP at 1 year after transplantation, the lower is the rate of allograft survival (Mange et al., 2004). Among children with ESRD, transplantation provides a better chance of survival than dialysis (McDonald et al., 2004), but the persistence of elevated blood pressure is associated with evidences of smoldering atherosclerosis (Mitsnefes et al., 2004).

### Causes

Table 9–7 lists a number of causes of posttransplantation hypertension beyond persistence of primary hypertension, to which should be added the presence of $AT_1$-receptor activating antibodies (Dragun et al., 2005).

### Cyclosporine and Tacrolimus

Cyclosporine and tacrolimus can cause both nephrotoxicity and hypertension. In one study of 24 transplant recipients, conversion from cyclosporine to tacrolimus resulted in lower blood pressure (Hillebrand et al., 2004). A CCB has been widely used to overcome the vasoconstrictive effect of the calcineurin-inhibitors, but other antihypertensive agents may be as effective (Remuzzi & Perico, 2002).

### Posttransplantation Renal Artery Stenosis

Renal artery stenosis, often at the suture line, is found in approximately 1% to 5% of patients with posttransplantation hypertension (Bruno et al., 2004) and should be suspected by appearance of a bruit.

---

### TABLE 9–7

## Causes of Post-Transplantation Hypertension

Immunosuppressive therapy
   Steroids
   Cyclosporine, tacrolimus
Allograft failure
   Chronic rejection
   Recurrent disease
Potentially surgically remediable causes
   Allograft renal artery stenosis
   Native kidneys
Volume expansion
   Erythrocytosis
   Sodium retention
Speculative cause
   Recurrent essential hypertension
     As a primary cause of ESRD
     From a hypertensive or prehypertensive donor
Other pressor mechanisms including:
   Endothelin
   Transforming growth factor β
   Decreased nitric oxide

---

The diagnosis should be suspected if hypertension suddenly appears or rapidly progresses or if allograft function deteriorates after an ACEI or ARB is begun. Duplex sonography with measurement of the resistive index is the preferred way to begin; if a stenosis is seen, arteriography followed by angioplasty with stenting are the usual corrective maneuvers (Bruno et al., 2004).

### Native Kidney Hypertension

If graft stenosis is excluded and the allograft is functioning well, the native kidneys may be responsible for the hypertension. If hypertension persists despite intensive medical therapy including ACEIs or ARBs, the native kidneys may have to be removed (Fricke et al., 1998).

### Management

Although CCBs have been the most widely used antihypertensive drugs (Kasiske et al., 2004), Remuzzi and Perico (2002) argue that renin-angiotensin inhibitors may be better. The immediate use of an ACEI or ARB after transplantation has been found to be both safe and effective in reducing the time to graft recovery (Lorenz et al., 2004). In patients with biopsy-proven allograft nephropathy, treatment with an ACEI or an ARB was followed by a slower decline in renal function (Zaltzman et al., 2004). In those with refractory allograft rejection who have $AT_1$-receptor activating antibodies, an ARB should be particularly beneficial (Dragun et al., 2005).

An additional benefit of these drugs is their ability to prevent the posttransplant erythrocytosis that is seen in about half of patients and which can contribute to thromboembolic events (Wang et al., 2002).

However, in an uncontrolled study of 1,662 kidney transplant recipients, the use of a CCB as initial therapy was associated with an improved rate of graft survival except in those with levels of systolic BP above 152 mm Hg and proteinuria. In such patients, ACEI/ARBs were more effective (Premasathian et al., 2004).

Other drugs including diuretics, α-blockers, and β-blockers may be needed to control posttransplant hypertension that is not related to discernible and correctable causes. However it is done, the intensive control of hypertension to below 130/80 is necessary to protect the kidney (Klassen, 2000) while close attention is directed toward all other treatable cardiovascular risk factors.

Now that normal parenchymal diseases have been examined, hypertension caused by renovascular diseases will be considered.

## REFERENCES

ACE Inhibitors in Diabetic Nephropathy Trialist Group. Should all patients with type 1 diabetes mellitus and microalbuminuria receive angiotensin-converting enzyme inhibitors? *Ann Intern Med* 2001;134:370–379.

Adler AL, Stevens RJ, Manley SE, et al. Development and progression of nephropathy in type 2 diabetes: the United Kingdom Prospective Diabetes Study (UKPDS 64). *Kidney Int* 2003;63:225–232.

Adler S. Diabetic nephropathy: linking histology, cell biology, and genetics. *Kidney Int* 2004;66:2095–2106.

Agarwal R. Hypertension and survival in chronic hemodialysis patients: past lessons and future opportunities. *Kidney Int* 2005;67:1–13.

Agarwal R, Nissenson AR, Batlle D, et al. Prevalence, treatment, and control of hypertension in chronic hemodialysis patients in the United States. *Am J Med* 2003;115: 291–297.

Agodoa LY, Appel L, Bakris GL, et al. Effect of ramipril vs amlopidine on renal outcomes in hypertensive nephrosclerosis. *JAMA* 2001;285:2719–2728.

Amar J, Vernier I, Rossignol E, et al. Nocturnal blood pressure and 24-hour pulse pressure are potent indicators of mortality in hemodialysis patients. *Kidney Int* 2000;57: 2485–2491.

American Diabetes Association. Nephropathy in diabetes. *Diabetes Care* 2004;27(Suppl 1):S79–S83.

Anderson MJ, Khawandi W, Agarwal R. Pathogenesis and treatment of kidney disease and hypertension: home blood pressure monitoring in CKD. *Am J Kidney Dis* 2005; published online June 3, 2005.

Andersen NH, Mogensen CE. Dual blockade of the renin angiotensin system in diabetic and nondiabetic kidney disease. *Curr Hypertens Rep* 2004;6:369–376.

Anderson S, Brenner BM. Progressive renal disease: a disorder of adaptation. *QJM* 1989;70:185–189.

Atkins RC, Briganti EM, Lewis JB, et al. Proteinuria reduction and progression to renal failure in patients with type 2 diabetes mellitus and overt nephropathy. *Am J Kidney Dis* 2005;45:281–287.

Augustyniak RA, Tuncel M, Zhang W, et al. Sympathetic overactivity as a cause of hypertension in chronic renal failure. *J Hypertens* 2002;20:3–9.

Bakris GL, Smith A. Effects of sodium intake on albumin excretion in patients with diabetic nephropathy treated with long-acting calcium antagonists. *Ann Intern Med* 1996; 125:201–204.

Bakris GL, Weir MR, Secic M, et al. Differential effects of calcium antagonist subclasses on markers of nephropathy progression. *Kidney Int* 2004;65:1991–2002.

Bakris GL, Weir MR, Shanifar S, et al. Effects of blood pressure level on progression of diabetic nephropathy: results from the RENAAL study. *Arch Intern Med* 2003; 163:1555–1565.

Bakris GL, Williams M, Dworkin L, et al. Preserving renal function in adults with hypertension and diabetes: a consensus approach. *Am J Kidney Dis* 2000;36:646–661.

Barai S, Bandopadhayaya GP, Bhowmik D, et al. Prevalence of vesicoureteral reflux in patients with incidentally diagnosed adult hypertension. *Urology* 2004;63:1045–1049.

Barnett AH, Bain SC, Bouter P, et al. Angiotensin-receptor blockade versus converting-enzyme inhibition in type 2 diabetes and nephropathy. *N Engl J Med* 2004;351:1952–1961.

Bennett WM, Porter GA. Efficacy and safety of metolazone in renal failure and the nephrotic syndrome. *Clin Pharmacol* 1973;13:357–364.

Berka JL, Alcorn D, Bertram JF, et al. Effects of angiotensin converting enzyme inhibition on glomerular number, juxtaglomerular cell activity and renin content in experimental unilateral hydronephrosis. *J Hypertens* 1994;12: 735–743.

Berkman J, Rifkin H. Unilateral nodular diabetic glomerulosclerosis (Kimmelstiel-Wilson): report of a case. *Metabolism* 1973;22:715–722.

Berl T, Hunsicker LG, Lewis JB, et al. Cardiovascular outcomes in the Irbesartan Diabetic Nephropathy Trial of patients with type 2 diabetes and overt nephropathy. *Ann Intern Med* 2003;138:542–549.

Bianchi S, Bigazzi R, Caiazza A, Campese VM. A controlled, prospective study on the effects of atorvastatin on proteinuria and progression of kidney disease. *Am J Kidney Dis* 2003:41:565–570.

Bianchi S, Bigazzi R, Campese VM. Antagonists of aldosterone and proteinuria in patients with CKD: an uncontrolled pilot study. *Am J Kidney Dis* 2005; published online June 3, 2005.

Bidani AK, Griffin KA. Pathophysiology of hypertensive renal disease: implications for therapy. *Hypertension* 2004; 44:595–601.

Bochud M, Elston RC, Maillard M, et al. Heritability of renal function in hypertensive families of African descent in the Seychelles (Indian Ocean). *Kidney Int* 2005; 67:61–69.

Braden GL, O'Shea MH, Mulhern JG, Germain MJ. Acute renal failure and hyperkalemia associated with cyclooxygenase-2 inhibitors. *Nephrol Dial Transplant* 2004;19: 1149–1153.

Brater DC. Use of diuretics in chronic renal insufficiency and nephrotic syndrome. *Semin Nephrol* 1988;8:333–341.

Brenner BM, Cooper ME, de Zeeuw D, et al. Effects of losartan on renal and cardiovascular outcomes in patients with type 2 diabetes and nephropathy. *N Engl J Med* 2001; 345:861–869.

Bruno S, Rumuzzi G, Ruggenenti P. Transplant renal artery stenosis. *J Am Soc Nephrol* 2004;15:134–141.

Campbell R, Sangalli F, Perticucci E, et al. Effects of combined ACE inhibitor and angiotensin II antagonist treatment in human chronic nephropathies. *Kidney Int* 2003; 63:1094–1103.

Campese VM. Neurogenic factors and hypertension in renal disease. *Kidney Int* 2000;57:S2–S6.

Chadban SJ, Atkins RC. Glomerulonephritis. *Lancet* 2005; 365:1797–1806.

Cheung AK, Sarnak MJ, Yan G, et al. Atherosclerotic cardiovascular disease risks in chronic hemodialysis patients. *Kidney Int* 2000;58:353–362.

Chobanian AV, Bakris GL, Black HR, et al. Seventh report of the Joint National Committee on the Prevention, Detection, Evaluation, and Treatment of High Blood Pressure. *Hypertension* 2003;42:1206–1252.

Christensen PK, Larsen S, Horn T, et al. Causes of albuminuria in patients with type 2 diabetes without diabetic retinopathy. *Kidney Int* 2000;58:1719–1731.

Cooper ME. Pathogenesis, prevention, and treatment of diabetic nephropathy. *Lancet* 1998;352:213–219.

Coresh J, Astor BC, Greene T, et al. Prevalence of chronic kidney disease and decreased kidney function in the adult US population: Third National Health and Nutrition Examination Survey. *Am J Kidney Dis* 2003;41:1–12.

Coresh J, Wei L, McQuillan G, et al. Prevalence of high blood pressure and elevated serum creatinine level in the United States. *Arch Intern Med* 2001;161:1207–1216.

Contreras G, Greene T, Agodoa LY, et al. Blood pressure control, drug therapy, and kidney disease. *Hypertension* 2005;45:1119–1125.

Dastoor H, Bernieh B, Boobes Y, et al. Plasma BNP in patients on maintenance hemodialysis: a guide to management? *J Hypertens* 2005;23:23–28.

De Nicola L, Minutolo R, Bellizzi V, et al. Achievement of target blood pressure levels in chronic kidney disease: a salty question? *Am J Kidney Dis* 2004;43:782–795.

de Zeeuw D, Remuzzi G, Parving H-H, et al. Albuminuria, a therapeutic target for cardiovascular protection in type 2 diabetic patients with nephropathy. *Circ* 2004;110: 921–927.

Deferrari G, Ravera M, Berruti V, et al. Optimizing therapy in the diabetic patient with renal disease: antihypertensive treatment. *J Am Soc Nephrol* 2004;15:S6–S11.

Deinum J, Rønn B, Mathiesen E, et al. Increase in serum prorenin precedes onset of microalbuminuria in patients with insulin-dependent diabetes mellitus. *Diabetologia* 1999;42:1006–1010.

de Jong PE, Brenner BM. From secondary to primary prevention of progressive renal disease: the case for screening for albuminuria. *Kidney Int* 2004;66:2109–2118.

Dragun D, Müller DN, Bräsen JH, et al. Angiotensin II type 1-receptor activating antibodies in renal-allograft rejection. *N Engl J Med* 2005;352:558–569.

Efrati S, Zaidenstein R, Dishy V, et al. ACE inhibitors and survival of hemodialysis patients. *Am J Kidney Dis* 2002; 40:1023–1029.

El-Dahr SS, Dipp S, Gee J, et al. Ureteral obstruction activates renin-angiotensin and suppresses kallikrein-kinin systems [Abstract]. *J Am Soc Nephrol* 1992;3:737.

Fanos V, Cataldi L. Antibiotics or surgery for vesicoureteric reflux in children. *Lancet* 2004;364:1720–1722.

Fernández Lucas M, Quereda C, Teruel JL, et al. Effect of hypertension before beginning dialysis on survival of hemodialysis patients. *Am J Kidney Dis* 2003;41:814–821.

Foley RN, Herzog CA, Collins AJ. Blood pressure and long-term mortality in United States hemodialysis patients USRDS Waves 3 and 4 study. *Kidney Int* 2002;62: 1784–1790.

Fouque D, Wang P, Laville M, Boissel J-P. Low protein diets delay end-stage renal disease in non-diabetic adults with chronic renal failure. *Nephrol Dial Transplant* 2000;15: 1986–1992.

Fox CS, Larson MG, Leip EP, et al. Predictors of new-onset kidney disease in a community-based population. *JAMA* 2004;291:844–850.

Fricke L, Doehn C, Steinhoff J, et al. Treatment of posttransplant hypertension by laparoscopic bilateral nephrectomy? *Transplantation* 1998;65:1182–1187.

Fujihara CK, Velho M, Malheiros DM, Zatz R. An extremely high dose of losartan affords superior renoprotection in the remnant model. *Kidney Int* 2005;67:1913–1924.

Gæde P, Tarnow L, Vedel P, et al. Remission of normoalbuminuria during multifactorial treatment preserves kidney function in patients with type 2 diabetes and microalbuminuria. *Nephrol Dial Transplant* 2004;19:2784–2788.

Ghose RR, Harindra V. Unrecognised high pressure chronic retention of urine presenting with systemic arterial hypertension. *BMJ* 1989;298:1626–1628.

Go AS, Chertow GM, Fan D, et al. Chronic kidney disease and the risks of death, cardiovascular events, and hospitalization. *N Engl J Med* 2004;351:1296–1305.

Goodship THJ, Stoddart JT, Martinek V, et al. Long-term follow-up of patients presenting to adult nephrologists with chronic pyelonephritis and "normal" renal function. *QJM* 2000;93:799–803.

Gridelli B, Remuzzi G. Strategies for making more organs available for transplantation. *N Engl J Med* 2000;343: 404–410.

Griffin KA, Picken MM, Bakris GL, Bidani AK. Class differences in the effects of calcium channel blockers in the rat remnant kidney model. *Kidney Int* 1999;44:1849–1860.

Guidi E, Cozzi MG, Minetti E, et al. Effect of familial hypertension on glomerular hemodynamics and tubuloglomerular feedback after uninephrectomy. *Am J Hypertens* 2001; 14:121–128.

Hammond JJ, Raffaele J, Liddel N, et al. A prospective study to evaluate the effects of extra corporeal shock wave lithotripsy (ESWL) on blood pressure (BP), renal function (RF) and glomerular filtration (GFR) [Abstract]. *J Am Coll Cardiol* 1993;21:257.

Heeg JE, de Jong PE, van der Hem GK, de Zeeuw D. Efficacy and variability of the antiproteinuric effect of ACE inhibition by lisinopril. *Kidney Int* 1989;36:272–279.

Hillebrand U, Gerhardt U, Suwelack B. Conversion from cyclosporine A to tacrolimus has beneficial effects on blood pressure in long-term renal transplant recipients [Abstract]. *Am J Hypertens* 2004;17:92A.

Hollenberg NK. Aldosterone in the development and progression of renal injury. *Kidney Int* 2004;66:1–9.

Hollenberg NK, Price DA, Fisher NDL, et al. Glomerular hemodynamics and the renin-angiotensin system in patients with type 2 diabetes mellitus. *Kidney Int* 2003;63: 172–178.

Hollenberg NK, Stevanovic R, Agarwal A, et al. Plasma aldosterone concentration in the patient with diabetes mellitus. *Kidney Int* 2004;65:1435–1439.

Hovind P, Tarnow L, Rossing P, et al. Predictors for the development of microalbuminuria and macroalbuminuria in patients with type 1 diabetes: inception cohort study. *BMJ* 2004;328:1105–1109.

Hsu C-Y, Lin F, Vittinghoff E, Shlipak MG. Racial differences in the progression from chronic renal insufficiency to end-stage renal disease in the United States. *J Am Soc Nephrol* 2003;14:2902–2907.

Hsu C-Y, MuCulloch CE, Darbinian J, et al. Elevated blood pressure and risk of end-stage renal disease in subjects without baseline kidney risk. *Arch Intern Med* 2005;165: 923–928.

Hsu C-Y, Vittinghoff E, Lin F, Shlipak MG. The incidence of end-stage renal disease is increasing faster than the prevalence of chronic renal insufficiency. *Ann Intern Med* 2004;141:95–101.

Huerta C, Castellsague J, Varas-Lorenzo C, Garcia Rodriguez LA. Nonsteroidal anti-inflammatory drugs and risk of ARF in the general population. *Am J Kidney Dis* 2005;45: 531–539.

Imanishi M, Yoshioka K, Okumura M, et al. Sodium sensitivity related to albuminuria appearing before hypertension in type 2 diabetic patients. *Diabetes Care* 2001;24:111–116.

Jafar TH, Stark PC, Schmid CH, et al. Progression of chronic kidney disease; the role of blood pressure control, proteinuria, and angiotensin-converting enzyme inhibition: a patient-level meta-analysis. *Ann Intern Med* 2003;139: 244–252.

Jafar TH, Stark PC, Schmid CH, et al. The effect of angiotensin-converting-enzyme inhibitors on progression of advanced polycystic kidney disease. *Kidney Int* 2005; 67:265–271.

Jardine AG. Angiotensin II and glomerulonephritis. *J Hypertens* 1995;13:487–493.

Jones CA, Krolewski AS, Rogus J, et al. Epidemic of end-stage renal disease in people with diabetes in the United States population: do we know the cause? *Kidney Int* 2005;67:1684–1691.

Jones DA, George NJR, O'Reilly PH, Barnard RJ. Reversible hypertension associated with unrecognised high pressure chronic retention of urine. *Lancet* 1987;1:1052–1054.

Jones M, Ibels L, Schenkel B, et al. Impact of epoetin alfa on clinical end points in patients with chronic renal failure: a meta-analysis. *Kidney Int* 2004;65:757–767.

Kalantar-Zadeh K, Kilpatrick R, McAllister CJ, Kopple JD. Reverse epidemiology of hypertension in dialysis patients: bad gone good? [Abstract] *Hypertension* 2004; 44:507.

Kappel J, Calissi P. Nephrology: 3. Safe drug prescribing for patients with renal insufficiency. *CMAJ* 2002;166: 473–477.

Kasiske BL, Anjum S, Shah R, et al. Hypertension after kidney transplantation. *Am J Kidney Dis* 2004;43:1071–1081.

Kasiske BL, Ma JZ, Louis TA, Swan SK. Long-term effects of reduced mass in humans. *Kidney Int* 1995;48:814–819.

Kestenbaum B, Gillen DL, Sherrard DJ, et al. Calcium channel blocker use and mortality among patients with end-stage renal disease. *Kidney Int* 2002;61:2157–2164.

Khosla UM, Johnson RJ. Hypertension in the hemodialysis patient and the "lag phenomenon": insights into pathophysiology and clinical management. *Am J Kidney Dis* 2004; 43:739–751.

Kimmelstiel P, Wilson C. Intercapillary lesions in the glomeruli of the kidney. *Am J Pathol* 1936;12:83–97.

Kincaid-Smith P. Hypothesis: obesity and the insulin resistance syndrome play a major role in end-stage renal failure attributed to hypertension and labelled 'hypertensive nephrosclerosis.' *J Hypertens* 2004;22:1051–1055.

Kiss I, Farsang C, Rodicio JL. Treatment of hypertension in dialysed patients. *J Hypertens* 2005;23:222–226.

Klag MJ, Whelton PK, Randall B, et al. End-stage renal disease in African-American and white men. *JAMA* 1997; 277:1293–1298.

Klassen DK. How aggressively should blood pressure be treated in renal transplant recipients? *Curr Hypertens Rep* 2000;2:473–477.

Knauf H, Mutschler E. Diuretic effectiveness of hydrochlorothiazide and furosemide alone and in combination in chronic renal failure. *J Cardiovasc Pharmacol* 1995; 26:394–400.

Knoll GA, Sahgal A, Nair RC, et al. Renin-angiotensin system blockade and the risk of hyperkalemia in chronic hemodialysis patients. *Am J Med* 2002;112:110–114.

Kvetny J, Gregersen G, Pedersen RS. Randomized placebo-controlled trial of perindopril in normotensive, normoalbuminuric patients with type 1 diabetes mellitus. *Q J Med* 2001;94:89–94.

Lassila M, Cooper ME, Jandeleit-Dahm K. Antiproteinuric effect of RAS blockade: new mechanisms. *Curr Hypertens Rep* 2004;6:383–392.

Laverman GD, Andersen S, Rossing P, et al. Renoprotection with and without blood pressure reduction. *Kidney Int* 2005;67(Suppl 94):S54–S59.

Lazarus JM, Bourgoignie JJ, Buckalew VM, et al. Achievement and safety of a low blood pressure goal in chronic renal disease. The modification of diet in renal disease study group. *Hypertension* 1997;29:641–650.

Lea J, Greene T, Hebert L, et al. The relationship between magnitude of proteinuria reduction and risk of end-stage renal disease: results from the AASK trial. *Arch Intern Med* 2005;165:947–953.

Levey AS. Nondiabetic kidney disease. *N Engl J Med* 2003; 347:1505–1511.

Levey AS, Coresh J, Balk E, et al. National Kidney Foundation practice guidelines for chronic kidney disease: evaluation, classification, and stratification. *Ann Intern Med* 2003;139:137–147.

Levin SR, Coburn JW, Abraira C, et al. Effect of intensive glycemic control on microalbuminuria in type 2 diabetes. *Diabetes Care* 2000;23:1478–1485.

Lewis EJ, Hunsicker LG, Clarke WR, et al. Renoprotective effect of the angiotensin-receptor antagonist irbesartan in patients with nephropathy due to type 2 diabetes. *N Engl J Med* 2001;345:851–860.

Li PK-T, Chow K-M, Wong TY-H, et al. Effects of an angiotensin-converting enzyme inhibitor on residual renal function in patients receiving peritoneal dialysis: a randomized, controlled study. *Ann Intern Med* 2003;139: 105–112.

Lingeman JE, Woods JR, Nelson DR. Commentary on ESWL and blood pressure. *J Urol* 1995;154:2–4.

Liu Y, Coresh J, Eustace JA, et al. Association between cholesterol level and mortality in dialysis patients: role of inflammation and malnutrition. *JAMA* 2004;291: 451–459.

Locatelli F, Covic A Chazot C, et al. Hypertension and cardiovascular risk assessment in dialysis patients. *Nephrol Dial Transplant* 2004;19:1058–1068.

Locatelli F, del Vecchio L, Pozzoni P, et al. Is it the agent or the blood pressure level that matters for renal and vascular protection in chronic nephropathies? *Kidney Int* 2005;67: S15–S19.

Lorenz M, Billensteiner E, Bodingbauer M, et al. The effect of ACE inhibitor and angiotensin II blocker therapy on early posttransplant kidney graft function. *Am J Kidney Dis* 2004;43:1065–1070.

Lurbe E, Redon J, Kesani A, et al. Increase in nocturnal blood pressure and progression to microalbuminuria in type 1 diabetes. *N Engl J Med* 2002;347:797–805.

MacGregor GA. Blood pressure: importance of the kidney and the need to reduce salt intake. *Am J Kidney Dis* 2001; 37(Suppl 2):S34–S38.

Madaio MP, Harrington JT. Acute glomerulonephritis and the nephrotic syndrome. *Arch Intern Med* 2001;161:25–34.

Mange KC, Feldman HI, Joffe MM, et al. Blood pressure and the survival of renal allografts from living donors. *J Am Soc Nephrol* 2004;15:187–193.

Mann JFE, Gerstein HC, Pogue J, et al. Renal insufficiency as a predictor of cardiovascular outcomes and the impact of ramipril. *Ann Intern Med* 2001;134:629–636.

Marshall MR, Song Q, Ma TM, et al. Evolving connectionist system versus algebraic formulas for prediction of renal function from serum creatinine. *Kidney Int* 2005;67: 1944–1954.

Mauer SM, Steffes MW, Connett J, et al. The development of lesions in the glomerular basement membrane and mesangium after transplantation of normal kidneys to diabetic patients. *Diabetes* 1983;32:948–952.

McCall AL. Hypertension management in patients with diabetic nephropathy. *Curr Hypertens Rep* 2004;6:272–278.

McClellan MM, Chertow GM. Beyond Framingham: cardiovascular risk profiling in ESRD. *J Am Soc Nephrol* 2005;16:1539–1541.

McCullough PA, Bakris GL, Owen WF Jr, et al. Slowing the progression of diabetic nephropathy and its cardiovascular consequences. *Am Heart J* 2004;148:243–251.

McDonald SP, Craig JC. Long-term survival of children with end-stage renal disease. *N Engl J Med* 2004;350: 2654–2662.

Mentari E, Rahman M. Blood pressure and progression of chronic kidney disease: importance of systolic, diastolic, and diurnal variation. *Curr Hypertens Rep* 2004;6: 400–404.

Mezzano S, Droguett A, Burgos E, et al. Renin-angiotensin system activation and interstitial inflammation in human diabetic nephropathy. *Kidney Int* 2003;64:S64–S70.

Mitra S, Chandna SM, Farrington K. What is hypertension in chronic haemodialysis? The role of interdialytic blood pressure monitoring. *Nephrol Dial Transplant* 1999;14: 2915–2921.

Mitsnefes MM, Kimball TR, Witt SA, et al. Abnormal carotid artery structure and function in children and adolescents with successful renal transplantation. *Circulation* 2004;110: 97–101.

Mogensen CE. Progression of nephropathy in long-term diabetes with proteinuria and effect of initial hypertensive treatment. *Scand J Clin Lab Invest* 1976;36: 383–388.

Mogensen CE. Microalbuminuria, blood pressure and diabetic renal disease: origin and development of ideas. *Diabetologia* 1999;42:263–285.

Mogensen CE, Viberti G, Halimi S, et al. Effect of low-dose perindopril/indapamide on albuminuria in diabetes: Preterax in Albuminuria Regression: PREMIER. *Hypertension* 2003;41:1063–1071.

Nakao N, Yoshimura A, Morita H, et al. Combination treatment of angiotensin-II receptor blocker and angiotensin-converting-enzyme inhibitor in non-diabetic renal disease (COOPERATE): a randomised controlled trial. *Lancet* 2003;361:117–124.

National Kidney Foundation. K/DOQI clinical practice guidelines on hypertension and antihypertensive agents in chronic kidney disease: executive summary. *Am J Kidney Dis* 2004; 43:S14–S33.

Nelson RG, Bennett PH, Beck GJ, et al. Development and progression of renal disease in Pima Indians with non-insulin-dependent diabetes mellitus. *N Engl J Med* 1996;334: 1636–1642.

Neumann J, Ligtenberg G, Klein II, et al. Sympathetic hyperactivity in chronic kidney disease: pathogenesis, clinical relevance, and treatment. *Kidney Int* 2004;65:1568–1576.

Nitta K, Uchida K, Nihei H. Spironolactone and angiotensin receptor blocker in nondiabetic renal diseases. *Am J Med* 2004;117:444–445.

Parulkar AA, Pendergrass ML, Granda-Ayala R, et al. Nonhypoglycemic effects of thiazolidinediones. *Ann Intern Med* 2001;134:61–71.

Parving H-H, Lehnert H, Bröchner-Mortensen J, et al. The effect of irbesartan on the development of diabetic nephropathy in patients with type 2 diabetes. *N Engl J Med* 2001; 345:870–878.

Parving H-H, Smidt UM, Andersen AR, Svendsen PAA. Early aggressive antihypertensive treatment reduces rate of decline in kidney function in diabetic nephropathy. *Lancet* 1983;I:1175–1179.

Pereira BJG. Optimization of pre-ESRD care: the key to improved dialysis outcomes. *Kidney Int* 2000;57:351–365.

Perez GO, Lespier L, Knowles R, et al. Potassium homeostasis in chronic diabetes mellitus. *Arch Intern Med* 1977; 137:1018–1022.

Perkins BA, Ficociello LH, Silva KH, et al. Regression of microalbuminuria in type 1 diabetes. *N Engl J Med* 2003;348: 2285–2293.

Pohl MA, Blumenthal S, Cordonnier DJ, et al. The independent and additive impact of blood pressure control and angiotensin II receptor blockade on renal outcomes in the Irbesartan Diabetic Nephropathy Trial (IDNT): clinical implications and limitations. *J Am Soc Nephrol* 2005; (in press).

Popovic-Rolovic M, Kostic M, Antic-Peco A, et al. Medium- and long-term prognosis of patients with acute poststreptococcal glomerulonephritis. *Nephron* 1991;58:393–399.

Port FK, Hulbert-Shearon TE, Wolfe RA, et al. Predialysis blood pressure and mortality risk in a national sample of maintenance hemodialysis patients. *Am J Kidney Dis* 1999; 33:507–517.

Praga M, Hernández E, Herrero JC, et al. Influence of obesity on the appearance of proteinuria and renal insufficiency after unilateral nephrectomy. *Kidney Int* 2000; 58:2111–2118.

Premasathian NC, Muehrer R, Brazy PC, et al. Blood pressure control in kidney transplantation: therapeutic implications. *J Human Hypertens* 2004;18:871–877.

Rachmani R, Levi Z, Slavachevsky I, et al. Effect of an α-adrenergic blocker, and ACE inhibitor and hydrochlorothiazide on blood pressure and on renal function in type 2 diabetic patients with hypertension and albuminuria; a randomized cross-over study. *Nephron* 1998;80:175–182.

Rahman M, Brown CD, Coresh J, et al. The prevalence of reduced glomerular filtration rate in older hypertensive patients and its association with cardiovascular disease: a report from the Antihypertensive and Lipid-Lowering Treatment to Prevent Heart Attack trial. *Arch Intern Med* 2004;164:969–976.

Rahman M, Fu P, Sehgal AR, Smith MC. Interdialytic weight gain, compliance with dialysis regimen, and age are independent predictors of blood pressure in hemodialysis patients. *Am J Kidney Dis* 2000;35:257–265.

Ravid M, Brosh D, Levi Z, et al. Use of enalapril to attenuate decline in renal function in normotensive, normoalbuminuric patients with type 2 diabetes mellitus. *Ann Intern Med* 1998;128:982–988.

Remuzzi G, Perico N. Routine renin-angiotensin system blockade in renal transplantation? *Curr Opin Nephrol Hypertens* 2002;11:1–10.

Remuzzi G, Schieppati A, Ruggenenti P. Nephropathy in patients with type 2 diabetes. *N Engl J Med* 2002;346: 1145–1151.

Ritz E. Renal dysfunction as a novel risk factor: microalbuminuria and cardiovascular risk. *Kidney Int* 2005;67: S25–S29.

Robinson FO, Johnston SR, Atkinson AB. Accelerated hypertension caused by severe phimosis. *J Hum Hypertens* 1992;6:165–166.

Rossing K, Christensen PK, Hovind P, et al. Progression of nephropathy in type 2 diabetic patients. *Kidney Int* 2004; 66:1596.

Ruggenenti P, Perna A, Lanzoni M, Remuzzi G. In non-diabetic chronic nephropathies urinary protein excretion rate accurately predicts progression to end stage renal failure (ESRF) [Abstract]. *J Am Soc Nephrol* 1996;7:1324.

Ruggenenti P, Perna A, Lesti M, et al. Pretreatment blood pressure reliably predicts progression of chronic nephropathies. *Kidney Int* 2000;58:2093–2101.

Ruggenenti P, Perna A, Loriga G, et al. Blood-pressure control for renoprotection in patients with non-diabetic chronic renal disease (REIN-2): multicentre, randomised controlled trial. *Lancet* 2005;365:939–946.

Ruilope LM, Salvetti A, Jamerson K, et al. Renal function and intensive lowering of blood pressure in hypertensive participants of the Hypertension Optimal Treatment (HOT) study. *J Am Soc Nephrol* 2001;12:218–225.

Rule AD, Larson TS, Bergstralh EJ, et al. Using serum creatinine to estimate glomerular filtration rate: accuracy in good health and in chronic kidney disease. *Ann Intern Med* 2004;141:929–937.

Rule AD, Lieber MM, Jacobsen SJ. Is benign prostatic hyperplasia a risk factor for chronic renal failure? *J Urol* 2005;173:691–696.

Russo LM, Bakris GL, Comper WD. Renal handling of albumin: a critical review of basic concepts and perspective. *Am J Kidney Dis* 2002;39:899–919.

Safian RD, Textor SC. Renal-artery stenosis. *N Engl J Med* 2001;344:431–442.

Sarnak MJ, Greene T, Wang X, et al. The effect of a lower target blood pressure on the progression of kidney disease: long-term follow-up of the modification of diet in renal disease study. *Ann Intern Med* 2005;142:342–351.

Sarnak MJ, Levey AS, Schoolwerth AC, et al. Kidney disease as a risk factor for development of cardiovascular disease: AHA Scientific Statement. *Circulation* 2003;108: 2154–2169.

Sato A, Hayashi K, Naruse M, Satura T. Effectiveness of aldosterone blockade in patients with diabetic nephropathy. *Hypertension* 2003;41:64–68.

Sato A, Hayashi K, Saruta T. Antiproteinuric effects of mineralocorticoid receptor blockade in patients with chronic renal disease. *Am J Hypertens* 2005;18:44–49.

Schieppati A, Remuzzi G. The future of renoprotection: frustration and promises. *Kidney Int* 2003;64:1947–1955.

Schrier RW, Estacio RO, Esler A, Mehler P. Effects of aggressive blood pressure control in normotensive type 2 diabetic patients on albuminuria, retinopathy and strokes. *Kidney Int* 2002;61:1086–1097.

Scribner BH. Can antihypertensive medications control BP in haemodialysis patients: yes or no? *Nephrol Dial Transplant* 1999;14:2599–2601.

Segura J, Campo C, Gil P, et al. Development of chronic kidney disease and cardiovascular prognosis in essential hypertensive patients. *J Am Soc Nephrol* 2004;15:1616–1622.

Steen VD, Medsger TA Jr. Long-term outcomes of scleroderma renal crisis. *Ann Intern Med* 2000;133:600–603.

Stevens LA, Levey AS. Clinical implications of estimating equations for glomerular filtration rate. *Ann Intern Med* 2004;141:959–961.

Strippoli GFM, Craig M, Deeks JJ, et al. Effects of angiotensin converting enzyme inhibitors and angiotensin II receptor antagonists on mortality and renal outcomes in diabetic nephropathy: systematic review. *BMJ* 2004; 329: 828–831.

Suzuki H, Kanno Y, Sugahara S, et al. Effects of an angiotensin II receptor blocker, valsartan, on residual renal function in patients on CAPD. *Am J Kidney Dis* 2004;43:1056–1064.

Szczech LA, Lazar IL. Projecting the United States ESRD population: issues regarding treatment of patients with ESRD. *Kidney Int* 2004;66:S3.

Tarnow L, Rossing P, Jensen C, et al. Long-term renoprotective effect of nisoldipine and lisinopril in type 1 diabetic patients with diabetic nephropathy. *Diabetes Care* 2000;23: 1725–1730.

Tee JB, Acott PD, McLellan DH, Crocker JFS. Phenotypic heterogeneity in pediatric autosomal dominant polycystic kidney disease at first presentation: a single-center, 20-year review. *Am J Kidney Dis* 2004;43:296–303.

Textor SC, Taler SJ, Driscoll N, et al. Blood pressure and renal function after kidney donation from hypertensive living donors. *Transplantation* 2004;78(2):276–282.

Tolins JP, Raij L. Antihypertensive therapy and the progression of chronic renal disease. are there renoprotective drugs? *Semin Nephrol* 1991;11:538–548.

Tonelli M, Isles C, Curhan GC, et al. Effect of pravastatin on cardiovascular events in people with chronic kidney disease. *Circulation* 2004;110:1557–1563.

Toto RD, Mitchell HC, Smith RD, et al. "Strict" blood pressure control and progression of renal disease in hypertensive nephrosclerosis. *Kidney Int* 1995;48:851–859.

U.K. Prospective Diabetes Study (UKPDS) Group. Efficacy of atenolol and captopril in reducing risk of macrovascular and microvascular complications in type 2 diabetes: UKPDS 39. *BMJ* 1998;317:713–720.

United States Renal Data System 2003 Annual Data Report (ADR). Available online at: http://www.usrds.org/slides.htm. Accessed May 9, 2005.

Valmadrid CT, Klein R, Moss SE, Klein BEK. The risk of cardiovascular disease mortality associated with microalbuminuria and gross proteinuria in persons with older-onset diabetes mellitus. *Arch Intern Med* 2000;160:1093–1100.

Vidt DG. Cholesterol emboli: a common cause of renal failure. *Annu Rev Med* 1997;48:375–385.

Walser M, Mitch WE, Maroni BJ, Kopple JD. Should protein intake be restricted in predialysis patients? *Kidney Int* 1999;55:771–777.

Wang AYM, Yu AYY, Lam CWK, et al. Effects of losartan or enalapril on hemoglobin, circulating erythropoietin, and insulin-like growth factor-1 in patients with and without posttransplant erythrocytosis. *Am J Kidney Dis* 2002;39: 600–608.

Watts RA, Hoffbrand BI. Hypertension following renal trauma. *J Hum Hypertens* 1987;1:65–71.

Weinberg MS, Kaperonis N, Bakris GL. How high should an ACE inhibitor or angiotensin receptor blocker be dosed in patients with diabetic nephropathy? *Curr Hypertens Rep* 2003;5:418–425.

Weiner DE, Tighiouart H, Amin MG, et al. Chronic kidney disease as a risk factor for cardiovascular disease and all-cause mortality: a pooled analysis of community-based studies. *J Am Soc Nephrol* 2004;15:1307–1315.

Weir MR, Fink JC. Salt intake and progression of chronic kidney disease: an overlooked modifiable exposure? A commentary. *Am J Kidney Dis* 2005;45:176–178.

White KE, Bilous RW. Type 2 diabetic patients with nephropathy show structural-functional relationships that are similar to type 1 disease. *J Am Soc Nephrol* 2000;11:1667–1673.

Wright JT Jr, Bakris G, Greene T, et al. Effect of blood pressure lowering and antihypertensive drug class on progression of hypertensive kidney disease: results of the AASK trial. *JAMA* 2002;288:2421–2431.

Writing Team for the Diabetes Control and Complications Trial/Epidemiology of Diabetes Interventions and Complications Research Group. Sustained effect of intensive treatment of type 1 diabetes mellitus on development and progression of diabetic nephropathy: the Epidemiology of Diabetes Interventions and Complications (EDIC) study. *JAMA* 2003;290:2159–2167.

Young CJ, Gaston RS. Renal transplantation in black Americans. *N Engl J Med* 2000;343:1545–1552.

Zaltzman JS, Nash M, Chiu R, Prasad R. The benefits of renin-angiotensin blockade in renal transplant recipients with biopsy-proven allograft nephropathy. *Nephrol Dial Transplant* 2004;19:940–944.

Zandbergen AAM, Baggen MGA, Lamberts SWJ, et al. Effect of losartan on microalbuminuria in normotensive patients with type 2 diabetes mellitus: a randomized clinical trial. *Ann Intern Med* 2003;139:90–96.

Zhang Z, Shahinfar S, Keane WF, et al. Importance of baseline distribution of proteinuria in renal outcomes trials: Lessons from the Reduction of Endpoints in NIDDM with the Angiotensin II Antagonist Losartan (RENAAL) Study. *J Am Soc Nephrol* 2005;16:1775–1780.

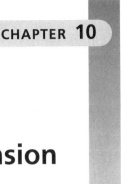

# Renovascular Hypertension

Of all of the fairly common identifiable causes of hypertension, renovascular hypertension (RVHT) remains the most puzzling: Although its pathophysiology seems clear, uncertainty remains as to its prevalence, natural history, diagnosis, and treatment.

These uncertainties reflect a confluence of factors:

- Structural renovascular disease is becoming more prevalent as the population becomes older, hypertensive, and atherosclerotic.
- The presence of structural renovascular disease is being more frequently recognized, particularly by "drive by" renal arteriography done in patients having coronary angiography.
- Revascularization by percutaneous angioplasty/stenting of structural renovascular disease that has not been documented to be the cause of functional renovascular hypertension, though technically easy and financially rewarding, has not been found to be helpful in most patients.
- With increasing scrutiny, tests to document functional renovascular hypertension (such as renal vein sampling) have been found to have poor predictability.

- Data are currently not available to prove the superiority of medical therapy, balloon angioplasty and/or stenting, or surgical repair of those with functional renovascular hypertension.

The dilemma is obvious: More patients have structural renovascular disease that can induce hypertension and renal ischemia but uncertainty remains as to how to diagnose and treat them (Salifu et al., 2005). The dilemma has been described in two contrasting comments: On the one hand, "Indiscriminate testing for renovascular stenosis or fortuitous documentation of lesions leads to procedures laden with morbidity, high cost, and mortality" (Weinrauch & D'Elia, 2004); on the other, "Waiting until revascularization no longer offers the potential for either blood pressure benefit or renal functional recovery serves our patients poorly" (Textor, 2003).

In this chapter, a more conservative approach is recommended than the common practice of immediate angioplasty/stenting whenever a "significant" renal artery stenosis is identified, a practice being performed even in patients with easily controlled hypertension and normal renal function. Long-term cost-benefit advantages may follow such "prophylactic" revascularization (Axelrod et al., 2003), but in view of complications seen even under the best of circumstances (Ivanovic et al., 2003), caution seems advisable. Such caution for most hypertensive patients is recommended by clinicians worldwide (Hartman et al., 2003; Sutton, 2003; Zuchelli, 2002).

On the other hand, patients with refractory hypertension and/or worsening renal function should be evaluated for RVHT and appropriately treated. In such patients, it is important to consider this disease because, if identified, it can be relieved; if left untreated, it may destroy the kidneys. The presence of bilateral renal artery stenosis should be considered in all patients with unexplained chronic or progressive renal insufficiency, because ischemic nephropathy may be involved in one fourth of such patients (Textor, 2004a). Even in patients with end-stage renal disease, relief of renal artery stenoses may prevent or at least delay the need for dialysis (Korsakas et al., 2004).

## RENOVASCULAR DISEASE VERSUS RENOVASCULAR HYPERTENSION

*Renovascular hypertension* refers to hypertension caused by renal ischemia. It is important to realize that renovascular *disease* may or may not cause sufficient hypoperfusion to set off the processes that lead to hypertension. The problem is simply that renovascular disease is much more common than is RVHT. For example, arteriography revealed some degree of renal artery stenosis in 32% of 303 normotensive patients and in 67% of 193 hypertensives with an increasing prevalence with advancing age (Eyler et al., 1962) (Table 10–1). Note that in Table 10–1 almost half of *normotensive* patients older than 60 had atherosclerotic lesions in their renal vessels.

More recent studies show similar data. Among patients having coronary angiograms whose average blood pressure was 143/80 and serum creatinine was 1.1 mL/dL, 47% had renovascular disease by renal angiography (Rihal et al., 2002).

Before procedures were available to prove the functional significance of stenotic lesions, surgery was frequently performed on hypertensive patients with a unilateral small kidney but who did not

> ## TABLE 10–1
>
> ### Prevalence of Renal Arterial Lesions in Normotensive and Hypertensive Patients

| Age, Years | Normotensive Normal | Normotensive Lesion | Hypertensive Normal | Hypertensive Lesion |
|---|---|---|---|---|
| 31–40 | 7 | 3 | 6 | 10 |
| 41–50 | 26 | 8 | 14 | 22 |
| 51–60 | 99 | 35 | 28 | 50 |
| 60+ | 69 | 56 | 15 | 48 |

Data from Eyler WR, Clark MD, Garman JE, et al. Angiography of the renal areas including a comparative study of renal arterial stenoses in patients with and without hypertension. *Radiology* 1962;78:879–892.

have reversible RVHT. Homer Smith (1956) recognized this as early as 1948 as a misguided application of Goldblatt's experimental model of hypertension induced by clamping the renal artery. Smith reported that only 25% of patients were relieved of their hypertension by nephrectomy and warned that only about 2% of all hypertensives probably could be helped by surgery.

## PREVALENCE OF RENOVASCULAR HYPERTENSION

Smith's (1956) estimate of the true prevalence of RVHT may be right. The prevalence varies with the nature of the hypertensive population:

- In nonreferred patient populations, the prevalence is likely less than 1% (see Chapter 1, Table 1–7).
- In patients with suggestive clinical features, the prevalence is higher; 7.3% of 837 patients with suggestive clinical features had at least a 70% stenosis of one or both renal arteries by renal angiography (Buller et al., 2004).
- Among patients with accelerated-malignant hypertension, the prevalence is even higher; of 123 adults with diastolic blood pressure (BP) greater than 125 mm Hg and grade III or IV retinopathy, 4% of Blacks and 32% of Whites had RVHT (Davis et al., 1979).
- High-grade renal artery stenosis also is seen more frequently in hypertensive patients with atherosclerotic disease in peripheral (Leertouwer et al., 2001), carotid, or coronary arteries (Buller et al., 2004); in elderly patients with heart failure (Missouris et al., 2000); and in patients with severe hypertension and rapidly progressing renal insufficiency, particularly if it develops after institution of angiotensin-converting enzyme inhibitor (ACEI) or angiotensin II receptor blocker (ARB) therapy (Krijnen et al., 2004).
- On the other hand, RVHT is less common in Blacks; in one series, it was found in 12% of Blacks versus 28% of Whites (Hansen et al., 1998). However, these same investigators found an equal prevalence of renovascular disease by duplex sonography among Blacks and non-Blacks in a less selected group of elderly people (Edwards et al., 2003).
- Diabetics, even though they have a higher prevalence of renal artery disease (Freedman et al., 2004), have less RVHT (Valabhji et al., 2000).
- Renovascular hypertension has been recognized in neonates (Tapper et al., 1987), children (Liang et al., 1996), and pregnant women (Keely, 1998).

# MECHANISMS OF HYPERTENSION

## Animal Models

Although Franz Volhard and his students supported a pressor role for renal ischemia even earlier (Wolf, 2000), the pathophysiology of RVHT was first identified by Goldblatt et al. (1934) who, looking not for RVHT but for a renal cause for primary hypertension, put clamps on both renal arteries of dogs. The clamps were inserted on separate occasions so that they could observe the effect of unilateral obstruction (Figure 10–1). However, with the modest degree of constriction that they used, unilateral clamping caused only transient hypertension. For permanent hypertension, both renal arteries had to be clamped, or one clamped and the contralateral kidney removed (Goldblatt, 1975).

After significant renal ischemia and the initial marked rise in renin secretion, renin levels fall but remain inappropriately high and are largely responsible for the hemodynamic changes (Welch, 2000). Figure 10–2 shows a stepwise scheme for the hemodynamic and hormonal changes that underlie RVHT.

Other factors may be involved that interrelate to these primary mechanisms, including the following:

- Activation of the sympathetic nervous system (Petersson et al., 2002)
- Progressive structural thickening of small arteries both inside (Anderson et al., 2000) and outside (Rizzoni et al., 2000) the kidney
- Increased lipoxygenases (Romero et al., 1997) and thromboxane (Martinez-Maldonado, 1991), likely involved in the significant fall in blood pressure noted in patients with RVHT who were given aspirin (Imanishi et al., 1989)

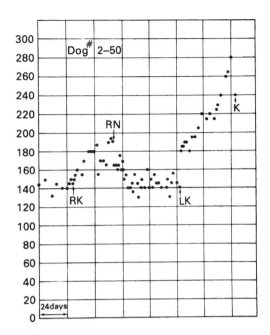

**FIGURE 10–1** ● Results from one of Goldblatt's original experiments. The graph shows the mean blood pressure of a dog whose right kidney was first moderately constricted (RK), with subsequent hypertension that was relieved after right nephrectomy (RN). After severe constriction of the left renal artery (LK), more severe hypertension occurred, and the animal was sacrificed (K). (Reprinted from Hoobler SW. History of experimental renovascular hypertension. In: Stanley JC, Ernst CB, Fry WJ, eds. *Renovascular hypertension*. Philadelphia: Saunders, 1984:12–19, with permission.)

- Increased levels of atrial natriuretic factor, kallikrein (Martinez-Maldonado, 1991), vasodilative prostaglandins (Milot et al., 1996), and nitric oxide (Nakamoto et al., 1995), which may counter

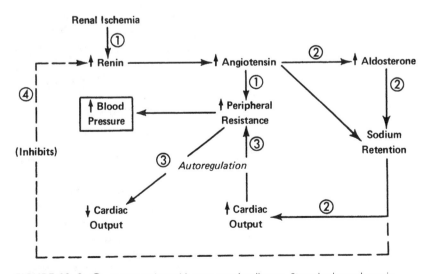

**FIGURE 10–2** ● Hypertension with renovascular disease. Stepwise hemodynamic changes in the development of renovascular hypertension.

the effects of the activated renin-angiotensin system.

## Studies in Humans

As in the animal models, RVHT in humans is caused by increased renin release from the ischemic kidney (Welch, 2000). Simon (2000) suggests that the stenosis must obstruct at least 80% of the arterial lumen to set off the process. The resultant high level of angiotensin II increases renal vascular resistance, causing a shift in the pressure-natriuresis curve; thus, fluid volume is maintained despite markedly elevated BP (Granger & Schnackenberg, 2000). Chronically, the ischemic kidney continues to secrete excess renin and BP falls when angiotensin inhibitors are given. When the stenosis is relieved, hypertension recedes by a fall in peripheral resistance and fluid volume (Valvo et al., 1987).

As in animal models, humans may enter into a third phase, wherein removal of the stenosis or the entire affected kidney will not relieve the hypertension because of arteriolar damage and contralateral glomerulosclerosis, i.e., atherosclerotic nephropathy (Farmer et al., 1999). This phenomenon is clinically relevant: The sooner an arterial lesion that is causing RVHT is removed, the greater the chance of relieving the hypertension. Among 110 patients, corrective surgery for unilateral RVHT was successful in 78% of those with hypertension of less than 5 years' duration but in only 25% of those with hypertension of longer duration (Hughes et al., 1981).

## CLASSIFICATION AND COURSE

The most common cause of RVHT is atherosclerotic stenosis of the main renal artery; most of the remaining cases are fibroplastic, but a number of both intrinsic and extrinsic lesions can induce RVHT (Table 10–2). The general features of the most common types of renal artery stenosis are listed in Table 10–3.

## Atherosclerotic Lesions

As compared to patients with primary hypertension, patients with atherosclerotic RVHT are older and have higher systolic pressure, more extensive renal damage, and vascular disease elsewhere (Buller et al., 2004); more extensive left ventricular hypertrophy; ischemic heart disease; renal insufficiency (Zoccali et al., 2002); and, not surprisingly, lower probability of survival (Conlon et al., 2000).

The atherosclerotic lesions in the renal artery are part of systemic atherosclerosis. Why the process progresses enough to set off renovascular hypertension only in some patients is unknown, but

## TABLE 10–2

### Types of Lesions Associated With Renovascular Hypertension

Intrinsic lesions
  Atherosclerosis
  Fibromuscular dysplasia
    Intimal
    Medial
      Dissection (Edwards et al., 1982)
      Segmental infarction (Salifu et al., 2000)
    Adventitial
  Aneurysm (English et al., 2004)
  Emboli (Dupont et al., 2000)
  Arteritis
    Large artery vasculitis (Slovut & Olin, 2004)
    Takayasu's (Weaver et al., 2004)
  Arteriovenous malformation or fistula (Lekuona et al., 2001)
  Renal artery (Kolhe et al., 2004) or aortic dissection (Rackson et al., 1990)
  Angioma (Farreras-Valenti, 1965)
  Neurofibromatosis[a] (Watano et al., 1996)
  Tumor thrombus (Jennings et al., 1964)
  Thrombosis with the antiphospholipid syndrome (Riccialdelli et al., 2001)
  Thrombosis after antihypertensive therapy (Dussol et al., 1994)
  Rejection of renal transplant (Kasiske et al., 2004)
  Injury to the renal artery
    Stenosis after transplantation (Bruno et al., 2004)
    Trauma (Monstrey et al., 1989)
    Radiation (Shapiro et al., 1977)
    Lithotripsy (Smith et al., 1991)
  Intrarenal cysts (Torres et al., 1991)
  Congenital unilateral renal hypoplasia[a] (Ask-Upmark kidney) (Steffens et al., 1991)
  Unilateral renal infection (Siamopoulos et al., 1983)
Extrinsic lesions
  Pheochromocytoma or paraganglioma (Nakano et al., 1996)
  Congenital fibrous band[a] (Silver & Clements, 1976)
  Pressure from diaphragmatic crus[a] (Martin, 1971)
  Tumors (Restrick et al., 1992)
  Subcapsular or perirenal hematoma (Nomura et al., 1996)
  Retroperitoneal fibrosis (Castle, 1973)
  Perirenal pseudocyst (Kato et al., 1985)
  Stenosis of celiac axis with steal of renal blood flow (Alfidi et al., 1972)

[a]More common in children.

## TABLE 10–3

### Features of the Two Major Forms of Renal Artery Stenosis

| Renal Artery Disease History | Incidence, % | Age, Years | Location of Lesion in Renal Artery | Natural History |
|---|---|---|---|---|
| Atherosclerosis | 90 | >50 | Ostia and proximal 2 cm | Progression is common, sometimes to occlusion |
| Fibromuscular dysplasias | | | | |
| Intimal | 1–2 | Children, young adults | Middle main renal artery | Progression in most |
| Medial | 10 | 15–50 | Distal main renal artery and branches | Progression in 33% |
| Adventitial | <1 | 15–30 | Mid to distal main renal artery | Progression in most |

evidence for two possibilities has been provided: infectious and genetic. The genetic associations are uncertain: Olivieri et al. (2002) reported a 2.25-fold increased odds ratio with the DD variant of the ACE I/D polymorphism; van Onna et al. (2004) found no association with the polymorphism but rather a 44% increased odds ratio with endothelial nitric oxide synthase gene polymorphism. As for infection, a sixfold greater odds ratio of renovascular disease was found in 100 patients clinically suspected of this disease if antibodies to *Chlamydia pneumonia* were present (van der Ven et al., 2002). Obviously, the issue is unsettled. Genetic factors may be responsible for a lower prevalence of RVHT in Blacks. However, when present, the disease is associated with even more severe hypertension and extrarenal vascular disease than are seen in non-Blacks with RVHT (Novick et al., 1994).

### Natural History

The natural history of atherosclerotic renal artery stenosis has been ascertained by repeated renal artery duplex scans in a total of 295 kidneys in 170 patients over a mean of 33 months (Caps et al., 1998a). As seen in Figure 10–3, progression was common in those with initially high-grade (≥60%) stenoses accompanied by a 21% incidence of renal atrophy, defined as a 1.0 cm or greater decrease in renal length (Caps et al., 1998b). Progression was associated with a systolic BP above 160 mm Hg, diabetes mellitus, and high-grade stenoses in either the ipsilateral or the contralateral kidney.

A less progressive loss of renal function has been observed in two studies of patients with at least a 50% renal artery stenosis, recognized incidentally during angiography for coronary (Conlon et al., 2000) or peripheral (Leertouwer et al., 2001) vascular disease. Even though the degree of renal artery stenosis was at least 70% in a significant portion of these patients, end-stage renal failure developed in only 1 of the 188 with coronary disease over 4 years and in none of the 126 with peripheral vascular disease over 10 years. Therefore, as Leertouwer et al. (2001) wrote, "The current trend toward aggressive interventional treatment of incidentally found renal artery stenosis may need careful reappraisal." At the least, a clear distinction should be made between the likelihood of progression of renal artery disease identified in patients with clinically suggestive features of RVHT and evidence of renal ischemia, on the one hand, and patients with no clinical or functional evidence of RVHT, on the other. Even in the presence of high-grade bilateral disease, the progress of renal damage can be slowed without revascularization if the hypertension is intensively treated: 85% of 68 such patients treated medically had stable renal function through 3 years of follow-up (Chábová et al., 2000).

Segmental lesions, usually stenosis of only a small branch supplying a portion of one kidney, were found in 11% of the patients in the large Cooperative Study of Renovascular Hypertension (Bookstein, 1968).

### Fibromuscular Dysplasia

As seen in Figure 10–4, three types of fibromuscular stenoses were defined by investigators at the Mayo Clinic (Lüscher et al., 1987). Of these, medial fibroplasia is the most common, whereas focal fibroplastic lesions are more common in children (Stanley et al., 1978).

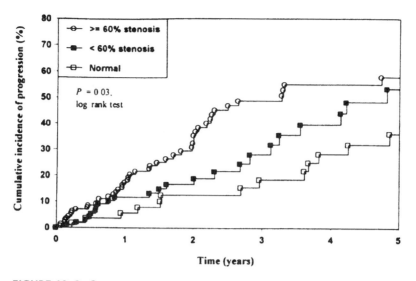

**FIGURE 10–3** ● Cumulative incidence of renal disease progression stratified according to baseline degree of renal artery narrowing. Standard errors were <10% for all plots through 5 years. (Reprinted from Caps MT, Perissinotto C, Zierler E, et al. Prospective study of atherosclerotic disease progression in the renal artery. *Circulation* 1998a;98:2866–2872, with permission.)

Medial fibromuscular dysplasia is usually noted in young women but has been found in older patients, often incidentally (Pascual et al., 2005). The process often involves multiple other arteries, most frequently the carotid and vertebral vessels. Intracranial aneurysms are not infrequent, but most cerebrovascular involvement is asymptomatic (Slovut & Olin, 2004). With high-resolution echograms, Boutouyrie et al. (2003) found abnormal patterns of the carotid artery and thickness of the radial artery in most of 70 patients with renal fibromuscular dysplasia.

The cause of fibromuscular dysplasia remains unknown, though cigarette smoking and hypertension are associated with an increased risk, as is the presence of the disease in first-degree relatives (Slovut & Olin, 2004). Other vascular diseases, in particular large-artery vasculitis, may require intravascular ultrasonography to be distinguished from fibromuscular dysplasia (Gowda et al., 2003).

Patients with the less common but more sharply localized fibroplastic lesions—intimal and adventitial—usually show rapid progression, so severe stenosis and hypertension are frequently observed (Pickering, 1989).

## Other Causes

Of the myriad causes of renovascular hypertension listed in Table 10–2, a few deserve additional comment.

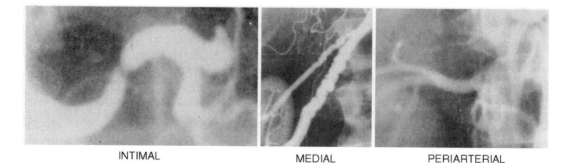

INTIMAL                    MEDIAL                    PERIARTERIAL

**FIGURE 10–4** ● Representative radiographs of the three major types of fibromuscular dysplasia. (Reprinted with permission from Lüscher TF, Lie JT, Stanson AW, et al. Arterial fibromuscular dysplasia. *Mayo Clin Proc* 1987;62:931–952.)

## Aneurysm

Aneurysms are common with medial fibroplasia. Saccular aneurysms, usually at the bifurcation of the renal artery, may induce hypertension by various mechanisms. They rarely rupture and need not be ablated if less than 2.0 cm in diameter in the absence of symptoms or severe hypertension (English et al., 2004).

## Emboli

Most commonly seen as a complication of angiography or vascular surgery, renal cholesterol emboli can induce subacute renal failure or RVHT (Dupont et al., 2000). Cutaneous and other visceral lesions are usually seen, but the diagnosis may be documented only by renal biopsy.

## Arteritis

Progressive aortic arteritis (Takayasu's arteritis) is seen infrequently in North America and Europe but is a common cause of RVHT in China, India, Japan, Mexico, and Brazil (Numano et al., 2000; Weaver et al., 2004).

Renovascular hypertension is common in various vasculitic syndromes with renal involvement, including Wegener's granulomatosis (Woodrow et al., 1990), systemic lupus erythematosus (Ward & Studenski, 1992), and the antiphospholipid syndrome (Riccialdelli et al., 2001). These patients may enter into an acute, severe hypertensive phase, usually associated with markedly elevated plasma renin levels, likely reflecting intrarenal stenoses from multiple arteriolar lesions. The hypertension can sometimes be rather remarkably reversed by ACEI therapy (Coruzzi & Novarini, 1992).

## Aortic Dissection

Renovascular hypertension was found in nearly 20% of patients with aortic dissection (Rackson et al., 1990).

## CLINICAL FEATURES

### General

Clinical features suggestive of renovascular disease as the cause of hypertension are presented in Table 10–4 (McLaughlin et al., 2000). Some of these features were identified in a cooperative study involving 2,442 hypertensive patients, 880 with renovascular disease (Maxwell et al., 1972). Of the 880, surgery was performed on 502; of these, 60% had atherosclerotic lesions and 35% had fibromuscular disease. Table 10–5 compares the clinical characteristics of 131 patients with surgically cured renovascular disease and a carefully

### TABLE 10–4

**Clinical Clues for Renovascular Hypertension**

History
  Onset of hypertension before age 30 in women with no family history (fibromuscular dysplasia)
  Abrupt onset or worsening of hypertension
  Severe or resistant hypertension
  Symptoms of atherosclerotic disease elsewhere
  Smoker
  Worsening renal function with ACE inhibition or AII-receptor blockade
  Recurrent flash pulmonary edema
Examination
  Abdominal bruits
  Other bruits
  Advanced hypertensive retinopathy
Laboratory
  Secondary aldosteronism
    Higher plasma renin
    Low serum potassium
    Low serum sodium
  Proteinuria, usually moderate
  Elevated serum creatinine
  >1.5 cm difference in kidney size on sonography
  Cortical atrophy on CT angiography

matched group with essential hypertension (Simon et al., 1972).

Of the clinical features more common in patients with RVHT, only an abdominal bruit was of clear discriminatory value, heard in 46% of those with RVHT but in only 9% of those with essential hypertension. The bruit was heard over the flank in 12% of those with RVHT and in only 1% of those with essential hypertension. As nicely reviewed by Turnbull (1995), most systolic bruits are innocent, but systolic-diastolic bruits in hypertensives are suggestive of RVHT.

### Additional Features

*Hyperaldosteronism*
Patients with RVHT occasionally have profound secondary aldosteronism with hypokalemia due to urinary potassium wasting but low serum sodium (Agarwal et al., 1999)—all reversed with relief of RVHT.

## TABLE 10–5

### Clinical Characteristics of 131 Patients with Proved Renovascular Hypertension Compared with a Matched Group of Patients with Essential Hypertension

| Characteristics | Essential Hypertension, % | Renovascular Hypertension, % |
|---|---|---|
| Duration of hypertension < 1 yr | 12 | 24 |
| Age at onset after 50 | 9 | 15 |
| Family history of hypertension | 71 | 46 |
| Grade 3 or 4 funduscopic changes | 7 | 15 |
| Abdominal bruit | 9 | 46 |
| Blood urea nitrogen > 20 mg/100 mL | 8 | 15 |
| Serum K < 3.4 mEq/L | 8 | 16 |
| Urinary casts | 9 | 20 |
| Proteinuria | 32 | 46 |

Reprinted with permission from Simon N, Franklin SS, Bleifer KH, et al. Clinical characteristics of renovascular hypertension. *JAMA* 1972;220:1209.

*Nephrotic Syndrome*

Proteinuria is common, and a few patients with RVHT have nephrotic-range proteinuria, usually with more severe renal damage and, often, renal artery thrombosis (Halimi et al., 2000).

*Polycythemia*

Polycythemia has been seen occasionally in patients with RVHT, but elevated peripheral and renal venous erythropoietin levels without polycythemia are much more common (Grützmacher et al., 1989).

*Dyslipidemia*

Not surprisingly, those with atherosclerotic RVHT may have dyslipidemia, in particular low apolipoprotein $A_1$ levels (Scoble et al., 1999). Correction of dyslipidemia may reverse RVHT (Khong et al., 2001).

*Cortical Atrophy*

Cortical atrophy demonstrable by computed tomography (CT) angiography may be an even earlier morphological marker of ischemic damage than overall renal length (Mounier-Vehier et al., 2002).

## Ischemic Nephropathy

Ischemic nephropathy is defined as renal dysfunction secondary to ischemia, usually from bilateral renal artery stenoses or unilateral stenosis with a solitary kidney (Textor, 2004a). Bilateral stenosis develops within 2 years in up to 18% of patients with unilateral atherosclerotic renal artery stenosis (Safian & Textor, 2001) and was present in 28% of the patients in the cooperative study (Bookstein et al., 1977). Such bilateral disease was estimated to be responsible for 38% of end-stage renal disease in the elderly (Gómez Campderá et al., 1998). Although unilateral RVHT is often associated with an elevated serum creatinine, presumably because of nephrosclerosis in the contralateral kidney, an increase to more than 2 mg/dL in a patient with known unilateral RVHT suggests the development of bilateral stenoses (Safian & Textor, 2001).

Such patients with ischemic nephropathy may be difficult to distinguish from the larger number with primary hypertension or primary renal parenchymal disease who progress into renal failure (Textor & Wilcox, 2000). The recognition is important, because surgical repair or angioplasty may occasionally relieve the hypertension and more frequently slow the progression of renal failure (Textor, 2003).

Although the evidence that unilateral renovascular disease is a common cause of renal failure is tenuous at best (Main & Wroe, 2004), the possibility of bilateral renovascular disease should be considered in the following groups:

- Young women with severe hypertension, in whom fibroplastic disease is common.
- Older patients with extensive atherosclerotic disease who suddenly have a worsening of renal function (Conlon et al., 2000).

- Azotemic hypertensives who develop multiple episodes of acute pulmonary edema (Missouris et al., 2000).
- Any hypertensive who develops rapidly progressive renal failure without evidence of obstructive uropathy (Baboolal et al., 1998).
- Patients in whom renal function quickly deteriorates after treatment with an ACEI or ARB (van der Ven et al., 1998).

Such patients, if they are candidates for intervention, should have an appropriate workup to determine the presence of occlusive disease, but no controlled trials in such patients have been performed to determine the best strategy. However, among 59 patients who had angioplasty, better improvement in renal function was seen in those whose serum creatinine levels had rapidly increased before the procedure (Muray et al., 2002).

## Variants

### Hypertension from Contralateral Ischemia

Hypertension may start with renal stenosis on one side but may persist because of damage to the non-stenotic kidney by the hypertension and high renin (Thal et al., 1963).

### Hypertension After Renal Transplantation

As described in Chapter 9, patients who develop severe hypertension after renal transplantation should be evaluated for stenosis of the renal artery. Posttransplant stenoses have been reported in from 1% to 23% of all renal allografts (Bruno et al., 2004).

### Hypertension and the Hypoplastic Kidney

As described in Chapter 9, those patients with a small kidney but without a stenotic lesion who respond to nephrectomy usually have increased levels of plasma renin activity from the venous blood draining the diseased kidney, suggesting a renovascular etiology (Mizuiri et al., 1992). Similarly, in patients with a small kidney and totally occluded renal artery, the presence of increased levels of renin from the occluded kidney is highly predictive of relief of hypertension by nephrectomy (Rossi et al., 2002).

## DIAGNOSTIC TESTS

Before any tests are performed for the diagnosis of renovascular hypertension, the clinician should consider whether, if renovascular disease is present, revascularization would be indicated to provide likely benefit despite the possible complications

(Hartman et al., 2003; Textor, 2003). As listed on the right side of Table 10–6, for those patients with stable renal function and longstanding, stable hypertension that is responsive to easily tolerated antihypertensive drugs, revascularization would likely provide no benefit; therefore, no tests should be performed in them. On the other hand, in those with one or more factors that make a favorable response to revascularization more likely, listed on the left side of Table 10–6, testing should be performed to define the extent of renovascular disease and its functional significance. In those with a high likelihood of RVHT, catheter-directed angiography and, if significant stenoses are seen, immediate revascularization are appropriate.

## Clinical Prediction Rule

Beyond the listing in Table 10–6, more formal protocols have been proposed to grade the clinical features into degrees of likelihood to guide the decision for additional workup for renovascular hypertension. Mann and Pickering (1992) provided an Index of Clinical Suspicion, dividing patients into *low* (who should *not* be further tested), *moderate* (who should have noninvasive testing), or *high* (who may be considered for proceeding directly to renal arteriography) (Table 10–7).

Subsequently, Krijnen and co-workers (1998) performed logistic regression analysis of data from 477 hypertensive patients who underwent renal angiography because of suspicion of RVHT on the basis of drug-resistant hypertension or increases in serum creatinine after ACE inhibition. Their scoring model included age, gender, presence of atherosclerotic vascular disease, recent onset of hypertension, body mass index, presence of abdominal bruit, serum creatinine and cholesterol levels, and smoking. The probability of renal artery stenosis sharply increased as total score rose above 10, reaching almost 100% with sum scores of 25. In these patients, the diagnostic accuracy of their model was similar to that of renal scintigraphy.

Although the predictive power of these clinical indices have not been validated by the results of revascularization, their application would sharply reduce the number of workups that might otherwise be performed in patients with little likelihood of having RVHT. Only those patients with clinical features indicating the presence of RVHT that would likely respond favorably to revascularization would undergo diagnostic testing. The algorithm shown in Figure 10–5 starts with tests that can confirm the clinical likelihood of the presence of RVHT that would likely respond favorably to revascularization and then proceeds to an imaging study.

## TABLE 10–6

### Factors Indicative of Response to Revascularization for Atherosclerotic RVHT

| Favorable | Nonfavorable |
|---|---|
| Blood pressure response likely<br>  —Treatment-resistant hypertension<br>  —Recent onset/progression of hypertension<br>  —Hypertension aggravating acute coronary syndromes<br>  —Impaired cardiac function/"flash" pulmonary edema | Blood pressure response less likely<br>  —Longstanding stable hypertension<br>  —Acceptable blood pressures/tolerable medication<br>    regimen |
| Renal functional response likely<br>  —Entire renal mass affected: solitary functioning<br>    kidney/bilateral RAS<br>  —Recent fall in GFR<br>  —Viable kidneys: blood flow preserved on<br>    nephrogram/favorable resistance index by Doppler<br>    ultrasound<br>  —Acute renal failure during antihypertensive therapy,<br>    especially with angiotensin-converting enzyme<br>    inhibitors/angiotensin receptor blockers | Renal function less likely to benefit<br>  —Unilateral RAS with normal contralateral circulation<br>  —Bilateral parenchymal disease (elevated resistance index<br>    in contralateral kidney)<br>  —Stable kidney function |
| Patient considered viable with reasonable life expectancy | Patient with limited viability<br>  —Severe comorbid disease likely to limit life expectancy |

Modified from Textor SC. Stable patients with atherosclerotic renal artery stenosis should be treated first with medical management. *Am J Kidney Dis* 2003;42:858–863.

As noted in Table 10–7, those patients with a high index of clinical suspicion, in whom it is essential to identify RVHT if it is present, should start with catheter-directed contrast angiography and, if a significant stenosis is found, have immediate angioplasty/stenting.

## Tests to Predict the Response to Revascularization

### Renin Measurements

According to the pathophysiology described earlier, renovascular hypertension should be associated with hypersecretion of renin from a kidney that is significantly hypoperfused.

#### Peripheral Blood

Although increased levels of plasma renin activity (PRA) are found in some patients with RVHT, they are not elevated in many (Rudnick & Maxwell, 1984), in keeping with the experimental evidence that secretion of renin from the clipped kidney falls to "normal" soon after RVHT is induced, whereas renin release from the contralateral kidney is suppressed.

On the other hand, low-normal peripheral blood renin levels may be an accurate predictor of no benefit from revascularization (Hasbak et al., 2002).

Various maneuvers have been used to augment renin release in the hope that patients with curable disease would show a hyperresponsiveness, thereby improving the discriminatory value of PRA levels (Wilcox, 2000). The most widely used maneuver, response of PRA to captopril, has been found to have limited value as a screening study (Vasbinder et al., 2001).

#### Comparison of Renal Vein Renins

The comparison of renin levels in blood from each renal vein, obtained by percutaneous catheterization, has been used to establish both the diagnosis and reversibility of RVHT with a ratio greater than 1.5:1.0 between the two renal veins considered abnormal or lateralizing. In initial reports, an abnormal ratio was 92% predictive of curability; however, 65% of those whose renal vein PRA level ratio did not lateralize also were improved by surgery (Rudnick & Maxwell, 1984). More recently, the procedure has been found to have poor

# FACTORS INDICATIVE OF RESPONSE TO REVASCULARIZATION (Table 10.6)

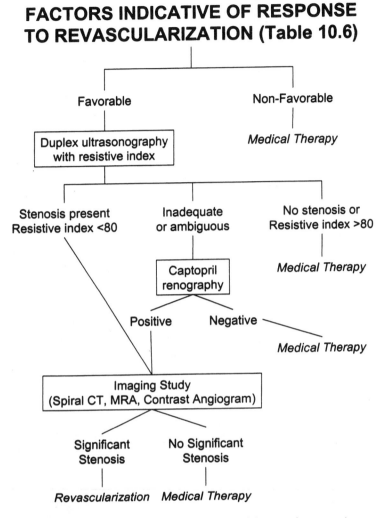

**FIGURE 10–5** ● An algorithm for evaluation and therapy of renovascular hypertension based on the presence of factors indicative of a response to revascularization (shown in Table 10–6).

predictive value (Hasbak et al., 2002) except in the relatively few patients with total occlusion of one renal artery (Rossi et al., 2002).

## Renal Scans

Even more than with renin levels, it seems logical that hypoperfusion of the affected kidney would be seen with RVHT. However, at least two factors may be involved in reducing the discriminatory power of renal perfusion studies. First, for reasons that are not apparent, considerable asymmetry of renal blood flow is present in the absence of RVHT. Asymmetry, defined as a 25% or greater difference between the two kidneys, was found in 51% of 148 hypertensive patients whose renal arteries were patent by angiography (van Onna et al., 2003). Not

surprisingly, the presence of asymmetry increased the rate of false-positive results of renal scintigraphy.

The second factor that may play a role is the frequent development of either bilateral renovascular disease or atherosclerotic nephropathy in the contralateral kidney, both leading to a decreased differential of blood flow. Nonetheless, renal perfusion scans may serve to predict the response to revascularization.

Renography may be done with radiolabeled agents that are excreted either by glomerular filtration—technetium-99 diethylenetriamine pentaacetic acid ($^{99}$Tc-DTPA)—or partially by filtration but mainly by tubular secretion to measure renal blood flow—$^{131}$I-hippurate, or $^{99}$Tc-mercaptoacetyltriglycine ($^{99}$Tc-MAG$_3$). When used alone, isotopic

## TABLE 10–7

**Testing for Renovascular Hypertension: Clinical Index of Suspicion as a Guide to Selecting Patients for Workup**

### Index of Clinical Suspicion

Low (should not be tested)

Borderline, mild to moderate hypertension, in the absence of clinical clues

Moderate (noninvasive tests recommended)

Severe hypertension (DBP > 120 mm Hg)

Hypertension refractory to standard therapy excluding ACE inhibitors and AII-blockers

Abrupt onset of sustained, moderate to severe hypertension at age <20 or >50

Hypertension with a suggestive abdominal or flank bruit

Moderate hypertension (DBP > 105 mm Hg) in a smoker, a patient with evidence of occlusive vascular disease (cerebrovascular, coronary, peripheral vascular), or a patient with unexplained but stable elevation of serum creatinine

Normalization of blood pressure by an ACE inhibitor in a patient with moderate to severe hypertension (particularly a smoker or a patient with recent onset of hypertension)

High (may consider proceeding directly to arteriography)

Severe hypertension (DBP > 120 mm Hg) with either progressive renal insufficiency or refractoriness to aggressive treatment, particularly in a patient who has been a smoker or has other evidence of occlusive arterial disease

Accelerated or malignant hypertension (grade III or IV retinopathy)

Hypertension with recent elevation of serum creatinine, either unexplained or reversibly induced by an ACE inhibitor or AII-receptor blocker

Moderate to severe hypertension with incidentally detected asymmetry of renal size

Modified from Mann SJ, Pickering TG. Detection of renovascular hypertension. State of the art: 1992. *Ann Intern Med* 1992;117:845–853.

renograms provided about 75% sensitivity and specificity for the diagnosis of RVHT (Pickering, 1991).

Soon after the observation that renal function in an ischemic kidney could abruptly be reduced further after a single dose of the ACEI captopril (Hricik et al., 1983), the effect of captopril on renal uptake of $^{99}$Tc-DTPA was reported (Wenting et al., 1984). Either a reduction of the uptake of $^{99}$Tc-DTPA or a slowing of the excretion of $^{131}$I-hippurate or $^{99}$Tc-MAG$_3$ can be used to identify the effect of the ACEI in removing the protective actions of the high levels of angiotensin II on the autoregulation of glomerular filtration and on the maintenance of renal blood flow, respectively (Figure 10–6).

To reduce the cost and time of the workup, the postcaptopril renal scan should be done first. If the result is negative (as it will be most of the time), there is no need for a precaptopril renogram. If the test is positive, the procedure should be repeated the next day without captopril to ensure that the differences are related to reversible vascular disease and not parenchymal damage.

As reviewed by Taylor (2000), ACEI renography is highly accurate in patients with a moderate likelihood of RVHT and normal renal function, wherein sensitivity and specificity are approximately 90%. By combining data from 10 studies that evaluated the effects of revascularization in 291 patients, the mean positive predictive value of ACEI renography was 92%. Less impressive results have been reported more recently in patients who had angioplasty (van Jaarsveld & Deinum, 2001; Soulez et al., 2003). As expected, the test is less sensitive in patients with renal insufficiency; as many as half will have an "indeterminate" test. The test can be done in patients taking various antihypertensive drugs although sensitivity is reduced in patients who are on ACEI or ARB therapy (Pedersen, 2000), which should be discontinued at least 3 days before renography.

### Resistive Index by Duplex Ultrasonography

In some centers, duplex ultrasonography has been found to be an excellent screening test (Olin et al.,

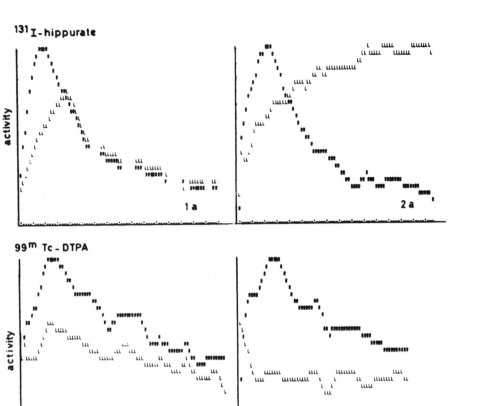

**FIGURE 10–6** ● Renography in a 42-year-old man with hypertension and stenosis of the left renal artery. L, left kidney; R, right kidney. After percutaneous transluminal angioplasty (PTA), his hypertension was cured. The upper half of the figure shows $^{131}$I-hippurate (a) and the lower half shows $^{99m}$Tc-diethylenetriamine pentaacetic acid (DTPA) (b) time-activity curves in two different circumstances: (1) before PTA without any medication (control) and (2) before PTA but with 25 mg captopril taken orally 1 hour before the investigation. Captopril slowed down the excretion of $^{131}$I-hippurate and reduced the uptake of $^{99m}$Tc-DTPA in only the left kidney. (Reprinted from Geyskes GG, Oei HY, Puylaert BAJ, et al. Renovascular hypertension identified by captopril-induced changes in the renogram. *Hypertension* 1987;9:451–458, with permission.)

1995), but some have found it to be technically difficult and relatively insensitive (de Haan et al., 2002). However, the estimation of the resistance index from the end-diastolic and maximal systolic velocities has been shown to predict the clinical response to revascularization.

Patients may not respond to technically effective revascularization because of structural damage to the poststenotic vasculature, either because their underlying disease was primary hypertension leading to nephrosclerosis or because of the development of atherosclerotic nephropathy. To measure the degree of vascular resistance beyond the stenosis, the velocities of blood flow within the renal artery have been estimated by Doppler ultrasonography (Cohn et al., 1998; Frauchiger et al., 1996). Radermacher et al. (2000) defined the resistive

index with this equation: [1 minus (end-diastolic velocity ÷ maximal systolic velocity)] x 100.

The resistive index was measured in 138 patients with renovascular disease before revascularization by angioplasty or surgery (Radermacher et al., 2001). In the 35 who had a resistive index value of 80 or higher, only one had a subsequent 10 mm Hg or greater fall in blood pressure. In the 96 patients with a resistive index value of less than 80, the mean blood pressure in 90 fell by at least 10 mm Hg. The index also predicted postrevascularization changes in renal function better than any other clinical or laboratory finding.

In another study involving 74 patients, a resistive index of below 75 when combined with kidney length of over 93 mm provided the best prediction of a favorable response to angioplasty

(Soulez et al., 2003). In 12 patients with post-transplant RVHT, a low resistive index was found before successful angioplasty (Bruno et al., 2003). Obviously, additional experience with this measure of intrarenal vascular resistance will be needed to prove its predictive ability.

## Tests Imaging the Renal Arteries

### Catheter-Directed Renal Arteriography

For many years, catheter-directed arteriography was the only procedure available to visualize the renal vessels. As noninvasive imaging became available, arteriography has been utilized less except as a "drive-by" procedure in patients having coronary angiography (Rihal et al., 2002).

Part of the resistance to arteriography arises from the potential for contrast media nephropathy, particularly in patients with underlying renal insufficiency. The likelihood of such nephropathy has been considerably reduced by current procedures, including selective injections of small volumes of low- or iso-osmolar contrast media (Morcos, 2004) and preventive hydration (Merten et al., 2004).

Arteriography is still necessary before revascularization either by surgery or angioplasty/stent and to rule out peripheral or branch renal arterial disease (Reidy, 2002).

Although renal arteriography is almost always successful in diagnosing renal artery stenosis, it is of relatively little value in determining curability of RVHT. In the cooperative study, the degree of stenosis, the presence of poststenotic dilatation, and the presence of collateral circulation were of no significant discriminatory value in predicting success or failure of surgery (Bookstein et al., 1972). Moreover, even in the best of hands, there is substantial interobserver variability in the grading of stenosis (Reidy, 2002). The addition of Doppler measurements during arteriography may provide a better indicator of reversibility by revascularization (Mounier-Vehier et al., 2004).

### Spiral Computed Tomography and Magnetic Resonance Imaging

Both spiral computed tomography (CT) and magnetic resonance imaging (MRI) are being increasingly used to visualize the renal arteries, to reduce the dangers of contrast media nephropathy and cholesterol embolization while providing excellent sensitivity (Textor, 2004b). The most important advantages of spiral computed tomographic angiography are the injection of contrast medium intravenously rather than directly into the renal arteries, the ability to visualize both the arterial lumen

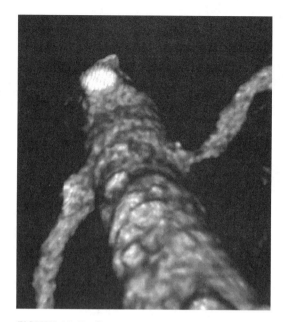

**FIGURE 10–7** ● An upward view of a spiral computed tomographic angiogram demonstrating proximal left renal artery atherosclerotic stenosis.

and wall in three dimensions, and the ability to visualize accessory and distal vessels (Figure 10–7).

Magnetic resonance imaging with gadolinium enhancement involves no ionizing radiation or potentially nephrotoxic contrast media. Moreover, in addition to imaging the renal arteries, MRI can provide useful data on total renal length and volume. In the future, newer procedures such as electron beam CT may provide separate measurements of renal hemodynamics and function (Juillard et al., 2004). Moreover, free-breathing rapid renal MRI has been developed that does not require a contrast media (Katoh et al., 2004).

Despite the increasing acceptance of CT and MRI as noninvasive techniques to visualize the renal arteries, Vasbinder et al. (2004) reported both procedures to have poor specificity and selectivity compared to digital subtraction angiography. As Textor (2004b) noted, their study has numerous weaknesses and should not detract from the appropriate use of either CT or MRI.

## Conclusion

The algorithm shown in Figure 10–5 recommends testing for atherosclerotic RVHT only in those patients who are more likely to have a favorable response to revascularization. No accurate estimates of the numbers of such patients are available, but they likely make up less than 5% of the total hypertensive population and even less than that percentage of hypertensives over age 65. The algorithm can be applied to patients with fibromuscular dysplasia. Being younger, they are usually easier to identify on clinical grounds, less likely to have renal insufficiency or extensive atherosclerosis, and, as will be seen, more likely to have a favorable response to medical therapy or revascularization.

Except in those relatively few patients with such high likelihood of RVHT in whom immediate direct angiography is indicated, the algorithm starts with a study to confirm the clinical evidence for a favorable response to revascularization. Only those likely to respond would then have an imaging study to visualize the extent of renovascular disease, thereby pointing to the appropriate mode of revascularization.

Since Doppler ultrasonography with measurement of the resistive index can both identify renovascular disease and, according to still limited experience, ascertain the likelihood of a response to revascularization, this procedure is a logical way to begin. If duplex sonography is unavailable or technically inadequate, captopril renography is recommended.

Current clinical practice often starts with a noninvasive imaging study and, if that portrays a stenosis considered significant—varying in published series from >50% to >80%—angioplasty/stent is recommended. However, such intervention without predictive testing has provided no benefit in up to 40% of patients (Morganti et al., 2002). Moreover, only those who have significant bilateral stenoses appear to need immediate intervention (Krijnen et al., 2004). Therefore, this more conservative approach as recommended by radiologists at the Mayo Clinic (Hartman et al., 2003) seems appropriate.

In an initial report, plasma levels of brain natriuretic peptide (BNP) were found to be a good predictor of BP response to stent revascularization: 17 of 22 with BNP >80 pg/mL responded whereas none of the five with <80 pg/mL improved (Silva et al., 2005).

## THERAPY

Once a lesion is found and proved to be functionally significant, three choices are available for the treatment of RVHT: medical therapy, angioplasty, and surgical revascularization. In addition, intensive control of all concomitant cardiovascular risk factors is mandatory.

Over the past few years, angioplasty with stenting has far surpassed surgery when revascularization is deemed necessary (Murphy et al., 2004).

At the same time, as the limitations of revascularization have become obvious, more patients are being treated medically, at least until they show evidence of progression of renal damage.

## Patients with Renal Insufficiency

The presence of renal insufficiency when RVHT is identified poses additional risks but also the potential for important benefits by revascularization (Textor, 2004a). In a series of 261 patients treated by angioplasty with stenting, the presence of renal insufficiency at baseline and follow-up was associated with increased mortality, primarily from cardiac causes, after adjusting for other known variables (Kennedy et al., 2003). On the other hand, survival was significantly improved in those whose renal function improved after revascularization.

About one fourth of patients with RVHT and renal insufficiency die within the next 2 to 3 years without revascularization (Chábová et al., 2000), and similar mortality rates have been noted in those revascularized by angioplasty (Kennedy et al., 2003) or surgery (Hallett et al., 1995).

The lack of clear reductions in mortality in the few comparative studies of revascularization versus medical therapy (Nordmann et al., 2003) and the potential adverse effects of either angioplasty or surgery have tempered the enthusiasm for revascularization in patients with RVHT and renal insufficiency. However, as Textor (2003) notes:

> What should not be lost in this debate [over whether to treat medically or by revascularization] is the major advantage accrued to the subset of patients who do, in fact, have major improvements in both blood pressure control and renal function. Our own series of patients revascularized with renal insufficiency (serum creatinine levels ≥2.0 mg/dL [≥177 μmol/L]) indicated that 27% had a major clinical improvement (defined as a fall in serum creatinine of at least 1.0 mg/dL [88 μmol/L]) (Hallett et al., 1995). Similar data appear consistently throughout reported series in the literature, regardless of the exact criteria to define improvement in renal function.

Uncertainty continues as to the choice of therapy (Plouin, 2003; Textor, 2003). As noted by Textor (2003), there is

> a window of opportunity for revascularization. If one intervenes too early or too broadly, many patients with easily controlled pressures and normal renal function will gain little and unnecessarily accrue the risks and expense of vascular procedures. If one intervenes too late or in cases of too advanced renal dysfunction, some patients miss the benefits of improved blood pressures and

recovery of renal function and face increased mortality risks. . . . The practical challenge for the responsible clinician, then, is to realistically evaluate measures of progression and the adequacy of arterial pressure control and stability of renal function over a period. Some of the compelling factors that guide this decision and favor moving ahead with renal revascularization are summarized in the table [Table 10–6]. This process requires a commitment to follow (1) accurate measures of blood pressure control and medication requirements and (2) serial assessment of kidney function and vascular disease progression, particularly when the entire renal mass is affected (e.g., with bilateral disease or disease to a solitary functioning kidney).

What are the risks of early intervention? These consist mainly of (1) treatment failure and/or (2) deterioration of renal function (occasionally with other systems involved, such as aortic dissection or atheroemboli). Rather than rely only on immediate complications attributed to the procedures themselves (which appear to be improving), I favor providing the patient with a realistic estimate of the risks of failure to obtain benefit and long-term clinical events. . . . Realistically, [in] at least 20% of patients . . . renal function will deteriorate after revascularization procedures. While this may be higher than many in the interventional world recognize, most series support this figure, including the one published by Kennedy et al. (2003). However, the presence of the conditions [listed on the left side of Table 10–6] commonly makes the risks of not undertaking renal revascularization even higher. As physicians, we must not fail to recognize and provide the benefits of restoring the renal circulation in such patients. The task of the clinician is to recognize when a patient with atherosclerotic RAS faces a combined risk of progressive renal disease, cardiovascular mortality, and poorly controlled blood pressure sufficient to accept the risks of revascularization. While this is a challenge, the penalties for delaying too long are even more severe, carrying the combined price of accelerated cardiovascular mortality and the need for renal replacement therapy. Until prospective trials outline more specific criteria, [clinicians] must weigh these factors carefully for each patient, with close follow-up over time.

## Medical Therapy

Although all classes of antihypertensive drugs have been used to treat RVHT, the largest experience has been with an ACEI (Plouin, 2003). In the largest published analysis, captopril was effective for at least 3 months in more than 80% of 269 patients with RVHT; progressive renal failure mandating the discontinuation of therapy occurred in only 5% (Hollenberg, 1988).

As noted earlier, the use of an ACEI (or an ARB) may markedly decrease blood flow to the kidney beyond the stenosis, and, if that is the only kidney or if there is bilateral renovascular disease, the result may be rapid, although usually reversible, renal failure. This occurs because of the removal of angiotensin II support of autoregulation and the preferential dilation of renal efferent vessels that together lead to reduced glomerular filtration and renal perfusion (van der Ven et al., 1998). Fortunately, return of renal function is usual when the ACEI is stopped. Nonetheless, complete occlusions of markedly stenotic renal arteries after ACEI therapy may occur (Dussol et al., 1994).

Calcium channel blockers (CCBs) may provide equal control of hypertension and less impairment of renal function than do ACEIs, as they maintain blood flow better because of their preferential preglomerular vasodilative effect, but there are no data documenting their long-term effectiveness. Extra caution is obviously needed in treating those with bilateral RVHT. Even without ACEIs, progression to end-stage renal disease may occur, particularly if the BP is not well controlled (Krijnen et al., 2004).

Preliminary evidence suggests a role of oxidative stress in the renal damage induced by ischemia and protection by large doses of antioxidants (Chade et al., 2003).

## Angioplasty

After the first report of successful treatment of RVHT by percutaneous transluminal renal angioplasty (Grüntzig et al., 1978), the technical aspects have continually improved, including the use of filtering devices to recapture debris that could otherwise induce atheroembolization (Holden & Hill, 2003). The high rate of restenosis with balloon angioplasty has led to increasing use of stents, particularly in those with atherosclerotic ostial lesions (Zeller et al., 2003) or posttransplant RVHT (Bruno et al., 2003).

The study by Zeller et al. (2003) and many other uncontrolled observational studies have shown benefit in both lowering of blood pressure and improvement in renal function in most patients after angioplasty with stenting (Sivamurthy et al., 2004). However, there are only limited data from controlled trials comparing it against medical therapy (Nordmann et al., 2003). In three trials involving 210 patients with 50% or greater renovascular stenosis and poorly controlled hypertension, angioplasty (without stents) provided better control of blood pressure (by an average of 7/3 mm Hg) than did medical therapy but had similar effects on renal function

(Plouin et al., 1998; van Jaarsveld et al., 2000; Webster et al., 1998). Even these small studies were flawed by exclusions and crossovers. The large-scale randomized trial comparing medical therapy with or without stenting that is now in progress (Textor, 2003) will hopefully provide definitive data.

## Surgery

As with angioplasty, there are many uncontrolled observational studies showing benefits for both blood pressure and renal function by surgery (Cherr et al., 2002; Marone et al., 2004). Despite the increasing likelihood that patients who are referred for surgical repair will either have failed to respond to angioplasty or have extensive atherosclerotic disease in the aorta or mesenteric vessels that also needs repair, the overall results with surgery seem generally comparable to those seen with technically successful angioplasty (Aurell & Jensen, 1997; Hallett et al., 1995). Postoperative mortality is higher, averaging about 5% in the first month (Cherr et al., 2002).

Surgery may be the only choice for patients with major renal artery involvement by arteritis (Weaver et al., 2004). In addition, nephrectomy may be appropriate for patients with refractory hypertension and an atrophic, nonfunctioning kidney (Canzanello, 2004).

### The Choice of Therapy

In reviewing the recent literature, a number of points become obvious:

- There are no properly controlled, large-scale, long-term studies of the relative value of the three modes of therapy. A multicenter, randomized trial comparing medical therapy with or without endovascular stenting for intensive medical therapy for preserving renal function, the Cardiovascular Outcomes for Renal Atherosclerotic Lesions (CORAL) trial, is now in progress but results will not be known for 5 or more years.
- Patients with fibroplastic disease do better than do those with atherosclerotic disease when treated medically or by revascularization (Slovut & Olin, 2004). Those who do not respond to medical therapy should have angioplasty, usually without a stent. Angioplasty cures or improves 70% to 90% (Slovut & Olin, 2004).
- For atherosclerotic RVHT, *medical therapy,* usually with an ACEI or ARB and often with a CCB, may be effective over many years (Chábová et al., 2000; Plouin, 2003).
- *Angioplasty,* usually with a stent, has become the initial therapy in most patients who do not tolerate

or respond to medical therapy or who have progressive renal impairment (Textor, 2003).
- *Surgical revascularization* is less commonly indicated, except when angioplasty with stenting is not feasible or is unsuccessful or when abdominal vascular surgery is required. Nonetheless, in experienced hands, surgery provides equal, if not better, preservation of renal function and amelioration of hypertension as compared to other procedures (Cherr et al., 2002).
- Revascularization or angioplasty is being increasingly performed for ischemic nephropathy, even in older patients with significant renal insufficiency, more to preserve renal function than to control hypertension (Korsakas et al., 2004; Marone et al., 2004).

Obviously, uncertainties remain about both the diagnosis and treatment of RVHT. The separation of patients with atherosclerotic renovascular disease, who comprise about 90% of those with RVHT, into those who are either likely or unlikely to have a favorable response to revascularization (shown in Table 10–6) should be of considerable help. However, the uncertainties that remain seem so formidable that clinicians experienced with the management of RVHT should almost always be involved in the evaluation and treatment of these patients.

## RENIN-SECRETING TUMORS

Renin-secreting tumors are not common. Since the recognition of the first case in 1967 (Robertson et al., 1967), only about 50 have been reported, but since it has been so well described (Corvol et al., 1994; Haab et al., 1995), fewer will be deemed worthy of publication. Most such tumors are relatively small and are composed of renin-secreting juxtaglomerular cells (i.e., hemangiopericytomas). Other causes of hypertension and high renin levels include:

- Wilms's tumor in children, usually associated with high levels of prorenin (Leckie et al., 1994).
- Renal cell carcinoma (Moein & Dehghani, 2000); tumors of various extrarenal sites, including lung, ovary, liver, pancreas, sarcomas, and teratomas (Pursell & Quinlan, 2003), and adrenal paraganglionoma (Arver et al., 1999).
- Large intrarenal tumors that compress renal vessels.
- Unilateral juxtaglomerular cell hyperplasia (Kuchel et al., 1993).

Most of the renin-secreting tumors of renal origin fit a rather typical pattern:

- Severe hypertension in relatively young patients: The oldest reported has been 53 (Haab et al., 1995), but most are younger than 25.

- Secondary aldosteronism, usually manifested by hypokalemia.
- Very high prorenin and renin levels in the peripheral blood; even higher levels from the kidney harboring the tumor (Koriyama et al., 1999).
- Tumor recognizable by CT scan.
- Morphologically, a hemangiopericytoma arising from the juxtaglomerular apparatus.

Now that the renal causes of hypertension have been covered, we turn to those seen during pregnancy and with the use of oral contraceptives.

## REFERENCES

Agarwal M, Lynn KL, Richards AM, Nicholls MG. Hyponatremic-hypertensive syndrome with renal ischemia. *Hypertension* 1999;33:1020–1024.

Alfidi RJ, Tarar R, Fosmoe RJ, et al. Renal splanchnic steal and hypertension. *Radiology* 1972;102:545–549.

Anderson WP, Kett MM, Stevenson KM, et al. Renovascular hypertension: structural changes in the renal vasculature. *Hypertension* 2000;36:648–652.

Arver S, Jacobsson H, Cedermark B, et al. Malignant human renin producing paraganglionoma—localization with [123]I-MIBG and treatment with [131]I-MIBG. *Clin Endocrinol* 1999;51:631–635.

Aurell M, Jensen G. Treatment of renovascular hypertension. *Nephron* 1997;75:373–383.

Axelrod DA, Fendrick AM, Carlos RC, et al. Percutaneous stenting of incidental unilateral renal artery stenosis: decision analysis of costs and benefits. *J Endovasc Ther* 2003; 10:546–556.

Baboolal K, Evans C, Moore RH. Incidence of end-stage renal disease in medically treated patients with severe bilateral atherosclerotic renovascular disease. *Am J Kidney Dis* 1998;31:971–977.

Bookstein JJ, Abrams HL, Buenger RE, et al. Radiologic aspects of renovascular hypertension. Part 3. Appraisal of arteriography. *JAMA* 1972;221:368–374.

Bookstein JJ, Maxwell MH, Abrams HL, et al. Cooperative study of radiologic aspects of renovascular hypertension. Bilateral renovascular disease. *JAMA* 1977;237:1706–1709.

Bookstein JJ. Segmental renal artery stenosis in renovascular hypertension. *Radiology* 1968;90:1073–1083.

Boutouyrie P, Gimenez-Roqueplo A-P, Fine E, et al. Evidence for carotid and radial artery wall subclinical lesions in renal fibromuscular dysplasia. *J Hypertens* 2003;21:2287–2295.

Bruno S, Ferrari S, Remuzzi G, Ruggenenti P. Doppler ultrasonography in posttransplant renal artery stenosis: a reliable tool for assessing effectiveness of revascularization? *Transplantation* 2003;76:147–153.

Bruno S, Remuzzi G, Ruggenenti P. Transplant renal artery stenosis. *J Am Soc Nephrol* 2004;15:134–141.

Buller CE, Norareda JG, Ramanathan K, et al. The profile of cardiac patients with renal artery stenosis. *J Am Coll Cardiol* 2004;43:1606–1613.

Canzanello VJ. Medical management of renovascular hypertension. In: G.A. Mansoor, ed. *Secondary Hypertension: Clinical Presentation, Diagnosis, and Treatment.* Totowa, NJ: Humana Press Inc., 2004.

Caps MT, Perissinotto C, Zierler RE, et al. Prospective study of atherosclerotic disease progression in the renal artery. *Circulation* 1998a;98:2866–2872.

Caps MT, Zierler RE, Polissar NL, et al. Risk of atrophy in kidneys with atherosclerotic renal artery stenosis. *Kidney Int* 1998b;53:735–742.

Castle CH. Iatrogenic renal hypertension: two unusual complication of surgery for familial pheochromocytoma. *JAMA* 1973;225:1085–1088.

Chábová V, Schirger A, Stanson AW, et al. Outcomes of atherosclerotic renal artery stenosis managed without revascularization. *Mayo Clin Proc* 2000;75:437–444.

Chade AR, Rodriguez-Porcel M, Herrmann J, et al. Beneficial effects of antioxidant vitamins on the stenotic kidney. *Hypertension* 2003;42:605–612.

Cherr GS, Hansen KJ, Craven TE, et al. Surgical management of atherosclerotic renovascular disease. *J Vasc Surg* 2002;35:236–245.

Cohn EJ, Benjamin ME, Sandager GP, et al. Can intrarenal duplex waveform analysis predict successful renal artery revascularization? *J Vasc Surg* 1998;28:471–481.

Conlon PJ, O'Riordan E, Kalra PA. New insights into the epidemiologic and clinical manifestations of atherosclerotic renovascular disease. *Am J Kidney Dis* 2000;35:573–587.

Coruzzi P, Novarini A. Which antihypertensive treatment in renal vasculitis? *Nephron* 1992;62:372.

Corvol P, Pinet F, Plouin P-F, et al. Renin-secreting tumors. *Endocrinol Metab Clin North Am* 1994;23:255–270.

Davis BA, Crook JE, Vestal RE, Oates JA. Prevalence of renovascular hypertension in patients with grade III or IV hypertensive retinopathy. *N Engl J Med* 1979;301:1273–1276.

de Haan MW, Kroon AA, Flobbe K, et al. Renovascular disease in patients with hypertension: detection with duplex ultrasound. *J Human Hypertens* 2002;16:501–507.

Dupont PJ, Lightstone L, Clutterbuck EJ, et al. Cholesterol emboli syndrome. *BMJ* 2000;321:1065–1067.

Dussol B, Nicolino F, Brunet P, et al. Acute transplant artery thrombosis induced by angiotensin-converting inhibitor in a patient with renovascular hypertension. *Nephron* 1994;66:102–104.

Edwards BS, Stanson AW, Holley KE, Sheps SG. Isolated renal artery dissection. Presentation, evaluation, management, and pathology. *Mayo Clin Proc* 1982;57:564–571.

Edwards MS, Hansen KJ, Craven TE, et al. Relationships between renovascular disease, blood pressure, and renal function in the elderly: a population-based study. *Am J Kidney Dis* 2003;41:990–996.

English WP, Pearce JD, Craven TE, et al. Surgical management of renal artery aneurysms. *J Vasc Surg* 2004; 40:53–60.

Eyler WR, Clark MD, Garman JE, et al. Angiography of the renal areas including a comparative study of renal arterial stenoses in patients with and without hypertension. *Radiology* 1962;78:879–892.

Farmer CK, Cook GJ, Blake GM, et al. Individual kidney function in atherosclerotic nephropathy is not related to the presence of renal artery stenosis. *Nephrol Dial Transplant* 1999;14:2880–2884.

Farreras-Valenti P, Rozman C, Jurado-Grau J, et al. Gröblad-Strandberg-Touraine syndrome with systemic hypertension due to unilateral renal angioma. *Am J Med* 1965; 39:355–360.

Frauchiger B, Zierler R, Bergelin RO, et al. Prognostic significance of intra renal resistance indices in patients with renal artery interventions: a preliminary duplex sonographic study. *Cardiovasc Surg* 1996;4:324–330.

Freedman BI, Hsu F-C, Langefeld CD, et al. Renal artery calcified plaque associations with subclinical renal and cardiovascular disease. *Kidney Int* 2004;65:2262–2267.

Geyskes GG, Oei HY, Puylaert BAJ, et al. Renovascular hypertension identified by captopril-induced changes in the renogram. *Hypertension* 1987;9:451–458.

Goldblatt H, Lynch J, Hanzal RF, Summerville WW. Studies on experimental hypertension. I. The production of persistent elevation of systolic blood pressure by means of renal ischemia. *J Exp Med* 1934;59:347–378.

Goldblatt H. Reflections. *Urol Clin North Am* 1975;2: 219–221.

Gómez Campderá FJ, Luño J, García de Vinuesa S, Valderrábano F. Renal vascular disease in the elderly. *Kidney Int* 1998;54(Suppl 68):S73–S77.

Gowda MS, Loeb AL, Crouse LJ, Kramer PH. Complementary roles of color-flow duplex imaging and intravascular ultrasound in the diagnosis of renal artery fibromuscular dysplasia: should renal arteriography serve as the "gold standard"? *J Am Coll Cardiol* 2003;41:1305–1311.

Granger JP, Schnackenberg CG. Renal mechanisms of angiotensin II-induced hypertension. *Semin Nephrol* 2000; 20:417–425.

Grüntzig A, Kuhlmann U, Vetter W, et al. Treatment of renovascular hypertension with percutaneous transluminal dilatation of a renal-artery stenosis. *Lancet* 1978;1: 801–802.

Grützmacher P, Radtke HW, Stahl RA, et al. Renal artery stenosis and erythropoietin [Abstract]. *Kidney Int* 1989; 35:326.

Haab F, Duclos JM, Guyenne T, et al. Renin secreting tumors: diagnosis, conservative surgical approach and long-term results. *J Urol* 1995;153:1781–1784.

Halimi J-M, Ribstein J, Du Cailar G, Mimran A. Nephrotic-range proteinuria in patients with renovascular disease. *Am J Med* 2000;108:120–126.

Hallett JW, Textor SC, Kos PB, et al. Advanced renovascular hypertension and renal insufficiency: trends in medical comorbidity and surgical approach from 1970 to 1993. *J Vasc Surg* 1995;21:750–760.

Hansen KJ, Deitch JS, Dean RH. Renovascular disease in blacks: prevalence and result of operative management. *Am J Med Sci* 1998;315:337–342.

Hartman RP, Kawashima A, King BF Jr. Evaluation of renal causes of hypertension. *Radiol Clin NA* 2003;41: 909–929.

Hasbak P, Jensen LT, Ibsen H, et al. Hypertension and renovascular disease: follow-up of 100 renal vein renin samplings. *J Human Hypertens* 2002;16:275–280.

Holden A, Hill A. Renal angioplasty and stenting with distal protection of the main renal artery in ischemic nephropathy: early experience. *J Vasc Surg* 2003;38:962–968.

Hollenberg NK. Medical therapy for renovascular hypertension. A review. *Am J Hypertens* 1988;1:338S–343S.

Hoobler SW. History of experimental renovascular hypertension. In: Stanley JC, Ernst CB, Fry WJ, eds. *Renovascular hypertension.* Philadelphia: Saunders, 1984.

Hricik DE, Browning PJ, Kopelman R, et al. Captopril-induced functional renal insufficiency in patients with bilateral renal-artery stenoses or renal-artery stenosis in a solitary kidney. *N Engl J Med* 1983;308:373–376.

Hughes JS, Dove HG, Gifford RW Jr, Feinstein AR. Duration of blood pressure elevation in accurately predicting surgical cure of renovascular hypertension. *Am Heart J* 1981;101:408–413.

Imanishi M, Kawamura M, Akabane S, et al. Aspirin lowers blood pressure in patients with renovascular hypertension. *Hypertension* 1989;14:461–468.

Ivanovic V, McKusick MA, Johnson CM III, et al. Renal artery stent placement: complications at a single tertiary care center. *J Vasc Interv Radiol* 2003;14:217–225.

Jennings RC, Shaikh VAR, Allen WMC. Renal ischaemia due to thrombosis of renal artery resulting in metastases from primary carcinoma of bronchus. *BMJ* 1964;2:1053–1054.

Juillard L, Textor SC, Diaz ME, et al. Electron beam computed tomography measurements of changes in renal hemodynamics and function induced by renal artery stenosis [Abstract]. *Hypertension* 2004;43:1351.

Kasiske BL, Anjum S, Shah R, et al. Hypertension after kidney transplantation. *Am J Kidney Dis* 2004;43:1071–1081.

Kato K, Takashi M, Narita H, Kondo A. Renal hypertension secondary to perirenal pseudocyst: resolution by percutaneous drainage. *J Urol* 1985;134:942–943.

Katoh M, Buecker A, Stuber M, et al. Free-breathing renal MR angiography with steady-state free-precession (SSFP) and slab-selective spin inversion: initial results. *Kidney Int* 2004;66:1272–1278.

Keely E. Endocrine causes of hypertension in pregnancy—when to start looking for zebras. *Semin Perinatol* 1998; 22:471–484.

Kennedy DJ, Colyer WR, Brewster PS, et al. Renal insufficiency as a predictor of adverse events and mortality after renal artery stent placement. *Am J Kidney Dis* 2003;42: 926–935.

Khong TK, Mossouris CG, Belli AM, MacGregor GA. Regression of atherosclerotic renal artery stenosis with aggressive lipid lowering therapy. *J Human Hypertens* 2001;15: 431–433.

Kolhe N, Downes M, O'Donnell P, et al. Renal artery dissection secondary to medial hyperplasia presenting as loin pain haematuria syndrome. *Nephrol Dial Transplant* 2004; 19:495–497.

Koriyama N, Kakei M, Yaekura K, et al. A case of renal juxtaglomerular cell tumor: usefulness of segmental sampling to prove autonomic secretion of the tumor. *Am J Med Sci* 1999;318:194–197.

Korsakas S, Mohaupt MG, Dinkel HP, et al. Delay in dialysis in end-stage renal failure: prospective study on percutaneous renal artery interventions. *Kidney Int* 2004;65: 251–258.

Krijnen P, van Jaarsveld BC, Deinum J, et al. Which patients with hypertension and atherosclerotic renal artery stenosis benefit from immediate intervention? *J Human Hypertens* 2004;18:91–96.

Krijnen P, van Jaarsveld BC, Steyerberg EW, et al. A clinical prediction rule for renal artery stenosis. *Ann Intern Med* 1998;129:705–711.

Kuchel O, Horky K, Cantin M, et al. Unilateral juxtaglomerular hyperplasia, hyperreninism and hypokalaemia relieved by nephrectomy. *J Hum Hypertens* 1993;7:71–78.

Leckie BJ, Birnie G, Carachi R. Renin in Wilms' tumor: prorenin as an indicator. *J Clin Endocrinol Metab* 1994; 79:1742–1746.

Leertouwer TC, Pattynama PMT, van den Berg-Huysmans A. Incidental renal artery stenosis in peripheral vascular disease. *Kidney Int* 2001;59:1480–1483.

Lekuona I, Laraudogoitia E, Salcedo A, et al. Congestive heart failure in a hypertensive patient. *Lancet* 2001;357:358.

Liang C-D, Huang S-C, Chen W-F. Renal artery stenosis complicated by hypertensive heart disease in a young child: successful therapy by balloon angioplasty. *Am Heart J* 1996;132:1077–1079.

Lüscher TF, Lie JT, Stanson AW, et al. Arterial fibromuscular dysplasia. *Mayo Clin Proc* 1987;62:931–952.

Main J, Wroe C. Atherosclerotic renal artery stenosis in patients starting dialysis: an emperor with no clothes. *Nephrol Dial Transplant* 2004;19:260–261.

Mann SJ, Pickering TG. Detection of renovascular hypertension. State of the art: 1992. *Ann Intern Med* 1992;117: 845–853.

Marone LK, Clouse WD, Dorer DJ, et al. Preservation of renal function with surgical revascularization in patients with atherosclerotic renovascular disease. *J Vasc Surg* 2004; 39:322–329.

Martin DC Jr. Anomaly of the right crus of the diaphragm involving the right renal artery. *Am J Surg* 1971;121:351–354.

Martinez-Maldonado M. Pathophysiology of renovascular hypertension. *Hypertension* 1991;17:707–719.

Maxwell MH, Bleifer KH, Franklin SS, Varady PD. Demographic analysis of the study. *JAMA* 1972;220: 1195–1204.

McLaughlin K, Jardine AG, Moss JG. Renal artery stenosis. *BMJ* 2000;320:1124–1127.

Merten GJ, Burgess P, Gray LV, et al. Prevention of contrast-induced nephropathy with sodium bicarbonate: a randomized controlled trial. *JAMA* 2004;291:2328–2334.

Milot A, Lambert R, Lebel M, et al. Prostaglandins and renal function in hypertensive patients with unilateral renal artery stenosis and patients with essential hypertension. *J Hypertens* 1996;14:765–771.

Missouris CG, Belli A-M, MacGregor GA. "Apparent" heart failure: a syndrome caused by renal artery stenoses. *Heart* 2000;83:152–155.

Mizuiri S, Amagasaki Y, Hosaka H, et al. Hypertension in unilateral atrophic kidney secondary to ureteropelvic junction obstruction. *Nephron* 1992;61:217–219.

Moein MR, Dehghani VO. Hypertension: a rare presentation of renal cell carcinoma. *J Urol* 2000;164:2019.

Monstrey SJM, Beerthuizen GIJM, vander Werken CHR, et al. Renal trauma and hypertension. *J Trauma* 1989;29:65–70.

Morcos SK. Prevention of contrast media nephrotoxicity— the story so far. *Clin Radiol* 2004;59:381–389.

Morganti A, Bencini C, del Vecchio C, et al. Treatment of atherosclerotic renal artery stenosis. *J Am Soc Nephrol* 2002; 13:S187–S189.

Mounier-Vehier C, Cocheteux B, Haulon S, et al. Changes in renal blood flow reserve after angioplasty of renal artery stenosis in hypertensive patients. *Kidney Int* 2004; 65:245–250.

Mounier-Vehier C, Lions C, Devos P, et al. Cortical thickness: an early morphological marker of atherosclerotic renal disease. *Kidney Int* 2002;61:591–598.

Muray S, Martín M, Amoedo ML, et al. Rapid decline in renal function reflects reversibility and predicts the outcome after angioplasty in renal artery stenosis. *Am J Kidney Dis* 2002;39:60–66.

Murphy TP, Soares G, Kim M. Increase in utilization of percutaneous renal artery interventions by Medicare beneficiaries, 1996–2000. *Am J Radiol* 2004;183:561–568.

Nakamoto H, Ferrario CM, Fuller SB, et al. Angiotensin-(1-7) and nitric oxide interaction in renovascular hypertension. *Hypertension* 1995;25(Part 2):796–802.

Nakano S, Kigoshi T, Uchida K, et al. Hypertension and unilateral renal ischemia (Page kidney) due to compression of a retroperitoneal paraganglioma. *Am J Nephrol* 1996; 16:91–94.

Nomura S, Hashimoto A, Shutou K, et al. Page kidney in a hemodialyzed patient. *Nephron* 1996;72:106–107.

Nordmann AJ, Woo K, Parkes R, Logan AG. Balloon angioplasty or medical therapy for hypertensive patients with atherosclerotic renal artery stenosis? A meta-analysis of randomized controlled trials. *Am J Med* 2003;114:44–50.

Novick AC, Zaki S, Goldfarb D, Hodge EE. Epidemiologic and clinical comparison of renal artery stenosis in black patients and white patients. *J Vasc Surg* 1994;20:1–5.

Numano F, Okawara M, Inomata H, Kobayashi Y. Takayasu's arteritis. *Lancet* 2000;356:1023–1025.

Olin JW, Piedmonte MR, Young JR, et al. The utility of duplex ultrasound scanning of the renal arteries for diagnosing significant renal artery stenosis. *Ann Intern Med* 1995;122:833–838.

Olivieri O, Grazioli S, Pizzolo F, et al. Different impact of deletion polymorphism of gene on the risk of renal and coronary artery disease. *J Hypertens* 2002;20:37–43.

Pascual A, Bush HS, Copley JB. Renal fibromuscular dysplasia in elderly persons. *Am J Kidney Dis* 2005;45:E63.

Pedersen EB. New tools in diagnosing renal artery stenosis. *Kidney Int* 2000;57:2657–2677.

Petersson MJ, Rundqvist B, Johansson M, et al. Increased cardiac sympathetic drive in renovascular hypertension. *J Hypertens* 2002;20:1181–1187.

Pickering TG. Renovascular hypertension: etiology and pathophysiology. *Semin Nucl Med* 1989;19:79–88.

Pickering TG. The role of laboratory testing in the diagnosis of renovascular hypertension. *Clin Chem* 1991;37: 1831–1837.

Plouin P-F, Chatellier G, Darne B, et al. Blood pressure outcome of angioplasty in atherosclerotic renal artery stenosis: a randomized trial. Multicentrique Medicaments vs Angioplastie (EMMA) Study Group. *Hypertension* 1998;31:822–829.

Plouin P-F. Stable patients with atherosclerotic renal artery stenosis should be treated first with medical management. *Am J Kidney Dis* 2003;42:851–857.

Pursell RN, Quinlan PM. Secondary hypertension due to a renin-producing teratoma. *Am J Hypertens* 2003;16:5 92–595.

Rackson ME, Lossef SV, Sos TA. Renal artery stenosis in patients with aortic dissection: increased prevalence. *Radiology* 1990;177:555–558.

Radermacher J, Chavan A, Bleck A, et al. Use of Doppler ultrasonography to predict the outcome of therapy for renal-artery stenosis. *N Engl J Med* 2001;344:410–417.

Radermacher J, Chavan A, Schäffer J, et al. Detection of significant renal artery stenosis with color Doppler sonography: combining extrarenal and intrarenal approaches to minimize technical failure. *Clin Nephrol* 2000;53:333–343.

Reidy JF. New diagnostic techniques for imaging the renal arteries. *Curr Opin Nephrol Hypertens* 2002;11:635–639.

Restrick LJ, Ledermann JA, Hoffbrand BI. Primary malignant retroperitoneal germ cell tumour presenting with accelerated hypertension. *J Hum Hypertens* 1992;6:243–244.

Riccialdelli L, Arnaldi G, Giacchetti G, et al. Hypertension due to renal artery occlusion in a patient with antiphospholipid syndrome. *Am J Hypertens* 2001;14:62–65.

Rihal CS, Textor SC, Breen JF, et al. Incidental renal artery stenosis among a prospective cohort of hypertensive patients undergoing coronary angiography. *Mayo Clin Proc* 2002;77:309–316.

Rizzoni D, Porteri E, Guefi D, et al. Cellular hypertrophy in subcutaneous small arteries of patients with renovascular hypertension. *Hypertension* 2000;35:931–935.

Robertson PW, Klidjian A, Harding LK, et al. Hypertension due to a renin-secreting renal tumour. *Am J Med* 1967; 43:963–976.

Romero JC, Feldstein AE, Rodriguez-Porcel MG, Cases-Amenos A. New insights into the pathophysiology of enovascular hypertension. *Mayo Clin Proc* 1997;72:251–260.

Rossi GP, Cesari M, Chiesura-Corona M, et al. Renal vein renin measurements accurately identify renovascular hypertension caused by total occlusion of the renal artery. *J Hypertens* 2002;20:975–984.

Rudnick MR, Maxwell MH. Limitations of renin assays. In: Narins RG, ed. *Controversies in Nephrology and Hypertension.* New York: Churchill Livingstone, 1984:123–160.

Safian RD, Textor SC. Renal-artery stenosis. *N Engl J Med* 2001;344:431–442.

Salifu MO, Gordon DH, Friedman EA, Delano BG. Bilateral renal infarction in a black man with medial fibromuscular dysplasia. *Am J Kidney Dis* 2000;36:184–189.

Salifu MO, Haria DM, Bardero O, et al. Challenges in the diagnosis and management of renal artery stenosis. *Curr Hypertens Rep* 2005;7:219–227.

Scoble JE, de Takats D, Ostermann ME, et al. Lipid profiles in patients with atherosclerotic renal artery stenosis. *Nephron* 1999;83:117–121.

Shapiro AL, Cavallo T, Cooper W, et al. Hypertension in radiation nephritis. Report of a patient with unilateral disease, elevated renin activity levels, and reversal after unilateral nephrectomy. *Arch Intern Med* 1977;137:848–851.

Siamopoulos K, Sellars L, Mishra SC, et al. Experience in the management of hypertension with unilateral chronic pyelonephritis: results of nephrectomy in selected patients. *QJM* 1983;52:349–362.

Silva JA, Chan AW, White CJ, et al. Elevated brain natriuretic peptide predicts blood pressure response after stent revascularization in patients with renal artery stenosis. *Circulation* 2005;111:328–333.

Silver D, Clements JB. Renovascular hypertension from renal artery compression by congenital bands. *Ann Surg* 1976;183:161–166.

Simon G. What is critical renal artery stenosis? *Am J Hypertens* 2000;13:1189–1193.

Simon N, Franklin SS, Bleifer KH, et al. Clinical characteristics of renovascular hypertension. *JAMA* 1972;220:1209–1218.

Sivamurthy N, Surowiec SM, Culakova E, et al. Divergent outcomes after percutaneous therapy for symptomatic renal artery stenosis. *J Vasc Surg* 2004;39:565–574.

Slovut DP, Olin JW. Fibromuscular dysplasia. *N Engl J Med* 2004;350:1862–1871.

Smith HW. Unilateral nephrectomy in hypertensive disease. *J Urol* 1956;76:685–701.

Smith LH, Drach G, Hall P, et al. National High Blood Pressure Education Program (NHBPEP) review paper on complications of shock wave lithotripsy for urinary calculi. *Am J Med* 1991;91:635–641.

Soulez G, Therasse E, Qanadli SD, et al. Prediction of clinical response after renal angioplasty: respective value of renal Doppler sonography and scintigraphy. *AJR* 2003;181:1029–1035.

Stanley P, Gyepes MT, Olson DL, Gates GF. Renovascular hypertension in children and adolescents. *Radiology* 1978;129:123–131.

Steffens J, Mast GJ, Braedel HU, et al. Segmental renal hypoplasia of vascular origin causing renal hypertension in a 3-year-old girl. *J Urol* 1991;146:826–829.

Sutton D. The kidneys and ureters. In: *Textbook of Radiology and Imaging,* volume II. London: Churchill Livingtone, 2003.

Tapper D, Brand T, Hickman R. Early diagnosis and management of renovascular hypertension. *Am J Surg* 1987;153:495–500.

Taylor A. Functional testing: ACEI renography. *Semin Nephrol* 2000;20:437–444.

Textor SC. Ischemic nephropathy: where are we now? *J Am Soc Nephrol* 2004a;15:1974–1982.

Textor SC. Pitfalls in imaging for renal artery stenosis. *Ann Intern Med* 2004b;141:730–731.

Textor SC. Stable patients with atherosclerotic renal artery stenosis should be treated first with medical management. *Am J Kidney Dis* 2003;42:858–863.

Textor SC, Wilcox CS. Ischemic nephropathy/azotemic renovascular disease. *Semin Nephrol* 2000;20:489–502.

Thal AP, Grage TB, Vernier RL. Function of the contralateral kidney in renal hypertension due to renal artery stenosis. *Circulation* 1963;27:36–43.

Torres VE, Wilson DM, Burnett JC Jr, et al. Effect of inhibition of converting enzyme on renal hemodynamics and sodium management in polycystic kidney disease. *Mayo Clin Proc* 1991;66:1010–1017.

Turnbull JM. Is listening for abdominal bruits useful in the evaluation of hypertension? *JAMA* 1995;274:1299–1301.

Valabhji J, Robinson S, Poulter C, et al. Prevalence of renal artery stenosis in subjects with type 2 diabetes and coexistent hypertension. *Diabetes Care* 2000;23:539–543.

Valvo E, Bedogna V, Gammaro L, et al. Systemic haemodynamics in renovascular hypertension: changes after revascularization with percutaneous transluminal angioplasty. *J Hypertens* 1987;5:629–632.

van der Ven AJAM, Hommels MJ, Kroon AA, et al. *Clamydia pneumoniae* seropositivity and systemic and renovascular atherosclerotic disease. *Arch Intern Med* 2002;162:786–790.

van der Ven PJG, Beutler JJ, Kaatee R, et al. Angiotensin converting enzyme inhibitor-induced renal dysfunction in atherosclerotic renovascular disease. *Kidney Int* 1998;53:986–993.

van Jaarsveld BC, Deinum J. Evaluation and treatment of renal artery stenosis: impact on blood pressure and renal function. *Curr Opin Nephrol Hypertens* 2001;10:399–404.

van Jaarsveld BC, Krijnen P, Pieterman H, et al. The effect of balloon angioplasty on hypertension in atherosclerotic renal-artery stenosis. *N Engl J Med* 2000;342:1007–1014.

van Onna M, Houben JHM, Kroon AA, et al. Asymmetry of renal blood flow in patients with moderate to severe hypertension. *Hypertension* 2003;41:108–113.

van Onna M, Kroon AA, Houben AJHM, et al. Genetic risk of atherosclerotic renal artery disease: the Candidate Gene Approach in a Renal Angiography cohort. *Hypertension* 2004;44:448–453.

Vasbinder GBC, Nelemans PJ, Kessels AGH, et al. Accuracy of computed tomographic angiography and magnetic resonance angiography for diagnosing renal artery stenosis. *Ann Intern Med* 2004;141:674–682.

Vasbinder GBC, Nelemans PJ, Kessels AGH, et al. Diagnostic tests for renal artery stenosis in patients suspected of having renovascular hypertension. *Ann Intern Med* 2001;135:401–411.

Ward MM, Studenski S. Clinical prognostic factors in lupus nephritis. The importance of hypertension and smoking. *Arch Intern Med* 1992;152:2082–2088.

Watano K, Okamoto H, Takagi C, et al. Neurofibromatosis complicated with XXX syndrome and renovascular hypertension. *J Intern Med* 1996;239:531–535.

Weaver FA, Kumar SR, Yellin AE, et al. Renal revascularization in Takayasu arteritis-induced renal artery stenosis. *J Vasc Surg* 2004;39:749–757.

Webster J, Marshall F, Abdalla M, et al. Randomised comparison of percutaneous angioplasty vs continued medical therapy for hypertensive patients with atheromatous renal artery stenosis. *J Human Hypertens* 1998;12:329–335.

Weinrauch LA, D'Elia JA. Renal artery stenosis: "Fortuitous diagnosis," problematic therapy. *J Am Coll Cardiol* 2004;43:1614–1616.

Welch WJ. The pathophysiology of renin release in renovascular hypertension. *Semin Nephrol* 2000;20:394–401.

Wenting GJ, Tan-Tjiong H, Derkx FHM, et al. Split renal function after captopril in unilateral renal artery stenosis. *BMJ* 1984;288:886–890.

Wilcox CS. Functional testing: renin studies. *Semin Nephrol* 2000;20:432–436.

Wolf G. Franz Volhard and his students' tortuous road to renovascular hypertension. *Kidney Int* 2000;57:2156–2166.

Woodrow G, Cook JA, Brownjohn AM, Turney JH. Is renal vasculitis increasing in incidence? *Lancet* 1990;336:1583.

Zeller T, Frank U, Müller C, et al. Predictors of improved renal function after percutaneous stent-supported angioplasty of severe atherosclerotic ostial renal artery stenosis. *Circulation* 2003;108:2244–2249.

Zoccali C, Mallamaci F, Finocchiaro P. Atherosclerotic renal artery stenosis: epidemiology, cardiovascular outcomes, and clinical prediction rules. *J Am Soc Nephrol* 2002;13:S179–S183.

Zucchelli PC. Hypertension and atherosclerotic renal artery stenosis: diagnostic approach. *J Am Soc Nephrol* 2002;13:S184–S186.

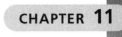
# Hypertension with Pregnancy and the Pill

Hypertension occurs in approximately 10% of first pregnancies and 8% of all pregnancies (Roberts et al., 2003). Preeclampsia, defined as new onset of hypertension with proteinuria, is a leading cause of maternal and neonatal mortality worldwide. Even though maternal mortality from preeclampsia has fallen in developed countries, it remains a common cause of preterm delivery of low-birth-weight babies from intrauterine growth retardation. (Sibai et al., 2005). When such babies become adults, they have an increased risk of hypertension and cardiovascular disease as well as an increased likelihood of preeclampsia in their own pregnancies (Dempsey et al., 2003). Moreover, the rate of preeclampsia is increasing, likely from increasing maternal age and multiple births (Paulson et al., 2002).

Hypertension is seen more often in users of oral contraceptives, although the absolute risk is small (Chobanian et al., 2003). Although the causes of neither pregnancy-related nor pill-induced hypertension are completely known, if these forms of hypertension are recognized early and handled appropriately, the morbidity and mortality they cause can hopefully be diminished (Wilson et al., 2003).

## TYPES OF HYPERTENSION DURING PREGNANCY

### Classification

The classification provided in the 2000 report of the National HBPEP Working Group (2000) is as follows:

- *Chronic hypertension:* Hypertension, defined as a blood pressure (BP) in excess of 140 mm Hg systolic or 90 mm Hg diastolic (taken as the disappearance of sound or Korotkoff phase V), present before pregnancy or diagnosed before the twentieth week of gestation or that persists beyond 6 weeks' postpartum.
- *Gestational hypertension (GH):* Hypertension detected for the first time after the twentieth week of gestation, without proteinuria. Some will develop preeclampsia; if not, and the BP returns to normal postpartum, the diagnosis of *transient hypertension of pregnancy* can be assigned; if the BP remains elevated postpartum, the diagnosis is *chronic hypertension.*
- *Preeclampsia (PE):* Hypertension detected for the first time after the twentieth week of gestation (or earlier with trophoblastic diseases) with proteinuria of at least 300 mg in a 24-hour specimen. A single-voided protein/creatinine ratio may not be reliable (Durnwald & Mercer, 2003).
- *Eclampsia:* Preeclampsia with seizures that cannot be attributed to other causes. Seizures may appear 2 or more days after delivery (Matthys et al., 2004).
- *Preeclampsia superimposed on chronic hypertension:* In women with chronic hypertension,

sudden increases of BP together with the appearance of proteinuria, thrombocytopenia, or abnormal liver function tests.

## Problems in Diagnosing Preeclampsia

There are problems inherent in diagnosing a syndrome of unknown cause on the basis of only highly nonspecific signs (Higgins & de Swiet, 2001). For example, as will be noted, the BP in normal pregnancy usually falls during the first and middle trimester, only to return toward the prepregnant level during the third trimester. Because women with chronic hypertension have an even greater fall early on, their subsequent rise in later pregnancy may give the appearance of the onset of PE. In addition, those with chronic hypertension may have previously unrecognized proteinuria: If seen only after midterm, the diagnosis of PE looks even more certain.

The distinction between chronic hypertension and PE is of more than academic interest: In the former, hypertension is the major problem, whereas "preeclampsia is more than hypertension; it is a systemic syndrome and several of its 'nonhypertensive' complications can be life-threatening when blood pressure elevations are quite mild" (National HBPEP Working Group, 2000). The management of the hypertension and the pregnancy, as well as the prognosis for future pregnancies, varies with the diagnosis. The bottom line, however, is clear: When in doubt, diagnose PE and institute its treatment, because even mild PE may rapidly progress. If PE is correctly diagnosed and managed, the risks to both mother and baby can be largely overcome.

Obviously, women should be evaluated before conception. If hypertensive, therapy should be revised to exclude ACEIs or ARBs. If renal disease is present, more careful observation is needed since there is an increased risk of adverse outcomes (Fischer et al., 2004). Foreknowledge of blood pressure and renal function is essential.

## BLOOD PRESSURE MONITORING DURING PREGNANCY

The various guidelines described in Chapter 2 should be followed in measuring the BP during pregnancy. For the diastolic level, the disappearance of sound (phase 5) is more accurate, reliable, and more easily ascertained than its muffling (phase 4) (Higgins & de Swiet, 2001).

With office readings, the diagnosis of hypertension either without proteinuria (i.e., gestational hypertension) or with proteinuria (i.e., PE) was clearly associated with significantly increased risks of maternal and fetal complications (Steer et al., 2004).

Until (and if) at-home BP monitoring and ambulatory BP monitoring (ABPM) become widely available and further documented to be more predictive than office BPs, most women will be monitored by occasional readings in the office. The definitions given earlier in this chapter are based on office readings with the caveat that, unless the woman is in serious trouble, repeated readings be taken before diagnosing any form of hypertension.

## Home Blood Pressure Recording

Patients may accurately monitor their own BP with the semiautomatic, inexpensive devices described in Chapter 2 (Waugh et al., 2003). The average home readings are similar to those recorded by ambulatory monitoring but with more variation (Brown et al., 2004).

## Ambulatory Blood Pressure Monitoring

In normal pregnancy, lower pressures are found in the midportion, with rises to nonpregnant levels near term (Brown et al., 1998; Ferguson et al., 1994) (Figure 11–1).

### Prospective Data

These data were from single sets of ABPM measurements in a cross-sectional study. Even more impressive are data from a longitudinal, prospective study in 403 women who started with normal casual BP during the first trimester and who had repeated ABPM recordings made every 4 weeks (Hermida et al., 2004). A highly significant higher level of both daytime and sleep BPs was noted *during the first trimester* in the 128 women who later developed GH and the 40 who later developed PE, in comparison to the 235 who remained normotensive. These data suggest that ABPM may provide the best tool now available for the early identification of women who are predisposed to GH or PE. Moreover, those who developed PE had a greater blunting of the nighttime dipping of BP during the third trimester as compared to those who only had GH, so the procedure may provide additional warning of the impending development of PE. Obviously, more such careful study of ABPM during pregnancy is needed.

## CIRCULATORY CHANGES IN NORMAL PREGNANCY

Serial measurements begun before conception have portrayed the evolution of the profound changes of normal pregnancy. In ten women, nine nulliparous, who were studied before and repeatedly during

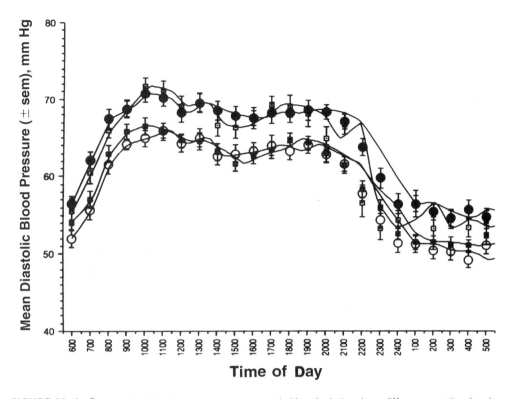

**FIGURE 11–1** ● Diastolic blood pressure patterns recorded hourly during three different gestational periods and in nonpregnant women. Mean diastolic blood pressure (± sem) was recorded in millimeters of mercury. *Open squares with dot,* nonpregnant; *open circles,* 18–22 weeks pregnant; *solid squares,* 30–32 weeks pregnant; *solid circles,* 36–38 weeks pregnant. (Adapted from Ferguson JH, Neubauer BL, Shaar CJ. Ambulatory blood pressure monitoring during pregnancy. Establishment of standards of normalcy. *Am J Hypertens* 1994;7:838–843.)

pregnancy, significant decreases in systemic vascular resistance resulted in a fall in BP, despite an increase in cardiac output, even before placentation (Chapman et al., 1998) (Figure 11–2). As the authors note, "Therefore, it is likely that maternal factors, possibly related to changes in ovarian function or extended function of the corpora lutea, are responsible for the initial peripheral vasodilation found in human pregnancy" (Chapman et al., 1998).

The progressive rise in plasma and blood volume are likely adaptations, via renal sodium retention, to the vasodilation and fall in BP. The low pressure and underfilled circulation provoke an increase in renin secretion and, secondarily, a rise in aldosterone levels. The somewhat later rise in plasma atrial natriuretic peptide is evidence that, despite the increased blood volume, the central circulation is not overexpanded. As a consequence of renal vasodilation, renal plasma flow and glomerular filtration increase and renal vascular resistance decreases.

At the same time as various forces raise levels of renin-angiotensin-aldosterone, normal pregnancy brings forth numerous mechanisms to protect the circulations of both mother and fetus from the intense vasoconstriction, volume retention, and potassium wastage that high angiotensin II and aldosterone levels would ordinarily engender. These include relative resistance to the pressor effects of angiotensin II, reflecting downregulation of angiotensin II receptors by the high levels of circulating angiotensin II (Baker et al., 1992) and antagonism by endothelium-derived prostacyclin and nitric oxide (NO) (Magness et al., 1996).

The large amounts of potent mineralocorticoids present during pregnancy would be expected to increase sodium reabsorption at the cost of progressive renal wastage of potassium, yet pregnant women are normokalemic. This appears to be the result of the high level of progesterone, which acts as an aldosterone antagonist (Brown et al., 1986).

Normal pregnancy, then, is a low BP state associated with marked vasodilation that reduces peripheral resistance, along with an expanded fluid volume that increases cardiac output. Renal blood flow is markedly increased, and the renin-aldosterone system is activated but with blunted effects.

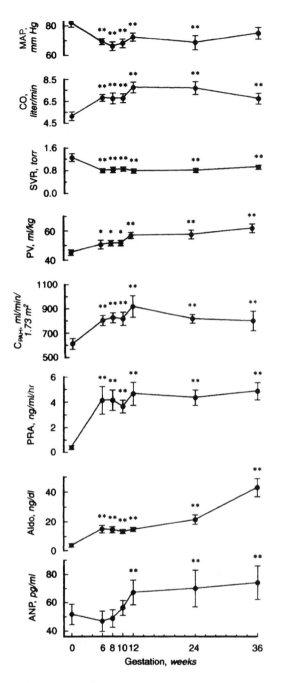

**FIGURE 11–2** ● Changes in mean arterial pressure (MAP), cardiac output (CO), systemic vascular resistance (SVR), plasma volume (PV), effective renal plasma flow measured by para-aminohippurate clearance ($C_{PAH}$), plasma renin activity (PRA), plasma aldosterone (Aldo), and atrial natriuretic peptide (ANP) in ten women studied in the midfollicular phase of the menstrual cycles and at weeks 6, 8, 10, 12, 24, and 36 of gestation. $*p < .05$; $**p < .01$. (Adapted from Chapman AB, Abraham WT, Zamudio S, et al. Temporal relationships between hormonal and hemodynamic changes in early human pregnancy. *Kidney Int* 1998;54:2056–2063.)

## PREECLAMPSIA

Almost all of these various hemodynamic, renal, and hormonal changes of normal pregnancy are altered in PE (Ganzevoort et al., 2004; Sibai et al., 2005).

Preeclampsia is a systemic syndrome of which hypertension is only its most obvious manifestation. As noted in the preamble to the report of the National HBPEP Working Group (2000):

> The maternal disease is characterized by vasospasm, activation of the coagulation system, and perturbations in many humoral and autacoid systems related to volume and BP control. Oxidative stress and inflammatory-like responses may also be important in the pathophysiology of preeclampsia. The pathologic changes in this disorder are primarily ischemic in nature and affect the placenta, kidney, liver, and brain.

Marked changes in hemodynamics occur: The previously elevated cardiac output plummets; the reduced peripheral resistance markedly rises (Ganzevoort et al., 2004) as does aortic stiffness (Elvan-Taşpinar et al., 2004). Blood volume shrinks (Rang et al., 2004), presumably reflecting the vasoconstricted vasculature. Adaptation to the elevated BP by the heart leads to increases in left ventricular mass and end-systolic and -diastolic volumes with reductions in left ventricular ejection fraction (Borghi et al., 2000). Glomerular filtration falls from reductions in endothelial cell fenestral density and size and fibrinoid deposition (Lafayette, 2005).

### Epidemiology

The cause of PE must explain the following features, as delineated by Chesley (1985):

- It occurs almost exclusively during the first pregnancy; nulliparas are six to eight times more susceptible than are multiparas. Older primigravida are more susceptible than younger.
- It occurs more frequently in those with multiple fetuses, hydatidiform mole, or diabetes.
- The incidence increases as term approaches; it is unusual before the end of the second trimester.
- The features of the syndrome are hypertension, edema, proteinuria and, when advanced, convulsions and coma.
- There is characteristic hepatic and renal pathology (Gärtner et al., 1998).
- The syndrome has a hereditary tendency; in the families of women who had PE, the syndrome developed in 25% of their daughters and

granddaughters but in only 6% of their daughters-in-law (Chesley, 1980).

- It rapidly disappears when the pregnancy is terminated.

As listed in Table 11–1, multiple risk factors for PE have been identified (Duckitt & Harrington, 2005). What remains elusive is the initiating mechanism, the trigger that sets off the oftentimes explosive course of this malady that disturbs up to one in ten first pregnancies and is rarely seen again. The difficulty in identifying a specific cause is related to the likely presence of multiple mechanisms (Roberts & Cooper, 2001) and the lack of an experimental model for PE. Another difficulty is the inability to identify the early pathogenetic mechanisms, which remain invisible to current technology. Most of what is recognized are late manifestations of a process that is initiated much earlier. As will be noted, no clinically useful screening test to predict the development of PE is currently available (Conde-Agudelo et al., 2004).

## Genetic Predisposition

In Sweden, the odds ratio for PE was increased 3.3 times between full sisters and 2.6 times between mothers and daughters with heredity estimated to contribute 31% of the risk (Nilsson et al., 2004). In the words of Broughton Pipkin and Roberts (2000):

> Rather than a single gene, there are likely the combined effects of several polymorphisms, probably in several different combinations, interacting with their environment and eventually precipitating a final common pathway of hypertension and proteinuria.

A number of candidate genes have been proposed, including ones associated with endothelial NO synthase (Serrano et al., 2004), thrombophilias (Kupferminc et al., 1999), factor V Leiden mutation (Dizon-Townson et al., 1996), tumor necrosis factor-$\alpha$ (Williams et al., 1999), angiotensinogen (Lévesque et al., 2004), lipoprotein-lipase (Hubel et al., 1999), and diabetes (Qiu et al., 2003). None has been consistently found (Roberts et al., 2004).

## Immunologic Mechanisms

A number of associations suggest an immunologic mechanism that involves the duration and degree of exposure to antigens in the father's sperm. Women who develop PE tend to have had shorter durations of cohabitation than women who do not have hypertension during pregnancy, suggesting that repeated exposure to male ejaculate may prevent PE

---

## TABLE 11–1

### Risk Factors for Preeclampsia

Preconceptional or chronic risk factors

Partner-related risk factors

Nulliparity, primipaternity

Limited sperm exposure, teenage pregnancy, donor insemination

Partner who fathered a preeclamptic pregnancy in another woman

Either parent the product of a pregnancy complicated by preeclampsia

Maternal-specific risk factors

History of previous preeclampsia

Increasing maternal age

Shorter interval between pregnancies

Family history

Black or Hispanic race

Patient requiring oocyte donation

Physical inactivity

Presence of specific underlying disorders

Chronic hypertension and renal disease

Obesity, insulin resistance, low maternal birthweight

Gestational diabetes, type 1 diabetes mellitus

Activated protein C resistance (factor V Leiden), protein S deficiency

Antiphospholipid antibodies

Hyperhomocysteinemia

Exogenous factors

Smoking (decreases risk)

Stress, work-related psychosocial strain

Inadequate diet

Pregnancy-associated risk factors

Multiple pregnancy

Urinary tract infection

Structural congenital anomalies

Hydrops fetalis

Chromosomal anomalies (trisomy 13, triploidy)

Hydatidiform moles

---

Modified from Dekker G, Sibai B. Primary, secondary, and tertiary prevention of pre-eclampsia. *Lancet* 2001;357:209–215.

(Robillard & Hulsey, 1996). When pregnancy occurs with a new father, the risk is increased from either the longer interpregnancy interval or the exposure to new paternal antigens (Basso et al., 2001). Similarly, the risk is greater for former users of contraceptives that block exposure to sperm (Klonoff-Cohen et al., 1989). In addition, the risk of PE is reduced among women with prior miscarriages, abortion (Eras et al., 2000), or previous blood transfusions, all of which may alter maternal immune reactions (Clark, 1994). These associations suggest that repeated exposure to sperm may correct a defect in trophoblast invasion, as will be described in the next section.

Beyond this hypothesis, antibodies capable of activating angiotensin II type 1 (AT1) receptors are found (Thway et al., 2004).

## Pathophysiology

Whatever is fundamentally responsible, as stated by Walker (2000): "Preeclampsia is the result of an initial placental trigger, which has no adverse effect on the mother, and a maternal systemic reaction that produces the clinical signs and symptoms of the disorder." The pathogenesis of PE can logically be divided into two stages: first, defective placental perfusion, and second, the maternal systematic reaction. The bridge between the two stages is increasingly being ascribed to oxidative stress (Roberts & Hubel, 2004).

### Deficient Trophoblastic Migration

The current leading hypothesis for the placental trigger is poor placental perfusion, first proposed more than 50 years ago (Page, 1948) and now related to deficient trophoblastic migration and invasion. As noted by Redman and Sargent (2000):

It is now taken for granted that pre-eclampsia originates with deficient placentation occurring during the first half of pregnancy. The critical process is invasion of the placental bed by extravillous cytotrophoblasts, which penetrate deep into the myometrium. They also infiltrate the spiral arteries, which are transformed into large structureless conduits, which can supply the hugely expanded blood flow of the third-trimester placenta [Figure 11–3]. In pre-eclampsia, cytotrophoblast invasion is abnormally shallow, so that only the decidual segments of the spiral arteries are modified and the distal myometrial segments remain small and muscular

### Uteroplacental Hypoperfusion

The consequences of deficient trophoblastic migration with retention of musculoelastic media in spiral arteries could explain the major phenomenon that is usually held responsible for the pathophysiology of PE: uteroplacental hypoperfusion. Uteroplacental hypoperfusion fits with the recognized clinical circumstances wherein PE is most common: *reduced placental mass relative to need* (first pregnancies in young women, twins, hydatidiform mole) and *compromised uterine vasculature* (diabetes and pre-existing hypertension). The maternal vascular disease referred to as *acute atherosis,* an obstructive lesion of the spiral arteries, could reduce placental perfusion even in the absence of poor placentation.

### The Placental Stimulus

The path between placental hypoperfusion and the maternal syndrome is uncertain. As seen in Figure 11–4, one hypothesis is the release of trophoblastic debris into the maternal circulation, which causes increased endothelial cell activation and inflammatory

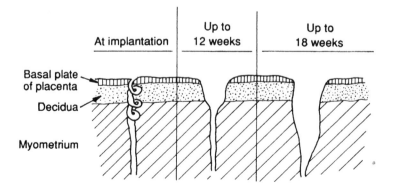

**FIGURE 11–3** ● The normal invasion of spiral arteries by the trophoblast converts them into deltas and so improves blood flow. This invasion is defective in preeclampsia. (Adapted from Chamberlain G. Raised blood pressure in pregnancy. *BMJ* 1991;302:1454–1458.)

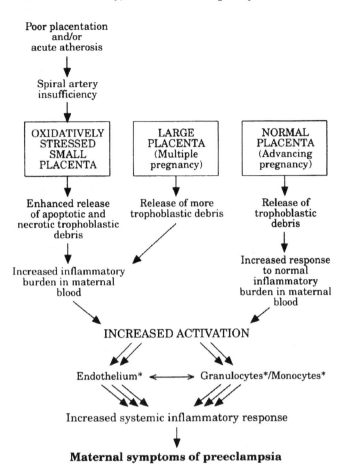

**FIGURE 11–4** ● Redman-Sargent model for the maternal symptoms of preeclampsia based on the release of trophoblastic debris into the maternal circulation. *, Activated cells. (Modified from Redman CWG, Sargent IL. Placental debris, oxidative stress and pre-eclampsia. *Placenta* 2000;21:597–602.)

responses (Freeman et al., 2004; Myers et al., 2005; Redman & Sargent, 2000). Cell-free fetal DNA has been identified in maternal blood before onset of PE, documenting the shedding of debris from syncytial trophoblasts (Levine et al., 2004b). Such "debris" may be accompanied by a number of stimuli from hyperperfused placenta, including:

- Factors that diminish endothelial barrier function (Y Wang et al., 2004).
- Increased expression of vascular endothelial growth factor (Chung et al., 2004).
- Increased expression of intercellular adhesion molecules (X Wang et al., 2004).
- Increased levels of soluble fms-like tyrosine kinase 1 which antagonize the angiogenic and vasodilatory effects of vascular endothelial growth factor and placental growth factor (Levine et al., 2004a) and decreased levels of placental growth factor (Levine et al., 2005).
- Increased production of uric acid (Kang et al., 2004).

Beyond these possible specific stimuli, the role of oxidative stress has been emphasized. As stated by Roberts et al. (2003):

The oxidative stress hypothesis proposes that hypoxia at the fetal-maternal interface results in the generation of free radicals that may lead to oxidative stress dependent on the maternal constitution. Abundant evidence of oxidative stress in blood and tissues of women with preeclampsia support the hypothesis [Roberts & Hubel, 2004]. Further support comes from a small study in which antioxidants were administered from early gestation to women at high risk of preeclampsia. The goal of the study was to determine if prophylactic antioxidants could prevent evidence of endothelial activation . . . In addition, and even more important from a clinical standpoint, the frequency of preeclampsia was reduced in the treated women [Chappell et al., 1999]. This study, although encouraging, was quite small, and thus the efficacy and safety of antioxidant treatment for the infant require confirmation in larger studies. . . .

If oxidative stress provides this linkage, how do the evanescent free radicals formed in the intervillous space result in systemic endothelial activation? There are numerous candidates proposed as intermediaries in this process, including stable products of lipid peroxidation (eg, malondialdehyde), and neutrophils or monocytes activated directly in the intervillous space or by material (placental fragments or cytokines) from the hypoxic placenta. Furthermore, the identification of angiotensin antibodies with the capability to activate NADPH oxidase with subsequent free radical formation in women with preeclampsia suggests a very different origin for oxidative stress [Dechend et al., 2003]. In addition, the role of oxidative stress, although attractive, can only be shown to be causally important by the demonstration in clinical trials that preventing oxidative stress prevents preeclampsia. It must be borne in mind that preeclampsia has been characterized as the "disease of theories," none of which has stood the test of time.

The larger studies of antioxidants called for by Roberts are underway (Raijmakers et al., 2004).

### The Maternal Syndrome

In Figure 11–4, the maternal features of PE are shown to be secondary to diffuse endothelial cell dysfunction. Some women are more sensitive to endothelial dysfunction or have pre-existing dysfunction secondary to hypertension or diabetes (Barden et al., 2004). Such dysfunction is one aspect of a generalized systemic maternal inflammatory response. As Redman and Sargent (2000) state:

> . . . this inflammatory response is detected in normal pregnancy when it is not intrinsically different from that in pre-eclampsia except that it is milder. We have proposed that pre-eclampsia develops when the systemic inflammatory process causes one or other maternal system to decompensate. In other words, the disorder is not a separate condition but simply the extreme end of a range of maternal systemic inflammatory responses engendered by pregnancy itself. This, the continuum theory of pre-eclampsia, implies that any factor that would increase the maternal system inflammatory response to pregnancy would predispose to pre-eclampsia. There are three possible such factors, and there is evidence that all are relevant: a large placenta; an abnormal stimulus from a small placenta; or an excessive maternal sensitivity to such stimuli [Figure 11–4].

### Diagnosis

As described previously, hypertension developing after the twentieth week of gestation with proteinuria in a young nullipara is probably PE, particularly if she has a positive family history for the syndrome. Because patients usually have no symptoms, prenatal care is crucial to detect the signs early and prevent the dangerous sequelae of the fully developed syndrome (Milne et al., 2005).

### Early Detection

In keeping with the known risk factors (Table 11–1), young primigravidas and women with these features should be more closely monitored: a family history of PE, multiple fetuses, pre-existing hypertension, heart disease, renal disease, obesity, PE in a previous pregnancy, or antiphospholipid syndrome.

A number of clinical and laboratory tests have been used in an attempt to recognize PE before it develops and to differentiate it from primary hypertension. After review of 87 relevant studies from over 7,000 articles published between 1966 and 2003, Conde-Agudelo et al. (2004) concluded: "As of 2004, there is no clinically useful screening test to predict the development of preeclampsia." Nonetheless, the search goes on and may be more fruitful when multiple tests are done, in one study with maternal plasma factor II:C and uterine artery Doppler testing (Florio et al., 2005).

### Hypertension

The BP criterion is based on readings of 140/90 mm Hg or higher recorded on at least two occasions, 6 hours or more apart. Obviously, it is not possible to reconfirm the pressure levels over many weeks, as is recommended in nonpregnant patients.

#### Overdiagnosis

Despite the greater overall perinatal mortality with even transient elevations in pressure, for the individual patient there is a significant chance of overdiagnosing PE on the basis of these values, which have been found to have only a 23% to 33% positive predictive value and an 81% to 85% negative predictive value (Dekker & Sibai, 2001). Higher ambulatory BP and heart rate are present at 18 weeks' gestation in those who later developed PE; but those signs, too, have low predictive value (Brown et al., 2001). Therefore, multiple readings and careful follow-up over at least a few days or weeks are needed for women who have BP above 140/90 but below 160/100 after 20 weeks' gestation in the absence of any other suggestive features.

#### Consequences

On the other hand, the level of pressure may not be inordinately high for it to have serious consequences: Women may convulse because of hypertensive encephalopathy with pressures of only 160/110 mm Hg. As noted in the report of the National HBPEP Working Group (2000):

> The clinical spectrum of preeclampsia ranges from mild-to-severe forms. In most women, progression through this spectrum is slow, and the disorder

may never proceed beyond mild preeclampsia. In others, the disease progresses more rapidly, changing from mild to severe in days or weeks. In the most serious cases, progression may be fulminant, with mild preeclampsia evolving to severe preeclampsia or eclampsia within days or even hours. Thus, for clinical management, preeclampsia should be overdiagnosed, because a major goal in managing preeclampsia is the prevention of maternal or perinatal morbidity and mortality, primarily through timing of delivery.

### Proteinuria

Proteinuria is defined as more than 300 mg of protein in a 24-hour urine collection or 300 mg/L in two random, cleanly voided specimens collected at least 4 hours apart. The protein-creatinine ratio in a random urine sample may not exclude the presence of significant proteinuria (Durnwald & Mercer, 2003).

### Differential Diagnosis

Most women with typical features of *de novo* hypertension in pregnancy with no other obvious disorders turn out to have PE (Reiter et al., 1994). The recognition of PE superimposed on chronic hypertension may be more difficult. As described in the report of the National HBPEP Working Group (2000): "Preeclampsia may occur in [15% to 25% of] women already hypertensive (i.e., who have chronic hypertension). . . . [T]he diagnosis of superimposed preeclampsia is highly likely with the following findings:

• In women with hypertension and no proteinuria early in pregnancy (<20 weeks), new-onset proteinuria, defined as the urinary excretion of 0.3 g protein or greater in a 24-hour specimen.

• In women with hypertension and proteinuria before 20 weeks gestation.
• Sudden increase in proteinuria.
• A sudden increase in BP in a woman whose hypertension has previously been well controlled.
• Thrombocytopenia (platelet count <100,000 cells per mm$^3$).
• An increase in ALT [alanine aminotransferase] or AST [aspartate aminotransferase] to abnormal levels."

The presence of hypertensive retinopathy, described in Chapter 4, or left ventricular hypertrophy would also favor chronic hypertension.

## Manifestations of More Severe Disease

### Intravascular Coagulation

As seen in Figure 11–5, activation of intravascular coagulation and subsequent fibrin deposition may be responsible for much of the eventual organ damage seen in severe PE. Increased plasma levels of indicators of platelet activation (β-thromboglobulin), coagulation (thrombin-antithrombin III complexes), and endothelial cell damage (fibronectin and laminin) have been measured up to 4 weeks before the onset of clinical features of PE (Ballegeer et al., 1992). Various inflammatory markers are found after the process has begun (Freeman et al., 2004).

### HELLP Syndrome

A few women develop a more serious complication of PE: the HELLP syndrome, which involves *h*emolysis, *e*levated *l*iver enzymes, and *l*ow *p*latelet counts. The syndrome shares many features with the hemolytic uremic syndrome and thrombotic thrombocytopenic purpura (Sibai et al., 2005). In one series

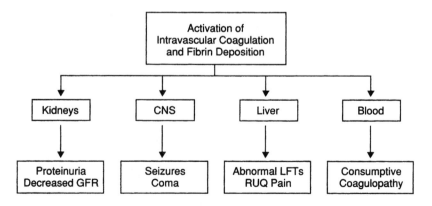

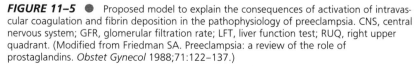

**FIGURE 11–5** ● Proposed model to explain the consequences of activation of intravascular coagulation and fibrin deposition in the pathophysiology of preeclampsia. CNS, central nervous system; GFR, glomerular filtration rate; LFT, liver function test; RUQ, right upper quadrant. (Modified from Friedman SA. Preeclampsia: a review of the role of prostaglandins. *Obstet Gynecol* 1988;71:122–137.)

of 454 pregnancies, with increasing degrees of thrombocytopenia of fewer than 150,000 platelets per mL, maternal and perinatal mortality increased and one in six patients developed eclampsia (Martin & Magann, 1996). Corticosteroids are helpful (Sibai et al., 2005).

## Cerebral Blood Flow

As will be noted, convulsions may occur (i.e., eclampsia) with or without prior manifestations of PE, suggesting that a continuum may or may not be in play. Many women with PE develop headaches; a few develop cortical blindness (Apollon et al., 2000) and other neurologic features of hypertensive encephalopathy. As described in Chapter 8, hypertensive encephalopathy reflects breakthrough hyperperfusion on the background of vasospasm. Similar findings have been described in PE: both vasospasm (Brackley et al., 2000) and brain edema (Schwartz et al., 2000) that reflects an increase in cerebral blood flow with a failure of autoregulation (Riskin-Mashiah & Belfort, 2005).

As will be noted in the next section, prophylactic magnesium sulfate is now recognized to be essential for prevention of eclampsia.

## Management

The report of the National HBPEP Working Group (2000) provides these three tenets for management:

1. Delivery is always appropriate therapy for the mother but may not be so for the fetus. . . . The cornerstone of obstetric management of preeclampsia is based on whether the fetus is more likely to survive without significant neonatal complications *in utero* or in the nursery.
2. The pathophysiologic changes of severe preeclampsia indicate that poor perfusion is the major factor leading to maternal physiologic derangement and increased perinatal morbidity and mortality. Attempts to treat preeclampsia by natriuresis or by lowering blood pressure may exacerbate the important pathophysiologic changes.
3. The pathogenic changes of preeclampsia are present long before clinical diagnostic criteria are manifest. . . . These findings suggest that irreversible changes affecting fetal well-being may be present before the clinical diagnosis. If there is a rationale for management other than delivery, it would be to palliate the maternal condition to allow fetal maturation and cervical ripening.

## Nonpharmacologic Management

### Monitoring
After an initial in-hospital evaluation, highly motivated women who have mild GH or PE remote from term may be safely followed as outpatients if they are able to monitor their BP with home semiautomatic devices, weigh themselves, check fetal movements, and measure urinary protein (Barton et al., 1994). Daycare is equally safe for such women and provides greater patient satisfaction than hospitalization (Turnbull et al., 2004).

### Modified Bed Rest
The value of bed rest has been widely accepted but has not been shown to be beneficial (Allen et al., 1999).

### Diet
Current evidence favors maintenance of usual sodium intake to avoid further reducing placental perfusion (Knuist et al., 1998). Calcium supplements, although claimed to be effective for prevention of PE in high-risk populations, have not proved useful in developed countries (Sibai et al., 2005) but have been associated with lower BP in the offspring at 6 months of age (Gillman et al., 2004). Because caffeine increases the risk of first-trimester abortion, it seems reasonable to restrict its intake even more in women with PE (Cnattingius et al., 2000).

## Pharmacologic Therapy

The Seventh Joint National Committee (JNC-7) (Chobanian et al., 2003) report states:

> Antihypertensive therapy should be prescribed only for maternal safety; it does not improve perinatal outcomes and may adversely affect uteroplacental blood flow. Selection of antihypertensive agents and route of administration depends on anticipated timing of delivery. If delivery is likely more than 48 hours off, oral methyldopa is preferred because of its safety record. Oral labetalol is an alternative, and other β-blockers and calcium antagonists are also acceptable on the basis of limited data. If delivery is imminent, parenteral agents are practical and effective [Table 11–2]. Antihypertensives are administered before induction of labor for persistent DBPs [diastolic BP] of 105 to 110 mm Hg or higher, aiming for levels of 95 to 105 mm Hg.

The preference given to hydralazine in both the 2003 JNC-7 report and the 2000 National HBPEP Group report is likely not warranted. As noted in a meta-analysis of all 21 randomized controlled trials published between 1966 and 2002 involving 893 women given short-acting antihypertensives for severe hypertension in pregnancy, hydralazine was associated with more maternal and fetal side effects

## TABLE 11–2

## Treatment of Acute Severe Hypertension in Preeclampsia

| | |
|---|---|
| Hydralazine | 5 mg IV bolus, then 10 mg every 20 to 30 minutes to a maximum of 25 mg, repeat in several hours as necessary. |
| Labetalol (second-line) | 20 mg IV bolus, then 40 mg 10 minutes later, 80 mg every 10 minutes for two additional doses to a maximum of 220 mg. |
| Nifedipine (controversial) | 10 mg PO, repeat every 20 minutes to a maximum of 30 mg. Caution when using nifedipine with magnesium sulfate, can see precipitous BP drop. Short-acting nifedipine is not approved by U.S. Food and Drug Administration for managing hypertension. |
| Sodium nitroprusside (rarely when others fail) | 0.25 µg/kg per min to a maximum of 5 µg/kg per min. Fetal cyanide poisoning may occur if used for more than 4 hours. |

From Chobanian AV, Bakris GL, Black HR, et al. Seventh report of the Joint National Committee on prevention, detection, evaluation, and treatment of high blood pressure. *Hypertension* 2003;42:1206–1252, with permission.

than nifedipine, isradipine, or labetalol (Magee et al., 2003).

Magnesium sulfate has been conclusively documented to be needed to prevent eclamptic convulsions, both when compared to placebo (Magpie Trial Collaborative Group, 2002) or a calcium channel blocker (CCB) (Belfort et al., 2003). In addition, its use provides neuroprotection to infants delivered before 30 weeks' gestation, as may be needed in women with severe preeclampsia (Crowther et al., 2003).

The decision to deliver is based upon the presence of fetal distress, signs of intrauterine growth retardation, or progressive maternal risk (Table 11–3).

### Long-Term Consequences

In a 47-year follow-up of 189 primigravida who had had eclampsia (to ensure a more accurate diagnosis than preeclampsia), Chesley (1980) found that, in 466 subsequent pregnancies, only 25% had recurrent hypertension and only four had a second episode of eclampsia. Their remote prognosis was excellent with a distribution of blood pressure identical to that of the general population (Chesley et al, 1976). However, Chesley reported a marked increase in both hypertension and cardiovascular events in women who had eclampsia in pregnancies other than the first, with the assumption that

## TABLE 11–3

### Indications for Delivery in Preeclampsia

| Maternal | Fetal |
|---|---|
| Gestational age ≥38 wk[a] | Severe fetal growth restriction |
| Platelet count <100,000 cells/mm$^3$ | Nonreassuring fetal testing results |
| Progressive deterioration in hepatic function | Oligohydramnios |
| Progressive deterioration in renal function | |
| Suspected abruptio placentae | |
| Persistent severe headaches or visual changes | |
| Persistent severe epigastric pain, nausea, or vomiting | |

[a]Delivery should be based on maternal and fetal conditions as well as on gestational age. Reprinted from National High Blood Pressure Education Program Working Group on High Blood Pressure in Pregnancy. Report of the National High Blood Pressure Education Program Working Group on high blood pressure in pregnancy. *Am J Obstet Gynecol* 2000;183:S1–S22, with permission.

preeclampsia in later pregnancies was caused be pre-existing cardiovascular disease.

Moreover, in a population-based cohort study of over 31,000 women who had been diagnosed as having pregnancy-related hypertension, an increased risk for subsequent cardiovascular events was seen both in those diagnosed with "mild" preeclampsia (2.2-fold) and in those diagnosed with "severe" preeclampsia (3.3-fold) (Kestenbaum et al., 2003). These increased risks are likely related to a greater prevalence of features of the metabolic syndrome in these women which may contribute to their persistent impaired vasodilatory state (Pouta et al., 2004; Wolf et al., 2004).

## Prevention

Dekker and Sibai (2001) have divided prevention into three stages:

1. *Primary* prevention will obviously be difficult without knowledge of the cause. However, avoidance of the known risk factors (Table 11–1) should help. In particular, avoiding teenage pregnancy, reducing obesity and insulin resistance, providing adequate nutrition, and avoiding multiple births during assisted pregnancies should be protective. In an intriguing report of 80 pregnant women with prior PE, the half given daily injections of low molecular weight heparin had a much lower rate of recurrence of PE during the second pregnancy (Mello et al., 2005).
2. *Secondary* prevention involves identifying the syndrome as early as possible and using strategies that are thought to influence pathogenic mechanisms. These include low-dose aspirin (Duley et al., 2001) and calcium supplementation in women with low baseline calcium intake (Hatton et al., 2003). Fish-oil supplements have been tested in six multicenter trials and been found to reduce preterm delivery but not to affect any other outcomes (Olsen et al., 2000). In addition, reduction of oxidative stress by antioxidants is being investigated.
3. *Tertiary* prevention involves the various lifestyle changes and therapies described under "Management."

## ECLAMPSIA

Eclampsia is defined by the occurrence of seizures due to hypertensive encephalopathy on the background of PE. This serious complication is becoming less common as better prenatal care is given.

The present incidence in North America and Europe is estimated to be approximately 1 case in every 2,000 deliveries (Mattar & Sibai, 2000).

## Clinical Features

Eclampsia is a form of hypertensive encephalopathy which, on the basis of MRI scanning, is characterized by an initial, reversible vasogenic edema that may lead to irreversible cerebral ischemia and infarction (Zeeman et al., 2004). The features were well defined among the 383 confirmed cases occurring throughout the United Kingdom during 1992 (Douglas & Redman, 1994): Eighty-five percent of the convulsions occurred within 1 week of the woman's last visit to a practitioner; 77% occurred in hospital; 38% occurred before proteinuria and hypertension had been documented; 38% occurred antepartum; 18% of the women died; and 35% had at least one major complication; the rate of stillbirths was 22/1,000; and the rate of neonatal deaths was 34/1,000.

## Management

Delivery is delayed until convulsions are stopped, the BP is controlled, and reasonable fluid and electrolyte balance has been established. With the following standardized treatment of 245 consecutive cases of eclampsia, only one maternal death occurred, and all but one of the fetuses survived who were alive when treatment was started and who weighed 1,800 g or more at birth (Pritchard et al., 1984):

- Magnesium sulfate to control convulsions
- Control of severe hypertension (diastolic BP, 110 mm Hg) with intermittent intravenous injections of hydralazine
- Avoidance of diuretics and hyperosmotic agents
- Limitation of fluid intake, unless fluid loss was excessive
- Delivery once convulsions are arrested and consciousness is regained

## CHRONIC HYPERTENSION AND PREGNANCY

As more women in developed countries delay pregnancies until they are in their 30s and 40s, the prevalence of pre-existing hypertension will likely reach 5% (Roberts et al., 2003).

Pregnant women may have any of the other types of hypertension listed in Table 1–6. Because the BP usually falls during the first half of pregnancy, pre-existing hypertension may not be recognized if the woman is first seen during that time. If the pressure is high during the first 20 weeks, however, chronic hypertension rather than PE is almost always the cause.

Pregnancy seems to bring out latent primary hypertension in certain women whose pressures return to normal between pregnancies but eventually remain elevated. In most patients, such "transient hypertension" appears late in gestation, is not accompanied by significant proteinuria or edema, and recedes within 10 days after delivery. Transient hypertension usually recurs during subsequent pregnancies and is often the basis for the misdiagnosis of PE in multiparous women (National HBPEP Working Group, 2000).

To elucidate the true nature of hypertension seen during a pregnancy, it is often necessary to follow up with the patient postpartum. By 3 months, complete resolution of the various changes seen in pregnancy will have resolved so that, if indicated, further studies to elucidate the cause of the hypertension can be obtained.

### Risks to Mother and Fetus

Women with chronic hypertension have an increased risk for superimposed PE and placental abruption, and their babies have a threefold greater risk for perinatal mortality (Ferrer et al., 2000) and for having intrauterine growth retardation (Haelterman et al., 1997). Even without superimposed PE, women with chronic hypertension have more complicated pregnancies with more intrauterine growth retardation and perinatal mortality (Vanek et al., 2004). These risks are even greater for Black women in the United States, for those with a diastolic BP above 110 mm Hg during the first trimester, and for those with proteinuria early in pregnancy (Sibai et al., 2005). For those with serum creatinine exceeding 2.0 mg/dL, a one-in-three chance of entering end-stage renal failure after pregnancy has been reported (Epstein, 1996), so that these women should be strongly advised against pregnancy. Nonetheless, successful pregnancies have been reported in most women who conceive during chronic dialysis therapy (Bagon et al., 1998).

### *Management*

Women with mild to moderate hypertension should be watched closely, warned about signs of early PE, and delivered at 37 weeks' gestation. They should be cautioned not to exercise intensively, told not to drink alcohol or smoke, and advised to restrict dietary sodium to 100 mmol per day (National HBPEP Working Group, 2000).

Uncertainty remains both about the decision to use (or continue) antihypertensive drugs and about which drugs to choose among those available (Table 11–4). As stated by Roberts et al. (2003):

> Clinicians do not have sufficient evidence to know which pharmacological therapy is best, when to begin treatment, how vigorously to treat, or whether to stop treatment and hope that the hypotensive effect of normal pregnancy will be enough to control blood pressure. The only trial for treatment of hypertension during pregnancy with adequate infant follow-up (7.5 years) was performed over 25 years ago with a drug (α-methyldopa) now rarely used in nonpregnant patients [Cockburn et al., 1982]. Past clinical trials also have not supported a beneficial effect on pregnancy outcome of treating mild hypertension. There has been no reduction in perinatal mortality, placental abruption, or superimposed preeclampsia. . . . Because of the unknown long-term effects on the infant of any treatment, these studies have led to recommendations to treat only on the basis of blood pressure sufficiently elevated to pose potential acute risk to the mother [National HBPEP Working Group, 2000]. Whether this is the appropriate strategy is not clear. . . . Even for women with blood pressure elevation sufficient to justify therapy for their own benefit,

## TABLE 11–4

### Drugs for Treatment of Chronic Hypertension in Pregnancy

| Agent | Comments |
|---|---|
| Methyldopa | Preferred on the basis of long-term follow-up studies supporting safety |
| β-blockers | Reports on intrauterine growth retardation (atenolol) |
| Labetalol | Increasingly preferred to methyldopa because of reduced side effects |
| Clonidine | Limited data |
| Calcium antagonists | Limited data<br>No increase in major teratogenicity with exposure |
| Diuretics | Not first-line agents<br>Probably safe |
| ACEIs, angiotensin II receptor antagonists | Contraindicated<br>Reported fetal toxicity and death |

Modified from Chobanian AV, Bakris GL, Black HR, et al. Seventh report of the Joint National Committee on prevention, detection, evaluation, and treatment of high blood pressure. *Hypertension* 2003;42:1206–1252.

it is not clear whether treatment is beneficial or detrimental for the fetus. In several studies, treatment of hypertensive women resulted in an increased risk of growth restriction in their infants [von Dadelszen et al., 2000]. It is not known whether this is the inevitable consequence of lowering blood pressure during pregnancy or whether it is due to excessive blood pressure decreases or to specific drugs.

## Other Causes of Hypertension During Pregnancy

Identifiable secondary forms of hypertension occur rarely during pregnancy (Lindsay et al., 2005; Shehata & Ahmed, 2004). Their diagnosis may be confounded by the multiple changes in the renin-aldosterone and other hormonal systems that occur during pregnancy, and their therapy may be made difficult by adverse effects on the fetus. Coverage of these various identifiable forms of hypertension during pregnancy is provided in the respective chapters.

## POSTPARTUM SYNDROMES

In women who were preeclamptic, continued close monitoring is needed after delivery. As noted earlier, PE and eclampsia may appear after delivery. Depending on the BP, the doses of antihypertensive drugs should be reduced and they may not be needed for some weeks. If BP remains elevated at 6 weeks' postpartum, further investigation for other causes of hypertension should be provided. The use of nonsteroidal anti-inflammatory drugs may contribute to postpartum hypertension (Makris et al., 2004).

*Peripartum cardiomyopathy* is a rare but serious form of left ventricular systolic dysfunction that appears in the last month of pregnancy or within 5 months after delivery in the absence of identifiable causes or prior recognizable heart disease (Elkayam et al., 2005). Endomyocardial biopsy often reveals myocarditis (Felker et al., 2000).

## Hypertension and Lactation

Breast-feeding does not raise the mother's BP (Robson et al., 1989) and may protect the baby from subsequent hypertension (Singhal & Lucas, 2004). All antihypertensive drugs taken by mothers enter their breast milk; most are present in very low concentrations, except most β-blockers other than propranolol (Ito, 2000). Thorough reviews of drugs for pregnant and lactating women are available (Briggs et al., 2002; Weiner & Buhimschi, 2004).

## HYPERTENSION WITH ORAL CONTRACEPTIVES

Oral contraceptives (OCs) have been used by millions of women since the early 1960s. Oral contraceptives are safe for most women, but their use carries some risk (Baillargeon et al., 2005).

### Incidence of Hypertension

The BP rises a little in most women who take estrogen-containing OCs (Kotchen & Kotchen, 2003) (Figure 11–6). In a prospective cohort study of almost 70,000 nurses covering the 4 years between 1989 and 1993, the overall relative risk for hypertension was 50% higher for current OC users as compared to never-users and 10% higher as compared to former users (Chasan-Taber et al., 1996). The 50% increase in relative risk translated to 41 cases per 10,000 person-years of OC use.

### Predisposing Factors

In the prospective U.S. Nurses Study, the risk for hypertension was not significantly modified by age, family history of hypertension, ethnicity, or body mass index (Chasan-Taber et al., 1996). Women with prior preeclampsia (PE) seem to carry little additional risk: Only 9 of 180 women who had PE had a rise in diastolic BP beyond 90 mm Hg after 6 months to 2 years of OC use (Pritchard & Pritchard, 1977).

### Clinical Course

In most women who develop hypertension while taking an OC, the disease is mild and, in more than half, the BP returns to normal when the OC is stopped (Weir, 1978). In a few women, the hypertension is severe, rapidly accelerating into a malignant phase and causing irreversible renal damage (Lim et al., 1987). Even in patients with reversible hypertension, proteinuria may persist (Ribstein et al., 1999).

Among nulliparous women who had recently stopped OCs and became pregnant, the risk for developing GH was reduced, but the risk for PE was slightly increased (Thadhani et al., 1999).

### Mechanism

Whether OCs cause hypertension *de novo* or simply uncover the propensity toward primary hypertension that would eventually appear spontaneously is unknown. The mechanism for OC-induced hypertension is also unknown, particularly because estrogen appears to be vasodilative (Lee et al., 2000).

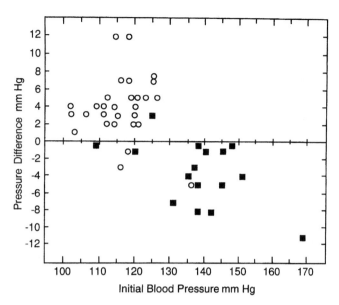

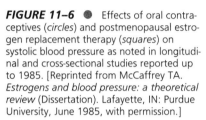

**FIGURE 11–6** ● Effects of oral contraceptives (*circles*) and postmenopausal estrogen replacement therapy (*squares*) on systolic blood pressure as noted in longitudinal and cross-sectional studies reported up to 1985. [Reprinted from McCaffrey TA. *Estrogens and blood pressure: a theoretical review* (Dissertation). Lafayette, IN: Purdue University, June 1985, with permission.]

Changes in endothelial function (Virdis et al., 2003), renin-angiotensin-aldosterone (Ribstein et al., 1999), and insulin sensitivity (Godsland et al., 1992) have been identified.

### Risks in Perspective

A meta-analysis of 14 studies published from 1980 to 2003 found a 1.8-fold increased relative risk of MI and a 2.1-fold increased relative risk of ischemic stroke in current users of low-dose OCs. The relative

risk for both MI and stroke was increased with second generation OCs, whereas third generation OC use increased only the relative risk for stroke (Baillargeon et al., 2005).

It is important to recognize that the reported increases in relative risk translate into only small increases in absolute risk. As seen in Table 11–5, the number of excess cases of myocardial infarction and stroke rises with age, smoking, and pre-existing hypertension but still remains considerably lower than the mortality seen with pregnancy (Petitti, 2003).

## TABLE 11–5

### Age-Specific Estimates of the Excess Rates of Myocardial Infarction and Ischemic Stroke Attributable to the Use of Low-Estrogen Oral Contraceptives and Pregnancy-Related Mortality

| Variable | Age | | |
|---|---|---|---|
| | 20–24 | 30–34 | 40–44 |
| No. of excess cases of myocardial infarction and ischemic stroke attributable to oral contraceptive use (per 100,000 woman-yr of use) | | | |
|    Among nonsmokers | 0.4 | 0.6 | 2 |
|    Among smokers | 1 | 2 | 20 |
|    Among women with hypertension | 4 | 7 | 29 |
| No. of pregnancy-related deaths (per 100,000 live births) | 10 | 12 | 45 |

Modified from Petitti DB. Clinical practice. Combination estrogen-progestin oral contraceptives. *N Engl J Med* 2003;349:1443–1450.

## TABLE 11-6

### Summary of Guidelines for the Use of Combination Estrogen-Progestin Oral Contraceptives in Women With Characteristics That Might Increase the Risk of Adverse Effects

| Variable | ACOG Guidelines | WHO Guidelines |
|---|---|---|
| Smoker, >35 yrs of age | | |
|   <15 cigarettes per day | Risk unacceptable | Risk usually outweighs benefit |
|   ≥15 cigarettes per day | Risk unacceptable | Risk unacceptable |
| Hypertension | | |
|   Blood pressure controlled | Risk acceptable; no definition of blood-pressure control | Risk usually outweighs benefit if systolic blood pressure is 140–159 mm Hg and diastolic blood pressure is 90–99 mm Hg |
|   Blood pressure uncontrolled | Risk unacceptable; no definition of uncontrolled blood pressure | Risk unacceptable if systolic blood pressure is ≥160 mm Hg or diastolic blood pressure is ≥100 mm Hg |
| History of stroke, ischemic heart disease, or venous thromboembolism | Risk unacceptable | Risk unacceptable |
| Diabetes | Risk acceptable if no other cardiovascular risk factors and no end-organ damage | Benefit outweighs risk if no end-organ damage and diabetes is of ≤20 yr duration |
| Hypercholesterolemia | Risk acceptable if LDL cholesterol <160 mg/dL and no other cardiovascular risk factors | Benefit-risk ratio is dependent on the presence or absence of other cardiovascular risk factors |

Modified from Petitti DB. Clinical practice. Combination estrogen-progestin oral contraceptives. *N Engl J Med* 2003;349:1443–1450.

## Guidelines for Use of Oral Contraceptives

Guidelines published by the American College of Obstetrics and Gynecology (ACOG, 2001) and the World Health Organization (2000) agree with the use of OCs in women with controlled hypertension, but not in those with uncontrolled hypertension above 160/100 mm Hg (Table 11–6).

When OCs are used, the following precautions should be taken:

- The lowest effective dose of estrogen and progestogen should be dispensed.
- The BP should be taken at least every 6 months and whenever the woman feels ill.
- If the BP rises significantly, the pill should be stopped and another form of contraceptive should be provided.
- If the BP does not become normal within 3 months, appropriate workup and therapy should be provided.
- If no alternative form of contraception is feasible, and OCs must be continued, antihypertensive therapy may be needed to control the BP.

## HYPERTENSION AND ESTROGEN REPLACEMENT THERAPY

After a major reassessment of the safety and benefits of postmenopausal estrogen replacement therapy (ERT), many fewer women will likely be using ERT (Hulley & Grady, 2004). Nonetheless it may turn out to be helpful in the immediate postmenopausal period, and many women may continue to use ERT since nothing else will effectively prevent hot flushes (Medical Letter, 2004).

In view of the known prohypertensive effect of estrogens given in superphysiologic doses for contraception, there are concerns that the smaller doses for replacement might also raise the BP, adding to the frequent rise in BP after menopause related to increased body weight and aging (Reckelhoff & Fortepiani, 2004). Although hypertension has been reported with high doses of postmenopausal estrogen use (Crane et al., 1971), most controlled trials find either no difference or a *decrease* in ambulatory BP and a greater dipping of nocturnal BP in ERT users (Kotchen & Kotchen, 2003), particularly in the initial period of ERT use (Brownley et al., 2004).

Women who are already hypertensive may have a fall in BP with transdermal estradiol (Mercuro et al., 1998; Modena et al., 1999) that may provide benefits not seen with oral estrogen (Vongpatanasin et al., 2004).

The often lower pressures with ERT may reflect a number of antihypertensive effects of estrogen replacement, including the following:

- Improved endothelium-dependent vasodilation (Higashi et al., 2001) that reflects increased endothelium-mediated nitric oxide activity (Jokela et al., 2003).
- Improved baroreceptor sensitivity (De Meersman et al., 1998).
- Reduced muscle sympathetic nerve activity (Vongpatanasin et al., 2001) and plasma normetanephrine levels (Brownley et al., 2004).
- Inhibition of vascular smooth muscle cell-dependent adventitial fibroblast migration (Li et al., 1999).

Despite these apparently beneficial vascular effects, ERT has been associated with worsening of angiographically defined coronary atherosclerosis and the profile of inflammatory markers in women with abnormal glucose tolerance, of whom 75% were hypertensive (Howard et al., 2004). These deleterious effects, however, were not translated into an increased risk of coronary heart disease among women given only estrogen without progestin in the massive Women's Health Initiative Clinical Trial (Langer et al., 2004). On the other hand, a 29% increase in the relative risk for ischemic strokes was noted among women taking either estrogen alone or combined estrogen plus progesterone in a meta-analysis of 28 trials (Bath & Gray, 2005). Thus, while hypertension should not be a concern for women taking estrogen replacement therapy, cardiovascular complications may be more common.

We will turn next to less common causes of secondary hypertension involving the adrenal glands; although relatively rare, they often must be excluded.

## REFERENCES

ACOG Committee on Practice Bulletins-Gynecology. ACOG Practice Bulletin. The use of hormonal contraception in women with coexisting medical conditions. Number 18, July 2000. *Int J Gynaecol Obstet* 2001;75:93–106.

Allen C, Glasziou P, Del Mar C. Bed rest: a potentially harmful treatment needing more careful evaluation. *Lancet* 1999;354:1229–1233.

Apollon KM, Robinson JN, Schwartz RB, Norwitz ER. Cortical blindness in severe preeclampsia: computer tomography, magnetic resonance imaging, and single-photon-emission computed tomography findings. *Obstet Gynecol* 2000;95:1017–1019.

Bagon JA, Vernaeve H, De Muylder X, et al. Pregnancy and dialysis. *Am J Kidney Dis* 1998;31:756–765.

Baillargeon JP, McClish DK, Essah PA, Nestler JE. Association between the current use of low-dose oral contraceptives and cardiovascular arterial disease: a meta-analysis. *J Clin Endocrinol Metab* 2005;90:3863–3870.

Baker PN, Broughton Pipkin F, Symonds EM. Longitudinal study of platelet angiotensin II binding in human pregnancy. *Clin Sci* 1992;82:377–381.

Ballegeer VC, Spitz B, De Baene LA, et al. Platelet activation and vascular damage in gestational hypertension. *Am J Obstet Gynecol* 1992;166:629–633.

Barden A, Singh R, Walters BN, et al. Factors predisposing to pre-eclampsia in women with gestational diabetes. *J Hypertens* 2004;22:2371–2378.

Barton JR, Stanziano GJ, Sibai BM. Monitored outpatient management of mild gestational hypertension remote from term. *Am J Obstet Gynecol* 1994;170:765–769.

Basso O, Christensen K, Olsen J. Higher risk of pre-eclampsia after change of partner. An effect of longer interpregnancy intervals? *Epidemiology* 2001;12:624–629.

Bath PMW, Gray LJ. Association between hormone replacement therapy and subsequent stroke: a meta-analysis. *BMJ* 2005;330:342–345.

Belfort MA, Anthony J, Saade GR, et al. Nimodipine Study Group. A comparison of magnesium sulfate and nimodipine for the prevention of eclampsia. *N Engl J Med* 2003;348:304–311.

Borghi C, Esposti DD, Immordino V, et al. Relationship of systemic hemodynamics, left ventricular structure and function, and plasma natriuretic peptide concentrations during pregnancy complicated by preeclampsia. *Am J Obstet Gynecol* 2000;183:140–147.

Brackley KJ, Ramsay MM, Broughton Pipkin F, et al. The maternal cerebral circulation in pre-eclampsia: investigations using Laplace transform analysis of Doppler waveforms. *Br J Obstet Gynaecol* 2000;107:492–500.

Briggs GG, Freeman RG, Yaffe SJ. *Drugs in Pregnancy and Lactation. A Reference Guide to Fetal and Neonatal Risk.* 6th Ed. Philadelphia: Lippincott Williams & Wilkins, 2002.

Broughton Pipkin F, Roberts JM. Hypertension in pregnancy. *J Hum Hypertens* 2000;14:705–724.

Brown MA, Bowyer L, McHugh L, et al. Twenty-four-hour automated blood pressure monitoring as a predictor of preeclampsia. *Am J Obstet Gynecol* 2001;185:618–622.

Brown MA, McHugh L, Mangos G, Davis G. Automated self-initiated blood pressure or 24-hour ambulatory blood pressure monitoring in pregnancy? *BJOG* 2004;111:38–41.

Brown MA, Robinson A, Bowyer L, et al. Ambulatory blood pressure monitoring in pregnancy: what is normal? *Am J Obstet Gynecol* 1998;178:836–842.

Brown MA, Sinosich MJ, Saunders DM, Gallery EDM. Potassium regulation and progesterone-aldosterone interrelationships in human pregnancy: a prospective study. *Am J Obstet Gynecol* 1986;155:349–353.

Brownley KA, Hinderliter AL, West SG, et al. Cardiovascular effects of 6 months of hormone replacement therapy versus placebo: differences associated with years since menopause. *Am J Obstet Gynecol* 2004;190:1052–1058.

Chamberlain G. Raised blood pressure in pregnancy. *BMJ* 1991;302:1454–1458.

Chapman AB, Abraham WT, Zamudio S, et al. Temporal relationships between hormonal and hemodynamic changes in early human pregnancy. *Kidney Int* 1998;54:2056–2063.

Chappell LC, Seed PT, Briley AL, et al. Effect of antioxidants on the occurrence of pre-eclampsia in women at increased risk: a randomized trial. *Lancet* 1999;354:810–816.

Chasan-Taber L, Willett WC, Manson JE, et al. Prospective study of oral contraceptives and hypertension among women in the United States. *Circulation* 1996;94:483–489.

Chesley LC, Annitto JE, Cosgrove RA. The remote prognosis of eclamptic women. *Am J Obstet Gynecol* 1976;124:446–459.

Chesley LC. Diagnosis of preeclampsia. *Obstet Gynecol* 1985;65:423–425.

Chesley LC. Hypertension in pregnancy: definitions, familial factor, and remote prognosis. *Kidney Int* 1980;18:234–240.

Chobanian AV, Bakris GL, Black HR, et al. Seventh report of the Joint National Committee on prevention, detection, evaluation, and treatment of high blood pressure. *Hypertension* 2003;42:1206–1252.

Chung JY, Song Y, Wang Y, et al. Differential expression of vascular endothelial growth factor (VEGF), endocrine gland derived-VEGF, and VEGF receptors in human placentas from normal and preeclamptic pregnancies. *J Clin Endocrinol Metab* 2004;89:2484–2490.

Clark DA. Does immunological intercourse prevent preeclampsia? *Lancet* 1994;344:969–970.

Cnattingius S, Signorello LB, Annerén G, et al. Caffeine intake and the risk of first-trimester spontaneous abortion. *N Engl J Med* 2000;343:1839–1845.

Cockburn J, Moar VA, Ounsted M, Redman CW. Final report of study on hypertension during pregnancy: the effects of specific treatment on the growth and development of the children. *Lancet* 1982;1:647–649.

Conde-Agudelo A, Villar J, Lindheimer M. World Health Organization systematic review of screening tests for preeclampsia. *Obstet Gynecol* 2004;104:1367–1391.

Crane MG, Harris JJ, Winsor W III. Hypertension, oral contraceptive agents, and conjugated estrogens. *Ann Intern Med* 1971;74:13–21.

Crowther CA, Hiller JE, Doyle LW, Haslam RR. Australasian Collaborative Trial of Magnesium Sulphate (ACTOMg SO4) Collaborative Group. Effect of magnesium sulfate given for neuroprotection before preterm birth: a randomized controlled trial. *JAMA* 2003;290:2669–2676.

De Meersman RE, Zion AS, Giardina V, et al. Estrogen replacement, vascular distensibility, and blood pressures in postmenopausal women. *Am J Physiol* 1998;274:H1539–H1544.

Dechend R, Viedt C, Muller DN, et al. AT$_1$ receptor agonistic antibodies from preeclamptic patients stimulate NADPH oxidase. *Circulation* 2003;107:1632–1639.

Dekker G, Sibai B. Primary, secondary, and tertiary prevention of pre-eclampsia. *Lancet* 2001;357:209–215.

Dempsey JC, Williams MA, Luthy DA, et al. Weight at birth and subsequent risk of preeclampsia as an adult. *Am J Obstet Gynecol* 2003;189:494–500.

Dizon-Townson DS, Nelson LM, Easton K, Ward K. The factor V Leiden mutation may predispose women to severe preeclampsia. *Am J Obstet Gynecol* 1996;175:902–905.

Douglas KA, Redman CWG. Eclampsia in the United Kingdom. *BMJ* 1994;309:1395–1400.

Duckitt K, Harrington D. Risk factors for pre-eclampsia at antenatal booking: systematic review of controlled studies. *BMJ* 2005;330:565–572.

Duley L, Henderson-Smart D, Knight M, King J. Antiplatelet drugs for prevention of pre-eclampsia and its consequences. *BMJ* 2001;322:329–333.

Durnwald C, Mercer B. A prospective comparison of total protein/creatinine ratio versus 24-hour urine protein in women with suspected preeclampsia. *Am J Obstet Gynecol* 2003;189:848–852.

Elkayam U, Akhter MW, Singh H, Khan S, et al. Pregnancy-associated cardiomyopathy: clinical characteristics and a comparison between early and late presentation. *Circulation* 2005;111:2050–2055.

Elvan-Taşpinar A, Franx A, Bots ML, et al. Central hemodynamics of hypertensive disorders in pregnancy. *Am J Hypertens* 2004;17:941–946.

Epstein FH. Pregnancy and renal disease. *N Engl J Med* 1996;335:277–278.

Eras JL, Saftlas AF, Triche E, et al. Abortion and its effects on risk of preeclampsia and transient hypertension. *Epidemiology* 2000;11:36–43.

Felker GM, Jaeger CJ, Klodas E, et al. Myocarditis and long-term survival in peripartum cardiomyopathy. *Am Heart J* 2000;140:785–791.

Ferguson JH, Neubauer BL, Shaar CJ. Ambulatory blood pressure monitoring during pregnancy. Establishment of standards of normalcy. *Am J Hypertens* 1994;7:838–843.

Ferrer RL, Sibai BM, Mulrow CD, et al. Management of mild chronic hypertension during pregnancy: a review. *Obstet Gynecol* 2000;96:849–860.

Fischer MJ, Lehnerz SD, Hebert JR, Parikh CR. Kidney disease is an independent risk factor for adverse fetal and maternal outcomes in pregnancy. *Am J Kidney Dis* 2004;43:415–423.

Florio P, D'Aniello G, Sabatini L, et al. Factor II:C activity and uterine artery Doppler evaluation to improve the early prediction of pre-eclampsia on women with gestational hypertension. *J Hypertens* 2005;23:141–146.

Freeman DJ, McManus F, Brown EA, et al. Short- and long-term changes in plasma inflammatory markers associated with preeclampsia. *Hypertension* 2004;43:708–714.

Friedman SA. Preeclampsia: a review of the role of prostaglandins. *Obstet Gynecol* 1988;71:122–137.

Ganzevoort W, Rep A, Bonsel GJ, et al. Plasma volume and blood pressure regulation in hypertensive pregnancy. *J Hypertens* 2004;22:1235–1242.

Gärtner HV, Sammoun A, Wehrmann M, et al. Preeclamptic nephropathy—an endothelial lesion. A morphological study with a review of the literature. *Eur J Obstet Gynecol* 1998;77:11–27.

Gillman MW, Rifas-Shiman SL, Kleinman KP, et al. Maternal calcium intake and offspring blood pressure. *Circulation* 2004;110:1990–1995.

Godsland IF, Walton C, Felton C, et al. Insulin resistance, secretion, and metabolism in users of oral contraceptives. *J Clin Endocrinol Metab* 1992;74:64–70.

Haelterman B, Bréart G, Paris-Llado J, et al. Effect of uncomplicated chronic hypertension on the risk of small-for-gestational age birth. *Am J Epidemiol* 1997;145:689–695.

Hatton DC, Harrison-Hohner J, Coste S, et al. Gestational calcium supplementation and blood pressure in the offspring. *Am J Hypertens* 2003;16:801–805.

Hermida RC, Ayala DE, Fernandez JR, et al. Reproducibility of the tolerance-hyperbaric test for diagnosing hypertension in pregnancy. *J Hypertens* 2004;22:565–572.

Higashi Y, Sanada M, Sasaki S, et al. Effect of estrogen replacement therapy on endothelial function in peripheral resistance arteries in normotensive and hypertensive postmenopausal women. *Hypertension* 2001;37:651–657.

Higgins JR, de Swiet M. Blood-pressure measurement and classification in pregnancy. *Lancet* 2001;357:131–135.

Howard BV, Hsia J, Ouyang P, et al. Postmenopausal hormone therapy is associated with atherosclerosis progression in women with abnormal glucose tolerance. *Circulation* 2004;110:201–206.

Hubel CA, Roberts JM, Ferrell RE. Association of pre-eclampsia with common coding sequence variations in the lipoprotein lipase gene. *Clin Genet* 1999;56:289–296.

Hulley SB, Grady D. The WHI estrogen-alone trial—do things look any better? *JAMA* 2004;291:1769–1771.

Ito S. Drug therapy for breast-feeding women. *N Engl J Med* 2000;343:118–126.

Jokela H, Dastidar P, Rontu R, et al. Effects of long-term estrogen replacement therapy versus combined hormone replacement therapy on nitric oxide-dependent vasomotor function. *J Clin Endocrinol Metab* 2003;88:4348–4354.

Kang DH, Finch J, Nakagawa T, et al. Uric acid, endothelial dysfunction and pre-eclampsia: searching for a pathogenetic link. *J Hypertens* 2004;22:229–235.

Kestenbaum B, Seliger SL, Easterling TR, et al. Cardiovascular and thromboembolic events following hypertensive pregnancy. *Am J Kidney Dis* 2003;42:982–989.

Klonoff-Cohen HS, Savitz DA, Cefalo RC, et al. An epidemiologic study of contraception and preeclampsia. *JAMA* 1989;262:3143–3147.

Knuist M, Bonsel GJ, Zondervan HA, et al. Low sodium diet and pregnancy-induced hypertension: a multi-centre randomised controlled trial. *Br J Obstet Gynecol* 1998; 105:430–434.

Kotchen JM, Kotchen TA. Impact of female hormones on blood pressure: review of potential mechanisms and clinical studies. *Curr Hypertens Rep* 2003;5:505–512.

Kupferminc MJ, Eldor A, Steinman N, et al. Increased frequency of genetic thrombophilia in women with complications in pregnancy. *N Engl J Med* 1999;340:9–13.

Lafayette R. The kidney in preeclampsia. *Kidney Int* 2005;67: 1194–1203.

Langer RD, Hsia J, Pettinger M, et al. Conjugated equine estrogens-alone and the risk of coronary heart disease: results of the Women's Health Initiative Clinical Trial [Abstract]. *Circulation* 2004;110(Suppl 3):III–791.

Lee AFC, McFarlane LC, Struthers AD. Ovarian hormones in man: their effects on resting vascular tone, angiotensin converting enzyme activity and angiotensin II-induced vasoconstriction. *Br J Clin Pharmacol* 2000;50:73–76.

Lévesque S, Moutquin JM, Lindsay C, et al. Implication of an AGT haplotype in a multigene association study with pregnancy hypertension. *Hypertension* 2004;43:71–78.

Levine RJ, Maynard SE, Qian C, et al. Circulating angiogenic factors and the risk of preeclampsia. *N Engl J Med* 2004;350:672–683.

Levine RJ, Qian C, LeShane ES, et al. Two-stage elevation of cell-free fetal DNA in maternal sera before onset of preeclampsia. *Am J Obstet Gynecol* 2004b;190:707–713.

Levine RJ, Thadhani R, Qian C, et al. Urinary placental growth factor and risk of preeclampsia. *JAMA* 2005;293: 77–85.

Li G, Chen Y-F, Greene GL, et al. Estrogen inhibits vascular smooth muscle cell-dependent adventitial fibroblast migration *in vitro*. *Circulation* 1999;100:1639–1645.

Lim KG, Isles CG, Hodsman GP, et al. Malignant hypertension in women of childbearing age and its relation to the contraceptive pill. *BMJ* 1987;294:1057–1059.

Lindsay JR, Jonklaas J, Oldfield EH, Nieman LK. Cushing's syndrome during pregnancy: personal experience and review of the literature. *J Clin Endocrinol Metab* 2005;90: 3077–3083.

Magee LA, Cham C, Waterman EJ, et al. Hydralazine for treatment of severe hypertension in pregnancy: meta-analysis. *BMJ* 2003;327:955–960.

Magness RR, Rosenfeld CR, Hassan A, Shaul PW. Endothelial vasodilator production by uterine and systemic arteries. I. Effects of ANG II on PGI$_2$ and NO in pregnancy. *Am J Physiol* 1996;270:H1914–H1923.

Magpie Trial Collaboration Group. Do women with pre-eclampsia, and their babies, benefit from magnesium sulphate? The Magpie Trial: a randomised placebo-controlled trial. *Lancet* 2002;359:1877–1890.

Makris A, Thornton C, Hennessy A. Postpartum hypertension and nonsteroidal analgesia. *Am J Obstet Gynecol* 2004; 190:577–578.

Martin JN Jr, Magann EF. HELLP syndrome: current principles and recommended practices. In: Lee RV, Garner PR, Barron WM, Coustan DR, eds. *Current Obstetric Medicine*. St. Louis: Mosby, 1996.

Mattar F, Sibai BM. Eclampsia. Risk factors for maternal morbidity. *Am J Obstet Gynecol* 2000;182:307–312.

Matthys LA, Coppage KH, Lambers DS, et al. Delayed postpartum preeclampsia: an experience of 151 cases. *Am J Obstet Gynecol* 2004;190:1464–1466.

McCaffrey TA. *Estrogens and blood pressure: a theoretical review* [Dissertation]. Lafayette, IN: Purdue University, June 1985.

Medical Letter. Treatment of menopausal vasomotor symptoms. *The Medical Letter* 2004;46:98–99.

Mello G, Parretti E, Fatini C. Low-molecular-weight heparin lowers the recurrence rate of preeclampsia and restores the physiological vascular changes in angiotensin-converting enzyme DD women. *Hypertension* 2005;45:86–91.

Mercuro G, Zoncu S, Piano D, et al. Estradiol-17β reduces blood pressure and restores the normal amplitude of the circadian blood pressure rhythm in postmenopausal hypertension. *J Hypertens* 1998;11:909–913.

Milne F, Redman C, Walker J, et al. The pre-eclampsia community guideline (PRECOG): how to screen for and detect onset of pre-eclampsia in the community. *BMJ* 2005;330: 576–580.

Modena MG, Molinari R, Muia N Jr, et al. Double-blind randomized placebo-controlled study of transdermal estrogen replacement therapy on hypertensive postmenopausal women. *Am J Hypertens* 1999;12:1000–1008.

Myers J, Mires G, Macleod M, et al. In preeclampsia, the circulating factors capable of altering *in vitro* endothelial function precede clinical disease. *Hypertension* 2005;45: 258–263.

National High Blood Pressure Education Program Working Group on High Blood Pressure in Pregnancy. Report of the National High Blood Pressure Education Program Working Group on high blood pressure in pregnancy. *Am J Obstet Gynecol* 2000;183:S1–S22.

Nilsson E, Salonen Ros H, Cnattingius S, et al. The importance of genetic and environmental effects for pre-eclampsia and gestational hypertension: a family study. *Br J Obstet Gynaecol* 2004;111:200–206.

Olsen S, Secher NJ, Tabor A, et al. Randomised clinical trials of fish oil supplementation in high risk pregnancies. *Br J Obstet Gynaecol* 2000;107:382–395.

Page EW. Placental dysfunction in eclamptogenic toxemias. *Obstet Gynecol Survey* 1948;3:615–628.

Paulson RJ, Boostanfar R, Saadat P, et al. Pregnancy in the sixth decade of life: obstetric outcomes in women of advanced reproductive age. *JAMA* 2002;288:2320–2323.

Petitti DB. Clinical practice. Combination estrogen-progestin oral contraceptives. *N Engl J Med* 2003;349:1443–1450.

Pouta A, Hartikainen AL, Sovio U, et al. Manifestations of metabolic syndrome after hypertensive pregnancy. *Hypertension* 2004;43:825–831.

Pritchard JA, Cunningham FG, Pritchard SA. The Parkland Memorial Hospital protocol for treatment of eclampsia: evaluation of 245 cases. *Am J Obstet Gynecol* 1984;148: 951–963.

Pritchard JA, Pritchard SA. Blood pressure response to estrogen-progestin oral contraceptive after pregnancy-induced hypertension. *Am J Obstet Gynecol* 1977;129:733–739.

Qiu C, Williams MA, Leisenring WM, et al. Family history of hypertension and type 2 diabetes in relation to preeclampsia risk. *Hypertension* 2003;41:408–413.

Raijmakers MTM, Dechend R, Poston L. Oxidative stress and preeclampsia: rationale for antioxidant clinical trials. *Hypertension* 2004;44:374–380.

Rang S, Wolf H, Montfrans GA, Karemaker JM. Serial assessment of cardiovascular control shows early signs of developing pre-eclampsia. *J Hypertens* 2004;22:369–376.

Reckelhoff JF, Fortepiani LA. Novel mechanisms responsible for postmenopausal hypertension. *Hypertension* 2004; 43:918–923.

Redman CWG, Sargent IL. Placental debris, oxidative stress and pre-eclampsia. *Placenta* 2000;21:597–602.

Reiter L, Brown MA, Whitworth JA. Hypertension in pregnancy: the incidence of underlying renal disease and essential hypertension. *Am J Kidney Dis* 1994;24:883–887.

Ribstein J, Halimi J-M, du Cailar G, Mimran A. Renal characteristics and effect of angiotensin suppression in oral contraceptive use. *Hypertension* 1999;33:90–95.

Riskin-Mashiah S, Belfort MA. Cerebrovascular hemodynamics in chronic hypertensive pregnant women who later develop superimposed preeclampsia. *J Soc Gynecol Investig* 2005;12:28–32.

Roberts CB, Rom L, Moodley J, Pegoraro RJ. Hypertension-related gene polymorphisms in pre-eclampsia and gestational hypertension in black South African women. *J Hypertens* 2004;22:945–948.

Roberts JM, Cooper DW. Pathogenesis and genetics of pre-eclampsia. *Lancet* 2001;357:53–56.

Roberts JM, Hubel CA. Oxidative stress in preeclampsia. *Am J Obstet Gynecol* 2004;190:1177–1178.

Roberts JM, Pearson G, Cutler J, Lindheimer M. NHLBI Working Group on Research on Hypertension During Pregnancy. Summary of the NHLBI Working Group on Research on Hypertension During Pregnancy. *Hypertension* 2003;41:437–445.

Robillard P-Y, Hulsey TC. Association of pregnancy-induced hypertension, preeclampsia, and eclampsia with duration of sexual cohabitation before conception. *Lancet* 1996; 347:619.

Robson SC, Dunlop W, Hunter S. Haemodynamic effects of breast-feeding. *Br J Obstet Gynaecol* 1989;96:1106–1108.

Schwartz RB, Feske SK, Polak JF, et al. Preeclampsia-eclampsia: clinical and neuroradiographic correlates and insights into the pathogenesis of hypertensive encephalopathy. *Radiology* 2000;217:371–376.

Serrano NC, Casas JP, Días LA, et al. Endothelial NO synthase genotype and risk of preeclampsia: a multicenter case-control study. *Hypertension* 2004;44:702–707.

Shehata HA, Ahmed K. Other endocrine disorders in pregnancy. *Curr Obstet Gynecol* 2004;14:387–394.

Sibai B, Dekker G, Kupferminc M. Pre-eclampsia. *Lancet* 2005;365:785–799.

Singhal A, Lucas A. Early origins of cardiovascular disease: is there a unifying hypothesis? *Lancet* 2004;363:1642–1645.

Steer PJ, Little MP, Kold-Jensen T, et al. Maternal blood pressure in pregnancy, birth weight, and perinatal mortality in first births: prospective study. *BMJ* 2004;329:1312–1318.

Thadhani R, Stampfer MJ, Chasan-Taber L, et al. A prospective study of pregravid oral contraceptive use and risk of

hypertensive disorders of pregnancy. *Contraception* 1999; 60:145–150.

Thway TM, Shlykov S, Day M-C, et al. Antibodies from preeclamptic patients stimulate increased intracellular Ca2+ mobilization through angiotensin receptor activation. *Circulation* 2004;110:1612–1619.

Turnbull DA, Wilkinson C, Gerard K, et al. Clinical, psychosocial, and economic effects of antenatal day care for three medical complications of pregnancy: a randomised controlled trial of 395 women. *Lancet* 2004;363:1104–1109.

Vanek M, Sheiner E, Levy A, Mazor M. Chronic hypertension and the risk for adverse pregnancy outcome after superimposed pre-eclampsia. *Int J Gynecol Obstet* 2004;86:7–11.

Virdis A, Pinto S, Versari D, et al. Effect of oral contraceptives on endothelial function in the peripheral microcirculation of healthy women. *J Hypertens* 2003;21:2275–2280.

von Dadelszen P, Ornstein MP, Bull SB, et al. Fall in mean arterial pressure and fetal growth restriction in pregnancy hypertension: a meta-analysis. *Lancet* 2000;355:87–92.

Vongpatanasin W, Abbas AA, Wang Z, et al. Differential effects of oral vs. transdermal estrogen replacement therapy on serum amyloid A in postmenopausal women [Abstract]. *Am J Hypertens* 2004;17:245A.

Vongpatanasin W, Tuncel M, Mansour Y, et al. Transdermal estrogen replacement therapy decreases sympathetic activity in postmenopausal women. *Circulation* 2001;103:2903–2908.

Walker JJ. Pre-eclampsia. *Lancet* 2000;356:1260–1265.

Wang X, Athayde N, Trudinger B. Microvascular endothelial cell activation is present in the umbilical placental microcirculation in fetal placental vascular disease. *Am J Obstet Gynecol* 2004;190:596–601.

Wang Y, Lewis DF, Gu Y, et al. Placental trophoblast-derived factors diminish endothelial barrier function. *J Clin Endocrinol Metab* 2004;89:2421–2428.

Waugh J, Habiba MA, Bosio P, et al. Patient initiated home blood pressure recordings are accurate in hypertensive pregnant women. *Hypertens Pregnancy* 2003;22:93–97.

Weiner CP, Buhimschi C. *Drugs for Pregnant and Lactating Women.* Philadelphia: Churchill Livingstone, 2004.

Weir RJ. When the pill causes a rise in blood pressure. *Drugs* 1978;16:522–527.

Williams MA, Farrand A, Mittendorf R, et al. Maternal second trimester serum tumor necrosis factor-α-soluble receptor p55 (sTNFp55) and subsequent risk of preeclampsia. *Am J Epidemiol* 1999;149:323–329.

Wilson BJ, Watson MS, Prescott GJ, et al. Hypertensive diseases of pregnancy and risk of hypertension and stroke in later life: results from cohort study. *BMJ* 2003;326:845–849.

Wolf M, Hubel CA, Lam C, et al. Preeclampsia and future cardiovascular disease: potential role of altered angiogenesis and insulin resistance. *J Clin Endocrinol Metab* 2004; 89:6239–6243.

World Health Organization. *Improving Access to Quality Care in Family Planning: Medical Eligibility Criteria for Contraceptive Use.* 2nd Ed. Geneva: World Health Organization, 2000.

Zeeman GG, Fleckenstein JL, Twickler DM, et al. Cerebral infarction in eclampsia. *Am J Obstet Gynecol* 2004;190: 714–720.

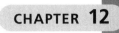

# Pheochromocytoma (with a Preface About Incidental Adrenal Masses)

## THE INCIDENTAL ADRENAL MASS

Before considering adrenal causes of hypertension in this and the subsequent two chapters, the management of incidentally discovered adrenal masses will be covered. Such masses are being found increasingly during abdominal computed tomography (CT) and magnetic resonance imaging (MRI) in patients undergoing imaging for an unrelated reason and who have no clinical evidence of adrenal hyperfunction. The masses must be evaluated, both because they may be functionally active and because they may be malignant (Barzon et al., 2003; Grumbach et al., 2003). If the evaluation is negative, the patient should be reassured about the low likelihood of future trouble; a repeat imaging procedure and screening for adrenal hyperfunction should be done after 1 year, but repeated evaluations are rarely indicated in the continued absence of clinical abnormalities. Logically, only those masses that are neither malignant nor hyperfunctioning should be called "*incidentalomas.*"

## Prevalence

Presumed adrenal incidentalomas were found in 2.3% of 71,206 autopsies (Barzon et al., 2003). In 82,483 adrenal scans performed up to 1994, the prevalence was 0.64%, but likely more are being recognized with improved technology.

The prevalence increases progressively with age. As noted in Chapter 13, increasing adrenal nodularity is also noted with age (Tracy & White, 2002), so that the differentiation and evaluation of discrete adenomas will pose an even greater challenge with advanced scanning technology.

## Evaluation

In patients without known primary cancers, about 90% of incidental adrenal masses are benign; in patients without clinical evidence of adrenal hyperfunction, about 85% are nonfunctional. Nonetheless, every adrenal mass should be evaluated to rule out both malignancy and hypersecretion using procedures that are readily available and relatively inexpensive.

## Workup for Malignancy

### Imaging

Masses that are small, smooth, round, and have a high-fat content are usually benign adenomas or, less commonly, myelolipomas (Udelsman & Fishman, 2000). These high-fat lesions have a low density on CT and are isointense to liver on $T_2$-weighted MRI. Chemical shift MRI can also demonstrate lipid within the adrenal mass (Haider et al., 2004). The ability of noncontrast CT attenuation value, expressed as Hounsfield Unit (HU), to differentiate benign adrenal adenomas or hyperplasia from adrenal cancer, metastases, or pheochromocytomas was analyzed from the findings of 299 adrenalectomies done at the Cleveland Clinic (Hamrahian et al., 2005). A noncontrast CT attenuation value of 10 HU was found to be a safe cutoff value to differentiate benign tumors from nonadenomas.

Grumbach et al. (2003) recommend excision of all tumors larger than 6 cm, 25% of which have been found to harbor an adrenal carcinoma. However, Copeland (2004) recommends that surgery not be done if the ≥6 cm tumor is smooth, homogenous, low density (<2 HU), and nonfunctional. All agree that lesions less than 4 cm and defined as low risk of malignancy by imaging criteria should not be resected whereas those between 4 and 6 cm have either close follow-up or adrenalectomy (Grumbach et al., 2003).

### Adrenal Scintigraphy

Adrenal scintigraphy with an iodinated cholesterol derivative (NP-59) that localizes in functioning adrenal cortical tissue but not in most malignant adrenal masses has been used by Gross et al. (1994) in 229 euadrenal patients with unilateral masses found on CT scans. Adrenal masses that took up the NP-59 were almost always benign; those that did not take up the NP-59 were mostly malignant, either metastatic or primary. In a series of 43 patients with a unilateral adrenal mass on scans, noncholesterol scintigraphy had a 100% sensitivity but only a 71% specificity for identifying a benign adrenal adenoma (Maurea et al., 2002).

### Biopsy

Fine needle aspiration (FNA) biopsy is rarely needed since imaging characteristics can usually be relied upon to exclude malignancy (Young, 2000).

### Hormonal Levels

In one series of 129 adrenal cancers, 40 had manifestations of endocrinopathy, most commonly of excess cortisol or androgen (Crucitti et al., 1996). High levels of plasma dehydroepiandrosterone sulfate (DHEA-S) are seen in some adrenocortical cancers, whereas low levels are seen in about two thirds of benign adenomas (Terzolo et al., 1996).

### Workup for Hyperfunction

Table 12–1 lists the suggestive clinical features and scanning tests for adrenal hyperfunction. In 26 published series reporting a total of 3,868 patients, the percentages with hormonal hypersecretions were 7.9% with preclinical Cushing's syndrome, 5.6% with pheochromocytoma (pheo), and 1.2% with primary aldosteronism (Barzon et al., 2003).

All patients should have an overnight 1 mg dexamethasone suppression test. Normal suppression is defined as an 8 a.m. plasma cortisol below 150 nmol/L, but perhaps additional testing should be done in those with levels between 50 and 150 nmol/L (Grumbach et al., 2003). These same experts recommend routine measure of plasma free metanephrines. However, Copeland (2004) correctly cautions about the 11% to 15% false-positive results with that procedure and recommends that no testing for pheo is needed for those without clinical or imaging evidence of a pheo.

### Management

Whereas subclinical pheos and aldosteronomas should usually be resected, uncertainty remains about the management of subclinical Cushing's

## TABLE 12–1

### Evaluation of Incidental Adrenal Masses

| Diagnosis | Suggestive Clinical Features | Laboratory Screening Tests |
|---|---|---|
| Pheochromocytoma | Paroxysmal hypertension; spells of sweating, headache, palpitations | Plasma or urine metanephrine |
| Cushing's syndrome | Truncal obesity, thin skin, muscle weakness, glucose intolerance | 8 A.M. plasma cortisol after 1 mg dexamethasone at bedtime |
| Primary aldosteronism | Hypertension, hypokalemia | Urinary potassium excretion, plasma aldosterone and renin |
| Adrenocortical carcinoma | Virilization or feminization | Plasma dehydroepiandrosterone, testosterone, or estrogens |

syndrome. As these patients have been closely examined, most turn out to have obesity, hypertension, glucose intolerance, and osteopenia (Chiodini et al., 2004), all of which can be relieved by adrenalectomy (Bernini et al., 2003). The presence of these multiple abnormalities questions the label of "subclinical." but, obviously, removal of the adenoma may be indicated in some of these patients.

The wisdom of simply observing the majority is supported by the absence of malignancy over an average follow-up of 50 months in 238 patients with tumors that averaged 2.5 cm in size (Young, 2000). Enlargement or hyperfunction may occur so that continued observation is needed (Barzon et al., 2003), but if no growth or hyperfunction is noted after 1 year, only routine follow-up is needed.

## OVERVIEW OF ADRENAL HYPERFUNCTION

Beyond the need to evaluate patients with incidentally discovered adrenal masses, an adrenal cause for hypertension will need to be considered much more frequently than the low prevalence—likely less than 2%—of these causes would suggest. The presence of adrenal hyperfunction is often considered in the evaluation of hypertensive patients because many of the symptoms and signs of adrenal hyperfunction are nonspecific and are encountered in patients with normal adrenal function. Recurrent spells suggestive of pheochromocytoma, hypokalemia pointing to primary aldosteronism, and cushingoid features are all encountered in many more patients than the relatively few who turn out to have these diseases. Of all of these, consideration of a pheochromocytoma is likely most important.

## PHEOCHROMOCYTOMA

The presence of a pheo should be considered in all hypertensives since, if not recognized, a pheo may provoke fatal hypertensive crises during anesthesia and other stresses (Manger & Eisenhofer, 2004; Prys-Roberts, 2000). Pheos are often unrecognized: At the Mayo Clinic from 1928 to 1977, of 54 pheos found at autopsy, only 13 had been diagnosed during life (Lie et al., 1980). Of the 41 previously unrecognized, death was related to the manifestations of the tumor in 30 patients. This experience with unrecognized pheos should be contrasted to the excellent results obtained at the same Mayo Clinic on 138 patients with demonstrated pheos who underwent surgery during these years; the survival curve of those with a benign pheo was similar to that of the normal population (Sheps et al., 1990).

In subsequent years, no perioperative mortality occurred in 143 patients, all but three diagnosed preoperatively (Kinney et al., 2000).

### Prevalence

Pheos are rare, with one found per 2,031 autopsies (McNeil et al., 2000). The prevalence of pheos diagnosed during life or at autopsy among the residents of Rochester, Minnesota—the location of the Mayo Clinic—was found to be 0.95 cases per 100,000 person-years (Beard et al., 1983). This figure, the most accurate estimate of the incidence of the tumor now available, suggests that, if 20% of the adult population is hypertensive, only about five pheos would be expected to be found among 100,000 hypertensives each year. However, about 10% of all pheos are found incidentally (Young, 2000), and about 5% of all incidentalomas are pheos (Barzon et al., 2003).

### Pathophysiology

#### Development

The cells of the sympathetic nervous system arise from the primitive neural crest as primordial stem cells, called *sympathogonia* (Figure 12–1). The sympathogonia migrate out of the central nervous system to occupy a place behind the aorta. These stem cells may differentiate into either sympathoblasts, which give rise to sympathetic ganglion cells, or pheochromoblasts, which give rise to chromaffin cells. As seen in Figure 12–1, tumors may arise from each of these cell lines, often sharing histologic and biochemical characteristics. These include highly malignant neuroblastomas, arising from sympathoblasts, and ganglioneuromas, which are usually more benign. These tumors are rarely seen after adolescence and are usually recognized by the excretion of large amounts of homovanillic acid (HVA), the urinary metabolite of dopamine (Figure 12–2).

The chromaffin cells, which have the capacity to synthesize and store catecholamines, therefore staining brown on treatment with chromium, are found mainly in the adrenal medulla. They also appear in the sympathetic ganglia and paraganglia that lie along the sympathetic chain and organ of Zuckerkandl, located anteriorly at the bifurcation of the aorta. In a developmental sense, the adrenal medulla may be considered a sympathetic ganglion that lacks postsynaptic fibers. In a functional sense, its chromaffin cells differ from the rest by having the capacity to convert norepinephrine (NE) to epinephrine (Epi) (Figure 12–2).

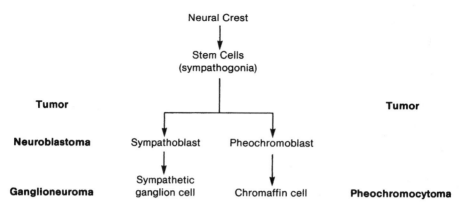

FIGURE 12–1 ● Developmental pathway for sympathetic ganglion and chromaffin cells and the tumors that may arise from them.

### Location and Tumor Nomenclature

Table 12–2 shows where chromaffin cell tumors, i.e., pheochromocytomas, have been found. As many as 15% of pheos in adults and 40% in children are extra-adrenal; they may be located anywhere along the sympathetic chain and, rarely, in aberrant sites (Whalen et al., 1992). Those functioning tumors arising outside the adrenal medulla are best termed *extra-adrenal pheochromocytomas* (Whalen et al., 1992), whereas nonsecreting extra-adrenal tumors are termed *paragangliomas* (Fonseca & Bouloux, 1993). Paragangliomas that arise from

the specialized chemoreceptor tissue in the carotid body, glomus jugulare, and aortic body have been separately classified as *chemodectomas,* and they may secrete catecholamines (Erickson et al., 2001).

In their review, Whalen et al. (1992) noted that at least 85% of extra-adrenal pheos have been below the diaphragm, about half in the superior para-aortic areas. The inferior para-aortic area, below the kidneys to the aortic bifurcation, is the next most common site, with most of these being in the organs of Zuckerkandl. Some are in the wall of the urinary bladder (Garovic et al., 2004). A few arise in the

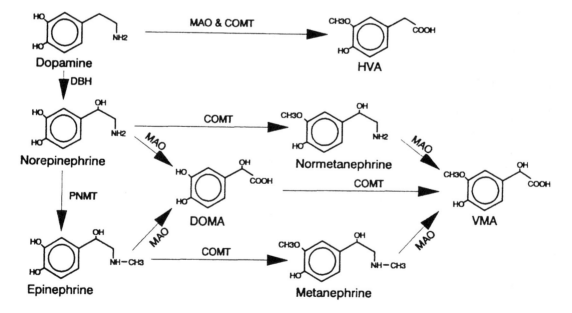

FIGURE 12–2 ● Pathways and enzymes of catacholamine metabolism. The excretory products are shown on the right of the biosynthetic pathway. DBH, dopamine β-hydroxylase; PNMT, phenylethanolamine N-methyltransferase; MAO, monoamine oxidase; COMT, catechol O-methyltransferase.

## TABLE 12–2

### Location of Pheochromocytoma

| Location | Percent |
|---|---|
| Intra-abdominal | 95 |
| Single adrenal tumor | 50–70 |
| Single extra-adrenal tumor | 10–20 |
| Multiple tumors[a] | 15–40 |
| Bilateral adrenal tumors | 5–25 |
| Multiple extra-adrenal tumors | 5–15 |
| Outside the abdomen | 5 |
| Intrathoracic | 2 |
| In the neck | <1 |

[a]More common in children and in familial syndromes.

head and neck; about 10% in the thorax, including almost 40 cases in the heart (Lin et al., 1999). Extra-adrenal pheos are more likely malignant compared to adrenal pheos (Bravo & Tagle, 2003). A larger proportion of extra-adrenal and multicentric pheos occur in children than in adults (Kohane et al., 2005).

On the other hand, the majority of the 297 benign paragangliomas seen over a 20-year interval at the Mayo Clinic were located in the head and neck (Erickson et al., 2001). Of the 49 of these tumors that were hyperfunctioning, i.e., extra-adrenal pheos, 36 were below the diaphragm, but nine were in the head and neck and four in the thorax.

### Chromaffin Cell Secretion

The chromaffin cells synthesize catecholamines from the dietary amino acid tyrosine, which is converted into dopa and then dopamine. As seen in Figure 12–2, NE is the end product, except in the adrenal medulla, where over 75% of the NE is methylated into Epi. Most adrenal medullary pheos secrete some Epi; but a few, usually small in size and having a rapid turnover of catecholamines, secrete only NE (Crout & Sjöerdsma, 1964). On the other hand, extra-adrenal pheos only rarely secrete Epi (Blumenfeld et al., 1993).

When catecholamines are released by exocytosis from adrenal storage vesicles, there is a coupled, proportional release of the enzyme dopamine β-hydroxylase and the soluble proteins chromogranin A, B, and C. Plasma chromogranin A and B levels are elevated in patients with pheos and other neuroendocrine tumors and may serve as sensitive

markers (Granberg et al., 1999). Plasma chromogranin A levels are usually markedly elevated with malignant pheos and may be used to monitor the response to therapy (Rao et al., 2000).

*Patterns of Catechol Secretion*
Secretion from pheos varies considerably. Small pheos tend to secrete larger proportions of active catecholamines; larger pheos, with the capacity to store and metabolize large quantities of catecholamines, tend to secrete less of their content, and most of that may be secreted in inactive forms.

The frequency and severity of symptoms and signs may relate to the secretory pattern of the pheo. Those that continuously release large amounts of catecholamines may induce sustained hypertension with few paroxysms, since the adrenergic receptors become desensitized after prolonged exposure to their agonists (Valet et al., 1988); those that are less active but cyclically release their catecholamine stores may induce striking paroxysms of hypertension with the classic symptoms of a pheo, since the receptors are more responsive.

Despite the logical assumption that the hypertension and symptoms of pheo are solely the consequences of the elevated circulating catecholamines that would suppress the sympathetic nervous system (SNS), Bravo and Tagle (2003) review evidence that the SNS remains active and may be involved. This evidence includes the poor correlation between blood pressure and levels of plasma catechols as well as the ability of the centrally acting SNS depressant clonidine to lower blood pressure without changes in circulating catechols. These authors postulate that the SNS may be involved in a number of the features of pheo: the potential for hypertensive crises when stimuli release NE from sympathetic nerve terminals; on one hand, the occurrence of marked symptoms with only small increments in circulating catechols while, on the other hand, blood pressure being normal despite high levels of catechols.

*Dopa and Dopamine*
Pheos that secrete large amounts of the vasodilating precursors dopa and dopamine may not manifest hypertension (Eisenhofer et al., 2005a). This could explain the rarity of symptoms in patients with neuroblastomas and in some patients with malignant pheos who hypersecrete dopa and dopamine.

*Other Secretions*
Table 12–3 lists various peptide hormones that may be released concomitantly with catecholamines from pheos; their secretion may be associated with various clinical manifestations (Fonseca & Bouloux, 1993). Neuropeptide Y may be involved in hypertension occurring in pheo patients despite α-blockade (Bravo & Tagle, 2003).

# TABLE 12–3

## Secretory Peptides from Pheochromocytomas and Their Manifestation

| Peptide | Manifestation |
|---|---|
| Adrenomedullin | Vasodilatation |
| Angiotensin-converting enzyme | Hypertension |
| Atrial natriuretic factor | Polyuria, hypotension? |
| Calcitonin | |
| Calcitonin gene-related peptide (CGRP) | Vasodilatation |
| Chromogranin A | |
| Corticotrophin-releasing factor, adrenocorticotrophin | Hypercortisolism |
| Endothelin | Vasoconstriction |
| Enkephalins | Constipation |
| Erythropoietin-like factor | Polycythemia |
| Human growth hormone releasing hormone | Acromegaly |
| Insulin-like growth factor II | Related to tumor growth? |
| Interleukin 6 | Pyrexia |
| Motilin | Diarrhea |
| Neurone-specific enolase | |
| Neuropeptide Y | Vasoconstriction |
| Parathormone | Hypercalcemia |
| Parathormone-related peptide | Hypercalcemia |
| Pituitary adenylate cyclase activating polypeptide | Vasodilatation, Interleukin 6 release |
| Renin | Vasoconstriction |
| Somatostatin | Constipation |
| Substance P | Flushing |
| Vasoactive intestinal peptide | Flushing, diarrhea |

Modified from Fonseca V, Bouloux P-M.
   Phaeochromocytoma and paraganglioma. *Baillière's Clin Endocrinol Metab* 1993;7:509–545.

## *Hemodynamics*

The hemodynamics in 24 patients with a pheo were little different from those in age-, sex-, and weight-matched patients with essential hypertension, despite the tenfold higher plasma NE levels in the pheo patients (Bravo, 1994). The major finding in both was an increased peripheral resistance, whereas the pheo patients had lower blood volumes. Heart rate is usually around 90 beats per minute, even when the blood pressure (BP) is not high,

but cardiac output is usually normal, except during surges of Epi release.

With ambulatory BP monitoring, pheo patients usually do not have a nocturnal fall in BP (Zelinka et al., 2004).

## Clinical Features

Table 12–4 summarizes the varied and often dramatic symptoms and signs of catecholamine excess. Most patients have headache, sweating, and palpitations; many have all three occurring in paroxysms. Some are asymptomatic, and others have their symptoms attributed to concomitant

# TABLE 12–4

## Symptoms and Signs of Pheochromocytoma

Common (>33% of patients)
   Hypertension (probably >90%)
      Paroxysmal (50%)
      Sustained (30%)
      Paroxysms superimposed (about 50%)
   Hypotension, orthostatic (10%–50%)
   Headache (40%–80%)
   Sweating (40%–70%)
   Palpitations and tachycardia (45%–70%)
   Pallor (40%–45%)
   Anxiety and nervousness (20%–40%)
   Nausea and vomiting (20%–40%)
   Funduscopic changes (50%–70%)
   Weight loss (60%–80%)
Less common (<33% of patients)
   Tremor
   Abdominal pain
   Chest pain
   Polydipsia, polyuria
   Acrocyanosis, cold extremities
   Flushing
   Dyspnea
   Dizziness, syncope
   Convulsions
   Bradycardia
   Fever
   Thyroid swelling

Data from 378 reported cases; analyzed by Ross and Griffith (1989) and Werbel and Ober (1995).

conditions (Cohen et al., 2005). Although most have lost weight, 8 of 22 patients in one series were 10% or more overweight, and 4 were definitely obese (Lee & Rousseau, 1967).

## Symptoms

### Paroxysmal Hypertension

The paroxysms represent the classic picture of the disease, but exclusively paroxysmal hypertension with intervening normotension is relatively uncommon. Most patients have sustained hypertension with superimposed paroxysms. The paroxysm can be brought on in multiple ways, including exercise, bending over, urination, defecation, an enema, induction of anesthesia, smoking, dipping snuff, palpation of the abdomen, or pressure from an enlarging uterus during pregnancy. Episodes may follow use of multiple drugs acting in various ways:

- Block vasodilatory β-receptors, e.g., β-blockers (Brown et al., 2005)
- Increase catecholamine synthesis, e.g., ACTH (Jan et al., 1990)
- Increase catecholamine release, e.g., histamine, opiates, or nicotine (McPhaul et al., 1984)
- Antagonize dopamine, e.g., droperidol (Montiel et al., 1986)
- Inhibit catechol reuptake, e.g., tricyclic antidepressants (Achong & Keane, 1981)
- Inhibit serotonin reuptake (Seelen et al., 1997)

Wide episodic fluctuations of BP may occur spontaneously. The episodes vary in frequency, duration, and severity. They may occur many times per day or only every few months. Patients are often considered psychoneurotic, particularly if they describe a sensation of tightness starting in the abdomen and rising into the chest and head, anxiety, tremors, sweating, and palpitations, followed by marked weakness. On the other hand, pheolike symptoms and paroxysms of marked hypertension may be seen with emotional reactions and panic attacks (Mann, 1999) as well as obstructive sleep apnea (Hoy et al., 2004).

Pheo episodes, sometimes with BP above 250/150 mm Hg, may lead to myocardial ischemia (Brown et al., 2005), cardiomyopathy with acute congestive heart failure (Sardesai et al., 1990), or arrhythmias (Shimizu et al., 1992). Rarely, the presentation may be as an acute abdomen from spontaneous rupture of the tumor (Tanaka et al., 1994), sudden death after minor abdominal trauma (Primhak et al., 1986), lactic acidosis (Bornemann et al., 1986), or high fever and encephalopathy (Newell et al., 1988). Tumors arising in the wall of the bladder may cause symptoms only with micturition and, in about half of such cases, produce painless hematuria (Thrasher et al., 1993).

In patients with predominant Epi secretion, β-blockers can raise the BP by blocking the β₂-mediated vasodilator action of Epi, leaving the α-mediated vasoconstrictor action unopposed. Those with NE-producing pheos likely will not have a pressor response to β-blockers, since NE has little action on vasodilatory β₂-receptors (Plouin et al., 1979).

### Hypotension

Patients with a pheo secreting predominantly Epi may rarely present with cardiogenic shock, presumably from decreased cardiac contractibility from downregulation of β-receptors in the heart after prolonged exposure to high Epi levels and from hypocalcemia of uncertain origin (Olson et al., 2004). Prolonged hypotension may also occur by spontaneous necrosis of the tumor (Atuk et al., 1977) or after administration of an α-blocker (Watson et al., 1990). Much more commonly, patients have modest postural hypotension associated with tachycardia and dizziness. Postural hypotension in an untreated nonelderly hypertensive may be a clue to the presence of a pheo.

## Other Associated Diseases

Other associated diseases include the following:

- *Cholelithiasis,* seen in up to 30% of patients (Gifford et al., 1994).
- *Diabetes,* with fasting glucose levels above 125 mg/dL in 14 of 60 patients (Stenström et al., 1984).
- *Hypercalcemia* in the absence of hyperparathyroidism (Kimura et al., 1990).
- *Polycythemia* due to increased erythropoietin production (Jacobs & Wood, 1994). More frequently, a high hematocrit is related to a contracted plasma volume.
- *Renovascular hypertension,* likely by compression of a renal artery by the pheo (Gill et al., 2000).
- *Adrenocortical hyperfunction* may arise from ACTH secretion from the pheo (Chen et al., 1995) or from a coincidental cortisol-secreting adenoma in the other adrenal (Ooi & Dardick, 1988) or bilateral hyperplasia (Amos & McRoberts, 1998). Hyperaldosteronism has been noted rarely (Tan et al., 1996).
- *Rhabdomyolysis,* which has occurred with renal failure (Shemin et al., 1990).
- *Megacolon,* reported in 17 cases (Sweeney et al., 2000).

## Conditions Simulating a Pheochromocytoma

Most patients with hypertension and one or more of the manifestations of pheo turn out *not* to have that diagnosis. Table 12–5 lists conditions that may

## TABLE 12–5

### Conditions That May Simulate Pheochromocytoma

**Cardiovascular**
  Hyperdynamic, labile hypertension
  Paroxysmal tachycardia
  Angina, coronary insufficiency
  Acute pulmonary edema
  Eclampsia
  Hypertensive crisis during or after surgery
  Rebound hypertension after abrupt cessation of clonidine and other antihypertensives

**Psychological**
  Anxiety with hyperventilation
  Panic attacks

**Neurological**
  Migraine and cluster headaches
  Brain tumor
  Basilar artery aneurysm
  Stroke
  Diencephalic seizures
  Porphyria
  Lead poisoning
  Familial dysautonomia
  Acrodynia
  Autonomic hyperreflexia, as with quadriplegia
  Baroreceptor dysfunction
  Fatal familial insomnia

**Endocrine**
  Menopausal symptoms
  Thyrotoxicosis
  Diabetes mellitus
  Hypoglycemia
  Carcinoid
  Mastocytosis

**Drug Induced**
  Monamine oxidase inhibitor + selective serotonin reuptake inhibitor
  Ephedrine + tricyclic antidepressant

**Factitious: ingestion of sympathomimetics**

simulate a pheo. Perhaps most common are repetitive episodes of acute anxiety or panic attacks that may induce both a hyperkinetic circulation and paroxysmal hypertension (Mann, 1999). Some are associated with increased sympathetic activity from such diverse causes as baroreceptor dysfunction (Kuchel et al, 1987), central nervous system (CNS) lesions (Wortsman et al., 1980), drug interactions (Lefebvre et al., 1995), or obstructive sleep apnea (Hoy et al., 2004). On the other hand, increased thyroid function may be caused by a pheo, so the possibility should be considered before giving a β-blocker to control thyrotoxic symptoms (Ober, 1991).

### Pheochromocytoma During Pregnancy

The association of pheochromocytoma and pregnancy may be greater than could be attributed to chance: More than 200 cases have been reported (Keely, 1998). When pheos are not recognized before delivery, the maternal mortality rate is about 25%, and the infant mortality rate is about 30%. If diagnosed during the first or second trimester, the pheo should be resected after the usual medical preparation (Finkenstedt et al., 1999). If in the third trimester, medical therapy is usually preferred with removal of the pheo at the time of elective cesarean section (Keely, 1998).

### Pheochromocytoma in Children

The younger the patient, the more likely it is that the syndrome is familial, the pheos multiple and extra-adrenal, and the hypertension persistent (Kohane et al., 2005; Stackpole et al., 1963). The youngest patient in the series by Stackpole et al. was only 1 month old. Many pheos found in screening of children for familial syndromes are silent (Weise et al., 2002).

### Familial Syndromes

Pheos are inherited as an autosomal dominant trait alone or in part of one of the syndromes listed in Table 12–6. The likelihood of a familial pheo has been generally estimated to be about 10% of all pheos. However, a screening of two large cohorts in Germany and Poland with a total of 271 apparently nonfamilial, sporadic pheos revealed 66 (24%) to have germ-line mutations of one of four susceptible genes for pheo (Neumann et al., 2002). Of these 66, 30 had mutations of the tumor-suppressor gene VHL (associated with von Hippel-Lindau disease), 13 of the proto-oncogene RET (associated with multiple endocrine neoplasia type 2 or MEN-2), 11 mutations of the succinate dehydrogenase subunit D (SDHD), and 12 of the succinate dehydrogenase subunit B (SDHB), both of which predispose to pheos and familial paragangliomas of the neck (glomus tumors) (Neumann et al., 2004). Of interest, 61 of the 66 patients with these mutations had no signs or symptoms associated with these familial syndromes, but the pheo patients who

## TABLE 12–6

### Familial Syndromes With Pheochromocytoma

| Type | Tumors (partial list) | Site of Genetic Mutations |
|---|---|---|
| Multiple endocrine neoplasia 2A (MEN 2A) | Medullary thyroid carcinoma (95%) Pheochromocytoma (50%) Hyperparathyroidism (20%) | Chromosome 10 q 11.2 codon 634, Cys→Arg in ~ 85% |
| Multiple endocrine neoplasia 2B (MEN2B) | Medullary thyroid carcinoma Pheochromocytoma Mucosal neuromas | Chromosome 10 q 11.2 codon 918, Met→Thy in >95% |
| von Hippel-Lindau, type 2 (VHL) | Pheochromocytoma (10–20%) Retinal angioma CNS hemangioblastoma Renal cysts and carcinoma Neuroendocrine tumors | Chromosome 3 p 25–26 codon 167 in ~ 40% |
| von Recklinghausen's disease (Neurofibromatosis 1) | Neurofibroma Optic glioma Pheochromocytoma (2–5%) Carcinoid tumors | Chromosome 17 q 11.2 in 90% |
| Familial carotid body tumors | Paraganglioma | Chromosome 11 q 21–23 |

carried the mutations tended to be younger and to have more multifocal and extra-adrenal tumors.

Bravo and Tagle (2003) recommend that patients with presumed sporadic pheos routinely have analyses of mutations of the four pheo-susceptibility genes. Such searches have revealed polymorphisms in the RET proto-oncogene (McWhinney et al., 2003) but not in the SDHB genes (Benn et al., 2003).

Obviously, all patients found to have a pheo should be suspect for a familial syndrome, particularly if young and with extra-adrenal tumors. In addition to a careful family history of component tumors in first-degree relatives, the physical exam should include a search for cutaneous or mucosal neurofibromas, a thyroid mass, carotid-body tumor, or retinal angioma (Dluhy, 2002). The best screening of close family members of patients with one of the familial syndromes seems to be the measurement of plasma free metanephrines, found to be elevated in 74 of 76 patients with hereditary pheos (Lenders et al., 2002b).

The treatment of familial syndromes in patients with pheos increasingly involves laparoscopic adrenocortical-sparing surgery (Walther, 2002). The recommendations agreed upon by the majority of experts at a 1998 workshop (Lips, 1998) have been confirmed by subsequent experience.

### Multiple Endocrine Neoplasia-2 (MEN-2)

Family members of a patient with medullary thyroid cancer should have DNA diagnosis before age 10, and if a germline RET gene mutation is found, total thyroidectomy should be done immediately. As for the diagnosis of pheo, plasma metanephrine levels should be measured every 6 months and an MRI obtained if levels are elevated (Eisenhofer et al., 1999). If a pheo is present in only one adrenal, unilateral adrenalectomy should be done. With bilateral tumors, found in about half of the 50% of patients who develop a pheo, adrenal sparing procedures should be attempted (Walther, 2002).

### von Hippel-Lindau Syndrome (VHL)

In family members, DNA analysis should be done before age 5 (Hes et al., 2003). Given the markedly variable expressions of the syndrome, with tumors reported in as many as 14 organs, diagnostic tests likely should be limited to MRI of the brain using gadolinium and plasma normetanephrine testing every year (Lonser et al., 2003).

Since a third of patients with VHL-pheos are asymptomatic and normotensive and have normal catacholamine levels (Eisenhofer et al., 2001), abdominal CT scanning and MIBG uptake should be done initially and repeated if blood pressure or cate-cholamine levels rise. Laparoscopic partial adrenal-ectomy may be feasible (Lonser et al., 2003).

### von Recklinghausen's Disease

In review of 118 articles, hypertension was noted in only about 2% of patients with von Reckling-hausen's disease, but, in those with hypertension, a pheo was identified in over one third (Walther et al., 1999a). In the 148 patients reported to have a pheo, the mean age was 42 years, 84% had a soli-tary adrenal tumor, 10% bilateral adrenal tumors, and 6% ectopic pheos. In 11.5%, the pheos were malignant, and 8.8% had coexisting gastrointesti-nal carcinoid tumors. Almost 80% of these pa-tients had symptoms of pheo or hypertension and had increased catecholamine excretion and MIBG uptake.

Since pheos are relatively rare, only those with hypertension should have yearly urinary cate-cholamines and abdominal CT scans. Genetic test-ing of family members has little value.

## Malignant Pheochromocytoma

As many as 10% of sporadic adrenal pheos and 40% of extra-adrenal pheos are malignant (Ilias & Pacak, 2004). Most metastases are to skeleton, lymph nodes, liver, and lungs. Tumor growth is often slow, and long survival is possible, likely en-hanced by intensive medical and surgical therapy as will be described at the end of this chapter.

To be classified as malignant, metastases have to be found in areas where chromaffin tissue nor-mally is not located, since benign pheos often show dysplasia and invasion of capsule and ves-sels. Routine histology is of little value, and analy-sis of nuclear DNA content is not always helpful, since the normal diploid pattern has been seen in patients with invasive, malignant tumors (Heaney et al., 1996).

A number of approaches have been taken to separate benign from malignant pheos. Thompson (2002) studied 50 benign and 50 malignant pheos and proposed a Pheo of the Adrenal Scaled Score (PASS) based on 12 pathologic and immunophe-notypic features to identify those with malignant behavior. The expression of telomerase subunits has been found to mark more aggressive tumors (Boltze et al., 2003). Markedly elevated urinary homovanil-lic acid or plasma chromagranin A levels are often seen with metastatic disease (Rao et al., 2000). In addition, somatostatin receptor scintigraphy with la-beled octreotide and positron emission tomography (PET) have been used to identify malignant tumors (Ilias et al., 2003).

### Death from Pheochromocytoma

Most deaths are related to failure to consider the dis-ease in patients undergoing severe stress, such as surgery or delivery. Many deaths are unexpected and sudden; this is likely related to catecholamine-induced effects on the cardiac muscle and conduction system. At least seven deaths have followed acute hemorrhagic necrosis of a pheo, most of them after phentolamine administration (van Way et al., 1976).

## Biochemical Diagnosis

Significant technical advances have made the bio-chemical diagnosis of pheo much more sensitive so that only a very few active tumors should be missed but, with greater sensitivity, less specificity, i.e., more false positives, becomes more of a problem. To avoid false positives and the need for additional test-ing, routine screening in hypertensives without sug-gestive symptoms is *not* recommended. When screening is done, assays for catecholamine deriva-tives can be done either in plasma or urine (Table 12–7). Currently, there is uncertainty as to what is the best test.

### Rationale

The greater sensitivity and specificity for assays of plasma metanephrines has been explained by Eisenhofer et al. (1998). They found that the large amounts of membrane-bound catechol-O-methyltransferase (COMT) in adrenal chromaffin cells have much higher affinity for catecholamines than does the soluble COMT present elsewhere. Therefore, the adrenal glands contribute more than 90% of metanephrine (derived from Epi) and 24% to 40% of normetanephrine (derived from NE) in plasma, whereas only 7% of plasma NE comes from the adrenals, the rest from sympathetic nerves.

These investigators showed that the elevated plasma levels of free metanephrines in patients with pheo are derived from catecholamines produced and metabolized within the tumor. Whereas some tu-mors do not secrete catecholamines, they all metab-olize the parent amines to free metanephrine (see Figure 12–2). This explains why some patients with a pheo have normal plasma Epi and NE levels but elevated metanephrines.

In most pheos, levels of both plasma free metanephrine and normetanephrine will be elevat-ed, reflecting increased production of both Epi and NE, respectively. However, in most extra-adrenal tumors which lack the phenylethanolamine N-methyltransferase (PNMT) enzyme needed for con-version of NE to Epi, and, for reasons not yet understood, from adrenal tumors seen as part of the

## TABLE 12-7

### Biochemical Tests of Catecholamine Excess for Diagnosis of Pheochromocytoma

| Biochemical Test (assay method) | Upper Reference Limits (true negatives » false negatives) | Tumor Possible (false positives > true positives) | Tumor Likely (true positives » false positives) |
|---|---|---|---|
| Urine tests | | | |
| 1. Catecholamines (HPLC) | | | |
|    Norepinephrine (µg/24 hr) | 80 | >80 and <300 | >300 |
|    Epinephrine (µg/24 hr) | 20 | >20 and <50 | >50 |
| 2. Fractionated metanephrines (HPLC) | | | |
|    Normetanephrine (µg/24 hr) | 540/310 | >540 and <1400 | >1400 |
|    Metanephrine (µg/24 hr) | 240/140 | >240 and <1000 | >1400 |
| 3. Total metanephrines (spectrophotometry) | | | |
|    Sum of NMN and MN (mg/24 hr) | 1.2 | >1.2 and <2 | >10 |
| 4. Vanillymandelic acid (spectrophotometry) | | | |
|    VMA (mg/24 hr) | 7.9 | >7.9 and <12 | >12 |
| Blood Tests | | | |
| 5. Catecholamines (HPLC) | | | |
|    Norepinephrine (ng/L) | 498 | >498 and <2000 | >2000 |
|    Epinephrine (ng/L) | 83 | >83 and <400 | >400 |
| 6. Free metanephrines (HPLC) | | | |
|    Normetanephrine (ng/L) | 112 | >112 and <400 | >400 |
|    Metanephrine (ng/L) | 61 | >61 and <236 | >236 |

*To convert values for plasma concentrations to nanomoles per liter or urinary levels to micromoles per 24 hour, divide by 183 for normetanephrine, by 169 for norepinephrine, by 197 for metanephrine, and by 183 for epinephrine.*
Modified from Lenders JW, Pacak K, Eisenhofer G, et al. New advances in the biochemical diagnosis of pheochromocytoma: moving beyond catecholamines. *Ann NY Acad Sci* 2002a;970:29–40.

von Hippel-Lindau syndrome, Epi production is not increased so that only normetanephrine levels are elevated (Eisenhofer et al., 1999).

### Technique

Whereas levels of free catecholamines are increased by even minimal anxiety and stress, levels of metanephrines are much less affected. Nonetheless, Eisenhofer et al. (2003) recommend that blood samples be obtained only after the patient has been supine for at least 20 minutes after insertion of an indwelling cannula in the forearm. The Mayo Clinic obtains the sample from seated ambulatory patients by standard venupuncture and finds similar results as in blood obtained from supine indwelling cannulas (Kudva et al., 2003). Patients should be fasted overnight, particularly avoiding caffeinated beverages. Acetaminophen should be avoided for 5 days prior to sampling since it may interfere with the analysis using high performance liquid chromatography (HPLC) with electrochemical detection.

Increasingly the measurement of urinary total metanephrines by spectrophotometry is being replaced by fractionation of metanephrines by liquid chromatography-tandem mass spectrometry (Kudva et al., 2003). To provide greater specificity, the Mayo Clinic laboratory uses a diagnostic cut-off approximately twofold higher than the normal population reference range. Therefore, a 24-hour urinary total metanephrine of 1.3 mg or higher should be considered highly suspicious of a pheo (Kudva et al., 2003).

Urinary vanillylmandelic acid (VMA) assays have a poor sensitivity since less than 20% of VMA comes from hepatic metabolism of circulating catecholamines and metanephrines; the remaining 80% comes from metabolites of NE from sympathetic neurons. Thus, to increase urinary VMA excretion from a pheo requires large increases in plasma catechols and metanephrines.

### Interferences

A variety of medications have been reported to alter measurements of catecholamines and metabolites (Table 12–8). Patients taking sympathomimetic drugs likely will have elevated levels. Patients under considerable stress (e.g., perioperatively, acute myocardial infarction, or severe congestive heart failure) may have high catechol levels, and they should be tested only after the stress has subsided for 5 to 7 days.

### Patients with End-Stage Disease

Patients with end-stage renal disease (ESRD) may be anuric so urine measurements are not feasible. In ESRD patients on dialysis, plasma norepinephrine, dopamine, and metanephrine levels are usually elevated one- to twofold but rarely more than threefold whereas plasma epinephrine levels are usually within normal limits (Godfrey et al., 2001).

---

## TABLE 12–8

### Medications That May Interfere with Biochemical Tests for Pheochromocytoma

---

Acetaminophen

Buspirone

Tricyclic antidepressants and antipsychotics

Labetalol, sotalol, β-blockers

Levodopa

I.V. dopamine

α-blockers

Phenoxybenzamine

Sympathomimetics, e.g., cocaine

Withdrawal from clonidine

Ethanol withdrawal

Acute stress: MI, CVA, CHF, sleep apnea, surgery

---

Plasma metanephrines are relatively independent of renal function and are rarely increased in non-pheo patients with renal insufficiency or on dialysis (Eisenhofer et al., 2005b).

### Chromogranin A Levels

Plasma chromogranin A levels are usually elevated in parallel with plasma NE levels but may be of additional value in identifying and following the course of malignant pheos (Rao et al., 2000) and in the presence of renal insufficiency (Canale & Bravo, 1994).

### Which Test Is Best

Investigators from the Mayo Clinic (Kudva et al., 2003) recommend an approach based on the pretest probability of a pheo. In those with a low likelihood—the large majority of hypertensive patients—no screening test should be done since routine testing would cost a tremendous amount of money and could lead to unnecessary surgery in those with false-positive readings (Sawka et al., 2004). In those patients who have a low probability of pheo but who deserve screening—truly resistant hypertensives, those with spells that include sweating and palpitations but with flushing rather than pallor, the presence of an adrenal incidentaloma with nonpheo characteristics—the Mayo Clinic investigators recommend a test with high *specificity* and acceptable sensitivity to minimize the number of false-positives, i.e., 24-hour urinary metanephrines and catecholamines (Kudva et al., 2003). In those patients with a higher degree of clinical suspicion—patients with spells that include pallor, a personal or family history of a pheo, a familial syndrome that includes pheo, and/or an adrenal mass with pheolike characteristics—these investigators recommend a test with higher *sensitivity* but lesser specificity, i.e., fractionated plasma free metanephrines.

On the other hand, investigators at the National Institutes of Health (NIH) recommend the assay of plasma free metanephrines as the best approach (Eisenhofer et al., 2003; Goldstein et al., 2004) (Figure 12–3). In their extensive experience, the findings of plasma normetanephrine below 112 ng/L and metanephrine below 61 ng/L virtually exclude pheo so that no additional testing is needed. On the other hand, when plasma normetanephrine is above 400 ng/L or metanephrine above 236 ng/L, the probability of pheo is so high that localization of the tumor should immediately be attempted.

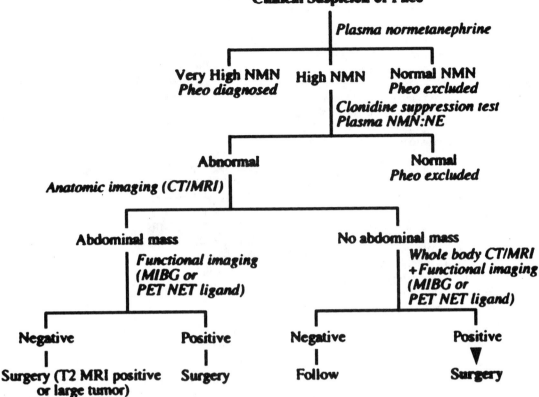

**FIGURE 12–3** ● Algorithm for diagnostic evaluation of a norepinephrine-producing pheochromocytoma. (Adapted from Goldstein DS, Eisenhofer G, Flynn JA, et al. Diagnosis and localization of pheochromocytoma. *Hypertension* 2004;43:907–910.)

The NIH investigators deal with the problem of false positives wherein metanephrine levels are between the highly unlikely and the highly likely by first excluding the presence of a number of medications that can give rise to false-positive assays (Table 12–8). In a series of 648 patients without a pheo, 51 had false-positive tests for plasma metanephrine or epinephrine and 121 false-positive tests for plasma normetanephrine or normetanephrine. In these patients, intake of phenoxybenzamine or tricyclic antidepressants accounted for 43% of false-positive normetanephrine and norepinephrine results.

Also shown in Figure 12–3, if repeat assays are in the indeterminate range after elimination of interfering medications, a clonidine suppression test is then used. This procedure will be described in the next section.

Investigators at the Cleveland Clinic (Bravo & Tagle, 2003) find that the combination of resting plasma NE plus E above 2,000 pg/mL and urinary metanephrine (NMN plus NM) above 1.8 mg/24hr provide a diagnostic accuracy of 98% in both sporadic and familial pheos. These investigators recommend the measurement of plasma free metanephrine as the best currently available screening test but conclude "because pheochromocytomas are a heterogeneous group of hormone-secreting tumors with variable metabolism, it is prudent to recommend that, for 100% diagnostic accuracy, multiple tests be performed" (Bravo & Tagle, 2003).

This advice seems appropriate, but if cost and convenience dictate only one test, it should be the plasma metanephrine. Though the choice of urine metanephrines in low likelihood patients and plasma metanephrines in high likelihood patients advocated by the Mayo Clinic investigators (Kudva et al., 2003) may reduce the number of false-positive results, the strategy shown in Figure 12–3 should distinguish true positives from false positives and give the fewest false-negative results. As noted by Eisenhofer (2003): "A false negative result in a patient with a pheochromocytoma could have serious consequences. An appropriately sensitive biochemical test, therefore, represents the first choice for diagnosis of pheochromocytoma."

## Pharmacologic Tests

### Provocative Tests

In view of the availability of accurate plasma and urinary assays, there is little need to subject patients to the discomfort and hazard of provocative tests. At the Mayo Clinic, histamine and glucagon stimulation tests have been performed on 542 patients who were suspect for a pheo despite normal urinary tests; not one patient had a positive stimulation test (Young, 1997).

The only rational use of the best of these provocative procedures, the glucagon-stimulation test, is to identify bilateral medullary hyperplasia in patients with medullary carcinoma of the thyroid whose control urine metanephrine assays are normal or to diagnose a pheo in the extremely rare patient with normal plasma and urine catecholamine levels. However, it has proven insensitive in familial forms of pheo (Walther et al., 1999b).

### Suppression Tests

Suppression tests by nature seem more physiologic and safer than provocative tests. The most widely used test uses the effect of the centrally acting sympathetic inhibitor clonidine on plasma catechols (Bravo et al., 1981). Plasma NE and Epi are measured before and 2 and 3 hours after a single oral 0.3-mg dose of clonidine; NE and Epi levels fall to below the normal range in patients without a pheo but remain high in those with a pheo. A normal response (i.e., an absolute fall of plasma NE and Epi to below 500 pg/mL and a relative fall of at least 40% from the basal level) was found in all 47 nonpheo hypertensives, but in only 1 of 40 patients with a pheo (Bravo, 1994). The 2-hour sample almost always gives the best discrimination. To save money, the 3-hour sample can be frozen and analyzed only if the 2-hour sample is equivocal.

Even more accurate results have been found by the NIH investigators with measurement of plasma normetanephrines rather than catecholamines (Eisenhofer et al., 2003). Their criterion for a positive response of plasma normetanephrine is a fall of less than 40% of the basal level.

## LOCALIZING THE TUMOR

Only after biochemical studies have confirmed the diagnosis of a catecholamine-producing tumor should localization be attempted. Figure 12–4 is the algorithm recommended by the NIH investigators (Ilias & Pacak, 2004). They begin with anatomical imaging, either CT or MRI, and follow, in most patients, with functional imaging. As seen in Figure 12–5, the imaging characteristics of a pheo include irregular, large (>2 cm) masses with cystic or hemorrhagic changes, enhancement with IV contrast medium on CT, and high signal intensity on $T_2$-weighted MRI. In children or during pregnancy, MRI is preferred, but ultrasonography is another option (Kann et al., 2004).

Both CT and MRI provide high sensitivity but about one third of the abnormal scans will be non-pheo lesions, most an incidental adrenal tumor, as noted at the beginning of this chapter. Computed tomography and MRI can identify extra-adrenal tumors and metastatic disease and have been of considerable help in evaluating patients with the MEN or VHL syndromes who may be normotensive and difficult to assess by biochemical tests.

According to Ilias and Pacak (2004):

Negative CT or MRI imaging of the adrenals, abdomen, and pelvis should be followed by additional CT scans, except where this modality [is] contraindicated, such as in children and during pregnancy, where MRI is preferred. If all CT scans are negative, little is to be gained by performing MRI, except in patients with previous surgery that may result in distorted anatomy.

The presence of pheo should always be ruled out or confirmed with functional imaging (even if CT and MRI are negative but pheo is biochemically proven). The functional imaging test of choice is [123I]MIBG, or, if this is not available, then [131I]MIBG should be performed. If the MIBG scan is negative, PET studies should be performed with specific ligands, preferably [18F]DA or [18F]DOPA. If these are also negative, the patient probably has an unusual type of pheo (in which tumor cells do not express the norepinephrine transfer system or may have a low number of catecholamine storage granules) or malignant pheo, and scintigraphy with nonspecific ligands, such as somatostatin receptor scintigraphy with Octreoscan or FDG PET, should be carried out. Venous sampling coupled with measurement of catecholamines or, preferably, metanephrines to localize the tumor through the discovery of a secretory gradient is an ultimate modality to be used with caution in selected cases where all imaging methods have failed. This is technically demanding and is best conducted at specialized centers. If access to such centers is not feasible, then a repeat noninvasive localization work-up after 2–6 months is a more attractive and preferable choice.

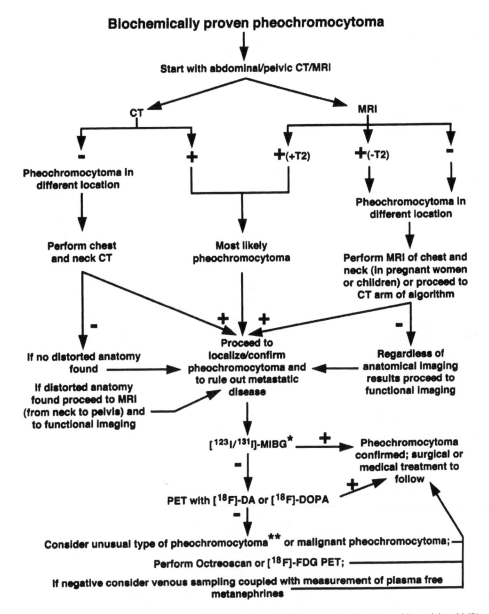

**FIGURE 12–4** ● Algorithm for diagnostic localization of PHEO. $+_{(+T2)}$, Positive $T_1$- and $T_2$-weighted MRI examinations; $+_{(-T2)}$, positive $T_1$- and negative $T_2$-weighted MRI examinations; +, examination positive for tumor; −, examination negative for tumor; *, [$^{123}$I]MIBG scintigraphy preferred over [$^{131}$I]MIBG scintigraphy, where available; **, unusual types of PHEOs may not express the norepinephrine transporter system or may have a low number of catecholamine storage granules. (From Ilias I, Pacak K. Current approaches and recommended algorithm for the diagnostic localization of pheochromocytoma. *J Clin Endocrinol Metab* 2004;89:479–491.)

## MANAGEMENT

The symptoms of pheo can be controlled medically, but, if possible, surgery should be done with the expectation that all symptoms will be relieved in the majority of patients who have benign tumors and in the hope that metastatic spread will be limited in the minority with malignant ones. Although excellent results of surgery *without* preoperative α-blockade have been reported (Ulchaker et al., 1999), most authorities recommend that the patient be treated medically for at least 1 week, preferably until hypertension and spells are controlled (Prys-Roberts, 2000; Walther, 2001). In those who cannot be cured by surgery, medical therapy can be used chronically.

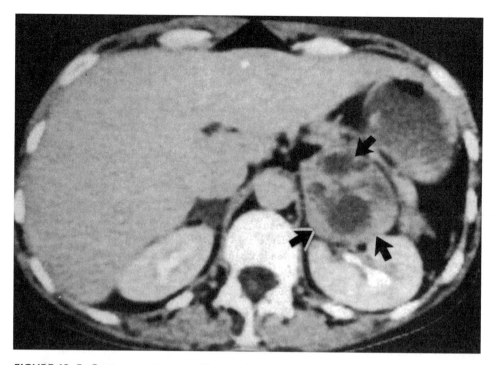

**FIGURE 12–5** ● Computed tomographic scan of a 40-year-old woman with a large left adrenal pheochromocytoma outlined by the *arrows*. Note the multiple cystic areas within the tumor.

## Benign Pheochromocytomas

### Medical Therapy

In the past, the nonspecific $\alpha$-blockers phentolamine and phenoxybenzamine (POB) were recommended, the first for intravenous use to control hypertensive crisis, the second for oral use to prepare for surgery. However, phentolamine is no longer available and selective $\alpha$-blockers and calcium channel blockers (CCBs) have been found to control the manifestations of pheo without the reflex tachycardia and other side effects of POB (Bravo & Tagle, 2003).

#### Selective $\alpha_1$-Blockers

Oral prazosin, terazosin, or doxazosin will preferentially block the postsynaptic $\alpha_1$-receptors on the vessel wall but will leave the presynaptic $\alpha_2$-receptors on the neuronal surface open. Thus the feedback inhibition of neuronal release of NE is preserved, unlike the situation with phenoxybenzamine. Tachycardia should be less of a problem, so that a $\beta$-blocker may not be needed (Prys-Roberts, 2000).

#### $\beta$-Blockers

$\beta$-blockers may be given to control tachycardia and arrhythmias but *only* after $\alpha$-blockers have been started. If inadvertently used alone, $\beta$-blockers may cause either a pressor response, since the $\beta$-blockade of the $\beta_2$-mediated vasodilator actions of Epi leaves the $\alpha$-mediated vasoconstrictor actions

unopposed, or pulmonary edema, presumably by removal of $\beta$-adrenergic drive to the heart (Prys-Roberts, 2000).

The combined $\alpha$- and $\beta$-blocking drugs labetalol or carvedilol may be used, but only after the diagnostic tests are obtained since false-positive catecholamine assays have been reported with labetalol (Eisenhofer et al., 2003).

#### Calcium Channel Blockers

Calcium channel blockers will control the hypertension and other manifestations of a pheo by inhibiting catecholamine-mediated release of intracellular calcium. They have been used alone or, in more resistant cases, with selective $\alpha_1$-receptor blockers to successfully manage pheo patients (Bravo & Tagle, 2003). In an intravenous formulation, CCBs have been used to control BP during resection of a pheo (Bravo & Tagle, 2003).

As Bravo and Tagle (2003) note: "Appropriately used calcium channel antagonists and selective $\alpha_1$-selective blockers are effective and safe without the adverse effects associated with nonspecific, complete, and prolonged $\alpha$-blockade using POB."

### Surgical Therapy

Nonetheless, even with adequate preoperative control and intraoperative management, perioperative morbidity and mortality still occur (Plouin et al., 2001).

*Anesthesia*

Certain anesthetic agents have been advocated because they tend not to cause a release of catecholamines or to sensitize the myocardium. However, in the extensive experience of Prys-Roberts (2000), the type of anesthetic agent was of secondary importance to the control of operative hypotension by replacement of fluid volume, and use of either phentolamine, labetalol, or nicardipine (Colson et al., 1998) to control hypertensive surges after tumor manipulation.

*Surgical Procedure*

In the past, most surgeons preferred an upper abdominal incision long enough to expose both adrenals, the entire periaortic sympathetic chain, and the urinary bladder because as many as 20% of patients have multiple pheos, particularly in familial cases.

There is now less need for such extensive exploration with the availability of CT and MRI scans. With accurate localization of a unilateral tumor, laparoscopy has been widely used (Walther et al., 2000), although catecholamine release may occur as with other procedures (Davies et al., 2004).

After removal of the pheo, the BP may fall precipitously for one or more reasons (Figure 12–6). The principal factor seems to be the shrunken blood volume, which is no longer supported by intense vasoconstriction.

*Postoperative Care*

Patients may become hypoglycemic in the immediate postoperative period, presumably because the sudden decrease in catecholamines leads to an increase in insulin secretion while simultaneously decreasing the formation of glucose from glycogen and fat.

If the pressure remains high, some of the tumor may have been inadvertently left behind. Less commonly, a renal artery may have been damaged, with induction of renovascular hypertension. Re-exploration should await repeated biochemical testing and appropriate imaging or scintigraphy.

*Long-Term Follow-Up*

The prognosis is usually excellent for benign pheos. In a long-time follow-up of 192 patients, 178 with benign tumors, recurrences were found in 29 (Amar et al., 2005). The likelihood of recurrence was 3.4-fold higher with a familial disease, 3.1-fold higher with a right rather than a left adrenal tumor, and 11.2-fold higher with extra-adrenal tumors.

If the pheo is not totally resectable or the patient is a high surgical risk, long-term medical therapy can provide excellent control (Pelegri et al., 1989). If the patient has one of the familial syndromes described earlier in this chapter, repeated catechol assays in conjunction with blood calcitonin levels and palpation of the neck for medullary thyroid cancer should be continued for life.

## Malignant Pheochromocytomas

As noted earlier in this chapter, malignancy is found in about 10% of sporadic and 40% of familial pheos. Metastases may appear many years after resection of an apparently benign tumor, and there is at present no certain way to predict malignancy.

The prognosis is obviously not as good for those with metastatic disease. As much tumor mass as can be reached should be resected, and medical therapy should be provided to shrink the tumor and

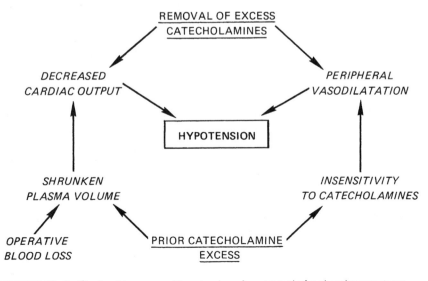

**FIGURE 12–6** ● Possible causes of hypotension after removal of a pheochromocytoma.

control the symptoms. Shrinkage of tumor mass has been reported with the inhibitor of catecholamine synthesis, metyrosine (Serri et al., 1984), streptozocin (Feldman, 1983), and [131]I-MIBG (Sisson, 2002); skeletal metastases may respond to irradiation (Scott et al., 1982) or radiofrequency ablation (Pacak et al., 2001). The best response has been reported with chemotherapy combining cyclophosphamide, vincristine, and dacarbazine (Averbuch et al., 1988; Tato et al., 1997). Long-term control of symptoms is possible with α-blockers and CCBs. With such intensive therapy, long-term survival is possible. The response to therapy may be gauged by levels of plasma chromagranin A (Rao et al., 2000).

We will next examine primary aldosteronism, another fascinating adrenal cause of hypertension that may be more common than previously thought.

# REFERENCES

Achong MR, Keane PM. Pheochromocytoma unmasked by desipramine therapy. *Ann Intern Med* 1981;94:358–359.

Amar L, Servais A, Gimenez-Roqueplo AP, et al. Year of diagnosis, features at presentation, and risk of recurrence in patients with pheochromocytoma or secreting paraganglioma. *J Clin Endocrinol Metab* 2005;90:2110–2116.

Amos AM, McRoberts JW. Cushing's syndrome associated with a pheochromocytoma. *Urology* 1998;52:331–335.

Atuk NO, Teja K, Mondzelewski J, et al. Avascular necrosis of pheochromocytoma followed by spontaneous remission. *Arch Intern Med* 1977;137:1073–1075.

Averbuch SD, Steakley CS, Young RC, et al. Malignant pheochromocytoma: effective treatment with a combination of cyclophosphamide, vincristine, and dacarbazine. *Ann Intern Med* 1988;109:267–273.

Barzon L, Sonino N, Fallo F, et al. Prevalence of natural history of adrenal incidentalomas. *Euro J Endocrinol* 2003; 149:273–285.

Beard CM, Sheps SG, Kurland LT, et al. Occurrence of pheochromocytoma in Rochester, Minnesota, 1950 through 1979. *Mayo Clin Proc* 1983;58:802–804.

Benn DE, Croxson MS, Tucker K, et al. Novel succinate dehydrogenase subunit B *(SDHB)* mutations in familial phaeochromocytomas and paragangliomas, but an absence of somatic *SDHB* mutations in sporadic phaeochromocytomas. *Oncogene* 2003;22:1358–1364.

Bernini G, Moretti A, Iocconi P, et al. Anthropometric, haemodynamic, humoral and hormonal evaluation in patients with incidental adrenocortical adenomas before and after surgery. *Eur J Endocrinol* 2003;148:213–219.

Blumenfeld J, Cohen N, Anwar M, et al. Hypertension and a tumor of the glomus jugulare region: evidence for epinephrine biosynthesis. *Am J Hypertens* 1993;6:382–387.

Boltze C, Mundschenk J, Unger N, et al. Expression profile of the telomeric complex discriminates between benign and malignant pheochromocytoma. *J Clin Endocrinol Metab* 2003;88:4280–4286.

Bornemann M, Hill SC, Kidd GS II. Lactic acidosis in pheochromocytoma. *Ann Intern Med* 1986;105:880–882.

Bravo EL, Tagle R. Pheochromocytoma: state-of-the-art and future prospects. *Endocr Rev* 2003;24:539–553.

Bravo EL, Tarazi RC, Fouad FM, et al. Clonidine-suppression test. A useful aid in the diagnosis of pheochromocytoma. *N Engl J Med* 1981;305:623–626.

Bravo EL. Evolving concepts in the pathophysiology, diagnosis, and treatment of pheochromocytoma. *Endocrinol Rev* 1994;15:356–368.

Brown H, Goldberg PA, Selter JG, et al. Hemorrhagic pheochromocytoma associated with systemic corticosteroid therapy and presenting as myocardial infarction with severe hypertension. *J Clin Endocrin Metab* 2005;90:563–569.

Canale MP, Bravo EL. Diagnostic specificity of serum chromogranin-A for pheochromocytoma in patients with renal dysfunction. *J Clin Endocrinol Metab* 1994;78: 1139–1144.

Chen H, Doppman JL, Chrousos GP, et al. Adrenocorticotropic hormone-secreting pheochromocytomas: the exception to the rule. *Surgery* 1995;118:988–995.

Chiodini I, Guglielmi G, Battista C, et al. Spinal volumetric bone mineral density and vertebral fractures in female patients with adrenal incidentalomas: the effects of subclinical hypercortisolism and gonadal status. *J Clin Endocrinol Metab* 2004;89:2237–2241.

Cohen DL, Fraker D, Townsend RR. Lack of symptomatology in patients with histological evidence of pheochromocytoma: a diagnostic challenge [Abstract]. *Am J Hypertens* 2005;18(suppl):238A.

Colson P, Ryckwaert F, Ribstein J, et al. Haemodynamic heterogeneity and treatment with the calcium channel blocker nicardipine during phaeochromocytoma surgery. *Acta Anaesthesiol Scand* 1998;42:1114–1119.

Copeland PM. Management of the clinically inapparent adrenal mass. *Ann Intern Med* 2004;140:401.

Crout JR, Sjöerdsma A. Turnover and metabolism and catecholamines in patients with pheochromocytoma. *J Clin Invest* 1964;43:94–102.

Crucitti F, Bellantone R, Ferrante A, et al. The Italian registry for adrenal cortical carcinoma: analysis of a multiinstitutional series of 129 patients. *Surgery* 1996;119:161–170.

Davies MJ, McGlade DP, Banting SW. A comparison of open and laparoscopic approaches to adrenalectomy in patients with phaeochromocytoma. *Anaeth Intensive Care* 2004;32:224–229.

Dluhy RG. Pheochromocytoma—Death of an axiom. *N Engl J Med* 2002;346:1486–1488.

Eisenhofer G. Editorial: Biochemical diagnosis of pheochromocytoma—is it time to switch to plasma-free metanephrines? *J Clin Endocrinol Metab* 2003;88:550–552.

Eisenhofer G, Goldstein DS, Sullivan P, et al. Biochemical and clinical manifestations of dopamine-producing paragangliomas: utility of plasma methoxytyramine. *J Clin Endocrinol Metab* 2005a;90:2068–2075.

Eisenhofer G, Goldstein DS, Walther MM, et al. Biochemical diagnosis of pheochromocytoma: how to distinguish true- from false-positive test results. *J Clin Endocrinol Metab* 2003;88:2656–2666.

Eisenhofer G, Huysmans F, Pacak K, et al. Plasma metanephrines in renal failure. *Kidney Int* 2005b;67:668–677.

Eisenhofer G, Keiser H, Friberg P, et al. Plasma metanephrines are markers of pheochromocytoma produced by catechol-O-methyltransferase within tumors. *J Clin Endocrinol Metab* 1998;83:2175–2185.

Eisenhofer G, Lenders JWM, Linehan WM, et al. Plasma normetanephrine and metanephrine for detecting pheochromocytoma in von Hippel-Lindau disease and multiple endocrine neoplasia type 2. *N Engl J Med* 1999;340: 1872–1879.

Erickson D, Kudva YC, Ebersold MJ, et al. Benign paragangliomas: clinical presentation and treatment outcomes in 236 patients. *J Clin Endocrinol Metab* 2001;86:5210–5216.

Feldman JM. Treatment of metastatic pheochromocytoma with streptozocin. *Arch Intern Med* 1983;143:1799–1800.

Finkenstedt G, Gasser RW, Höfle G, et al. Pheochromocytoma and sub-clinical Cushing's syndrome during pregnancy: diagnosis, medical pre-treatment and cure by laparoscopic unilateral adrenalectomy. *J Endocrinol Invest* 1999;22:551–557.

Fonseca V, Bouloux P-M. Phaeochromocytoma and paraganglioma. *Baillière's Clin Endocrinol Metab* 1993;7: 509–545.

Garovic VD, Hogan MC, Kanakiriya SK, et al. Labile hypertension, increased metanephrines and imaging misadventures. *Nephrol Dial Transplant* 2004;19:1004–1006.

Gifford RW Jr, Manger WM, Bravo EL. Pheochromocytoma. *Endocrinol Metab Clin North Am* 1994;23:387–404.

Gill IS, Meraney AM, Bravo EL, Novick AC. Pheochromocytoma coexisting with renal artery lesions. *J Urol* 2000; 164:296–301.

Godfrey JA, Rickman OB, Williams AW, et al. Pheochromocytoma in a patient with end-stage renal disease: case report and literature review. *Mayo Clin Proc* 2001;76:953–957.

Goldstein DS, Eisenhofer G, Flynn JA, et al. Diagnosis and localization of pheochromocytoma. *Hypertension* 2004;43: 907–910.

Goldstein DS, Stull R, Eisenhofer G, et al. Plasma 3,4-dihydroxyphenylalanine (dopa) and catecholamines in neuroblastoma or pheochromocytoma. *Ann Intern Med* 1986; 105:887–888.

Granberg D, Stridsberg M, Seensalu R, et al. Plasma chromogranin A in patients with multiple endocrine neoplasia type 1. *J Clin Endocrinol Metab* 1999;84:2712–2717.

Gross MD, Shapiro B, Francis IR, et al. Scintigraphic evaluation of clinically silent adrenal masses. *J Nucl Med* 1994; 35:1145–1152.

Grumbach MM, Biller BM, Braunstein GD, et al. Management of the clinically inapparent adrenal mass ("incidentaloma"). *Ann Intern Med* 2003;138:424–429.

Haider MA, Ghai S, Jhaveri K, Lockwood G. Chemical shift MR imaging of hyperattenuating (>10 HU) adrenal masses: does it still have a role? *Radiology* 2004;231:711–716.

Hamrahian AH, Ioachimescu AG, Remer EM, et al. Clinical utility of nonconstrast CT attenuation value (HU) to differentiate adrenal adenomas/hyperplasias from nonadenomas: Cleveland Clinic experience. *J Clin Endocrinol Metab* 2005;90:871–877.

Heaney AP, O'Rourke D, Arthur K, et al. Flow cytometric analysis does not reliably differentiate benign from malignant phaeochromocytoma. *Clin Endocrinol* 1996;44: 233–238.

Hes FJ, Hoppener JW, Lips CJ. Clinical review 155: pheochromocytoma in Von Hippel-Lindau disease. *J Clin Endocrinol Metab* 2003;88:969–974.

Hoy LJ, Emery M, Wedzicha JA, et al. Obstructive sleep apnea presenting as pheochromocytoma: a case report. *J Clin Endocrinol Metab* 2004;89:2033–2038.

Ilias I, Pacak K. Current approaches and recommended algorithm for the diagnostic localization of pheochromocytoma. *J Clin Endocrinol Metab* 2004;89:479–491.

Ilias I, Yu J, Carrasquillo JA, Chen CC, et al. Superiority of 6-[$^{18}$F]-fluorodopamine positron emission tomography *versus* [$^{131}$I]-metaiodobenzylguanidine scintigraphy in the localization of metastatic pheochromocytoma. *J Clin Endocrinol Metab* 2003;88:4083–4087.

Jacobs P, Wood L. Recurrent benign erythropoietin-secreting pheochromocytomas. *Am J Med* 1994;97:307–308.

Jan T, Metzger BE, Baumann G. Epinephrine-producing pheochromocytoma with hypertensive crisis after corticotropin injection. *Am J Med* 1990;89:824–825.

Kann PH, Wirkus B, Behr T, et al. Endosonographic imaging of benign and malignant pheochromocytomas. *J Clin Endocrinol Metab* 2004;89:1694–1697.

Keely E. Endocrine causes of hypertension in pregnancy—when to start looking for zebras. *Seminars in Perinatology* 1998;22:471–484.

Kimura S, Nishimura Y, Yamaguchi K, et al. A case of pheochromocytoma producing parathyroid hormone-related protein and presenting with hypercalcemia. *J Clin Endocrinol Metab* 1990;70:1559–1563.

Kinney MAO, Warner ME, vanHeerden JA, et al. Perianesthetic risks and outcomes of pheochromocytoma and paraganglioma resection. *Anest Analg* 2000;91:1118–1123.

Kohane DS, Ingelfinger JR, Nimkin K, Wu CL. Case records of the Massachusetts General Hospital. Case 16-2005. A nine-year-old girl with headaches and hypertension. *N Engl J Med* 2005;352:2223–2231.

Kuchel O, Cusson JR, Larochelle P, et al. Posture- and emotion-induced severe hypertensive paroxysms with baroreceptor dysfunction. *J Hypertens* 1987;5:277–283.

Kudva YC, Sawka AM, Young WF Jr, et al. The laboratory diagnosis of adrenal pheochromocytoma: the Mayo Clinic experience. *J Clin Endocrinol Metab* 2003;88:4533–4539.

Lee RE, Rousseau P. Pheochromocytoma and obesity. *J Clin Endocrinol Metab* 1967;27:1050–1052.

Lefebvre H, Noblet C, Moore N, Wolf LM. Pseudophaeochromocytoma after multiple drug interactions involving the selective monoamine oxidase inhibitor selegiline. *Clin Endocrinol* 1995;42:95–99.

Lenders JW, Pacak K, Eisenhofer G, et al. New advances in the biochemical diagnosis of pheochromocytoma: moving beyond catecholamines. *Ann NY Acad Sci* 2002a;970:29–40.

Lenders JW, Pacak K, Walther MM, et al. Biochemical diagnosis of pheochromocytoma: which test is best? *JAMA* 2002b;287:1427–1434.

Lie JT, Olney BA, Spittel JA. Perioperative hypertensive crisis and hemorrhagic diathesis: fatal complication of clinically unsuspected pheochromocytoma. *Am Heart J* 1980; 100:716–722.

Lin CL, Palafox BA, Jackson HA, et al. Cardiac pheochromocytoma: resection after diagnosis by 111-indium octreotide scan. *Ann Thorac Surg* 1999;67:555–558.

Lips CJM. Clinical management of the multiple endocrine neoplasia syndromes: results of a computerized opinion poll at the Sixth International Workshop on Multiple Endocrine Neoplasia and von Hippel-Lindau disease. *J Intern Med* 1998;243:589–594.

Lonser RR, Glenn GM, Walther M, et al. von Hippel-Lindau disease. *Lancet* 2003;361:2059–2067.

Manger WM, Eisenhofer G. Pheochromocytoma: diagnosis and management update. *Curr Hypertens Rep* 2004;6: 477–484.

Mann SJ. Severe paroxysmal hypertension (pseudopheochromocytoma). *Arch Intern Med* 1999;159:670–674.

Maurea S, Klain M, Caraco C, et al. Diagnostic accuracy of radionuclide imaging using $^{131}$I nor-cholesterol or *meta*-iodobenzylguanidine in patients with hypersecreting or non-hypersecreting adrenal tumours. *Nucl Med Commun* 2002;23:951–960.

McNeil AR, Blok BH, Koelmeyer TD, et al. Phaeochromocytomas discovered during coronial autopsies in Sydney, Melbourne and Auckland. *Aust NZ J Med* 2000;30: 648–652.

McPhaul M, Punzi HA, Sandy A, et al. Snuff-induced hypertension in pheochromocytoma. *JAMA* 1984;252:2860–2862.

McWhinney SR, Boru G, Binkley PK, et al. Intronic single nucleotide polymorphisms in the *RET* protooncogene are associated with a subset of apparently sporadic pheochromocytoma and may modulate age of onset. *J Clin Endocrinol Metab* 2003;88:4911–4916.

Montiel C, Artalejo AR, Bermejo PM, Sanchez-Garcia P. A dopaminergic receptor in adrenal medulla as a possible site of action for the droperidol-evoked hypertensive response. *Anesthesiology* 1986;65:474–479.

Neumann HP, Bausch B, McWhinney SR, et al. for the Freiburg-Warsaw-Columbus Pheochromocytoma Study Group. Germ-line mutations in nonsyndromic pheochromocytoma. *N Engl J Med* 2002;346:1459–1466.

Neumann HP, Pawlu C, Pęczkowska M, et al. Distinct clinical features of paragangioma syndromes associated with SDHB and SDHD gene mutations. *JAMA* 2004;292:943–951.

Newell K, Prinz RA, Braithwaite S, Brooks M. Pheochromocytoma crisis. *Am J Hypertens* 1988;1:189S–191S.

Ober KP. Pheochromocytoma in a patient with hyperthyroxinemia. *Am J Med* 1991;90:137–138.

Olson SW, Deal LE, Piesman M. Epinephrine-secreting pheochromocytoma presenting the cardiogenic shock and profound hypocalcemia. *Ann Intern Med* 2004;140: 849–851.

Ooi TC, Dardick I. Coexisting pheochromocytomas and adrenocortical tumour discovered incidentally. *Can Med Assoc J* 1988;139:869–871.

Pacak K, Linehan WM, Eisenhofer G, et al. Recent advances in genetics, diagnosis, localization, and treatment of pheochromocytoma. *Ann Intern Med* 2001; 134: 315–329.

Pelegri A, Romero R, Reguant M, Aisa L. Non-resectable phaeochromocytoma: long term follow-up. *J Hum Hypertens* 1989;3:145–147.

Plouin P, Duclos J, Soppelsa F, et al. Factors associated with perioperative morbidity and mortality in patients with pheochromocytoma. *J Clin Endocrinol Metab* 2001;86: 1480–1486.

Plouin P-F, Menard J, Corvol P. Noradrenaline producing phaeochromocytomas with absent pressor response to beta-blockade. *Br Heart J* 1979;42:359–361.

Primhak RA, Spicer RD, Variend S. Sudden death after minor abdominal trauma: an unusual presentation of phaeochromocytoma. *BMJ* 1986;292:95–96.

Prys-Roberts C. Phaeochromocytoma—recent progress in its management. *Br J Anaesth* 2000;85:44–57.

Rao F, Keiser HR, O'Connor DT. Malignant pheochromocytoma. *Hypertension* 2000;36:1045–1052.

Ross EJ, Griffith DNW. The clinical presentation of phaeochromocytoma. *Quart J Med* 1989;266:485–496.

Sardesai SH, Mourant AJ, Sivathandon Y, et al. Phaeochromocytoma and catecholamine induced cardiomyopathy presenting as heart failure. *Br Heart J* 1990;63:234–237.

Sawka AM, Gafni A, Thabane L, Young WF Jr. The economic implications of three biochemical screening algorithms for pheochromocytoma. *J Clin Endocrinol Metab* 2004;89:2859–2866.

Scott HW, Reynolds V, Green N, et al. Clinical experience with malignant pheochromocytomas. *Surg Gynecol Obstet* 1982;154:801–818.

Seelen MAJ, De Meijer PHEM, Meinders AE. Serotonin reuptake inhibitor unmasks a pheochromocytoma [Letter]. *Ann Intern Med* 1997;126:333.

Serri O, Comtois R, Bettez P, et al. Reduction in the size of a pheochromocytoma pulmonary metastasis by metyrosine therapy. *N Engl J Med* 1984;310:1264–1265.

Shemin D, Cohn PS, Zipin SB. Pheochromocytoma presenting as rhabdomyolysis and acute myoglobinuric renal failure. *Arch Intern Med* 1990;150:2384–2385.

Sheps SG, Jiang N-S, Klee GG, van Heerden JA. Recent developments in the diagnosis and treatment of pheochromocytoma. *Mayo Clin Proc* 1990;65:88–95.

Shimizu K, Miura Y, Meguro Y, et al. QT prolongation with torsade de pointes in pheochromocytoma. *Am Heart J* 1992; 124:235–239.

Sisson JC. Radiopharmaceutical treatment of pheochromocytomas. *Ann NY Acad Sci* 2002;970:54–60.

Stackpole RH, Melicow MM, Uson AC. Pheochromocytoma in children. *J Pediatr* 1963;63:315–336.

Stenström G, Sjöström L, Smith U. Diabetes mellitus in phaeochromocytoma. Fasting blood glucose levels before and after surgery in 60 patients with phaeochromocytoma. *Acta Endocrinol* 1984;106:511–515.

Sweeney AT, Malabanan AO, Blake MA, et al. Megacolon as the presenting feature in pheochromocytoma. *J Clin Endocrinol Metab* 2000;85:3968–3972.

Tan GH, Carney JA, Grant CS, Young WF Jr. Coexistence of bilateral adrenal phaeochromocytoma and idiopathic hyperaldosteronism. *Clin Endocrinol* 1996;44:603–609.

Tanaka K, Noguchi S, Shuin T, et al. Spontaneous rupture of adrenal pheochromocytoma: a case report. *J Urol* 1994;151: 120–121.

Tato A, Orte L, Diz P, et al. Malignant pheochromocytoma, still a therapeutic challenge. *Am J Hypertens* 1997;10: 479–481.

Terzolo M, Osella G, Alí A, et al. Different patterns of steroid secretion in patients with adrenal incidentaloma. *J Clin Endocrinol Metab* 1996;81:740–744.

Thompson LD. Pheochromocytoma of the Adrenal gland Scaled Score (PASS) to separate benign from malignant neoplasms: a clinicopathologic and immunophenotypic study of 100 cases. *Am J Surg Pathol* 2002;26:551–566.

Thrasher JB, Humphrey PA, Rajan RR, et al. Pheochromocytoma of urinary bladder: contemporary methods of diagnosis and treatment options. *Urology* 1993;41:435–439.

Tracy RE, White S. A method for quantifying adrenocortical nodular hyperplasia at autopsy: some use of the method in illuminating hypertension and atherosclerosis. *Ann Diagn Pathol* 2002;6:20–29.

Udelsman R, Fishman EK. Radiology of the adrenal. *Endocrinol Metab Clin NA* 2000;29:27–42.

Ulchaker JC, Goldfarb DA, Bravo EL, Novick AC. Successful outcomes in pheochromocytoma surgery in the modern era. *J Urol* 1999;161:764–767.

Valet P, Damase-Michel C, Chamontin B, et al. Platelet $\alpha_2$ and leucocyte $\beta_2$-adrenoceptors in phaeochromocytoma: effect of tumour removal. *Eur J Clin Invest* 1988;18:481–485.

van Way CE III, Faraci RP, Cleveland HC, Foster JF, Scott HW Jr. Hemorrhagic necrosis of pheochromocytoma associated with phentolamine administration. *Ann Surg* 1976; 184:26–30.

Walther MM, Herring J, Choyke PL, Linehan WM. Laparoscopic partial adrenalectomy in patients with hereditary forms of pheochromocytoma. *J Urol* 2000;164: 14–17.

Walther MM, Herring J, Enquist E, et al. Von Recklinghausen's disease and pheochromocytoma. *J Urology* 1999a; 162:1582–1586.

Walther MM, Reiter R, Keiser HR, et al. Clinical and genetic characterization of pheochromocytoma in von Hippel-Lindau families: comparison with sporadic pheochromocytoma gives insight into natural history of pheochromocytoma. *J Urol* 1999b;162:659–664.

Walther MM. Management of pheochromocytoma. *Ann Intern Med* 2001;134:323–325.

Walther MM. New therapeutic and surgical approaches for sporadic and hereditary pheochromocytoma. *Ann NY Acad Sci* 2002;970:41–53.

Watson JP, Hughes EA, Bryan RL, et al. A predominantly adrenaline-secreting phaeochromocytoma. *Q J Med* 1990; 76: 747–752.

Weise M, Merke DP, Pacak K, et al. Utility of plasma free metanephrines for detecting childhood pheochromocytoma. *J Clin Endocrinol Metab* 2002;87:1955–1960.

Werbel SS, Ober KP. Pheochromocytoma. Update on diagnosis, localization, and management. *Med Clin NA* 1995; 79:131–153.

Whalen RK, Althausen AF, Daniels GH. Extra-adrenal pheochromocytoma. *J Urol* 1992;147:110.

Wortsman J, Burns G, Van Beek AL, Couch J. Hyperadrenergic state after trauma to the neuroaxis. *JAMA* 1980;243: 1459–1460.

Young WF Jr. Management approaches to adrenal incidentalomas. *Endocrinol Metab Clin NA* 2000;29:159–185.

Young WF Jr. Pheochromocytoma and primary aldosteronism: diagnostic approaches. *Endocrinol Metab Clin NA* 1997;26:801–827.

Zelinka T, Štrauch B, Pecen L, Widimsk J Jr. Diurnal blood pressure variation in pheochromocytoma, primary aldosteronism and Cushing's syndrome. *J Hum Hypertens* 2004;18: 107–111.

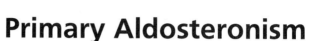

# Primary Aldosteronism

Until recently, primary aldosteronism was held to be a relatively rare cause of hypertension, present in fewer than 1% of all patients. However, over the past few years, the prevalence of this condition has been reported to be much higher, reaching 40% in highly selected groups (Girerd et al., 2003) and close to 20% in referred patients (Mulatero et al., 2004; Stowasser et al., 2003). These figures are almost certainly inflated by the confounding effect of referral and selection (Kaplan, 2004), but the availability of a simple screening test has led to an increased recognition of the milder forms of this condition, particularly related to bilateral adrenal hyperplasia (Olivieri et al., 2004).

I do not believe that the incidence of primary aldosteronism is rapidly growing. Rather, increased screening has uncovered many patients with either mild aldosteronism or, more likely, low-renin primary hypertension who have bilateral adrenal hyperplasia. This is a scientific advance but it usually complicates clinical practice with little, if any, help for the patient (Plouin et al., 2004).

This chapter will cover those syndromes listed in Table 13–1 in which secretion of the physiologic mineralocorticoid aldosterone is primarily increased.

The next chapter will cover syndromes caused by increased secretion of other mineralocorticoids (e.g., congenital adrenal hyperplasias) or by cortisol acting on mineralocorticoid receptors (e.g., apparent mineralocorticoid excess).

As milder degrees of primary aldosteronism have been recognized by the wider application of the plasma aldosterone to renin ratio (ARR), computed tomography (CT) and magnetic resonance imaging (MRI) have made it abundantly clear that the majority of patients with a positive screening test do not have a solitary adrenal adenoma (Magill et al., 2001; Rossi et al., 2001). Therefore, bilateral adrenal venous sampling (AVS), a procedure that requires considerable expertise in performance and is only 80% conclusive even in the best of circumstances, is now being advocated for confirmation of the type of pathology (Magill et al., 2001; Phillips et al., 2000; Rossi et al., 2001; Stowasser et al., 2003; Young et al., 2004).

The need to establish the type of pathology is critical: Adenomas usually should be surgically removed; bilateral hyperplasia should never be surgically attacked but will almost always respond to medical therapy (Lim et al., 2001).

The clinician is left in a dilemma: As the diagnosis of primary aldosteronism has become easier, the recognition of the type of pathology has become more difficult. Since CT and MRI are often misleading and AVS requires considerable expertise, patients increasingly need referral to a center for definitive testing, which is often difficult and always expensive.

To avoid this dilemma, this text will present a more conservative view: The ARR screening study should not be done except in patients with unexplained hypokalemia or resistance to three-drug therapy, particularly with low plasma renin (Eide et al.,

## TABLE 13–1

### Syndromes of Mineralocorticoid Excess

Adrenal origin

  Aldosterone excess (primary)

    Aldosterone-producing adenoma

    Bilateral hyperplasia

    Primary unilateral adrenal hyperplasia

    Glucocorticoid-remediable aldosteronism

      (Familial hyperaldosteronism, type I)

    Adrenal carcinoma

    Extra-adrenal tumors

  Deoxycorticosterone excess

    DOC-secreting tumors

    Congenital adrenal hyperplasia

      11β-hydroxylase deficiency

      17α-hydroxylase deficiency

  Cortisol excess

    Cushing's syndrome from ACTH-producing tumor

    Glucocorticoid receptor resistance

Renal origin

  Activating mutation of mineralocorticoid receptor

  Pseudohypoaldosteronism, type II (Gordon's)

  11β-hydroxysteroid dehydrogenase deficiency

    Congenital: Apparent mineralocorticoid excess

    Acquired: Licorice, carbenoxolone

---

2004), or after finding of an adrenal incidentaloma (as described in Chapter 12). Even if primary aldosteronism is thereby missed, medical therapy—in particular the aldosterone receptor blockers spironolactone or eplerenone—will almost always control the hypertension and, if present, the hypokalemia and all of the additional harmful effects of aldosterone excess since they are mediated through the mineralocorticoid receptor (White, 2003). Thereby, the patient will be protected while expensive laboratory procedures, invasive diagnostic tests, and unnecessary surgery will be avoided.

This view, which will be detailed in the remainder of this chapter, may be too conservative. However, as of now, it seems to be the best balance between the multiple costs of diagnosis and the limited benefits of invasive therapy.

## DEFINITIONS

Primary aldosteronism is the syndrome resulting from the autonomous hypersecretion of aldosterone, almost always from the adrenal cortex, usually by a solitary adenoma or by bilateral hyperplasia, rarely by variants of these two (Ferrari & Bonny, 2003) (Table 13–1).

Most aldosteronism seen in clinical practice is secondary to an increase in renin-angiotensin activity. A classification of the various forms of secondary aldosteronism by mechanism is virtually the same as the right side of Table 3–4, Chapter 3. The ability to measure plasma renin activity (PRA) has made the differentiation much easier, since renin is elevated in secondary aldosteronism and suppressed in primary aldosteronism.

## INCIDENCE

Soon after the first cases were described, apparently by a Polish physician writing in an obscure journal (Litynski, 1953), Conn (1955) fully characterized this fascinating syndrome. Over the next decade, Conn et al. (1965) broadened the scope of primary aldosteronism so that it covered almost 20% of the hypertensive patients at the University of Michigan. This high prevalence was subsequently shown to reflect the nature of the patients referred to that center, highly selected and suspected of having the disease. In most series of unselected patients, classic primary aldosteronism was found in fewer than 0.5% of hypertensives (Gifford, 1969; Kaplan, 1967; Sinclair et al., 1987).

On the other hand, using a relatively simple screening test—the plasma aldosterone-to-plasma renin ratio (ARR)—one group of investigators in Brisbane, Australia, have found almost 100 patients with primary aldosteronism per year (Stowasser, 2000). Others have found an abnormal ARR in 4% to 39% of hypertensives (Kaplan, 2004), but, as I will indicate later, that alone does not establish the diagnosis. Though the incidence of primary aldosteronism is likely higher than previously thought, it is very unlikely to be as common as some now believe.

## CLINICAL FEATURES

The disease is usually seen in patients between the ages of 30 and 50 (though cases have been found in patients from age 3 to 75), and in women more frequently than in men. The syndrome has been recognized during pregnancy in hypokalemic patients with even higher aldosterone levels than expected and, most important, suppressed PRA (Solomon et al., 1996).

The classic clinical features of primary aldosteronism are hypertension, hypokalemia, excessive urinary potassium excretion, hypernatremia, and metabolic alkalosis (Figure 13–1). The usual presence of these features reflects the pathophysiology of aldosterone excess.

## Hypertension

Patients with primary aldosteronism are hypertensive, with very few exceptions (Suzuki et al., 1999; Vantyghem et al., 1999). The blood pressure (BP) may be quite high—the mean in one series of 136 patients was 205/123 (Ferriss et al., 1978b). In another series of 140 patients, 28 had severe, resistant hypertension (Bravo et al., 1988). More than a dozen cases have had malignant hypertension (Kaplan, 1963; Zarifis et al., 1996). The blood pressure decline (dip) during the night is usually attenuated (Zelinka et al., 2004).

Looked at in another way, increased levels of aldosterone may be seen before hypertension becomes manifest. Among 1,688 hypertensive participants in the Framingham Offspring Study, more of the subjects in the quartile with the highest plasma aldosterone levels (mean of 19 ng/dL) developed hypertension over the next 4 years (17.9%) than did those in the lowest quartile of plasma aldosterone (11.9%) (Vasan et al., 2004). Some of the new hypertensives may have had early primary aldosteronism, but no further evaluations were performed.

## Complications

Aldosterone levels inappropriate to sodium status exert deleterious effects on various tissues (Rocha & Funder, 2002). Aldosterone exerts rapid, nongenomic

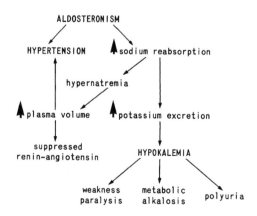

*FIGURE 13–1* ● Pathophysiology of primary aldosteronism. (Reprinted with permission from Kaplan NM. Primary aldosteronism. In: EB Astwood, CE Cassidy, eds. *Clinical Endocrinology*, Vol. 2. New York: Grune & Stratton, 1968.)

effects through its interaction with the mineralocorticoid receptor which leads to endothelial stiffness (Oberleithner, 2005) and vascular damage (Schmidt et al., 2003) and stimulates fibrosis in the heart (GP Rossi et al., 2002) and kidney (Ciraku et al., 2000) so that cardiovascular complications reflect more than the accompanying hypertension (Milliez et al., 2005). Moreover, aldosterone may be synthesized in the heart (White, 2003), providing a direct path to cardiac pathology. Nonetheless, left ventricular structure and function by echocardiography were similar in patients with primary aldosteronism or essential hypertension (Goldkorn et al., 2002).

### Hemodynamics

In addition to multiple direct effects, aldosterone induces hypertension by increasing renal sodium retention (Sosa León et al., 2002). The hypertension is hemodynamically characterized by a slightly expanded plasma volume, an increased total body and exchangeable sodium content, and an increased peripheral resistance (Bravo, 1994; Williams et al., 1984). When 10 patients with primary aldosteronism, previously well controlled on spironolactone, were studied 2 weeks after the drug was stopped and the hypertension reappeared, cardiac output and sodium content (both plasma volume and total exchangeable sodium) rose initially (Wenting et al., 1982) (Figure 13–2). Between weeks 2 and 6, the hemodynamic patterns separated into two types: in five patients, the hypertension was maintained through increased cardiac output; in the other five, cardiac output and blood volume returned to their initial values, but total peripheral resistance rose markedly. Total body sodium space remained expanded in both groups, though more so in those with increased cardiac output (Man in't Veld et al., 1984). After surgery, the cardiac output fell in the high-flow patients, and the peripheral resistance fell in the high-resistance patients.

### Mechanism of Sodium Retention

The pressor actions of aldosterone are generally related to its effects on sodium retention via its action on renal mineralocorticoid receptors (Baxter et al., 2004). The human kidney mineralocorticoid receptor is equally receptive to glucocorticoids and to mineralocorticoids (Arriza et al., 1987; Farman & Rafestin-Oblin, 2001). Relatively small concentrations of aldosterone are able to bind to the mineralocorticoid receptor in the face of much higher concentrations of glucocorticoids (mainly cortisol) because of the action of the 11β-hydroxysteroid dehydrogenase enzyme, which converts the cortisol (with its equal affinity) into cortisone, which does not bind to the receptor (Walker, 1993).

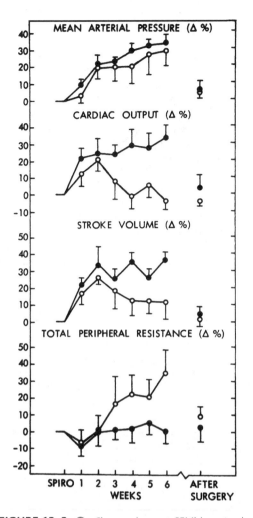

**FIGURE 13–2** ● Changes (mean ± SEM) in systemic hemodynamics after discontinuation of spironolactone treatment (SPIRO) and after surgery in 10 patients with primary aldosteronism. Note the fall in stroke volume and cardiac output after 2 weeks in the five patients with high-resistance hypertension (*open circles*) compared to the five with high-flow hypertension (*closed circles*). (Reprinted with permission from Wenting GJ, Man in't Veld AJ, Derkx FHM, Schalekamp MADH. Recurrence of hypertension in primary aldosteronism after discontinuation of spironolactone. Time course of changes in cardiac output and body fluid volumes. *Clin Exp Hypertens* 1982;4:1727–1748.)

Aldosterone stimulates sodium reabsorption through complex genomic effects that collectively act to increase the activity of the epithelial sodium channel (ENaC) in the apical membrane (Stokes, 2000). After a certain amount of volume expansion, the increases in renal perfusion pressure and natriuretic factors inhibit sodium reabsorption so that "escape" from progressive sodium retention occurs, despite continued aldosterone excess (Kato et al., 2005; Yokota et al., 1994).

## Hypokalemia

### Incidence

Although normokalemia was found occasionally in classic cases of aldosterone-producing adenomas (Conn et al., 1965), hypokalemia was usual in series reported prior to the early 1990s. In the Medical Research Council (MRC) series, hypokalemia occurred in all 62 patients with a proved adenoma and was persistent in 53; among the 17 with hyperplasia, plasma potassium was persistently normal in only three patients (Ferriss et al., 1983). On the other hand, most patients recently diagnosed by the finding of an elevated ARR are normokalemic (Stowasser et al., 2003), likely reflecting the presence of less elevated aldosterone levels, particularly related to the more common finding of bilateral adrenal hyperplasia in such patients.

Patients with glucocorticoid-remediable aldosteronism are often normokalemic, attributable to their mild degree of hyperaldosteronism with minimal potassium wasting from the lack of stimulation of aldosterone synthesis in the zona fasciculata by dietary potassium (Litchfield et al., 1997).

### Significance

Although persistent hypokalemia is less common in patients diagnosed early in the course of the disease, the argument can be made that the search for primary aldosteronism need only be undertaken in those with hypokalemia or other suggestive features (Stewart, 1999). The few who might initially be missed because of a normal potassium level will likely show up subsequently with diuretic-induced or spontaneous hypokalemia. In the interim, a few patients may have had a delay in their diagnosis, but many more will be saved the expense and discomfort of unnecessary workups. On the other hand, in hypertensives with *unprovoked* hypokalemia, perhaps half will turn out to have primary aldosteronism; thus, they must have a complete evaluation.

### Mechanism

Considering the effects of persistent aldosterone excess, hypokalemia is certainly to be expected. Whereas with continued exposure to excessive mineralocorticoids the renal retention of sodium escapes, the renal wastage of potassium is unrelenting (Giebisch, 1998). There are multiple reasons why hypokalemia is not seen. Renal potassium wastage may have been ameliorated by dietary sodium restriction, but it is more likely that blood potassium levels have fallen during the course of the disease but not yet to the level defined as hypokalemia. A fall from 4.8 to 3.5 mmol/L reflects a significant loss of body potassium. As noted under "Screening Tests," there are multiple other factors that may mask hypokalemia.

### Consequences

The effects of hypokalemia include easy fatigability and muscle weakness, even to paralysis (Huang et al., 1996); polyuria from a loss of renal-concentrating ability; a high incidence of renal cysts (Torres et al., 1990); increased ventricular ectopy (Coca et al., 2005); blunting of circulatory reflexes with postural falls in pressure without compensatory tachycardia; impaired insulin secretion with decreased carbohydrate tolerance (Shimamoto et al., 1994), and suppression of aldosterone synthesis, even from presumably autonomous adenomas (Kaplan, 1967). Beyond these rather obvious effects, chronic potassium depletion may accelerate atherosclerosis and vascular injury (Young & Ma, 1999).

### Suppression of Renin Release

As a consequence of the initial expansion of vascular volume and the elevated BP, the baroreceptor mechanism in the walls of the renal afferent arterioles suppresses the secretion of renin to the point that renin mRNA may be undetectable in the kidney (Shionoiri et al., 1992). Patients with primary aldosteronism almost all have low levels of PRA that respond poorly to upright posture and diuretics, two maneuvers that usually raise PRA (Montori et al., 2001). Rarely, concomitant renal damage may stimulate renin release (Oelkers et al., 2000), but renin levels are almost always suppressed, even in those with malignant hypertension (Wu et al., 2000). The presence of a low renin in patients with therapy-resistant hypertension is a clue to the presence of primary aldosteronism (Eide et al., 2004).

### Other Effects

- Hypernatremia is usual, unlike most forms of edematous secondary aldosteronism in which the sodium concentration is often quite low or with diuretic-induced hypokalemia in which a slightly low serum sodium is usually found; thus the serum sodium concentration provides a useful clinical separation between primary and secondary aldosteronism.
- Hypomagnesemia from excessive renal excretion of magnesium may produce tetany.
- Sodium retention and potassium wastage may be demonstrable wherever such exchange is affected by aldosterone: sweat, saliva, and stool.
- Natriuretic peptide levels are appropriately elevated for a state of volume expansion (Kato et al., 2005; Opocher et al., 1992).

## DIAGNOSIS

The diagnosis of primary aldosteronism is easy to make in patients with unprovoked hypokalemia and other manifestations of the fully expressed syndrome. Unprovoked hypokalemia must be thoroughly evaluated, by following the scheme shown in Figure 13–3. Although a surprisingly high prevalence of possible primary aldosteronism has been uncovered in normokalemic hypertensives by the use of the ARR (Stowasser et al., 2003), I believe the ratio should not be a routine procedure (Kaplan, 2004). Admittedly, the fact that hypokalemia was present in most patients in large series published before 1990 may reflect the failure to look for the syndrome in normokalemic hypertensives. However, as will be detailed under "Screening Tests," there

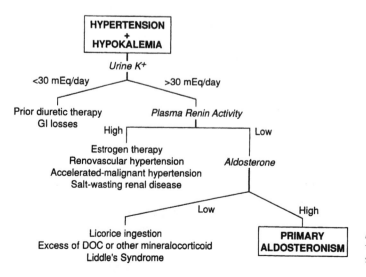

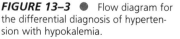

FIGURE 13–3 ● Flow diagram for the differential diagnosis of hypertension with hypokalemia.

is a significant potential for medical mischief and the wasteful spending of considerable money if the ARR is routinely performed on all hypertensives, as advocated by Stowasser et al. (2003). As Grimes and Schulz (2002) note: "Screening has a darker side that is often overlooked. It can be inconvenient, unpleasant, and expensive. . . . A second wave of injury can arise after the initial screening insult: false-positive results and true-positive results leading to dangerous interventions."

Therefore, I still screen for primary aldosteronism by the measurement of plasma renin and aldosterone only with unexplained hypokalemia or hypokalemia induced by diuretics but resistant to correction, in hypertensive family members of patients with familial aldosteronism, patients with an adrenal incidentaloma, and in some patients with difficult to control hypertension.

## Screening Tests

### Plasma Potassium

Caution should be used to ensure that hypokalemia is not inadvertently missed. A number of factors may cause a temporary and spurious rise in plasma potassium (Wiederkehr & Moe, 2000) including:

- A difficult and painful venipuncture causes plasma potassium to rise for multiple reasons: If the patient hyperventilates, the respiratory alkalosis causes potassium to leave cells; repeated fist clenching causes potassium to leave the exercising muscles; if the tourniquet is left on, plasma potassium rises from venous stasis. In a series of 152 patients with primary aldosteronism, serum potassium was above 3.6 mmol/L in only 10.5% in samples obtained without fist clenching but in 69.1% after fist-clenching with a tourniquet in place (Abdelhamid et al., 2003).
- Any degree of hemolysis.
- Efflux of potassium from blood cells if separation of plasma by centrifugation is delayed or if the sample is placed on ice.
- Release of potassium from red cells during clot formation if serum is analyzed, raising the average level by 0.2 mmol/L (Hyman & Kaplan, 1985).
- Efflux of potassium from blood with high counts of white cells or platelets.

### Urine Potassium

If hypokalemia is present, a 24-hour urine sample should be collected for sodium and potassium levels before starting potassium-replacement therapy but 3 to 4 days after diuretics have been stopped. If the urine sodium is above 100 mmol per 24 hours (to ensure that enough sodium is present to allow potassium wastage to express itself), the presence of a potassium level above 30 mmol per 24 hours indicates a driven wastage of potassium through the kidneys. In addition to the action of excess mineralocorticoid in the syndromes of primary aldosteronism, a number of other conditions may require consideration, conditions in which hypokalemia is coupled with renal potassium wastage (Table 13–2). If the urine potassium is less than 30 mmol per 24 hours, mineralocorticoid excess is much less likely, and other causes of hypokalemia may be responsible (Table 13–3).

If the collection of a 24-hour urine is difficult, measurement of either the fractional excretion of potassium (FEK+) or the transtubular potassium gradient (TTKG) in a single voided specimen will separate renal from nonrenal causes of hypokalemia (Halperin & Kamel, 1998).

Once the renal origin of hypokalemia is recognized, it may be preferable to correct the hypokalemia with potassium supplements, 40 to 80 mmol per day, after discontinuation of diuretics before performing additional workup. To restore total body potassium deficits after prolonged diuretic

## TABLE 13–2

### Causes of Hypokalemia Due to Renal Loss of Potassium

I. High flow rate of potassium in the cortical collecting duct (CCD)
  A. Increased sodium excretion, e.g., diuretics
  B. Increased organic osmoles
    1. Glucose
    2. Urea
    3. Mannitol
II. High potassium concentration in the CCD
  A. With expanded intravascular volume (low plasma renin)
    1. Primary mineralocorticoid excess (see Table 13–1)
    2. Liddle's syndrome
    3. Amphotericin B
  B. With contracted intravascular volume (high plasma renin)
    1. Bartter's syndrome
    2. Giletman's syndrome
    3. Magnesium depletion
    4. Increased bicarbonate excretion
    5. Secondary aldosteronism, e.g., nephrotic syndrome

## TABLE 13-3

### Causes of Hypokalemia Without Urinary Potassium Wastage

Prior diuretic use

Cellular shifts

    Rapid tumor growth

    Alkalosis (e.g., hyperventilation)

    Hormones; insulin, β-agonists

    Periodic paralysis

Decreased intake: starvation

Increased nonrenal loss

    Gastrointestinal

        Vomiting and drainage

        Diarrhea and laxatives

    Skin

        Sweating

        Burns

use, a minimum of 3 weeks is needed, and it may take months. After a suitable interval, the supplemental potassium should be stopped for at least 3 days and the plasma potassium level should be rechecked. If plasma potassium is normal, plasma renin and aldosterone levels should be measured.

A more rapid screening protocol may be used: Once hypokalemia is recognized, measure plasma renin and aldosterone. If renin is low and aldosterone is high, the diagnosis of primary aldosteronism is strongly supported. However, hypokalemia will suppress aldosterone secretion even from an adenoma, so the plasma aldosterone level may not be elevated. As a reasonable compromise, the blood for renin and aldosterone could be drawn, the plasma separated and frozen, and the analyses done only if the 24-hour urine sample displays excessive potassium wastage. Regardless, if the plasma aldosterone is not definitely elevated in the presence of hypokalemia, it may need to be repeated after potassium replenishment.

### Plasma Aldosterone-Renin Ratio (ARR)

The ARR is derived by dividing the plasma aldosterone (normal = 5 to 20 ng/dL) by the plasma renin activity (normal = 1 to 3 ng/mL per hour). The normal ratio would be around 10, whereas patients with primary aldosteronism are usually well above 20, in fact, usually above 50 (Kaplan, 2004). If plasma aldosterone is measured in picomoles per liter and

PRA in nanograms per liter, the values should be 27.7-fold higher, i.e., a ratio of 20 equals a ratio of 555 in SI units.

Now that measurement of actual plasma renin concentration (PRC)—also called "direct" or "active" renin assay—is being performed by automated immunoassays in commercial labs, ARR results will increasingly be reported as plasma aldosterone in pmol/L divided by PRC in mU/L (PA/PRC). The PRC values are approximately seven times the PRA values. An abnormal ARR (PA/PRC), based on results in 76 normal patients and 28 patients with primary aldosteronism, is considered to be above 71 pmol/mU (Perschel et al., 2004). Others use a cutoff of 64 pmol/mU (Plouin et al., 2004).

The blood sample should be obtained without stasis in the morning after the patient is seated for 5 to 15 minutes in the absence of most antihypertensive medications (Lamarre-Cliche et al., 2005), particularly aldosterone receptor blockers (Gordon, 2004). Differences in time of day and patient's posture can cause threefold differences in the same patients (Tiu et al., 2005).

With the knowledge that plasma aldosterone levels were high and plasma renin levels were suppressed in primary aldosteronism, Dunn and Espiner (1976) first reported the use of the ARR as a screening test with much stronger support for its use provided in the data from 348 untreated hypertensives by Hiramatsu et al. (1981). The first evidence that the ARR identified far more patients with primary aldosteronism than the small percentage previously recognized came from Richard Gordon and colleagues from the Greenslopes Hospital in Brisbane, Australia (Gordon et al., 1993). The Brisbane group's findings of a high prevalence of an elevated ARR have been replicated by a number of investigators in various countries throughout the world, mostly on referred patients with resistant hypertension or hypokalemia (Table 13–4).

As noted in Table 13–4, there are considerable differences in the definition of an elevated ARR, with most of the ARR threshold levels representing the upper values obtained in patients presumed to have essential hypertension. The reported prevalence of an elevated ARR in hypertensive patients varies from 6% to as high as 39% in those referred because of resistant hypertension (Girerd et al., 2003). However, in 287 presumably unselected hypertensives, an elevated ARR was found in 32.4%, using a PA/PRC cutoff of 32 pg/mL (Olivieri et al., 2004).

As seen in Table 13–4, as few as half of those with an elevated ARR fail to suppress plasma or urinary aldosterone levels after intravenous or oral salt loading, the usual procedure used to document

## TABLE 13-4

### The Prevalence of Autonomous Hyperaldosteronism and Aldosterone-Producing Adenomas (APA) in Patients Tested by Plasma Aldosterone to Plasma-Renin Activity Ratio (ARR)*

| Reference | No. Patients | ARR Threshold* | Raised ARR | Abnormal Suppression by Salt Loads | Proven APA |
|---|---|---|---|---|---|
| Hiramatsu, 1981 | 348 | 40 | 7.4% | NA† | 2.6% |
| Gordon, 1993 | 199 | 30 | 20.0% | 8.5% | 2.5% |
| Lim, 1999 | 125 | 27 | 14.0% | NA | NA |
| Lim, 2000 | 495 | 27 | 16.6% | 9.2% | 0.4% |
| Nishikawa, 2000 | 1,020 | 20 | 6.4% | NA | 4.2% |
| Loh, 2000 | 350 | 20+ PA >15 | 18.0% | 4.6% | 1.7% |
| Rayner, 2000 | 216 | 36+ PA >18 | 32.0% | NA | 2.3% |
| Fardella, 2000 | 305 | 25 | 9.5% | 4.9% | 0.3% |
| Douma, 2001 | 978 | 30+ PA‡↑ | 21.2% | 13.8% | NA |
| E. Rossi, 2002 | 1,046 | 35 | 12.8% | 6.3% | 1.5% |
| Hood, 2002 | 835 | 40 | 12.3% | NA | 0.7% |
| Mulatero, 2002 | 2,160 | 50 | 10.6% | 7.0% | 1.6% |
| Calhoun, 2002 | 88 | 20 | NA | 20.4% | NA |
| Girerd, 2003 | 143 | NA | 39.0% | NA | 6.0% |
| Fogari, 2003 | 750 | 25 | 12.0% | 6.0% | 2.0% |
| Strauch, 2003 | 403 | 50 | 21.6% | 19.0% | 6.5% |
| Stowasser, 2003 | ~300 | 30 | 18.6% | 17.7% | 5.0% |
| Mosso, 2003 | 609 | 25 | 10.2% | 6.1% | 0% |

PA, plasma aldosterone.
*ARR expressed as plasma aldosterone in ng/dL, divided by PRA in ng/mL per hour.
† NA, not available.
‡ ↑, increased.

autonomous hyperaldosteronism, as noted under "Confirmatory Tests."

Despite the widespread use of the ARR to make important diagnostic and therapeutic decisions, very little study has been made of its test characteristics, i.e., sensitivity, specificity, and likelihood ratios at different cutoff values. At the conclusion of a systematic review of all of the literature on the ARR published from January 1966 to October 2001, Montori and Young (2002) state: "There are no published valid estimates of the test characteristics of the aldosterone-renin ratio when used as a screening test for primary aldosteronism in patients with presumed essential hypertension."

Subsequent to that review, limited data have been published about the test characteristics. Hirohara et al. (2001) reported a specificity of an ARR level of 32 or higher to be only 61% among 114 patients whose adrenal status was clearly defined,

of whom 35 had an aldosterone-producing adenoma (APA). In the study by Schwartz et al. (2002) on 505 adults with presumed essential hypertension but whose adrenal status was not otherwise determined, the sensitivity of the test was 66% and the specificity was 67% for identifying patients whose aldosterone levels were increased relative to the level of renin. These authors conclude that the ARR "lacks sensitivity and specificity and has only a modest predictive value [34%] for combinations of renin and aldosterone that are compatible with primary aldosteronism." In another analysis of data from 497 of these patients, two observations were made: First, the ratio varied considerably in the same patients whose posture changed from supine to standing and even more so after diuretic therapy (25 mg of hydrochlorothiazide daily) for 4 weeks; second, the ratio was "strongly and inversely dependent on the PRA level," leading to the conclusion that "the aldosterone-renin ratio does not provide a renin-independent measure of circulating aldosterone that is suitable for determining whether plasma aldosterone concentration is elevated relative to PRA. . . . Elevation of the ARR is predominantly an indicator of low PRA" (Montori et al., 2001).

Further concern over the sensitivity of the ARR has been raised by the data on repeated studies in 71 patients with a proven unilateral APA (Tanabe et al., 2003). The ARR was normal (below 35) in 31% of these patients on at least one occasion and only 37% had an abnormal ARR on all occasions.

The confounding effect of diuretic therapy noted by Montori et al. (2001) may also apply to other antihypertensive medications. β-blockers, by reducing PRA more than plasma aldosterone, can markedly increase the number of false-positive ARRs (Mulatero et al., 2002; Seifarth et al., 2002) and an angiotensin receptor blocker may cause false-negative results (Mulatero et al., 2002). Fortunately, the protocol followed by the Brisbane (Gordon, 2004) and Mayo Clinic (Schwartz et al., 2002) investigators required cessation of most drugs, but many other studies were performed while usual medications were being taken (Montori & Young, 2002).

Gordon (2004) identified another probable source of inaccuracy with the ARR: the potential errors introduced by the increasing use of commercial renin activity and aldosterone assay kits in nonresearch labs. This problem may be reduced by use of a direct measure of active renin (Ferrari et al., 2004). Moreover, the ARR varied between 13 to 35, depending upon the time of day and posture of the patients (Tiu et al., 2005).

The most common reasons for false-positive ARRs is the presence of a low level of PRA as often found in the elderly, the Black, and the hypertensive (Alderman et al., 2004). With a not-unusual low PRA level of 0.3 ng/mL per hour, the presence of a normal plasma aldosterone level of 12 ng/dL would provide an ARR of 40 which by most investigators' current criteria (see Table 13–4) would be abnormal.

To reduce this source of false-positive tests, some require an absolutely elevated plasma aldosterone level of 16 ng/dL or higher to call the ARR abnormal (Young, 2002). However, the Brisbane group do not, since in a recent description of 54 patients with documented primary aldosteronism, 20 had plasma aldosterone levels of 15 ng/dL or lower (Stowasser et al., 2003). The wisdom of requiring an elevated plasma aldosterone has been documented in recent series, reducing false positives from 30% to 3% in one series (Seiler et al., 2004).

Beyond the error that could be induced by a low PRA or PRC when aldosterone levels are normal, an elevated ARR is found in patients with a polymorphism of the CYP-11β2 gene that gives rise to impaired adrenal 11β-hydroxylation and, in turn, low levels of cortisol, compensatory increased adrenocorticotropic hormone (ACTH), and then increased aldosterone secretion (Barbato et al., 2004; Freel & Connell, 2004; Lim et al., 2002a; Nicod et al., 2003).

For all of these reasons, the ARR should not be used. Rather, if screening is indicated, a plasma renin and a plasma aldosterone level should be measured, preferably in the absence of all antihypertensive drugs. A low-renin and a high-aldosterone level are suggestive of primary aldosteronism.

## Confirmatory Tests

### Elevated and Nonsuppressible Aldosterone

If the PRA or PRC is low and the aldosterone is high, the presence of an inappropriately elevated and nonsuppressible aldosterone secretion should be documented. This was first demonstrated with the saline suppression test of plasma aldosterone (Kem et al., 1971). Plasma aldosterone is measured before and after the infusion of 2 L of normal saline over 4 hours. Patients with primary aldosteronism have higher basal levels but, more importantly, fail to suppress these levels after saline to below 10 ng/dL. Some patients with adrenal hyperplasia may suppress to a level between 5 and 10 ng/dL after saline, so that the normal level may need to be set at 5 ng/dL when screening is done for hyperplasia (Holland et al., 1984).

Most prefer to measure urine aldosterone levels after 3 days of oral sodium loading, with an abnormal level being above 12 (Young, 2002) or 14 μg per 24 hours (Bravo, 1994). However, the Brisbane group has found that both the intravenous and oral salt loading tests are often inaccurate and it utilizes a high-salt diet plus large doses of the mineralocorticoid Florinef over a 4-day hospitalization, the FST test (Stowasser et al., 2003).

#### Captopril Suppression

Whereas plasma aldosterone levels were markedly suppressed 3 hours after oral intake of 1 mg captopril per kilogram of body weight in patients with essential hypertension or renovascular hypertension, they remained elevated in patients with primary hyperaldosteronism (Thibonnier et al., 1982). An ARR above 26 obtained 2 hours after 25 mg captopril has been reported to be a useful confirmatory test, including a few patients with a normal routine ARR (Castro et al., 2002). In a larger group of patients, measurement of ARR 90 minutes after 50 mg captopril provided better sensitivity and specificity than routine ARR testing (E Rossi et al., 2002).

### *Response to Spironolactone*

Spark and Melby (1968) showed that patients with primary aldosteronism had a fall of at least 20 mm Hg in their diastolic BP after 5 weeks of spironolactone, 100 mg 4 times a day. Although the procedure is no longer needed as a diagnostic test, the response to spironolactone may have prognostic value, since the response to spironolactone in patients with an adenoma closely resembled their subsequent response to surgery (Ferriss et al., 1978a).

### *Rule Out Glucocorticoid-Remediable Aldosteronism (GRA)*

As will be described in the next section, GRA should be considered in the absence of an adenoma, particularly if other family members have aldosteronism. This is most easily confirmed by demonstrating the hybrid gene in a blood sample, as noted later in this chapter.

### Excluding Other Diseases

Various causes of secondary aldosteronism are easily excluded by the presence of edema and high levels of peripheral blood PRA. In addition, there are a number of inherited renal tubular disorders, some associated with hypertension and hypokalemia, that should not be confused with primary aldosteronism (Ferrari & Bonny, 2003) (Table 13–5). Others are associated with either hyperkalemia or normotension, so the distinction should be obvious.

Those listed under Hypertension and Hypokalemia also have suppressed, low PRA but all have low aldosterone levels, either because of the secretion of other mineralocorticoids (glucocorticoid-remediable hyperaldosteronism, to be covered later in this chapter), because of increased cortisol acting as a mineralocorticoid (apparent mineralocorticoid excess, to be covered in Chapter 14), or increased sodium reabsorption from activated sodium channels (Liddle's syndrome), or increased activity of mineralocorticoid receptors (Geller et al., 2000).

## TABLE 13–5

### Inherited Renal Tubular Disorders

| Disorder | Inheritance | Consequence of Mutant Gene |
|---|---|---|
| **Hypertension and Hypokalemia** | | |
| Glucocorticoid-remediable aldosteronism (familial hyperaldosteronism, type I) | Dominant | Increased mineralocorticoids from chimeric 11-β-hydroxylase and aldosterone synthase genes |
| Apparent mineralocorticoid excess | Recessive | Reduced inactivation of cortisol due to 11-β-HSD deficiency |
| Mutation of mineralocorticoid receptor | Dominant | Increased activity of mineralocorticoid receptor |
| Liddle's syndrome | Dominant | Increased activity of epithelial sodium channel |
| **Hypertension and Hyperkalemia** | | |
| Pseudohypoaldosteronism, type II (Gordon's syndrome) | Dominant | Increased chloride reabsorption in distal tubule |
| **Normotension and Hypokalemia** | | |
| Bartter's syndrome | Recessive | Decreased sodium chloride reabsorption in thick ascending Henle's loop (five types of defect) |
| Gitelman's syndrome | Recessive | Decreased sodium chloride cotransport in distal convoluted tubule |
| **Normotension and Hyperkalemia** | | |
| Pseudohypoaldosteronism, type I | Recessive | Reduced activity of epithelial sodium channel |
| | Dominant | Reduced activity of mineralocorticoid receptor |

### Excessive Renal Sodium Conservation

*Liddle's Syndrome*

Liddle et al. (1963) described members of a family with hypertension, hypokalemic alkalosis, and negligible aldosterone secretion, apparently resulting from an unusual tendency of the kidneys to conserve sodium and excrete potassium even in the virtual absence of mineralocorticoids. Such patients have a mutation of the $\beta$ or $\gamma$ subunits of the renal epithelial sodium channel, which causes increased sodium reabsorption in the distal nephron (Furuhashi et al., 2005). As will be noted in Chapter 14, these clinical features are also seen in apparent mineralocorticoid excess caused by mutations in 11$\beta$-hydroxysteroid dehydrogenase, preventing conversion of cortisol to cortisone.

An activating mutation of the renal epithelial chloride channel C1C-Kb has been found in 22% of Africans and 12% of Caucasians (Jeck et al., 2004). The mutation is associated with hypertension and higher plasma sodium but not lower plasma potassium levels. The authors suggest that this common mutation may predispose to primary hypertension.

*Activation of Mineralocorticoid Receptor*

Geller et al. (2000) have identified a mutation in the mineralocorticoid receptor that causes early-onset hypertension that is markedly exacerbated in pregnancy. The exacerbation is a consequence of the altered receptor specificity so that the high levels of progesterone and other steroids lacking 21-hydroxyl groups become potent agonists.

*Gordon's Syndrome*

Another syndrome has been described with increased renal sodium and chloride retention that causes hypertension and suppression of the renin-aldosterone mechanism but with hyperkalemia (Gordon, 1986). The syndrome known as pseudohypoaldosteronism, type II, is inherited as an autosomal dominant with at least three loci having been recognized (Disse-Nicodème et al., 2000). An elevated ARR has been noted with aldosterone stimulated by hyperkalemia and renin suppressed by volume expansion (Stowasser, 2000).

### Decreased Renal Sodium Conservation

No diagnostic confusion should occur with the two rare normotensive hypokalemic salt-losing tubulopathies caused by inactivating mutations in genes wherein volume contraction leads to secondary hyperaldosteronism from increased renin secretion (Bichet & Fujiwara, 2004). Bartter's syndrome (Bartter et al., 1962) is usually recognized in early childhood and runs a severe clinical course with marked hypokalemia. Gitelman's syndrome (Gitelman et al., 1966) tends to appear later and run a milder course but is associated with a reduced quality of life (Cruz et al., 2001). Multiple mutations in the thiazide-sensitive Na-Cl cotransporter gene have been identified in patients with Gitelman's syndrome (Lin et al., 2005; Maki et al., 2004).

### Iatrogenic Mineralocorticoid Excess

As with Cushing's syndrome induced by exogenous glucocorticoids, aldosteronism may be induced by exogenous mineralocorticoids, even when absorbed through the skin in an ointment for the treatment of dermatitis (Lauzurica et al., 1988).

This long listing of various diseases, most involving hypokalemia and many with hypertension, should not imply the need for a long and complicated workup to diagnose primary aldosteronism. By following the flow diagram shown in Figure 13–4, one can usually make the correct diagnosis with relative ease.

### During Pregnancy

Normal pregnancy is associated with elevated plasma aldosterone but also elevated renin activity. In 18 reported cases of primary aldosteronism diagnosed during pregnancy, usually presenting with marked hypokalemia, renin levels were reduced (Keely, 1998). Moreover, pre-existing hypertension due to primary aldosteronism may be ameliorated during pregnancy, perhaps by antagonism of the effects of elevated aldosterone by the high progesterone levels (Murakami et al., 2000). Management is complicated by the inability to use most medical therapies and laparoscopic adrenalectomy may be the preferred treatment.

Even more cases have been reported of pregnancy in women with glucocorticoid remediable aldosteronism, 35 pregnancies in 16 patients (Wyckoff et al., 2000). Most of the pregnancies were successful, although hypertension often exacerbated.

## TYPES OF ADRENAL PATHOLOGY

Once the diagnosis of primary aldosteronism is made, the type of adrenal pathology must be ascertained, since the choice of therapy is different: surgical for an adenoma, medical for hyperplasia. This need is even greater today than in the past as recognition of patients with milder manifestations of presumed aldosteronism is so much easier and more frequently performed. At the Mayo Clinic, an adenoma was found in 68% of patients with primary aldosteronism up to 1985; in 1999, only 28% of such patients had an adenoma (Young, 2003).

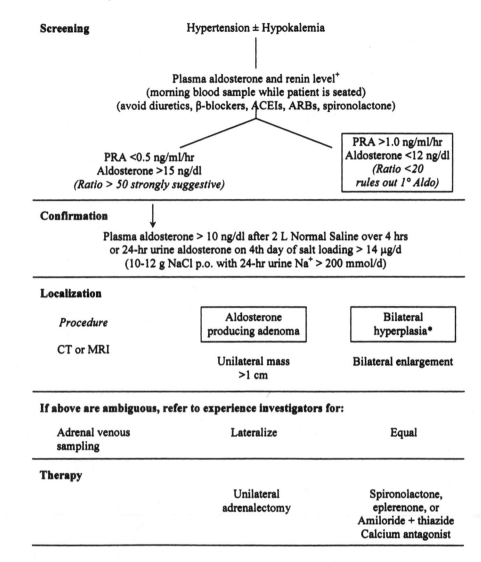

Screening            Hypertension ± Hypokalemia

Plasma aldosterone and renin level[+]
(morning blood sample while patient is seated)
(avoid diuretics, β-blockers, ACEIs, ARBs, spironolactone)

PRA <0.5 ng/ml/hr
Aldosterone >15 ng/dl
*(Ratio > 50 strongly suggestive)*

PRA >1.0 ng/ml/hr
Aldosterone <12 ng/dl
*(Ratio <20
rules out 1° Aldo)*

**Confirmation**

Plasma aldosterone > 10 ng/dl after 2 L Normal Saline over 4 hrs
or 24-hr urine aldosterone on 4th day of salt loading > 14 µg/d
(10-12 g NaCl p.o. with 24-hr urine Na$^+$ > 200 mmol/d)

**Localization**

*Procedure*

CT or MRI

| Aldosterone producing adenoma | Bilateral hyperplasia* |
|---|---|
| Unilateral mass >1 cm | Bilateral enlargement |

**If above are ambiguous, refer to experience investigators for:**

Adrenal venous sampling      Lateralize      Equal

**Therapy**

Unilateral adrenalectomy

Spironolactone, eplerenone, or Amiloride + thiazide Calcium antagonist

**FIGURE 13–4** ● A diagnostic flow chart for evaluating and treating patients with primary aldosteronism. 1° Aldo, primary aldosteronism; ACEI, angiotensin-converting enzyme inhibitor; ARB, angiotensin II-receptor blocker; CT, computed tomography; MRI, magnetic resonance imaging. *Consider glucocorticoid remediable hyperaldosteronism in young with family history of aldosteronism; confirm by genetic testing. [+]Different values will be used with PRC or active renin assays.

## Aldosterone-Producing Adenomas

Solitary benign adenomas (Figure 13–5) are almost always unilateral and most are small, weighing less than 6 g and measuring less than 3 cm in diameter. In various series, from 20% to 85% are smaller than 1 cm (Rossi et al., 2001). Histologically, most adenomas are composed of lipid-laden cells arranged in small acini or cords, similar in appearance and arrangement to the normal zona fasciculata, the middle zone of the adrenal cortex. Moreover, focal or diffuse hyperplasia, as seen in Figure 13–5, is

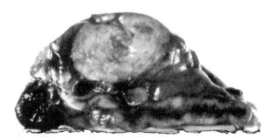

**FIGURE 13–5** ● Solitary adrenal adenoma with diffuse hyperplasia removed from a patient with primary aldosteronism.

usually present in both the remainder of the adrenal with the adenoma and the contralateral gland (Lack et al., 1990).

Gordon et al. (1995) postulate that such histologic hyperplasia outside the adenoma "suggests a genetic abnormality not limited to the adenoma cells." These investigators have also identified 57 patients among 23 families with two or more members who had adenomas that were not suppressed by glucocorticoids and which were biochemically and morphologically identical to nonfamilial primary aldosteronism (Stowasser & Gordon, 2000). Of these 57 patients with "familial hyperaldosteronism, type II," only 15 were hypokalemic and 2 were normotensive. Inheritance is consistent with an autosomal dominant pattern, and a genome-wide search of a single large kindred identified polymorphic gene markers on chromosome 7 (Jackson et al., 2002).

Thus genetics may be involved in more of primary aldosteronism than is now appreciated. Nonetheless, most patients with an adenoma do not have a family history or features that indicate a genetic basis for their condition (Pilon et al., 1999). Since most of these benign adenomas are monoclonal in origin (Gicquel et al., 1994), their origin is more likely from proliferation of aldosterone-producing cells rather than from dysregulation of its synthesis as may be seen in patients with bilateral hyperplasia (Mulatero et al., 2000).

## Bilateral Adrenal Hyperplasia (Idiopathic Hyperaldosteronism)

In the late 1960s, reports of hyperaldosteronism with no adenoma but rather with bilateral adrenal hyperplasia (BAH) began to appear (Davis et al., 1967) and was referred to as idiopathic hyperaldosteronism (IHA) (Biglieri et al., 1970). These patients tend to have milder biochemical and hormonal abnormalities that are less obvious than those seen with adenomas. The wide availability of hormonal assays and adrenal imaging techniques have made it much easier to recognize hyperplasia, and as more patients have been screened by the ARR, the proportion of primary aldosteronism related to BAH has steadily increased from less than one-third in the 1970s to more than two-thirds in the 1990s (Stowasser et al., 2003; Young, 2003).

However, the better detail provided by newer imaging procedures may lead to confusion: Because the hyperplasia that often accompanies an adenoma can now be recognized, bilateral hyperplasia may be mistakenly diagnosed on the one hand; because nodularity is often seen with hyperplasia, an adenoma may be mistakenly diagnosed on the other

(Glodny et al., 2000; Magill et al., 2001). Moreover, the clear separation between adenoma and hyperplasia may also be blurred by the recognition that, in response to suppression or stimulation tests, a solitary adenoma occasionally behaves like bilateral hyperplasia (Phillips et al., 2000), and bilateral hyperplasia occasionally mimics the responses of a solitary adenoma (Biglieri, 1991). Therefore, anatomic evidence must be correlated with functional data to ensure the correct diagnosis (Magill et al., 2001; McAlister & Lewanczuk, 1998; Young et al., 2004).

The presence of bilateral hyperplasia suggests a secondary response to some stimulatory mechanism rather than a primary neoplastic growth, but none has been identified. Lim et al. (2002b) postulate that, in susceptible hypertensives, an increased sensitivity to angiotensin II may gradually induce adrenal hyperplasia that become autonomous, i.e., "tertiary aldosteronism."

In view of the known polymorphism in the aldosterone synthase gene ($CYP11\beta2$) that is responsible for glucocorticoid-remediable aldosteronism, to be described shortly, such genetic polymorphisms have been sought in patients with bilateral hyperplasia that is not glucocorticoid-remediable (Lim et al., 2002a). One group has found a variation in this gene in about half of 90 patients with bilateral hyperplasia (Mulatero et al., 2000) whereas another found increased aldosterone synthase activity and mRNA expression but no mutations in the gene in nine patients with bilateral hyperplasia (Takeda et al., 1999).

It should be recalled that, soon after the description of hyperaldosteronism associated with bilateral adrenal hyperplasia, members of the MRC Blood Pressure Unit at the Western Infirmary in Glasgow published a series of papers with convincing evidence that this condition was totally different from Conn's syndrome of aldosterone-producing adenoma (Table 13–6) (Ferriss et al., 1970). They referred to bilateral adrenal hyperplasia as simply a form of "low-renin essential hypertension" (McAreavey et al., 1983).

Moreover, there is a progressive increase in adrenal nodular hyperplasia with age having no relationship to hypertension (Tracy & White, 2002). Therefore, the increased frequency of cases with hyperplasia may simply reflect natural changes with age: increased adrenal nodular hyperplasia, progressively lower renin but maintained aldosterone levels (Guthrie et al., 1976), giving rise to an elevated aldosterone-renin ratio without hyperaldosteronism. This scenario is in keeping with the Medical Research Council investigators' belief that these patients have "low-renin essential hypertension" (McAreavey et al., 1983).

## TABLE 13 – 6

**Differences Between Aldosterone Producing Adenoma, Bilateral Adrenal Hyperplasia, and Low-Renin Hypertension***

| | Aldosterone Producing Adenoma | Bilateral Adrenal Hyperplasia | Low-Renin Essential Hypertension |
|---|---|---|---|
| Clinical Features | | | |
|   Age | Middle-aged | Older | Older |
|   Hypokalemia | Frequent | Less common | Uncommon |
| Hemodynamics | | | |
|   Body sodium content | Increased | Normal | Normal |
|   Plasma aldosterone in response to standing | Fall | Rise | Rise |
| Hormonal | | | |
|   Plasma renin levels | Very low | Low | Low |
|   Plasma aldosterone levels | Very high | High-normal | Normal |
|   Aldosterone secretion | Autonomous | Responsive to AII† | Responsive to AII† |
|   Aldosterone suppressibility to volume loads | Minimal | Partial | Complete |
|   Aldosterone to angiotensin relation | Inverse | Direct | Direct |
|   Hybrid steroids | Present | Absent | Absent |
| Relief by surgical removal | Usual | Extremely rare | Never |

*Based on data included in Ferriss JB, Brown JJ, Fraser R, et al. Hypertension with aldosterone excess and low plasma-renin: preoperative distinction between patients with and without adrenocortical tumour. *Lancet* 1970;2:995–1000 and McAreavey D, Murray GD, Lever AF, et al. Similarity of idiopathic aldosteronism and essential hypertension. *Hypertension* 1983;5:116–121.

† AII, angiotensin II.

## Unilateral Hyperplasia

Even more difficult to explain than the presence of bilateral hyperplasia are the 18 reported cases of hyperaldosteronism that apparently are caused by hyperplasia of only one adrenal gland (Mansoor et al., 2002).

## Glucocorticoid-Remediable Aldosteronism (Familial Hyperaldosteronism, Type I)

### Early Observations

In 1966, Sutherland and coworkers described a father and son with classic features of primary aldosteronism whose entire syndrome was completely relieved by dexamethasone, 0.5 mg 4 times a day (i.e., glucocorticoid remediable). Subsequently, the syndrome was shown to follow an autosomal dominant mode of inheritance. In the early 1980s, Ulick et al. (1983) and Gomez-Sanchez et al. (1984) found increased levels of 18-hydroxylated cortisol in such patients. This led Ulick et al. (1990) to postulate that

the syndrome was the result of the acquisition of aldosterone synthase activity by cells of the zona fasciculata. This would explain the high levels of 18-hydroxylated steroids, which can be suppressed by exogenous glucocorticoid, which in turn suppresses ACTH, the normal stimulus to synthetic activity within the zona fasciculata.

### Genetic Confirmation

The correctness of Ulick et al.'s postulate was proven in a striking manner by Lifton et al. (1992). Using restriction fragment length polymorphism analysis of cells from eight affected members of a large kindred, these investigators found "complete linkage of glucocorticoid-remediable aldosteronism to a gene duplication arising from unequal crossing over, fusing the 5' regulatory region of 11-beta-hydroxylase to the 3' coding sequences of aldosterone synthase" (Lifton et al., 1992) (Figure 13–6). The two genes lie next to each other on human chromosome 8 and are 94% identical, likely explaining the propensity to cross-over (Dluhy & Lifton, 1999).

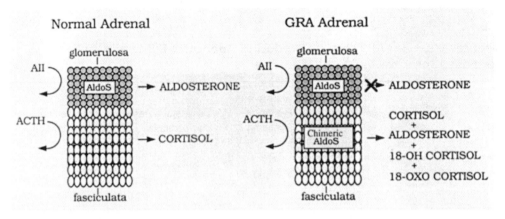

**FIGURE 13–6** ● Regulation of aldosterone production in the zona glomerulosa and cortisol production in the zona fasciculata in the normal adrenal, and model of the physiologic abnormalities in the adrenal cortex in GRA. Ectopic expression of aldosterone synthase enzymatic activity in the adrenal fasciculata results in GRA. (Reprinted with permission from Lifton RP, Dluhy RG, Powers M, et al. Hereditary hypertension caused by chimaeric gene duplications and ectopic expression of aldosterone synthase. *Nature Genet* 1992;2:66–74.)

## Clinical and Laboratory Features

As more patients with GRA have been identified, variations in both genotype and phenotype have been identified. Different sites of gene cross-over do not seem to influence the phenotype, but patients who inherited GRA from their mothers have higher plasma aldosterone concentrations and blood pressures than those who inherited the chimeric gene from their fathers (Jamieson et al., 1995). Moreover, considerably different phenotypes have been seen within a single family that are not accounted for by different genotypes (Fallo et al., 2004).

In their review of this syndrome, Dluhy and Lifton (1999) noted that cases have been reported worldwide but not in Blacks. The hyperaldosteronism is usually evident at birth with inheritance as an autosomal dominant trait, occurring equally among men and women. The hypertension is often severe, poorly responsive to usual antihypertensive therapy, but some affected subjects in pedigrees are normotensive. An increased prevalence of strokes, particularly cerebral hemorrhage from intracranial aneurysm, has prompted the recommendation for MRI beginning at puberty and every 5 years thereafter in all family members.

These authors confirm the earlier observation that about half of affected patients are normokalemic so that measurement of serum potassium is not a sensitive screening test. The absence of hypokalemia may be related to a number of factors, including a lesser mineralocorticoid activity of the 18-hydroxylated steroids and to the inability of dietary potassium to stimulate aldosterone secretion when it arises from the zona fasciculata (Litchfield et al., 1997).

## Diagnosis

Initially, the definitive diagnosis was based on dexamethasone suppression of aldosterone, but, now that genetic testing is so readily available, this is the preferred procedure. The genetic test can be obtained by contacting the International Registry for GRA, phone 800-722-5520, extension 25011, or fax 617-732-5764.

It is possible that variants of GRA are more common than now recognized. Lim et al. (2002a) found an increased frequency of variations at the aldosterone synthase gene locus in 91 hypertensives with an elevated ARR whose condition was otherwise not defined. However, no GRA mutations were found in genetic testing of 300 randomly chosen hypertensives so that the investigators recommended that screening should be targeted to those with a family history of early onset of hypertension associated with intracranial hemorrhage or a personal history of hypertension of early onset that is difficult to control or associated with hypokalemia (Gates et al., 2001).

## Treatment

Suppressive doses of exogenous glucocorticoid will usually control the hypertension even if all the hormonal pertubations are not normalized (Stowasser et al., 2000). Spironolactone with or without a thiazide diuretic has been used without glucocorticoid suppression (Dluhy & Lifton, 1999).

## Significance

Elucidation of this mutation represents the first description of a genetic basis of a form of hypertension in otherwise phenotypically normal humans. Beyond this rather limited population, polymorphic variability in the aldosterone synthase (CYP11B2) gene has been found in patients with "essential" hypertension by some investigators but not by others (Davies & Kenyon, 2003; Rajput et al., 2005). Indeed, Freel and Connell (2004) attribute bilateral adrenal hyperplasia with elevated ARR to such genetic polymorphisms. The search will go on, spurred by the old observations that adrenal suppression with dexamethasone will lower blood pressure in some "essential" hypertensives (Hamilton et al., 1979).

## Other Pathologies

### Carcinoma

Aldosterone-producing carcinomas are rare, with only 68 having been reported since 1955 (Seccia et al., 2003). Most are associated with concomitant hypersecretion of other adrenal hormones, but a few may hypersecrete only aldosterone (Touitou et al., 1992). Genetic markers may be useful in differentiating malignancies from benign tumors and in determining prognosis (Kanauchi et al., 2003).

### Associated Conditions

Patients have been reported with primary aldosteronism caused by an adrenal adenoma in association with acromegaly (Dluhy & Williams, 1969), primary hyperparathyroidism, the multiple endocrine neoplasia I syndrome (Gordon et al., 1995), neurofibromatosis (Biagi et al., 1999), familial adenomatous polyposis (Alexander et al., 2000), and renal artery stenosis (Mansoor et al., 2002). An aldosterone-producing adenoma may co-exist with a nonfunctioning contralateral adrenal tumor (Hollak et al., 1991).

### Extra-adrenal Tumors

Single ectopic aldosterone-producing tumors have been found in the kidney (Abdelhamid et al., 1996) and ovary (Kulkarni et al., 1990).

## DIAGNOSING THE TYPE OF ADRENAL PATHOLOGY

Various procedures have been used to diagnose the type of adrenal pathology (Table 13–7). This list is much shorter than in previous editions of this book because of the ascendancy of adrenal venous sampling (AVS) when any ambiguity is noted on CT or MRI. Increasingly, investigators recommend AVS even when there is no apparent ambiguity because of the vagaries of adrenal pathology (Espiner et al., 2003; Magill et al., 2001; Phillips et al., 2000; Stowasser et al., 2003; Young et al., 2004).

### Ancillary Procedures

In general, autonomous lesions that can be cured by surgery (adenomas and the rare primary adrenal hyperplasia) display their autonomy from the normal control of aldosterone production by the renin-angiotensin mechanism by having (a) high levels of aldosterone and its precursor 18-OH-corticosterone along with more severe clinical features of aldosteronism, (b) little or no response to stimulation of renin-angiotensin such as during an upright posture test, and (c) the production of hybrid steroids such as 18-OH-cortisol.

## TABLE 13–7

**Techniques to Differentiate Adrenal Adenoma from Bilateral Hyperplasia**

| Technique | Adenoma | Hyperplasia | Discriminatory Value |
|---|---|---|---|
| Basal plasma 18-OHB | >65 ng/dL | <65 ng/dL | Fair |
| Basal 18-oxo-F, 18-OHF | Increased | Normal[a] | Fair |
| Upright posture (rise in PA) | <30% | >30% | Fair |
| Adrenal CT and MRI | Unilateral mass | Bilaterally enlarged | Fair |
| Adrenal venous aldosterone: cortisol ratio | Increased on side of adenoma | Equal | Excellent |
| Adrenal scintiscan with [131I]cholesterol + dex | Unilateral persistent uptake | Bilateral suppressed uptake | Good |

18-oxo-F, 18-oxycortisol; 18-OHF, 18-hydroxy-cortisol; PA, plasma aldosterone.
[a]Markedly elevated in glucocorticoid-remediable aldosteronism.

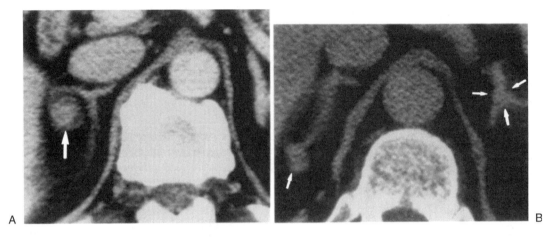

**FIGURE 13–7** ● Computed tomographic scans of two patients with clinical features of primary aldosteronism. **Left**, a 1.5-cm solitary adenoma in the right adrenal. The diagnosis of aldosteronoma was confirmed with relief of the syndrome by resection of the gland. **Right**, several 9-mm nodules (*arrows*) in both adrenal glands, which are hyperplastic. The patient's hypokalemia and hypertension were controlled medically. (Reprinted with permission from Radin DR, Manoogian C, Nadler JL. Diagnosis of primary hyperaldosteronism: importance of correlating CT findings with endocrinologic studies. *Am J Roentgenol* 1992;158:553–557.)

## Other Adrenal Steroids

Most adenomas, but not hyperplastic glands, secrete excess amounts of both normal precursors (e.g., 18-OH-B), and hybrid steroids (e.g., 18-oxo-cortisol; 18-oxo-F) (Ulick et al., 1993). However, the diagnostic accuracy of 18-OH-B levels was only 82%, and there seems no current role for this measure (Young, 2002).

## Response to Upright Posture

This test depends on changes in plasma aldosterone in response to variations in endogenous stimuli during 2 to 4 hours of upright posture (Ganguly et al., 1973). The premise is that adenomas are not responsive to postural increases in angiotensin (which stay suppressed anyway) but are exquisitely sensitive to the diurnal fall in plasma ACTH, whereas hyperplasia is responsive to even small postural rises in angiotensin. Thus patients with hyperplasia should have an even greater than normal *rise* in plasma aldosterone after 4 hours of standing, whereas patients with an adenoma show an anomalous *fall* in plasma aldosterone, in parallel with the falling plasma ACTH levels during the early morning hours.

Although a fall in plasma aldosterone after posture has been found to have good specificity for the diagnosis of an adenoma, the procedure has low sensitivity and little value (Espiner et al., 2003; Phillips et al., 2000).

## Adrenal Computed Tomography or Magnetic Resonance Imaging

Most aldosterone-producing adenomas (APA) are visible by CT or MRI scans even though they may be less than 1 cm in size (Figure 13–7). However, two developments have lead to a lesser role of these imaging techniques in establishing the cause of primary aldosteronism. On the one hand, with improved ability to identify milder degrees of hyperaldosteronism, the diagnosis is being made in patients with smaller solitary adenomas and, even more, with minor degrees of bilateral hyperplasia, neither of which may be identified with even the most advanced CT or MRI technology. On the other hand, with such technology, areas of hyperplasia that often co-exist with solitary functioning adenomas (see Figure 13–5) are being identified as multiple nodules or bilateral adrenal hyperplasia.

Numerous reports attest to the ambiguities of current CT scanning, with findings that only half of adenomas, proven by AVS and surgical relief, are thereby identified, giving the procedure an unacceptably low sensitivity (Espiner et al., 2003; Loh et al., 2000; Nishikawa et al., 2000; Stowasser et al., 2003). Stowasser et al. (2003) also found misleading CT scans, demonstrating a unilateral mass in patients subsequently proven to have bilateral hyperplasia.

Young et al. (2004) continues to rely on the presence by CT scan of a solitary unilateral macroadenoma, larger than 1 cm, with normal contralateral adrenal morphology in patients below age 40 with primary aldosteronism (who are much more likely to have an adenoma than BAH) to recommend surgery without further testing. However, they too recognize the frequent need for further testing in most patients whose CT findings are less certain.

## Adrenal Venous Sampling

Guidelines on the performance and interpretation of AVS have been provided by Rossi et al. (2001) who reported their findings in 104 patients with primary aldosteronism and equivocal CT or MRI findings, as defined by the absence of a solitary adrenal mass larger than 1.8 cm. Adrenal venous sampling was feasible in 97.1% of attempts and, in 80.6% of cases, bilateral samples were obtained almost simultaneously. Without ACTH stimulation, they found that the greatest selectivity in defining AVS accuracy was a plasma cortisol in the adrenal venous sample 1.1 times or higher than in the inferior vena caval sample. With bilateral selective AVS, a value of aldosterone/cortisol of one side over the contralateral side of 2.0 or greater identified a unilateral source of excess aldosterone in 80% of the patients. They also noted that unilateral sampling of the left adrenal vein (which is easier to catheterize than the right) was of no value in identifying the type of pathology. More definite data in a larger percentage of patients have been reported when ACTH stimulation is utilized (Espiner et al., 2003). Moreover, Espiner et al. (2003) found that, when bilateral access was not possible, lateralization was usually successful when only the contralateral adrenal vein was sampled.

These data are encouraging in one sense since good discrimination was provided by AVS in most patients despite ambiguous findings on CT or MRI. On the other hand, even in the hands of such experienced investigators, 20% of patients could not be correctly characterized by AVS, although better results have been reported in more recent series (Espiner et al., 2003; Stowasser et al., 2003; Young et al., 2004).

All who perform AVS or who wish to interpret data from the procedure should read the report of Rossi et al. (2001) and the previous review by Doppman and Gill (1996).

## Adrenal Scintigraphy

Adrenal scintiscans with the isotope, $6-\beta-[^{131}I]$-iodomethyl-19-norcholesterol (NP-59), have been claimed to provide discrimination almost as good as found by adrenal vein sampling, with less discomfort (Francis et al., 1992). Results are better with suppression scintiscans using 0.5 or 1 mg of dexamethasone every 6 hours to discriminate between adenomas, which remain visible, and bilateral hyperplasia, which fades after a few days of dexamethasone (Shapiro et al., 1994).

Since small adenomas with relatively low uptake of the tracer may give false-negative results (Nakahama et al., 2003) and spironolactone may increase bilateral uptake (Shapiro et al., 1994), this procedure will rarely need to be utilized.

## Overall Plan

As seen in Figure 13–4, once the presence of primary aldosteronism has been confirmed, a CT or MRI scan of the adrenals should be obtained. If a solitary adrenal mass ≥1 cm is seen with normal contralateral morphology, unilateral adrenalectomy may be recommended. If the scans show clear bilateral hyperplasia, medical therapy should be recommended, with the realization that even if a unilateral adenomatous source is missed, the patient will still be protected.

If the CT or MRI findings are ambiguous or if an adrenal mass smaller than 1 cm is present, AVS should be performed in a center with considerable experience with the procedure. If the results remain equivocal, the patient should be treated medically and the evaluation repeated in 6 to 12 months.

Remember that young patients and particularly those with a family history of aldosteronism should be evaluated for glucocorticoid-remediable aldosteronism, as described earlier in this chapter. The problem of excluding adrenal hyperfunction in adrenal glands found incidentally to have a mass by abdominal CT done for other reasons is addressed in the first portion of Chapter 12.

## THERAPY

Once the type of adrenal pathology has been ascertained, surgery should be done if the diagnosis is *adenoma,* and medical therapy is indicated if the diagnosis is *bilateral hyperplasia.* Although there are reports of relief of aldosteronism by removal of a unilaterally hyperplastic gland (Mansoor et al., 2002) or one of two hyperplastic glands (Irony et al., 1990), surgery should be performed only if a solitary adrenal adenoma >1 cm is visualized by scan or if adrenal venous sampling clearly defines a unilateral source of the aldosterone hypersecretion.

## Surgical Treatment

### Preoperative Management

Once the diagnosis of adenoma is made, a 3- to 5-week course of spironolactone or eplerenone may be given to normalize the various disturbances of electrolyte composition and fluid volume, easing operative management.

### Surgical Technique

With improved preoperative diagnosis of an adenoma, laparoscopic adrenalectomy has become the procedure of choice (Meria et al., 2003) even in very obese patients (Fazeli-Matin et al., 1999) and can be done as an outpatient procedure (Gill et al., 2000).

If hyperplasia is found at surgery despite the preoperative diagnosis of an adenoma, only a unilateral adrenalectomy should be done. In view of the poor overall results with bilateral adrenalectomy and its complications, one gland should be left intact.

### Postoperative Complications

#### Hypoaldosteronism

Even if an aldosterone blocker is given preoperatively, hypoaldosteronism may develop with an inability to conserve sodium and excrete potassium. This may persist for some time analogous to the slowness of the return of cortisol production after prolonged ACTH suppression by exogenous glucocorticoids.

The aldosterone deficiency is usually not severe or prolonged and can be handled simply by providing adequate salt without the need for exogenous glucocorticoid or mineralocorticoid therapy. However, of 37 patients who underwent unilateral adrenalectomy for an adenoma, five were symptomatically hypotensive 1 year later, some with low plasma cortisol, others with low plasma aldosterone and epinephrine levels (Gordon et al., 1989).

#### Sustained Hypertension

The hypertension may persist for some time; a few patients require years for return of normal BP. In six series published between 1987 and 2001, 52% of 420 patients who had unilateral adrenalectomy for APA were improved or cured of hypertension (Plouin et al., 2004). In the series of 93 adrenalectomies, 57 laparoscopically, performed at the Mayo Clinic from 1993 to 1999 for primary aldosteronism, hypertension was improved in 95% and cured in 33% (Sawka et al., 2001). Cure was independently predicted by a negative family history of hypertension, relatively mild preoperative hypertension, and a very high preoperative ARR.

If the BP fails to respond, hyperfunctioning adrenal tissue may have been left. More likely is the presence of coincidental primary hypertension, as would be expected in at least 20% of cases, or the occurrence of significant renal damage from the prolonged secondary hypertension (Proye et al., 1998). Few patients with bilateral hyperplasia respond to unilateral (Groth et al., 1985) or even to bilateral adrenalectomy (Ferriss et al., 1978b).

### Medical Treatment

Chronic medical therapy with spironolactone or eplerenone or, if those are not tolerated, amiloride with or without a thiazide diuretic is the treatment of choice for patients with hyperplasia, patients with an adenoma who are unable or unwilling to have surgery, patients who remain hypertensive after surgery, and patients with equivocal findings (Ghose et al., 1999; Lim et al., 2001).

Spironolactone, 100 to 200 mg a day, may be needed initially, but a satisfactory response may then be maintained with as little as 50 mg a day (Ferriss et al., 1978a). The combination with a thiazide diuretic may provide better control and allow for smaller doses of spironolactone. With lower doses, side effects are generally minor, and in only 3 of 95 cases were they severe enough to lead to withdrawal of the drug (Ferriss et al., 1978a). The more selective aldosterone receptor antagonist, eplerenone, produces fewer side effects than spironolactone (Baxter et al., 2004), and it will likely be the medical therapy of choice. If additional antihypertensive therapy is needed, CCBs or angiotensin-converting enzyme inhibitors may be used (Lim et al., 2001).

The addition of an aldosterone blocker will often control resistant hypertension whether primary aldosteronism is present or not (Eide et al., 2004).

In patients with adrenal cancer, various inhibitors of steroidogenesis are useful. These are described in the next chapter in the section "Treatment of Cushing's Syndrome."

## CONCLUSIONS

Primary aldosteronism remains a fascinating disease that is more common than previously thought but less common than some now claim. Other mineralocorticoid induced forms of hypertension are covered in the next chapter.

## REFERENCES

Abdelhamid S, Blomer R, Hommel G, et al. Urinary tetrahydroaldosterone as a screening method for primary aldosteronism: a comparative study. Am J Hypertens 2003;16: 522–530.

Abdelhamid S, Müller-Lobeck, Pahl S, et al. Prevalence of adrenal and extra-adrenal Conn syndrome in hypertensive patients. Arch Intern Med 1996;156:1190–1195.

Alderman MH, Cohen HW, Sealey JE, Laragh JH. Plasma renin activity levels in hypertensive persons: their wide range and lack of suppression in diabetic and in most elderly patients. Am J Hypertens 2004;17:1–7.

Alexander GL, Thompson GB, Schwartz DA. Primary aldosteronism in a patient with familial adenomatous polyposis. Mayo Clin Proc 2000;75:636–637.

Arriza JL, Weinberger C, Cerelli G, et al. Cloning of human mineralocorticoid receptor complementary DNA: structural and functional kinship with the glucocorticoid receptor. Science 1987;237:268–275.

Barbato A, Russo P, Siani A, et al. Aldosterone synthase gene (CYP11B2) C-344T polymorphism, plasma aldosterone, renin activity and blood pressure in a multi-ethnic population. J Hypertens 2004;22:1895–1901.

Bartter FC, Pronove P, Gill JR Jr, MacCardle RC, et al. Hyperplasia of the juxtaglomerular complex with hyperaldosteronism and hypokalemic alkalosis. *Am J Med* 1962;33: 811–828.

Baxter JD, Funder JW, Apriletti JW, Webb P. Towards selectively modulating mineralocorticoid receptor function: lessons from other systems. *Mol Cell Endocrinol* 2004;217: 151–165.

Biagi P, Alessandri M, Campanella G, et al. A case of neurofibromatosis type 1 with an aldosterone-producing adenoma of the adrenal. *J Intern Med* 1999;246:509–512.

Bichet DG, Fujiwara TM. Reabsorption of sodium chloride—lessons from the chloride channels. *N Engl J Med* 2004;350: 1281–1283.

Biglieri EG, Schambelan M, Slaton PE Jr, Stockigt JR. The intercurrent hypertension of primary aldosteronism. *Circ Res* 1970;26/27(Suppl I):I195–I202.

Biglieri EG. Spectrum of mineralocorticoid hypertension. *Hypertension* 1991;17:251–261.

Bravo EL, Fouad-Tarazi FM, Tarazi RC, et al. Clinical implications of primary aldosteronism with resistant hypertension. *Hypertension* 1988;11(Suppl 1):207–211.

Bravo EL. Primary aldosteronism. Issues in diagnosis and management. *Endocrinol Metab Clin NA* 1994;23:271–283.

Calhoun DA, Nishizaka MK, Zaman MA, et al. Hyperaldosteronism among black and white subjects with resistant hypertension. *Hypertension* 2002;40:892–896.

Castro OL, Yu X, Kem DC. Diagnostic value of the post-captopril test in primary aldosteronism. *Hypertension* 2002; 39:935–938.

Ciraku I, Kailasam MT, O'Connor DT, Parmer RJ. Renal aldosterone excretion predicts early renal injury in human essential hypertension [Abstract]. *J Am Soc Nephrol* 2000; 11:345A.

Coca SG, Perazella MA, Buller GK. The cardiovascular implications of hypokalemia. *Am J Kidney Dis* 2005;45:233-247.

Conn JW, Cohen ED, Rovner DR, Nesbit RM. Normokalemic primary aldosteronism. A detectable cause of curable "essential" hypertension. *JAMA* 1965;193:200–206.

Conn JW. Part I. Painting background. Part II. Primary aldosteronism, a new clinical syndrome. *J Lab Clin Med* 1955; 43:317.

Cruz DN, Shaer AJ, Bia MJ, et al. Gitelman's syndrome revisited. *Kidney Int* 2001;59:710–717.

Davies E, Kenyon CJ. CYP11β2 polymorphisms and cardiovascular risk factors. *J Hypertens* 2003;21:1249–1253.

Davis WW, Newsome HH Jr, Wright LD Jr, et al. Bilateral adrenal hyperplasia as a cause of primary aldosteronism with hypertension, hypokalemia and suppressed renin activity. *Am J Med* 1967;42:642–647.

Disse-Nicodème S, Achard JM, Desitter I, et al. A new locus on chromosome 12p13.3 for pseudohypoaldosteronism type II, an autosomal dominant form of hypertension. *Am J Hum Genet* 2000;67:302–310.

Dluhy RG, Lifton RP. Glucocorticoid-remediable aldosteronism. *J Clin Endocrinol Metab* 1999;84:4341–4344.

Dluhy RG, Williams GH. Primary aldosteronism in a hypertensive acromegalic patient. *J Clin Endocrinol* 1969;29: 1319–1324.

Doppman JL, Gill JR Jr. Hyperaldosteronism: sampling of adrenal veins. *Radiology* 1996;198:309–312.

Douma S, Petidis K, Vogiatzis K, Zamboulis C. The aldosterone/PRA ratio (ARR) application in the diagnosis of primary aldosteronism [Abstract]. *J Hypertens* 2001;19 (Suppl 2): S12.

Dunn PJ, Espiner EA. Outpatient screening tests for primary aldosteronism. *Aust NZ J Med* 1976;6:131–135.

Eide IK, Torjesen PA, Drolsum A, et al. Low-renin status in therapy-resistant hypertension: a clue to efficient treatment.

*J Hypertens* 2004;22:2217–2226.

Espiner EA, Ross DG, Yandle TG, et al. Predicting surgically remedial primary aldosteronism: role of adrenal scanning, posture testing, and adrenal vein sampling. *J Clin Endocrinol Metab* 2003;88:3637–3644.

Fallo F, Pilon C, Williams TA, et al. Coexistence of different phenotypes in a family with glucocorticoid-remediable aldosteronism. *J Human Hypertens* 2004;18:47–51.

Fardella CE, Mosso L, Gomez-Sanchez C, et al. Primary aldosteronism in essential hypertensives: prevalence, biochemical profile and molecular biology. *J Clin Endocrinol Metab* 2000;85:1863–1867.

Farman N, Rafestin-Oblin M-E. Multiple aspects of mineralocorticoid sensitivity. *Am J Physiol Renal Physiol* 2001; 280:F181–F192.

Fazeli-Matin S, Gill IS, Hsu THS, et al. Laparoscopic renal and adrenal surgery in obese patients: comparison to open surgery. *J Urol* 1999;162:665–669.

Ferrari P, Bonny O. Forms of mineralocorticoid hypertension. *Vitamins & Hormones* 2003;66:113–156.

Ferrari P, Shaw SG, Nicod J, et al. Active renin versus plasma renin activity to define aldosterone-to-renin ratio for primary aldosteronism. *J Hypertens* 2004;22:377–381.

Ferriss JB, Beevers DG, Boddy K, et al. The treatment of low-renin ("primary") hyperaldosteronism. *Am Heart J* 1978a; 96:97–109.

Ferriss JB, Beevers DG, Brown JJ, et al. Clinical, biochemical and pathological features of low-renin ("primary") hyperaldosteronism. *Am Heart J* 1978b;95:375–388.

Ferriss JB, Brown JJ, Fraser R, et al. Primary aldosterone excess: Conn's syndrome and similar disorders. In: JIS Robertson, ed. *Handbook of Hypertension*. Vol. 2, Clinical Aspects of Secondary Hypertension. New York: Elsevier, 1983.

Ferriss JB, Brown JJ, Fraser R, et al. Hypertension with aldosterone excess and low plasma-renin: preoperative distinction between patients with and without adrenocortical tumour. *Lancet* 1970;2:995–1000.

Fogari R, Preti P, Mugellini A, et al. Prevalence of primary aldosteronism among hypertensive patients [Abstract]. *J Hypertens* 2003;21(Suppl 4):S142.

Francis IR, Gross MD, Shapiro B, et al. Integrated imaging of adrenal disease. *Radiology* 1992;184:113.

Freel EM, Connell JM. Mechanisms of hypertension: the expanding role of aldosterone. *J Am Soc Nephrol* 2004;15: 1993–2001

Furuhashi M, Kitamura K, Adachi M, et al. Liddle's syndrome caused by a novel mutation in the proline-rich PY motif of the epithelial sodium channel β-subunit. *J Clin Endocrinol Metab* 2005;90:340–344.

Ganguly A, Dowdy AJ, Luetscher JA, Melada GA. Anomalous postural response of plasma aldosterone concentration in patients with aldosterone-producing adrenal adenoma. *J Clin Endocrinol Metab* 1973;36:401–404.

Gates LJ, Benjamin N, Haites NE, et al. Is random screening of value in detecting glucocorticoid-remediable aldosteronism within a hypertensive population? *J Hum Hypertens* 2001;15:173–176.

Geller DS, Farhl A, Pinkerton N, et al. Activating mineralocorticoid receptor mutation in hypertension exacerbated by pregnancy. *Science* 2000;289:119–123.

Ghose RP, Hall PM, Bravo EL. Medical management of aldosterone-producing adenomas. *Ann Intern Med* 1999;131: 105–108.

Gicquel C, Leblond-Francillard M, Bertagna X, et al. Clonal analysis of human adrenocortical carcinomas and secreting adenomas. *Clin Endocrinol (Oxf)* 1994;40:465–477.

Giebisch G. Renal potassium transport: mechanisms and regulation. *Am J Physiol* 1998;274:F817–F833.

Gifford RW Jr. Evaluation of the hypertensive patient with emphasis on detecting curable causes. *Milbank Mem Fund Q* 1969;47:170–186.

Gill IS, Hobart MG, Schweizer D, Bravo EL. Outpatient adrenalectomy. *J Urol* 2000;163:717–720.

Girerd X, Villeveuve F, Lemaire A, et al. A clinical prediction rule for primary aldosteronism in drug-resistant hypertensive patients referred to an hypertension clinic [Abstract]. *J Hypertens* 2003;21(Suppl 4):S145.

Gitelman HJ, Graham JB, Welt LG. A new familial disorder characterized by hypokalemia and hypomagnesemia. *Trans Assoc Am Phys* 1966;79:221–235.

Glodny B, Kühle C, Cromme S, et al. An assessment of diagnostic procedures preparatory to retroperitoneoscopic removal of adenoma in cases of primary hyperaldosteronism. *Endo J* 2000;47:657–665.

Goldkorn R, Yurenev A, Blumenfeld J, et al. Echocardiographic comparison of left ventricular structure and function in hypertensive patients with primary aldosteronism and essential hypertension. *Am J Hypertens* 2002;15:340–345.

Gomez-Sanchez CE, Montgomery M, Ganguly A, et al. Elevated urinary excretion of 18-oxocortisol in glucocorticoid-suppressible aldosteronism. *J Clin Endocrinol Metab* 1984;59:1022–1024.

Gordon RD, Hawkins PG, Hamlet SM, et al. Reduced adrenal secretory mass after unilateral adrenalectomy for aldosterone-producing adenoma may explain unexpected incidence of hypotension. *J Hypertens* 1989;7(Suppl 6):210–211.

Gordon RD, Klemm SA, Stowasser M, et al. How common is primary aldosteronism? Is it the most frequent cause of curable hypertension? *Curr Sci* 1993;11(Suppl 5):S310–S311.

Gordon RD, Stowasser M, Klemm SA, Tunny TJ. Primary aldosteronismsome genetic, morphological, and biochemical aspects of subtypes. *Steroids* 1995;60:35–41.

Gordon RD. Syndrome of hypertension and hyperkalemia with normal glomerular filtration rate. *Hypertension* 1986;8:93–102.

Gordon RD. The challenge of more robust and reproducible methodology in screening for primary aldosteronism. *J Hypertens* 2004;22:251–255.

Grimes DA, Schulz KF. Uses and abuses of screening tests. *Lancet* 2002;359:881–884.

Groth H, Vetter W, Stimpel M, et al. Adrenalectomy in primary aldosteronism: a long-term follow-up study. *Cardiology* 1985;72(Suppl 1):107–116.

Guthrie GP Jr, Genest J, Nowaczynski W, et al. Dissociation of plasma renin activity and aldosterone in essential hypertension. *J Clin Endocrinol Metab* 1976;43:446–448.

Halperin ML, Kamel KS. Potassium. *Lancet* 1998;352:135–140.

Hamilton BP, Zadik Z, Edwin CM, et al. Effect of adrenal suppression with dexamethasone in essential hypertension. *J Clin Endocrinol Metab* 1979;48:848–853.

Hiramatsu K, Yamada T, Yukimura Y, et al. A screening test to identify aldosterone-producing adenoma by measuring plasma renin activity. Results in hypertensive patients. *Arch Intern Med* 1981;141:1589–1593.

Hirohara D, Nomura K, Okamoto T, et al. Performance of the basal aldosterone to renin ratio and of the renin stimulation test by furosemide and upright posture in screening for aldosterone-producing adenoma in low renin hypertensives. *J Clin Endocrinol Metab* 2001;86:4292–4298.

Hollak CEM, Prummel MF, Tiel-Van Buul MMC. Bilateral adrenal tumours in primary aldosteronism: localization of a unilateral aldosteronoma by dexamethasone suppression scan. *J Intern Med* 1991;229:545–548.

Holland OB, Brown H, Kuhnert L, et al. Further evaluation of saline infusion for the diagnosis of primary aldosteronism. *Hypertension* 1984;6:717–723.

Hood S, Cannon J, Scanlon M, Brown MJ. Prevalence of primary hyperaldosteronism measured by aldosterone to renin ratio and spironolactone testing: Pharst study [Abstract]. *J Hypertens* 2002;20(Suppl 4):S119.

Huang Y-Y, Hsu BR-S, Tsai J-S. Paralytic myopathy—a leading clinical presentation for primary aldosteronism in Taiwan. *J Clin Endocrinol Metab* 1996;81:4038–4041.

Hyman D, Kaplan NM. The difference between serum and plasma potassium. *N Engl J Med* 1985;313:642.

Irony I, Kater CE, Biglieri EG, Shackleton CHL. Correctable subsets of primary aldosteronism. Primary adrenal hyperplasia and renin responsive adenoma. *Am J Hypertens* 1990;3:576–582.

Jackson RV, Lafferty A, Torpy DJ, Stratakis AC. New genetic insights in familial hyperaldosteronism. *Ann NY Acad Sci* 2002;970:77–88.

Jamieson A, Slutsker L, Inglis GC, et al. Glucocorticoid-suppressible hyperaldosteronism: effects of crossover site and parental origin of chimaeric gene on phenotypic expression. *Clin Sci* 1995;88:563–570.

Jeck N, Waldegger S, Lampert A, et al. Activating mutation of the renal epithelial chloride channel C1C-Kb predisposing to hypertension. *Hypertension* 2004;43:1175–1181.

Kanauchi H, Wada N, Ginzinger DG, et al. Diagnostic and prognostic value of fas and telomeric-repeat binding factor-1 genes in adrenal tumors. *J Clin Endocrinol Metab* 2003;88:3690–3693.

Kaplan NM. Primary aldosteronism with malignant hypertension. *N Engl J Med* 1963;269:1282–1286.

Kaplan NM. Hypokalemia in the hypertensive patient. With observation on the incidence of primary aldosteronism. *Ann Intern Med* 1967;66:1079–1090.

Kaplan NM. Primary aldosteronism. In: EB Astwood, CE Cassidy, eds. *Clinical Endocrinology,* Vol. 2. New York: Grune & Stratton, 1968.

Kaplan NM. The current epidemic of primary aldosteronism: causes and consequences. *J Hypertens* 2004;22:863–869.

Kato J, Etoh T, Kitamura K, Eto T. Atrial and brain natriuretic peptides as markers of cardiac load and volume retention in primary aldosteronism. *Am J Hypertens* 2005;18:354–357.

Keely E. Endocrine causes of hypertension in pregnancy—when to start looking for zebras. *Sem Perinatol* 1998;22:471–484.

Kem DC, Weinberger MH, Mayes DM, Nugent CA. Saline suppression of plasma aldosterone in hypertension. *Arch Intern Med* 1971;128:380–386.

Kulkarni JN, Mistry RC, Jamat MR, et al. Autonomous aldosterone-secreting ovarian tumor. *Gynecol Oncol* 1990;37:284–289.

Lack EE, Travis WD, Oertel JE. Adrenal cortical nodules, hyperplasia, and hyperfunction. In: EE Lack, ed. *Contemporary Issues in Surgical Pathology.* Vol. 14, Pathology of the Adrenal Glands. New York: Churchill Livingstone, 1990.

Lamarre-Cliche M, de Champlain J, Lacourcière Y, et al. Effects of circadian rhythms, posture, and medication on renin-aldosterone interrelations in essential hypertensives. *Am J Hypertens* 2005;18:56–64.

Lauzurica R, Bonal J, Bonet J, et al. Rhabdomyolysis, oedema and arterial hypertension: different syndromes related to topical use of 9-alpha-fluoroprednisolone. *J Hum Hypertens* 1988;2:183–186.

Liddle GW, Bledsoe T, Coppage WS Jr. A familial renal disorder simulating primary aldosteronism but with negligible aldosterone secretion. *Trans Assoc Am Phys* 1963;76: 199–213.

Lifton RP, Dluhy RG, Powers M, et al. Hereditary hypertension caused by chimaeric gene duplications and ectopic expression of aldosterone synthase. *Nature Genet* 1992;2: 66–74.

Lim PO, Brennan G, Jung RT, MacDonald TM. High prevalence of primary aldosteronism in the Tayside hypertension clinic population. *J Hum Hypertens* 2000;14:311–315.

Lim PO, MacDonald TM, Holloway C, et al. Variation of the aldosterone synthase (CYP11β2) locus contributes to hypertension in subjects with a raised aldosterone-to-renin ratio. *J Clin Endocrinol Metab* 2002a;87:4398–4402.

Lim PO, Rodgers P, Cardale K, et al. Potentially high prevalence of primary aldosteronism in a primary-care population. *Lancet* 1999;353:40.

Lim PO, Struthers AD, MacDonald TM. The neurohormonal natural history of essential hypertension: towards primary or tertiary aldosteronism? *J Hypertens* 2002b;20:11–15.

Lim PO, Young WF, MacDonald TM. A review of the medical treatment of primary aldosteronism. *J Hypertens* 2001;19: 353–361.

Lin SH, Shiang JC, Huang CC, et al. Phenotype and genotype analysis in Chinese patients with Gitelman's syndrome. *J Clin Endocrinol Metab* 2005;90:2500–2507.

Litchfield WR, Coolidge C, Silva P, et al. Impaired potassium-stimulated aldosterone production: a possible explanation for normokalemia in glucocorticoid-remediable aldosteronism. *J Clin Endocrinol Metab* 1997;82:1507–1510.

Litynski M. Nadcisnienie tetnicze wywolane guzami korowo-nad-nerczowymi. *Pol Tyg Lek* 1953;8:204–208.

Loh K-C, Koay ES, Khaw M-C, et al. Prevalence of primary aldosteronism among Asian hypertensive patients in Singapore. *J Clin Endocrinol Metab* 2000;85:2854–2859.

Magill SB, Raff H, Shaker JL, et al. Comparison of adrenal vein sampling and computed tomography in the differentiation of primary aldosteronism. *J Clin Endocrinol Metab* 2001;86:1066–1071.

Maki N, Komatsuda A, Wakui H, et al. Four novel mutations in the thiazide-sensitive Na-Cl co-transporter gene in Japanese patients with Gitelman's syndrome. *Nephrol Dial Transplant* 2004;19:1761–1766.

Man in't Veld AJ, Wenting GJ, Schalekamp MADH. Distribution of extracellular fluid over the intra- and extravascular space in hypertensive patients. *J Cardiovasc Pharmacol* 1984;6:S143–S150.

Mansoor GA, Malchoff CD, Arici MH, et al. Unilateral adrenal hyperplasia causing primary aldosteronism: limitations of I-131 norcholesterol scanning. *Am J Hypertens* 2002;15:459–464.

McAlister FA, Lewanczuk RZ. Primary hyperaldosteronism and adrenal incidentaloma: an argument for physiologic testing before adrenalectomy. *Can J Surg* 1998;41:299–305.

McAreavey D, Murray GD, Lever AF, Robertson JIS. Similarity of idiopathic aldosteronism and essential hypertension. *Hypertension* 1983;5:116–121.

Meria P, Kempf BF, Hermieu JF, et al. Laparoscopic management of primary hyperaldosteronism: clinical experience with 212 cases. *J Urol* 2003;169:32–35.

Milliez P, Girerd X, Plouin PF, et al. Evidence for an increased rate of cardiovascular events in patients with primary aldosteronism. *J Am Coll Cardiol* 2005;45:1243–1248.

Montori VM, Schwartz GL, Chapman AB, et al. Validity of the aldosterone-renin ratio used to screen for primary aldosteronism. *Mayo Clin Proc* 2001;76:877–882.

Montori VM, Young WF Jr. Use of plasma aldosterone concentration-to-plasma renin activity ratio as a screening

test for primary aldosteronism: a systematic review of the literature. *Endocrinol Metab Clin NA* 2002;31:619–632.

Mosso L, Carvajal C, Gonzalez A, et al. Primary aldosteronism and hypertensive disease. *Hypertension* 2003;42:161–165.

Mulatero P, Rabbia F, Milan A, et al. Drug effects on aldosterone/plasma renin activity ratio in primary aldosteronism. *Hypertension* 2002;40:897–902.

Mulatero P, Schiavone D, Fallo F, et al. CYP11B2 gene polymorphisms in idiopathic hyperaldosteronism. *Hypertension* 2000;35:694–698.

Mulatero P, Stowasser M, Loh K-C, et al. Increased diagnosis of primary aldosteronism, including surgically correctable forms, in centers from five continents. *J Clin Endocrinol Metab* 2004;89:1045–1050.

Murakami T, Ogura EW, Tanaka Y, Yamamoto M. High blood pressure lowered by pregnancy. *Lancet* 2000;356:1980.

Nakahama H, Fukuchi K, Yoshihara F, et al. Efficacy of screening for primary aldosteronism by adrenocortical scintigraphy without discontinuing antihypertensive medication. *Am J Hypertens* 2003;16:725–728.

Nicod J, Bruhin D, Auer L, et al. A biallelic gene polymorphism of CYP11β2 predicts increased aldosterone to renin ratio in selected hypertensive patients. *J Clin Endocrinol Metab* 2003;88:2495–2500.

Nishikawa T, Omura T. Clinical characteristics of primary aldosteronism: its prevalence and comparative studies on various causes of primary aldosteronism in Yokohama Rosai Hospital. *Biomed Pharmacother* 2000;54(Suppl 1):83–85.

Nishizaka MK, Zaman MA, Green SA, et al. Impaired endothelin-dependent flow-mediated vasodilation in hypertensive subjects with hyperaldosteronism. *Circulation* 2004; 109:2857–2861.

Oberleithner H. Aldosterone makes human endothelium stiff and vulnerable. *Kidney Int* 2005;67:1680–1682.

Oelkers W, Diederich S, Bähr V. Primary hyperaldosteronism without suppressed renin due to secondary hypertensive kidney damage. *J Clin Endocrinol Metab* 2000;85: 3266–3270.

Olivieri O, Ciacciarelli A, Signorelli D, et al. Aldosterone to renin ratio in a primary care setting: the Bussolengo study. *J Clin Endocrinol Metab* 2004;89:4221–4226.

Opocher G, Rocco S, Carpenéa G, et al. Usefulness of atrial natriuretic peptide assay in primary aldosteronism. *Am J Hypertens* 1992;5:811–816.

Perschel FH, Schemer R, Seiler L, et al. Rapid screening test for primary hyperaldosteronism: ratio of plasma aldosterone to renin concentration determined by fully automated chemiluminescence immunoassays. *Clin Chem* 2004;50: 1650–1655.

Phillips JL, Walther MM, Pezzullo JC, et al. Predictive value of preoperative tests in discriminating bilateral adrenal hyperplasia from an aldosterone-producing adrenal adenoma. *J Clin Endocrinol Metab* 2000;85:4526–4533.

Pilon C, Mulatero P, Barzon L, et al. Mutations in CYP11B1 gene converting 11β-hydroxylase into an aldosterone-producing enzyme are not present in aldosterone-producing adenomas. *J Clin Endocrinol Metab* 1999;84:4228–4231.

Plouin P-F, Amar L, Chatellier G. Trends in the prevalence of primary aldosteronism, aldosterone-producing adenomas, and surgically correctable aldosterone-dependent hypertension. The COMETE-Conn Study Group. *Nephrol Dial Transplant* 2004;19:774–777.

Proye CAG, Mulliez EAR, Carnaille BML, et al. Essential hypertension: first reason for persistent hypertension after unilateral adrenalectomy for primary aldosteronism? *Surgery* 1998;124:1128–1133.

Radin DR, Manoogian C, Nadler JL. Diagnosis of primary hyperaldosteronism: importance of correlating CT findings with endocrinologic studies. *Am J Roentgenol* 1992; 158:553–557.

Rajput C, Makhijani K, Norboo T, et al. CYP11B2 gene polymorphisms and hypertension in highlanders accustomed to high salt intake. *J Hypertens* 2005;23:79–86.

Rayner BL, Opie LH, Davidson JS. The aldosterone/renin ratio as a screening test for primary aldosteronism. *S Afr Med J* 2000;90:394–400.

Rocha R, Funder JW. The pathophysiology of aldosterone in the cardiovascular system. *Ann NY Acad Sci* 2002;970: 89–100.

Rossi E, Regolisti G, Negro A, et al. High prevalence of primary aldosteronism using postcaptopril plasma aldosterone to renin ratio as a screening test among Italian hypertensives. *Am J Hypertens* 2002;15:896–902.

Rossi GP, Di Bello V, Banzaroli C, et al. Excess aldosterone is associated with alterations of myocardial texture in primary aldosteronism. *Hypertension* 2002;40:23–27.

Rossi GP, Sacchetto A, Chiesura-Corona M, et al. Identification of the etiology of primary aldosteronism with adrenal vein sampling in patients with equivocal computed tomography and magnetic resonance findings. *J Clin Endocrinol Metab* 2001;86:1083–1090.

Sawka AM, Young WF Jr, Thompson GB, et al. Primary aldosteronism: factors associated with normalization of blood pressure after surgery. *Ann Intern Med* 2001;135:258–261.

Schmidt BMW, Oehmer S, Delles C, et al. Rapid nongenomic effects of aldosterone on human forearm vasculature. *Hypertension* 2003;42:156–160.

Schwartz GL, Chapman AB, Boerwinkle E, et al. Screening for primary aldosteronism: implications of an increased plasma aldosterone/renin ratio. *Clin Chem* 2002;48:1919–1923.

Seccia TM, Fassina A, Nussdorfer GG, et al. Conn's syndrome caused by aldosterone-producing adrenocortical carcinoma: report of two divergent cases and a meta-analysis of all reported cases since 1955 [Abstract]. *Am J Hypertens* 2003;16(5 patient 2):167A–168A.

Seifarth C, Trenkel S, Schobel H, et al. Influence of antihypertensive medication on aldosterone and renin concentration in the differential diagnosis of essential hypertension and primary aldosteronism. *Clin Endocrinol* 2002;57:457–465.

Seiler L, Rump LC, Schulte-Mönting J, et al. Diagnosis of primary aldosteronism: value of different screening parameters and influence of antihypertensive medication. *Eur J Endocrinol* 2004;150:329–337.

Shapiro B, Grekin R, Gross MD, Freitas JE. Interference by spironolactone on adrenocortical scintigraphy and other pitfalls in the location of adrenal abnormalities in primary aldosteronism. *Clin Nucl Med* 1994;19:441–445.

Shimamoto K, Shiiki M, Ise T, et al. Does insulin resistance participate in an impaired glucose tolerance in primary aldosteronism? *J Hum Hypertens* 1994;8:755–759.

Shionoiri H, Hirawa N, Ueda S-I, et al. Renin gene expression in the adrenal and kidney of patients with primary aldosteronism. *J Clin Endocrinol Metab* 1992;74:103–107.

Sinclair AM, Isles CG, Brown I, et al. Secondary hypertension in a blood pressure clinic. *Arch Intern Med* 1987;147: 1289–1293.

Solomon CG, Thiet M-P, Moore F Jr, Seely EW. Primary hyperaldosteronism in pregnancy. A case report. *J Reprod Med* 1996;41:255–258.

Sosa León LA, McKinley MJ, McAllen RM, May CN. Aldosterone acts on the kidney, not the brain, to cause mineralocorticoid hypertension in sheep. *J Hypertens* 2002;20: 1203–1208.

Spark RF, Melby JC. Aldosteronism in hypertension. The spironolactone response test. *Ann Intern Med* 1968;69: 685–691.

Stewart PM. Mineralocorticoid hypertension. *Lancet* 1999; 353:1341–1347.

Stokes JB. Understanding how aldosterone increases sodium transport. *Am J Kidney Diseases* 2000;36:866–870.

Stowasser M, Bachmann, AW, Huggard PR, et al. Treatment of familial hyperaldosteronism type I: only partial suppression of adrenocorticotropin required to correct hypertension. *J Clin Endocrinol Metab* 2000;85:3313–3318.

Stowasser M, Gordon RD. Primary aldosteronism: learning from the study of familial varteties. *J Hypertens* 2000;18: 1165–1176.

Stowasser M, Gordon RD, Gunasekera TG, et al. High rate of detection of primary aldosteronism, including surgically treatable forms, after "non-selective" screening of hypertensive patients. *J Hypertens* 2003;21:2149–2157.

Stowasser M. How common is adrenal-based mineralocorticoid hypertension? *Curr Opin Endocrinol Diabetes* 2000; 7:143–150.

Strauch B, Zelinka T, Hampf M, et al. Prevalence of primary hyperaldosteronism in moderate to severe hypertension in the Central Europe region. *J Human Hypertens* 2003;17: 349–352.

Sutherland DJA, Ruse JL, Laidlaw JC. Hypertension, increased aldosterone secretion and low plasma renin activity relieved by dexamethasone. *Can Med Assoc J* 1966;95: 1109–1119.

Suzuki Y, Nakada T, Izumi T, et al. Primary aldosteronism due to aldosterone producing adenoma without hypertension. *J Urol* 1999;161:1272.

Takeda Y, Furukawa K, Inaba S, et al. Genetic analysis of aldosterone synthase in patients with idiopathic hyperaldosteronism. *J Clin Endocrinol Metab* 1999;84:1633–1637.

Tanabe A, Naruse M, Takagi S, et al. Variability in the renin/aldosterone profile under random and standardized sampling conditions in primary aldosteronism. *J Clin Endocrinol Metab* 2003;88:2489–2494.

Thibonnier M, Sassano P, Joseph A, et al. Diagnostic value of a single dose of captopril in renin- and aldosterone-dependent, surgically curable hypertension. *Cardiovasc Rev Rep* 1982;3:1659–1667.

Tiu S-C, Choi C-H, Shek C-C, et al. The use of aldosterone-renin ratio as a diagnostic test for primary hyperaldosteronism and its test characteristics under different conditions of blood sampling. *J Clin Endocrinol Metab* 2005;90:72–78.

Torres VE, Young WF Jr, Offord KP, Hattery RR. Association of hypokalemia, aldosteronism, and renal cysts. *N Engl J Med* 1990;322:345–351.

Touitou Y, Boissonnas A, Bogdan A, Auzéby A. Concurrent adrenocortical carcinoma and Conn's adenoma in a man with primary hyperaldosteronism. *In vivo* and *in vitro* studies. *Acta Endocrinol* 1992;127:189–192.

Tracy RE, White S. A method of quantifying adrenocortical nodular hyperplasia at autopsy: some use of the method in illuminating hypertension and atherosclerosis. *Ann Diagn Pathol* 2002;6:20–29.

Ulick S, Blumenfeld JD, Atlas SA, et al. The unique steroidogenesis of the aldosteronoma in the differential diagnosis of primary aldosteronism. *J Clin Endocrinol Metab* 1993; 76:873–878.

Ulick S, Chan CK, Gill JR Jr, et al. Defective fasciculata zone function as the mechanism of glucocorticoid-remediable aldosteronism. *J Clin Endocrinol Metab* 1990;71:1151–1157.

Ulick S, Chu MD, Land M. Biosynthesis of 18-oxocortisol by aldosterone-producing adrenal tissue. *J Biol Chem* 1983; 258:5498–5502.

Vantyghem M-C, Ronci N, Provost F, et al. Aldosterone-producing adenoma without hypertension: a report of two cases. *Eur J Endocrinol* 1999;141:279–285.

Vasan RS, Evan JC, Larson MG, et al. Serum aldosterone and the incidence of hypertension in nonhypertensive persons. *N Engl J Med* 2004;351:33–41.

Walker BR. Defective enzyme-mediated receptor protection: novel mechanisms in the pathophysiology of hypertension. *Clin Sci* 1993;85:257–263.

Wenting GJ, Man in't Veld AJ, Derkx FHM, Schalekamp MADH. Recurrence of hypertension in primary aldosteronism after discontinuation of spironolactone. Time course of changes in cardiac output and body fluid volumes. *Clin Exp Hypertens* 1982;4:1727–1748.

White PC. Aldosterone: direct effects on and production by the heart. *J Clin Endocrinol Metab* 2003;88:2376–2383.

Wiederkehr MR, Moe OW. Factitious hyperkalemia. *Am J Kidney Diseases* 2000;36:1049–1053.

Williams ED, Boddy K, Brown JJ, et al. Body elemental composition, with particular reference to total and exchangeable sodium and potassium and total chlorine, in untreated and treated primary hyperaldosteronism. *J Hypertens* 1984;2:171–176.

Wu F, Bagg W, Drury PL. Progression of accelerated hypertension in untreated primary aldosteronism. *Aust NZ J Med* 2000;30:91.

Wyckoff JA, Seely EW, Hurwitz S, et al. Glucocorticoid-remediable aldosteronism and pregnancy. *Hypertension* 2000; 35:668–672.

Yokota N, Bruneau BG, Kuroski de Bold ML, de Bold AJ. Atrial natriuretic factor significantly contributes to the mineralocorticoid escape phenomenon: evidence of a guanylate cyclase-mediated pathway. *J Clin Invest* 1994;94: 1938–1946.

Young DB, Ma G. Vascular protective effects of potassium. *Sem Nephrol* 1999;19:477–486.

Young WF Jr. Primary aldosteronism: management issues. *Ann NY Acad Sci* 2002;970:61–76.

Young WF Jr. Minireview: primary aldosteronism—changing concepts in diagnosis and treatment. *Endocrinology* 2003;144:2208–2213.

Young WF Jr, Stanson AW, Thompson GB, et al. Role for adrenal venous sampling in primary aldosteronism. *Surgery* 2004;136:1227–1235.

Zarifis J, Lip GY, Leatherdale B, Beevers G. Malignant hypertension in association with primary aldosteronism. *Blood Pressure* 1996;5:250–254.

Zelinka T, Štrauch B, Pecen L, Widimský J Jr. Diurnal blood pressure variation in pheochromocytoma, primary aldosteronism and Cushing's syndrome. *J Human Hypertens* 2004; 18:107–111.

# Hypertension Induced by Cortisol or Deoxycorticosterone

T he preceding chapter described the syndromes of hypertension induced by primary aldosterone excess. This chapter will cover syndromes in which hypertension is induced by other adrenal steroids: *cortisol,* either in excess (Cushing's syndrome) or with increased binding to mineralocorticoid receptors (apparent mineralocorticoid excess and licorice ingestion); or *deoxycorticosterone* (congenital adrenal hyperplasias).

## CUSHING'S SYNDROME

### Significance

Although Cushing's syndrome is rare, it often must be suspected in the growing number of patients with the metabolic syndrome who have abdominal obesity, glucose intolerance, and hypertension (Findling et al., 2004). Moreover, as milder and cyclical forms of Cushing's syndrome have been recognized (van Aken et al., 2005), the laboratory confirmation of the diagnosis has become more difficult despite the availability of better hormonal assays (Arnaldi et al., 2003).

When present, Cushing's syndrome is a serious disease. Hypertension is present in more than 80%

of patients with Cushing's syndrome (Arnaldi et al., 2003), is often difficult to treat (Fallo et al., 1993), and contributes to a mortality rate, even after successful therapy, that is almost four times above that of an age- and sex-matched population (Lindholm et al., 2001).

### Pathophysiology

Cushing's syndrome is caused either by excess endogenous cortisol with the idiopathic form or excess exogenous steroids in the iatrogenic form. The idiopathic disease may be either adrenocorticotropic hormone (ACTH) dependent or independent (Table 14–1; Figure 14–1). The most common type, termed Cushing's disease, is due to overproduction of ACTH from a pituitary microadenoma with resultant diffuse bilateral adrenal hyperplasia. Ectopic ACTH production may come from multiple types of tumors, the largest number being malignant small-cell carcinomas of the lung (Boscaro et al., 2001). In addition, adrenocortical cells may harbor "illegitimate" receptors, responding to unusual ligands (Lacroix et al., 2001).

ACTH-independent forms are mostly benign adrenal adenomas or malignant carcinomas, but various forms of hyperplasia may pose diagnostic difficulty. As noted in Chapter 12, the number of adrenal tumors found incidentally by abdominal computed tomography (CT) or magnetic resonance imaging (MRI) is increasing. As many as 20% of these "incidentalomas" secrete cortisol in a partially unregulated manner, often in association with

## TABLE 14–1

### Prevalence of Various Types of Cushing's Syndrome in Three Separate Series (in percentages)

| Reference:<br>No. Patients: | Orth, 1995<br>630 | Newell-Price, et al., 1998<br>306 | Boscaro et al., 2000<br>302 |
|---|---|---|---|
| **ATCH–dependent** | | | |
| Pituitary ACTH (Cushing's disease) | 68 | 68 | 66 |
| Ectopic ACTH syndrome | 12 | 10 | 7 |
| Ectopic CRH syndrome | <1 | 5 | <1 |
| Macronodular adrenal hyperplasia | | | 2 |
| **ACTH–independent** | | | |
| Adrenal adenoma | 10 | 8 | 18 |
| Adrenal carcinoma | 8 | 7 | 6 |
| Micronodular hyperplasia | 1 | 2 | <1 |
| Adrenal hyperplasia from other stimuli<br>(e.g., gastric inhibitory polypeptide) | <1 | | <1 |
| Exogenous glucocorticoid intake | | | |

hypertension, diabetes, and generalized obesity (Rossi et al., 2000).

A number of interesting variants have been reported, including:

- Spontaneously remitting disease (Ishibashi et al., 1993);
- Cyclic or periodic disease (Boscaro et al., 2000; van Aken et al., 2005);
- Association with overt hypothalamic disorders (Stewart et al., 1992);
- Transition from pituitary-dependent to pituitary-independent disease (Hermus et al., 1988);
- ACTH-independent bilateral macronodular hyperplasia, which is often massive (Doppman et al., 2000), may be familial (Lieberman et al., 1994), and may be associated with the expression of ectopic receptors for various hormones including the gastric inhibitory polypeptide (GIP), vasopressin, β-adrenergic agonists, LH/human CG or serotonin 5-HT$_4$ (Lacroix et al., 2001). Such receptors are occasionally found in adrenal adenomas as well.
- Pigmented micronodular dysplasia, in most cases as part of the autosomal dominant familial syndrome with cardiac and skin myxomas, the Carney complex (Malchoff, 2000);
- Association with pheochromocytoma (Amos & McRoberts, 1998), chemodectoma, and carcinoid tumors (Tremble et al., 2000); and

- Increased sensitivity of peripheral glucocorticoid receptors causing clinical features without increased levels of cortisol (van Rossum & Lamberts, 2004).

### Hypertension with Glucocorticoid Excess

Hypertension is present in about 80% of patients with Cushing's syndrome. It may be severe; in the series of Ross and Linch (1982), 10 of 70 patients had blood pressure (BP) exceeding 200/120 mm Hg, and all but one of these patients died, despite treatment of the Cushing's syndrome. Among all 70 patients, 55% had an abnormal electrocardiogram and 28% had cardiomegaly. The severity of the hypertension may be related to the abolition of the normal nocturnal fall in BP seen after exogenous glucocorticoid administration and in patients with Cushing's syndrome (Zelinka et al., 2004). The longer the duration of hypertension, the greater the likelihood that it will persist after relief of the syndrome (Suzuki et al., 2000).

Hypertension is relatively rare in patients who take exogenous glucocorticoids (Sato et al., 1995), because of the use of steroid derivatives with less mineralocorticoid activity than cortisol. However, significant rises of BP can occur within 5 days of fairly high doses of cortisol (Whitworth et al., 2000) or dexamethasone (Brotman et al., 2005).

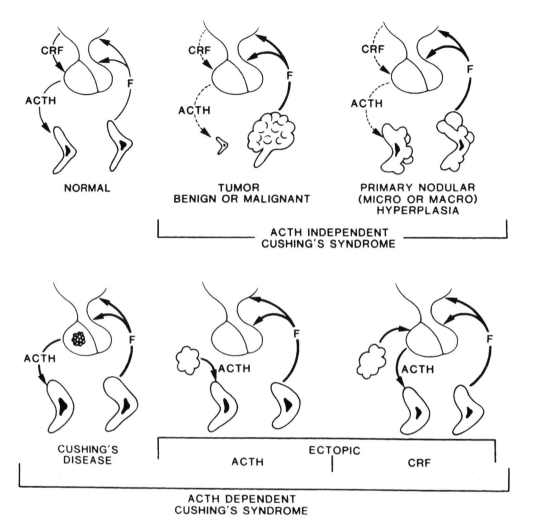

**FIGURE 14–1** ● Causes of endogenous Cushing's syndrome. The lesions of the *top* arise within the adrenal. Those in the *bottom* arise within the pituitary (Cushing's disease) or from ectopic production of ACTH or corticotropin-releasing factor (CRF). F, cortisol. (Reprinted with permission from Carpenter PC. Diagnostic evaluation of Cushing's syndrome. *Endocrinol Metab Clin NA* 1988;17:445–472.)

## Mechanisms for the Hypertension

Multiple mechanisms may be responsible for the hypertension so common in Cushing's syndrome (Whitworth et al., 2000). The mechanisms may include:

- A sodium-retaining action of the high levels of *cortisol*, through binding to either mineralocorticoid receptors or nonreceptor mechanisms (Montrella-Waybill et al., 1991). Although cortisol is 300 times less potent a mineralocorticoid than is aldosterone, 200 times more cortisol is normally secreted; and this level is increased by two times or more in Cushing's syndrome. With high levels of cortisol, the 11β-hydroxysteroid dehydrogenase 2 (11β-HSD2) capacity to convert cortisol to

cortisone is overwhelmed, allowing cortisol to act on mineralocorticoid receptors (Quinkler & Stewart, 2003). However, when the mineralocorticoid antagonist spironolactone was given along with cortisol, the mineralocorticoid effects such as weight gain and potassium wastage were blunted, but the BP still rose, suggesting that mineralocorticoid effects are not totally responsible for cortisol-induced hypertension (Whitworth et al., 2000).

- Increased production of *mineralocorticoids*. Though usually noted only in patients with adrenal tumors, increased levels of 19-nor-deoxycorticosterone (Ehlers et al., 1987), deoxycorticosterone (DOC), and less commonly, aldosterone (Cassar et al., 1980) have been found in patients with all forms of the syndrome.

- Stimulation of glucocorticoid receptors in the dorsal hindbrain (Scheuer et al., 2004).
- Reduced activity of various vasodepressor mechanisms (Saruta, 1996), in particular, endothelial nitric oxide (Mangos et al., 2000).
- Increased levels of *renin* substrate and an increased responsiveness to various *pressors* (Pirpiris et al., 1992).
- Increased erythropoieten (Whitworth et al., 2000) or endothelin (Kirilov et al., 2003).
- Sleep apnea (Sacerdote et al., 2005).

## Clinical Features

Many more patients with cushingoid features are seen than the relatively few who have the syndrome. The syndrome is more likely in patients with the clinical features shown in Table 14–2 ( Arnaldi et al.,

## TABLE 14–2

### Clinical Features of Cushing's Syndrome

| Clinical Features | Approximate Incidence, % |
|---|---|
| General | |
|   Obesity | 80–95 |
|     Truncal | 45–95[a] |
|   Hypertension | 70–90 |
|   Headache | 10–50 |
| Skin | |
|   Facial plethora | 70–90 |
|   Hirsutism | 70–80 |
|   Purple striae | 50–70[a] |
|   Bruising | 30–70[a] |
| Neuropsychiatric | 60–95 |
| Gonadal dysfunction | |
|   Menstrual disorders | 75–95 |
|   Impotence or decreased libido | 65–95 |
| Musculoskeletal | |
|   Osteopenia | 75–85 |
|   Weakness from myopathy | 30–90[a] |
| Metabolic | |
|   Glucose intolerance/diabetes | 40–90 |
|   Kidney stones | 15–20 |

Modified from Danese RD, Avon DC. Cushing's syndrome and hypertension. *Endocrinol Metab Clin NA* 1994;23:299–324.
[a]Most discriminatory features.

2003; Boscaro et al., 2001). In addition, significant hypokalemia is usually noted with the ectopic ACTH syndrome from the very high levels of cortisol (Torpy et al., 2002).

Cushing's syndrome in children is usually manifested by weight gain and growth retardation, with systolic hypertension noted in 93% of 63 young patients (Magiakou et al., 1997). Fortunately, they usually become normotensive within a few months of surgical cure, and they are able to catch up their linear growth (Lebrethon et al., 2000).

### Pseudo-Cushing's Syndrome

As many as 50% to 80% of patients with Cushing's syndrome meet the criteria for major depression and may have persistent psychological and cognitive problems even after surgical remission (Arnaldi et al., 2003). On the other hand, patients with endogenous *depression* without Cushing's syndrome may have poorly suppressible hypercortisolism related to increased ACTH pulse frequency (Mortola et al., 1987), but their basal cortisol levels are usually normal and they do not hyperrespond to corticotrophin-releasing hormone (CRH) (Yanovski et al., 1998). Moreover, depressed patients usually have a normal rise in cortisol during an insulin tolerance test and a normal suppression after the opiate agonist loperamide, unlike most patients with Cushing's syndrome (Newell-Price et al., 1998).

*Alcoholics* often display numerous features suggestive of Cushing's syndrome, including hypertension and a failure to suppress plasma cortisol after overnight dexamethasone (Stewart et al., 1993), which likely reflects increased secretion of corticotrophin-releasing factor (Groote Veldman & Meinders, 1996). On the other hand, 20% of patients with Cushing's syndrome have hepatic steatosis by CT scans (Rockall et al., 2003).

*Pregnant women* often have features suggestive of Cushing's syndrome; the rare appearance of Cushing's syndrome during pregnancy may pose diagnostic dilemmas (Keely, 1998).

### Laboratory Diagnosis

Two somewhat contradictory scenarios exist in relation to the diagnosis of Cushing's syndrome. First, the disease is being looked for in more patients with suggestive clinical features such as poorly controlled obese diabetics; in one study, 4% were found to have Cushing's syndrome (Leibowitz et al., 1996). This scenario requires screening tests with high specificity, i.e., few false positives—so that fewer suspects will have to be put through extensive confirmatory testing.

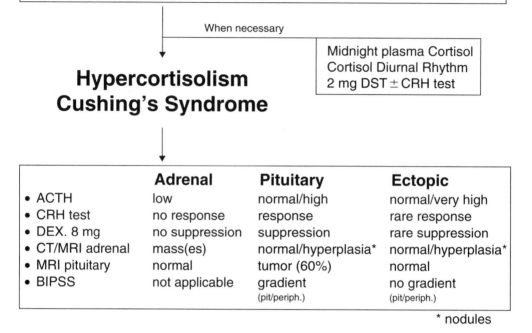

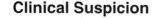

**Clinical Suspicion**

- Increased Urinary Free Cortisol (three 24h collections)
- Lack of cortisol suppression after low-dose dexamethasone testing
- Increased "Late-Evening" Salivary Cortisol (test incompletely evaluated)

When necessary

**Hypercortisolism
Cushing's Syndrome**

Midnight plasma Cortisol
Cortisol Diurnal Rhythm
2 mg DST ± CRH test

|  | **Adrenal** | **Pituitary** | **Ectopic** |
|---|---|---|---|
| • ACTH | low | normal/high | normal/very high |
| • CRH test | no response | response | rare response |
| • DEX. 8 mg | no suppression | suppression | rare suppression |
| • CT/MRI adrenal | mass(es) | normal/hyperplasia* | normal/hyperplasia* |
| • MRI pituitary | normal | tumor (60%) | normal |
| • BIPSS | not applicable | gradient (pit/periph.) | no gradient (pit/periph.) |

\* nodules

**FIGURE 14–2** ● Pathways to the diagnosis of Cushing's syndrome. Dex, dexamethasone; DST, dexamethasone suppression test; BIPSS, bilateral inferior petrosal sinus sampling. (Modified from Arnaldi G, Angeli A, Atkinson AB, et al. Diagnosis and complications of Cushing's syndrome: a consensus statement. *J Clin Endocrinol Metab* 2003;88:5593–5602.)

The second scenario relates to the usually long duration between onset of symptoms and the time of diagnosis, averaging 29 months in a multicenter study from Italy (Invitti et al., 1999). This scenario requires confirmatory tests with high sensitivity, i.e., few false negatives—so that all patients can be correctly identified as early as possible. In view of the serious nature and the often irreversibility of the complications of the disease, the best balance is likely to be with a number of tests done over a short interval to achieve maximal predictive power.

### Screening Tests

The extent of the workup of patients suspected of having Cushing's syndrome varies with the clinical situation. An overnight 1-mg dexamethasone suppression test will be adequate for most patients with only minimally suggestive features; patients with highly suggestive features should have repeated 24-hour urinary cortisol and midnight salivary cortisol

(Arnaldi et al., 2003; Raff & Findling, 2003) (Figure 14–2).

*Urinary Free Cortisol*

The 24-hour urinary cortisol provides an integrated measure of the unbound circulating cortisol. High-performance liquid chromatography coupled with mass spectrometry provides better specificity than immunoassays but carbamazepine may cause interference (Ma et al., 2005). The upper range of normal is 40–50 ug per day (110–138 nmol per day) and a value four times greater is usually diagnostic (Raff & Findling, 2003). The level may be lowered in patients with renal damage or raised with increased urinary volumes by reducing the fraction of filtered cortisol that is metabolized to cortisone or reabsorbed. Three daily specimens are usually assayed.

*Overnight Plasma Suppression*

For screening, the single bedtime 1-mg dose dexamethasone suppression test, measuring the plasma cortisol at 8 a.m. the next morning, has worked well, but, to provide adequate sensitivity, the cut-off value should be 1.8 ug/dL, rather than the previously recommended 5 ug/dL (Findling et al., 2004). However, at the lower level, false-positive results are seen in about 10% of non-Cushing's patients and false-negative results are seen in about 20% of patients with Cushing's disease (Findling et al., 2004). Drugs that induce CYP3A4 enzymes that metabolize dexamethasone may cause false-positive tests (Ma et al., 2005).

*Late-Night Salivary Cortisol*

An elevated late-night cortisol level is the earliest and most sensitive marker for Cushing's syndrome (Raff & Findling, 2003). Rather than the inconvenience of obtaining blood samples, measurement of salivary cortisol levels in easily obtained samples has rapidly been accepted as a valid screening test (Yaneva et al., 2004). Levels above 0.25 ug/dL (7.0 nmol/L) are diagnostic (Raff & Findling, 2003).

*Low-Dose Dexamethasone Suppression (DST) and Combined DST-CRH*

Dexamethasone suppression tests may give anomalous results because hormone hypersecretion may be cyclic or variable. Pseudo-Cushing's states, including depression, may be more accurately excluded by adding a CRH stimulation test 2 hours after completion of the low-dose dexamethasone test (Yanovski et al., 1998). The plasma cortisol level value 15 minutes after CRH (1 ug/kg) is above 1.4 ug/dL in patients with Cushing's syndrome but remains suppressed in normals and patients with pseudo-Cushing's.

## Establishing the Cause of Cushing's Syndrome

Once Cushing's syndrome has been diagnosed, the anatomic cause needs to be accurately determined to guide therapy (Figure 14–2).

### Corticotropin (ACTH) Assay

Measurement of plasma ACTH is the first step, using two-site immunometric assays that are sensitive, specific, and reliable, able to reliably detect values below 10 pg/mL (2 pmol/L). A suppressed ACTH concentration, below 5 pg/mL, indicates adrenal-dependent Cushing's syndrome; normal or elevated plasma ACTH, above 20 pg/mL, indicate an ACTH-secreting neoplasia, either pituitary or ectopic. When values are between 10 and 20 pg/mL, a CRH stimulation test is indicated (Arnaldi et al., 2003).

### Corticotrophin-Releasing Hormone Stimulation Test

Most pituitary tumors respond to IV CRH (1 ug/kg) with a release of plasma ACTH whereas adrenal tumors do not. Unfortunately, some ectopic ACTH-secreting tumors express the CRH receptor and

also respond, so the test has not been found useful in separating the type of ACTH-dependent Cushing's syndrome (Raff & Findling, 2003).

### High-Dose Dexamethasone Suppression

Using the criterion of suppression of urinary free cortisol to less than 10% of baseline for the diagnosis of pituitary-dependent Cushing's disease, the high-dose (2 mg four times a day for 2 days) dexamethasone suppression test provides 70% to 80% sensitivity and close to 100% specificity (Boscaro et al., 2001). However, the results do not clearly separate ectopic ACTH from pituitary tumors, and this test is no longer recommended (Raff & Findling, 2003).

### Pituitary Magnetic Resonance Imaging

In most patients, the measurement of plasma ACTH will be followed by a pituitary MRI with gadolinium enhancement. Thereby, a discrete pituitary adenoma will be seen in about 60% of patients; if the tumor is greater than 6 mm in size, no further studies are required and the patients may be referred to a pituitary neurosurgeon (Arnaldi et al., 2003). It should be remembered that at least 10% of the general population harbor incidental pituitary tumors, although most are below 5 mm in diameter. Since some patients with an ectopic ACTH-secreting tumor have abnormal pituitary MRI findings, bilateral inferior petrosal sinus sampling is indicated in those with clinical features suggesting an ectopic tumor, such as rapid onset of symptoms or hypokalemia (Raff & Findling, 2003).

### Inferior Petrosal Sinus Sampling

Bilateral simultaneous sampling of the inferior petrosal sinuses (IPSS) is a powerful means of confirming whether or not the source of corticotropin is the pituitary, especially if imaging is negative (Ilias et al., 2005). Ratio of central to peripheral ACTH of >3 after CRH provides a sensitivity of 95% to 97% and specificity of 100% in diagnosing pituitary-dependent Cushing's disease (Arnaldi et al., 2003). Less discrimination was found in a series of 185 IPSS procedures with a 99% positive predictive power but only a 20% negative predictive power (Swearingen et al., 2004). In view of the technical difficulty with IPSS, sampling of the internal jugular vein may be performed and only patients with a negative result referred for IPSS (Ilias et al., 2004).

If clinical and lab data point to an ectopic ACTH-secreting tumor, CT and/or MRI of the neck, thorax, and abdomen and, for occult tumors, scintigraphy with the somatostatin analog [111]In-pentetreotide are currently used to locate the tumor (de Herder & Lamberts, 1999).

## TABLE 14–3

**Therapies for Cushing's Syndrome**

| Class | Site | Therapy |
|---|---|---|
| Surgery | Pituitary | Transphenoidal microsection; transfrontal hypophysectomy |
| | Adrenal | Unilateral adrenalectomy; bilateral adrenalectomy |
| Radiation | External | High-voltage x-ray (cobalt) with or without mitotane (etc.), α-particle, proton beam (cyclotron) |
| | Internal | Implants of yttrium-90, gold 198 |
| Drugs | Acting at hypothalamic-pituitary | Serotonin antagonists (cyproheptadine, ritanserin) |
| | | Dopamine agonists (bromocriptine, lisuride) |
| | | GABA agonists (sodium valproate) |
| | | Somatostatin analogues (octreotide) |
| | Inhibitors of adrenocortical steroid synthesis | Mitotane |
| | | Metyrapone |
| | | Aminoglutethimide |
| | | Ketoconazole |
| | | Etomidate |
| | Glucocorticoid antagonist | Mifepristone |

In view of all the clinical vagaries and laboratory pitfalls that often confuse the differential diagnosis of the etiology of Cushing's syndrome, referral to a medical facility with experience in dealing with such patients is almost always appropriate.

## Treatment

### Treatment of the Hypertension

Until definitive therapy is provided, the hypertension that accompanies Cushing's syndrome can temporarily be treated with the usual antihypertensive agents described in Chapter 7 (Sacerdote et al., 2005). Since excess fluid volume is likely involved, a diuretic, perhaps in combination with an aldosterone antagonist, spironolactone or eplerenone, is an appropriate initial choice. After definitive therapy, hypertension usually improves, but atherosclerotic risk factors often persist, likely because of residual abdominal obesity and insulin resistance (Arnaldi et al., 2003).

### Treatment of the Syndrome in General

In view of the long-term morbidity associated with Cushing's syndrome, the condition must be treated as rapidly as possible after the diagnosis has been established. The choice of definitive therapy depends on the cause of the syndrome (Table 14–3).

- In the majority of patients who have a pituitary tumor, transphenoidal microsurgical removal is the treatment of choice (Hammer et al., 2004). In some circumstances, unilateral adrenalectomy followed by external pituitary irradiation has been successful (Nagesser et al., 2000).
- Benign adrenal tumors should be surgically removed, increasingly by laparoscopy.
- For adrenal cancers and ectopic ACTH tumors that cannot be resected, removal of the adrenal may be helpful, but chemotherapy is usually needed (Morris & Grossman, 2002).
- The drugs listed in Table 14–3 are mainly used to quickly overcome severe complications, either in preparation for surgery or whenever definitive treatment must be delayed (Morris & Grossman, 2002).

### Follow-up

With definitive therapy, remission rates of 70% to 80%—defined as normal plasma and urinary cortisol levels and resolution of clinical stigmata—have been noted (Arnaldi et al., 2003; Hammer et al., 2004). However, as many as 25% of pituitary-dependent Cushing's patients have recurrences at

10 years after transspenoidal surgery, so close and long-term follow-up is necessary.

## SYNDROMES WITH INCREASED ACCESS OF CORTISOL TO MINERALOCORTICOID RECEPTORS

Less common than Cushing's syndrome caused by cortisol excess are a variety of fascinating syndromes wherein normal or increased levels of cortisol exert a mineralocorticoid effect by binding to the renal mineralocorticoid receptors. As depicted in Figure 14–3, the normal renal mineralocorticoid receptor (MCR) is as receptive to glucocorticoids as it is to mineralocorticoids. The 11β-hydroxysteroid dehydrogenase type 2 isoform (11β-HSD2) enzyme in the renal tubules upstream to these receptors normally converts the large amounts of fully active cortisol to the inactive cortisone, thereby leaving the mineralocorticoid receptors open to the effects of aldosterone (Quinkler & Stewart, 2003).

However, there are both congenital and acquired deficiencies of the 11β-HSD2 enzyme, so that the normal levels of cortisol remain fully active, flooding the mineralocorticoid receptor and inducing the full syndrome of mineralocorticoid excess: sodium retention, potassium wastage, and hypertension with virtually complete suppression of renin and aldosterone secretion (Stewart, 2003).

### 11β-HSD2 Deficiency: Apparent Mineralocorticoid Excess

Apparent mineralocorticoid excess (AME) is an autosomal recessive disorder that has now been identified in about 75 patients. The syndrome clinically is characterized by familial consanguinity, low birth weight, failure to thrive, onset of severe hypertension in early childhood with extensive target organ damage, hypercalciuria, nephrocalcinosis, and renal failure (Chemaitilly et al., 2003). As noted, sodium retention, hypokalemia, low aldosterone, and low-renin levels are present.

### Genetics

Soon after the first case was described (Werder et al., 1974), Ulick et al. (1979) recognized that these children did not metabolize cortisol normally. Some years later, Stewart et al. (1988), in studies on a 20-year-old with the syndrome, recognized a defect in the renal cortisol-cortisone shuttle and demonstrated the deficiency of the 11β-HSD2 enzyme. A number of mutations in the 11β-HSD gene have now been identified in patients with AME (Carvajal et al., 2003; Cerame & New, 2000; Lin-Su et al., 2004).

Some of these mutations result in only partial inhibition of the 11β-HSD2 enzyme as evidenced by a higher ratio of urinary cortisone to cortisol metabolites and a milder clinical course with larger birth weight, later age of presentation (Nunez et al., 1999), and in at least one patient, only mild low-renin hypertension (Wilson et al., 1998). Not surprisingly, mutations resulting in less inhibition of the enzyme have been sought in patients with "essential" hypertension. Some have found them, but most have not (Quinkler & Stewart, 2003). A role of impaired 11β-HSD2 activity has also been proposed for sodium sensitivity (Ferrari et al., 2001), intrauterine growth retardation (McTernan et al., 2001), and preeclampsia (Schoof et al., 2001).

#### Variant

A few patients with the features of AME have a defect not in the cortisol to cortisone shuttle but in the ring A reduction of cortisol to inactive metabolites because of a deficiency of the 5β-reductase enzyme (Ulick et al., 1992a). The resultant high levels of cortisol keep the mineralocorticoid receptors flooded in the same manner as when 11β-HSD2 is deficient. In one family with classical AME, some affected patients also had reduced 5β-reductase activity (Morineau et al., 1999).

### Therapy

Therapy is usually based on competitive blockade of the mineralocorticoid receptor with spironolactone (Dave-Sharma et al., 1998) or the more selective blocker eplerenone (Funder, 2000). Suppression of endogenous cortisol with dexamethasone has also been used (Quinkler & Stewart, 2003). Cure has been reported on one patient after transplantation of

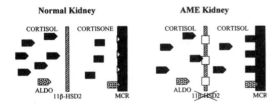

**Normal Kidney**          **AME Kidney**

**FIGURE 14–3** ● Enzyme-mediated receptor protection. Normally, 11β-dehydrogenase (11-β-HSD2) converts cortisol to inactive cortisone in the more proximal nephron, protecting mineralocorticoid receptors (MCR) from cortisol and allowing selective access for aldosterone. When 11β-dehydrogenase is defective, e.g., in congenital deficiency (AME kidney) or after licorice administration, cortisol gains inappropriate access to mineralocorticoid receptors, resulting in sodium retention and potassium wasting. (Modified from Cerame BI, New MI. Hormonal hypertension in children: 11β-hydroxylase deficiency and apparent mineralocorticoid excess. *J Ped Endocrinol Metab* 2000;13:1537–1547.)

a kidney with normal 11β-HDS2 activity (Palermo et al., 1998).

## 11β-HSD2 Inhibition: Glycyrrhetinic Acid (Licorice)

Since the early 1950s, glycyrrhizin acid, the active ingredient in licorice extract, has been known to cause hypertension, sodium retention, and potassium wastage. Stewart et al. (1987) and Edwards et al. (1988) recognized the similarities between the syndrome induced by licorice and the syndrome of apparent mineralocorticoid excess and documented that licorice inhibited the same renal 11β-HSD2 enzyme that was deficient in AME. These effects are accompanied by a fall in cortisone and a rise in cortisol excretion, reflecting the inhibition of renal 11β-HSD2 activity.

Relatively small amounts of confectionary licorice, as little as 50 g daily for 2 weeks, produce a rise in BP in normal people (Sigurjonsdottir et al., 2001). The syndrome also has been induced by the licorice extracts in chewing tobacco and gum (Rosseel & Schoors, 1993). Of interest is the preliminary report of the ability of glycyrrhizin to inhibit replication of SARS-associated coronavirus (Cinati et al., 2003) which could herald a much greater exposure to this agent. Not surprisingly, aldosterone receptor blockers (spironolactone and eplerenone) have been shown to relieve all of the effects of licorice-induced hypertension (Quaschning et al., 2001).

### Massive Cortisol Excess

The capacity of the 11β-HSD-directed cortisol-cortisone shuttle and of 5β-reductase inactivation may be overcome by massive amounts of cortisol. Ulick et al. (1992b) have shown this to be the mechanism responsible for the significant features of mineralocorticoid excess—profound hypokalemia and hypertension—that are seen in patients with ectopic ACTH tumors wherein cortisol levels are much higher than in other causes of Cushing's syndrome (Torpy et al., 2002).

## Glucocorticoid Resistance

Both sporadic and familial forms of glucocorticoid receptor resistance, ascribed to various mutations in the receptor gene (Charmandari et al., 2005), have increased levels of circulating cortisol but without typical Cushing's stigmata (Kino et al., 2002). Many of these patients have hypertension that may mimic mineralocorticoid excess. Moreover, among 60 hypertensive patients under age 36, increased levels of urinary glucocorticoid metabolites were seen

in 45, suggesting partial resistance of glucocorticoid receptors with subsequent increased mineralocorticoid effects (Shamim et al., 2001).

## DEOXYCORTICOSTERONE EXCESS: CONGENITAL ADRENAL HYPERPLASIA

Excessive amounts of the mineralocorticoid DOC may cause hypertension (Ferrari & Bonny, 2003), arising either from hyperplastic adrenals with enzymatic deficiencies or from rare DOC-secreting tumors (Gröndal et al., 1990).

Defects in all of the enzymes involved in adrenal steroid synthesis have been recognized (Figure 14–4). These defects are inherited in an autosomal recessive manner and their manifestations result from inadequate levels of the end products of steroid synthesis—in particular, cortisol. The low levels of cortisol call forth increased secretion of ACTH, further increasing the accumulation of the precursor steroids proximal to the enzymatic block and stimulating steroidogenesis in pathways that are not blocked (Table 14–4).

The clinical manifestations of congenital adrenal hyperplasia (CAH), often obvious at birth, vary with the degree of enzymatic deficiency and the mix of steroids secreted by the hyperplastic adrenal glands. The most common type, the 21-hydroxylase deficiency, responsible for perhaps 90% of all CAH, is not associated with hypertension but is accompanied by a high prevalence of benign adrenal tumors (Speiser & White, 2003).

The two forms of CAH in which hypertension occurs are caused by deficiency of the 11β-hydroxylase (CYP11β1) or 17-hydroxylase (CYP-17A) enzymes. Though these are rare causes of hypertension, partial enzymatic deficiencies have been observed in hirsute women (Lucky et al., 1986), so some hypertensive adults may have unrecognized, subtle forms of CAH.

## 11-Hydroxylase Deficiency

Particularly in the Middle East, this is the second most common form of CAH and is usually recognized in infancy because, as shown in Figure 14–4, the defect sets off production of excessive androgens. The enzyme deficiency prevents the hydroxylation of 11-deoxycortisol, resulting in cortisol deficiency and prevents the conversion of DOC to corticosterone and aldosterone. The high levels of DOC induce hypertension and hypokalemia, the expected features of mineralocorticoid excess. Thus the syndrome features virilization of the infant, hypertension, and hypokalemia.

TABLE 14-4

## Syndromes of Congenital Adrenal Hyperplasia

| Enzyme | Site of Defect | | Steroid Levels | | | Clinical Features | |
|---|---|---|---|---|---|---|---|
| | Increased Precursor | Decreased Product | 17-OH-P or P' triol | DOC | Aldo | Virilization | Hypertension |
| 21-hydroxylase | | | | | | | |
|   Nonsalt wasting | 17-hydroxyprogesterone | 11-deoxycortisol, cortisol | ↑↑↑ | N | N | Marked | No |
|   Salt wasting | Progesterone | 11-deoxycorticosterone, cortisol | ↑↑↑ | ↓ | ↓↓ | Marked | No |
| 11-hydroxylase | 11-deoxycortisol 11-deoxycorticolsteroid | Cortisol Cortisterone | N, ↑ | ↑↑ | ↓↓,N | Marked | Yes |
| 17-hydroxylase | Progesterone Pregnenolone | Cortisol 17-hydroxypregnenolone | ↓↓ | ↑↑ | ↓,N, ↑ | Absent | Yes |
| 3β-ol-dehydrogenase | Pregnenolone | Progesterone, cortisol | N, ↑ ↓↓ | N, ↓ ↓↓ | ↓,N ↓↓ | Sight | No |
| STAR protein | Cholesterol | All steroids | ↓↓ | ↓↓ | ↓↓ | Absent | No |

17-KS, 17-ketosteroids; 17-OH-P, 17-hydroxyprogesterone; P' triol, pregnanetriol; Aldo, aldosterone; N, normal; ↑, increased by varying degrees; ↓, decreased by varying degrees.

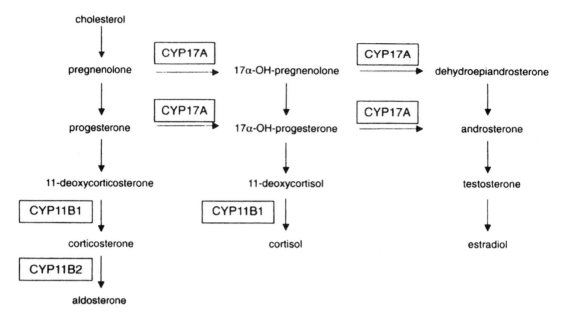

**FIGURE 14–4** ● The adrenal steroid pathway.

The enzyme deficiency has been attributed to various mutations in the *CYP 11B1* gene (Krone et al., 2005). The syndrome is diagnosed by finding high levels of 11-deoxycortisol and DOC in urine and plasma. Treatment, as for all of the syndromes of CAH, is with glucocorticoid, which should relieve the hypertension and hypokalemia and allow the child to develop normally. Prenatal diagnosis and treatment have been shown to prevent virilization (Cerame & New, 2000).

### 17-Hydroxylase Deficiency

Unlike the 21-hydroxylase and 11-hydroxylase deficiencies, CAH caused by a 17-hydroxylase deficiency is typically associated with an absence of sex hormones, leading to incomplete masculinization in males and primary amenorrhea in females in addition to hypertension and hypokalemia (Figure 14–4, Table 14–4). The first hypertensive disorder of steroidogenesis identified (Biglieri et al., 1966), nearly 40 different mutations in CYP17 have now been described, and there is considerable variability in the clinical and hormonal features. This is the second most common form of CAH in Brazil and, among 24 affected patients, the severity of hypertension, hypokalemia, 17-deoxysteroid excess, and sex steroid deficiency varied, even among those with completely inactive CYP17 proteins (Costa-Santos et al., 2004).

Now that the various renal and adrenal causes of hypertension have been covered, we shall turn to an even larger variety of less common forms.

### REFERENCES

Amos AM, McRoberts JW. Cushing's syndrome associated with a pheochromocytoma. *Urology* 1998;52:331–335.

Arnaldi G, Angeli A, Atkinson AB, et al. Diagnosis and complications of Cushing's syndrome: a consensus statement. *J Clin Endocrinol Metab* 2003;88:5593–5602.

Biglieri EG, Herron MA, Brust N. 17-Hydroxylation deficiency in man. *J Clin Invest* 1966;45:1946–1954.

Boscaro M, Barzon L, Fallo, F, Sonino N. Cushing's syndrome. *Lancet* 2001;357:783–791.

Boscaro M, Barzon L, Sonino N. The diagnosis of Cushing's syndrome: atypical presentations and laboratory shortcomings. *Arch Intern Med* 2000;160:3045–3053.

Brotman DJ, Girod JP, Garcia MJ, et al. Effects of short-term glucocorticoids on cardiovascular biomarkers. *J Clin Endocrinol Metab* 2005;90:3202–3208.

Carvajal CA, Gonzalez AA, Romero DG, et al. Two homozygous mutations in the 11β-hydroxysteroid dehydrogenase type 2 gene in a case of apparent mineralocorticoid excess. *J Clin Endocrinol Metab* 2003;88:2501–2507.

Cassar J, Loizou S, Kelly WF, Joplin GF. Deoxycorticosterone and aldosterone excretion in Cushing's syndrome. *Metabolism* 1980;29:115–119.

Cerame BI, New MI. Hormonal hypertension in children: 11β-hydroxylase deficiency and apparent mineralocorticoid excess. *J Ped Endocrinol Metab* 2000;13:1537–1547.

Charmandari E, Raji A, Kino T, et al. A novel point mutation in the ligand-binding domain (LBD) of the human glucocorticoid receptor (hGR) causing generalized glucocorticoid resistance: the important of the C terminus of hGR LBD in conferring transactivational activity. *J Clin Endocrinol Metab* 2005;90:3696–3705.

Chemaitilly W, Wilson RC, New MI. Hypertension and adrenal disorders. *Curr Hypertens Rep* 2003;5:498–504.

Cinati J, Morgenstern B, Bauer G, et al. Glycyrrhizin, an active component of liquorice roots, and replication of SARS-associated coronavirus. *Lancet* 2003;361:2045–2046.

Costa-Santos M, Kater CE, Auchus RJ. Two prevalent *CYP17* mutations and genotype-phenotype correlations in

24 Brazilian patients with 17-hydroxylase deficiency. *J Clin Endocrinol Metab* 2004;89:49–60.

Dave-Sharma S, Wilson RC, Harbison MD, et al. Examination of genotype and phenotype relationships in 14 patients with apparent mineralocorticoid excess. *J Clin Endocrinol Metab* 1998;83:2244–2254.

Doppman JL, Chrousos GP, Papanicolaou DA, et al. Adrenocorticotropin-independent macronodular adrenal hyperplasia: an uncommon cause of primary adrenal hypercortisolism. *Radiology* 2000;216:797–802.

Edwards CRW, Burt D, McIntyre MA, et al. Localisation of 11β-hydroxysteroid dehydrogenase-tissue specific protector of the mineralocorticoid receptor. *Lancet* 1988;2:986–989.

Ehlers ME, Griffing GT, Wilson TE, Melby JC. Elevated urinary 19-nor-deoxycorticosterone glucuronide in Cushing's syndrome. *J Clin Endocrinol Metab* 1987;64:926–930.

Fallo F, Paoletta A, Tona F, et al. Response of hypertension to conventional antihypertensive treatment and/or steroidogenesis inhibitors in Cushing's syndrome. *J Intern Med* 1993; 234:595–598.

Ferrari P, Bonny O. Forms of mineralocorticoid hypertension. *Vitamins & Hormones* 2003;66:113–156.

Ferrari P, Sansonnens A, Dick B, Frey FJ. In vivo 11β-HSD-2 activity; variability, salt-sensitivity, and effect of licorice. *Hypertension* 2001;38:1330–1336.

Findling JW, Raff H, Aron DC. The low-dose dexamethasone suppression test: a reevaluation in patients with Cushing's syndrome. *J Clin Endocrinol Metab* 2004;89:1222–1226.

Funder JW. Eplerenone, a new mineralocorticoid antagonist: *in vitro* and *in vivo* studies. *Curr Opin Endocrinol Diabetes* 2000;7:138–142.

Gröndal S, Eriksson B, Hagenäs L, et al. Steroid profile in urine: a useful tool in the diagnosis and follow up of adrenocortical carcinoma. *Acta Endocrinol (Copenh)* 1990;122: 656–663.

Groote Veldman R, Meinders AE. On the mechanism of alcohol-induced pseudo-Cushing's syndrome. *Endo Rev* 1996;17:262–268.

Hammer GD, Tyrrell JB, Lamborn KR, et al. Transsphenoidal microsurgery for Cushing's disease: initial outcome and long-term results. *J Clin Endocrinol Metab* 2004;89: 6348–6357.

Hermus AR, Pieters GF, Smals AG, et al. Transition from pituitary-dependent to adrenal-dependent Cushing's syndrome. *N Engl J Med* 1988;318:966–970.

Ilias I, Chang R, Pacak K, et al. Jugular venous sampling: an alternative to petrosal sinus sampling for the diagnostic evaluation of adrenocorticotropic hormone-dependent Cushing's syndrome. *J Clin Endocrinol Metab* 2004;89:3795–3800.

Ilias I, Torpy DJ, Pacak K, et al. Cushing's Syndrome due to ectopic corticotropin secretion: twenty years' experience at the National Institutes of Health. *J Clin Endocrinol Metab* 2005;(published online May 24).

Invitti C, Giraldi FP, de Martin M, et al. Diagnosis and management of Cushing's syndrome: results of an Italian multicentre study. *J Clin Endocrinol Metab* 1999;84:440–448.

Ishibashi M, Shimada K, Abe K, et al. Spontaneous remission in Cushing's disease. *Arch Intern Med* 1993;153:251–255.

Keely E. Endocrine causes of hypertension in pregnancy— when to start looking for zebras. *Sem Perinatol* 1998;22: 471–484.

Kino T, Vottero A, Charmandari E, Chrousos GP. Familial/sporadic glucocorticoid resistance syndrome and hypertension. *Ann NY Acad Sci* 2002;970:101–111.

Kirilov G, Tomova A, Dakovska L, et al. Elevated plasma endothelin as an additional cardiovascular risk factor in patients with Cushing's syndrome. *Eur J Endocrinol* 2003; 149:549–553.

Krone N, Riepe FG, Götze D, et al. Congenital adrenal hyperplasia due to 11-hydroxylase deficiency: functional characterization of two novel point mutations and a three-base pair deletion in the CYP11B1 gene. *J Clin Endocrinol Metab* 2005;90:3724–3730.

Lacroix A, N'Diaye N, Tremblay J, Hamet P. Ectopic and abnormal hormone receptors in adrenal Cushing's syndrome. *Endocrine Rev* 2001;22:75–110.

Lebrethon M-C, Grossman AB, Afshar F, et al. Linear growth and final height after treatment for Cushing's disease in childhood. *J Clin Endocrinol Metab* 2000;85:3262–3265.

Leibowitz G, Tsur A, Chayen SD, et al. Pre-clinical Cushing's syndrome: an unexpected frequent cause of poor glycaemic control in obese diabetic patients. *Clin Endocrinol* 1996;44:717–722.

Lieberman SA, Eccleshall TR, Feldman DA. ACTH-independent massive bilateral adrenal disease (AIMBAD): a subtype of Cushing's syndrome with major diagnostic and therapeutic implications. *Eur J Endocrinol* 1994;131:67–73.

Lin-Su K, Zhou P, Arora N, et al. *In vitro* expression studies of a novel mutation Δ299 in a patient affected with apparent mineralocorticoid excess. *J Clin Endocrinol Metab* 2004;89:2025–2027.

Lindholm J, Juul S, Lørgensen JOL, et al. Incidence and late prognosis of Cushing's syndrome. *J Clin Endocrinol Metab* 2001;86:117–123.

Lucky AW, Rosenfield FL, McGuire J, et al. Adrenal androgen hyperresponsiveness to adrenocorticotropin in women with acne and/or hirsutism: adrenal enzyme defects and exaggerated adrenarche. *J Clin Endocrinol Metab* 1986;62: 840–848.

Ma RC, Chan WB, So WY, et al. Carbamazepine and false positive dexamethasone suppression tests for Cushing's syndrome. *BMJ* 2005;330:299–300.

Magiakou MA, Mastorakos G, Zachman K, Chrousos GP. Blood pressure in children and adolescents with Cushing syndrome before and after surgical cure. *J Clin Endocrinol* 1997;82:1734–1738.

Malchoff CD. Carney complex—clarity and complexity. *J Clin Endocrinol Metab* 2000;85:4010–4012.

Mangos GJ, Walker BR, Kelly JJ, et al. Cortisol inhibits cholinergic vasodilatation in the human forearm. *Am J Hypertens* 2000;13:1155–1160.

McTernan CL, Draper N, Nicholson H, et al. Reduced placental 11β-hydroxysteroid dehydrogenase type 2 mRNA levels in human pregnancies complicated by intrauterine growth reduction: an analysis of possible mechanisms. *J Clin Endocrinol Metab* 2001;86:4979–4983.

Montrella-Waybill M, Clore JN, Schoolwerth AC, Watlington CO. Evidence that high dose cortisol-induced Na+ retention in man is not mediated by the mineralocorticoid receptor. *J Clin Endocrinol Metab* 1991;72:1060–1066.

Morineau G, Marc J-M, Boudi A, et al. Genetic, biochemical, and clinical studies of patients with A328V or R213C mutations in 11βHSD2 causing apparent mineralocorticoid excess. *Hypertension* 1999;34:435–441.

Morris D, Grossman A. The medical management of Cushing's syndrome. *Ann NY Acad Sci* 2002;970:119–113.

Mortola JF, Liu JH, Gillin JC, et al. Pulsatile rhythms of adrenocorticotropin (ACTH) and cortisol in women with endogenous depression: evidence for increased ACTH pulse frequency. *J Clin Endocrinol Metab* 1987;65:962–968.

Nagesser SK, van Seters AP, Kievit J, et al. Treatment of pituitary-dependent Cushing's syndrome: long-term results of unilateral adrenalectomy followed by external pituitary irradiation compared to transsphenoidal pituitary surgery. *Clin Endocrinol* 2000;52:427–435.

Newell-Price J, Trainer P, Besser M, Grossman A. The diagnosis and differential diagnosis of Cushing's syndrome and pseudo-Cushing's states. *Endocrine Rev* 1998;19:647–672.

Nunez BS, Rogerson FM, Mune T, et al. Mutant of 11β-hydroxysteroid dehydrogenase (11-HSD2) with partial activity. *Hypertension* 1999;34:638–642.

Orth DN. Cushing's syndrome. *N Engl J Med* 1995;332: 791–803.

Palermo M, Cossu M, Shackleton CHL. Cure of apparent mineralocorticoid excess by kidney transplantation. *N Engl J Med* 1998;329:1782–1788.

Pirpiris M, Sudhir K, Yeung S, et al. Pressor responsiveness in corticosteroid-induced hypertension in humans. *Hypertension* 1992;19:567–574.

Quaschning T, Ruschitzka FT, Shaw S, Lüscher TF. Aldosterone receptor antagonism normalizes vascular function in liquorice-induced hypertension. *Hypertension* 2001;37: 801–805.

Quinkler M, Stewart PM. Hypertension and the cortisol-cortisone shuttle. *J Clin Endocrinol Metab* 2003;88: 2384–2392.

Raff H, Findling JW. A physiologic approach to diagnosis of the Cushing syndrome. *Ann Intern Med* 2003;138:980–991.

Rockall AG, Sohaib SA, Evans D, et al. Hepatic steatosis in Cushing's syndrome: a radiological assessment using computer tomography. *Eur J Endocrinol* 2003;149:543–548.

Ross EJ, Linch DC. Cushing's syndrome—killing disease: discriminatory value of signs and symptoms aiding early diagnosis. *Lancet* 1982;2:646–649.

Rosseel M, Schoors D. Chewing gum and hypokalaemia. *Lancet* 1993;341:175.

Rossi R, Tauchmanova L, Luciano A, et al. Subclinical Cushing's syndrome in patients with adrenal incidentaloma: clinical and biochemical features. *J Clin Endocrinol Metab* 2000;85:1440–1448.

Sacerdote A, Weiss K, Tran T, et al. Hypertension in patients with Cushing's disease: pathophysiology, diagnosis, and management. *Curr Hypertens Rep* 2005;7:212–218.

Saruta T. Mechanism of glucocorticoid-induced hypertension. *Hypertens Res* 1996;19:18.

Sato A, Funder JW, Okubo M, et al. Glucocorticoid-induced hypertension in the elderly. Relation to serum calcium and family history of essential hypertension. *Am J Hypertens* 1995;8:823–828.

Scheuer DA, Bechtold AG, Shank SS, Akana SF. Glucocorticoids act in the dorsal hindbrain to increase arterial pressure. *Am J Physiol Heart Circ Physiol* 2004;286:H458–H467.

Schoof E, Girsti M, Frobenius W, et al. Decreased gene expression of 11β-hydroxysteroid dehydrogenase type 2 and 15-hydroxyprostaglandin dehydrogenase in human placenta of patients with preeclampsia. *J Clin Endocrinol Metab* 2001;86:1313–1317.

Shamim W, Yousufuddin M, Francis DP, et al. Raised urinary glucocorticoid and adrenal androgen precursors in the urine of young hypertensive patients: possible evidence for partial glucocorticoid resistance. *Heart* 2001;86:139–144.

Sigurjonsdottir HA, Manhem K, Wallerstedt S. Liquorice-induced hypertension—a linear dose-response relationship. *J Human Hypertens* 2001;15:549–552.

Speiser PW, White PC. Congenital adrenal hyperplasia. *N Engl J Med* 2003;349:776–788.

Stewart PM. Tissue-specific Cushing's syndrome, 11β-hydroxysteroid dehydrogenases and the redefinition of corticosteroid hormone action. *Eur J Endocrinol* 2003;149: 163–168.

Stewart PM, Burra P, Shackleton CHL, et al. 11β-hydroxysteroid dehydrogenase deficiency and glucocorticoid status in patients with alcoholic and non-alcoholic chronic liver disease. *J Clin Endocrinol Metab* 1993;76:748–751.

Stewart PM, Corrie JET, Shackleton CHL, Edwards CRW. Syndrome of apparent mineralocorticoid excess. A defect in the cortisol-cortisone shuttle. *J Clin Invest* 1988;82:340–349.

Stewart PM, Penn R, Gibson R, et al. Hypothalamic abnormalities in patients with pituitary-dependent Cushing's syndrome. *Clin Endocrinol* 1992;36:453–458.

Stewart PM, Wallace AM, Valentino R, et al. Mineralocorticoid activity of liquorice: 11-beta-hydroxysteroid dehydrogenase deficiency comes of age. *Lancet* 1987;2:821–824.

Suzuki T, Shibata H, Ando T, et al. Risk factors associated with persistent postoperative hypertension in Cushing's syndrome. *Endocrine Res* 2000;26:791–795.

Swearingen B, Katznelson L, Miller K, et al. Diagnostic errors after inferior petrosal sinus sampling. *J Clin Endocrinol Metab* 2004;89:3752–3763.

Torpy DJ, Mullen N, Ilias J, Nieman LK. Association of hypertension and hypokalemia with Cushing's syndrome caused by ectopic ACTH secretion: a series of 58 cases. *Ann NY Acad Sci* 2002;970:134–144.

Tremble JM, Buxton-Thomas M, Hopkins D, et al. Cushing's syndrome associated with a chemodectoma and a carcinoid tumour. *Clin Endocrinol* 2000;52:789–793.

Ulick S, Levine LS, Gunczler P, et al. A syndrome of apparent mineralocorticoid excess associated with defects in the peripheral metabolism of cortisol. *J Clin Endocrinol Metab* 1979;49:757–764.

Ulick S, Tedde R, Wang JZ. Defective ring A reduction of cortisol as the major metabolic error in the syndrome of apparent mineralocorticoid excess. *J Clin Endocrinol Metab* 1992a;74:593–599.

Ulick S, Wang JZ, Blumenfeld JD, Pickering TG. Cortisol inactivation overload: a mechanism of mineralocorticoid hypertension in the ectopic adrenocorticotropin syndrome. *J Clin Endocrinol Metab* 1992b;74:963–967.

van Aken MO, Pereira AM, van Thiel SW, et al. Irregular and frequent cortisol secretory episodes with preserved diurnal rhythmicity in primary adrenal Cushing's syndrome. *J Clin Endocrinol Metab* 2005;90:1570–1577.

van Rossum EFC, Lamberts SWJ. Polymorphisms in the glucocorticoid receptor gene and their associations with metabolic parameters and body composition. *Recent Prog Hormone Res* 2004;59:333–357.

Werder E, Zachmann M, Völlmin JA, et al. Unusual steroid excretion in a child with low-renin hypertension. *Res Steroids* 1974;6:385–395.

Whitworth JA, Mangos GJ, Kelly JJ. Cushing, cortisol, and cardiovascular disease. *Hypertension* 2000;36:912–916.

Wilson RC, Dave-Sharma S, Wei J-Q, et al. A genetic defect resulting in mild low-renin hypertension. *Proc Natl Acad Sci USA* 1998;95:10200–10205.

Yaneva M, Mosnier-Pudar H, Dugué M-A, et al. Midnight salivary cortisol for the initial diagnosis of Cushing's syndrome of various causes. *J Clin Endocrinol Metab* 2004; 89:3345–3351.

Yanovski JA, Cutler Jr. GB, Chrousos GP, Nieman LK. The dexamethasone-suppressed corticotropin-releasing hormone stimulation test differentiates mild Cushing's disease from normal physiology. *J Clin Endocrinol Metab* 1998;83: 348–352.

Zelinka T, Štrauch B, Pecen L, Widimský J Jr. Diurnal blood pressure variation on pheochromocytoma, primary aldosteronism, and Cushing's syndrome. *J Human Hypertens* 2004;18:107–111.

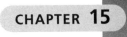
# Other Forms of Identifiable Hypertension

As described in Chapter 3, the pathogenesis of primary (essential) hypertension likely involves multiple mechanisms. Beyond the involvement of obvious players such as renal sodium handling, renin-angiotensin, and the sympathetic nervous system, whose altered roles may be genetically determined, lurk a number of environmental factors. Of those factors, sodium and potassium intake, weight gain, and stress most likely are causal. Others, such as smoking and alcohol, may raise the blood pressure (BP), but they are generally considered to be contributory rather than causal, since, when they are discontinued, their pressor effect disappears.

As described in Chapters 9 through 14, a number of secondary or identifiable causes of hypertension have been characterized. In addition to those, which primarily reflect renal and adrenal hormonal abnormalities, a number of other, generally less common, forms of hypertension have been identified and will be covered in this chapter. Additional coverage of hypertension in childhood is provided in Chapter 16.

## COARCTATION OF THE AORTA

Constriction of the lumen of the aorta may occur anywhere along its length but is seen most commonly just beyond the origin of the left subclavian artery, at or below the insertion of the ligamentum arteriosum. This lesion makes up approximately 7% of all congenital heart disease. Hypertension in the upper extremities with diminished or absent femoral pulses is the usual presentation (Table 15–1).

The traditional separation into infantile (preductal) and adult (postductal) types is now considered inappropriate, with many preductal lesions not identified until adult life. As Jenkins and Ward (1999) state:

> A spectrum of lesions is now recognized, and it is only those with the most severe obstruction (e.g., aortic arch atresia or interruption) or associated cardiac defects who invariably present in infancy. Most other cases are now identified at routine medical examination. Otherwise, age at presentation is related to the severity rather than the site of obstruction, as a result of cardiac failure or occasionally cerebrovascular accident (CVA), aortic dissection, or endocarditis.

### Pathophysiology

If the coarctation is proximal to the ductus arteriosus, pulmonary hypertension, congestive failure, and cyanosis of the lower half of the body occur early in life. Before surgery was possible, 45% to 84% of infants found to have coarctation died during their first year of life (Campbell, 1970).

Patients with less severe postductal lesions may have no difficulties during childhood. However, they almost always develop premature cardiovascular disease; in the two largest series of autopsied cases seen

## TABLE 15–1

### Symptoms and Signs of Coarctation

Symptoms
  Headache
  Cold feet
  Pain in legs with exercise
Signs
  Hypertension
  Hyperdynamic apical impulse
  Murmurs in front or back of chest
  Pulsations in neck
  Weak femoral pulse

---

before the advent of effective surgery, the mean age of death was 34 years (Campbell, 1970). The causes of death reflected the pressure load on the heart and the associated cardiac and cerebral lesions.

Beyond the obvious obstruction to blood flow, coarctation likely involves a wider abnormality with defects found in the vascular media both proximal and distal (Niwa et al., 2001) that may, in turn, reflect an innate cellular defect (Swan et al., 2002). The presence of intracranial aneurysm in 10% of adults with coarctation (Connolly et al., 2003) may reflect such underlying vascular weakness. Moreover, after the initial insult of coarctation, a number of secondary processes such as left ventricular hypertrophy are initiated and may persist even after repair. Therefore, early detection and repair are critical (Daniels, 2001).

### Recognition of Coarctation

Hypertension in the arms with weak femoral pulses in a young person strongly suggests coarctation. With minimal constriction, symptoms may not appear until late in life. Often the heart is large and shows left ventricular strain on the electrocardiogram. The chest radiograph can be diagnostic, demonstrating the "three" sign from dilation of the aorta above and below the constriction, and notching of the ribs by enlarged collateral vessels. The diagnosis is now usually made by echocardiography and color Doppler flow mapping.

Atypical aortic coarctation in adults most likely represents Takayasu's arteritis, or pulseless disease, which usually affects the aortic arch and may also involve the descending aorta (Numano et al., 2000) or renal arteries (Weaver et al., 2004). This large-vessel

vasculitis may be successfully treated with balloon angioplasty (Tyagi et al., 1992) but usually improves with corticosteroids (Numano et al., 2000).

### Management

Early repair by surgery or angioplasty (Macdonald et al., 2003) is now recommended with very low rates of re-coarctation being encountered (Pearl et al., 2004). If repair is delayed until adulthood, there is a greater likelihood of persistent hypertension, which may be severe. Nonetheless, repair usually improves the hypertension (Vriend et al., 2004). Even in those with normal resting blood pressures, there may be an exaggerated blood pressure response to exercise, but Vriend et al. (2004) found no independent relationship of this response to left ventricular mass.

Obviously, patients after repair need to be closely followed, and any degree of hypertension intensively treated.

## HORMONAL DISTURBANCES

### Hypothyroidism

Hypertension, particularly diastolic, may be more common in hypothyroid patients. Among 40 patients prospectively followed over the time who became hypothyroid after radioiodine therapy for thyrotoxicosis, 16 (40%) developed a diastolic BP higher than 90 mm Hg (Streeten et al., 1988). However, others found no differences in diastolic BP in 122 elderly patients with elevated thyroid-stimulating hormone levels, averaging 13.8 mU/L, as compared to the BPs in euthyroid controls (Bergus et al., 1999).

Hypothyroid patients tend to have a low cardiac output with a decrease in contractility and impaired diastolic relaxation (Danzi & Klein, 2003). To maintain tissue perfusion, peripheral resistance increases, from a combination of increased responsiveness of α-adrenergic receptors, increased levels of sympathetic nervous activity (Fletcher & Weetman, 1998), and aldosterone (Fommei & Iervasi, 2002). These would tend to raise diastolic BPs more than systolic BPs, the usual pattern seen in hypothyroidism (Saito & Saruta, 1994).

A hormonal status pointing toward incipient hypothyroidism was found among apparently healthy, community-dwelling subjects: The 194 hypertensives had higher TSH levels (1.7 vs 1.5) and lower free thyroxine index (6.8 vs 7.8) than the 90 normotensives (Gumieniak et al., 2004).

### Hyperthyroidism

An elevated systolic but lowered diastolic BP is usual in patients with hyperthyroidism. This pattern is associated with a high cardiac output and reduced peripheral resistance (Danzi & Klein, 2003).

## Hyperparathyroidism

Primary hyperparathyroidism (PHPT), once seen only as a symptomatic disease with significant hypercalcemia, is now most commonly recognized in asymptomatic patients with minimally elevated serum calcium levels (Bilezikian & Silverberg, 2004). Often the hypercalcemia is noted only after thiazide therapy is started.

Hypertension is common in PHPT (Toft, 2000) and, if present, contributes to the increased risk of cardiovascular events that, along with the BP, may not be ameliorated by parathyroidectomy (Vestergaard & Mosekilde, 2003). Since no correlation was found between serum calcium or parathyroid hormone levels and BP in 194 PHPT patients (Lumachi et al., 2000), it is perhaps not surprising that hypertension usually does not recede after surgical relief (Silverberg, 2000), although left ventricular hypertrophy usually regresses (Stefenelli et al., 1997). The ability of the oral calcimimetic cinacalcet to relieve hypertension has not yet been reported (Peacock et al., 2005).

## Acromegaly

Hypertension is found in approximately 35% of patients with acromegaly and is a risk factor for their increased rate of mortality (Holdaway et al., 2004). The hypertension is related to a number of factors: sodium retention (Gomberg-Maitland & Frishman, 1996), increased sympathetic vasoconstriction and reduced endothelium-dependent vasodilation (Maison et al., 2000), and hypertrophic remodeling of resistance arteries (Rizzoni et al., 2004). Left ventricular hypertrophy and impaired systolic function are usual, a consequence of a specific acromegalic cardiomyopathy that is aggravated by hypertension (Colao et al., 2000). Cardiovascular risks are further increased by a high prevalence of sleep apnea (Weiss et al., 2000).

## OBSTRUCTIVE SLEEP APNEA

One of the reasons people in the United States are getting so fat is that they don't get enough sleep (Vorona et al., 2005). But there is an even worse problem: obstructive sleep apnea (OSA), which is common, infrequently diagnosed, and likely responsible for a significant incidence of hypertension (Baguet et al., 2005). In two large population studies in the U.S., about 20% of adults had mild OSA, defined as an apnea-hypopnea index of at least five episodes lasting 10 seconds or more per

hour of sleep, and 1 in 15 adults had OSA of a more severe degree (Young et al., 2004). Over a 5-year follow-up of subjects initially with a normal sleep study, 16% developed OSA, with 7.5% of moderate to severe degree (Tishler et al., 2003). Young et al. (2004) estimate that 75% to 80% of OSA patients who could benefit from treatment remain undiagnosed. Young children may have abnormal breathing patterns during sleep that are relieved by adenotonsillectomy (Guilleminault et al., 2004).

More than poor sleep may afflict OSA patients: Their relative likelihood of sudden cardiac death occurring between midnight and 6 a.m. was 2.6 times greater than seen among the general population (Gami et al., 2005).

### Clinical Features and Diagnosis

Obstructive sleep apnea should be considered in patients with the clinical features of increasing obesity, loud snoring, fitful sleep, and daytime sleepiness (Table 15–2). Although OSA is common in patients who are morbidly obese, most afflicted are not "Pickwickian." A 10% increase in weight was associated with a sixfold increased risk of developing OSA among subjects initially free of OSA (Peppard et al., 2000a). Virtually all with OSA will snore, but only approximately half of people who snore for more than half the night have sleep apnea (Ferini-Strambi et al., 1999). The diagnosis can be made by a sleep study at home (Tishler et al., 2003) but with more certainty by overnight polysomnography in a sleep laboratory, with continuous recordings of respiration, electroencephalogram, electromyogram, eye movements, electrocardiogram, $O_2$ saturation, and BP (Caples et al., 2005).

### Association with Hypertension

#### Incidence

Multiple cross-sectional and observational studies have unequivocally shown a higher prevalence and incidence of systemic hypertension in direct proportion to the severity of sleep apnea (Sjöström et al., 2002). The odds ratio (OR) for hypertension among patients with sleep apnea has been found to vary from as little as 1.37 (Nieto et al., 2000) to 2.89 (Peppard et al., 2000a) to 4.15 (Grote et al., 1999). Increasing ORs are seen with increasing levels of sleep apnea. Lavie et al. (2000) found that each apneic event per hour of sleep increased the odds for hypertension by 1%, whereas each 10% decrease in $O_2$ saturation increased the odds by 13%.

A history of snoring, by itself, has been associated with an increased incidence of hypertension. Among 73,000 U.S. female nurses followed for

## TABLE 15–2

### Clinical Features of Obstructive Sleep Apnea

History
  Snoring[a]
  Apnea during sleep
  Arousals or awakenings
  Choking spells
  Nocturnal diaphoresis or enuresis
  Abnormal motor activity during sleep
  Excessive daytime sleepiness[a]
  Headaches
  Loss of memory and concentration
  Personality changes, depression
  Angina
  Diminished libido, impotence
Physical Examination
  Hypertension[a]
  Overweight, particularly visceral[a]
Oral Cavity Abnormalities
  Enlarged tonsils
  Thickened uvula
  Long and redundant soft palate
Cardiovascular Findings
  Increased heart rate variability
  Left ventricular hypertrophy
  Arrhythmias
  Conduction disturbances

[a]Most useful in considering diagnosis.

8 years, the risk of developing hypertension increased by 29% in those who snored occasionally and by 55% in those who snored regularly as compared to those who said they did not snore (Hu et al., 1999). The association was independent of age, body mass index, waist circumference, and other lifestyle factors.

The risk of hypertension is greater for younger subjects than for those older than 60 years (Haas et al., 2005) and is independent of all other relevant risk factors (Lavie et al., 2000). Moreover, the prevalence of sleep apnea is even higher both in patients with uncontrolled hypertension (Grote et al., 2000; Logan et al., 2003) and in patients after stroke (Mohsenin, 2001).

### Mechanisms of Hypertension

A number of possible mechanisms for persistent hypertension as a consequence of OSA have been proposed (Caples et al., 2005). Increased sympathetic nervous activity (Wolk et al., 2003), increased levels of endothelin-1 (Phillips et al., 1999), and erythropoietin (Winnicki et al., 2004) have been measured along with a blunted vasodilation in response to various stimuli (Duchna et al., 2000). Low levels of plasma renin activity and increased levels of urinary aldosterone were noted in half of 72 patients with resistant hypertension and features suggestive of OSA (Calhoun et al., 2004).

### Treatment

Weight loss—even as little as 10% of body weight (Peppard et al., 2000b)—and regular exercise (Sherrill et al., 1998) will help over the long term; avoiding the supine position during sleep by taping a tennis ball to the back may help in the short-term (Berger et al., 1997). The best relief is by nasal continuous positive airway pressure, which has been shown in controlled trials to relieve symptoms (Patel et al., 2003) and lower day and night blood pressure by about 10 mm Hg (Becker et al., 2003).

These effects on BP are accompanied by decreases in daytime sympathetic nerve traffic (Narkiewicz et al., 1999) and improved vasodilator responses (Leuenberger et al., 2000).

If the hypertension persists, antihypertensive drugs should be used. In a sequential study of one agent each from five classes of drugs, each given for 6 weeks to 40 hypertensives with obstructive sleep apnea, atenolol, 50 mg per day, provided greater lowering of both office and 24-hour ambulatory BP than did amlodipine, enalapril, losartan, or hydrochlorothiazide (Kraiczi et al., 2000). This better response to a β-blocker is in keeping with the known involvement of increased sympathetic nervous activity in the causation of obstructive sleep apnea-induced hypertension. No effects on sleep-disordered breathing or daytime well-being were noted with any of the drugs.

As will be noted in the next chapter, OSA is increasingly being recognized in obese children (Wing et al., 2003). Among them, adenotonsillectomy may provide considerable relief (Tarasiuk et al., 2004).

## NEUROLOGIC DISORDERS

Beyond stroke, the most common neurological disease associated with hypertension *may* be Alzheimer's. More certainly, a number of seemingly different disorders of the central and peripheral nervous system may cause hypertension. Many may do so by a common mechanism involving sympathetic nervous system discharge from the vasomotor centers in response to an increased intracranial pressure. The rise in systemic pressure is necessary to restore cerebral perfusion.

As noted in Chapters 4 and 7, patients with acute stroke may have transient marked elevations in BP. Rarely, episodic hypertension suggestive of a pheochromocytoma may occur after cerebral infarction (Funck-Brentano et al., 1987).

### Alzheimer's Disease

As noted by Casserly and Topol (2004), the late-onset disease, which accounts for 90% to 95% of all cases, appears to be linked to both vascular risk factors including hypertension and atherosclerosis. Prospective analyses of large populations have provided mixed results in regard to a connection to prior hypertension: Some find no association (Lindsay et al., 2002); most do (Kivipelto et al., 2001; Qiu et al., 2003). The presence of hypertension in late midlife (age 68) was associated with a decline in cognitive function in those retested at age 81 (Reinprecht et al., 2003). However, a causal connection between hypertension and Alzheimer's remains speculative (de la Torre, 2002). Once developed, Alzheimer's is usually accompanied by *less* hypertension, blood pressure apparently receding as the process worsens even without weight loss (Morris et al., 2000).

### Brain Tumors

Intracranial tumors, especially those arising in the posterior fossa, may cause hypertension (Pallini et al., 1995). In some patients, paroxysmal hypertension and other features that suggest catecholamine excess may point mistakenly to the diagnosis of pheochromocytoma. The problem may be confounded by the increased incidence of neuroectodermal tumors, some within the central nervous system, in patients with pheochromocytoma. Unlike patients with a pheochromocytoma who always have high catechol levels, patients with a brain tumor may have increased catecholamine levels during a paroxysm of hypertension but normal levels at other times.

### Quadriplegia

Patients with transverse lesions of the cervical spinal cord above the origins of the thoracolumbar sympathetic neurons lose central control of their sympathetic outflow. Stimulation of nerves below the injury, as with bladder or bowel distension, may cause reflex sympathetic activity via the isolated spinal cord, inducing hypertension, sweating, flushing, piloerection, and headache, a syndrome described as *autonomic hyperreflexia*. Such patients have markedly exaggerated pressor responses to various stimuli (Krum et al., 1992). The hypertension may be severe and persistent enough to cause cerebrovascular accidents and death. An α-blocker effectively controlled the syndrome (Chancellor et al., 1994).

### Severe Head Injury

Immediately after severe head injury, the BP may rise because of a hyperdynamic state mediated by excessive sympathetic nervous activity (Simard & Bellefleur, 1989). If the hypertension is persistent and severe, a short-acting β-blocker (e.g., esmolol) should be given. Caution is needed in the use of vasodilators such as hydralazine and nitroprusside, which may increase cerebral blood flow and intracranial pressure (Van Aken et al., 1989). Moreover, hypotension is an even greater threat (Winchell et al., 1996).

### Other Neurologic Disorders

Hypertension may be seen with:

- Guillain-Barré syndrome (Minami et al., 1995).
- Fatal familial insomnia, a prion disease with severe atrophy of the thalamus (Portaluppi et al., 1994).
- Baroreceptor failure (Robertson et al., 1993).
- Autonomic failure with orthostatic hypotension and supine hypertension, which may be helped by bedtime transdermal nitroglycerin (Shannon et al., 1996).
- Parkinson's disease, wherein severe postural hypotension may also be accompanied by nocturnal hypertension (Arias-Vera et al., 2003).

## FUNCTIONAL SOMATIC DISORDERS

Anxiety and depression are common in the general population and even more prevalent in patients with hypertension or cardiovascular disease (Davies et al., 2004). The incidence of psychiatric morbidity will certainly rise as a consequence of the persistent threat of terrorism (Hassett & Sigal, 2002) and the return of more soldiers from the Iraqi conflict (Clauw, 2003). Even before these provocations, 17.9% of postmeopausal women reported having panic attacks over a 6-month interval (Smoller et al., 2003).

As common as it is, anxiety and its manifestations are often not recognized as being responsible for a variety of symptoms. Because of the common failure to recognize the underlying nature of various functional syndromes (Wessely et al., 1999) (Table 15–3), patients and their physicians often enter into a vicious cycle: more and more testing, often with false-positive results; more and more incorrect "organic" disease diagnoses; more and more ineffective therapy; more and more anxiety; and more and more functional symptoms.

## Anxiety-Induced Hyperventilation

The problem is often encountered with hypertensive patients, either because of their concern over having "the silent killer" or because of their poor response to antihypertensive therapies. In 300 consecutive patients referred to me, usually because of hypertension that was difficult to control, 104 had symptoms attributable to anxiety-induced hyperventilation (Kaplan, 1997) (Figure 15–1). The symptoms and signs of panic attack encompass all these same manifestations but go beyond them to include fears of falling apart, losing control, or even more acute anxiety and are associated with

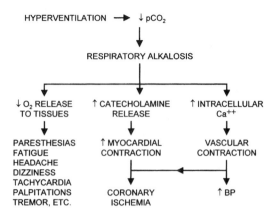

**FIGURE 15–1** ● The mechanisms by which acute hyperventilation may induce various symptoms, coronary ischemia, and a rise in blood pressure (BP). Ca, calcium; $pCO_2$, partial pressure of carbon dioxide.

increased reactivity of vasoconstricting sympathetic nerves (Lambert et al., 2002).

Many of these patients had been subjected to intensive workup for dizziness, headaches, chest pain, fatigue, and the like (Kaplan, 1997). In only a small number had the referring physicians considered the functional nature of their symptoms. When the symptoms are reproduced by voluntary overbreathing and relieved by rebreathing into a paper sack, the patient's recognition of the mechanism often provides immediate relief and opens the way to the appropriate use of rebreathing exercises, other cognitive therapy or, if needed, antianxiety medications.

My experience is not unique. Among 351 hypertensive patients randomly selected from one primary care practice in Sheffield, United Kingdom, panic attacks had occurred in 18% during the previous 6 months and in 37% over their lifetime (Davies et al., 1999). The reported diagnosis of hypertension usually antedated the onset of panic attacks. Anxiety and panic attacks were even more common among their patients who had nonspecific intolerance to multiple antihypertensive drugs (Davies et al., 2003). Mann (1999) described 21 patients with severe, symptomatic paroxysmal hypertension that had usually been attributed to a pheochromocytoma but that was emotionally provoked and was relieved by antianxiety therapies.

In patients who have experienced panic attacks, the BP rises significantly during voluntary hyperventilation, unlike a tendency for the BP to go down during hyperventilation in subjects who have not had panic attacks (Fontana et al., 2003; Martinez et al., 1998). Moreover, they tend to have more distress and slower recovery from hypocapnia during voluntary hyperventilation (Wilhelm et al., 2001).

## TABLE 15–3

## Functional Somatic Syndromes by Specialty

| Specialty | Syndrome |
| --- | --- |
| Gastroenterology | Irritable bowel syndrome, nonulcer dyspepsia |
| Gynecology | Premenstrual syndrome, chronic pelvic pain |
| Rheumatology | Fibromyalgia |
| Cardiology | Atypical or noncardiac chest pain |
| Respiratory medicine | Hyperventilation syndrome |
| Infectious diseases | Chronic (postviral) fatigue syndrome |
| Neurology | Tension headache |
| Dentistry | Temporomandibular joint dysfunction, atypical facial pain |
| Ear, nose, and throat | Globus syndrome |
| Allergy | Multiple chemical sensitivity |

Modified from Wessely S, Nimnuan C, Sharpe N. Functional somatic syndromes: one or many? *Lancet* 1999;354:936–939.

The scenario is obvious: Anxiety over hypertension may lead to more hypertension; failure to recognize the functional nature of the symptoms may lead to more anxiety, and on and on. A direct correlation between levels of anxiety, measured by the Spielberger Inventory Trait, and BP has been observed (Paterniti et al., 1999). As noted in Chapter 3, anxiety from psychological stress may be involved in the genesis of hypertension. Hypertension can also be responsible for more anxiety. Of further interest, Gratacòs et al. (2001) found a gene duplication on chromosome 15 in 90% of patients with anxiety disorders so that other connections with hypertension may be involved.

Depression may not be more common in uncomplicated hypertension, but it is frequently observed after heart attack or stroke (Gump et al., 2005). Selective serotonin reuptake inhibitor antidepressants do not affect blood pressure (Davies et al., 2004).

## ACUTE PHYSICAL STRESS

Hypertension may appear during various acute physical stresses, usually reflecting an intense sympathetic discharge and sometimes the contribution of increased renin-angiotensin from volume contraction. Problems related to anesthesia and surgery are covered in Chapter 7.

### Medical Conditions

Significant hypertension has been observed in patients with various acutely stressed medical conditions, including the following:

- Hypoglycemia, particularly if it develops in diabetics receiving noncardioselective β-blockers, wherein α-mediated vasoconstriction may be unopposed (Lloyd-Mostyn & Oram, 1975);
- Acute pancreatitis (Greenstein et al., 1987);
- Acute intermittent porphyria (Andersson et al., 2000); and
- Acute respiratory distress in patients with chronic obstructive pulmonary disease (Fontana et al., 2000).

### Surgical Conditions

#### Perioperative Hypertension

In addition to the reasons mentioned in the coverage of anesthesia and hypertension in Chapter 7, for numerous reasons hypertension may be a problem during and soon after surgery. In 60 patients with transient postoperative readings in excess of 190/100 mm Hg in the recovery room, the probable causes were pain (36%), hypoxia and hypercapnia (19%), and physical and emotional excitement (32%) (Gal

& Cooperman, 1975). As noted in Chapter 8, these causes should be managed rather than treating the BP with antihypertensives.

Marked rises in BP have been measured when pneumoperitoneum is performed for abdominal laparoscopic surgery (Joris et al., 1998). The rise in BP was accompanied by increases in blood catecholamines, cortisol, and vasopressin and was blunted by preoperative clonidine.

### Cardiovascular Surgery

Table 15–4 summarizes the causes of hypertension associated with surgery in a temporal fashion (Estafanous & Tarazi, 1980; Vuylsteke et al., 2000).
*Coronary Bypass*
Approximately one third of patients will have hypertension after coronary artery bypass grafting, usually starting within the first 2 hours after surgery and lasting 4 to 6 hours. Immediate therapy may be important to prevent postoperative heart

---

## TABLE 15–4

### Hypertension Associated with Cardiac Surgery

Preoperative
   Anxiety, angina
   Discontinuation of antihypertensive therapy
   Rebound from β-blockers in patients with coronary artery disease
Intraoperative
   Induction of anesthesia: tracheal intubation; nasopharyngeal, urethral, or rectal manipulation
   Before cardiopulmonary bypass (during sternotomy and chest retraction)
   Cardiopulmonary bypass
   After cardiopulmonary bypass (during surgery)
Postoperative
   Early (within 2 hours)
      Obvious cause: hypoxia, hypercapnia, ventilatory difficulties, hypothermia, shivering, arousal from anesthesia
      With no obvious cause: after myocardial revascularization; less frequently after valve replacement; after resection of aortic coarctation
   Late (weeks to months)
      After aortic valve replacement by homografts

Modified from Estafanous FG, Tarazi RC. Systemic arterial hypertension associated with cardiac surgery. *Am J Cardiol* 1980;46:685–694.

failure or myocardial infarction. In addition to deepening of anesthesia, various parenteral antihypertensives have been used, including nitroprusside and nitroglycerin (Vuylsteke et al., 2000).

*Other Cardiac Surgery*

Hypertension has been reported, although less frequently, after other cardiac surgery. Virtually all patients who undergo orthotopic heart transplantation develop hypertension (Taegtmeyer et al., 2004) and lose the usual nocturnal fall in BP, likely from a combination of effects, including the effects of immunosuppressive agents (see the section "Cyclosporine and Tacrolimus," later in this chapter), impaired baroreceptor control from cardiac denervation, and inability to excrete sodium normally (Eisen, 2003). The hypertension may be controlled by either angiotensin-converting enzyme inhibitors (ACEI) or calcium channel blockers (CCBs) as monotherapy, each effective in approximately half of patients (Brozena et al., 1996).

*Carotid Endarterectomy*

Postoperative hypertension may be particularly serious in patients with known cerebrovascular disease who have carotid endarterectomy, perhaps because of increased baroreceptor sensitivity (Hirschl et al., 1993). Treatment most logically should be with either of the short-acting β-blockers esmolol or labetalol (Orlowski et al., 1988) rather than with a vasodilator that might further increase cerebral blood flow.

## INCREASED INTRAVASCULAR VOLUME

If vascular volume is raised a significant degree over a short period, the renal natriuretic response may not be able to excrete the excess volume, particularly if renal function is also impaired.

### Erythropoietin Therapy

Recombinant human erythropoietin is now being widely used to correct the anemia of chronic renal failure. As the hematocrit rises, so do blood viscosity and BP; nearly one third of patients developed clinically important hypertension (Luft, 2000).

### Polycythemia and Hyperviscosity

Patients with primary polycythemia are often hypertensive, and some hypertensives have a relative polycythemia that may resolve when the BP is lowered (Chrysant et al., 1976). The hypertension seen in polycythemic states may reflect increased blood viscosity (de Simone et al., 2005). Significant falls in BP were seen in 12 hypertensive patients with polycythemia when blood viscosity was reduced without changing blood volume (Bertinieri et al., 1998).

### Inappropriate Antidiuretic Hormone

Hypertension has been reported in patients with inappropriate secretion of antidiuretic hormone, presumably related to an overexpanded vascular volume (Whitaker et al., 1979).

## CHEMICAL AGENTS THAT CAUSE HYPERTENSION

Table 15–5 lists various chemical agents that may cause hypertension, indicating their mechanism if known. Some of these substances, such as sodium-containing antacids, alcohol, insulin, licorice, oral contraceptives, and monoamine oxidase inhibitors, are covered elsewhere in this book because of their frequency or special features.

### Caffeine

Caffeine is likely the most widely consumed drug in the world, and its use will almost certainly increase with the amazing proliferation of Starbucks and its clones. Acting as a sympathomimetic, it acutely raises BP by increasing peripheral resistance by an increase in aortic stiffness (Vlachopoulos et al., 2003). Although tolerance to this pressor effect has been widely assumed, such tolerance was found in only half of regular consumers (Lovallo et al., 2004).

Increasingly strong evidence points to an effect of caffeine on BP, at least in those who remain tolerant. Acutely, about half of hypertensives given 250 mg of caffeine had significant rises in blood pressure that persisted for about 3 hours (Rachima-Maoz et al., 1998). Among older hypertensives, 24-hour ambulatory blood pressures rose an average of 4.8/3.0 mm Hg after ingestion of 300 mg of caffeine (Rakic et al., 1999).

Despite these effects, after a follow-up of 33 years, coffee drinkers had only a slightly higher blood pressure and an insignificant increase in the prevalence of hypertension (Klag et al., 2002). Moreover, long-term coffee consumption was associated with a significantly lower risk for type 2 diabetes (Salazar-Martinez et al., 2004). Despite some conflicting data, chronic caffeine ingestion has not been found to increase the risk for cardiovascular disease (Frishman et al., 2003).

Thus, the effects of caffeine on hypertension may, over the long term, be neutral but, at least acutely, a pressor effect may be noted. It may involve other components of coffee than caffeine (Corti et al., 2002), and tea may induce even larger immediate pressor effects (Hodgson et al., 1999). Perhaps the wisest course is to have patients check their home BPs before and within an hour after drinking their coffee or tea. Those who experience

| TABLE 15–5 |
|---|

## Hypertension Induced by Chemical Agents

| Mechanism | Examples |
|---|---|
| **Expansion of fluid volume** | |
| Increased sodium intake | Antacids, processed foods (Chapter 6) |
| Mineralocorticoid effects | Licorice (Chapter 13); cortisone (Chapter 14); anabolic steroids (Owens et al., 1998) |
| Stimulation of renin-angiotensin | Estrogens (oral contraceptives; Chapter 11) |
| Inhibition of prostaglandins | NSAIDs (Solomon, 2004) |
| **Stimulation of sympathetic nervous activity** | |
| Sympathomimetic agents | Caffeine (Lovallo et al., 2004); cocaine (Tuncel et al., 2002); ephedrine (Bent et al., 2003); methylenedioxymethamphetamine (MDMA, "ecstasy") (Lester et al., 2000); methylphenidate (Ritalin) (Ballard et al., 1976); modafinil (Taneja et al., 2005); nicotine (Halimi et al., 2002); phencyclidine (Sernulan) (Eastman & Cohen, 1975); phenylpropanolamine (Kernan et al., 2000) |
| Interactions with monoamine oxidase inhibitors | Foods with high tyramine content (e.g., red wines, aged cheese) (Liu & Rustgi, 1987) |
| Anesthetics | Ketamine (Broughton Pipkin & Waldron, 1983) |
| Ergot alkaloids | Ergotamine (Joyce & Gubbay, 1986) |
| Dopamine receptor agonist | Bromocriptine (Bakht et al., 1990) |
| Antidopaminergic | Metoclopramide (Roche et al., 1985) |
| Sandostatin analogue | Sandostatin LAR (Pop-Busui et al., 2000) |
| **Interference with antihypertensive drugs** | |
| Inhibition of prostaglandin synthesis | NSAIDs (Izhar et al., 2004) |
| Inhibition of neuronal uptake | Tricyclic antidepressants (Walsh et al., 1992) Sibutramine (Bray, 2002) |
| **Paradoxical response to antihypertensive drugs** | |
| Withdrawal, followed by ↑ catechols | Clonidine (Metz et al., 1987) |
| Unopposed α-adrenergic vasoconstriction | β-blockers (Drayer et al., 1976) |
| Intrinsic sympathomimetic activity | Pindolol (Collins & King, 1972) |
| Combination α- and β-blocker | Propranolol plus clonidine (Warren et al., 1979) |
| **Unknown mechanisms** | |
| Heavy metal poisoning | Lead (Nash et al., 2003); mercury (Velzeboer et al., 1997); thallium (Bank et al., 1972) |
| Chemicals | Carbon disulfide (Egeland et al., 1992); arsenic (Rahman et al., 1999) methyl chloride (Scharnweber et al., 1974); polychlorinated biphenyl (Kreiss et al., 1981); |
| Insecticides | Parathion (Tsachalinas et al., 1971) |

*(continued)*

## TABLE 15–5 (Continued)

### Hypertension Induced by Chemical Agents

| Mechanism | Examples |
|---|---|
| Insect bites | Spider (Weitzman et al., 1977); scorpion (Gueron & Yaron, 1970) |
| Diagnostic agents | Indigo carmine (Wu & Johnson, 1969); pentagastrin (Merguet et al., 1968); thyrotropin-releasing hormone (Rosenthal et al., 1987) |
| Therapeutic agents | Bevacizumab (Kabbinavar et al., 2005); Cyclosporine (Zhang & Victor, 2000); clozapine (Henderson et al., 2004); disulfiram (Volicer & Nelson, 1984); erythropoietin (Luft, 2000); herbal remedies (De Smet, 2002); indinavir (Cattelan et al., 2000); lithium (Michaeli et al., 1984) |
| Alcohol | Alcohol (Sierksma et al., 2004) |

Adapted from Grossman E, Messerli FH. High blood pressure. A side effect of drugs, poisons, and food. *Arch Intern Med* 1995;155:450–460.

a significant pressor effect should be advised to reduce or stop their caffeine consumption.

### Nicotine and Smoking

Almost 25% of U.S. adults are currently smokers, and almost one third started before age 16 (Schoenborn et al., 2003). Obviously, the profound dangers of smoking are not adequately impressed upon young people, and they are easily enticed to smoke by such seemingly benign provocations as viewing smoking in movies (Dalton et al., 2003).

Even in chronic smokers, each cigarette induces a pressor response (Figure 15–2) (Mahmud & Feely, 2003). As seen in Figure 15–2, whereas the peripheral blood pressure returns to near baseline within 15 minutes, pressure within the aorta remains higher. Moreover, the indices of large artery stiffness start higher in the chronic smokers and remain higher than in the nonsmokers. These data suggest that the hemodynamic consequences of smoking have been underestimated for two reasons: First, in the smoke-free environment where patients are seen, the BP is usually measured well after the acute effects are over; second, the arm (peripheral) blood pressure is usually deceptively lower in chronic smokers who have reduced aortic-brachial pressure amplification (Mahmud & Feely, 2003). A similar acute increase of larger artery stiffness has been seen with cigar smoking (Vlachopoulos et al., 2004).

Data on prevalence of persistent hypertension among smokers have not been consistent: Most find them to have higher BP recorded by ambulatory monitoring while they continue to smoke (Oncken et al., 2001; Verdecchia et al., 1995), but, if BP is taken while subjects are not smoking, little more hypertension is seen (Halimi et al., 2002; Primatesta et al., 2001). On the contrary, when chronic smokers quit smoking, their blood pressures tend to rise (Lee et al., 2001), in large part because of weight gain (Halimi et al., 2002).

Smoking has been found to have a profoundly deleterious effect on renal function (Orth & Ritz, 2002), particularly in patients with diabetic nephropathy (Chuahirun et al., 2003). Moreover, the 2,983 smokers enrolled in the massive Hypertension Optimal Treatment (HOT) trial were the only subgroup to experience an *increased* risk of major cardiovascular events when given more intensive therapy to achieve a lower BP (Zanchetti et al., 2003). As the authors note, these data "strengthen the need for concerted efforts to persuade patients to quit smoking."

Fortunately, the nicotine replacement therapies that help patients quit do not seem to have deleterious cardiovascular effects (Benowitz et al., 2002).

### Alcohol

Alcohol is a two-edged sword: In excess, it is a major cause of social disorder, trauma, and death; in moderation, it is a protector against heart attack,

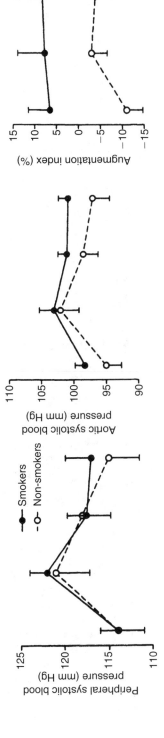
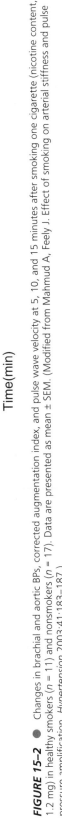
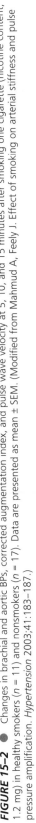

**FIGURE 15-2** ● Changes in brachial and aortic BPs, corrected augmentation index, and pulse wave velocity at 5, 10, and 15 minutes after smoking one cigarette (nicotine content, 1.2 mg) in healthy smokers (*n* = 11) and nonsmokers (*n* = 17). Data are presented as mean ± SEM. (Modified from Mahmud A, Feely J. Effect of smoking on arterial stiffness and pulse pressure amplification. *Hypertension* 2003;41:183–187.)

stroke, diabetes, and, likely, dementia (Rehm et al., 2003). Part of its diverse role involves hypertension: In excess, alcohol raises BP; in moderation, it may be protective against the development of hypertension.

### The Relation to Hypertension

When consumed in amounts equivalent to three usual portions—a usual portion being 12 ounces of beer, 4 ounces of wine, or 1.5 ounces of whiskey, which all contain about 12 g of ethanol—alcohol causes an immediate depressor effect and subsequently a pressor action (Rosito et al., 1999). These changes are reflected in measurements of arterial stiffness by pulse-wave velocity (Mahmud & Feely, 2002; Sierksma et al., 2004).

In large population studies, the incidence of hypertension is increased among those who drink more than three drinks per day, either in a liner dose-response relationship (Fuchs et al., 2001) or with a threshold wherein smaller quantities are associated with a modest decrease (Thadhani et al., 2002). The cessation of heavy drinking is usually followed by significant falls in BP (Aguilera et al., 1999).

The mechanisms for the pressor effect of large quantities of ethanol are not well defined, but in moderate amounts, multiple beneficial effects have been noted, which could translate into both antihypertensive actions and multiple protective effects. These effects include improvements in glucose tolerance and insulin sensitivity (Davies et al., 2002), reductions in lipoprotein(a) along with rises in HDL-cholesterol (Catena et al., 2003), and decreases in levels of inflammatory markers such as interleukin-6 and C-reactive protein (Volpato et al., 2004).

### Relations to Other Diseases

Light to moderate consumption, i.e., less than three drinks per day, has been shown to provide multiple significant benefits, including:

- Decreased risk of myocardial infarction (Mukamal et al., 2003a);
- Decreased complications after myocardial infarction (de Lorgeril et al., 2002);
- Decreased risk of congestive heart failure (Walsh et al., 2002);
- Decreased risk of stroke (Iso et al., 2004);
- Decreased complications after stroke (Jackson et al., 2003);
- Decreased risk of dementia in people over age 55 (Ruitenberg et al., 2002) or over age 65 (Mukamal et al., 2003b);
- Decreased risk of type 2 diabetes (Wannamethee et al., 2003) and a decreased risk of heart disease in those with diabetes (Howard et al., 2004); and

- Higher bone mineral density in elderly women (Rapuri et al., 2000).

This litany of benefits must be balanced by the potential for encouragement of alcohol abuse and a high prevalence of excessive drinking among the elderly (O'Connell et al., 2003). Gout is more common among even light drinkers (Choi et al., 2004). Moreover, alcohol consumption beyond 1.5 drinks per day was found to increase the risk of breast cancer in postmenopausal women (Chen et al., 2002), although a reduced mortality from cancer has been noted in wine drinkers (Grønbæk et al., 2000). And, despite the aforementioned decrease in dementia, brain atrophy has been found to increase linearly with alcohol intake (Ding et al., 2004).

### Conclusions

Those who choose to drink in moderation should be encouraged to continue. The type of alcohol-containing beverage is likely irrelevant; the putative greater benefits of wine (Di Castelnuovo et al., 2002) likely reflect a healthier lifestyle (Barefoot et al., 2002) and psychological functioning (Mortensen et al., 2001) among wine drinkers as opposed to beer and whiskey drinkers.

I have no hesitation in encouraging hypertensives to drink in moderation, but others do not believe that drinking alcohol should be recommended by physicians (Wilson, 2003).

### Nonsteroidal Anti-inflammatory Drugs (NSAIDs)

Nonsteroidal anti-inflammatory drugs are well known to blunt the antihypertensive effect of most antihypertensive agents (Izhar et al., 2004), with the apparent exception of CCBs. This interference likely reflects an inhibition of prostaglandin-dependent counter-regulatory mechanisms in the kidney that have been invoked by the antihypertensive drugs. Less well recognized is their propensity to increase the BP and precipitate hypertension (Grover et al., 2005).

Though this was noted with the first generation of nonspecific COX-1 inhibiting NSAIDs (Johnson et al., 1994), the most striking increased risk of new-onset hypertension has been noted with the selective COX-2 inhibitor rofecoxib (Vioxx) (Solomon et al., 2004). In this retrospective case-control study, the relative risk of new onset hypertension was 2.1 times higher with rofecoxib than with celecoxib (Celebrex). This finding coincides with the greater rise in BP and edema with this agent in osteoarthritic hypertensives (Aw et al., 2005; Whelton et al., 2002). As a consequence of an increased incidence of heart attack and stroke with rofecoxib, the drug has been withdrawn from the market (Chang & Harris, 2005).

## Cyclosporine and Tacrolimus

The introduction of cyclosporine in 1983 greatly improved the long-term survival of patients undergoing organ transplantation. However, major complications soon became obvious: nephrotoxicity and hypertension, which were assumed to be connected, and hepatotoxicity.

In 25% to 95% of patients given cyclosporine, hypertension develops after weeks or months, most commonly after heart transplantation (Eisen, 2003). Despite hopes that tacrolimus (FK506) would be less of a problem, it causes as much hypertension as does cyclosporine (Takeda et al., 1999).

### Mechanism

A number of abnormalities have been blamed for cyclosporine-induced hypertension (Eisen, 2003). The basic fault may involve a molecular mechanism that mediates both the immunosuppressive and the hypertensive actions of these drugs. Sander and co-workers (1996) noted that these agents bind to a recently discovered class of cytoplasmic receptors (immunophilins) present on various cells including T lymphocytes. Binding of cyclosporine to these receptors leads to inhibition of calcineurin, the calcium-calmodulin-dependent protein phosphatase. The inhibition of calcineurin was subsequently found to activate renal sympathetic afferent nerves (Zhang & Victor, 2000).

### Treatment

Whatever the mechanism, CCBs seem to prevent many of the adverse effects of cyclosporine (Sánchez-Lozada et al., 2000), but multiple drugs may be needed to overcome the hypertension (Taler et al., 1999).

## Other Agents

Perhaps the most commonly encountered form of chemically induced hypertension is that related to the use of foods and drugs containing large amounts of sodium. More dramatic effects are seen with the use of sympathomimetic agents. Large amounts of these drugs, available over the counter as herbal remedies (De Smet, 2002) and for use as nasal decongestants (e.g., pseudoephedrine) and, until recently, as appetite suppressants (e.g., phenylpropanolamine), may raise the BP enough to induce, on rare occasions, hypertensive encephalopathy, strokes, and heart attacks (Kernan et al., 2000). In usual doses, however, pseudoephedrine does not raise BP, even in patients receiving β-blockers

(Mores et al., 1999). The greatly increased risk of adverse reactions to ephedra (Bent et al., 2003) has led to restriction of its use in the United States. Perhaps the safest way to prevent these various interactions is to advise hypertensives to avoid all over-the-counter drugs and herbal remedies and to inform their physicians who prescribe other medications about their antihypertensive drug regimens.

## Street Drugs

Marijuana, or δ-9-tetrahydrocannabinol, in moderate amounts will increase the heart rate but may lower the BP (Frishman et al., 2003). More strikingly, although reported only in rats, endogenous cannabinoids acting at cannabinoid-1 receptors lower BP by reducing cardiac contractibility and vasodilating (Bátkai et al., 2004).

Cocaine (Tuncel et al., 2002) and amphetamines (Lester et al., 2000) may cause transient but significant hypertension that may cause strokes and serious cardiac damage. Most cocaine-related deaths are associated with myocardial injury similar to that seen from catecholamine excess and aggravated by acute hypertension (Lange & Hillis, 2001). Chronic cocaine abuse does not appear to induce hypertension (Brecklin et al., 1998) but may be associated with chronic renal disease (Vupputuri et al., 2004).

The next and last chapter looks further at hypertension in children and adolescents.

## REFERENCES

Aguilera MT, de la Sierra A, Coca A, et al. Effect of alcohol abstinence on blood pressure: assessment by 24-hour ambulatory blood pressure monitoring. *Hypertension* 1999; 33:653–657.

Andersson C, Lithner F, Wikberg A, Stegmayr B. Hypertension and renal impairment in patients with acute intermittent porphyria—a population-based study [Abstract]. *J Hypertens* 2000;18(Suppl 4):S98.

Arias-Vera JR, Mansoor GA, White WB. Abnormalities in blood pressure regulation in a patient with Parkinson's disease. *Am J Hypertens* 2003;16:612–613.

Aw TJ, Haas SJ, Liew D, Krum H. Meta-analysis of cyclooxygenase-2 inhibitors and their effects on blood pressure. *Arch Intern Med.* 2005;165:490–496.

Baguet JP, Hammer L, Lévy P, et al. Night-time and diastolic hypertension are common and underestimated conditions in newly diagnosed apnoeic patients. *J Hypertens* 2005;23:521–527.

Bakht FR, Kirshon B, Baker T, Cotton DB. Postpartum cardiovascular complications after bromocriptine and cocaine use. *Am J Obstet Gynecol* 1990;162:1065–1066.

Ballard JE, Boileau RA, Sleator EK, Massey BH, Sprague RL. Cardiovascular responses of hyperactive children to methylphenidate. *JAMA* 1976;236:2870–2874.

Bank WJ, Pleasure DE, Suzuki K, et al. Thallium poisoning. *Arch Neurol* 1972;26:456–464.

Barefoot JC, Grønbæk M, Feaganes JR, et al. Alcoholic beverage preference, diet, and health habits in the UNC Alumni Heart Study. *Am J Clin Nutr* 2002;76: 466–472.

Bátkai S, Pacher P, Osei-Hyiaman D, et al. Endocannabinoids acting at cannabinoid-1 receptors regulate cardiovascular function in hypertension. *Circulation* 2004;110:1996–2002.

Becker HF, Jerrentrup A, Ploch T, et al. Effect of nasal continuous positive airway pressure treatment on blood pressure in patients with obstructive sleep apnea. *Circulation* 2003;107:68–73.

Benowitz NL, Hansson A, Jacob P III. Cardiovascular effects of nasal and transdermal nicotine and cigarette smoking. *Hypertension* 2002;39:1107–1112.

Bent S, Tiedt TN, Odden MC, et al. The relative safety of ephedra compared with other herbal products. *Ann Intern Med* 2003;138:468–471.

Berger M, Oksenberg A, Silverberg DS, et al. Avoiding the supine position during sleep lowers 24 h blood pressure in obstructive sleep apnea (OSA) patients. *J Hum Hypertens* 1997;11:657–664.

Bergus GR, Mold JW, Barton ED, Randall CS. The lack of association between hypertension and hypothyroidism in a primary care setting. *J Hum Hypertens* 1999;13:231–235.

Bertinieri G, Parati G, Ulian L, et al. Hemodilution reduces clinic and ambulatory blood pressure in polycythemic patients. *Hypertension* 1998;31:848–853.

Bilezikian JP, Silverberg SJ. Clinical practice. Asymptomatic primary hyperparathyroidism. *N Engl J Med* 2004; 350:1746–1751.

Bray GA. Sibutramine and blood pressure: a therapeutic dilemma. *J Hum Hypertens* 2002;16:1–3.

Brecklin CS, Gopaniuk-Folga A, Kravetz T, et al. Prevalence of hypertension in chronic cocaine users. *Am J Hypertens* 1998;11:1279–1283.

Broughton Pipkin FB, Waldron BA. Ketamine hypertension and the renin-angiotensin system. *Clin Exp Hypertens* 1983;5:875–883.

Brozena SC, Johnson MR, Ventura H, et al. Effectiveness and safety of diltiazem or lisinopril in treatment of hypertension after heart transplantation. *J Am Coll Cardiol* 1996; 27:1707–1712.

Calhoun DA, Nishizaka MK, Zaman MA, Harding SM. Aldosterone excretion among subjects with resistant hypertension and symptoms of sleep apnea. *Chest* 2004;125: 112–117.

Campbell M. Natural history of coarctation of the aorta. *Br Heart J* 1970;32:633–640.

Caples SM, Gami AS, Somers VK. Obstructive sleep apnea. *Ann Intern Med* 2005;142:187–197.

Casserly I, Topol E. Convergence of atherosclerosis and Alzheimer's disease: inflammation, cholesterol, and misfolded proteins. *Lancet* 2004;363:1139–1146.

Catena C, Novello M, Dotto L, et al. Serum lipoprotein(a) concentrations and alcohol consumption in hypertension: possible relevance for cardiovascular damage. *J Hypertens* 2003;21:281–288.

Cattelan A, Trevenzoli M, Naso A, et al. Severe hypertension and renal atrophy associated with indinavir. *Clin Infect Dis* 2000;30:619–621.

Chancellor MB, Erhard MJ, Hirsch IH, Stass WE. Prospective evaluation of terazosin for the treatment of autonomic dysreflexia. *J Urol* 1994;151:111–113.

Chang IJ, Harris RC. Are all COX-2 inhibitors created equal? *Hypertension* 2005;45:178–180.

Chen WY, Colditz GA, Rosner B, et al. Use of postmenopausal hormones, alcohol, and risk for invasive breast cancer. *Ann Intern Med* 2002;137:798–804.

Choi HK, Atkinson K, Karlson EW, et al. Alcohol intake and risk of incident gout in men: a prospective study. *Lancet* 2004;363:1277–1281.

Chrysant SG, Frohlich ED, Adamopoulos PN, et al. Patho-physiologic significance of "stress" or relative poly-cythemia in essential hypertension. *Am J Cardiol* 1976;37: 1069–1072.

Chuahirun T, Khanna A, Kimball K, Wesson DE. Cigarette smoking and increased urine albumin excretion are interrelated predictors of nephropathy progression in type 2 diabetes. *Am J Kidney Dis* 2003;41:13–21.

Clauw D. The health consequences of the first Gulf war. *BMJ* 2003;327:1357–1358.

Colao A, Baldelli R, Marzullo P, et al. Systemic hypertension and impaired glucose tolerance are independently correlated to the severity of the acromegalic cardiomyopathy. *J Clin Endocrinol Metab* 2000;85:193–199.

Collins IS, King IW. Pindolol (Visken LB46): a new treatment for hypertension: report of a multicentric open study. *Curr Ther Res* 1972;14:37–194.

Connolly HM, Huston J III, Brown RD Jr, et al. Intracranial aneurysms in patients with coarctation of the aorta: a prospective magnetic resonance angiographic study of 100 patients. *Mayo Clin Proc* 2003;78:1491–1499.

Corti R, Binggeli C, Sudano I, et al. Coffee acutely increases sympathetic nerve activity and blood pressure independently of caffeine content: role of habitual versus nonhabitual drinking. *Circulation* 2002;106:2935–2940.

Dalton MA, Sargent JD, Beach ML, et al. Effect of viewing smoking in movies on adolescent smoking initiation: a cohort study. *Lancet* 2003;362:281–285.

Daniels SR. Repair of coarctation of the aorta and hypertension: does age matter? *Lancet* 2001;358:89.

Danzi S, Klein I. Thyroid hormone and blood pressure regulation. *Curr Hypertens Rep* 2003;5:513–520.

Davies MJ, Baer DJ, Judd JT, et al. Effects of moderate alcohol intake on fasting insulin and glucose concentrations and insulin sensitivity in postmenopausal women: a randomized controlled trial. *JAMA* 2002;287:2559–2562.

Davies SJC, Ghahramani P, Jackson PR, et al. Association of panic disorder and panic attacks with hypertension. *Am J Med* 1999;107:310–316.

Davies SJ, Jackson PR, Potokar J, Nutt DJ. Treatment of anxiety and depressive disorders in patients with cardiovascular disease. *BMJ* 2004;328:939–943.

Davies SJ, Jackson PR, Ramsay LE, Ghahramani P. Drug intolerance due to nonspecific adverse effects related to psychiatric morbidity in hypertensive patients. *Arch Intern Med* 2003;163:592–600.

de la Torre JC. Alzheimer disease as a vascular disorder: nosological evidence. *Stroke* 2002;33:1152–1162.

de Lorgeril M, Salen P, Martin JL, et al. Wine drinking and risks of cardiovascular complications after recent acute myocardial infarction. *Circulation* 2002;106:1465–1469.

de Simone G, Devereux RB, Chinali M, et al. Association of blood pressure with blood viscosity in American Indians: the Strong Heart Study. *Hypertension* 2005;45:625–630.

De Smet PA. Herbal remedies. *N Engl J Med* 2002;347: 2046–2056.

Di Castelnuovo A, Rotondo S, Iacoviello L, et al. Meta-analysis of wine and beer consumption in relation to vascular risk. *Circulation* 2002;105:2836–2844.

Ding J, Eigenbrodt ML, Mosley TH Jr, et al. Alcohol intake and cerebral abnormalities on magnetic resonance imaging in a community-based population of middle-aged adults: the Atherosclerosis Risk in Communities (ARIC) study. *Stroke* 2004;35:16–21.

Drayer JIM, Keim JH, Weber MA, et al. Unexpected pressor response to propranolol in essential hypertension: an interaction between renin-aldosterone and sympathetic activity. *Am J Med* 1976;60:887–893.

Duchna HW, Guilleminault C, Stoohs RA, et al. Vascular reactivity in obstructive sleep apnea syndrome. *Am J Respir Crit Care Med* 2000;161:187–191.

Eastman JW, Cohen SN. Hypertensive crisis and death associated with phencyclidine poisoning. *JAMA* 1975;231: 1270–1271.

Egeland GM, Burkhart GA, Schnorr TM, et al. Effects of exposure to carbon disulphide on low density lipoprotein cholesterol concentration and diastolic blood pressure. *Br J Indust Med* 1992;49:287–293.

Eisen HJ. Hypertension in heart transplant recipients: more than just cyclosporine. *J Am Coll Cardiol* 2003;41:433–434.

Estafanous FG, Tarazi RC. Systemic arterial hypertension associated with cardiac surgery. A*m J Cardiol* 1980;46: 685–694.

Ferini-Strambi L, Zucconi M, Castronovo V, et al. Snoring & sleep apnea: a population study in Italian women. *Sleep* 1999;22:859–864.

Fletcher AK, Weetman AP. Hypertension and hypothyroidism. *J Hum Hypertens* 1998;12:79–82.

Fommei E, Iervasi G. The role of thyroid hormone in blood pressure homeostasis: evidence from short-term hypothyroidism in humans. *J Clin Endocrinol Metab* 2002;87: 1996–2000.

Fontana F, Bernardi P, Lanfranchi G, et al. Blood pressure response to hyperventilation test reflects daytime pressor profile. *Hypertension* 2003;41:244–248.

Fontana F, Bernardi P, Tartuferi L, et al. Mechanisms of hypertension in patients with chronic obstructive pulmonary disease and acute respiratory failure. *Am J Med* 2000;109: 621–627.

Frishman WH, Del Vecchio A, Sanal S, Ismail A. Cardiovascular manifestations of substance abuse: part 2: alcohol, amphetamines, heroin, cannabis, and caffeine. *Heart Dis* 2003;5:253–271.

Fuchs FD, Chambless LE, Whelton PK, et al. Alcohol consumption and the incidence of hypertension: the Atherosclerosis Risk in Communities Study. *Hypertension* 2001; 37:1242–1250.

Funck-Brentano C, Pagny J-Y, Menard J. Neurogenic hypertension associated with an excessively high excretion rate of catecholamine metabolites. *Br Heart J* 1987;57:487–489.

Gal TJ, Cooperman LH. Hypertension in the immediate postoperative period. *Br J Anaesth* 1975;47:70–74.

Gami AS, Howard DE, Olson EJ, Somers VK. Day-night pattern of sudden death in obstructive sleep apnea. *N Engl J Med* 2005;352:1206–1214.

Gomberg-Maitland M, Frishman WH. Recombinant growth hormone: a new cardiovascular drug therapy. *Am Heart J* 1996;132:1244–1262.

Gratacòs M, Nadal M, Martín-Santos R, et al. A polymorphic genomic duplication on human chromosome 15 is a susceptibility factor for panic and phobic disorders. *Cell* 2001;106:367–379.

Greenstein RJ, Krakoff LR, Felton K. Activation of the renin system in acute pancreatitis. *Am J Med* 1987;82:401–404.

Grønbæk M, Becker U, Johansen D, et al. Type of alcohol consumed and mortality from all causes, coronary heart disease, and cancer. *Ann Intern Med* 2000;133: 411–419.

Grossman E, Messerli FH. High blood pressure. A side effect of drugs, poisons, and food. *Arch Intern Med* 1995;155: 450–460.

Grote L, Hedner J, Peter JH. Sleep-related breathing disorder is an independent risk factor for uncontrolled hypertension. *J Hypertens* 2000;18:679–685.

Grote L, Ploch T, Heitmann J, et al. Sleep-related breathing disorder is an independent risk factor for systemic hypertension. *Am J Respir Care Med* 1999;160:1875–1882.

Grover SA, Coupal L, Zowall H. Treating osteoarthritis with cyclooxygenase-2–specific inhibitors: what are the benefits of avoiding blood pressure destabilization? *Hypertension* 2005;45:92–97.

Gueron M, Yaron R. Cardiovascular manifestations of severe scorpion sting. *Chest* 1970;57:156–162.

Guilleminault C, Li K, Khramtsov A, et al. Breathing patterns in prepubertal children with sleep-related breathing disorders. *Arch Pediatr Adolesc Med* 2004;158: 153–161.

Gumieniak O, Perlstein TS, Hopkins PN, et al. Thyroid function and blood pressure homeostasis in euthyroid subjects. *J Clin Endocrinol Metab* 2004;89:3455–3461.

Gump BB, Matthews KA, Eberly LE, et al. Depressive symptoms and mortality in men: results from the Multiple Risk Factor Intervention trial. *Stroke* 2005;36:98–102.

Halimi JM, Giraudeau B, Vol S, et al. The risk of hypertension in men: direct and indirect effects of chronic smoking. *J Hypertens* 2002;20:187–193.

Haas DC, Foster GL, Nieto FJ, et al. Age-dependent associations between sleep-disordered breathing and hypertension: importance of discriminating between systolic/diastolic hypertension and isolated systolic hypertension in the Sleep Heart Health Study. *Circulation* 2005;111:614–621.

Hassett AL, Sigal LH. Unforeseen consequences of terrorism: medically unexplained symptoms in a time of fear. *Arch Intern Med* 2002;162:1809–1813.

Henderson DC, Daley TB, Kunkel L, et al. Clozapine and hypertension: a chart review of 82 patients. *J Clin Psychiatry* 2004;65:686–689.

Hirschl M, Kundi M, Hirschl MM, et al. Blood pressure responses after carotid surgery: relationship to postoperative baroreceptor sensitivity. *Am J Med* 1993;94:463–468.

Hodgson JM, Puddey IB, Burke V, et al. Effects on blood pressure of drinking green and black tea. *J Hypertens* 1999; 17:457–463.

Holdaway IM, Rajasoorya RC, Gamble GD. Factors influencing mortality in acromegaly. *J Clin Endocrinol Metab* 2004;89:667–674.

Howard AA, Arnsten JH, Gourevitch MN. Effect of alcohol consumption on diabetes mellitus: a systematic review. *Ann Intern Med* 2004;140:211–219.

Hu FB, Willett WC, Colditz GA, et al. Prospective study of snoring and risk of hypertension in women. *Am J Epidemiol* 1999;150:806–816.

Iso H, Baba S, Mannami T, et al. Alcohol consumption and risk of stroke among middle-aged men: the JPHC Study Cohort I. *Stroke* 2004;35:1124–1129.

Izhar M, Alausa T, Folker A, et al. Effects of COX inhibition on blood pressure and kidney function in ACE inhibitor-treated blacks and Hispanics. *Hypertension* 2004; 43:573–577.

Jackson VA, Sesso HD, Buring JE, Gaziano JM. Alcohol consumption and mortality in men with preexisting cerebrovascular disease. *Arch Intern Med* 2003;163:1189–1193.

Jenkins NP, Ward C. Coarctation of the aorta: natural history and outcome after surgical treatment. *QJM* 1999;92: 365–371.

Johnson AG, Nguyen TV, Day RO. Do nonsteroidal anti-inflammatory drugs affect blood pressure? A meta-analysis. *Ann Intern Med* 1994;121:289–300.

Joris JL, Chiche J-D, Canivet J-LM, et al. Hemodynamic changes induced by laparoscopy and their endocrine correlates: effects of clonidine. *J Am Coll Cardiol* 1998;32: 1389–1396.

Joyce DA, Gubbay SS. Arterial complications of migraine treatment with methysergide and parenteral ergotamine. *BMJ* 1986;285:260–261.

Kabbinavar FF, Schulz J, McCleod M, et al. Addition of bevacizumab to bolus fluorouracil and leucovorin in first-line metastatic colorectal cancer: results of a randomized phase II trial. *J Clin Oncol* 2005;23:3697–3705.

Kaplan NM. Anxiety-induced hyperventilation: a common cause of symptoms in patients with hypertension. *Arch Intern Med* 1997;157:945–948.

Kernan WN, Viscoli CM, Brass LM, et al. Phenylpropanolamine and the risk of hemorrhagic stroke. *N Engl J Med* 2000;343:1826–1832.

Kivipelto M, Helkala EL, Laakso MP, et al. Midlife vascular risk factors and Alzheimer's disease in later life: longitudinal, population based study. *BMJ* 2001;322: 1447–1451.

Klag MJ, Wang NY, Meoni LA, et al. Coffee intake and risk of hypertension: the Johns Hopkins precursors study. *Arch Intern Med* 2002;162:657–662.

Kraiczi H, Hedner J, Peker Y, Grote L. Comparison of atenolol, amlodipine, enalapril, hydrochlorothiazide, and losartan for antihypertensive treatment of patients with obstructive sleep apnea. *Am J Respir Crit Care Med* 2000; 161:1423–1428.

Kreiss K, Zack MM, Kimbrough RD, et al. Association of blood pressure and polychlorinated biphenyl levels. *JAMA* 1981;245:2505–2509.

Krum H, Louis WJ, Brow DJ, Howes LG. Pressor dose responses and baroreflex sensitivity in quadriplegic spinal cord injury patients. *J Hypertens* 1992;10:245–250.

Lambert EA, Thompson J, Schlaich M, et al. Sympathetic and cardiac baroreflex function in panic disorder. *J Hypertens* 2002;20:2445–2451.

Lange RA, Hillis LD. Cardiovascular complications of cocaine use. *N Engl J Med* 2001;345:351–358.

Lavie P, Herer P, Hoffstein V. Obstructive sleep apnoea syndrome as a risk factor for hypertension: population study. *BMJ* 2000;320:479–482.

Lee DH, Ha MH, Kim JR, Jacobs DR Jr. Effects of smoking cessation on changes in blood pressure and incidence of hypertension: a 4-year follow-up study. *Hypertension* 2001;37:194–198.

Lester SJ, Baggott M, Welm S, et al. Cardiovascular effects of 3,4-methylenedioxymethamphetamine: a double-blind, placebo-controlled trial. *Ann Intern Med* 2000;133:969–973.

Leuenberger UA, Sinoway LI, Imadojemu VA. Abnormal vasodilator responses in sleep apnea are improved with positive airway pressure therapy [Abstract]. *Circulation* 2000; 102(Suppl 2):II–515.

Lindsay J, Laurin D, Verreault R, et al. Risk factors for Alzheimer's disease: a prospective analysis from the Canadian Study of Health and Aging. *Am J Epidemiol* 2002; 156:445–453.

Liu L, Rustgi AK. Cardiac myonecrosis in hypertensive crisis associated with monoamine oxidase inhibitor therapy. *Am J Med* 1987;82:1060–1064.

Lloyd-Mostyn RH, Oram S. Modification by propranolol of cardiovascular effects of induced hypoglycemia. *Lancet* 1975;1:1213–1215.

Logan AG, Tkacova R, Perlikowski SM, et al. Refractory hypertension and sleep apnoea: effect of CPAP on blood pressure and baroreflex. *Eur Respir J* 2003;21:241–247.

Lovallo WR, Wilson MF, Vincent AS, et al. Blood pressure response to caffeine shows incomplete tolerance after short-term regular consumption. *Hypertension* 2004;43:760–765.

Luft FC. Erythropoietin and arterial hypertension. *Clin Nephrol* 2000;53(Suppl):S61–S64.

Lumachi F, Behboo R, Scarpa M, et al. The effect of serum calcium and serum PTH on arterial blood pressure in patients with primary hyperparathyroidism. Population based study in 194 patients undergoing parathyroidectomy [Abstract]. *Endo Soc* 2000;421.

Macdonald S, Thomas SM, Cleveland TJ, Gaines PA. Angioplasty or stenting in adult coarctation of the aorta? A

retrospective single center analysis over a decade. *Cardiovasc Interven Radiol* 2003;26:357–364.

Mahmud A, Feely J. Divergent effect of acute and chronic alcohol on arterial stiffness. *Am J Hypertens* 2002;15: 240–243.

Mahmud A, Feely J. Effect of smoking on arterial stiffness and pulse pressure amplification. *Hypertension* 2003;41: 183–187.

Maison P, Démolis P, Young J, et al. Vascular reactivity in acromegalic patients: preliminary evidence for regional endothelial dysfunction and increased sympathetic vasoconstriction. *Clin Endocrinol* 2000;53:445–451.

Mann SJ. Severe paroxysmal hypertension (pseudopheochromocytoma). *Arch Intern Med* 1999;159:670–674.

Martinez JM, Coplan JD, Browne ST, et al. Hemodynamic response to respiratory challenges in panic disorder. *J Psychosom Res* 1998;44:153–161.

Merguet P, Ewers HR, Brouwers HP. Blitdruck und Herzfrequenz von Normotonikern nach maximaler Stimulation der Magensekretion mit Pentagastrin. *Kongr Innere Med* 1968;80:561–564.

Metz S, Klein C, Morton N. Rebound hypertension after discontinuation of transdermal clonidine therapy. *Am J Med* 1987;82:17–19.

Minami N, Imai Y, Miura Y, Abe K. The mechanism responsible for hypertension in a patient with Guillain-Barré syndrome. *Clin Exp Hypertens* 1995;17:607–617.

Mohsenin V. Sleep-related breathing disorders and risk of stroke. *Stroke* 2001;32:1271–1278.

Mores N, Campia U, Navarra P, et al. No cardiovascular effects of single-dose pseudoephedrine in patients with essential hypertension treated with β-blockers. *Eur J Clin Pharmacol* 1999;55:251–254.

Morris MC, Scherr PA, Herbert LE, et al. The cross-sectional association between blood pressure and Alzheimer's disease in a biracial community population of older persons. *J Gerontol* 2000;55A:M130–M136.

Mortensen EL, Jensen HH, Sanders SA, Reinisch JM. Better psychological functioning and higher social status may largely explain the apparent health benefits of wine: a study of wine and beer drinking in young Danish adults. *Arch Intern Med* 2001;161:1844–1848.

Mukamal KJ, Conigrave KM, Mittleman MA, et al. Roles of drinking pattern and type of alcohol consumed in coronary heart disease in men. *N Engl J Med* 2003a;348:109–118.

Mukamal KJ, Kuller LH, Fitzpatrick AL, et al. Prospective study of alcohol consumption and risk of dementia in older adults. *JAMA* 2003b;289:1405–1413.

Narkiewicz K, Kato M, Phillips BG, et al. Nocturnal continuous positive airway pressure decreases daytime sympathetic traffic in obstructive sleep apnea. *Circulation* 1999; 100:2332–2335.

Nash D, Magder L, Lustberg M, et al. Blood lead, blood pressure, and hypertension in perimenopausal and postmenopausal women. *JAMA* 2003;289:1523–1532.

Nieto FJ, Young TB, Lind BK, et al. Association of sleep-disordered breathing, sleep apnea, and hypertension in a large community-based study. *JAMA* 2000;283: 1829–1936.

Niwa K, Perloff JK, Bhuta SM, et al. Structural abnormalities of great arterial walls in congenital heart disease: light and electron microscopic analyses. *Circulation* 2001;103: 393–400.

Numano F, Okawara M, Inomata H, Kobayashi Y. Takayasu's arthritis. *Lancet* 2000;356:1023–1025.

O'Connell H, Chin AV, Cunningham C, Lawlor B. Alcohol use disorders in elderly people—redefining an age old problem in old age. *BMJ* 2003;327:664–667.

Oncken CA, White WB, Cooney JL, et al. Impact of smoking cessation on ambulatory blood pressure and heart rate in postmenopausal women. *Am J Hypertens* 2001;14: 942–949.

Orlowski JP, Shiesley D, Vidt DG, et al. Labetalol to control blood pressure after cerebrovascular surgery. *Crit Care Med* 1988;16:765–768.

Orth SR, Ritz E. The renal risks of smoking: an update. *Curr Opin Nephrol Hypertens* 2002;11:483–488.

Owens P, Lyons S, O'Brien ET. Body beautiful? *J Hum Hypertens* 1998;12:485–487.

Pallini R, Lauretti L, Fernandez E. Chronic arterial hypertension as unique symptom of brainstem astrocytoma. *Lancet* 1995;345:1573.

Patel SR, White DP, Malhotra A, et al. Continuous positive airway pressure therapy for treating sleepiness in a diverse population with obstructive sleep apnea: results of a meta-analysis. *Arch Intern Med* 2003;163:565–571.

Paterniti S, Alpérovitch A, Ducimetière P, et al. Anxiety but not depression is associated with elevated blood pressure in a community group of French elderly. *Psychosom Med* 1999;61:77–83.

Peacock M, Bilezikian JP, Klassen PS, et al. Cinacalcet hydrochloride maintains long-term normocalcemia in patients with primary hyperparathyroidism. *J Clin Endocrinol Metab* 2005;90:135–141.

Pearl JM, Manning PB, Franklin C, et al. Risk of recoarctation should not be a deciding factor in the timing of coarctation repair. *Am J Cardiol* 2004;93:803–805.

Peppard PE, Young T, Palta M, et al. Longitudinal study of moderate weight change and sleep-disordered breathing. *JAMA* 2000b;284:3015–3021.

Peppard PE, Young T, Palta M, Skatrud J. Prospective study of the association between sleep-disordered breathing and hypertension. *N Engl J Med* 2000a;342:1378–1384.

Phillips BG, Narkiewicz K, Pesek CA, et al. Effects of obstructive sleep apnea on endothelin-1 and blood pressure. *J Hypertens* 1999;17:61–66.

Pop-Busui R, Chey W, Stevens MJ. Severe hypertension induced by the long-acting somatostatin analogue sandostatin LAR in a patient with diabetic autonomic neuropathy. *J Clin Endocrinol Metab* 2000;85:943–946.

Portaluppi F, Cortelli P, Avoni P, et al. Diurnal blood pressure variation and hormonal correlates in fatal familial insomnia. *Hypertension* 1994;23:569–576.

Primatesta P, Falaschetti E, Gupta S, et al. Association between smoking and blood pressure: evidence from the health survey for England. *Hypertension* 2001;37:187–193.

Qiu C, Winblad B, Viitanen M, Fratiglioni L. Pulse pressure and risk of Alzheimer disease in persons aged 75 years and older: a community-based, longitudinal study. *Stroke* 2003; 34:594–599.

Rachima-Maoz C, Peleg E, Rosenthal T. The effect of caffeine on ambulatory blood pressure in hypertensive patients. *Am J Hypertens* 1998;11:1426–1432.

Rahman M, Tondel M, Ahmad A, et al. Hypertension and arsenic exposure in Bangladesh. *Hypertension* 1999;33:74–78.

Rakic V, Burke V, Beilin LJ. Effects of coffee on ambulatory blood pressure in older men and women: a randomized controlled trial. *Hypertension* 1999;33:869–873.

Rapuri PB, Gallagher JC, Balhorn KE, Ryschon KL. Alcohol intake and bone metabolism in elderly women. *Am J Clin Nutr* 2000;72:1206–1213.

Rehm J, Room R, Graham K, et al. The relationship of average volume of alcohol consumption and patterns of drinking to burden of disease: an overview. *Addiction* 2003;98: 1209–1228.

Reinprecht F, Elmståhl S, Janzon L, André-Petersson L. Hypertension and changes of cognitive function in 81-year-old men: a 13-year follow-up of the population study "Men born in 1914," Sweden. *J Hypertens* 2003;21:57–66.

Rizzoni D, Porteri E, Giustina A, et al. Acromegalic patients show the presence of hypertrophic remodeling of subcutaneous small resistance arteries. *Hypertension* 2004; 43:561–565.

Robertson D, Hollister AS, Biaggioni I, et al. The diagnosis and treatment of baroreceptor failure. *N Engl J Med* 1993; 329:1449–1455.

Roche H, Hyman G, Nahas G. Hypertension and intravenous antidopaminergic drugs. *N Engl J Med* 1985;312: 1125–1126.

Rosenthal E, Najm YC, Maisey MN, Curry PVL. Pressor effects of thyrotrophin releasing hormone during thyroid function testing. *BMJ* 1987;294:806–807.

Rosito GA, Fuchs FD, Duncan BB. Dose-dependent biphasic effect of ethanol on 24-h blood pressure in normotensive subjects. *Am J Hypertens* 1999;12:236–240.

Ruitenberg A, van Swieten JC, Witteman JC, et al. Alcohol consumption and risk of dementia: the Rotterdam Study. *Lancet* 2002;359:281–286.

Saito I, Saruta T. Hypertension in thyroid disorders. *Endocrinol Metab Clin North Am* 1994;23:379–386.

Salazar-Martinez E, Willett WC, Ascherio A, et al. Coffee consumption and risk for type 2 diabetes mellitus. *Ann Intern Med* 2004;140:1–8.

Sánchez-Lozada LG, Gamba G, Bolio A, et al. Nifedipine prevents changes in nitric oxide synthase mRNA levels induced by cyclosporine. *Hypertension* 2000;36:642–647.

Sander M, Lyson T, Thomas GD, Victor RG. Sympathetic neural mechanisms of cyclosporine-induced hypertension. *Am J Hypertens* 1996;9:121S–138S.

Scharnweber HC, Spears GN, Cowles SR. Chronic methyl chloride intoxication in six industrial workers. *J Occup Med* 1974;16:112–113.

Schoenborn CA, Vickerie JL, Barnes PM. *Cigarette smoking behavior of adults: United States, 1997–98. Adv Data from vital and health statistics; no 331.* Hyattsville, MD: National Center for Health Statistics, 2003.

Shannon JR, Robertson RM, Biaggioni I. Treatment of hypertension in autonomic failure [Abstract]. *Circulation* 1996;94(Suppl 1):2676.

Sherrill DL, Kotchou K, Quan SF. Association of physical activity and human sleep disorders. *Arch Intern Med* 1998; 158:1894–1989.

Sierksma A, Muller M, van der Schouw YT, et al. Alcohol consumption and arterial stiffness in men. *J Hypertens* 2004; 22:357–362.

Silverberg SJ. Cardiovascular disease in primary hyperparathyroidism. *J Clin Endocrinol Metab* 2000;85:3513–3514.

Simard JM, Bellefleur M. Systemic arterial hypertension in head trauma. *Am J Cardiol* 1989;63:32C–35C.

Sjöström C, Lindberg E, Elmasry A, et al. Prevalence of sleep apnoea and snoring in hypertensive men: a population based study. *Thorax* 2002;57:602–607.

Smoller JW, Pollack MH, Wassertheil-Smoller S, et al. Prevalence and correlates of panic attacks in postmenopausal women: results from an ancillary study to the Women's Health Initiative. *Arch Intern Med* 2003;163:2041–2050.

Solomon DH, Schneeweiss S, Levin R, Avorn J. Relationship between COX-2 Specific inhibitors and hypertension. *Hypertension* 2004;44:140–145.

Stefenelli T, Abela C, Frank H, et al. Cardiac abnormalities in patients with primary hyperparathyroidism: implications for follow-up. *J Clin Endocrinol Metab* 1997;82:106–112.

Streeten DHP, Anderson GH Jr, Howland T, et al. Effects of thyroid function on blood pressure. Recognition of hypothyroid hypertension. *Hypertension* 1988;11:78–83.

Swan L, Ashrafian H, Gatzoulis MA. Repair of coarctation: a higher goal? *Lancet* 2002;359:977–978.

Taegtmeyer AB, Crook AM, Barton PJR, Banner NR. Reduced incidence of hypertension after heterotopic cardiac transplantation compared to orthotopic cardiac transplantation. *J Am Coll Cardiol* 2004;44:1254–1260.

Takeda Y, Miyamori I, Furukawa K, et al. Mechanisms of FK 506-induced hypertension in the rat. *Hypertension* 1999;33:130–136.

Taler SJ, Textor SC, Canzanello VJ, Schwartz L. Cyclosporin-induced hypertension: incidence, pathogenesis and management. *Drug Safety* 1999;20:437–449.

Taneja I, Diedrich A, Black BK, et al. Modafinil elicits sympathomedullary activation. *Hypertension* 2005;45:612–618.

Tarasiuk A, Simon T, Tal A, Reuveni H. Adenotonsillectomy in children with obstructive sleep apnea syndrome reduces health care utilization. *Pediatrics* 2004;113:351–356.

Thadhani R, Camargo CA Jr, Stampfer MJ, et al. Prospective study of moderate alcohol consumption and risk of hypertension in young women. *Arch Intern Med* 2002;162:569–574.

Tishler PV, Larkin EK, Schluchter MD, Redline S. Incidence of sleep-disordered breathing in an urban adult population: the relative importance of risk factors in the development of sleep-disordered breathing. *JAMA* 2003;289:2230–2237.

Toft AD. Surgery for primary hyperparathyroidism—sooner rather than later. *Lancet* 2000;355:1478–1479.

Tsachalinas D, Logaras G, Paradelis A. Observations on 246 cases of acute poisoning with parathion in Greece. *Eur J Toxicol Environ Hyg* 1971;4:46–49.

Tuncel M, Wang Z, Arbique D, et al. Mechanism of the blood pressure-raising effect of cocaine in humans. *Circulation* 2002;105:1054–1059.

Tyagi S, Kaul UA, Nair M, et al. Balloon angioplasty of the aorta in Takayasu's arteritis: initial and long-term results. *Am Heart J* 1992;124:876–882.

Van Aken H, Cottrell JE, Anger C, Puchstein C. Treatment of intraoperative hypertensive emergencies in patients with intracranial disease. *Am J Cardiol* 1989;63:43C–47C.

Velzeboer SCJM, Frenkel J, de Wolff FA. A hypertensive toddler. *Lancet* 1997;349:1810.

Verdecchia P, Schillaci G, Borgioni C, et al. Cigarette smoking, ambulatory blood pressure and cardiac hypertrophy in essential hypertension. *J Hypertens* 1995;13:1209–1215.

Vestergaard P, Mosekilde L. Cohort study on effects of parathyroid surgery on multiple outcomes in primary hyperparathyroidism. *BMJ* 2003;327:530–534.

Vlachopoulos C, Alexopoulos N, Panagiotakos D, et al. Cigar smoking has an acute detrimental effect on arterial stiffness. *Am J Hypertens* 2004;17:299–303.

Vlachopoulos C, Hirata K, O'Rourke MF. Effect of caffeine on aortic elastic properties and wave reflection. *J Hypertens* 2003;21:563–570.

Volicer L, Nelson KL. Development of reversible hypertension during disulfiram therapy. *Arch Intern Med* 1984;144:1294–1296.

Volpato S, Pahor M, Ferrucci L, et al. Relationship of alcohol intake with inflammatory markers and plasminogen activator inhibitor-1 in well-functioning older adults: the Health, Aging, and Body Composition study. *Circulation* 2004;109:607–612.

Vorona RD, Winn MP, Babineau TW, et al. Overweight and obese patients in a primary care population report less sleep than patients with a normal body mass index. *Arch Intern Med* 2005;165:25–30.

Vriend JW, van Montfrans GA, Romkes HH, et al. Relation between exercise-induced hypertension and sustained hypertension in adult patients after successful repair of aortic coarctation. *J Hypertens* 2004;22:501–509.

Vupputuri S, Batuman V, Muntner P, et al. The risk for mild kidney function decline associated with illicit drug use among hypertensive men. *Am J Kidney Dis* 2004;43:629–635.

Vuylsteke A, Feneck RO, Jolin-Mellgård Å, et al. Perioperative blood pressure control: a prospective study of patient management in cardiac surgery. *J Cardiothorac Vasc Anesth* 2000;14:269–273.

Walsh BT, Hadigan CM, Wong LM. Increased pulse and blood pressure associated with desipramine treatment of bulimia nervosa. *J Clin Psychopharmacol* 1992;12:163–168.

Walsh CR, Larson MG, Evans JC, et al. Alcohol consumption and risk for congestive heart failure in the Framingham Heart Study. *Ann Intern Med* 2002;136:181–191.

Wannamethee SG, Camargo CA Jr, Manson JE, et al. Alcohol drinking patterns and risk of type 2 diabetes mellitus among younger women. *Arch Intern Med* 2003;163:1329–1336.

Warren SE, Ebert E, Swerdlin A-H, et al. Clonidine and propranolol paradoxical hypertension. *Arch Intern Med* 1979;139:253.

Weaver FA, Kumar SR, Yellin AE, et al. Renal revascularization in Takayasu arteritis-induced renal artery stenosis. *J Vasc Surg* 2004;39:749–757.

Weiss V, Šonka K, Pretl M, et al. Prevalence of the sleep apnea syndrome in acromegaly population. *J Endocrinol Invest* 2000;23:515–519.

Weitzman S, Margulis G, Lehmann E. Uncommon cardiovascular manifestations and high catecholamine levels due to "black widow" bite. *Am Heart J* 1977;93:89–90.

Wessely S, Nimnuan C, Sharpe N. Functional somatic syndromes: one or many? *Lancet* 1999;354:936–939.

Whelton A, White WB, Bello AE, et al. Effects of celecoxib and rofecoxib on blood pressure and edema in patients ≥65 years of age with systemic hypertension and osteoarthritis. *Am J Cardiol* 2002;90:959–963.

Whitaker MD, McArthur RG, Corenblum B, et al. Idiopathic, sustained, inappropriate secretion of ADH with associated hypertension and thirst. *Am J Med* 1979;67: 511–515.

Wilhelm FH, Gerlach AL, Roth WT. Slow recovery from voluntary hyperventilation in panic disorder. *Psychosom Med* 2001;63:638–649.

Wilson JF. Should doctors prescribe alcohol to adults? *Ann Intern Med* 2003;139:711–714.

Winchell RJ, Simons RK, Hoyt DB. Transient systolic hypertension. *Arch Surg* 1996;131:533–539.

Wing YK, Hui SH, Pak WM, et al. A controlled study of sleep related disordered breathing in obese children. *Arch Dis Child* 2003;88:1043–1047.

Winnicki M, Shamsuzzaman A, Lanfranchi P, et al. Erythropoietin and obstructive sleep apnea. *Am J Hypertens* 2004; 17:783–786.

Wolk R, Shamsuzzaman AS, Somers VK. Obesity, sleep apnea, and hypertension. *Hypertension* 2003;42:1067–1074.

Wu CC, Johnson AJ. The vasopressor effect of indigo carmine. *Henry Ford Hosp Med J* 1969;17:131–134.

Young T, Skatrud J, Peppard PE. Risk factors for obstructive sleep apnea in adults. *JAMA* 2004;291:2013–2016.

Zanchetti A, Hansson L, Clement D, et al. Benefits and risks of more intensive blood pressure lowering in hypertensive patients of the HOT study with different risk profiles: does a J-shaped curve exist in smokers? *J Hypertens* 2003;21:797–804.

Zhang W, Victor RG. Calcineurin inhibitors cause renal afferent activation in rats: a novel mechanism of cyclosporine-induced hypertension. *Am J Hypertens* 2000;13:999–1004.

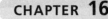

# CHAPTER 16

# Hypertension in Childhood and Adolescence

Joseph T. Flynn, M.D., M.S.

Until recently, hypertension had been considered relatively uncommon in children and adolescents. However, this may be changing, primarily because of the influence of the childhood obesity epidemic. This chapter will describe the features of hypertension in children and adolescents and will also examine a quantitatively larger issue: the increasingly strong evidence that the genesis of adult cardiovascular disease has its origins in childhood (Williams et al., 2002).

## PREVALENCE OF HYPERTENSION IN CHILDHOOD

Recognition that children and adolescents could manifest or develop hypertension began in the mid-1960s as a result of the work of Londe and others (Loggie, 1977). Using similar thresholds for defining hypertension as were in use for adults, it was established that hypertension was exceedingly rare in young children but could be seen in a small percentage of adolescents (Table 16–1). The performance of large-scale blood pressure (BP) screening programs, typically conducted in schools, confirmed that fewer than 2% of children were hypertensive (Fixler et al., 1979). These screening programs also

demonstrated the importance of performing repeated measures of BP before labeling a child as hypertensive: Studies that used just one BP determination found significantly higher "prevalences" of hypertension than studies in which repeated screenings were performed (Table 16–1).

More recent studies have generally confirmed a low prevalence of hypertension in children and adolescents. However, recent data from the Houston Screening Project (Sorof et al., 2002; Sorof et al., 2004a) have demonstrated that the increased prevalence of childhood obesity is associated with an increased prevalence of primary hypertension. In this study, over 5,000 primarily minority Houston public school children underwent BP and obesity screening. The prevalence of hypertension among these children after three screenings was 4.5%, significantly higher than in earlier studies. The significant effect of obesity on childhood BP will be discussed in detail later in this chapter.

## CHILDHOOD PRECURSORS OF ADULT HYPERTENSION

To determine childhood precursors of adult hypertension, BP levels and other known cardiovascular risk factors measured in childhood have been related to the subsequent development of hypertension or its cardiovascular manifestations in adult life.

### Blood Pressure Tracking

The pattern of BP over time, referred to as tracking, has been examined by a number of investigators, most notably in Muscatine, Iowa (Lauer et al., 1993), and Bogalusa, Louisiana (Berenson, 2002).

These studies have shown that systolic BP levels track from childhood better than diastolic BP. In all

## TABLE 16–1

## Prevalence of Hypertension in Children and Adolescents

| Study Location | Number Screened | Age (yrs) | Number of Screenings | Normative Criteria | Prevalence | Reference |
|---|---|---|---|---|---|---|
| Muscatine, IA, United States | 1,301 | 14–18 | 1 | 140/90 | 8.9% SHTN 12.2% DHTN | Lauer et al., 1975 |
| Edmonton, Canada | 15,594 | 15–20 | 1 | 150/95 | 2.2% | Silverberg et al., 1975 |
| Dallas, TX, United States | 10,641 | 14 | 3 | Ninety-fifth percentile | 1.2% SHTN 0.4% DHTN | Fixler et al., 1979 |
| Minneapolis, MN, United States | 14,686 | 10–15 | 1 | 1987 TF | 4.2% | Sinaiko et al., 1989 |
| Tulsa, OK, United States | 5,537 | 14–19 | 1 | 1987 TF | 6.0% | O'Quin et al., 1992 |
| Buraidah, Saudi Arabia | 3,299 | 3–18 | 1 | 1996 WG | 10.6% | Soyannwo et al., 1997 |
| Minneapolis, MN, United States | 14,686 | 10–15 | 2 | 1996 WG | 0.8% SHTN 0.4% DHTN | Adrogue & Sinaiko, 2001 |
| Houston, TX, United States | 5,102 | 12–16 | 3 | 1996 WG | 4.5% | Sorof et al., 2004a |

DHTN, diastolic hypertension; SHTN, systolic hypertension; TF, Second Task Force Report (Task Force on Blood Pressure Control in Children, 1987); WG, Working Group Report (National High Blood Pressure Education Program Working Group, 1996).

studies, the most predictive indicator of subsequently sustained elevated BP is an antecedent elevated level (Bao et al., 1995). Although an initially elevated level may not evolve into later sustained elevation, Lauer et al. (1993) found that 24% of young adults whose pressures ever exceeded the ninetieth percentile as children had adult BP greater than the ninetieth percentile, a percentage that is 2.4 times higher than expected. In the Bogalusa cohort, 40% of those with systolic BP and 37% of those with diastolic BP above the eightieth percentile at baseline continued to have BP above the eightieth percentile 15 years later (Bao et al., 1995).

Tracking is more consistent if the elevated childhood BP levels are combined with obesity, a parental history of hypertension, or increased left ventricular mass by echocardiography (Lauer et al., 1993; Shear et al., 1986).

In view of the higher prevalence of hypertension in Black adults than in White adults, comparisons of the tracking phenomenon in Black and White children have been made (Lane & Gill, 2004). Black children have significantly higher mean BP than White children even after adjustments for potential confounders such as weight gain (Bao et al., 1995), growth, or socioeconomic status (Dekkers et al., 2002). Dekkers et al. (2002) found that ethnic differences in systolic BP become manifest earlier in girls than in boys, and both systolic and diastolic differences tended to increase with age.

### Childhood Blood Pressure and Subsequent Cardiovascular Disease

There are no data at present that clearly document a relationship between childhood BP and cardiovascular (CV) morbidity and mortality in adulthood. However, a number of studies have shown that BP and other traditional cardiovascular risk factors in childhood predict the subsequent presence of carotid intimal-medial thickness (Davis et al., 2001; Li et al., 2003; Raitakari et al., 2003) and arterial stiffness (Li et al., 2004), two well-accepted surrogate markers for cardiovascular events. Presumably, with more time, adult morbidity and mortality will be more tightly connected with childhood precursors, particularly because lipid profiles and smoking in children are also predictive of adult vascular disease (Li et al., 2004).

### The Critical Role of Obesity

Obesity is growing at an alarming pace among children and adolescents in all developed societies, with—as in some other aberrant behaviors—the United States leading the way (Lissau et al., 2004). Unfortunately, adolescent obesity tracks closely with adult obesity (Kvaavik et al., 2003), setting the foundation for all of the consequences. The expanding waistlines of schoolchildren, measured by waist circumference, are a particularly ominous predictor of the metabolic syndrome that now afflicts the majority of U.S. adults (Rudolf et al., 2004).

The causes for the increasing obesity of children and adolescents involve both an increase in caloric intake from larger portions of fast foods (Bowman et al., 2004) and, perhaps even more importantly, a reduction in physical activity (Patrick et al., 2004). The American Academy of Pediatrics has issued a policy statement for restriction of the availability of soft drinks in schools (AAP Committee on School Health, 2004), but this move alone will do little if not combined with a multifaceted attack on the other factors involved (Wiehe et al., 2004).

Mainly as a consequence of increasing obesity, the mean BPs of U.S. children and adolescents has risen by 1.4/3.3 mm Hg from 1990 to 2000 (Muntner et al., 2004), a rise that translates into significant increases in childhood hypertension and a greater likelihood of adult hypertension. Those overweight children who have hypertension may also manifest more severe cardiovascular disease assessed by surrogate markers such as dyslipidemia (Flynn & Alderman, 2005) or increased left ventricular mass and carotid intimal-medial thickness (Sorof et al., 2004b). The combination of obesity, elevated BP, and other cardiovascular risk factors has led to the prediction that an epidemic of adult cardiovascular disease is on its way (Daniels, 1999).

In addition, an increased frequency of sleep-related disordered breathing and sleep apnea has been seen in obese children (Wing et al., 2003) and may, as they do in adults, raise BP. Such children may have less sleep apnea than adults, presenting more frequently with tachypnea and increased breathing effort (Guilleminault et al., 2004). In some of these children, relief may be provided by surgical removal of enlarged adenoids and tonsils (Tarasiuk et al., 2004), but others may require surgical procedures such as uvulopalatoplasty or even the use of nocturnal continuous positive airway pressure (CPAP) (Erler et al., 2004; Wiet et al., 1997).

### The Role of Early Childhood Growth

The dangers of excess weight appear to extend back into early childhood. Those children who were small at birth but who have accelerated weight gain either very early after birth (Singhal et al., 2003) or between ages 1 to 5 (Law et al., 2002) have more insulin resistance, obesity, and hypertension later in life. This association between rapid weight gain postnatally and higher BP has been prospectively documented in 8-year-olds (Burke et al., 2004) and 11- to 14-year-olds (Falkner et al., 2004).

Those infants who are breastfed and thereby have a lower rate of weight gain during infancy have lower BPs in later life than those who are fed enriched formula (Singhal et al., 2001). Although this protection against higher BP by breastfeeding may have been exaggerated by selective publication (Owen et al., 2003), the weight of evidence supports an association (Martin et al., 2004). Whether there is more to breastfeeding than a reduced rate of excess weight gain (Grummer-Strawn & Mei, 2004) is uncertain, but slower early growth appears to be beneficial for long-term cardiovascular health (Singhal et al., 2004).

*Low Birth Weight as a Precursor of Adult Hypertension*

These data have been used to argue that small for gestational age infants may develop more hypertension and cardiovascular disease not because of prenatal influences but rather because of rapid or excessive postnatal weight gain. As described in Chapter 3, the reduction in nephron development found in both animals and humans who are poorly nourished in late pregnancy and born small for gestational age has been incorporated into the "fetal origins" hypothesis of adult hypertension. As attractive as this hypothesis may be, more and more data deny an important relevance of birth weight to BPs in later life (Doyle et al., 2003; Falkner et al., 2004; Huxley et al., 2002). As Falkner et al. (2004) conclude from their own data and much more:

> The birth-weight hypothesis has been an interesting and novel concept for investigators on the origins of hypertension and cardiovascular disease. Despite the evidence from experimental studies that alterations in the intrauterine fetal environment can have effects on later life, the evidence in humans has been less clear. The number of reports

that support the birth-weight hypothesis outnumbers those reports that are not supportive. However, in those reports that do support the birth-weight hypothesis, the effect has been very small. Few studies have been longitudinal and most have relied on recall or other records for determination of birth weight. The results of this longitudinal investigation do not support the birth-weight or fetal programming theory.

### Other Factors That Determine Blood Pressure

Additional factors that correlate with BP levels during childhood, both cross-sectionally and over time, are being analyzed to identify which predict a subsequent rise in BP, with the hope that primary prevention of adult hypertension may become a realistic public health (as well as clinical) goal. Multiple factors have been reported to correlate with BP levels in children (Table 16–2).

---

### TABLE 16–2

### Factors Related to Blood Pressure Levels in Children and Adolescents

---

**Genetic**

  Ethnicity (Hohn et al., 1994; Sorof et al., 2004a)

  Parental and sibling BP levels (Schieken et al., 1993)

  Increased salt sensitivity in Blacks (Wilson et al., 1996)

  Obesity (Sorof et al., 2004a)

  Deletion of angiotensin converting enzyme (ACE) gene (Taittonen, 1999)

**Environmental**

  Birth weight (Huxley et al., 2002)

  Breast feeding (Martin et al., 2004)

  Neonatal weight gain (Singhal et al., 2004)

  Socioeconomic status (Dekkers et al., 2002)

  Pulse rate (Zhou et al., 2000)

  Exercise (Alpert, 2000)

**Mixed Genetic and Environmental**

  Height (Daniels et al., 1996)

  Weight (Sorof et al., 2004a)

  Body mass (Kvaavik et al., 2003)

  Somatic growth and sexual maturation (Daniels et al., 1996)

  Sodium and other nutrient intakes (Falkner et al., 2000)

  Sympathetic nervous system reactivity (Urbina et al., 1998)

  Stress (Saab et al., 2001)

---

The Montreal adoption study provided a statistical assessment of the contribution of various factors to the variability of BP in children (Mongeau, 1987). Some factors are either genetic or environmental, but most have contributions of both. Height, body mass, and somatic development depend not only on genetic influences but also on nutrition and exercise. Sodium intake may exert its effect on BP in those who are genetically predisposed to higher BP levels and are sodium sensitive, especially Blacks (Wilson et al., 1996). Obese adolescents also have heightened responsiveness to sodium intake (Rocchini et al., 1989). An association between BP and increased sympathetic nervous system activity in Whites and increased parasympathetic activity in Blacks has been noted (Urbina et al., 1998). Blood pressure reactivity to some forms of stress reflect heightened vascular reactivity in children and adolescents with BPs that are higher and more labile (Saab et al., 2001).

#### Genetic Factors

The influence of genetic factors on BP has been established by the findings of a correlation of BP levels between parents and their natural offspring but no correlation between parents and their adopted children (Mongeau, 1987). Genetic influences have been shown in comparisons of siblings (Wang et al., 1999) and twins (monozygotic and dizygotic) and their families (Schieken, 1993). Table 16–3 lists some of the differences reported among normotensive children with a positive family history versus those with a negative family history of hypertension. It is likely that yet-undiscovered genetic polymorphisms may account for the development of "primary" hypertension in families, and that these in combination with environmental factors may explain the early appearance of hypertension in some nonobese children and adolescents.

#### Environmental Factors

Of the environmental factors, increased body mass has increasingly been recognized as a major determinant of higher BP levels throughout childhood and adolescence (Luepker et al., 1999; Sorof et al., 2004a). The epidemic of childhood obesity may well produce an epidemic of hypertension in the not-so-distant future (Sorof & Daniels, 2002).

The relationship between sodium and BP was comprehensively reviewed in Chapter 3. A comprehensive review of the literature on diet and BP in children and adolescents suggested that sodium intake is related to higher BP in children and adolescents whereas data concerning potassium and calcium revealed no significant effect (Simons-Morton et al., 1997). In another study, Falkner et al. (2000), using folate as a surrogate for adequacy of micronutrient intake, concluded that Black adolescents with

## TABLE 16–3

### Characteristics of FH+ Normotensive Compared with FH– Normotensives

↑ Carotid artery stiffness (Meaney et al., 1999)

↑ Blood pressure reactivity (Lemne, 1998)

↑ Leptin and insulin levels (Makris et al., 1999)

↑ Pulse and DBP with dynamic exercise; ↑ pulse with isometric exercises (Mehta et al., 1996)

↑ SBP in African American male adolescents homozygous for the deletion polymorphism of the ACE gene (Taittonen et al., 1999)

↑ Rate of sodium-lithium countertransport (McDonald et al., 1987)

↑ Sleep BP in Black adolescents as measured with ABPM (Harshfield et al., 1994)

Cardiac indices:

   ↑ intravascular septum:posterior wall mass index ratio (deLeonardis et al., 1988)

   ↑ thickness of the interventricular septum during systole (Hansen et al., 1992)

   ↑ LVMI (van Hooft et al., 1993)

---

higher folate and micronutrient intakes had lower mean diastolic BP. Caffeine intake has also been associated with an elevated BP in adolescents, with the effect greater in Blacks than in Whites (Savoca et al., 2004).

### Prevention

Despite the absence of a specific marker in children for the subsequent development of hypertension, it is clear that the roots of hypertension may be traced to early childhood. The evidence includes tracking for the highest deciles of pressure from childhood to diagnosed hypertension in later years, which is even more pronounced in Blacks than in other populations (Lane & Gill, 2004).

The need for early recognition and appropriate management of elevated BP in children is being increasingly emphasized (Kavey et al., 2003). This need is heightened by the recognition that cardiac hypertrophy (Hanevold et al., 2004; Laird & Fixler, 1981) and decreased cognitive function (Lande et al., 2003) are often manifested in children with elevated BP.

Practitioners working with children and their families are in an ideal position to introduce preventive measures that will ensure future cardiovascular

health (Kavey et al., 2003). Children and their families need detailed information about optimal dietary intakes, with appropriate cultural orientation. Once the dietary needs for cholesterol and myelinization of the central nervous system have been met (typically by age 2 years), recommendations for a prudent intake of fat such as in the Dietary Approaches to Stop Hypertension (DASH) diet (Appel et al., 1997) should be provided. Family meals are an ideal setting to create lifetime healthful food habits.

Similarly, family activities that include age-appropriate exercise are helpful. Families must be informed of the deleterious effects of pressor agents—including tobacco, street drugs, and nonsteroidal anti-inflammatory drugs (NSAIDs)—and their potential to increase BP with chronic use. With these proactive steps, the health of children will be improved. Whether hypertension will be prevented remains unknown.

### CLASSIFICATION AND DIAGNOSIS OF HYPERTENSION IN CHILDREN AND ADOLESCENTS

Diagnostic criteria for elevated BP in childhood are based on the concept that BP in children increases with age and with body size, which makes it impossible to utilize a single BP level to define hypertension as is done in adults. This was recognized by early investigators of juvenile hypertension, who initially adopted the adult threshold of 140/90, but later realized that this represented a severe level of BP elevation, particularly in young children, and that population data were needed in order to better define what constitutes an elevated BP in the young (Loggie, 1977). Furthermore, the lack of cardiovascular end points in childhood necessitates that the definitions of normal and elevated BP be statistical criteria derived from large-scale, cross-sectional studies of BP in normal children.

Under the auspices of the National Heart, Lung and Blood Institute, consensus guidelines with recommendations for identification and management of elevated BP in childhood have been issued on four occasions over approximately the past 30 years. The most recent of these, "The Fourth Report on the Diagnosis, Evaluation, and Treatment of High Blood Pressure in Children and Adolescents" (National High Blood Pressure Education Program Working Group, 2004), is notable for its adaptation of terminology and staging criteria utilized in consensus guidelines for adult hypertension (Chobanian et al., 2003) to the problem of childhood hypertension, and for its emphasis on prevention of adult cardiovascular disease by early intervention in children and adolescents with elevated BP.

## Definitions and Classification of Elevated Blood Pressure

According to the Fourth Report, normal BP in childhood is defined as systolic and diastolic BP less than the ninetieth percentile for age, gender, and height, and hypertension is defined as systolic and/or diastolic BP persistently equal to or greater than the ninety-fifth percentile. These values are found in tables of BP percentiles for boys and girls ages 1 to 17 years (Tables 16–4, 16–5). Children with systolic or diastolic BP between the ninetieth and

## TABLE 16–4

### Blood Pressure Levels for Boys by Age and Height Percentile[a]

| Age (yr) | BP Percentile ↓ | Systolic BP (mm Hg) ←Percentile of Height→ | | | | | | | Diastolic BP (mm Hg) ←Percentile of Height→ | | | | | | |
|---|---|---|---|---|---|---|---|---|---|---|---|---|---|---|---|
| | | 5 | 10 | 25 | 50 | 75 | 90 | 95 | 5 | 10 | 25 | 50 | 75 | 90 | 95 |
| 1 | 50 | 80 | 81 | 83 | 85 | 87 | 88 | 89 | 34 | 35 | 36 | 37 | 38 | 39 | 39 |
| | 90 | 94 | 95 | 97 | 99 | 100 | 102 | 103 | 49 | 50 | 51 | 52 | 53 | 53 | 54 |
| | 95 | 98 | 99 | 101 | 103 | 104 | 106 | 106 | 54 | 54 | 55 | 56 | 57 | 58 | 58 |
| | 99 | 105 | 106 | 108 | 110 | 112 | 113 | 114 | 61 | 62 | 63 | 64 | 65 | 66 | 66 |
| 2 | 50 | 84 | 85 | 87 | 88 | 90 | 92 | 92 | 39 | 40 | 41 | 42 | 43 | 44 | 44 |
| | 90 | 97 | 99 | 100 | 102 | 104 | 105 | 106 | 54 | 55 | 56 | 57 | 58 | 58 | 59 |
| | 95 | 101 | 102 | 104 | 106 | 108 | 109 | 110 | 59 | 59 | 60 | 61 | 62 | 63 | 63 |
| | 99 | 109 | 110 | 111 | 113 | 115 | 117 | 117 | 66 | 67 | 68 | 69 | 70 | 71 | 71 |
| 3 | 50 | 86 | 87 | 89 | 91 | 93 | 94 | 95 | 44 | 44 | 45 | 46 | 47 | 48 | 48 |
| | 90 | 100 | 101 | 103 | 105 | 107 | 108 | 109 | 59 | 59 | 60 | 61 | 62 | 63 | 63 |
| | 95 | 104 | 105 | 107 | 109 | 110 | 112 | 113 | 63 | 63 | 64 | 65 | 66 | 67 | 67 |
| | 99 | 111 | 112 | 114 | 116 | 118 | 119 | 120 | 71 | 71 | 72 | 73 | 74 | 75 | 75 |
| 4 | 50 | 88 | 89 | 91 | 93 | 95 | 96 | 97 | 47 | 48 | 49 | 50 | 51 | 51 | 52 |
| | 90 | 102 | 103 | 105 | 107 | 109 | 110 | 111 | 62 | 63 | 64 | 65 | 66 | 66 | 67 |
| | 95 | 106 | 107 | 109 | 111 | 112 | 114 | 115 | 66 | 67 | 68 | 69 | 70 | 71 | 71 |
| | 99 | 113 | 114 | 116 | 118 | 120 | 121 | 122 | 74 | 75 | 76 | 77 | 78 | 78 | 79 |
| 5 | 50 | 90 | 91 | 93 | 95 | 96 | 98 | 98 | 50 | 51 | 52 | 53 | 54 | 55 | 55 |
| | 90 | 104 | 105 | 106 | 108 | 110 | 111 | 112 | 65 | 66 | 67 | 68 | 69 | 69 | 70 |
| | 95 | 108 | 109 | 110 | 112 | 114 | 115 | 116 | 69 | 70 | 71 | 72 | 73 | 74 | 74 |
| | 99 | 115 | 116 | 118 | 120 | 121 | 123 | 123 | 77 | 78 | 79 | 80 | 81 | 81 | 82 |
| 6 | 50 | 91 | 92 | 94 | 96 | 98 | 99 | 100 | 53 | 53 | 54 | 55 | 56 | 57 | 57 |
| | 90 | 105 | 106 | 108 | 110 | 111 | 113 | 113 | 68 | 68 | 69 | 70 | 71 | 72 | 72 |
| | 95 | 109 | 110 | 112 | 114 | 115 | 117 | 117 | 72 | 72 | 73 | 74 | 75 | 76 | 76 |
| | 99 | 116 | 117 | 119 | 121 | 123 | 124 | 125 | 80 | 80 | 81 | 82 | 83 | 84 | 84 |
| 7 | 50 | 92 | 94 | 95 | 97 | 99 | 100 | 101 | 55 | 55 | 56 | 57 | 58 | 59 | 59 |
| | 90 | 106 | 107 | 109 | 111 | 113 | 114 | 115 | 70 | 70 | 71 | 72 | 73 | 74 | 74 |
| | 95 | 110 | 111 | 113 | 115 | 117 | 118 | 119 | 74 | 74 | 75 | 76 | 77 | 78 | 78 |
| | 99 | 117 | 118 | 120 | 122 | 124 | 125 | 126 | 82 | 82 | 83 | 84 | 85 | 86 | 86 |
| 8 | 50 | 94 | 95 | 97 | 99 | 100 | 102 | 102 | 56 | 57 | 58 | 59 | 60 | 60 | 61 |
| | 90 | 107 | 109 | 110 | 112 | 114 | 115 | 116 | 71 | 72 | 72 | 73 | 74 | 75 | 76 |
| | 95 | 111 | 112 | 114 | 116 | 118 | 119 | 120 | 75 | 76 | 77 | 78 | 79 | 79 | 80 |
| | 99 | 119 | 120 | 122 | 123 | 125 | 127 | 127 | 83 | 84 | 85 | 86 | 87 | 87 | 88 |

*(continued)*

## TABLE 16–4 (Continued)

### Blood Pressure Levels for Boys by Age and Height Percentile

| Age (yr) | BP Percentile ↓ | Systolic BP (mm Hg) ←Percentile of Height→ | | | | | | | Diastolic BP (mm Hg) ←Percentile of Height→ | | | | | | |
|---|---|---|---|---|---|---|---|---|---|---|---|---|---|---|---|
| | | 5 | 10 | 25 | 50 | 75 | 90 | 95 | 5 | 10 | 25 | 50 | 75 | 90 | 95 |
| 9 | 50 | 95 | 96 | 98 | 100 | 102 | 103 | 104 | 57 | 58 | 59 | 60 | 61 | 61 | 62 |
| | 90 | 109 | 110 | 112 | 114 | 115 | 117 | 118 | 72 | 73 | 74 | 75 | 76 | 76 | 77 |
| | 95 | 113 | 114 | 116 | 118 | 119 | 121 | 121 | 76 | 77 | 78 | 79 | 80 | 81 | 81 |
| | 99 | 120 | 121 | 123 | 125 | 127 | 128 | 129 | 84 | 85 | 86 | 87 | 88 | 88 | 89 |
| 10 | 50 | 97 | 98 | 100 | 102 | 103 | 105 | 106 | 58 | 59 | 60 | 61 | 61 | 62 | 63 |
| | 90 | 111 | 112 | 114 | 115 | 117 | 119 | 119 | 73 | 73 | 74 | 75 | 76 | 77 | 78 |
| | 95 | 115 | 116 | 117 | 119 | 121 | 122 | 123 | 77 | 78 | 79 | 80 | 81 | 81 | 82 |
| | 99 | 122 | 123 | 125 | 127 | 128 | 130 | 130 | 85 | 86 | 86 | 88 | 88 | 89 | 90 |
| 11 | 50 | 99 | 100 | 102 | 104 | 105 | 107 | 107 | 59 | 59 | 60 | 61 | 62 | 63 | 63 |
| | 90 | 113 | 114 | 115 | 117 | 119 | 120 | 121 | 74 | 74 | 75 | 76 | 77 | 78 | 78 |
| | 95 | 117 | 118 | 119 | 121 | 123 | 124 | 125 | 78 | 78 | 79 | 80 | 81 | 82 | 82 |
| | 99 | 124 | 125 | 127 | 129 | 130 | 132 | 132 | 86 | 86 | 87 | 88 | 89 | 90 | 90 |
| 12 | 50 | 101 | 102 | 104 | 106 | 108 | 109 | 110 | 59 | 60 | 61 | 62 | 63 | 63 | 64 |
| | 90 | 115 | 116 | 118 | 120 | 121 | 123 | 123 | 74 | 75 | 75 | 76 | 77 | 78 | 79 |
| | 95 | 119 | 120 | 122 | 123 | 125 | 127 | 127 | 78 | 79 | 80 | 81 | 82 | 82 | 83 |
| | 99 | 126 | 127 | 129 | 131 | 133 | 134 | 135 | 86 | 87 | 88 | 89 | 90 | 90 | 91 |
| 13 | 50 | 104 | 105 | 106 | 108 | 110 | 111 | 112 | 60 | 60 | 61 | 62 | 63 | 64 | 64 |
| | 90 | 117 | 118 | 120 | 122 | 124 | 125 | 126 | 75 | 75 | 76 | 77 | 78 | 79 | 79 |
| | 95 | 121 | 122 | 124 | 126 | 128 | 129 | 130 | 79 | 79 | 80 | 81 | 82 | 83 | 83 |
| | 99 | 128 | 130 | 131 | 133 | 135 | 136 | 137 | 87 | 87 | 88 | 89 | 90 | 91 | 91 |
| 14 | 50 | 106 | 107 | 109 | 111 | 113 | 114 | 115 | 60 | 61 | 62 | 63 | 64 | 65 | 65 |
| | 90 | 120 | 121 | 123 | 125 | 126 | 128 | 128 | 75 | 76 | 77 | 78 | 79 | 79 | 80 |
| | 95 | 124 | 125 | 127 | 128 | 130 | 132 | 132 | 80 | 80 | 81 | 82 | 83 | 84 | 84 |
| | 99 | 131 | 132 | 134 | 136 | 138 | 139 | 140 | 87 | 88 | 89 | 90 | 91 | 92 | 92 |
| 15 | 50 | 109 | 110 | 112 | 113 | 115 | 117 | 117 | 61 | 62 | 63 | 64 | 65 | 66 | 66 |
| | 90 | 122 | 124 | 125 | 127 | 129 | 130 | 131 | 76 | 77 | 78 | 79 | 80 | 80 | 81 |
| | 95 | 126 | 127 | 129 | 131 | 133 | 134 | 135 | 81 | 81 | 82 | 83 | 84 | 85 | 85 |
| | 99 | 134 | 135 | 136 | 138 | 140 | 142 | 142 | 88 | 89 | 90 | 91 | 92 | 93 | 93 |
| 16 | 50 | 111 | 112 | 114 | 116 | 118 | 119 | 120 | 63 | 63 | 64 | 65 | 66 | 67 | 67 |
| | 90 | 125 | 126 | 128 | 130 | 131 | 133 | 134 | 78 | 78 | 79 | 80 | 81 | 82 | 82 |
| | 95 | 129 | 130 | 132 | 134 | 135 | 137 | 137 | 82 | 83 | 83 | 84 | 85 | 86 | 87 |
| | 99 | 136 | 137 | 139 | 141 | 143 | 144 | 145 | 90 | 90 | 91 | 92 | 93 | 94 | 94 |
| 17 | 50 | 114 | 115 | 116 | 118 | 120 | 121 | 122 | 65 | 66 | 66 | 67 | 68 | 69 | 70 |
| | 90 | 127 | 128 | 130 | 132 | 134 | 135 | 136 | 80 | 80 | 81 | 82 | 83 | 84 | 84 |
| | 95 | 131 | 132 | 134 | 136 | 138 | 139 | 140 | 84 | 85 | 86 | 87 | 87 | 88 | 89 |
| | 99 | 139 | 140 | 141 | 143 | 145 | 146 | 147 | 92 | 93 | 93 | 94 | 95 | 96 | 97 |

BP, blood pressure.

[a]To use the table, first plot the child's height on a standard growth curve (http://www.cdc.gov/growthcharts). The child's measured SBP and DBP are compared with the numbers provided in the table according to the child's age and height percentile.

Reproduced from National High Blood Pressure Education Program Working Group on High Blood Pressure in Children and Adolescents. The fourth report on the diagnosis, evaluation, and treatment of high blood pressure in children and adolescents. National Heart, Lung, and Blood Institute, Bethesda, Maryland. *Pediatrics* 2004;114:555–576.

## TABLE 16–5

### Blood Pressure Levels for Girls by Age and Height Percentile[a]

| Age (yr) | BP Percentile ↓ | Systolic BP (mm Hg) ←Percentile of Height→ | | | | | | | Diastolic BP (mm Hg) ←Percentile of Height→ | | | | | | |
|---|---|---|---|---|---|---|---|---|---|---|---|---|---|---|---|
| | | 5 | 10 | 25 | 50 | 75 | 90 | 95 | 5 | 10 | 25 | 50 | 75 | 90 | 95 |
| 1 | 50 | 83 | 84 | 85 | 86 | 88 | 89 | 90 | 38 | 39 | 39 | 40 | 41 | 41 | 42 |
| | 90 | 97 | 97 | 98 | 100 | 101 | 102 | 103 | 52 | 53 | 53 | 54 | 55 | 55 | 56 |
| | 95 | 100 | 101 | 102 | 104 | 105 | 106 | 107 | 56 | 57 | 57 | 58 | 59 | 59 | 60 |
| | 99 | 108 | 108 | 109 | 111 | 112 | 113 | 114 | 64 | 64 | 65 | 65 | 66 | 67 | 67 |
| 2 | 50 | 85 | 85 | 87 | 88 | 89 | 91 | 91 | 43 | 44 | 44 | 45 | 46 | 46 | 47 |
| | 90 | 98 | 99 | 100 | 101 | 103 | 104 | 105 | 57 | 58 | 58 | 59 | 60 | 61 | 61 |
| | 95 | 102 | 103 | 104 | 105 | 107 | 108 | 109 | 61 | 62 | 62 | 63 | 64 | 65 | 65 |
| | 99 | 109 | 110 | 111 | 112 | 114 | 115 | 116 | 69 | 69 | 70 | 70 | 71 | 72 | 72 |
| 3 | 50 | 86 | 87 | 88 | 89 | 91 | 92 | 93 | 47 | 48 | 48 | 49 | 50 | 50 | 51 |
| | 90 | 100 | 100 | 102 | 103 | 104 | 106 | 106 | 61 | 62 | 62 | 63 | 64 | 64 | 65 |
| | 95 | 104 | 104 | 105 | 107 | 108 | 109 | 110 | 65 | 66 | 66 | 67 | 68 | 68 | 69 |
| | 99 | 111 | 111 | 113 | 114 | 115 | 116 | 117 | 73 | 73 | 74 | 74 | 75 | 76 | 76 |
| 4 | 50 | 88 | 88 | 90 | 91 | 92 | 94 | 94 | 50 | 50 | 51 | 52 | 52 | 53 | 54 |
| | 90 | 101 | 102 | 103 | 104 | 106 | 107 | 108 | 64 | 64 | 65 | 66 | 67 | 67 | 68 |
| | 95 | 105 | 106 | 107 | 108 | 110 | 111 | 112 | 68 | 68 | 69 | 70 | 71 | 71 | 72 |
| | 99 | 112 | 113 | 114 | 115 | 117 | 118 | 119 | 76 | 76 | 76 | 77 | 78 | 79 | 79 |
| 5 | 50 | 89 | 90 | 91 | 93 | 94 | 95 | 96 | 52 | 53 | 53 | 54 | 55 | 55 | 56 |
| | 90 | 103 | 103 | 105 | 106 | 107 | 109 | 109 | 66 | 67 | 67 | 68 | 69 | 69 | 70 |
| | 95 | 107 | 107 | 108 | 110 | 111 | 112 | 113 | 70 | 71 | 71 | 72 | 73 | 73 | 74 |
| | 99 | 114 | 114 | 116 | 117 | 118 | 120 | 120 | 78 | 78 | 79 | 79 | 80 | 81 | 81 |
| 6 | 50 | 91 | 92 | 93 | 94 | 96 | 97 | 98 | 54 | 54 | 55 | 56 | 56 | 57 | 58 |
| | 90 | 104 | 105 | 106 | 108 | 109 | 110 | 111 | 68 | 68 | 69 | 70 | 70 | 71 | 72 |
| | 95 | 108 | 109 | 110 | 111 | 113 | 114 | 115 | 72 | 72 | 73 | 74 | 74 | 75 | 76 |
| | 99 | 115 | 116 | 117 | 119 | 120 | 121 | 122 | 80 | 80 | 80 | 81 | 82 | 83 | 83 |
| 7 | 50 | 93 | 93 | 95 | 96 | 97 | 99 | 99 | 55 | 56 | 56 | 57 | 58 | 58 | 59 |
| | 90 | 106 | 107 | 108 | 109 | 111 | 112 | 113 | 69 | 70 | 70 | 71 | 72 | 72 | 73 |
| | 95 | 110 | 111 | 112 | 113 | 115 | 116 | 116 | 73 | 74 | 74 | 75 | 76 | 76 | 77 |
| | 99 | 117 | 118 | 119 | 120 | 122 | 123 | 124 | 81 | 81 | 82 | 82 | 83 | 84 | 84 |
| 8 | 50 | 95 | 95 | 96 | 98 | 99 | 100 | 101 | 57 | 57 | 57 | 58 | 59 | 60 | 60 |
| | 90 | 108 | 109 | 110 | 111 | 113 | 114 | 114 | 71 | 71 | 71 | 72 | 73 | 74 | 74 |
| | 95 | 112 | 112 | 114 | 115 | 116 | 118 | 118 | 75 | 75 | 75 | 76 | 77 | 78 | 78 |
| | 99 | 119 | 120 | 121 | 122 | 123 | 125 | 125 | 82 | 82 | 83 | 83 | 84 | 85 | 86 |
| 9 | 50 | 96 | 97 | 98 | 100 | 101 | 102 | 103 | 58 | 58 | 58 | 59 | 60 | 61 | 61 |
| | 90 | 110 | 110 | 112 | 113 | 114 | 116 | 116 | 72 | 72 | 72 | 73 | 74 | 75 | 75 |
| | 95 | 114 | 114 | 115 | 117 | 118 | 119 | 120 | 76 | 76 | 76 | 77 | 78 | 79 | 79 |
| | 99 | 121 | 121 | 123 | 124 | 125 | 127 | 127 | 83 | 83 | 84 | 84 | 85 | 86 | 87 |

(continued)

## TABLE 16–5 (Continued)

### Blood Pressure Levels for Girls by Age and Height Percentile

| Age (yr) | BP Percentile ↓ | Systolic BP (mm Hg) ←Percentile of Height→ | | | | | | | Diastolic BP (mm Hg) ←Percentile of Height→ | | | | | | |
|---|---|---|---|---|---|---|---|---|---|---|---|---|---|---|---|
| | | 5 | 10 | 25 | 50 | 75 | 90 | 95 | 5 | 10 | 25 | 50 | 75 | 90 | 95 |
| 10 | 50 | 98 | 99 | 100 | 102 | 103 | 104 | 105 | 59 | 59 | 59 | 60 | 61 | 62 | 62 |
| | 90 | 112 | 112 | 114 | 115 | 116 | 118 | 118 | 73 | 73 | 73 | 74 | 75 | 76 | 76 |
| | 95 | 116 | 116 | 117 | 119 | 120 | 121 | 122 | 77 | 77 | 77 | 78 | 79 | 80 | 80 |
| | 99 | 123 | 123 | 125 | 126 | 127 | 129 | 129 | 84 | 84 | 85 | 86 | 86 | 87 | 88 |
| 11 | 50 | 100 | 101 | 102 | 103 | 105 | 106 | 107 | 60 | 60 | 60 | 61 | 62 | 63 | 63 |
| | 90 | 114 | 114 | 116 | 117 | 118 | 119 | 120 | 74 | 74 | 74 | 75 | 76 | 77 | 77 |
| | 95 | 118 | 118 | 119 | 121 | 122 | 123 | 124 | 78 | 78 | 78 | 79 | 80 | 81 | 81 |
| | 99 | 125 | 125 | 126 | 128 | 129 | 130 | 131 | 85 | 85 | 86 | 87 | 87 | 88 | 89 |
| 12 | 50 | 102 | 103 | 104 | 105 | 107 | 108 | 109 | 61 | 61 | 61 | 62 | 63 | 64 | 64 |
| | 90 | 116 | 116 | 117 | 119 | 120 | 121 | 122 | 75 | 75 | 75 | 76 | 77 | 78 | 78 |
| | 95 | 119 | 120 | 121 | 123 | 124 | 125 | 126 | 79 | 79 | 79 | 80 | 81 | 82 | 82 |
| | 99 | 127 | 127 | 128 | 130 | 131 | 132 | 133 | 86 | 86 | 87 | 88 | 88 | 89 | 90 |
| 13 | 50 | 104 | 105 | 106 | 107 | 109 | 110 | 110 | 62 | 62 | 62 | 63 | 64 | 65 | 65 |
| | 90 | 117 | 118 | 119 | 121 | 122 | 123 | 124 | 76 | 76 | 76 | 77 | 78 | 79 | 79 |
| | 95 | 121 | 122 | 123 | 124 | 126 | 127 | 128 | 80 | 80 | 80 | 81 | 82 | 83 | 83 |
| | 99 | 128 | 129 | 130 | 132 | 133 | 134 | 135 | 87 | 87 | 88 | 89 | 89 | 90 | 91 |
| 14 | 50 | 106 | 106 | 107 | 109 | 110 | 111 | 112 | 63 | 63 | 63 | 64 | 65 | 66 | 66 |
| | 90 | 119 | 120 | 121 | 122 | 124 | 125 | 125 | 77 | 77 | 77 | 78 | 79 | 80 | 80 |
| | 95 | 123 | 123 | 125 | 126 | 127 | 129 | 129 | 81 | 81 | 81 | 82 | 83 | 84 | 84 |
| | 99 | 130 | 131 | 132 | 133 | 135 | 136 | 136 | 88 | 88 | 89 | 90 | 90 | 91 | 92 |
| 15 | 50 | 107 | 108 | 109 | 110 | 111 | 113 | 113 | 64 | 64 | 64 | 65 | 66 | 67 | 67 |
| | 90 | 120 | 121 | 122 | 123 | 125 | 126 | 127 | 78 | 78 | 78 | 79 | 80 | 81 | 81 |
| | 95 | 124 | 125 | 126 | 127 | 129 | 130 | 131 | 82 | 82 | 82 | 83 | 84 | 85 | 85 |
| | 99 | 131 | 132 | 133 | 134 | 136 | 137 | 138 | 89 | 89 | 90 | 91 | 91 | 92 | 93 |
| 16 | 50 | 108 | 108 | 110 | 111 | 112 | 114 | 114 | 64 | 64 | 65 | 66 | 66 | 67 | 68 |
| | 90 | 121 | 122 | 123 | 124 | 126 | 127 | 128 | 78 | 78 | 79 | 80 | 81 | 81 | 82 |
| | 95 | 125 | 126 | 127 | 128 | 130 | 131 | 132 | 82 | 82 | 83 | 84 | 85 | 85 | 86 |
| | 99 | 132 | 133 | 134 | 135 | 137 | 138 | 139 | 90 | 90 | 90 | 91 | 92 | 93 | 93 |
| 17 | 50 | 108 | 109 | 110 | 111 | 113 | 114 | 115 | 64 | 65 | 65 | 66 | 67 | 67 | 68 |
| | 90 | 122 | 122 | 123 | 125 | 126 | 127 | 128 | 78 | 79 | 79 | 80 | 81 | 81 | 82 |
| | 95 | 125 | 126 | 127 | 129 | 130 | 131 | 132 | 82 | 83 | 83 | 84 | 85 | 85 | 86 |
| | 99 | 133 | 133 | 134 | 136 | 137 | 138 | 139 | 90 | 90 | 91 | 91 | 92 | 93 | 93 |

BP, blood pressure.

[a]To use the table, first plot the child's height on a standard growth curve (http://www.cdc.gov/growthcharts). The child's measured SBP and DBP are compared with the numbers provided in the table according to the child's age and height percentile.

Reproduced from National High Blood Pressure Education Program Working Group on High Blood Pressure in Children and Adolescents. The fourth report on the diagnosis, evaluation, and treatment of high blood pressure in children and adolescents. National Heart, Lung, and Blood Institute, Bethesda, Maryland. *Pediatrics* 2004;114:555–576.

ninety-fifth percentiles, who had previously been classified as having "high-normal" BP (Task Force on Blood Pressure Control in Children, 1987), are now classified as "prehypertensive," in keeping with the terminology used in the JNC-7 recommendations for adults (Chobanian et al., 2003). The prehypertension classification is also utilized for adolescents with BP ≥120/80.

The Fourth Report additionally provides guidelines for staging the severity of hypertension in children and adolescents, which can then be used clinically to guide evaluation and management (Table 16–6). Stage 1 hypertension is defined as BPs between the ninety-fifth percentile for age, gender, and height and the ninety-nineth percentile

plus 5 mm Hg, or approximately up to 10% above the ninety-fifth percentile, which is roughly similar to Stage 1 hypertension in adults (Chobanian et al., 2003). Stage 2 hypertension is any BP above the ninety-nineth percentile plus 5 mm Hg. Children or adolescents with stage 2 hypertension should be evaluated and treated more quickly and/or intensively than those with lower degrees of BP elevation.

## Assessment

### Confirmation of BP Elevation

The first step in evaluating the hypertensive child or adolescent is to make sure that the BP is truly elevated. As in the past, the BP distributions published

## TABLE 16–6

### Classification of Hypertension in Children and Adolescents, with Measurement Frequency and Therapy Recommendations

| | SBP or DBP Percentile* | Frequency of BP Measurement | Therapeutic Lifestyle Changes | Pharmacologic Therapy |
|---|---|---|---|---|
| Normal | <ninetieth | Recheck at next scheduled physical examination | Encourage healthy diet, sleep, and physical activity | — |
| Prehypertension | ninetieth to <ninety-fifth or if BP exceeds 120/80 even if below ninetieth percentile up to <ninety-fifth percentile[†] | Recheck in 6 months | Weight management counseling if overweight, introduce physical activity and diet management[§] | None unless compelling indications such as CKD, diabetes mellitus, heart failure, LVH |
| Stage 1 hypertension | ninety-fifth percentile to the ninety-nineth percentile plus 5 mm Hg | Recheck in 1 to 2 weeks or sooner if the patient is symptomatic; if persistently elevated on two additional occasions, evaluate or refer to source of care within 1 month | Weight management counseling if overweight, introduce physical activity and diet management[§] | Initiate therapy based on indications on page 479 if compelling indications as above |

BP, blood pressure; CKD, chronic kidney disease; DBP, diastolic blood pressure; LVH, left ventricular hypertrophy; SBP, systolic blood pressure.
*For sex, age, and height measured on at least three separate occasions; if systolic and diastolic categories are different, categorize by the higher value.
[†]This occurs typically at 12 years old for SBP and at 16 years old for DBP.
[§]Parents and children trying to modify the eating plan to the DASH eating plan (Appel et al., 1997) could benefit from consultation with a registered or licensed nutritionist to get them started.
Adapted from National High Blood Pressure Education Program Working Group on High Blood Pressure in Children and Adolescents. The fourth report on the diagnosis, evaluation, and treatment of high blood pressure in children and adolescents. National Heart, Lung, and Blood Institute, Bethesda, Maryland. Pediatrics 2004;114:555–576.

in the Fourth Report are based upon auscultated BPs. Given this, and given the inherent inaccuracies of oscillometric BPs and their variation from auscultated BPs in children and adolescents (Kaufmann et al., 1996; Park et al., 2001; Pickering et al., 2005), it is recommended that if a child's BP is found to be elevated using an automated device, it should be repeated by auscultation before entertaining the diagnosis of hypertension. Exceptions to this would include infants and young children who are unable to cooperate with manual BP determination. Furthermore, BP should be shown to be elevated on at least three occasions before making the diagnosis of hypertension (National High Blood Pressure Education Program Working Group, 2004).

Techniques for manual BP measurement recommended by the American Heart Association (Pickering et al., 2005) with respect to cuff size, patient position, etc., should be followed in children and adolescents whenever feasible. As in adults, the fifth Korotkoff sound should be reported as the diastolic BP, except in those children and adolescents in whom Korotkoff sounds can be heard down to "zero;" in such children, the fourth Korotkoff sound should be reported as the diastolic.

Ambulatory BP monitoring has now been endorsed as an appropriate technique for the evaluation of elevated BP in children and adolescents (National High Blood Pressure Education Program Working Group, 2004). Applications of ambulatory BP monitoring in children include identification of white coat hypertension, assessment of BP control in those treated with antihypertensive medications, and investigation of hypotensive episodes (Flynn, 2000; Lurbe et al., 2004). In at least one study, children with secondary hypertension have been found to have more significant nocturnal hypertension and greater daytime diastolic hypertension than those with primary hypertension (Flynn, 2002), suggesting that ambulatory monitoring can be used to identify children who need a more intensive evaluation for underlying causes of hypertension.

The importance of identifying children with white coat hypertension cannot be underestimated. White coat hypertension appears to be at least as common in children as it is in adults (Sorof & Portman, 2000). In adults, white coat hypertension is not felt to be associated with significant cardiovascular morbidity or mortality (Pickering et al., 1999), so pharmacologic treatment of such patients is not recommended. Therefore, proving that a child has white coat hypertension could help avoid unnecessary exposure to medications and reduce unnecessary diagnostic testing. However, children found to have white coat hypertension should have ongoing follow-up of their BP, as tracking studies would suggest that they may be at increased risk of development of hypertension in the future.

### Differential Diagnosis

Traditionally, most hypertension in children has been felt to be secondary to an underlying disorder.

## TABLE 16-7

### Causes of Childhood Hypertension by Age Group

| | Infants[a] | School-age | Adolescents |
|---|---|---|---|
| Primary/Essential | <1% | 15%–30% | 85%–95% |
| Secondary | 99% | 70%–85% | 5%–15%[b] |
| *Renal Parenchymal Disease* | 20% | 60%–70% | |
| *Renovascular* | 25% | 5%–10% | |
| *Endocrine* | 1% | 3%–5% | |
| *Aortic Coarctation* | 35% | 10%–20% | |
| *Reflux Nephropathy* | 0% | 5%–10% | |
| *Neoplastic* | 4% | 1%–5% | |
| *Miscellaneous* | 20% | 1%–5% | |

[a]Less than 1 year of age.
[b]Breakdown of causes is generally similar to that for school-age children.

As can be seen in Table 16–7, this is certainly the case for infants and young children. In hypertensive children in these age groups, renal disease, renovascular disease, and cardiac disease will often be found after an appropriate diagnostic evaluation. Primary hypertension in young children is therefore usually considered a diagnosis of exclusion (Arar et al., 1994).

In adolescents, however, hypertension is most likely to be primary in origin. This was clearly demonstrated over a decade ago in a study of over 1,000 hypertensive children evaluated at a Polish children's hospital (Wyszynska et al., 1992). In this series, the vast majority of adolescents with persistent BP elevation had no identifiable underlying cause. Other features that support the diagnosis of primary hypertension include normal growth (and/or obesity), lack of symptoms of hypertension, unremarkable past medical history, and a family history of hypertension (Flynn & Alderman, 2005). Hypertensive adolescents that fit this profile may not need as extensive an evaluation as those who do not.

### Diagnostic Evaluation

Hypertension in childhood and adolescence is typically asymptomatic. The most frequent symptom is headache, usually without distinguishing features that separate it from other etiologies. In adolescent athletes, headaches may occur after strenuous exercise. Symptoms such as seizures, nosebleeds, dizziness, and syncope are rare and, if present, suggest that the BP elevation has been exacerbated by ingested substances or by emotional upset. On the other hand, if these symptoms occur in conjunction with elevated BP in a younger child, they may be a clue to the presence of secondary hypertension. For this reason, it is important to include a systems review designed to elicit signs and symptoms of underlying conditions such as renal disease that may be causing the elevated BP.

The family history should include not only hypertension but also associated conditions and complications such as dyslipidemia, stroke, myocardial infarction, and diabetes. Many substances commonly used or abused in children and adolescents can elevate BP, including prescribed and over-the-counter medications (e.g., corticosteroids or decongestants) and street drugs such as amphetamines and cocaine.

The physical examination should begin with plotting of growth parameters, including body mass index (BMI), and measurement of BP in both arms and at least one leg. From there, the examination should be focused on detecting signs of secondary causes of hypertension, such as decreased femoral pulses, abdominal bruits, and cushingoid stigmata (Table 16–8).

Except in very young children, the likelihood that an asymptomatic child with persistently elevated BP will have an underlying cause for the elevation is remote. In children with an identifiable cause for their hypertension, the history and physical examination usually reveal suggestive evidence of the cause, so that detailed diagnostic evaluation of children without suggestive evidence is not warranted. Basic screening tests, including serum chemistries and lipids as well as a urinalysis, should be obtained in all patients. Specific specialized studies may be required in some children, particularly those with symptomatic hypertension or stage 2 hypertension (Flynn, 2001b; National High Blood Pressure Education Program Working Group, 2004).

Consideration should be given to including ambulatory BP monitoring (ABPM) in evaluation of all children and adolescents with persistent office BP evaluation, to identify both children with white coat hypertension who may need no further workup (Lurbe et al., 2004; Sorof et al., 2000) and children with possible secondary hypertension (Flynn, 2002). Given the high frequency of left ventricular hypertrophy in hypertensive children and adolescents (Flynn & Alderman, 2005; Hanevold et al., 2004; Sorof et al., 2004b), echocardiography should be considered part of the baseline evaluation, especially if pharmacologic intervention is required, so that reversal of abnormalities can be monitored and correlated with the adequacy of BP control.

## MANAGEMENT OF HYPERTENSION IN CHILDREN AND ADOLESCENTS

Treatment of hypertension in children and adolescents is still largely empiric, because there are no long-term studies of either dietary intervention or drug therapy (Kay et al., 2001). Even though more data are now available on safety and effectiveness of drug therapy than in the past (Flynn, 2003a), the decision as to whether a specific child should receive medication must be individualized, following the principles shown in Figure 16–1.

### Nonpharmacologic Management

Consensus reports emphasize that treatment of hypertension in children and adolescents should begin with nonpharmacologic measures (National High Blood Pressure Education Program Working Group, 2004). Although the magnitude of change in BP may be modest, weight loss, aerobic exercise, and dietary modifications have been shown to reduce BP in children and adolescents. For exercise, for example, sustained training over 3 to 6 months has been shown to result in a reduction of

## TABLE 16–8

### Physical Examination Findings and Etiology of Hypertension in Children and Adolescents

| | Finding | Possible Etiology |
|---|---|---|
| Vital Signs | Tachycardia | Hyperthyroidism, pheochromocytoma, Neuroblastoma, primary hypertension |
| | Diminished femoral pulses; BP lower in legs than arms | Aortic coarctation |
| Height/weight | Growth retardation | Chronic renal failure |
| | Obesity | Primary hypertension |
| | Truncal obesity | Cushing's syndrome |
| Head and Neck | Moon facies | Cushing's syndrome |
| | Elfin facies | Williams syndrome |
| | Webbed neck | Turner's syndrome |
| | Thyromegaly | Hyperthyroidism |
| Skin | Pallor, flushing, diaphoresis | Pheochromocytoma |
| | Acne, hirsutism, striae | Cushing's syndrome, anabolic steroid abuse |
| | Cafe-au-lait spots | Neurofibromatosis |
| | Adenoma sebaceum | Tuberous sclerosis |
| | Malar rash | Systemic lupus erythematosus |
| Chest | Widely spaced nipples/shield chest | Turner's syndrome |
| | Heart murmur | Aortic coarctation |
| | Friction rub | Systemic lupus erythematosus (pericarditis) |
| | Apical heave | Left ventricular hypertrophy/chronic hypertension |
| Abdomen | Mass | Wilms' tumor, neuroblastoma, pheochromocytoma |
| | Epigastric/flank bruit | Renal artery stenosis |
| | Palpable kidneys | Polycystic kidney disease, hydronephrosis, multicystic-dysplastic kidney |
| Genitalia | Ambiguous/virilization | Adrenal hyperplasia |
| Extremities | Edema | Acute glomerulonepdritis, chronic renal failure |
| | Joint swelling | Systemic lupus erythematosus |
| | Muscle weakness | Hyperaldosteronism, Liddle's syndrome |

6 to 12 mm Hg for systolic BP and 3 to 5 mm Hg for diastolic BP (Alpert, 2000). However, cessation of training is generally promptly followed by a rise in BP to pre-exercise levels. It is important to emphasize that aerobic exercise activities such as running, walking, or cycling are preferred to static forms of exercise in the management of hypertension (Alpert & Fox, 1995). Many children may already be participating in one or more appropriate activities and may only need to increase the frequency and intensity of these activities to see a benefit in terms of lower BP. Hypertension is *not* considered a contraindication to participation in competitive sports so long as the child's BP is "controlled" (AAP Committee on Sports Medicine and Fitness, 1997).

Several studies have demonstrated that weight loss in obese adolescents lowers BP (Figueroa-Colon et al., 1996; Rocchini et al., 1988). Weight loss not only decreases BP, but it also improves other cardiovascular risk factors such as dyslipidemia and insulin resistance (Williams et al., 2002). In studies where a reduction in BMI of about 10% was achieved, short-term reductions in BP were in the range of 8 to 12 mm Hg. Unfortunately, weight loss is notoriously difficult and usually unsuccessful,

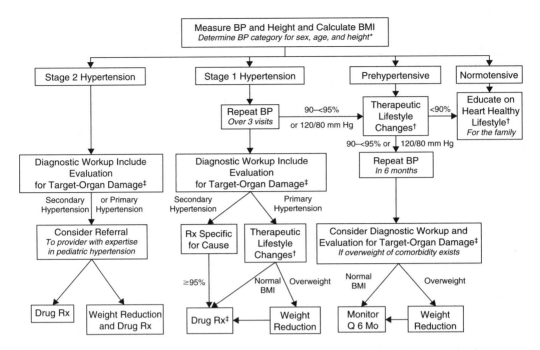

**FIGURE 16–1** ● Suggested Management Algorithm for Children and Adolescents with Elevated Blood Pressure. BMI, body mass index; Q, every; *, see Tables 16–4, 16–5, and 16–6; †, diet modification and physical activity; ‡, especially if younger, very high BP, little or no family history, diabetic, or other risk factors. Reproduced from National High Blood Pressure Education Program Working Group on High Blood Pressure in Children and Adolescents. The fourth report on the diagnosis, evaluation, and treatment of high blood pressure in children and adolescents. National Heart, Lung, and Blood Institute, Bethesda, Maryland. *Pediatrics* 2004;114:555–576.

especially in the primary care setting (Epstein et al., 1998). However, identifying a complication of obesity such as hypertension can perhaps provide the necessary motivation for patients and families to make the appropriate lifestyle changes.

The role of diet in the treatment of hypertension has received a great deal of attention, most of which has focused on sodium. Once hypertension has been established, "salt sensitivity" becomes more common, and reduction in sodium intake may be of benefit (Cutler, 1999; Weinberger, 1996). Other dietary constituents that have been examined in patients with hypertension include potassium and calcium, both of which have been shown to have antihypertensive effects (Cutler, 1999; Gillman et al., 1992). Therefore, a diet that is low in sodium and enriched in potassium and calcium may be even more effective than a diet that restricts sodium only. An example of such a diet is the so-called DASH diet, which has been shown to have a clear BP-lowering effect in adults with hypertension, even in those receiving antihypertensive medication (Appel et al., 1997). Although this diet has not been specifically studied in children, the basic elements of the DASH diet are logical to apply to the treatment of

hypertensive children. The DASH diet also incorporates measures designed to reduce dietary fat intake, an important strategy given the frequent presence of both hypertension and elevated lipids in children and adolescents and the imperative to begin prevention of adult cardiovascular disease at as early an age as possible (Gidding, 1993; Kavey et al., 2003; Williams et al., 2002).

### Pharmacologic Management

Experience in adults indicates that hypertension is a life-long condition in most patients, which implies that once a hypertensive patient is started on medication, he or she is likely to remain on medication for the rest of his or her life. This is usually readily accepted for an adult patient given the known long-term adverse consequences of untreated or under-treated hypertension (Chobanian et al., 2003; Klag et al., 1996). However, since the long-term consequences of untreated hypertension in an asymptomatic, otherwise healthy child or adolescent remain unknown (Kay et al., 2001), the decision to initiate pharmacologic therapy in the first or second decade of life is not to be undertaken lightly. The lack of data on the long-term effects of antihypertensive medications on the growth and development of children adds further uncertainty. Therefore, a definite indication for initiating pharmacologic therapy should be ascertained before medication is prescribed.

Reasonable indications for use of antihypertensive medications in children and adolescents include the following:

- Symptomatic hypertension
- Secondary hypertension
- Hypertensive target-organ damage
- Diabetes (Types I and II)
- Persistent hypertension despite nonpharmacologic measures

Pharmacologic reduction of BP for hypertensive children who fall into one of these categories is likely to result in health benefit.

Additional indications for use of antihypertensive medications have been proposed, all based upon the premise of reducing future cardiovascular risk and end stage renal disease. It is clearly established, for example, that the presence of multiple cardiovascular risk factors (elevated BP, hyperlipidemia, tobacco use, etc.) increases cardiovascular risk in an exponential rather than additive fashion (Kavey et al., 2003). Thus, it is suggested that antihypertensive therapy be instituted if the child or adolescent is known to have hyperlipidemia. Similarly, elevated nocturnal BP and/or blunted nocturnal dipping on ABPM increases the likelihood of developing hypertensive target-organ damage and other adverse cardiovascular outcomes (Clement et al., 2003).

The number of antihypertensive medications that have been systematically studied in children has increased markedly over the past 5 years due to incentives provided to the pharmaceutical industry under the auspices of the 1997 Food and Drug Modernization Act (FDAMA) and the Best Pharmaceuticals for Children Act (BPCA) of 2002 (Flynn, 2003a). Publication of the results of the industry-sponsored clinical trials can be used to guide prescribing of antihypertensive agents in children and adolescents who require pharmacologic treatment, thereby increasing the confidence of the practitioner who treats such children. The dosing recommendations contained in Table 16–9 incorporate data from many of these studies.

No studies comparing different classes of antihypertensive agents have been conducted in children; therefore, the choice of initial antihypertensive agent for use in children remains up to the preference of the individual practitioner. Diuretics and β-adrenergic blockers, which were recommended as initial therapy in the First and Second Task Force Reports (Blumenthal et al., 1977; Task Force on Blood Pressure Control in Children, 1987), have a long track record of safety and efficacy in hypertensive children and are considered appropriate for pediatric use. Similarly, newer classes of agents, including angiotensin-converting enzyme inhibitors (ACEI), calcium channel blockers (CCBs), and angiotensin receptor blockers (ARBs) (Flynn et al., 2004; Sakarcan et al., 2001; Wells et al., 2002), have been shown to be safe and well tolerated in hypertensive children in recent industry-sponsored trials and may be prescribed if indicated. Since many antihypertensive drugs now have specific FDA-approved pediatric labeling, generalists should restrict their choices to those agents.

Consideration should be given to using specific classes of antihypertensive medications in certain hypertensive children with specific underlying or concurrent medical conditions. The best example of this would be the use of ACEIs or angiotensin receptor antagonists in children with diabetes or proteinuric renal diseases, something that is already being done by many physicians who treat hypertensive children (Woroniecki & Flynn, 2005). This parallels the approach outlined in the JNC-7 report, which recommends that specific classes of antihypertensive agents be used in adults in certain high-risk categories (Chobanian et al., 2003).

Antihypertensive drugs in children are generally prescribed in a stepped-care manner: The child is initially started on the lowest recommended dose, then the dose is increased until the highest recommended dose is reached, or until the child experiences adverse effects from the medication, at which point a second drug from a different class should be added, until the desired goal BP is reached. For children with uncomplicated primary hypertension and no hypertensive target-organ damage, goal BP should be less than the ninety-fifth percentile for age, gender, and height, whereas for children with secondary hypertension, diabetes, or hypertensive target-organ damage, goal BP should be less than the ninetieth percentile for age, gender, and height (National High Blood Pressure Education Program Working Group, 2004).

Treatment of childhood hypertension obviously does not end when a prescription is written. There should be ongoing monitoring of BP, surveillance for medication side effects, periodic monitoring of electrolytes (in children treated with ACEIs or diuretics), counseling regarding other cardiovascular risk factors, and continued emphasis on therapeutic lifestyle changes. Hypertensive target organ damage such as left ventricular hypertrophy, if present, should be reassessed periodically.

## TABLE 16–9

### Dosing Recommendations for Selected Antihypertensive Agents for Use in Hypertensive Children and Adolescents

| Class | Drug | Starting Dose | Interval | Maximum Dose[a] |
|---|---|---|---|---|
| ACE inhibitors | Benazepril | 0.2 mg/kg per day up to 10 mg per day | QD | 0.6 mg/kg per day up to 40 mg qd |
| | Captopril | 0.3–0.5 mg/kg per dose | BID–TID | 6 mg/kg per day up to 450 mg per day |
| | Enalapril | 0.08 mg/kg per day | QD | 0.6 mg/kg per day up to 40 mg per day |
| | Fosinopril | 0.1 mg/kg per day up to 10 mg per day | QD | 0.6 mg/kg per day up to 40 mg per day |
| | Lisinopril | 0.07 mg/kg per day up to 5 mg per day | QD | 0.6 mg/kg per day up to 40 mg per day |
| | Quinapril | 5–10 mg per day | QD | 80 mg per day |
| ARBs | Candesartan | 4 mg per day | QD | 32 mg QD |
| | Irbesartan | 75–150 mg per day | QD | 300 mg per day |
| | Losartan | 0.75 mg/kg per day up to 50 mg per day | QD | 1.4 mg/kg per day up to 100 mg per day |
| α- and β-antagonists | Labetalol | 2–3 mg/kg per day | BID | 10–12 mg/kg per day up to 1.2 g per day |
| | Carvedilol | 6.25–12.5 mg BID | BID | 25 mg BID |
| β-antagonists | Atenolol | 0.5–1 mg/kg per day | QD–BID | 2 mg/kg per day up to 100 mg per day |
| | Bisoprolol/ HCTZ | 2.5/6.25 mg per day | QD | 10/6.25 mg qd |
| | Metoprolol | 1–2 mg/kg per day | BID | 6 mg/kg per day up to 200 mg per day |
| | Propranolol | 1 mg/kg per day | BID–TID | 16 mg/kg per day up to 640 mg per day |
| CCBs | Amlodipine | 0.06 mg/kg per day | QD | 0.3 mg/kg per day up to 10 mg per day |
| | Felodipine | 2.5 mg per day | QD | 10 mg per day |
| | Isradipine | 0.05–0.15 mg/kg/dose | TID–QID | 0.8 mg/kg per day up to 20 mg per day |
| | Extended-release nifedipine | 0.25–0.5 mg/kg per day | QD–BID | 3 mg/kg per day up to 120 mg per day |
| Central α-agonists | Clonidine | 5–10 mcg/kg per day | BID-TID | 25 mcg/kg per day up to 0.9 mg per day |
| | Methyldopa | 5 mg/kg per day | BID-QID | 40 mg/kg per day up to 3 g per day |
| Diuretics | Amiloride | 5–10 mg per day | QD | 20 mg per day |
| | Chlorthalidone | 0.3 mg/kg per day | QD | 2 mg/kg per day up to 50 mg per day |
| | Furosemide | 0.5–2.0 mg/kg/dose | QD-BID | 6 mg/kg per day |

*(continued)*

## TABLE 16–9 (Continued)

### Dosing Recommendations for Selected Antihypertensive Agents for Use in Hypertensive Children and Adolescents

| Class | Drug | Starting Dose | Interval | Maximum Dose[a] |
|---|---|---|---|---|
| Diuretics | HCTZ | 0.5–1 mg/kg per day | QD | 3 mg/kg per day up to 50 mg per day |
| | Sprionolactone | 1 mg/kg per day | QD-BID | 3.3 mg/kg per day up to 100 mg per day |
| | Triamterene | 1–2 mg/kg per day | BID | 3–4 mg/kg per day up to 300 mg per day |
| Peripheral | Doxazosin | 1 mg per day | QD | 4 mg per day |
| α-antagonists | Prazosin | 0.05–0.1 mg/kg per day | TID | 0.5 mg/kg per day |
| | Terazosin | 1 mg per day | QD | 20 mg per day |
| Vasodilators | Hydralazine | 0.25 mg/kg per dose | TID–QID | 7.5 mg/kg per day up to 200 mg per day |
| | Minoxidil | 0.1–0.2 mg/kg per day | BID–TID | 1 mg/kg per day up to 50 mg per day |

[a]The maximum recommended adult dose should never be exceeded.
BID, twice daily; HCTZ, hydrochlorothiazide; QD, once daily; QID, four times daily; TID, three times daily.

It may also be appropriate to consider "step-down" therapy in selected children and adolescents. This involves an attempt at gradual reduction in medication after an extended course of good BP control, with the eventual goal of completely discontinuing drug therapy. Children with uncomplicated primary hypertension, especially obese adolescents who successfully lose weight and maintain their weight loss, are the best candidates for the step-down approach. These children should receive continued BP monitoring after drug therapy is withdrawn, as well as continued nonpharmacologic treatment.

## SPECIAL TOPICS

### Hypertension in Infancy

In newborn and premature infants, systemic hypertension is best defined as systolic and/or diastolic BP that persistently exceeds the mean +2 standard deviations for infants of similar postconceptual age (Flynn, 2004a). The graphs published by Zubrow et al. are probably most useful in this regard (Zubrow et al., 1995). After 1 month of age, hypertension is defined as systolic and/or diastolic BP greater than the ninety-fifth percentile for that infant's age and gender (Task Force on Blood Pressure Control in Children, 1987).

Although one recent series found that 28% of infants with body weights (BWs) <1,500 grams had at least one elevated BP documented during their neonatal intensive care unit stay (Al-Aweel et al., 2001), the actual incidence of hypertension in neonates is very low, ranging from 0.2% in healthy newborns to between 0.7% and 2.5% in high-risk newborns (Flynn, 2004a). Certain categories of infants are at significantly higher risk, however. For example, hypertension is relatively common in patients with a history of umbilical artery catheterization and those with bronchopulmonary dysplasia. On the other hand, hypertension is so uncommon in otherwise healthy term infants that routine BP determination isn't even recommended (AAP Committee on Fetus and Newborn, 1993).

The differential diagnosis of hypertension in neonates and older infants is wide-ranging (Tables 16–7, 16–10). However, the most important categories of causes of neonatal hypertension include renovascular disease (most commonly umbilical artery related aortic or renal thromboembolism) (Bauer et al., 1975), renal parenchymal disease, and bronchopulmonary dysplasia (Alagappan et al., 1998). The most common cardiac cause is coarctation of the thoracic aorta, in which hypertension may persist or recur after surgical repair (O'Sullivan et al., 2002). For a more comprehensive

## TABLE 16–10

### Causes of Neonatal Hypertension

**Renovascular**
  Thromboembolism
  Renal artery stenosis
  Mid-aortic coarctation
  Renal venous thrombosis
  Renal artery compression
  Abdominal aortic aneurysm
  Idiopathic arterial calcification
  Congenital rubella syndrome

**Renal Parenchymal Disease**
  Congenital
    Polycystic kidney disease
    Multicystic-dysplastic kidney disease
    Tuberous sclerosis
    Ureteropelvic junction obstruction
    Unilateral renal hypoplasia
    Primary megaureter
    Congenital nephrotic syndrome
  Acquired
    Acute tubular necrosis
    Cortical necrosis
    Interstitial nephritis
    Hemolytic-uremic syndrome
    Obstruction (stones, tumors)

**Pulmonary**
  Bronchopulmonary dysplasia
  Pneumothorax

**Cardiac**
  Thoracic aortic coarctation

**Endocrine**
  Congenital adrenal hyperplasia
  Hyperaldosteronism
  Hyperthyroidism
  Pseudohypoaldosteronism type II
  (Gordon syndrome)

**Medications/Intoxications**
  Infant
    Dexamethasone
    Adrenergic agents
    Vitamin D intoxication
    Theophylline
    Caffeine
    Pancuronium
    Phenylephrine
  Maternal
    Cocaine
    Heroin

**Neoplasia**
  Wilms tumor
  Mesoblastic nephroma
  Neuroblastoma
  Pheochromocytoma

**Neurologic**
  Pain
  Intracranial hypertension
  Seizures
  Familial dysautonomia
  Subdural hematoma

**Miscellaneous**
  Total parenteral nutrition
  Closure of abdominal wall
  defect
  Adrenal hemorrhage
  Hypercalcemia
  Traction
  ECMO
  Birth asphyxia
  Primary HTN

---

ECMO, extracorporeal membrane oxygenation.

discussion, the reader is encouraged to consult other references (Flynn, 2004a).

Investigation of hypertensive infants should proceed in a similar fashion to evaluation of older children with hypertension. There may be significant variability between upper and lower limb BPs in neonates (Crossland et al., 2004), so it is important to be consistent in choice of extremity for BP measurement. A thorough review of the infant's history and a focused physical examination points to the underlying cause in most cases. Selected laboratory studies should be obtained as indicated. Renal ultrasonagraphy is particularly useful given the preponderance of renal causes (Table 16–10).

Therapy of neonatal hypertension should be tailored to the severity of the hypertension and the infant's overall clinical status. For example, critically ill infants with severe hypertension should be treated with an intravenous agent administered by continuous infusion, as this will allow the greatest control over the magnitude and rapidity of the BP reduction. On the other hand, relatively well infants with mild hypertension may be treated with oral antihypertensive agents. Recommended doses for antihypertensive drugs in infants can be found in Table 16–11. Unfortunately, few data on drug efficacy and safety exist for infants, and recent federal initiatives designed to expand the availability

## TABLE 16–11

### Recommended Doses for Selected Antihypertensive Agents for Treatment of Hypertensive Infants

| Class | Drug | Route | Dose | Interval |
|---|---|---|---|---|
| ACE Inhibitor | Captopril | Oral | <3m: 0.01–0.5 mg/kg per dose<br>Max 2 mg/kg per day<br>>3m: 0.15–0.3 mg/kg per dose<br>Max 6 mg/kg per day | TID |
|  | Enalapril | Oral | 0.08–0.6 mg/kg per day | QD-BID |
| α- and β-antagonist | Labetalol | Oral | 0.5–1.0 mg/kg per dose<br>Max 10 mg/kg per day | BID-TID |
|  |  | IV | 0.20–.0 mg/kg per dose | Q4–6hr |
|  |  |  | 0.25–3.0 mg/kg per hr | Infusion |
| β-antagonist | Esmolol | IV | 100–300 mcg/kg per min | Infusion |
|  | Propranolol | Oral | 0.5–1.0 mg/kg per dose<br>Max 8–10 mg/kg per day | TID |
| Calcium channel blocker | Amlodipine | Oral | 0.05–0.3 mg/kg per dose<br>Max 0.6 mg/kg per day | QD-BID |
|  | Isradipine | Oral | 0.05–0.15 mg/kg per dose<br>Max 0.8 mg/kg per day | QID |
|  | Nicardipine | IV | 1–4 mcg/kg per min | Infusion |
| Diuretic | Chlorothiazide | Oral | 5–15 mg/kg per dose | BID |
|  | Hydrochlorothiazide | Oral | 1–3 mg/kg per dose | QD |
|  | Spironolactone | Oral | 0.5–1.5 mg/kg per dose | BID |
| Vasodilator | Hydralazine | Oral | 0.25–1.0 mg/kg per dose<br>Max 7.5 mg/kg per day | TID - QID |
|  |  | IV | 0.15–0.6 mg/kg per dose | Qh4r |
|  | Minoxidil | Oral | 0.1–0.2 mg/kg per dose | BID - TID |
|  | Sodium nitroprusside | IV | 0.5–10 mcg/kg per min | Infusion |

BID, twice daily; IV, intravenous; Q, every; QD, once daily; QID, four times daily; TID, three times daily.

## TABLE 16–12

### Recommended Doses for Antihypertensive Agents Used for Hypertensive Emergencies and Urgencies in Children and Adolescents

| Drug | Class | Dose | Route | Comments |
|---|---|---|---|---|
| Clonidine | Central α-agonist | 0.05–0.1 mg/dose, may be repeated up to 0.8 mg total dose | Oral | Side effects include dry mouth and sedation. |
| Enalaprilat | ACE inhibitor | 0.05–0.10 mg/kg per dose up to 1.25 mg/dose | IV bolus | May cause prolonged hypotension and acute renal failure. |
| Esmolol | β-blocker | 100–500 mcg/kg per min | IV infusion | Very short-acting. May cause profound bradycardia. |
| Fenoldopam | Dopamine receptor agonist | 0.2–0.8 mcg/kg per min | IV infusion | Produced modest reductions in BP in a pediatric clinical trial in patients up to 12 years. |
| Hydralazine | Vasodilator | 0.2–0.6 mg/kg per dose | IV, IM | Should be given q 4 hr when given IV bolus. |
| Isradipine | CCB | 0.05–0.1 mg/kg per dose | Oral | Stable suspension can be compounded. |
| Labetalol | α- and β-blocker | Bolus: 0.20–1.0 mg/kg per dose up to 40 mg/dose Infusion: 0.25–3.0 mg/kg per hr | IV bolus or infusion | Asthma and overt heart failure are relative contraindications. |
| Minoxidil | Vasodilator | 0.1–0.2 mg/kg per dose | Oral | Most potent oral vasodilator; long acting. |
| Nicardipine | CCB | 1–3 mcg/kg per min | IV infusion | May cause reflex tachycardia. |
| Sodium Nitroprusside | Vasodilator | 0.53–10 mcg/kg per min | IV infusion | Monitor cyanide levels with prolonged (>72 hr) use or in renal failure; or co-administer with sodium thiosulfate. |

ACE, angiotensin-converting enzyme; IM, intramuscular; IV, intravenous.

of pediatric drug efficacy and safety information will not change this situation (Flynn, 2003a). Thus, choice of antihypertensive medications for use in neonates relies heavily on the experience of the individual practitioner.

### Hypertensive Emergencies

The pathophysiology, management, and outcome of severe hypertension in children and adolescents was last reviewed in detail several years ago (Adelman et al., 2000). Many aspects are similar to hypertensive emergencies in adults as reviewed in Chapter 8. However, a few unique aspects warrant consideration.

Underlying conditions that may produce a hypertensive emergency in a child or adolescent may include acute or chronic renal disease, organ transplantation, renal artery stenosis, or congenital renal disease such as autosomal recessive polycystic kidney disease. Hypertensive encephalopathy is frequent, particularly in younger children with severe hypertension, emphasizing the need for slow, controlled reduction in BP to prevent complications arising through loss of normal autoregulatory processes (Adelman et al., 2000). Less severe symptoms may include nausea, vomiting, or unusual irritability; since these may be somewhat nonspecific, especially in younger children, a high degree of clinical suspicion must be maintained.

Although evidence-based recommendations are lacking, the usual goal in treatment of a hypertensive emergency is to reduce the BP by no more than 25% over the first 8 hours, with a gradual return to normal/goal BP over 24 to 48 hours (Adelman et al., 2000). Treatment of hypertensive emergencies in children should be initiated with a continuous infusion of an intravenous antihypertensive, with nicardipine and labetalol finding the greatest popularity in many centers (Flynn et al., 2001a). The dopamine receptor agonist fenoldopam has also been reported effective (Strauser et al., 1999).

For less severe degrees of BP elevation, or if the child's symptoms permit, oral antihypertensive agents can be used. The choice of oral antihypertensives for use in management of severe hypertension remains a topic of debate among pediatric nephrologists (Calvetta et al., 2003), with short-acting nifedipine advocated as safe by some authors (Yiu et al., 2004), and as dangerous by others (Flynn, 2003b). A list of recommended doses for drugs used to treat severe hypertension in children and adolescents can be found in Table 16–12.

# REFERENCES

Adelman RD, Coppo R, Dillon MJ. The emergency management of severe hypertension. *Pediatr Nephrol* 2000;14:422–427.

Adrogue HE, Sinaiko AR. Prevalence of hypertension in junior high school-aged children: effect of new recommendations in the 1996 Updated Task Force Report. *Am J Hypertens* 2001;14(5 Pt 1):412–414.

Alagappan A, Malloy MH. Systemic hypertension in very low-birth weight infants with bronchopulmonary dysplasia: incidence and risk factors. *Am J Perinatol* 1998;15:3–8.

Al-Aweel I, Pursley DM, Rubin LP, et al. Variations in prevalence of hypotension, hypertension and vasopressor use in NICUs. *J Perinatol* 2001;12:272–278.

Alpert BS, Fox ME. Hypertension. In: Goldberg B, ed., *Sports and Exercise for Children with Chronic Health Conditions*. Champaign, IL; Human Kinetics, 1995.

Alpert BS. Exercise as a therapy to control hypertension in children. *Int J Sports Med* 2000;21(Suppl 2):S94–S96.

American Academy of Pediatrics Committee on Fetus and Newborn. Routine evaluation of blood pressure, hematocrit and glucose in newborns. *Pediatrics* 1993;92:474–476.

American Academy of Pediatrics Committee on School Health. Organizational principles to guide and define the child health care system and/or improve the health of all children. *Pediatrics* 2004;113:152–154.

American Academy of Pediatrics Committee on Sports Medicine and Fitness. Athletic participation by children and adolescents who have systemic hypertension. *Pediatrics* 1997;99:637–638.

Appel LJ, Moore TJ, Obarzanek E, et al. A clinical trial of the effects of dietary patterns on blood pressure. *N Engl J Med* 1997;336:1117–1124.

Arar MY, Hogg RJ, Arant BS Jr, et al. Etiology of sustained hypertension in children in the southwestern United States. *Pediatr Nephrol* 1994;8:186–189.

Bao W, Threefoot SA, Srinivasan SR, Bergenson GS. Essential hypertension predicted by tracking of elevated blood pressure from childhood to adulthood: the Bogalusa Heart Study. *Am J Hypertens* 1995;8:657–665.

Bauer SB, Feldman SM, Gellis SS, et al. Neonatal hypertension: a complication of umbilical-artery catheterization. *N Engl J Med* 1975;293:1032–1033.

Berenson GS. Childhood risk factors predict adult risk associated with subclinical cardiovascular disease: the Bogalusa Heart Study. *Am J Cardiol* 2002;90:3L–7L.

Blumenthal S, Epps RP, Heavenrich R, et al. Report of the task force on blood pressure control in children. *Pediatrics* 1977;59:797–820.

Bowman SA, Gortmaker SL, Ebbeling CB, et al. Effects of fast-food consumption on energy intake and diet quality among children in a national household survey. *Pediatrics* 2004;113:112–118.

Burke V, Beilin LJ, Blake KV, et al. Indicators of fetal growth do not independently predict blood pressure in 8-year-old Australians: a prospective cohort study. *Hypertension* 2004; 43:208–213.

Calvetta A, Martino S, von Vigier RO, et al. "What goes up must immediately come down!" Which indication for short-acting nifedipine in children with arterial hypertension? *Pediatr Nephrol* 2003;18:1–2.

Chobanian AV, Bakris GL, Black HR, et al. The seventh report of the Joint National Committee on Prevention, Detection, Evaluation, and Treatment of High Blood Pressure: the JNC 7 report. *JAMA* 2003;289:2560–2572.

Clement DL, De Buyzere ML, De Bacquer DA, et al. Prognostic value of ambulatory blood-pressure recordings in patients with treated hypertension. *N Engl J Med* 2003;348: 2407–2415.

Crossland DS, Furness JC, Abu-Harb M, et al. Variability of four limb blood pressure in normal neonates. *Arch Dis Child Fetal Neonatal Ed* 2004;89:F325–F327.

Cutler JA. The effects of reducing sodium and increasing potassium intake for control of hypertension and improving health. *Clin & Exp Hypertens* 1999;21:769–783.

Daniels SR, Obarzanek E, Barton BA, et al. Sexual maturation and racial differences in blood pressure in girls. *J Pediatr* 1996;129:208–213.

Daniels SR. Is there an epidemic of cardiovascular disease on the horizon? *J Pediatr* 1999;134:665–666.

Davis PH, Dawson JD, Riley WA, Lauer RM. Carotid intimal-medial thickness is related to cardiovascular risk factors measured from childhood through middle age: the Muscatine Study. *Circulation* 2001;104:2815–2819.

Dekkers JC, Snieder H, van den Oord EJCG, Treiber FA. Moderators of blood pressure development from childhood to adulthood: a 10-year longitudinal study. *J Pediatr* 2002;141:770–779.

deLeonardis V, DeScalzi M, Falchetti A, et al. Echocardiographic evaluation of children with and without family history of hypertension. *Am J Hypertens* 1988;1:305–308.

Doyle LW, Faber B, Callahan C, Morley R. Blood pressure in late adolescence and very low birth weight. *Pediatrics* 2003;111:252–257.

Epstein LH, Myers MD, Raynor HA, Saelens BE. Treatment of pediatric obesity. *Pediatrics* 1998;101:554–570.

Erler T, Paditz E. Obstructive sleep apnea syndrome in children: a state-of-the-art review. *Treat Respir Med* 2004; 3:107–122.

Falkner B, Hulman S, Kushner H. Effect of birth weight on blood pressure and body size in early adolescence. *Hypertension* 2004;43:203–207.

Falkner B, Sherif K, Michel S, et al. Dietary nutrients and blood pressure in urban minority adolescents at risk for hypertension. *Arch Pediatr Adolesc Med* 2000;154: 918–922.

Figueroa-Colon R, Franklin FA, Lee JY, et al. Feasibility of a clinic-based hypocaloric dietary intervention implemented in a school setting for obese children. *Obes Res* 1996;4: 419–429.

Fixler DE, Laird WP, Fitzgerald V, et al. Hypertension screening in schools: results of the Dallas study. *Pediatrics* 1979; 63:32–36.

Flynn JT. Impact of ambulatory blood pressure monitoring on the management of hypertension in children. *Blood Press Monitor* 2000;5:211–216.

Flynn, JT, Mottes TA, Brophy PB, et al. Intravenous nicardipine for treatment of severe hypertension in children. *J Pediatr* 2001a;139:38–43.

Flynn JT. Evaluation and management of hypertension in childhood. *Prog Ped Cardiol* 2001b;12:177–188.

Flynn JT. Differentiation between primary and secondary hypertension in children using ambulatory blood pressure monitoring. *Pediatrics* 2002;110:89–93.

Flynn JT. Successes and shortcomings of the FDA Modernization Act. *Am J Hypertens* 2003a;16:889–891.

Flynn JT. Safety of short-acting nifedipine in children with severe hypertension. *Expert Opin Drug Saf* 2003b;2:133–139.

Flynn JT. Neonatal hypertension. In: Portman R, Sorof J, Ingelfinger J, eds. *Pediatric Hypertension*. Totowa, NJ: Humana Press, 2004a.

Flynn JT, Newburger JW, Daniels SR, et al. A randomized, placebo-controlled trial of amlodipine in children with hypertension. *J Pediatr* 2004b;145:353–359.

Flynn JT, Alderman MH. Characteristics of children with primary hypertension seen at a referral center. *Pediatr Nephrol* 2005;20:961–966.

Gidding SS. Relationships between blood pressure and lipids in childhood. *Pediatr Clin North Am* 1993;40:41–49.

Gillman MW, Oliveria SA, Moore LL, et al. Inverse association of dietary calcium with systolic blood pressure in young children. *J Am Med Assoc* 1992;267:2340–2343.

Grummer-Strawn LM, Mei Z. Does breastfeeding protect against pediatric overweight? Analysis of longitudinal data from the Centers for Disease Control and Prevention Pediatric Nutrition Surveillance System. *Pediatrics* 2004;113: e81–e86.

Guilleminault C, Li K, Khramtsov A, et al. Breathing patterns in prepubertal children with sleep-related breathing disorders. *Arch Pediatr Adolesc Med* 2004;158:153–161.

Hanevold C, Waller J, Daniels S, et al. The effects of obesity, gender, and ethnic group on left ventricular hypertrophy and geometry in hypertensive children: a collaborative study of the International Pediatric Hypertension Association. *Pediatrics* 2004;113:328–333.

Hansen HS, Nielsen JR, Hyldebrandt N, Froberg K. Blood pressure and cardiac structure in children with a parental history of hypertension. *J Hypertens* 1992;10:677–682.

Harshfield GA, Pulliam DA, Alpert BS. Ambulatory blood pressure and renal function in healthy children and adolescents. *Am J Hypertens* 1994;7:282–285.

Hohn AR, Dwyer KM, Dwyer JH. Blood pressure in youth from four ethnic groups: the Pasadena Prevention Project. *J Pediatr* 1994;125:368–373.

Huxley R, Neil A, Collins R. Unravelling the fetal origins hypothesis: is there really an inverse association between birthweight and subsequent blood pressure? *Lancet* 2002; 360:659–665.

Kaufmann MA, Pargger H, Drop LJ. Oscillometric blood pressure measurements by different devices are not interchangeable. *Anesth Analg* 1996;82:377–381.

Kavey REW, Daniels SR, Lauer RM, et al. American Heart Association guidelines for primary prevention of atherosclerotic cardiovascular disease beginning in childhood. *Circulation* 2003;107:1562–1566.

Kay JD, Sinaiko AR, Daniels SR. Pediatric hypertension. *Am Heart J* 2001;142:422–432.

Klag MJ, Whelton PK, Randall BL, et al. Blood pressure and end-stage renal disease in men. *N Engl J Med* 1996; 334:13–18.

Kvaavik E, Tell GS, Klepp K-I. Predictors and tracking of body mass index from adolescence into adulthood. *Arch Pediatr Adolesc Med* 2003;157:1212–1218.

Laird WP, Fixler DE. Left ventricular hypertrophy in adolescents with elevated blood pressure: assessment by chest roentgenography, electrocardiography, and echocardiography. *Pediatrics* 1981;67:255–259.

Lande MB, Kaczorowski JM, Auinger P, et al. Elevated blood pressure and decreased cognitive function among school-age children and adolescents in the United States. *J Pediatr* 2003;143:720–724.

Lane DA, Gill P. Ethnicity and tracking blood pressure in children. *J Human Hypertens* 2004;18:223–228.

Lauer Rm, Clarke WR, Mahoney LT, Witt J. Childhood predictors for high adult blood pressure. *Pediatr Clin North Am* 1993;40:23–40.

Lauer RM, Connor WE, Leaverton PE, et al. Coronary heart disease risk factors in school children: the Muscatine study. *J Pediatr* 1975;86:697–706.

Law CM, Shiell AW, Newsome CA, et al. Fetal, infant, and childhood growth and adult blood pressure: a longitudinal study from birth to 22 years of age. *Circulation* 2002;105: 1088–1092.

Lemne CE. Increased blood pressure reactivity in children of borderline hypertensive fathers. *J Hypertens* 1998;16: 1243–1248.

Li S, Chen W, Srinivasan SR, Berenson GS. Childhood blood pressure as a predictor of arterial stiffness in young adults: the Bogalusa Heart Study. *Hypertension* 2004;43:541–546.

Li S, Chen W, Srinivasan SR, et al. Childhood cardiovascular risk factors and carotid vascular changes in adulthood: the Bogalusa Heart Study. *JAMA* 2003;290:2271–2276.

Lissau I, Overpeck MD, Ruan WJ, et al. Body mass index and overweight in adolescents in 13 European countries, Israel, and the United States. *Arch Pediatr Adolesc Med* 2004;158:27–33.

Loggie JM. Prevalence of hypertension and distribution of causes. In: New MI, Levine LS, eds. *Juvenile Hypertension*. New York, Raven Press, 1977.

Luepker RV, Jacobs DR, Prineas RJ, Sinaiko AR. Secular trends of blood pressure and body size in a multi-ethnic adolescent population: 1986 to 1996. *J Pediatr* 1999;134: 668–674.

Lurbe E, Sorof JM, Daniels SR. Clinical and research aspects of ambulatory blood pressure monitoring in children. *J Pediatr* 2004;144:7–16.

Makris TK, Stavroulakis GA, Krespi PG, et al. Elevated plasma immunoreactive leptin levels preexist in healthy offspring of patients with essential hypertension. *Am Heart J* 1999;138:922–925.

Martin RM, Ness AR, Gunnell D, et al. Does breast-feeding in infancy lower blood pressure in childhood? The Avon Longitudinal Study of Parents and Children (ALSPAC). *Circulation* 2004;109:1259–1266.

McDonald A, Trevisan M, Cooper R, et al. Epidemiological studies in sodium transport and hypertension. *Hypertension* 1987;10(Suppl 1):I42–I47.

Meaney E, Samaniego V, Alva F, et al. Increased arterial stiffness in children with a parental history of hypertension. *Pediatr Cardiol* 1999;20:203–205.

Mehta SK, Super DM, Anderson RL, et al. Parental hypertension and cardiac alterations in normotensive children and adolescents. *Am Heart J* 1996;131:81–88.

Mongeau JG. Heredity and blood pressure in humans: an overview. *Pediatr Nephrol* 1987;1:69–75.

Muntner P, He J, Cutler JA, et al. Trends in blood pressure among children and adolescents. *JAMA* 2004;291: 2107–2113.

National High Blood Pressure Education Program Working Group on Hypertension Control in Children and Adolescents (1996). Update on the 1987 task force report on high blood pressure in children and adolescents: a working group report from the National High Blood Pressure Education Program. *Pediatrics* 1996; 98:649–658.

National High Blood Pressure Education Program Working Group on High Blood Pressure in Children and Adolescents. The fourth report on the diagnosis, evaluation, and treatment of high blood pressure in children and adolescents. National Heart, Lung, and Blood Institute, Bethesda, Maryland. *Pediatrics* 2004;114:555–576.

O'Quin M, Sharma BB, Miller KA, Tomsovic JP. Adolescent blood pressure survey: Tulsa, Oklahoma, 1987 to 1989. *South Med J* 1992;85:487–490.

O'Sullivan JJ, Derrick G, Darnell R. Prevalence of hypertension in children after early repair of coarctation of the aorta: a cohort study using casual and 24 hour blood pressure measurement. *Heart* 2002; 88:163–166.

Owen CG, Whincup PH, Gilg JA, Cook DG. Effect of breast feeding in infancy on blood pressure in later life: systematic review and meta-analysis. *BMJ* 2003;327:1189–1195.

Park MK, Menard SW, Yuan C. Comparison of auscultatory and oscillometric blood pressures. *Arch Pediatr Adolesc Med* 2001;155:50–53.

Patrick K, Norman GJ, Calfas KJ, et al. Diet, physical activity, and sedentary behaviors as risk factors for overweight in adolescence. *Arch Pediatr Adolesc Med* 2004;158:385–390.

Pickering TG, Coats A, Mallion JM, et al. Blood Pressure Monitoring. Task force V: white-coat hypertension. *Blood Press Monit* 1999;4:333–341.

Pickering TG, Hall JE, Appel LJ, et al. Recommendations for blood pressure measurement in humans and experimental animals. Part 1: blood pressure measurement in humans. A statement for professionals from the Subcommittee of Professional and Public Education of the American Heart Association Council on High Blood Pressure Research. *Hypertension* 2005;45:142–161.

Raitakari OT, Juonala M, Kähönen M, et al. Cardiovascular risk factors in childhood and carotid artery intima-medial thickness in adulthood: the Cardiovascular Risk in Young Finns study. *JAMA* 2003;290:2277–2283.

Rocchini AP, Katch V, Anderson J, et al. Blood pressure in obese adolescents: effect of weight loss. *Pediatrics* 1988; 82:16–23.

Rocchini AP, Key J, Bondie D, et al. The effect of weight loss on the sensitivity of blood pressure to sodium in obese adolescents. *N Engl J Med* 1989;321:580–585.

Rudolf MCJ, Greenwood DC, Cole TJ, et al. Rising obesity and expanding waistlines in schoolchildren: a cohort study. *Arch Dis Child* 2004;89:235–237.

Saab PG, Liabre MM, Ma M, et al. Cardiovascular responsivity to stress in adolescents with and without persistently elevated blood pressure. *J Hypertens* 2001;19:21–27.

Sakarcan A, Tenney F, Wilson JT, et al. The pharmacokinetics of irbesartan in hypertensive children and adolescents. *J Clin Pharmacol* 2001;41:742–749.

Savoca MR, Evans CD, Wilson ME, et al. The association of caffeinated beverages with blood pressure in adolescents. *Arch Pediatr Adolesc Med* 2004;158:473–477.

Schieken RM. Genetic factors that predispose the child to develop hypertension. *Pediatr Clin North Am* 1993; 40:1–11.

Shear CL, Burke GL, Freedman DS, Berenson GS. Value of childhood blood pressure measurements and family history in predicting future blood pressure status: results from 8 years of follow-up in the Bogalusa Heart Study. *Pediatrics* 1986;77:862–869.

Silverberg DS, Nostrand CV, Juchli B, et al. Screening for hypertension in a high school population. *Can Med Assoc J* 1975;113:103–108.

Simons-Morton DG, Hunsberger SA, Van Horn L, et al. Nutrients intake and blood pressure in the dietary intervention study in children. *Hypertension* 1997;29:930–936.

Sinaiko AR, Gomez-Marin O, Prineas RJ. Prevalence of "significant" hypertension in junior high school-aged children: the Children and Adolescent Blood Pressure Program. *J Pediatr* 1989;114(4 Pt 1):664–669.

Singhal A, Cole TJ, Fewtrell M, et al. Is slower early growth beneficial for long-term cardiovascular health? *Circulation* 2004;109:1108–1113.

Singhal A, Cole TJ, Lucas A. Early nutrition in preterm infants and later blood pressure: two cohorts after randomised trials. *Lancet* 2001;357:413–419.

Singhal A, Fewtrell M, Cole TJ, Lucas A. Low nutrient intake and early growth for later insulin resistance in adolescents born preterm. *Lancet* 2003;361:1089–1097.

Sorof JM, Portman RJ. White coat hypertension in children with elevated casual blood pressure. *J Pediatr* 2000;137: 493–497.

Sorof JM, Poffenbarger T, Franco K, et al. Isolated systolic hypertension, obesity, and hyperkinetic hemodynamic states in children. *J Pediatr* 2002;140:660–666.

Sorof J, Daniels S. Obesity hypertension in children: a problem of epidemic proportions. *Hypertension* 2002;40:441–447.

Sorof JM, Lai D, Turner J, et al. Overweight, ethnicity, and the prevalence of hypertension in school-aged children. *Pediatrics* 2004a;113:475–482.

Sorof JM, Turner J, Martin DS, et al. Cardiovascular risk factors and sequelae in hypertensive children identified by referral versus school-based screening. *Hypertension* 2004b; 43:214–218.

Soyannwo MAO, Gadallah M, Kurashi NY, et al. Studies on preventative nephrology: systemic hypertension in the pediatric and adolescent population of Gassim, Saudi Arabia. *Ann Saudi Med* 1997;17:47–52.

Strauser LM, Pruitt RD, Tobias JD. Initial experience with fenoldopam in children. *Am J Ther* 1999;6:283–288.

Taittonen L, Uhari M, Kontula K, et al. Angiotensin converting enzyme gene insertion/deletion polymorphism, angiotensinogen gene polymorphisms, family history of hypertension, and childhood blood pressure. *Am J Hypertens* 199;858–866.

Tarasiuk A, Simon T, Tal A, Reuveni H. Adenotonsillectomy in children with obstructive sleep apnea syndrome reduces health care utilization. *Pediatrics* 2004;113:351–356.

Task Force on Blood Pressure Control in Children. Report of the Second Task Force on Blood Pressure Control in Children—1987. National Heart, Lung, and Blood Institute, Bethesda, Maryland. *Pediatrics* 1987;79:1–25.

Urbina Em, Bao W, Pickoff As, et al. Ethnic (black–white) contrasts in heart rate variability during cardiovascular reactivity testing in male adolescents with high and low blood pressure. *Am J Hypertens* 1998;11:196–202.

van Hooft IMS, Grobbee DE, Wall-Manning HJ, et al. Hemodynamic characteristics of the early phase of primary hypertension. *Circulation* 1993;87:1100–1106.

Wang X, Wang B, Chen C, et al. Familial aggregation of blood pressure in a rural Chinese community. *Am J Epidemiol* 1999;149:412–420.

Weinberger MH. Salt sensitivity of blood pressure in humans. *Hypertension* 1996;27:481–490.

Wells T, Frame V, Soffer B, et al. A double-blind, placebo controlled, dose-response study of the effectiveness and safety of enalapril for children with hypertension. *J Clin Pharmacol* 2002;42:870–880.

Wiehe S, Lynch H, Park K. Sugar high: the marketing of soft drinks to America's schoolchildren. *Arch Pediatr Adolesc Med* 2004;158:209–211.

Wiet GJ, Bower C, Seibert R, Griebel M. Surgical correction of obstructive sleep apnea in the complicated pediatric patient documented by polysomnography. *Int J Pediatr Otorhinolaryngol* 1997;41:133–143.

Williams CL, Hayman LL, Daniels SR, et al. Cardiovascular health in childhood: a statement for health professionals from the Committee on Atherosclerosis, Hypertension, and Obesity in the Young (AHOY) of the Council on Cardiovascular Disease in the Young, American Heart Association. *Circulation* 2002;106:143–160.

Wilson DK, Bayer L, Sica DA. Variability in salt sensitivity classifications in black male versus female adolescents. Hypertension 1996;28:250–255.

Wing JK, Hui SH, Pak WM, et al. A controlled study of sleep related disordered breathing in obese children. *Arch Dis Child* 2003;88:1043–1047.

Woroniecki RP, Flynn JT. How are hypertensive children evaluated and managed? A survey of North American pediatric nephrologists. *Pediatr Nephrol* 2005;20:791–797.

Wyszynska T, Cichocka E, Wieteska-Klimczak A, et al. A single center experience with 1025 children with hypertension. *Acta Pædiatrica* 1992;81:244–246.

Yiu V, Orrbine E, Rosychuk RJ, et al. The safety and use of short-acting nifedipine in hospitalized hypertensive children. *Pediatr Nephrol* 2004;19:644–650.

Zhou L, Ambrosius WT, Newman SA, et al. Heart rate as a predictor of future blood pressure in schoolchildren. *Am J Hypertens* 2000;13:1082–1087.

Zubrow AB, Hulman S, Kushner H, Falkner B. Determinants of blood pressure in infants admitted to neonatal intensive care units: a prospective multicenter study. *J Perinatol* 1995; 15:470–479.

# PATIENT INFORMATION

## WHAT IS HYPERTENSION?

For most people, a blood pressure above 140/90 is considered as hypertension. The upper number, the *systolic* pressure, is the highest pressure in the arteries when the heart beats and fills the arteries. The lower number, the *diastolic* pressure, is the lowest pressure in the arteries when the heart relaxes between beats.

As part of aging, blood vessels usually become stiff or rigid, so that they are less able to dilate when blood enters from the heart. Therefore the systolic pressure usually increases with age.

## WHAT CAUSES HYPERTENSION?

In most patients, no specific cause for hypertension can be found. In about 10%, a specific cause can be found and often relieved by either medical or surgical treatment.

The term used for the usual type of hypertension has been "essential," but "primary" is preferable. These factors are involved:

- Hereditary
- Obesity
- High sodium intake
- Psychological stress

In addition, a number of other factors sometimes play a role, including:

- Excessive alcohol drinking (more than two to three portions a day)
- Smoking
- Sleep apnea
- Herbal remedies
- Diet pills and other stimulants, such as ephedra
- Physical inactivity

## CAN HYPERTENSION BE CURED?

Not usually. Some people who lose considerable excess weight, reduce a high intake of sodium (or alcohol), and relieve stress may have a return of elevated blood pressure to a normal level.

## WHAT ARE THE CONSEQUENCES OF HYPERTENSION?

By placing a burden on the heart and blood vessels, hypertension in concert with other risk factors induces heart attacks, heart failure, strokes, and kidney damage. The other important cardiovascular risk factors are:

- Smoking
- Abnormal blood lipids (an elevated LDL cholesterol or a low HDL cholesterol)
- Diabetes

## HOW IS HYPERTENSION TREATED?

Treatment should always include an improvement in all the unhealthy lifestyle habits, including:

- Stopping smoking
- Losing excess weight
- Increasing physical activity
- Reducing sodium intake (easiest accomplished by reading labels on processed foods and avoiding any with more than 300 mg of sodium per portion)
- Drinking no more than a healthy quantity of alcohol:
  - One drink per day for women, two for men. (The portions are 12 ounces of beer, 4 ounces of wine, and 1.5 ounces of whiskey.)

Antihypertensive drugs are usually needed. These include three major types:

- **Diuretics,** which remove some of the excess sodium and fluid from the circulation
- **β-blockers**, which decrease the rate and strength of heart contraction
- **Vasodilators**, which open blood vessels.
  - This group includes angiotensin-converting enzyme inhibitors, angiotension blockers, and calcium channel blockers.

All of these may cause side effects, and your physician should be contacted if you feel unwell after starting one or more drugs. The action of most drugs can be reduced by weight gain, excessive sodium or alcohol and certain drugs such as nonsteroid anti-inflammatories (ibuprofen, naprosyn, celebrex, etc.). Inform your physician about all over-the-counter or prescription drugs you take. Take your pills every day at the same time, usually soon after awakening.

## HOW TO ENSURE GOOD CONTROL OF HYPERTENSION

In the past, only occasional readings in the physician's office were used to determine the degree of hypertension. Increasingly, home measurements with a battery-operated, semiautomatic device are being used to ensure adequate but not excessive treatment. With such a device, costing $40 to $100, you can monitor your blood pressure, particularly when changes in the type or doses of medications are made.

## GUIDELINES FOR HOME BLOOD PRESSURE MONITORING

### Equipment

The device should be checked against the mercury manometer in the physician's office to ensure its accuracy. The cuff should be large enough to encircle the upper arm. For most adults, a "large adult cuff" should be used. If the device comes with a smaller cuff, a larger one can be substituted.

### Procedure

Do not smoke or drink coffee for 30 minutes before. Sit with the back and arm supported, the arm at the level of the heart (middle of chest). After 3 to 5 minutes of quiet sitting, take two readings, a minute apart. If the two readings differ by more than 10 mm (points), take additional readings each minute until they are within 10 mm Hg.

Record the readings in this manner:

| Date | Time | First Reading | Second Reading | Circumstances |
|------|------|---------------|----------------|---------------|
| May 3 | 7am | 150/95 | 145/90 | Before breakfast |
| May 5 | 6pm | 135/85 | 130/80 | After exercise |
| May 7 | 8am | 110/70 | 105/60 | Dizzy after standing |

If the readings are being taken to diagnose hypertension, as many as possible, four or five a day, should be taken for a few weeks.

If the readings are being taken to monitor treatment, two or three readings one day a week may be adequate.

Take a reading if you feel unwell, such as being dizzy or light-headed or having a bad headache. You usually cannot tell when your pressure is rising, but the pressure can rise if you are anxious.

The readings may vary as much as 40 mm Hg from one time to another. They rarely remain the same. Take your diary with you on your next appointment.

More information can be obtained from the American Heart Association by phone, at (800) 242-8721 or on the web at http://www.american-heart.org.

# INDEX

*Note:* Page numbers followed by "f" indicate figures; those followed by "t" indicate tables.